Gary K. Stimac, Ph.D., M.D.
Imaging Network of Seattle and
First Hill Diagnostic Imaging Center
Seattle, Washington

Introduction to Diagnostic Imaging

W. B. SAUNDERS COMPANY
Harcourt Brace Jovanovich, Inc.
Philadelphia London Toronto Montreal Sydney Tokyo

W. B. SAUNDERS COMPANY
Harcourt Brace Jovanovich, Inc.

The Curtis Center
Independence Square West
Philadelphia, Pennsylvania 19106

Library of Congress Cataloging-in-Publication Data

Stimac, Gary K.

Introduction to Diagnostic Imaging/Gary K. Stimac.

p. cm.

ISBN 0–7216–1305–5

1. Radiology, Medical. 2. Radiography, Medical.
I. Stimac, Gary K.
[DNLM: 1. Diagnostic Imaging. WN 100 S858i]

RC78.S79 1992 616.07′54—dc20

DNLM/DLC 91–40448

INTRODUCTION TO DIAGNOSTIC IMAGING ISBN 0–7216–1305–5

Printed in the United States of America.

Last digit is the print number: 9 8 7 6 5 4 3 2 1

To the important teachers in my life,

especially

Lee, Helen, Leonid, and Andrew.

Contributors

Jonathan E. Briggs, BA, ELS

Publications Editor/Technical Editor, Department of Radiology, University of New Mexico, Albuquerque, New Mexico

Michael Davis, MD

Associate Professor, Department of Radiology, University of New Mexico; Chief, Gastrointestinal Radiology, University of New Mexico Hospital, Albuquerque, New Mexico

Alimentary Tract and Abdominal Radiology

Juleann Cottini Gandara, MD, EdM

Clinical Assistant Professor; Director of Mammography, University of Washington Medical Center, Seattle, Washington

Mammography

Michael F. Hartshorne, MD

Associate Professor, Department of Radiology, University of New Mexico; Chief, Joint Imaging Service, Veterans Administration Medical Center, Albuquerque, New Mexico

Chest Radiology
Cardiovascular Radiology
Nuclear Medicine

Charles A. Kelsey, PhD

Professor of Radiology, University of New Mexico, Albuquerque, New Mexico

Advanced Imaging Techniques

Fred A. Mettler Jr., MD, MPH

Professor and Chairman, Department of Radiology, University of New Mexico, Albuquerque, New Mexico

Genitourinary Radiology

William W. Orrison, Jr., MD

Professor, Department of Radiology, University of New Mexico; Chief, Neuroradiology and MRI, University of New Mexico Hospital and Veterans Administration Hospital, Albuquerque, New Mexico

Neuroimaging

Robert D. Rosenberg, MD

Associate Professor, Department of Radiology, University of New Mexico; Chief of Diagnostic Imaging, University of New Mexico Hospital, Albuquerque, New Mexico

Mammography

Gary K. Stimac, PhD, MD

President, Imaging Network of Seattle; Neuroradiologist, First Hill Diagnostic Imaging Center, Seattle, Washington

Advanced Imaging Techniques
Chest Radiology
Alimentary Tract and Abdominal Radiology
Genitourinary Radiology
Cardiovascular Radiology
Mammography
Musculoskeletal Radiology
Neuroimaging
Nuclear Medicine

Robert J. Telepak, MD

Associate Professor, Department of Radiology, University of New Mexico, Albuquerque, New Mexico

Cardiovascular Radiology

Michael R. Williamson, MD

Associate Professor, Department of Radiology, University of New Mexico; Chief, Diagnostic Ultrasound, University of New Mexico Hospital, Albuquerque, New Mexico

Alimentary Tract and Abdominal Radiology

Susan L. Williamson, MD

Associate Professor, Department of Radiology, University of New Mexico; Chief, Pediatric Radiology, University of New Mexico Hospital, Albuquerque, New Mexico

Chest Radiology
Alimentary Tract and Abdominal Radiology

Preface

This text, originally designed as a study guide for radiology residents in training, is applicable at many levels of medical education. It is intended to be a first resource and a core learning text in radiology that is more comprehensive than remedial texts currently available. All diseases of radiologic interest are covered, and essential clinical and radiographic information is included. For rare or unusual manifestations of diseases and experimental results, the reader is directed to the large textbooks, subspecialty works, and journals.

This book is recommended for medical students as a complete text in diagnostic radiology and as a valuable aid to learning general medicine and surgery. It includes essential material for radiology residency training and for board certification. It also will be of benefit for training and review by students in specialty areas of surgery and medicine. Practicing radiologists can use it for specific diseases and differential diagnosis. Selected parts, with instruction by a radiologist, will be of value to nurses, technologists, and other members of the health care system.

Because the goal of this text is to present the optimal methods for imaging particular conditions, it includes applications of many types of equipment, thus showing the unique advantages of each. With regard to MRI, this approach includes high-resolution and rapid-scanning sequences and high- and low-field strength applications. Although these methods may not be available to all radiology centers, they can serve as models for imaging strategy. All of these methods have been used extensively in clinical imaging. The images speak for themselves in the demonstration of anatomy and pathology.

The information in this text is of two types: factual descriptions of diseases, and suggested methods of evaluation. Knowledge from the pathology, medicine, and radiology literature is presented concurrently. The suggested approach to radiology is based on my training in physics, radiology, and medicine. Most of these methods represent my personal style, which is based on experience with a wide variety of resources. Several textbooks are listed as suggested readings at the end of each chapter rather than reference citations within the text, as such references often are not used by students.

This text is intended to cover most methods used in diagnostic radiology at a practical depth from which an advanced understanding can be gained through actual experience and study. Other procedures, including interventional angiography, biopsy and drainage techniques, cineradiographic cardiac evaluation, and most cardiovascular ultrasonography, are performed by specially trained radiologists or by neurosurgeons, cardiologists, and vascular surgeons and require specialized knowledge, the use of highly technical equipment, and much experience. Thus they are beyond the scope of this book.

HOW TO USE THIS BOOK

This text presents the essentials of modern radiology: the principles of radiologic technology and their effective use for evaluating all areas of the body, the clinical aspects and radiographic information of diseases, the radiographic appearance of individual diseases (as shown in diagrammatic or radiographic form), and the effective use of differential diagnosis. These essentials are presented in a systematic four-part approach.

First, Chapter 1 presents radiographic methods and discusses each imaging technique and its application. Subsequent chapters discuss the major anatomic areas and organ systems. The initial section, entitled *Basic Evaluation,* of Chapters 2 to 8 presents application of each imaging test to diseases in that organ system. Nuclear Medicine is presented as a separate chapter (Chapter 9) because of its special areas of application in various parts of the body.

Second, diseases in each radiologic subspeciality (grouped by organ system) are presented in a logical order under major subheadings (trauma, congenital, systemic, inflammatory, neoplastic, vascular, etc.) as the most basic approach to differential diagnosis. Diseases are discussed briefly in paragraph form, followed by a diagram and/or a radiographic image. Many rare diseases are mentioned in their appropriate categories, which ensures completeness for the student and provides additional diagnostic options for the clinician who has exhausted the common possibilities. The text presents the most advanced (but not experimental) radiographic considerations for imaging of each particular disease process. Optimal methods from several institutions are intended to provide a universal viewpoint of the imaging process and to emphasize the importance of scan quality and imaging technique.

Drawings are the third and key element of the book. The drawings are labeled with anatomy, radiographic findings, interpretation, and relevant clinical information. Carefully chosen facts are thus presented in pictorial form and are supported by short descriptive phrases; as a result, the information is more easily recalled than it would be from lists, tables, or text. These diagrams also assist in the recall of the spatial and density information contained in the radiographs.

To ensure that the true radiographic appearance is understood, photographs of actual examinations are used throughout, either in addition to or instead of a diagram. These examples were carefully chosen to represent application of the most modern diagnostic method, to clearly illustrate the disease process, and to reflect the diagnostic approach to the disease or technique. In some cases, the abnormalities on these photographs are marked with arrows. In most cases, their location is described in radiologic terms (as in an actual radiology report) to allow the reader to find the abnormalities without the crutch (and the clutter) of arrows.

Fourth, the last section of each chapter, entitled *Radiographic Differential Diagnosis,* provides a set of lists to further aid the student in summarizing related information and to give the radiologist and the clinician an overview of selected diagnostic problems. Each list is preceded by a short description of relevant facts. These lists are practical and easily remembered. Their value has been proved in daily clinical care, teaching conferences, and radiology board examinations.

The larger intent of this text is to provide an integrated understanding of diagnostic radiology for the radiology resident and the advanced medical student. It is hoped that the student will gain the ability to synthesize information by logical analysis of findings, application of clinical and radiographic knowledge, and comparison through the use of differential diagnosis. Diseases common to more than one organ system are usually mentioned in several chapters to provide the full spectrum of their evaluation. The text is cross-referenced so that diseases that affect more than one organ system are unified.

Clinical examples are used in the first chapter and in the *Basic Evaluation* sections of each chapter to demonstrate both radiographic principles and to augment the later presentation of particular disease processes. The student is advised to carefully consider the descriptions of scans for technical approach and diagnostic appearance. Different manifestations of the same disease or similar appearances of different diseases are frequently noted. These should be reviewed along with the content of the drawings and the *Radiographic Differential Diagnosis* lists. The *Basic Evaluation* sections describe an approach to evaluation that indicates the types of abnormalities that might be identified.

To summarize:

"Never produce a film you can't read,"
and
"You see what you look for;
you look for what you know."

—GARY K. STIMAC

Acknowledgments—The Origins of This Book

This book originated during my residency at the University of California, San Francisco, in the early 1980s and initially represented my synthesis of information provided by the radiology staff in addition to textbooks, journals, and clinical experience as I learned radiology. By the completion of my training, I had more than 500 sketches that summarized specific diseases in all parts of the body. Those drawings became the basis for this textbook. Continued research, study, and work with colleagues at several additional institutions have resulted in the integration of those drawings and other presentations of radiology information into this book.

This text reflects my personal approach to radiology, combining the best methods and the most advanced approaches that I have developed or have had the good fortune to learn from others. On the one hand, it could be viewed as my personal view of radiology, displaying my specific biases, knowledge, and diagnostic approach. On the other hand, it could be regarded as a selective presentation of the knowledge of hundreds of radiologists and clinicians. In either context, I am indebted to all of the radiologists and other physicians, fellows, students, and medical writers who have taught me medicine, physics, and radiology. It would be impossible to thank everyone for the assistance I have received in this project. In fact, I cannot even identify the origins of some of the material in this book, especially differential diagnostic lists, which have been handed down and modified by generations of radiologists. It is possible, however, to thank those who have had a major impact on my training, on my knowledge, and in the preparation of this text.

Alexander Margulis provided the initial incentive and has continued through the years to provide encouragement in the undertaking of this task. In addition to providing me with many resources in the preparation of this book, he influenced my view of gastrointestinal radiology by the example set by the faculty and fellows whom he trained, and most important, by his personal teaching. Two members of this faculty, Michael Federle and Brooke Jeffrey, provided my basis in general imaging of the gastrointestinal tract and the solid organs of the abdomen and pelvis as evaluated by CT, ultrasonography, and contrast examinations. My knowledge of the genitourinary system is founded on lectures, publications, and the direct clinical teaching of Alphonse Palubinskas, Faye Laing, and Brooke Jeffrey. I thank Harry Genant for establishing an unsurpassed program in bone radiology; Clyde Helms for teaching a practical approach to bone film analysis and for many examples that he has provided for the musculoskeletal chapter; and Hideyo Minagi for teaching me plain film diagnosis, especially in musculoskeletal disease. I thank Charles Gooding for teaching me a comprehensive and reliable approach to pediatric cardiac disease, and I thank both him and Robert Brasch for teaching me their approaches to pediatric radiology and for the use of many cases of pediatric diseases. I was fortunate to be at the University of California at a time when an unparalleled staff of neuroradiologists was present. I thank Hans Newton both for establishing such a fine program and for the personal attention and training that he provided me. Michael Brant-Zawadzki and David Norman provided me a basic knowledge of CT and MRI of the nervous system. I thank William Bank for intensive training in neuroangiography and for first demonstrating to me the excitement of neuroradiology. I thank Gordon Gamsu, Philip Goodman, and many others for instruction in chest radiology.

Since leaving the University of California, I have been fortunate to collaborate with several others who by their knowledge, attention, and experience provided unique approaches in radiology that I have incorporated into my personal approach and that are reflected in this text. I am especially indebted to Bruce Porter at the First Hill Diagnostic Imaging Center in Seattle for demonstrating powerful methods of abdominal, pelvic, and bone marrow imaging with MRI and CT. I thank Ellsworth Alvord for informative collaborations in neuropathology and for reviewing the neuroradiology chapter; Alfred Weber for our collaborative exchange in MRI of head and neck disease; and Justin Smith for valuable assistance in reviewing the chest and nuclear medicine chapters.

The completion of this text has been just as important as its origins. I am especially indebted to Fred Mettler for providing the personal and departmental support required for completing this project. Without the intensive support of his department, including chapter contributors from his faculty at the University of New Mexico, it would not have been possible to complete the individual chapters at the intended level of modern radiology. Substantial additional assistance has been provided by the administrative and technical staffs at the First Hill Diagnostic Imaging Center, Seattle, and the North Shore Magnetic Imaging Center, Boston. This includes collaborative evaluation of patients, assistance in producing and obtaining images and follow-up information, and research support. I especially thank Darrell McNabb for providing resources at the First Hill Diagnostic Imaging Center to complete this project.

The completion of this book has also required extensive support from the publisher, W.B. Saunders, and I thank Lisette Bralow for her continuing assistance. I received a great deal of initial training in medical publication and medical writing from the late Jo Wheeler, University of California, San Francisco, who helped me develop the structural organization for this text. The final text has been the result of the efficient, enjoyable collaboration with the Department of Radiology Publications Staff at the University of New Mexico School of Medicine, directed by Jonathan Briggs. I am also especially thankful to Sarah Langwell and Mike Norviel of the Medical Illustration Department at the University of New Mexico for working with me closely in the preparation of the fine, informative drawings in this text.

GARY K. STIMAC

Contents

1

Advanced Imaging Techniques

Gary K. Stimac
Charles A. Kelsey

The modern radiologist is a clinical consultant, a technical expert, a skilled examiner, and, occasionally, a treating physician. In order to perform these roles, an understanding of the theory and use of film radiography, computed tomography, ultrasonography, magnetic resonance, and digital imaging is essential. This chapter presents an introduction to the methods of modern diagnostic imaging. It includes the basic theory and the modern developments of each type of examination. Applications to each organ system are discussed, and the principles of interpretation are described. Specific use of each type of examination appropriate to each organ system is presented in the "Basic Evaluation" section of subsequent chapters. (Nuclear medicine is discussed separately in Chapter 9.) In addition to using diagnostic imaging methods effectively, the radiologist has a responsibility to consider the cost, the radiation exposure, and the risk, in comparison with the diagnostic value, of an examination (see Appendix 1–1).

FILM RADIOGRAPHY

The current techniques of film radiography permit radiographs of superior spatial resolution and contrast to be obtained on a routine basis. Computer-controlled x-ray tubes deliver the optimal x-ray energy in order to provide the best possible radiographic contrast. Modern machines also permit films to be obtained with very short exposure times, thereby reducing radiation exposure to the patient and image degradation caused by motion of the patient. Small focal-spot x-ray tubes provide the nearly point-source x-ray beam needed to produce images of exceptional spatial detail.

Basic Principles

In film radiography, an x-ray generator is used to produce a limited or collimated beam of x-rays of desired energy range that pass through the patient and expose a film (Fig. 1–1). Important aspects of the technique, which are under the direct control of the radiologist and the radiology technologist, allow optimization of the diagnostic quality of the film and minimization of the radiation dose. The most important of these factors are the x-ray beam energy, the total number of x-rays, the type of film and the photo-enhancing screen used, and

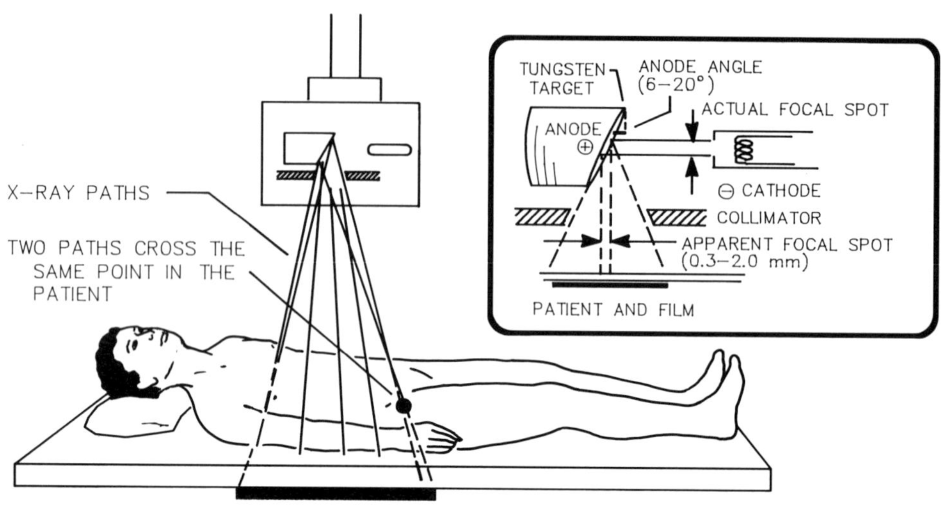

FIGURE 1–1. X-ray tube and plain-film radiography technique. The x-rays are produced when electrons bombard a spinning tungsten anode. Collimators permit the x-rays to travel through a defined portion of the patient and then expose the film. Because the anode is not a point source, x-rays from slightly different directions can pass through the same part of the patient and cause slight blurring of the image. The image is sharpest at the anode side because the x-rays emanate from a narrower angle.

the type and the amount of contrast material used.

X-Ray Production. The primary components of an x-ray tube are a filament (the cathode), which emits electrons, and a target (the anode), toward which the electrons are accelerated. Electrical current flows through the filament, causing electrons to boil off. A strong electric potential (60,000 to 100,000 V) accelerates movement of the electrons toward the anode. When the electrons reach the anode, they are slowed by electromagnetic interactions with the target material (usually tungsten). This deceleration of the electrons produces x-radiation, called "braking radiation" or bremsstrahlung, that travels in all directions. The energy of the x-rays varies from zero up to the maximal energy of the electrons, called the peak energy or kilovoltage peak (kVp).

The range of x-ray energies in the beam and the area of the patient that is irradiated is determined by the geometry of the anode and the use of collimators and absorbers. The anode angle (the angle between the surface of the anode and the plane perpendicular to the cathode-anode axis; Fig. 1–1) determines the area of the target from which x-rays emanate (the apparent focal spot). Ideally, the apparent focal spot would represent a point source, but such a small area would result in excessive heating (and melting) of the target for the number of x-rays required for radiographic exposures. The necessarily finite size of the focal spot results in a small amount of image blurring caused by x-rays that traverse the same abnormality but at slightly different angles. The use of rapidly rotating anodes composed of alloys that effectively dissipate heat allows reduction of the size of the focal spot to provide high-resolution radiographs. Such high resolution is particularly valuable in bone imaging and in angiography. A collimator that surrounds the tube limits the radiation to the desired area of exposure. Absorbers remove the lower energy x-rays from the beam before they reach the patient, which results both in decreased radiation dose to the patient and in improved contrast.

The kVp is determined by the electric potential between the cathode and the anode. The amount of radiation (i.e., the number of x-rays) depends on the current that flows through the filament and the duration of the exposure.

The radiologist or the technologist optimizes the kVp to provide the best image contrast and the lowest radiation dose to the patient. The objectives of this optimization are (1) adequate penetration of individual x-rays through the patient, (2) limitation of the overall dose, and (3) attainment of the more favorable x-ray interaction, called the photoelectric effect, as opposed to simple scattering of the x-rays (Compton scattering). A high kVp (above 75 kV) results in good penetration of the patient and reduced dose; however, it minimizes the probability of photoelectric interactions, resulting in reduced contrast differences among adjacent structures. Therefore, high-kVp films show a relatively uniform shade of gray (poor contrast) throughout a wide range of tissue density (wide latitude). Such films are advantageous when tissues of widely varying density are present, as in chest imaging (see Chapter 2). Obtaining low-kVp films requires a larger x-ray dose to the patient because of the poorer penetration of the low-energy x-rays. However, because the photoelectric interaction is favored and because there is greater variation among different tissues for the absorption of x-rays by this mechanism, a wide range of shading differences among different tissues is attainable. The use of low-kVp technique is particularly important when contrast material is administered.

The total exposure, expressed in milliampere seconds (mAs), determines, for a given kVp, the darkness of the film. This exposure is optimized when the tissue of most interest appears as a middle shade of gray on the film and when the varying densities of other structures are displayed as shades from black to white. The optimal exposure for a given patient at the desired kVp is determined from charts of calibrated exposure factors and the experience of the technologist and the radiologist. For some examinations (intravenous urography, angiography, and myelography), scout films are obtained before the procedure for preliminary evaluation and in order to ensure that the radiographic technique is optimal. An exposure of inadequate mAs produces a film in which all structures appear white and results in a film without diagnostic information. An overexposure results in a dark film, in which all structures are dark gray or black. Another consequence of overexposure is unnecessary radiation dose to the patient. The total required exposure is more easily estimated for the high-kVp technique because most of these high-energy x-rays pass through the patient. Determining the exposure for the low-kVp technique is difficult because of increased absorption of low-energy x-rays.

Film-Screen Combination. Photographic film is insensitive to x-rays, in comparison with its sensitivity to light (film is about 1000 times more sensitive to light photons), and so an x-ray system with only photographic film would require very large radiation doses (doses similar to those used in radiation therapy) to provide an image. To overcome this deficiency, a film-screen combination (Fig. 1–2) made up of photographic film sandwiched between thin sheets of phosphorescent material (the screens) is used. When x-rays collide with the crystals in the screens, many light photons are emitted, which then interact with the light-sensitive film.

Most screens are made of calcium tungstate, which efficiently converts x-rays to light photons and is inexpensive. A thick screen provides a large yield of light photons because it has a greater likelihood of absorbing the x-rays than does a thin screen. However, because the light photons spread out as they travel from their point of production (in the screen) to the film, a thick screen results in blurred images. Thus the thickness of the screen represents a compromise between greater yield of light photons and acceptable spatial resolution. High-speed screens (i.e., ones that produce more light per x-ray) allow either (1) rapid filming, thereby minimizing the effects of motion by the patient (which is important in angiographic studies, emergency room examinations, and portable examinations) or (2) the use of a thinner screen, thereby improving spatial resolution. These high-speed screens are made from rare-earth elements such as gadolinium and lanthanum.

Continued advances in photographic film also have greatly improved plain-film imaging. Wide-latitude films provide excellent contrast resolution of objects of markedly different densities, as, for example, in the chest radiograph, in which detail of the low-density lungs and the high-density mediastinum is desired. The increased sensitivity of modern film allows better spatial resolution, lower x-ray exposure, and a decrease in blurring caused by a patient's motion.

Contrast Material. Contrast materials are

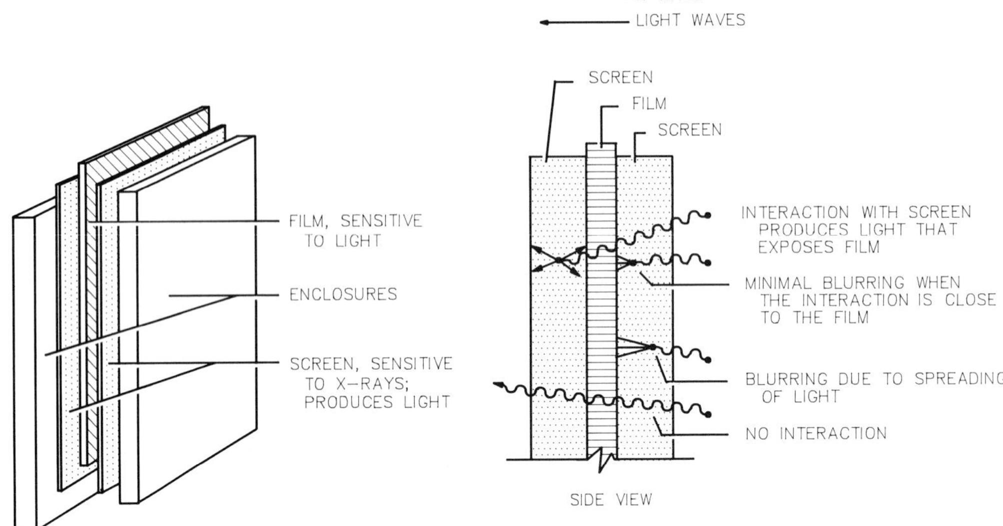

FIGURE 1–2. Film-screen combination. The x-ray film is sandwiched between light-emitting screens that are sensitive to x-rays. After x-rays interact with the screen, light photons emanate in all directions, exposing the film near the interaction. Interactions that occur close to the film result in the clearest image. Thin screens can enhance this effect but yield fewer interactions than do thicker screens.

available for intravenous, intrathecal, oral, and rectal use. They greatly improve and expand the application of plain-film examinations.

Many compounds are available for intravascular contrast enhancement (such as Conray, Renografin, and Angiovist). These are large-molecule, iodine-containing complexes that are introduced directly into the vascular system by bolus, infusion, or rapid high-pressure injection. Considering the large volumes (50 to 150 mL per injection) and the high osmolality of these materials (600 to 1200 mOsm/L), they are surprisingly safe. Adverse reactions to these agents, although infrequent, are serious and potentially fatal (such reactions and their treatment are discussed in Appendix 1–2). These adverse effects may be diminished by increased awareness of potential problems by both the radiologist and the referring physician, including the danger of inadequate hydration of the patient. Nonionic, iodinated contrast agents (iopamidol, iohexol, iotrolal, and others) have distinct safety advantages over the ionic agents but are much more expensive.

Water-soluble, nonionic iodinated contrast materials for intrathecal use (iopamidol, iohexol) are preferable to the oil-based contrast agent (iophendylate) and the initial nonionic agent (metrizamide) used in myelographic studies. The advantages of the nonionic agents are superior demonstration of nerve roots and sleeves, excretion by the kidneys, absence of long-term arachnoidal scarring, and enhancement of the subarachnoid spaces for computed tomography. The disadvantage of the nonionic agents in intrathecal use is that during their reabsorption into the venous system, they can cause changes in mental status, nausea and vomiting, and, in rare instances, seizures. These adverse effects are minimized by hydration of the patient. The newer nonionic, water-soluble agents have fewer and less severe side effects and are used routinely for intrathecal injections.

In gastrointestinal evaluation, barium sulfate is the primary contrast material. Modern methods of suspension result in improved coating of the lumen of the gastrointestinal tract and allow the simultaneous use of air to produce double-contrast examinations. These examinations have the unique ability to demonstrate the mucosal surface of the bowel. Water-soluble contrast material can be used when barium agents are contraindicated. Very dilute barium sulfate or water-soluble iodinated contrast material is also used to identify the gastrointestinal tract in CT examinations.

COMPUTED TOMOGRAPHY

Computed tomography (CT) produces exquisite anatomical detail with high-contrast resolution in all parts of the body. Thin, axial tomographic images (slices) of the head, neck, chest, abdomen, pelvis, and extremities are easily obtained and can be reformatted into sagittal, parasagittal, coronal, and oblique projections.

Principles

In CT, a collimated x-ray beam and a detector system are used to measure x-ray attenuation (absorption and scattering) for a series of projections of the beam through the patient (Fig. 1–3). A computer then uses mathematical reconstruction techniques to calculate a gray-scale value for each pixel of a slice. This information in turn is used to produce an electronic or a film image.

The CT x-ray tube is similar to that used in conventional radiographic studies except that it rotates around the axis of the patient. The kVp is fixed (usually between 120 and 140 kV), and heavy filtration results in a beam of predominantly high-energy x-rays. The x-rays are collimated to a fan-shaped beam that irradiates only a designated thin slice of the patient. Some of the x-rays are attenuated by the patient, and the remainder pass through to interact with an arc of detectors. The energy deposited in each detector is stored by computer. The x-ray tube and detectors then rotate 1 degree about the scan axis, and a second exposure is made. This process continues until a series of exposures at 300 to 600 different angles is made. The complete slice is produced in 1 to 4 sec. The patient is then advanced by the distance of the desired slice spacing (1 to 10 mm) and another slice is obtained in a similar manner. Scanning is continued until the area of interest has been imaged.

The intensity *(I)* of x-rays received by the detector is equal to the initial intensity (I_0) reduced by the fraction stopped by the patient according to the law of x-ray attenuation:

$$I = I_0\exp[-\mu L],$$

where μ is the linear attenuation coefficient (which depends on the type of tissue and the energy of the x-rays) and L is the x-ray path length. The body part to be scanned is divided into an array of boxes (voxels) approximately 1 mm on a side and of a thickness determined by the beam collimation (Fig. 1–4). The received intensity *(I)* at the detector is the initial intensity reduced by the attenuation that occurs in each voxel, given by

$$I = I_0\exp[-(\mu_1 + \mu_2 + \ . \ . \ . + \mu_n)dL],$$

where dL is the length and width of each voxel and the μ values are those of each voxel along the path. The simple addition of the attenuation coefficients in the exponent makes possible the determination of the tissue density in each voxel.

For a typical CT scanner, a complete scan yields approximately 40,000 equations in 40,000 unknowns (the attenuation coefficients). This set of equations can be solved analytically or by iteration to yield the normalized attenuation coefficients (called CT numbers).

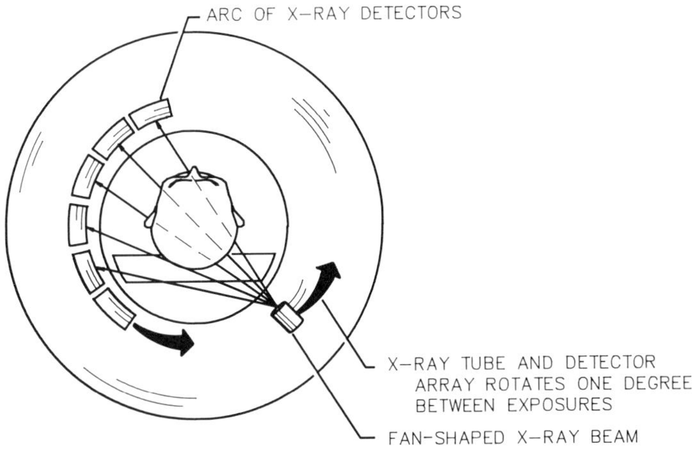

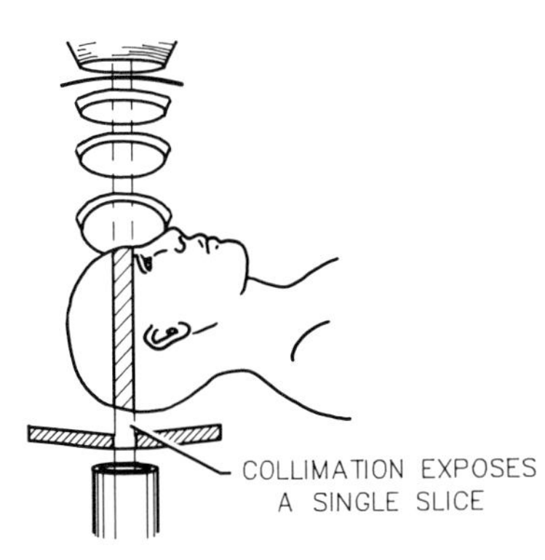

FIGURE 1–3. Principles of computed tomographic (CT) scanning. The x-ray tube produces a fan-shaped beam that passes through a section (slice) of the patient. This fan-shaped beam is received by a circular array of detectors at the opposite side. These detectors receive x-rays attenuated during passage along a specific path through the patient's body. The detector and x-ray source rotate around the axis, producing exposures at 1-degree intervals of rotation. Collimators (side view) allow exposure of slices varying from 1 to 10 mm in thickness.

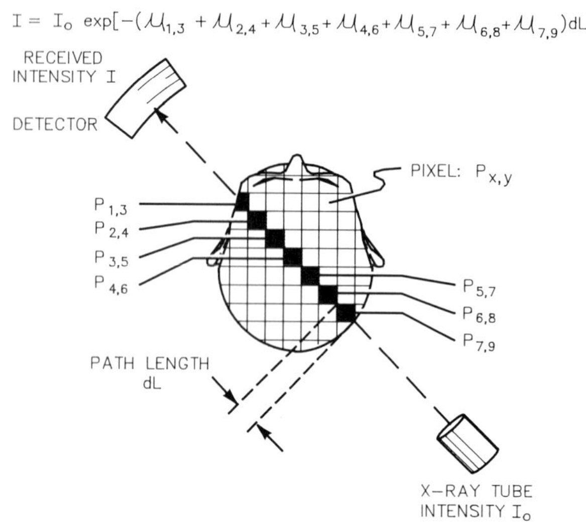

FIGURE 1–4. Principle of x-ray summation in CT. The path defined by the x-ray tube and the detector crosses a series of pixels within the slice. The attenuation within each pixel contributes to the total attenuation of that x-ray beam. Such information from a large number of paths through the patient's body allows determination of the attenuation within each pixel. This information is displayed in gray-scale format.

Rapid computation of this large data set results in nearly real-time display. Mathematical smoothing, calibration corrections, and filtering improve image production; additional software identifies and removes artifacts.

Clinical Imaging

Although in principle the actual attenuation coefficient could be calculated for each point in the scan, in practice each attenuation value is assigned a CT number on a scale defined by the attenuation values of air and water. In this assignment, the CT number of water is arbitrarily set to zero and that of air as −1000 units (called Hounsfield units, or HU). These CT numbers can be listed by the computer or displayed and photographed in gray-scale format on a viewing monitor.

Because the CT numbers are stored by the computer, the radiologist can choose to display the image in a manner in which the abnormalities are best depicted. Most viewing monitors have 256 shades of gray, varying from white (for most dense) to neutral gray (for average density) to black (for lowest density). The radiologist can set the average density (called the level) to any value (usually that of the average CT number of the tissue of most interest) so that the tissue of most interest appears medium gray. The range of CT numbers displayed (called the window) can be made narrow (as small as 60 HU) or wide (up to 4000 HU). For example, a wide window (1000 HU) that is set at a level of zero encompasses 500 HU above zero and 500 HU below zero. It has 128 gradations of gray above zero (progressively whiter) and 128 gradations of gray below zero (progressively blacker). Thus each shade of gray represents a density change of 4 HU. Narrower windows, centered at the average tissue CT number of interest, demonstrate more subtle variations in CT number, but any tissue whose CT number is above the range appears white, and any tissue below that range appears black. Often several level and window settings are viewed so as to optimally demonstrate all structures (Fig. 1–5).

The CT scan that results is a series of tomographic images (slices) of predetermined thickness, high spatial resolution, and high contrast resolution. Thin slices are especially helpful in the evaluation of small areas of the brain and the spinal cord. The spatial resolution, determined by the pixel size, can be made as small as 0.5 mm through high-resolution technique. The use of reconstruction algorithms that maximize contrast differences among various tissues allows detection of soft tissue contrast differences as small as 0.5%. Intravenously administered contrast agents can enhance vessels, vascular masses, or normal tissue and provide direct information about a

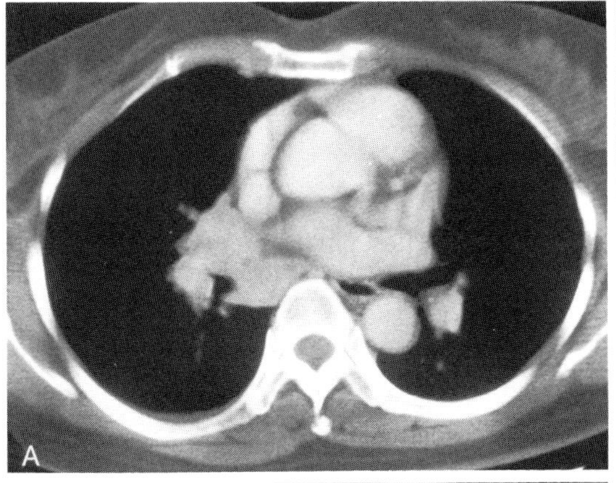

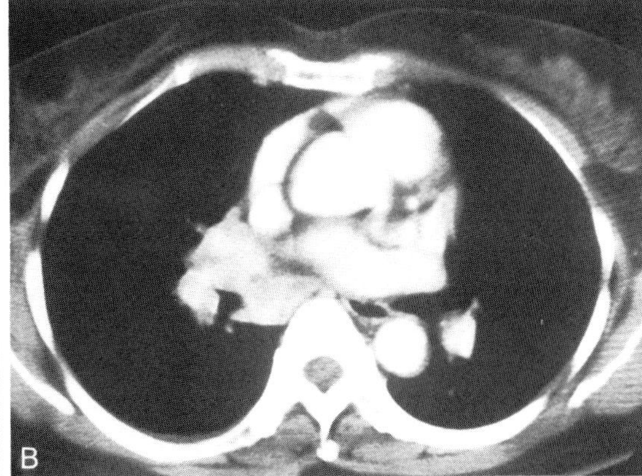

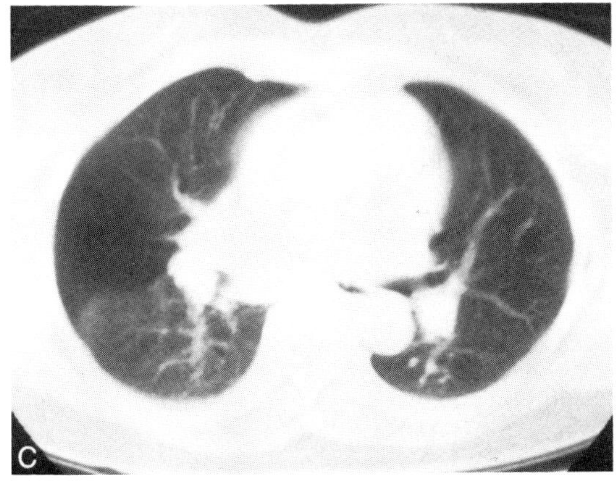

FIGURE 1–5. Window and level setting on CT scans. The use of window and level settings in the display of CT scans allows the radiologist to produce images that best demonstrate certain details. *A.* In a patient with a right hilar lung carcinoma and mediastinal adenopathy, the trabecular pattern and cortical margin of the bones can be best shown on bone windows (level 300, window 1200). *B.* The mediastinal and perihilar soft tissue can best be shown on mediastinal windows (level 40, window 400). *C.* The lung parenchyma can be best shown by lung windows (level −675, window 1650). (Courtesy of B. Porter, First Hill Diagnostic Imaging Center, Seattle.)

suspected abnormality or allow a nonenhancing structure to be better seen (Fig. 1–6). For images of the brain, inhaled xenon can assist in evaluating blood flow.

Interpretation

CT scans are interpreted by an evaluation of each slice first individually and then as a part of the whole scan for evidence of masses and compression or displacement of normal structures. The greater anatomical detail shown by CT than by conventional radiographs requires a thorough knowledge of normal cross-sectional anatomical structure and an understanding of the normal CT appearance of the each part of the body. Comparison of opposite sides can be especially valuable in the evaluation of paired or axially symmetrical organs.

Artificial streaks, lines, ghosts, dropout, and other alterations of the true image, called artifacts, occur in all areas of radiology, but they are most common in digitally processed examinations as a result of electronic and electromagnetic phenomena. A knowledge of artifacts that occur in CT scanning prevents misinterpretations. The most common artifacts are streaks of either low or high density. They occur in areas where there is a large, abrupt change in density, such as the location of a surgical clip, or where an airspace is adjacent to a bone. It is usually possible to follow the streaks to a point of intersection and identify their cause. Unfortunately, these streaks can obscure an area of clinical interest. In brain scans, streak artifacts are commonly caused by surgical clips, metal fragments, and dental hardware; air in the paranasal sinuses contrasts with the dense petrous bone, causing streaks that often degrade the images of the middle cranial fossa and the posterior fossa. Nasogastric tubes and surgical clips are the most common artifacts in chest scans and can limit the evaluation of the mediastinum. Tubes, clips, and barium are the most common causes of streak artifacts in abdominal scans. Some CT scanners have algorithms that reduce the effect of artifacts by identifying the high-density object and subtracting the streaks from the image (Fig. 1–7).

Motion by the patient causes a generalized degradation of the image and can make the

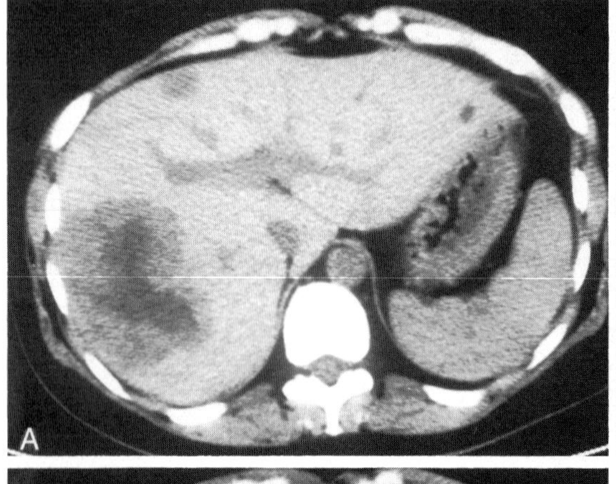

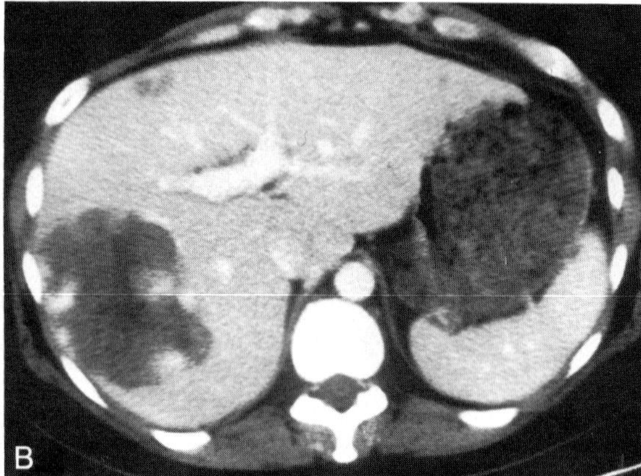

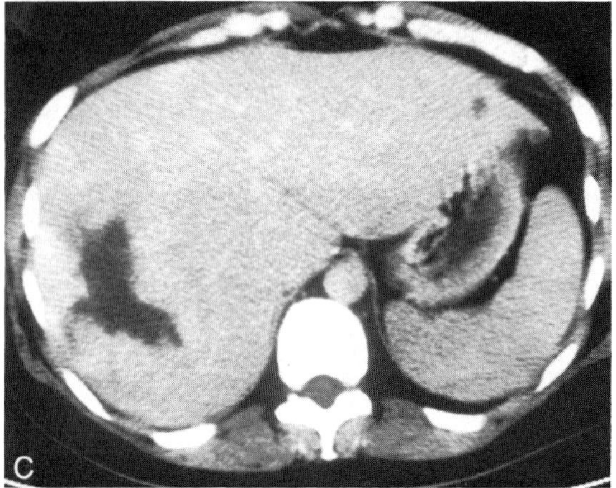

FIGURE 1–6. Intravenous contrast on CT scans. *A.* The precontrast scan shows a focal, low-density abnormality in the right lobe of the liver. *B.* During infusion of contrast, the hepatic vessels and aorta show marked enhancement. The periphery of the lesion shows early enhancement. *C.* A delayed scan shows gradual filling in of contrast enhancement in the lesion and generalized washout of the major vessels. This filling in of contrast enhancement over time is characteristic of cavernous hemangioma. (Courtesy of B. Porter, First Hill Diagnostic Imaging Center, Seattle.)

scan uninterpretable. A so-called blooming artifact is an apparent enlargement of an object when viewed at narrow windows; for example, neural foramina can appear small because of apparent enlargement of the surrounding bones when viewed through soft tissue windows. A beam-hardening artifact occurs when the beam passes through high-density bone, resulting in a higher average x-ray energy; the computer then assigns falsely low CT numbers to the intervening soft tissue. The most common locations of beam-hardening artifact are the brainstem between the petrous ridges (Fig. 1–8), the foramen magnum, and the spinal canal. A volume-averaging artifact occurs when the computer assigns an average CT number to a volume element that contains tissues of different densities. Volume averaging can usually be suspected when slices above and below the presumed abnormality show structures of different density at the same location.

Although the CT numbers for various body tissues and fluids are somewhat predictable (Table 1–1), absolute CT numbers cannot be reliably used for diagnosis because they vary. In addition, there is considerable overlap in CT numbers among fluids, blood, abscess, and tumor, and so CT numbers should be used as only general guides for interpretation. In any one study, comparison of CT numbers with those of other body parts in the same scan is reliable and reproducible.

TABLE 1–1. APPROXIMATE CT NUMBERS OF VARIOUS SUBSTANCES

Substance	Density (HU)
Air*	−1000
Fat	−50 to −300
Water*	0
Cerebrospinal fluid	0 to 10
Blood	30 to 60
Liver	60 to 80
Muscle	40 to 80
Bone	200 to 2000

CT, computed tomographic; HU = Hounsfield units (see text).

*CT numbers for air and water are set arbitrarily.

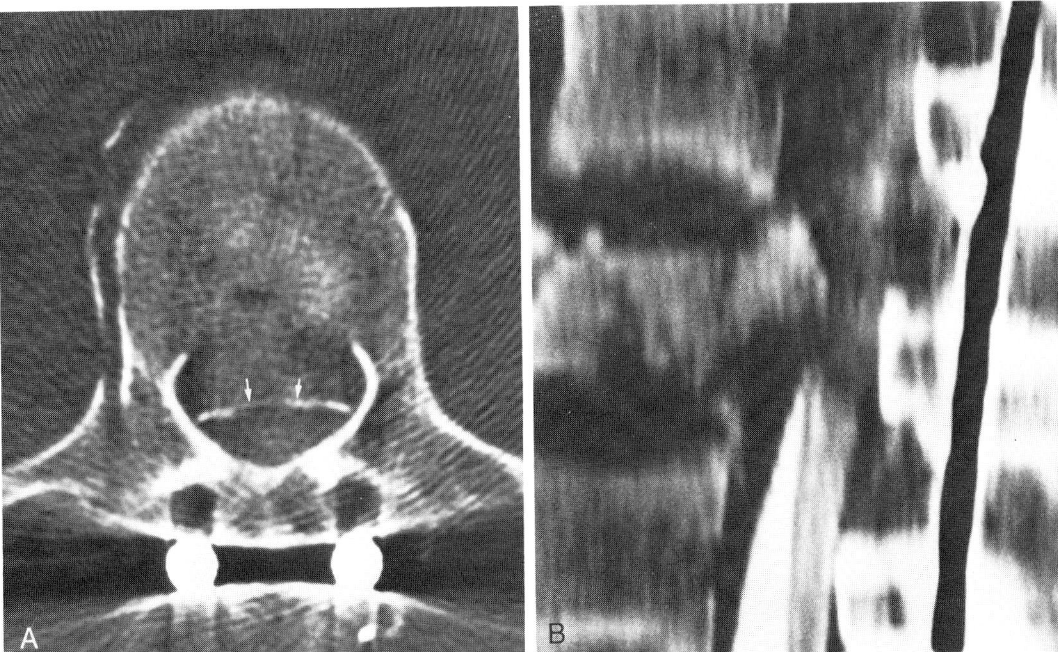

FIGURE 1–7. Reduction of streak artifact from metallic rod. The patient sustained a severe compression fracture of L-1 with retropulsion of fragments into the spinal canal. Initial stabilization with Harrington rods was performed, and an assessment of alignment was required. *A.* The axial image shows marked streak artifact and nonpenetration of the x-ray beam in the region of the rods. However, the compression of the vertebral body and especially the displaced bone fragment *(arrows)* severely compromising the canal are evident. *B.* The sagittal reconstruction obtained from the axial images shows a complete signal absence in the region of the rods but clearly demonstrates the crushed vertebral body and the retropulsed fragment.

FIGURE 1–8. Beam-hardening artifact in the posterior fossa. The x-rays that must pass through both petrous bones are attenuated more severely than those that pass through brain. The computer assigns a falsely low density to the part of the brainstem that lies between the petrous bones. The result is a series of low-density streaks through the anterior brainstem in the region between the petrous bones.

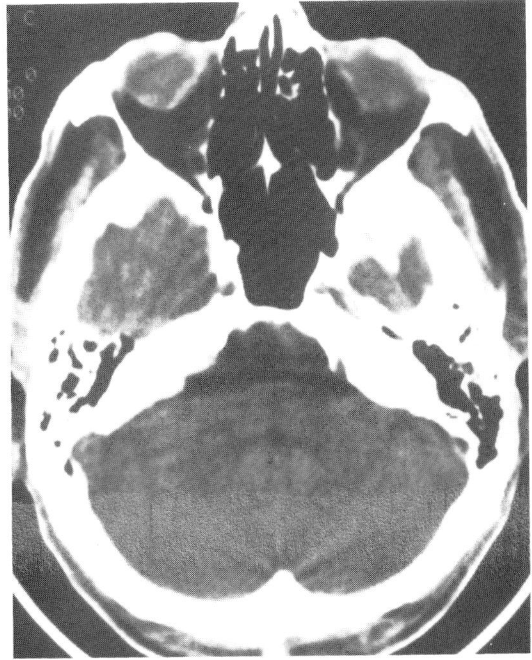

ULTRASONOGRAPHY

Ultrasonography provides diagnostic evaluation by reflections of focused, high-frequency sound waves from internal tissues. It is noninvasive and provides, without radiation risk, unique information about all parts of the body. In the chest, ultrasonography is used to evaluate fluid in the pleural spaces and the pericardium, competency of heart valves, and cardiac structure and function. In the abdomen, it provides both primary diagnosis and information that is complementary to that provided by other techniques in the evaluation of the liver, the gallbladder, the spleen, and the pancreas. In the genitourinary system, the kidneys, the bladder, and the reproductive organs are easily assessed. The brain of an infant can be studied by imaging directly through the thin skull or through the fontanelles to demonstrate tumors and congenital anomalies. In adults, brain and spinal cord masses can be located during surgery for biopsy or removal. In the extremities and the neck, vascular-occlusive disease can be evaluated by real-time and Doppler techniques.

Principles

The ultrasonographic transducer, an electrically driven vibrating crystal, both transmits and receives the high-frequency sound waves that are used to produce the image. The temporal and spatial distribution of the echoes of the sound waves are analyzed and displayed in a digitized, gray-scale format similar to that used in CT.

The sound waves used for imaging are generated by the longitudinal oscillations of the transducer against the tissue surface (usually the skin). The coupling of the transducer to the surface is improved by the application of a thin layer of aqueous gel. Sound waves of defined frequency (between 2 and 10 million oscillations per second, or 2 to 10 MHz) are created by the vibration of the transducer in short 1- to 20-μsec bursts. The intensity of these sound waves can be altered to optimize penetration. The sound waves propagate through the patient at speed *(v)*, given by the wave equation

$$v = \lambda f,$$

where f is the frequency of the oscillations and λ is the wavelength. The waves are partially reflected by internal tissue planes; some of these reflected sound waves are received by the transducer between transmissions. The speed of sound varies slightly for different types of tissues but (except for bone or air) is nearly 1500 m/sec. These variations in the speed of propagation can sometimes assist in the characterization of the tissue.

Clinical Imaging

Imaging is usually performed with real-time scanning. Real-time scanning employs a transducer that rotates from side to side, sending sound waves into an arc of about 30 degrees (Fig. 1–9) to produce a two-dimensional image that is viewed and recorded in real time (i.e., during the examination). The detection system records the transducer direction, time of arrival, and intensity of the reflected pulses. The transducer direction is the position along the arc (i.e., the angle) from which the reflections came, and the arrival time correlates with the depth (i.e., the sound waves that return early are plotted at the surface; those that return late are mapped deeper). The intensity of the echoes is depicted by the brightness of the image at the location prescribed by the direction and depth. Thus the image is formed by a mapping of the intensity of reflected sound waves in a two-dimensional plane.

Real-time scanning allows the examination to specifically address the clinical question and provides information about changes over time, such as pulsations of vessels, peristalsis, cardiac motion, and fetal activity. Real-time ultrasonography is also ideal for locating masses and fluid collections for biopsy or drainage procedures.

Ultrasonography is the primary technique in the evaluation of obstetric patients because it is noninvasive and does not involve the use of ionizing radiation. Elsewhere in the body, it is used in conjunction with CT, magnetic resonance imaging (MRI), and other examinations to provide unique and complementary diagnostic information. Ultrasonographic examinations are significantly less expensive than CT and MRI, and they can be directed to address the specific clinical question. Because the image is produced by the echoes from the internal structures (in comparison, for example, with the density displayed by CT), ultrasonography can demonstrate the complex internal structure of tumors and the location of tissue interfaces

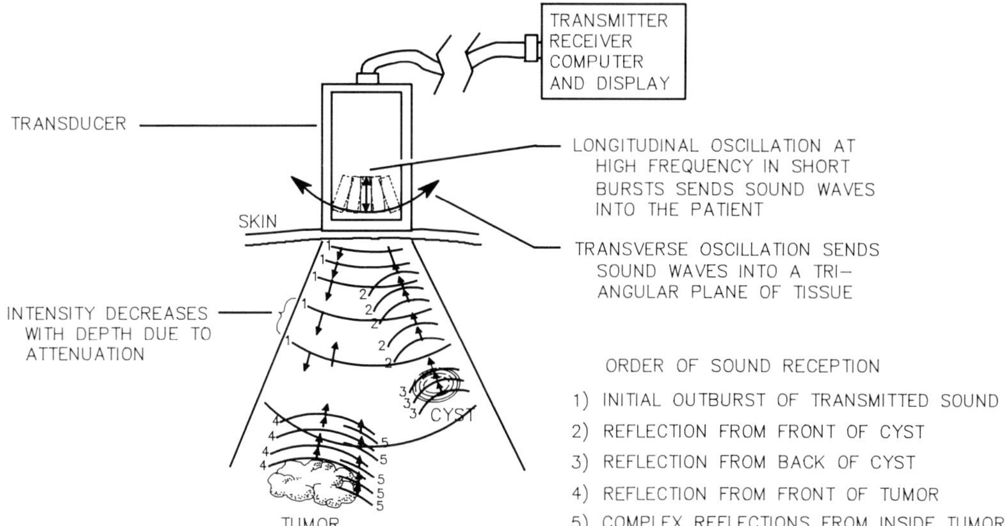

FIGURE 1–9. Principles of real-time ultrasonography. The element of the transducer oscillates in a longitudinal direction, transmitting sound waves into the patient's body. This element also rotates in an arc of approximately 30 degrees, sending the sound waves into a plane of the patient's body. The direction from which reflected sound waves are received and the time of return allow mapping of the surface from which they were reflected. The intensity of the reflected sound waves determines the brightness of the image.

and can distinguish fluid from solid masses (Fig. 1–10). The convenience of ultrasonography and its ability to precisely locate masses and fluid collections make this technique ideal for use in interventional procedures, such as fluid aspiration, abscess drainage, and percutaneous needle biopsy.

Interpretation

Ultrasonographic interpretation requires a precise knowledge of anatomical relationships because some landmarks such as bone or bowel are not easily seen. Structures must be identified by their echo characteristics and their

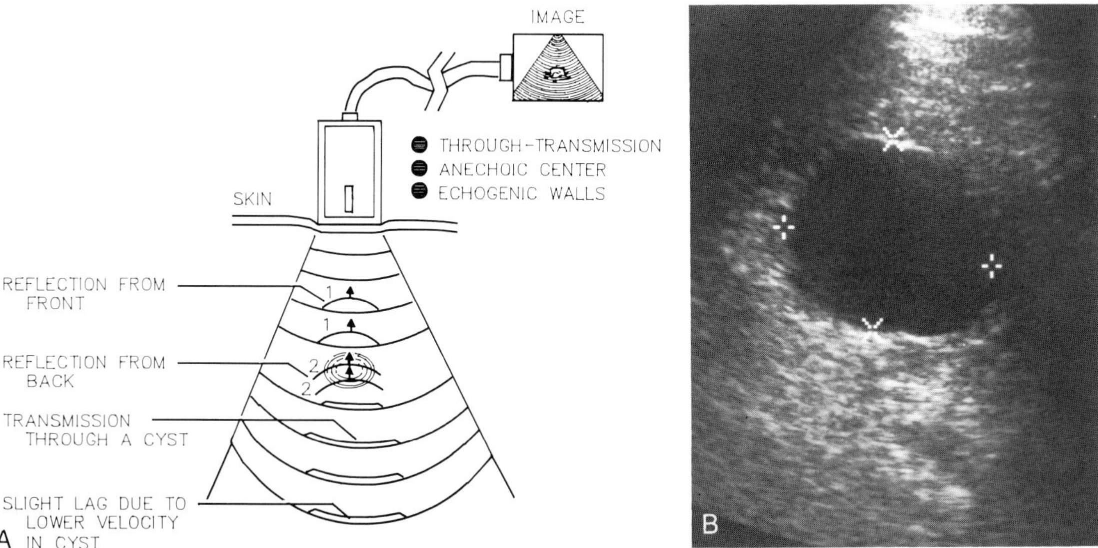

FIGURE 1–10. Ultrasonography of a cystic fluid collection. *A.* Diagram shows reflection from the front of the cyst (1), the back wall of the cyst (2), and through-transmission. *B.* The findings, in gray-scale format, show typical increased echoes in the margin of the cyst, near absence of echoes centrally, and dense echoes posterior to the cyst, indicating through-transmission. Note cursors placed for automated measurement of the cyst size.

spatial relationships to other identified structures (Fig. 1–11). Abnormalities can be either identified by their appearance or inferred from displacement of adjacent normal structures. Ultrasonography depends more than any other diagnostic examination on the skill and the observations of the diagnostician. In many instances, only the ultrasonographer can confidently explain the images because he or she possesses additional knowledge about the location and the orientation of the transducer and the appearance of nearby structures not shown on the image. In addition, he or she must determine when the area has been adequately evaluated. Therefore, the ultrasonographer bears a great responsibility to perform a thorough examination and to communicate the findings directly to the clinical staff.

The ultrasonic beam does not penetrate dense objects (such as bone and calcifications) and gas collections (such as air in the lungs and intestines), and it only poorly penetrates structures with complex architecture, such as fat. Although the failure of the beam to adequately penetrate such substances may limit the effectiveness of the examination, this lack of penetration is often an advantage. Dense calcifications cause a characteristic shadowing of the beam that allows easy identification of gallstones (Fig. 1–12) and renal calculi. The identification of gas in the bowel, the stomach, or the lungs precludes the presence of fluid or a mass; a change of body position or ingestion of fluid can sometimes confirm that the gas is within the bowel. The dense architecture of fat often assists in its identification. Fortunately, calcium, gas, and fat are well demonstrated on CT.

Echocardiography and Doppler Ultrasonography

Two specialized uses of ultrasonography are echocardiography and Doppler-flow measurements. The heart is evaluated by a variety of ultrasonographic techniques that are optimized for both structural and functional imaging of the chambers and valves. Most cardiac ultrasonography is performed by the cardiologist.

The Doppler effect, the frequency change of reflected sound waves from a moving object, can be used for the ultrasonographic evaluation of blood flow. An ultrasonic probe sends out sound waves at a constant rate (frequency). The waves that encounter stationary objects return at the same rate; those that encounter blood cells moving away from the transducer return at a lower rate; and those that encounter blood cells moving toward the transducer return at a higher rate. The frequency of the reflected sound waves is thus used to determine the flow rate and direction. This quantification of flow, in conjunction with ultrasonographic imaging of vessels to show anatomical features, provides noninvasive evaluation of the carotid bifurcation. The technique is also used to assess peripheral vascular disease and blood flow

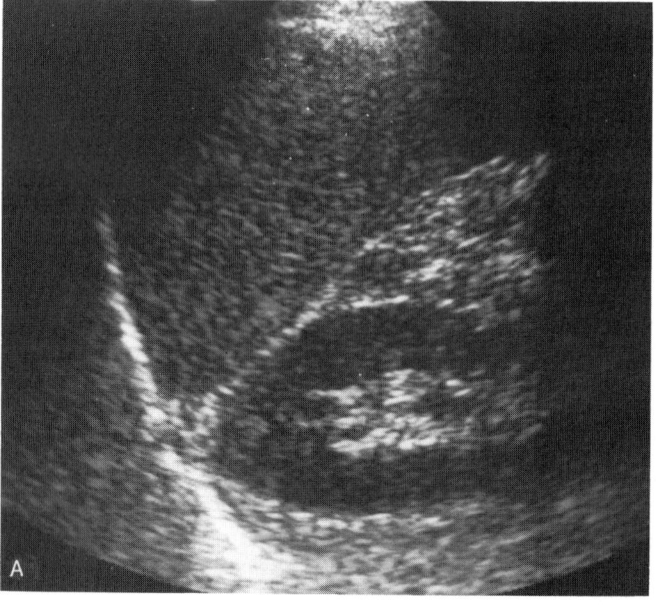

FIGURE 1–11. Distinguishing structures by echo texture and location. *A.* This scan demonstrates the different echo textures of the kidney and the liver. The renal cortex shows the lowest echo texture. The liver is slightly more echogenic. The renal pelvis shows increased echoes caused by the presence of fat.

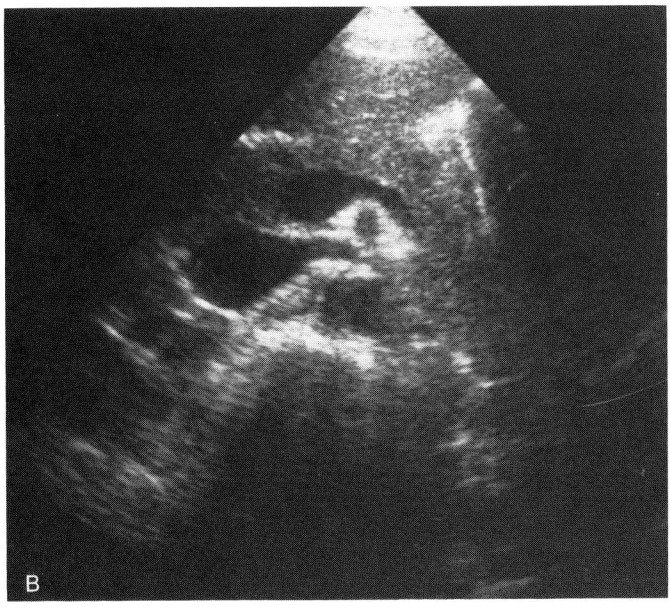

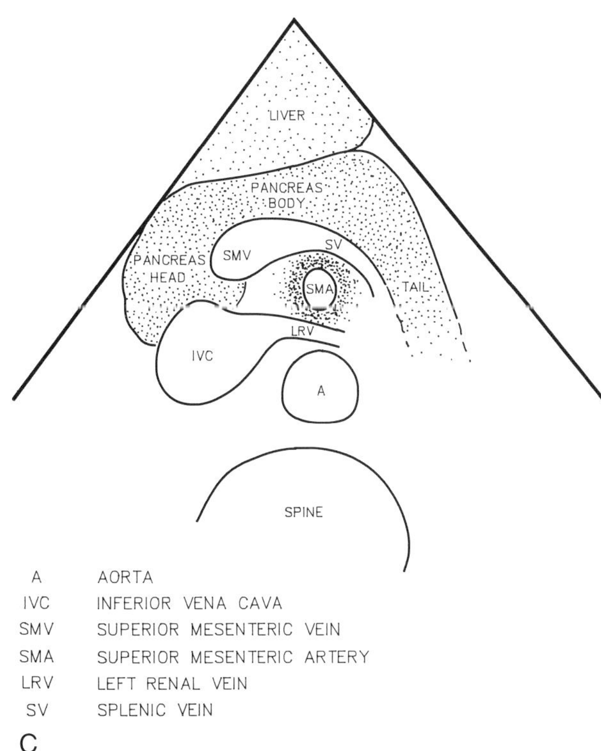

FIGURE 1–11 *Continued* Ultrasonogram *(B)* and matching diagram *(C)* of the midabdomen at the level of the pancreas show normal vascular anatomic structure. Posteriorly, the spine shows lack of echoes. Directly anterior to the spine is the aorta, and to its right is the inferior vena cava, shown with the entering left renal vein, which passes between the aorta and the more anteriorly located superior mesenteric artery (SMA). The SMA is surrounded by highly echogenic fat. To the right of the SMA is the superior mesenteric vein (SMV), shown at its confluence with the splenic vein (SV), which passes anterior to the SMA. Directly anterior and to the right of the SMV are the head and the body of the pancreas. Left and anterior to the splenic vein are the body and the tail of the pancreas. Anterior to the pancreas is the liver. These structures have a well-defined and constant relationship in the abdomen and allow for ultrasonographic evaluation of the pancreas and retroperitoneal structures. (Courtesy of Rebecca Hall, University of New Mexico.)

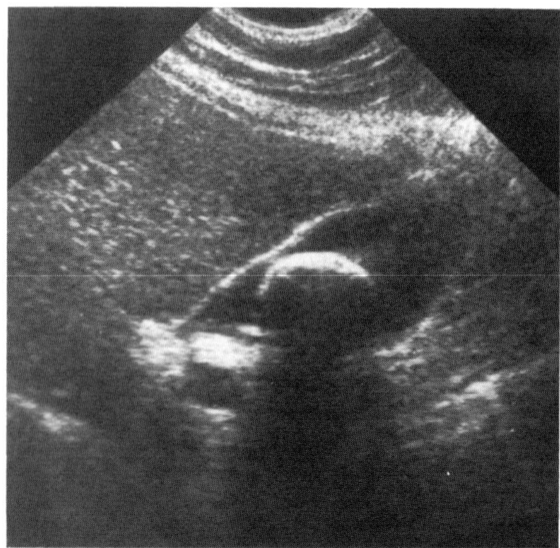

FIGURE 1–12. Acoustic shadowing of a gallstone. The gallbladder has a cystic appearance except for the focal area of nontransmission that is caused by a large gallstone. As a result, there is a shadow beyond this gallstone from which no return echoes are received.

in the eye. In color Doppler imaging, arterial flow is displayed in red and venous flow in blue.

MAGNETIC RESONANCE IMAGING

MRI is the newest and most powerful diagnostic imaging method. As in diagnostic ultrasonography, no ionizing radiation is used. The images are representations of the intensities of electromagnetic signals from hydrogen nuclei in the patient. These signals, the result of a resonance interaction between the nuclei and externally applied magnetic fields, can be spatially encoded to provide a mapping of the image area in two or three dimensions. The signal intensity depends on the density and the magnetic environment of the hydrogen nuclei (protons). The most important components of MRI are the protons, an external magnetic field, the interaction of the protons with the magnetic field, and excitation by radiofrequency and gradient pulses.

Principles

Magnetic Properties of the Proton. Protons (and many other nuclei) possess magnetic characteristics as a result of their charge distribution and intrinsic spin. Just as a current-carrying wire loop has an associated magnetic field along its axis (Fig. 1–13), a spinning proton has a magnetic moment directed along its axis of spin. The interaction of this nuclear magnetic moment with the magnetic field of the imager and with externally applied radiofrequency pulses affects the orientations of the protons within the body. The resultant changes in magnetization of the protons, which can be detected by sensitive electronic equipment, form the basis for imaging with magnetic resonance.

Externally Applied Magnetic Fields. Magnetic resonance imagers are equipped with large magnets to provide a strong, static, magnetic field, which preferentially aligns the proton magnetic moments. These magnets may be constructed from permanently magnetized materials, from coils made of resistive wire, or from coils made of superconducting materials (such as niobium-titanium alloy). The field strength of magnets used in imagers ranges from 0.06 to 2.00 T (0.6 to 20.0 kG). By

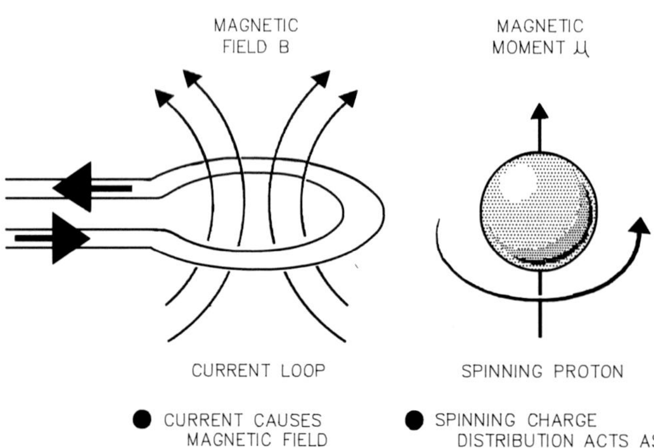

FIGURE 1–13. Magnetic moment of the proton. The spinning charge distribution of the proton results in a magnetic field similar to that induced in a current-carrying wire loop.

comparison, the magnetic field of the earth at the surface is 0.00005 T (0.5 G).

The strongest and most stable magnetic fields are produced by concentric coils of superconducting wires. Such coils produce a strong magnetic field along the axis of the coil (Fig. 1–14). Superconducting materials conduct electricity without resistive losses when maintained at liquid helium temperatures (4 degrees Kelvin). The magnetic fields produced by such coils can be homogeneous to within one part in 1,000,000 over a 30-cm-diameter cylindrical volume. Resistive and permanent magnets have practical advantages in terms of cost, siting, and the availability of hydroelectric power, helium, and other necessary materials. These magnets are generally of lower field strength and have important applications in trauma and tumor imaging. Low-field and midfield magnet systems provide higher tissue contrast than do high-field magnet systems and are less sensitive to respiratory and cardiac motion. Also, their lower cost allows their use in hospitals with limited resources or small numbers of patients.

Additional, variable magnetic fields (called gradient fields) in directions parallel (*z*-axis) and perpendicular (*x*- and *y*-axes) to the primary magnetic field are provided by separate coils called gradient coils. These gradient fields are much weaker (about 1 G/cm) than the large static magnetic field and are used to produce a slightly different field strength in each part of the patient's body. The ability to vary the field strength during imaging allows spatial mapping of the signals received from the protons. It also allows the behavior of the protons to be altered to produce information about their motion and chemical environment.

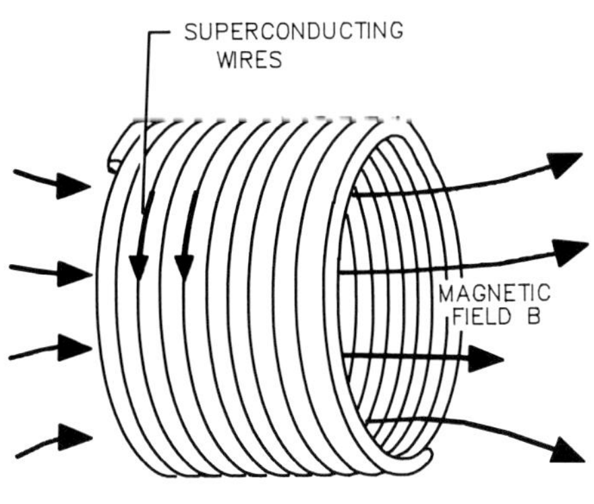

FIGURE 1–14. Magnetic field of a solenoid. Superconductive and resistive magnets are composed of circular coils of conducting wire. Each coil contributes a magnetic field along the axis of the solenoid. The field direction is most nearly axial in the center of the solenoid. The field strength is highly uniform (it varies by less than 1 part per 1,000,000) over a 30-cm diameter cylindrical volume. Magnets containing permanent magnetic materials create highly homogeneous magnetic fields perpendicular to their north and south poles.

Proton and Magnetic Field Interaction. The proton magnetic moment, in the presence of an external magnetic field, is analogous to a spinning top under the influence of gravity. Rather than align directly with the magnetic field, the spinning proton precesses about the magnetic axis, just as the spinning top precesses about the axis of the gravitational field. The angular speed (rotational frequency) of precession is, in both cases, directly proportional to the field strength. The spinning top eventually stops precessing because of frictional forces; the precession of the protons in magnetic resonance is altered by interactions with internal magnetic fields.

Because thermal interactions constantly disturb the alignment, some protons precess about the magnetic field axis (spin-up orientation, or lower energy state), and others precess about an axis exactly opposite the magnetic field axis (spin-down orientation, or higher energy state). Thermal collisions, which are thousands of times more energetic than the difference in the high and low energy states of the protons, constantly upset the alignment of protons with and against the magnetic field. Consequently, only a slight excess of protons is aligned with the field (about 10 protons per 1,000,000) at a given time. This small number of preferentially aligned protons provides the signal for MRI.

Excitation and Signal Detection. Although transitions between the spin-up and spin-down orientations are continuously and randomly induced by thermal interactions of adjacent atoms and molecules, they can be induced selectively and repeatedly by radiofrequency waves of appropriate energy. These induced transitions are the resonances that produce the images. This interaction of radiofrequency pulses with the precessing protons can be understood from two descriptions, the quantum mechanical and the classical descriptions. Both contribute to the understanding of MRI.

According to the quantum mechanical description, the radiofrequency excitation is caused by a single photon whose energy is proportional to the frequency of the radiation. If the energy of the photon is equal to the difference between the spin-up and the spin-down states, it can change a spin-up proton to the spin-down state. When this proton makes the return transition to the lower energy state, a photon of exactly the same energy is emitted and can be detected by the imager. Because the magnetic field can be adjusted (by means of the gradient coils) so that the frequency of excitation, emitted radiation, or both is unique to a particular volume element of the patient, the location of this interaction can be precisely determined.

According to the classical description, the protons can be made to precess in unison (that is, in phase) by an electromagnetic wave whose magnetic field is rotating at the precession frequency of the protons. When these protons precess together (in phase), their individual magnetizations sum to create a collective magnetization (which also precesses). The strength of this collective magnetization can be detected from the induction of current in the receiver coil. The magnetic field can be adjusted by means of the gradient coils in order to make the precession frequency unique to a particular volume element and therefore to determine the location of the interaction. Because local factors influence each individual proton, the phase coherence of these precessing protons is gradually lost and the detected signal is diminished; that is, some protons precess faster and others slower so that their magnetization is no longer additive. Because each type of tissue has different local factors, the rate at which this coherence is lost can be used to assess the tissue.

Imaging With Magnetic Resonance

Clinical MRI is made possible by three factors. First, protons of different tissues have different magnetic resonance characteristics as a result of differences in concentration, mobility of the protons, binding to adjacent atoms, and local magnetic environment. Second, different imaging technical factors (such as the rate of repeated excitations, the time at which the signal is received, or the type of excitation-detection sequence used) can provide different appearances for different tissues. Third, by variation in the magnetic field and the excitation pulses, the signal intensities of the protons can be mapped as a function of position.

The intensity of the magnetic resonance signal depends on the number of protons that participate in the resonance, on the magnetization of the protons, and on the phase coherence of their precession. The number of protons is characterized by the proton density; the degree of magnetization is characterized by a time, T1; and the coherence of these precessing protons is characterized by a time, T2. T1 and T2 are called relaxation times.

Proton Density. The concentrations of protons capable of participating in the resonance interaction are similar for most human tissues because most biological materials contain a predominance of hydrogen atoms; the effect of differences in proton density among most tissues is therefore small in comparison with the effect of differences in relaxation times. Some tissues, such as cortical bone, ligaments, and calcified tissues, either have a significantly lower proton density or possess protons that are unable to move about freely enough to participate in MRI. The magnetic resonance signal from such tissues is weak and cannot be directly differentiated from a decreased signal from air or rapidly flowing blood. The lack of a signal from cortical bone allows demonstration of the thin cortical line of the bones against the high intensity of bone marrow fat and the positive intensity of the cerebrospinal fluid or other external tissue (Fig. 1–15). As a result, bone tumor or infection can be detected easily.

Magnetization: T1 Effect. The degree to which protons in each tissue are magnetized at the time of the imaging influences the strength of the signals obtained. Several operator-chosen factors can be varied to enhance or suppress the signal difference between protons of different tissues. The primary measure of the magnetization of the protons of each tissue is the T1 relaxation time, the characteristic time interval required for return of the protons to full magnetization after excitation. T1 is an exponential time constant that depends on the molecular lattice structure of the tissue and on the thermal motion of adjacent atoms and molecules. The value of T1 depends on the magnetic field strength; it is generally between 0.1 and 3.0 sec for biological tissues.

The time between successive repeated excitations, called the repetition time (TR), can be chosen to enhance or diminish the difference in T1 between two types of tissue. For example, a short TR results in a large differ-

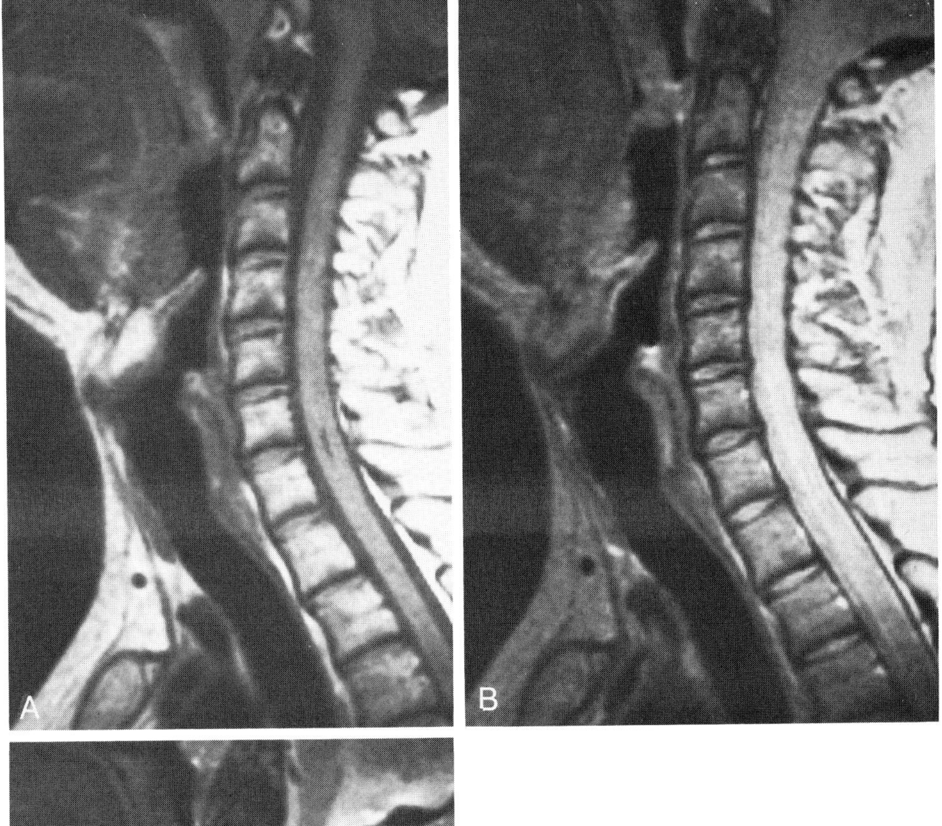

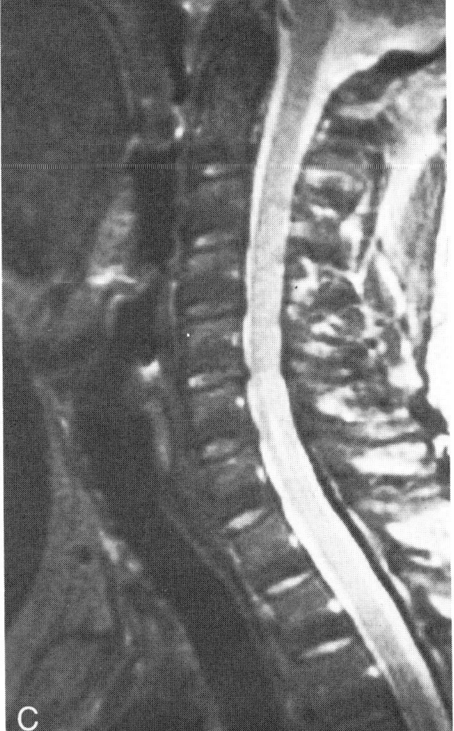

FIGURE 1–15. Effect of echo time (TE) on image appearance. *A.* T1-weighted spin echo scan shows fat in the soft tissues and in the bone marrow as white; spinal cord, muscle, and disc material as gray; and fluid (including a small traumatic syrinx at C-6 to C-7) as dark gray. *B.* The early echo (TE = 30 msec) of a 2250 repetition-time scan shows similar intensities for fluid and the spinal cord. The impressions of the lower cervical discs on the dural sac are evident. The syrinx is difficult to see. *C.* The late echo (TE = 80 msec) shows high-intensity fluid contrasted with a gray appearance of the spinal cord and brain. The normal disc is bright centrally on such scans, a finding that can be used to determine disc degeneration. The inhomogeneity of the vertebral bodies is caused by a chemical-shift artifact related to the technique used.

ence in magnetization and signal strength between two tissues with different T1 (assuming other factors are unimportant) (Fig. 1–15*A*). On the other hand, a long TR minimizes the effect of T1 because tissues of both long and short T1 become almost fully magnetized before each new excitation. The use of a long TR allows evaluation of factors other than T1.

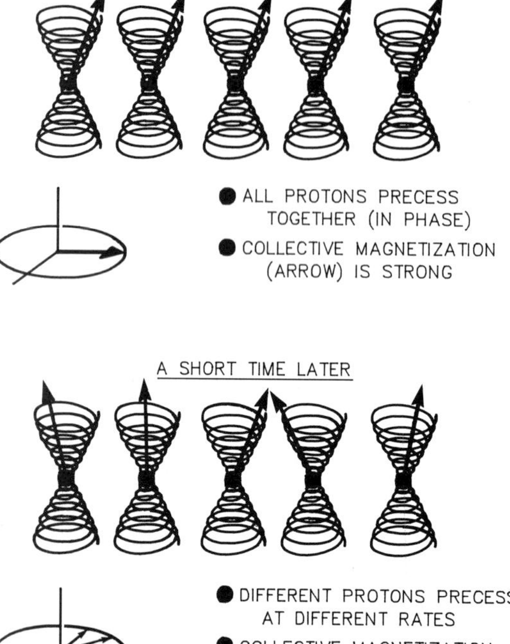

FIGURE 1–16. Phase coherence and tissue magnetization. Loss of phase coherence results in a decrease of the collective magnetization of the tissue. In the upper view, taken immediately after excitation, all protons are precessing in phase and their magnetic vectors *(inset)* align to provide maximal magnetization detected by the receiver coil. Because of local interactions, the protons precess at slightly different rates. In the lower view, taken within a brief time after excitation (about 20 msec), the proton magnetic vectors are becoming out of phase with one another and the collective magnetization is decreased *(inset).*

Precession Coherence: T2 Effect. The phase coherence of the precessing protons decreases as a result of local variations in the magnetic field that affect each proton. The most important causes of these variations are inhomogeneities of the externally applied magnetic field and interactions of neighboring atoms and electrons with the resonating protons. Both effects cause some protons to precess slightly faster and others slightly slower than their initial rate (Fig. 1–16). As a result, the collective magnetization of the protons is gradually lost. The interactions of the protons with neighboring atoms and molecules cause a different rate of loss of phase coherence for each type of tissue and, as a result, can provide distinctly different signal strengths for different tissues.

The measure of this loss of phase coherence is the T2 relaxation time, an exponential constant that characterizes the time required for the synchronously precessing protons to become out of phase with one another. If T2 is long (i.e., precession continues in phase long after excitation), the protons maintain a maximal collective magnetization and, consequently, provide a long-lasting magnetic resonance signal. The time after excitation at which the signal is detected (called the echo time, TE) can be chosen to be long to emphasize the long T2 of one tissue, in comparison with a shorter value of adjacent tissue (Fig. 1–15*B*, 1–15*C*). Substances with longer T2, such as fluid and tumors, maintain their phase coherence longer than other tissues and, therefore, appear bright on images that emphasize T2 effects (such images are called T2-weighted images). If T2 is short (i.e., the protons rapidly become out of phase with one another), the collective magnetization and, therefore, the magnetic resonance signal decrease rapidly. Tissues with short T2, such as muscle, appear dark on images that emphasize T2.

Mapping of Magnetic Resonance Signals. A variety of techniques are used to determine the location from which a given signal emanates. The basis for these techniques is the encoding of signals from different locations as a function of frequency. The most basic technique is two-dimensional Fourier transformation. In this technique a single slice of the patient is excited and then the various signal positions within that slice are mapped. For

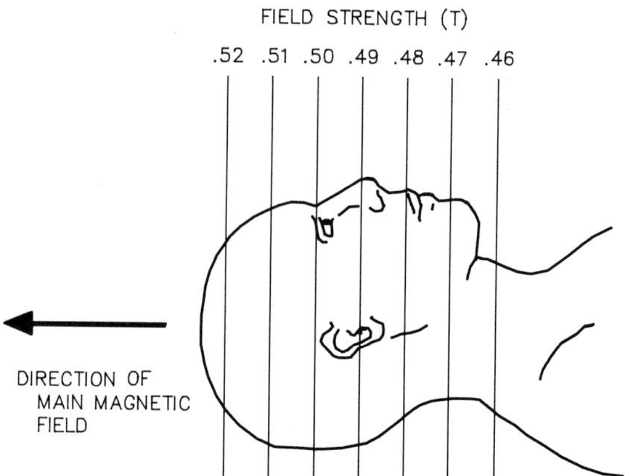

FIGURE 1–17. Slice excitation. Excitation of a single slice can be accomplished by employing a gradient field along the patient's axis that varies the magnetic field slightly. A specific frequency can be used to excite the protons in a single slice.

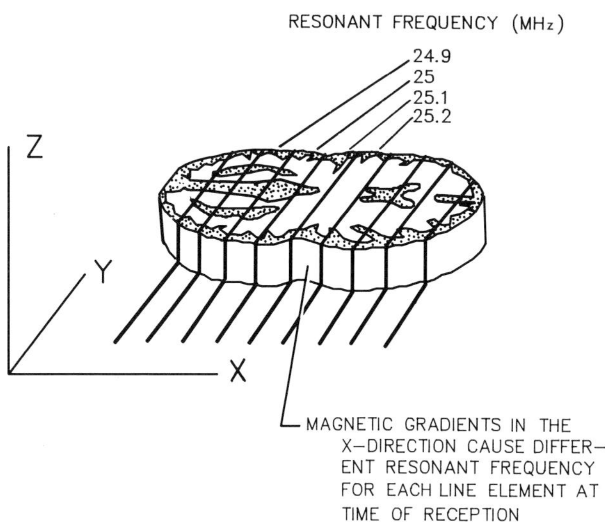

FIGURE 1–18. Locating image information. Spatial encoding is accomplished by altering the magnetic field in the *x–y* plane in such a way that each element resonates at a particular frequency and with a particular phase. Mathematical analysis allows assignment of an intensity to each pixel element (see text).

axial imaging, a small gradient magnetic field is added to the main axial magnetic field that causes each slice to have a different resonant frequency (Fig. 1–17). The slice is then excited by pulses of its preferred radiofrequency. Later, the use of a magnetic field gradient in the transverse plane (for example, in the *x*-direction) during the signal reception changes slightly the precession frequency of each linear segment of the plane (Fig. 1–18). The signal is then received as a function of intensity versus time. Mathematical transformation of the time information into frequency information (Fourier transformation) provides the signal strength for each frequency (corresponding to a particular linear strip of the slice). Finally, the information in the linear strip is separated by field gradients in the *y*-direction to encode the location of each segment of the line element. In other methods the entire volume is excited, and complex combinations of gradient and radiofrequency pulses are used to spatially encode in two or three dimensions.

Clinical MRI

The sequence of applied radiofrequency pulses determines the relative signal strengths received from the tissues and, consequently, the lesions that can be identified. An understanding of these operator-controlled imaging factors is important to the radiologist and the clinician for determining the best examination and for interpreting its results.

The three types of sequences most often used in clinical imaging are spin echo, inversion recovery, and gradient echo. These sequences differ by the combination of excitation pulse and read-out pulses. The excitation pulse, a short burst of resonant frequency radio waves of prescribed intensity and duration, changes the direction of the magnetization by 90 degrees (spin echo), 180 degrees (inversion recovery), or an intermediate angle (gradient echo) (Fig. 1–19). Later pulses (or gradient changes, or both) cause rephasing, spatial encoding, and artifact reduction in preparing the signal for reception (readout). Additional techniques entail variations of spin echo, inversion recovery, and gradient echo sequences and have special application in vascular imaging, three-dimensional acquisition, and artifact reduction.

Spin Echo. In the spin echo technique, a 90-degree excitation pulse is used to divert the magnetization from the axis of the main magnetic field and establish coherent precession in the transverse plane. The total transverse magnetization then decays as the protons return to their original polarization (a T1 effect) and as local interactions and magnetic field inhomogeneities decrease the phase coherence of the precessing protons (T2 effects).

The T1 effects and the true T2 effects (those caused by local interactions between atoms)

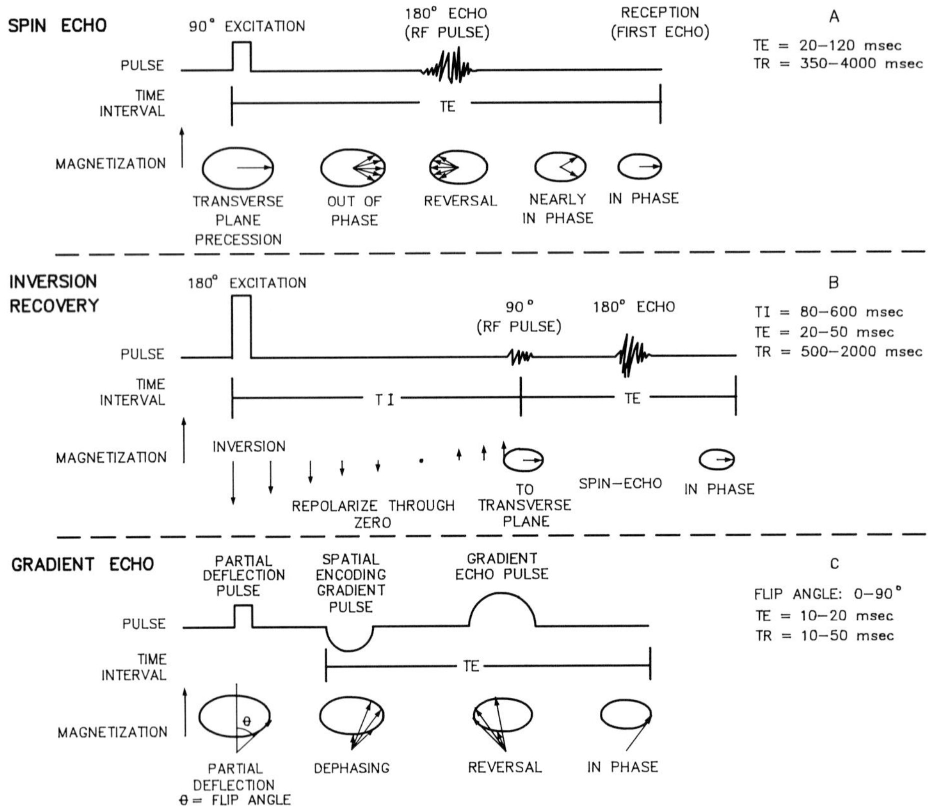

FIGURE 1–19. Applied radiofrequency pulses. The timing and the type of radiofrequency pulses influence the direction and the phase coherence of the magnetization, listed here for spin echo, inversion recovery, and gradient echo imaging sequences.

cause gradual decrease of signal and produce images that display T1 or T2 properties of tissue. The magnetization lost because of local magnetic field inhomogeneities is recovered through the use of a 180-degree echo pulse that maintains the precession in the transverse plane but changes the order of the precessing protons. This pulse places the more rapidly precessing protons behind and the more slowly precessing ones ahead; a short time later, the more rapidly precessing protons catch up and the more slowly precessing protons fall back so that all protons are again in phase with one another. At this time, called the echo time (TE), the net magnetization (diminished by true T2 effects) is maximized. The detected signal is called the first echo. A second echo can be obtained through the use of another echo pulse at a later time. Additional, later echoes can be obtained, although the overall signal strength continues to decay as a result of true T2 effects. Spin echo images are typically obtained at TE times of about 25, 50, 75, and 100 msec after the initial 90-degree excitation pulse.

The spin echo technique is especially sensitive to pathological disorders because it can emphasize a prolonged T2, which is found in most disease processes. It can also suggest tissue characteristics because it allows separate evaluation of T1 and T2 effects. The two operator-controlled factors in spin echo imaging are the repetition time (TR) and the echo time (TE); they can be varied to demonstrate different tissue properties (Tables 1–2, 1–3). TR for spin-echo varies from 0.2 to 4.0 sec for most imagers. A short TR selects those protons that remagnetize rapidly (i.e., those with short T1, such as fat). A long TR allows all protons to become nearly fully magnetized before each new excitation, thereby obscuring T1 differences and allowing separation of T2 effects by varying TE. A long TE selects protons that maintain phase coherence for a longer period than do protons of other tissues (i.e., protons with long T2, such as cerebrospinal fluid). A short TE can be used either in conjunction with a short TR to demonstrate T1 effects or with long TR when overall signal strength must be maximized and T2 information is unimpor-

TABLE 1–2. SUMMARY OF MRI INTERPRETATION

Definitions	
Relaxation times	Characteristic behavior of tissue magnetization (properties of the tissue)
T1	The characteristic time required for the protons to initially become aligned with the static magnetic field (or to become realigned after repetitive excitations)
T2	The characteristic time required for the protons to become out of phase with one another after radiofrequency (RF) excitation
Imaging times	Timing of instrument pulses used to excite and receive tissue RF signal (variables of the imaging technique)
TR	The time between successive RF *excitation* of the tissue (short TR selects protons with short T1)
TE	Spin echo imaging: the time at which tissue RF signal (spin echo) is *received* (long TE selects protons with long T2)
TI	Inversion recovery imaging: the time at which the recovering tissue magnetization is deflected for *reception* (tissue whose magnetization crosses zero at time TI produces zero intensity).
Flip angle	Gradient echo imaging: the angle through which the magnetization vector is rotated; a small flip angle allows more rapid imaging
Effects on Imaging	
T1	A *short* T1 allows remagnetization to occur *rapidly*, so the signal intensity is large (fat has a very short T1) and the tissue appears bright; tissue with *long* T1 (such as fluid) does not fully remagnetize between excitations and appears dark on the image; a T1-weighted spin echo technique employs short TR and short TE; inversion recovery with a TI that is similar to the T1 of a tissue results in a null signal for that tissue (fat can be nulled with the use of short TI); in gradient echo imaging, a large flip angle causes maximum change in longitudinal magnetization and can provide T1 weighting
T2	A *short* T2 causes precessing protons to become *rapidly* out of phase, which results in loss of signal; tissue with short T2 (such as muscle) appears dark on images obtained with a long TE; tissue with *long* T2 (such as fluid or tumor) maintains its phase coherence longer than other tissues and appears bright on images obtained using a long TE; a T2-weighted technique uses a long TR and long TE; in gradient echo imaging, a small flip angle causes minimal change in longitudinal magnetization and can provide T2 weighting; Spin echo and inversion recovery provide T2 weighting by the TE used in the echo pulse

MRI, magnetic resonance imaging.

tant. The 180-degree spin echo pulse is also used in other sequences, such as inversion recovery, to accomplish maximal in-phase precession before signal reception.

Inversion Recovery. The inversion recovery technique begins with an excitation pulse that inverts the magnetization of the sample, changing the excess of spin-up protons to an excess

TABLE 1–3. TISSUE APPEARANCE ON MRI SEQUENCES

		Spin Echo		Inversion Recovery		Gradient Echo		
Tissue	Relaxation Times	*T1-Weighted*	*T2-Weighted*	*Short TI (STIR)*	*Long TI*	*T1-Weighted**	*T2-Weighted†*	*T2-Fast‡*
Tumor/fluid	Long T1 and long T2	Dark	Bright	Bright	Dark	Dark	Bright	Dark
Muscle	Long T1 and short T2	Dark	Dark	Dark	Dark	Dark	Dark	Gray
Fat	Short T1 and long T2	Bright	Less bright	Black	Bright	Bright	Dark	Bright
Liver	Short T1 and short T2	Gray	Gray	Dark	Gray	Bright	Dark	Bright

The appearance of various tissues depends on the T1 and T2 of the tissue and on the imaging sequence. Four combinations of T1 and T2 are listed to show their appearances in the most common imaging sequences. The appearance also depends on field strength and, to some extent, the imaging software (particularly for gradient echo techniques).

*Short TE, 10 to 15 msec; moderate TR, 200 to 400; large angle, 45 to 90 degrees.

†Long TE, 30 to 60; moderate TR, 200 to 400; small angle, 5 to 45 degrees.

‡Short TE, 12 to 15, short TR, 20 to 50; mid-size angle, 30 to 60 degrees.

in the direction antiparallel to the main magnetic field. The protons gradually return to the lower energy state (parallel to the main magnetic field). As a result, the magnitude of the magnetization initially decreases to zero as the tissue attains equal populations of spin-up and spin-down protons and then increases toward its original value (Fig. 1–20). The time evolution of these changes depends on T1, and so each tissue has a different progression from antiparallel to zero to full magnetization. The time at which the protons are deflected into the transverse plane for detection, called the inversion time (TI), determines the signal intensity of each tissue. TI values range from 80 to 600 msec and are used with repetition times ranging from 500 to 2000 msec.

Two types of inversion recovery sequences are used in clinical imaging. In short TI inversion recovery (STIR) sequences, TI of 80 to 150 msec is used, depending on the field strength, to produce images when the signal from fat is passing through zero. Fluid and tumors have a strong negative signal on short TI scans and appear very bright. The contrast produced on STIR images is much higher than that of spin echo and gradient echo scans because (1) T1 differences (which are predominantly imaged by STIR) are greater than T2 effects for most tissues; (2) tumors, fluid, and adenopathy, findings of greatest clinical interest, have very long T1 and therefore a strong signal on STIR; (3) most other tissues such as fat, muscles, and connective tissue have low or zero intensity on STIR; and (4) T1 and T2 effects are additive. This high-contrast technique is ideal for abdominal imaging in detection of tumor, adenopathy, bone lesions (including tumor and soft tissue injury), bone marrow abnormalities, and head and neck lesions (Fig. 1–21).

Inversion recovery with a long TI (400 to 600 msec) is used for anatomical imaging of the brain and, because of its T1 weighting, can be used for scans enhanced with gadolinium. Gray and white matter can be clearly distinguished, and meningiomas are more easily distinguished from the brain. The major drawback of long TI inversion recovery is that tissues may have markedly different magnetization but attain similar intensity after the long TI interval.

Gradient Echo Imaging. In gradient echo imaging, excitation-deflection angles of less than 90 degrees are used. The echo rephasing is provided by a gradient reversal rather than the 180-degree radiofrequency pulse used in spin echo imaging. In gradient echo imaging and related sequences called by various acronyms (GRASS, GRE, FLASH), the smaller flip angle is used to reduce the time required for repolarization. This allows the use of very short TR (20 to 50 msec), resulting in thin-slice acquisition or volume acquisition.

T1-weighted images can be produced with the use of factors similar to those used in T1-weighted spin echo images (200- to 400-msec TR, 10- to 15-msec TE, and a flip angle of 45 to 90 degrees). T2-weighted images can be produced by use of short TR, short TE, and small flip angles. However, these T2-weighted images show less tissue contrast than do STIR

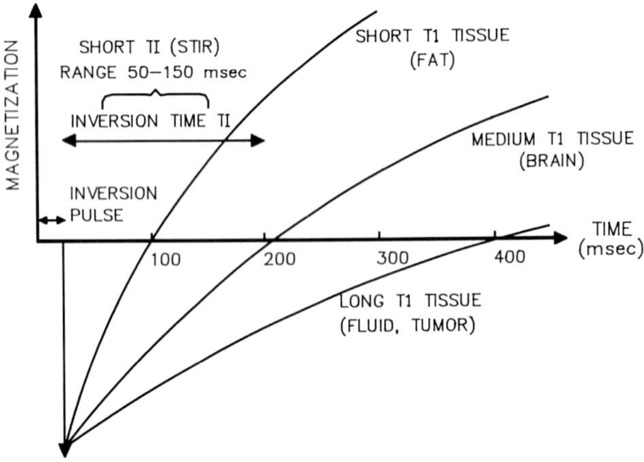

FIGURE 1–20. Inversion recovery. After the initial inversion of the magnetization, different tissues repolarize at different rates. At the time of deflection of the magnetization into the transverse plane for reception, the tissues have different magnitudes of magnetization. By appropriate choice of the inversion time, fat or other tissues will have zero magnitude.

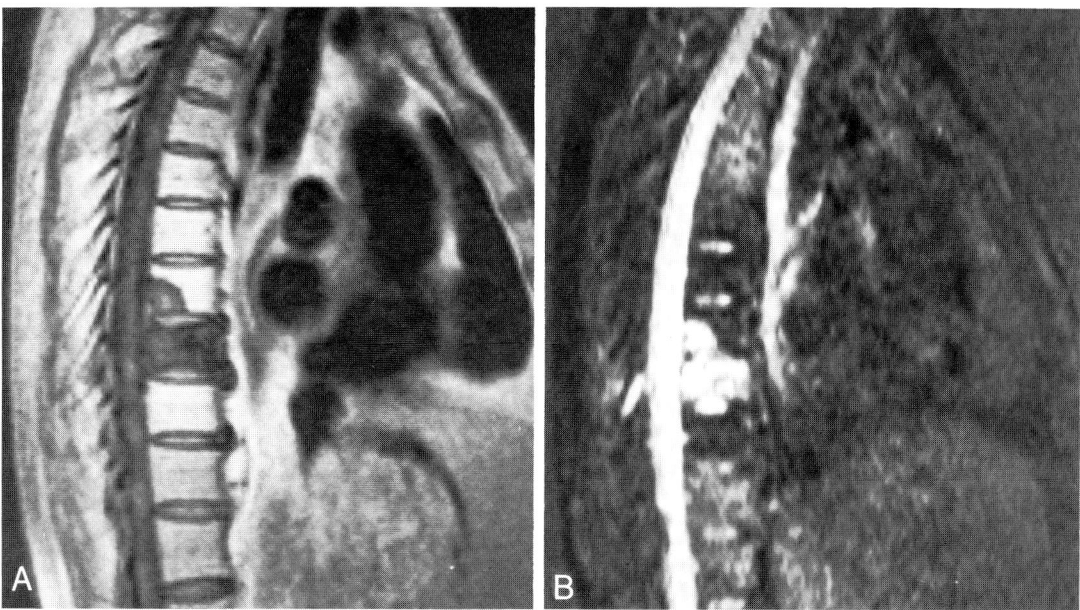

FIGURE 1–21. Bone invasion by metastatic prostate carcinoma. *A.* This T1-weighted spin echo image shows invasion of the bone marrow at T-7 and T-8, as evidenced by replacement of the normally high-intensity fatty marrow by tumor. Note the high intensity of the fatty marrow replacement at adjacent levels as a result of previous radiation therapy. *B.* Matching TI to inversion recovery (STIR) sequence suppresses the normal marrow fat and makes its low-intensity signal similar to that of cortical bone. The area of tumor abnormality has a high intensity and is clearly identified. The irradiated adjacent vertebral bodies show very low intensity as a result of fatty replacement. (*A* and *B* from Stimac GK, Porter BA, Olson DO, et al. Gadolinium-DTPA-enhanced MR imaging of spinal neoplasms: preliminary investigation and comparison with unenhanced spin-echo and STIR sequences. AJNR 1988; 9:839–846.)

images and T2-weighted spin echo images, and they are less effective in detecting altered tissue signals such as those seen in tumors, inflammation, necrosis, and demyelination. Gradient echo technique is used to image blood flow (Fig. 1–22) and cerebrospinal fluid pulsation and the musculoskeletal system, especially the spine and the large joints, and to reduce artifacts. The thin slices afforded by volume imaging sequences can provide rapid image acquisition with high spatial resolution in any plane.

Additional Techniques in MRI

Several additional applications enhance the diagnostic capacity of MRI. These include blood-flow imaging, intravascular paramagnetic pharmaceutical agents for use as contrast agents, and nuclear magnetic resonance spectroscopy.

Blood-Flow Imaging. Flowing blood has a magnetic resonance appearance different from that of stationary blood because the excitation-reception process is altered for moving protons. The most important factor is the speed of the flowing blood. For spin echo and inversion recovery imaging, rapidly flowing blood either enters the slice after excitation of that slice or leaves the slice before reception of the signal. In either case, no signal is received from the blood. Other factors that influence the appearance of flowing blood are the direction of flow, the initial magnetization of the blood as it enters the slice being imaged, the flow character (i.e., laminar flow, turbulent flow, or pulsatile flow), and the imaging technique. Gradient echo sequences are particularly effective in demonstrating blood flow because the blood experiences the gradient irrespective of the type of motion.

Blood in high-flow vessels such as the carotid arteries and their main branches, the aorta, and the large visceral vessels provides no magnetic resonance signal on spin echo and inversion recovery sequences because it fails to experience both the excitation and read-out pulses. It therefore appears black on scans. In most cases this lack of signal is an ideal contrast between the vessel and the surrounding tissues. MRI is ideally suited to evaluation of the heart and mediastinal vessels and of vascular lesions of the central nervous system. Other tech-

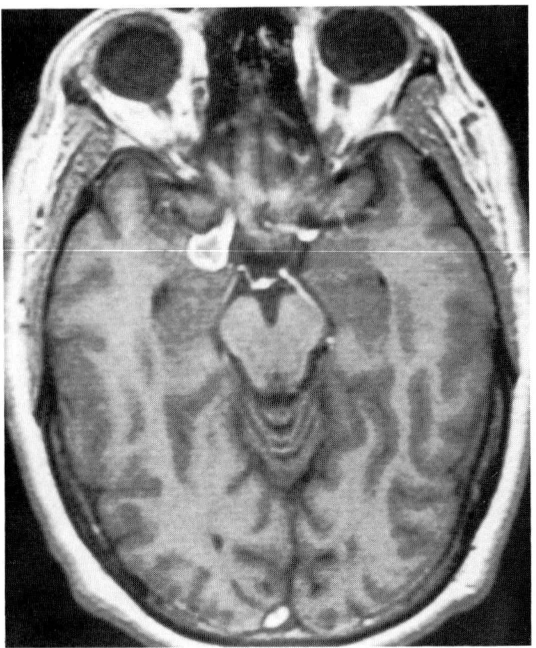

FIGURE 1–22. Vascular lesion shown on gradient echo scan. The choice of a small flip angle with short TR and short TE allows the demonstration of vascular flow in this carotid artery aneurysm. The flowing blood shows high intensity, whereas the rest of the brain shows relatively weak signal intensity. Note also the flow in other vessels at the base of the brain. (Courtesy of Robert Parry, North Shore Magnetic Imaging Center, Boston.)

niques provide a positive image of the vessels, producing a magnetic resonance angiogram.

Paramagnetic Agents. The inherent soft-tissue contrast in MRI is very high (up to 100 times that of CT). Nevertheless, some types of abnormalities such as meningiomas in the brain, tumors in the spinal cord, and scar tissue after lumbar spine surgery are not highly visible on MRI sequences. Additional enhancement can improve the sensitivity and the specificity of the examination. Contrast agents used in MRI are paramagnetic substances that create local variations in the magnetic field and cause a shortening of both T1 and T2. Depending on the dose and the imaging sequence used, the signal strength of the enhanced structure may be increased (on a T1-weighted scan) or reduced (on a T2-weighted scan). These agents are used primarily with T1-weighted, usually spin echo, images.

Paramagnetic substances are atoms or molecules that have one or more unpaired electrons. The unpaired electrons have a strong magnetic moment, 700 times the moment of unpaired protons. The most important of these paramagnetic substances in MRI is gadolinium (attached to a large molecule to render it biocompatible). Injectable gadolinium complexed to dimethylene triamine pentacetic acid (Gd-DTPA) or other molecules improves the radiologist's ability to diagnose many diseases in the brain and the spine (Fig. 1–23).

Nuclear Magnetic Resonance Spectroscopy. Local magnetic fields of atoms, especially their electrons, produce small spatial variations in the externally applied magnetic field. These variations result in a slightly different resonant frequency for protons in different parts of molecules. This change in the resonant frequency (typically between 1 and 200 parts per 1,000,000) is called the chemical shift. Nuclear magnetic resonance (NMR) spectroscopy, the detection of these frequency separations and their relative intensities, provides the ratios of protons in each environment. The technique has long been used in chemistry to identify molecules by their NMR signature.

NMR spectroscopy is also applied to detect the chemical shift of hydrogen, phosphorus, sodium, carbon, and potassium in biologically important molecules. The most important uses

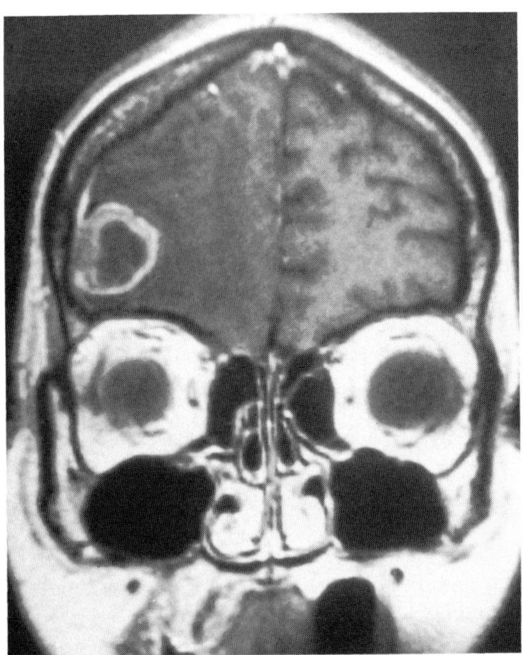

FIGURE 1–23. Brain tumor enhanced by gadolinium complexed to dimethylene triamine pentacetic acid (Gd-DTPA). This lesion, in a patient with lung carcinoma metastatic to the brain, shows rim enhancement after injection of paramagnetic contrast material. The center of the mass is necrotic and shows no enhancement. Note also right frontal lobe edema, effacing the sulci.

of NMR spectroscopy are the separation of lipid protons from water protons to describe the relative amounts of lipid and water in tissue, the characterization of lactic acid levels in ischemic states, and the comparison of the phosphorus atoms attached to adenosine triphosphate, adenosine diphosphate, phosphocreatine, and inorganic phosphate to assess the metabolic vitality of the tissue. NMR spectroscopy may be useful in the evaluation of ischemic and hypoxic brain disease, epilepsy, acid-base disturbances, and metabolic diseases. Some of the high-field strength imagers (about 1.5 T or greater) are capable of performing both imaging and spectroscopy. Low-field chemical shifts are small, and spectroscopy is consequently not practical for low-field MRI scanners.

MRI Interpretation

MRI interpretation requires the same attention to anatomical structure and the presence of masses and areas of abnormal intensity as required in CT interpretation. The greater contrast sensitivity and the many imaging sequences available with MRI provide greater sensitivity to disease and allow characterization of lesions by (1) location, (2) T1 and T2 relaxation times, (3) appearance on various imaging sequences, and (4) contrast enhancement. The ability to image in several planes is a further advantage in diagnosis and in treatment planning. The requirements of MRI diagnosis are knowledge of basic anatomical structure and pathological disorder, knowledge of the appearance of abnormalities in various imaging sequences, and the separation of real findings from artifacts.

In general, significant abnormalities such as tumors and fluid display high intensity on T2-weighted spin echo or STIR images. There are exceptions to this rule, which are discussed within the radiographic diagnoses throughout the text. Anatomical abnormalities are best shown on high-resolution scans such as T1-weighted spin echo and gradient echo sequences that depict cross-sectional anatomical structure. Cortical bone, ligaments, and fascial planes are of low intensity on all types of scans and assist greatly in identifying soft tissue boundaries.

Artifacts caused by complex pulse sequences, the effects of paramagnetic and diamagnetic substances, motion by the patient, and equipment or software occur in all types of images but are generally more troublesome with high-field-strength scanners. Metallic artifacts arise from termination of electromagnetic field lines on metal clips, shunt tubes, needles, monitoring wires, and so forth. These are easily identified because they cause a dropout and often a distortion of the signal in the area of the metal. Paramagnetic artifacts occur when a magnetic material alters the relaxation times of the tissue. Depending on the amount and the type of magnetic material (which includes endogenous iron and other metal, administered contrast material, and biological molecules) and the imaging sequence, the intensity may increase or decrease (Fig. 1–24). Equipment artifacts result from loose connectors, ineffective radiofrequency shielding, and improper choice of imaging parameters. These produce generalized degradation of images or a regular pattern of interference throughout the image.

Motion artifacts are especially difficult to deal with in MRI because they can cause general degradation of the images, can cause

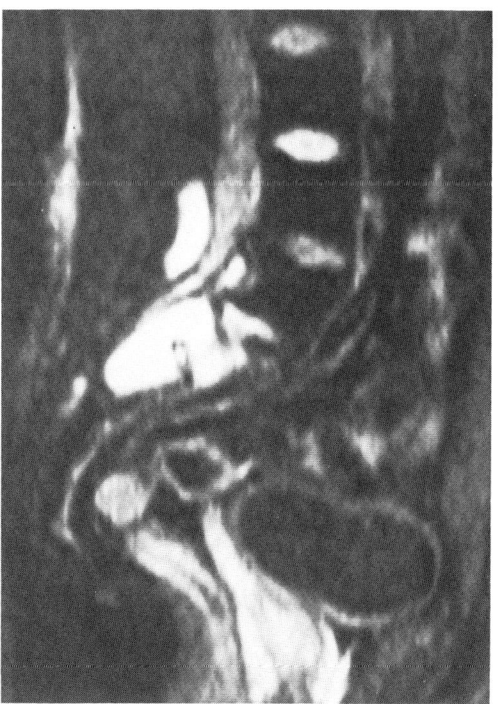

FIGURE 1–24. Magnetic resonance artifact from Gd-DTPA in the bladder. This post-Gd-DTPA STIR image shows a negative signal in the fluid in the bladder. (Fluid is normally high intensity on STIR images.) In this case, the shortening of T1 and T2 has resulted in a low-intensity appearance that allows identification of the bladder wall. The appearance of enhanced tumor in the lumbosacral spine was similar to that shown by the nonenhanced scan.

ghosting that suggests a lesion when none is present, and can place an object in the wrong location. Generalized motion by an uncooperative patient can be minimized by use of sedation and short imaging sequences. Pulsation artifact in the vessels or the cerebrospinal fluid that causes ghosting and blurring of adjacent soft tissue can be minimized by cardiac gating, judicious choice of the direction of phase encoding, and use of gradient pulses to eliminate or correct for the motion.

Software-generated artifacts pose a serious hazard because they often are not recognizable. Such artifacts can arise when phase angles of greater than 360 degrees are not distinguished from small angles, when signals from adjacent slices interfere with each other, and when algebraic sign changes occur when the magnitude of magnetization is near zero. Because each scanner has a different operating system, such problems can be identified and solved only by constant evaluation of image quality and machine function. Radiologists and MRI technologists must be familiar with such artifacts in order to eliminate them or to correctly interpret them.

DIGITAL IMAGING

Digital imaging, the recording of image information in binary format for later display, has developed with and made possible the image construction in CT, ultrasonography, MRI, and nuclear medicine. Such recording and display is applied to many examinations in which film-screen systems were previously used, including plain films of the chest and the gastrointestinal tract, and in angiography. Digitization allows storage, transfer, and manipulation of images, which result in improved diagnostic quality, more convenient image evaluation, decreased cost, and, in many cases, decreased risk to the patient.

In general, digital images are of superior contrast resolution and of slightly inferior (but adequate) spatial resolution in comparison with traditional film images. Many institutions photograph digital images for permanent storage, aided by the great flexibility in image formatting and electronic enhancement provided by laser camera photography. However, digital images can be used exclusively for clinical evaluation and consultation by display on monitors, and they can be stored on large memory devices (computer discs, laser discs, and magnetic tape systems), eliminating the need for hard copy films. Computer technology and data management are affecting all areas of diagnostic imaging by providing unprecedented image quality and ease of viewing.

Digital Cameras

Digital images from MRI, CT, and ultrasonography are often photographed onto conventional film with photographic cameras. Laser cameras project digital information by using bursts of infrared light. Specially developed film is sensitive to this infrared spectrum. Laser camera systems can enhance the contrast of the images electronically, allowing postprocessing of the data to improve image contrast or change the latitude of the system. These cameras can also print in a variable format and produce multiple copies.

Principles of Digital Imaging

A digital image is a numerical representation of the original analog image. Both the numerical values (which represent such qualities as optical density, photon intensity, or magnetic field intensity) and the locations to which they are assigned are characterized by discrete (rather than continuous) increments. The use of such values allows rapid and powerful manipulation of the images.

The digital image is represented in the computer (and on the display monitor) as a matrix of pixels of equal size; each element of the matrix is a number that represents the intensity of the image at that location. The size of the pixels determines the size of the smallest objects that can be detected (spatial resolution). An array of large pixels provides limited spatial delineation and, therefore, a squared-off image (Fig. 1–25). A finely divided matrix has small pixels and is therefore capable of demonstrating small objects. An array of very small pixels can appear to be continuous, like the true image; however, such factors as signal intensity per pixel, computer storage space, and data manipulation time restrict the range of pixel sizes.

Display screens used in medical imaging, computers, and television sets divide the image into arrays of 128 to 2048 segments in the vertical and horizontal directions. Larger arrays are available but have substantial data

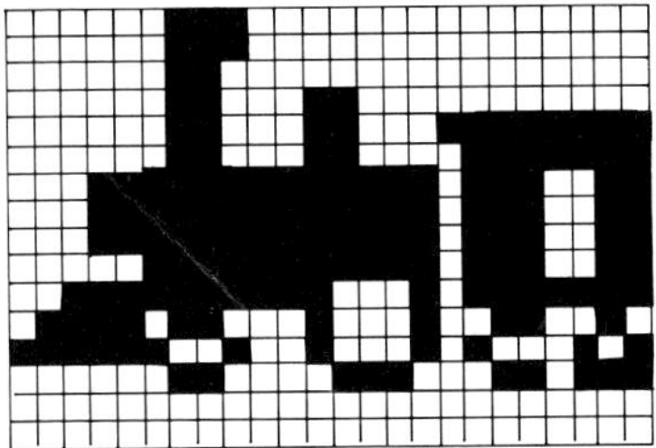

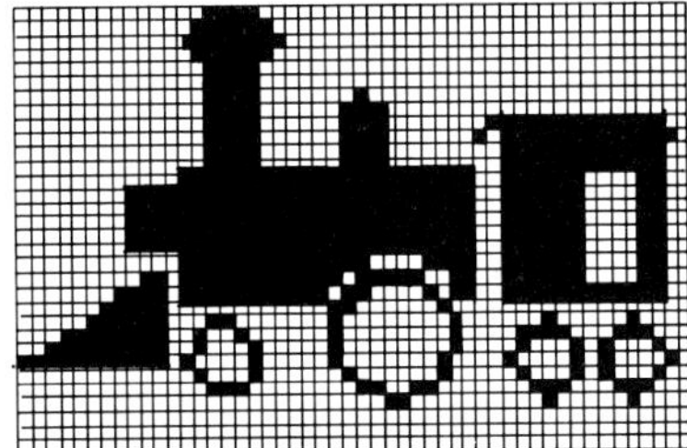

FIGURE 1–25. Image clarity is determined by the size of the matrix. The matrix with higher resolution (more elements) shows greater picture definition but requires greater overall signal (usually requiring longer acquisition time) and increased computation.

management and display requirements. The trade-off between pixel size and intensity per pixel is especially important in MRI, in which intensity is proportional to imaging time. As a result, MRI uses a matrix of 256 × 256 or fewer elements. The spatial resolution (the size of the smallest resolvable object) of an instrument depends on the size of the matrix and the size of the body part imaged. For CT, digital angiography, and chest radiography, this resolution is approximately 0.5 mm. For MRI, resolution is limited to approximately 1.0 mm.

The image intensity at each location is represented as a whole number: the result of rounding off the analog value of the optical density, the photon density, or the magnetic field intensity. The range of numbers stored in CT scanning is −1000 to +3000 HU. The images are displayed in gray-scale format to demonstrate the digitized information. For digital chest radiography and digital angiography, the x-ray density is divided into approximately 256 units for display on monitors, which allow changes in the window and the level that are similar to those of CT. Plain radiographs can be converted to digital format by dividing the optical density in each pixel into approximately 256 increments. The density differences per increment are just above the threshold of separation by the human eye.

Image Processing and Manipulation

A digital image can be processed to improve quality and diagnostic information. This processing can be done by the imaging device or by the laser camera used in photography. The most important data manipulations are subtraction, smoothing, and edge enhancement. The digital format allows mathematical processing through the use of high-speed computation techniques, many of which can be employed during the acquisition of the raw data. In most digital systems, some smoothing and edge-enhancement capabilities are built in; the radiologist can make additional changes retrospectively. Inherent in all these processes is the possibility that a lesion will be rendered less detectable or that a fictitious lesion will be displayed.

Image Subtraction. Digital image subtraction is the most important component of digital image processing for angiography. The detection scheme is illustrated in Figure 1–26. An image obtained before injection of contrast material (called the mask image) is subtracted from each successive postinjection image (Fig. 1–27). The resulting images contain, apart from a small amount of noise, only the image of the opacified vessels. The contrast shown on the subtracted images (the difference in density between the vessels and the parenchymal tissue) is very high. Consequently, structures of relatively small difference in contrast (as small as 5%) can be detected. This dramatic improvement in radiographic contrast resolution more than compensates for the slight loss of spatial resolution in digital angiography. Vessels as small as 0.2 mm in diameter can be detected; this is adequate spatial resolution for most vascular abnormalities in the neck, the face, and the brain and for some evaluations in the chest, the abdomen, and the extremities.

Additional techniques can further improve the quality of subtracted images. Several masks can be averaged to reduce the inherent noise in the mask; also, the contrast-enhanced images can be added, to result in a higher signal-to-noise ratio. Images can be compared with each other to maximize signal intensity and minimize radiographic noise. Finally, the image and mask can be displaced or rotated to eliminate the effects of motion by the patient

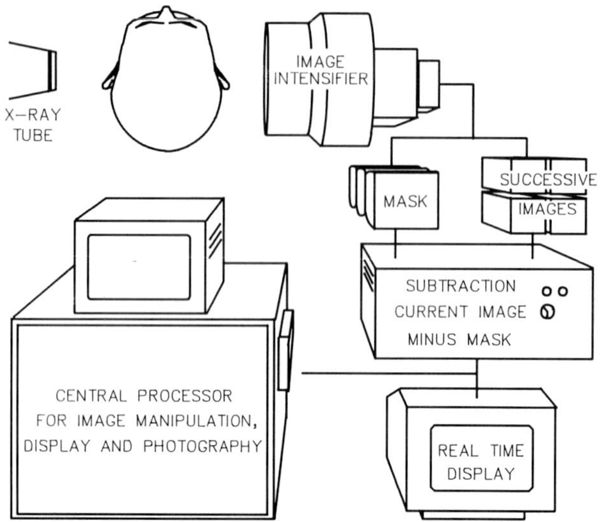

FIGURE 1–26. Scheme for digital subtraction angiography. The x-rays strike the image intensifier and produce sequential views. An early view, selected as a mask, is subtracted from each of the successive images, and these images are displayed in real time as the examination progresses. The data are also sent to a central processor for image manipulation, display, and photography.

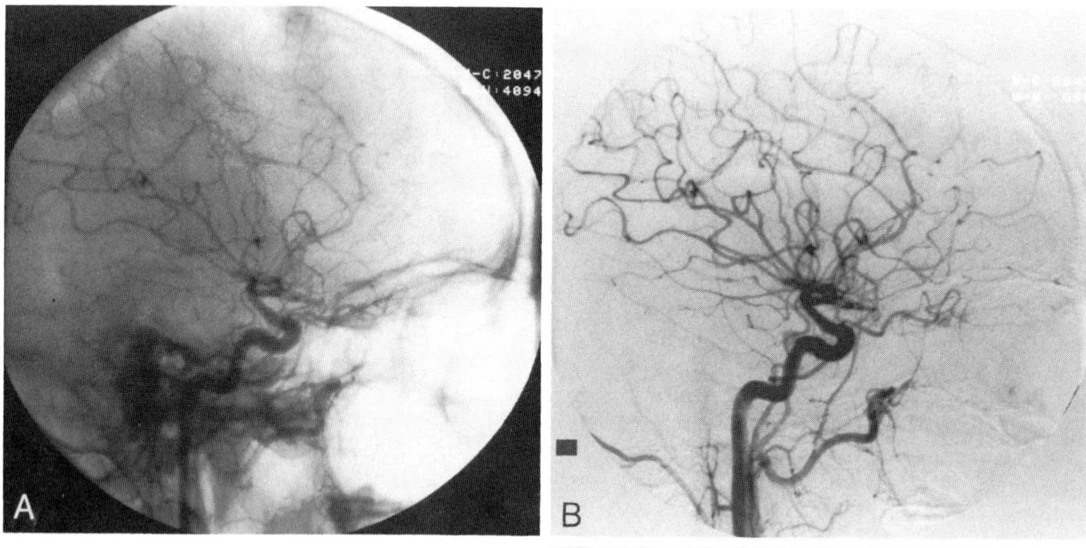

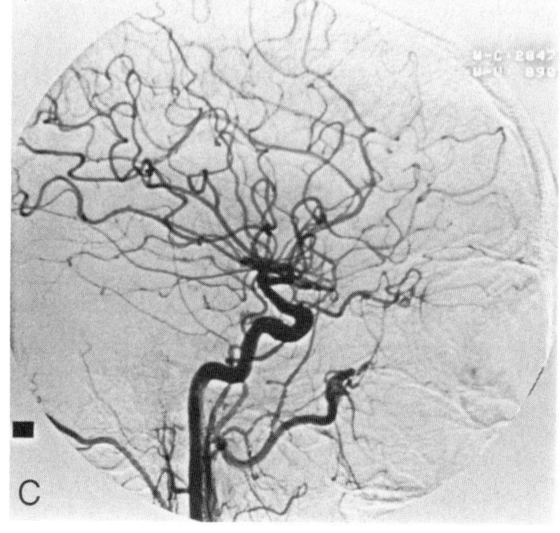

FIGURE 1–27. Manipulations of digital imaging. *A.* The unsubtracted image of a carotid angiogram shows the bones and the opacified vessels. *B.* In the subtracted image, the overlying density of bones and soft tissues is removed. The image can be smoothed or edged enhanced *(C)*, but these techniques can sometimes create the appearance of fictitious lesions or eliminate real ones. (Courtesy of Jerry King, University of New Mexico.)

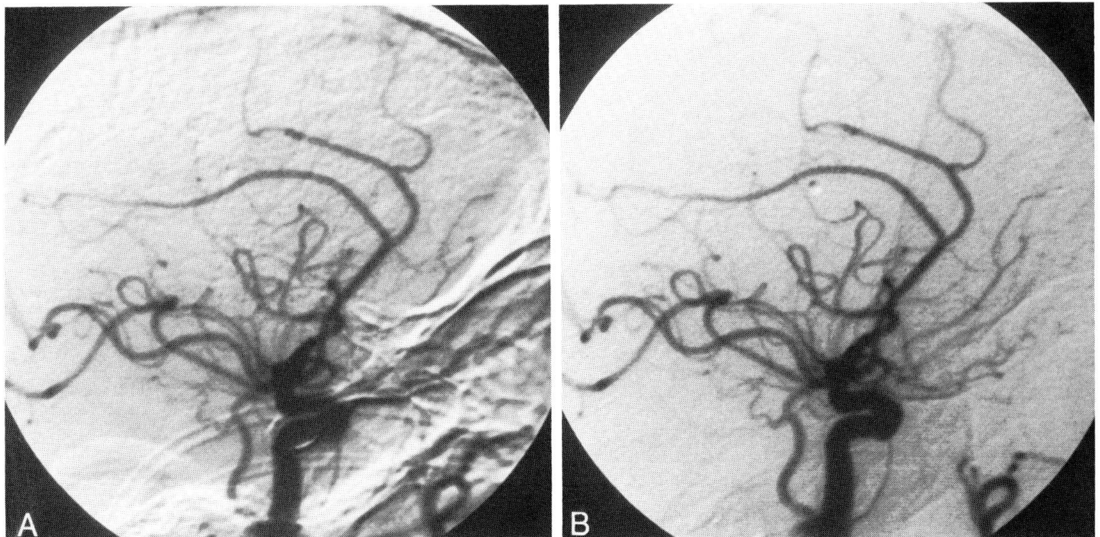

FIGURE 1–28. Reregistration of digital films. *A.* The original subtracted film shows bone and soft tissue margins as a result of motion by the patient between time when the mask was obtained and this film (the sixth in the series). *B.* After movement of the mask 10 pixels to the right and 16 pixels down, the subtraction is much improved. The vessels are more clearly demonstrated, and bone margins are eliminated.

(Fig. 1–28). Such reregistration can, at times, create fictitious abnormalities.

Smoothing. All images (digital or analog) contain a combination of structures that are sharply marginated and others that are poorly marginated. In some cases, it is desirable to partially eliminate sharp margins to make poorly marginated objects visible. This elimination is accomplished by smoothing the data—that is, averaging the values of each pixel with those of its immediate neighbors. Such an image is usually more pleasing to the eye and can demonstrate a large, poorly defined object (such as a large soft tissue mass) better than an unsmoothed image can; however, the altered image generally contains less information about sharply defined objects (such as bones and opacified arteries). Sometimes a subtle abnormality is rendered undetectable by image smoothing.

Edge Enhancement. It is more commonly desirable to sharpen the margins of adjacent structures to make them more readily seen. This edge enhancement is particularly important in angiography but can be important in digital radiography, CT, MRI, and ultrasonography. The edges are sharpened by means of filter functions that subtract from the low-intensity side of the margin and add to the high-intensity side (Fig. 1–27*C*). The human eye accomplishes the same edge enhancement by a similar process (lateral inhibition). Edge enhanced images generally have a sharper appearance, but because the process affects all points in the image, fictitious edges simulating lesions can be created by this technique.

POSITRON EMISSION TOMOGRAPHY

Positron emission tomography (PET) is an imaging technique capable of demonstrating physiological changes in tissue. The radiation from radioactive (positron-emitting) atoms attached to biologically active molecules is used to produce tomographic slices. Scans are obtained in a manner similar to that used in nuclear medicine examinations in that a radiopharmaceutical agent is injected into the patient and the radioactive decay products are detected by gamma cameras. The advantages of PET over traditional nuclear medicine techniques are the production of high-resolution, tomographic slices and the availability of a wide range of biologically active molecules that can be injected in order to study a variety of metabolic processes.

More than 100 compounds have been successfully labeled with radionuclides for use in PET. These radiopharmaceutical agents are organic substances combined with a positron-emitting radionuclide. Important substances that can be labeled include deoxyglucose (a glucose analog that is not rapidly degraded), carbon dioxide, oxygen, ammonia, numerous sugars, amino acids, fatty acids, and precursors of biological molecules. The most commonly used radionuclides are isotopes of carbon, oxygen, nitrogen, and fluorine (Table 1–4). Because these isotopes have short half-lives, they must be produced in a cyclotron near the PET scanner.

The principles of PET are summarized in Figure 1–29. The injected radiopharmaceutical agent becomes concentrated in target cells, and the radionuclide decays by positron emission. The positron travels a short distance (up to about 5 mm) before colliding with a free electron, a process that results in the annihilation of the electron and the positron and conversion of the mass of the particles into two gamma rays of equal energy (511 keV) and traveling in nearly opposite directions. The two gamma rays are received on opposite sides of the patient by a circular array of detectors. The locations of the two detectors and the difference in the time of detection determine the position of the decay of the positron to within about 6 mm. The number of decays in each pixel of a tomographic slice can be displayed in a gray-scale or color-intensity-scale format to produce an image of the metabolic process. The result is an image that shows the spatial concentration of the radiopharmaceutical agent in a series of slices at the time of image acquisition.

TABLE 1–4. ISOTOPES USED IN POSITRON EMISSION TOMOGRAPHY

Isotope	Half-Life (Minutes)
Carbon 11	20
Nitrogen 13	10
Oxygen 15	2
Fluorine 18	110

Because PET collects sequential data with excellent temporal resolution, it provides input for biomathematical modeling. Much investigation is directed toward demonstration of metabolic and physiological changes in the brain as reflected by glucose uptake, oxygen consumption, carbon dioxide production, and the incorporation of labeled precursors into molecules. Areas of application include the quantification of blood flow in ischemia, the anatomical mapping of brain functions, determination of sites of injury in diseases such as multiple sclerosis and Alzheimer's disease, the metabolic activity of tumors, and the identification of chemical mediators of central nervous system function and disease. PET is also used in cardiac evaluation to assess myocardial blood flow and infarction. Because of its ability to demonstrate metabolic changes in tissue, PET is valuable in the development of MRI by providing correlation of anatomical, physi-

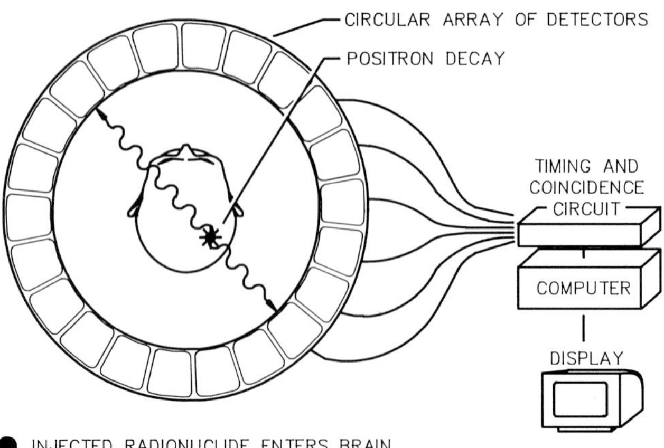

FIGURE 1–29. Principles of positron emission tomography.

ological, biophysical, and biochemical characteristics of tissue.

Important limitations of PET are the necessity of a nearby cyclotron to produce the short-lived radioisotopes and the consequent expense of obtaining and operating a PET imaging system. In addition, the spatial resolution is poor in comparison with other imaging techniques, and imaging times are long.

APPENDIX 1–1: COST, EXPOSURE, AND RISK OF RADIOGRAPHIC EXAMINATIONS

The radiologist must consider the cost and the risks of radiation exposure when recommending an evaluation (Tables 1–5, 1–6, 1–7). The most difficult to assess is the risk of a higher radiation dose in comparison with the benefit of the superior quality of the examination that may result. In most cases, the radiation from a single examination is about 0.01 Gy (1 rad), and the risk to the patient is very small. Exposure risk of diagnostic x-rays is best understood (and explained to the patient) through a comparison with other types of radiation exposure. The average yearly radiation dose from natural external sources (i.e., cosmic rays and naturally occurring radioactive elements in the environment) to each person is about 0.002 Gy (0.2 rad). The risk of radiation injury or the development of cancer from such low doses is believed to be insignificant. Only at very high doses, such as those used in radiation therapy, do radiation injury and inducement of cancer become apparent (8 to 50 Gy, or 800 to 5000 rad, usually administered over a period of several weeks). Many victims of the atomic bomb developed various types of cancer, but they had received doses of more than 8 Gy (800 rad) in a short period. The risk of causing defects in the developing fetus is high, especially during the first trimester, so pregnant women should not be exposed to x-rays unless it is absolutely necessary.

APPENDIX 1–2: ADVERSE EFFECTS OF IODINATED CONTRAST

Iodinated radiographic contrast, although safely used in the vast majority of patients, can cause renal toxicity, anaphylaxis, or hypotension. Despite the low incidence of these adverse effects, the referring physician and the radiologist must assess the relative risks and benefits of the use of these agents because reactions do occur in healthy patients and can be fatal. It is important to distinguish between anaphylaxis and hypotensive reaction. Because of the seriousness and the low probability of a reaction, many centers require patients to sign a consent form that details the risks of iodinated contrast and even the risks of the nonionic in comparison with the ionic agents.

Renal Toxicity. Renal toxicity occurs when the intravenously administered contrast material becomes concentrated in and injures the renal parenchyma cells. It occurs most commonly in patients who have renal failure. Patients who have myeloma, elevated uric acid, and diabetes are also at risk. Of patients with creatinine values greater than 2 mg/dL, 75% develop nephrotoxicity (which is usually reversible) after a contrast injection. Nearly all patients who have creatinine values greater than 5 mg/dL develop nephrotoxicity; in 60% of cases, this nephrotoxicity is irreversible. Good hydration is the key to the prevention of nephrotoxicity.

Anaphylaxis. Severe, systemic (anaphylactic) reaction to ionic contrast material occurs in 1 in 14,000 patients; it is fatal in 1 in 40,000. This allergic reaction is unpredictable. It can occur in patients who have had previous injections but no reaction; it often does not occur in patients who had a previous reaction. The only known risk factors of anaphylaxis are previous reaction to iodinated contrast material, allergy to penicillin, and asthma. Allergies to fish and to iodine are not risk factors.

Patients at risk for allergy to iodinated contrast material should be treated with steroids (such as 6 mg of dexamethasone orally every 6 hours for four doses) for 24 hours before the examination. In addition, 50 mg of diphenhydramine hydrochloride (such as Benadryl or Allerdryl) can be given orally or intravenously just before the injection. There is no firm evidence that either of these preventative measures is effective. The injection of iodinated contrast in a high-risk patient should be monitored by an anesthesiologist. The newer, nonionic materials carry a threefold lower incidence of anaphylaxis, but they are much more expensive.

Treatment of anaphylaxis consists of epinephrine and supportive measures. If the patient has good cardiac output, 0.3 mL of a 1:1000 concentration should be administered subcutaneously; if the patient is in shock, 5.0 mL of a 1:10,000 concentration should be given intravenously. Fifty milligrams of diphenhydramine and 100 mg of hydrocortisone can be added intravenously but will not be effective immediately. Aminophylline can be helpful in anaphylactic reactions to contrast material because it counteracts the slow-reacting substance of anaphylaxis. A mixture of 250 mg of aminophylline with 250 mL of normal saline should be given in the form of a 150-mL intravenous bolus. When bronchospasm is the only symptom, a sympathomimetic inhaler of metaproterenol sulfate (such as Alupent) is faster,

TABLE 1–5. RADIATION DOSE, COST, AND COMPLICATION RISK OF TYPICAL DIAGNOSTIC EXAMINATIONS

Examination	Dose* (Millirad)		Cost†	Risk‡ of Serious Complication
	To Skin	*To Midline*		
Skull series (4 views)	2000	350	130	None
Chest film (2 views)	100	15	90	None
Abdomen (2 views)	1500	250	90	None
Hand (3 views)	300	250	85	None
Lumbar spine films (4 views)	5500	650	150	None
Barium enema (double contrast)	5100	1300	250	1:1000
Intravenous urogram	7000	750	210	1:15,000
Abdominal angiogram (3 runs)	24,000	5000	500 to 1500	1:1000
Renogram	855	855	820	None
Lumbar myelogram	5500	650	670	1:1000
Cerebral angiogram (4 vessel)	54,000	9000	800 to 1500	1:500
CT (head)§	3400	1700	750	1:15,000
Ultrasonogram (abdomen)	None	None	280	None
MRI (head)	None	None	950	None

CT, computed tomogram; MRI, magnetic resonance image.

*One rad (for radiation absorbed dose) is 100 erg absorbed energy per gram of tissue. One gray, the SI unit of absorbed radiation, equals 100 rad.

†Costs (in dollars) at University of New Mexico Hospital, 1991.

‡Probabilities of complication vary widely, depending on the patient's condition and the type of examination. The most serious complication of barium enema is bowel perforation. Complications of intravenous urogram and CT scan are from anaphylaxis caused by intravenous contrast material. Nerve root injury and severe reaction to contrast material are the most serious complications of myelography. Stroke and arterial injury are the most serious complications of angiography.

§CT radiation is not additive for multiple slices because each slice is irradiated separately.

TABLE 1–6. MAXIMUM PERMISSIBLE YEARLY RADIATION DOSES

Organ or Body Part	Dose (in rem)
Total body (general population)	0.5
Total body (radiation worker)	5.0
Hands	75.0
Forearms	30.0
Gonads	5.0
Other (skin, thyroid)	15.0
Developing fetus (total gestation)	0.5

One roentgen is the amount of radiation that produces 0.000258 coulombs of ionized particles per kilogram of air. One rem (*r*oentgen *e*quivalent *m*an) is the dose in rads multiplied by a quality factor to take account of the size and charge of the particle in producing damage. This quality factor is unity for x-rays, gamma rays, and electrons; 5 for protons; 20 for alpha particles; 3 for slow neutrons; and 10 for fast neutrons.

TABLE 1–7. RADIATION INJURY TO VARIOUS ORGANS

Organ	Dose (in Roentgens)	Injury or Symptom
Total Body	0 to 200	None
	200 to 400	Nausea and vomiting
	400 to 600	Bone marrow depression (often fatal)
	600 to 1000	Gastrointestinal mucosa (death in 2 to 4 weeks)
	More than 1000	Central nervous system (death in hours)
Testes	400 to 600	Sterilization
Ovaries	300 to 400	Sterilization
Lens	200 to 500	Cataracts (children)
Lens	600 to 1000	Cataracts (adults)
Developing fetus	2	Leukemia

is more reliable, and produces fewer side effects than epinephrine.

Hypotension. Hypotension can occur as a result of a vasovagal response to the injection of contrast material. Patients do not experience bronchospasm, but they can exhibit signs of vascular insufficiency, including chest pain, dyspnea, and altered consciousness. Treatment requires fluids and, if response is not adequate, 0.4 mg of intravenously administered atropine.

Suggested Readings

Newell JD, Kelsey CA (eds): Digital Imaging in Diagnostic Radiology. New York: Churchill Livingstone, 1990.
Stark DD, Bradley WG Jr: Magnetic Resonance Imaging. St. Louis: CV Mosby, 1988.

2

Chest Radiology

Gary K. Stimac
Michael F. Hartshorne
Susan L. Williamson

BASIC EVALUATION

Plain Film Interpretation

The plain film of the chest remains the initial diagnostic chest examination because it is easily obtained and shows most chest abnormalities. It is the best radiographic examination for general screening and for the diagnosis of most lung diseases because it has high spatial resolution and displays a wide latitude of density. Evaluation of the chest begins with a view of the plain frontal and lateral radiographs (Fig. 2–1). Inexperienced observers should systematically assess chest films by first noting such factors as beam direction, position of the patient, degree of rotation of the patient, level of inspiration, and filming technique.

Beam direction determines the relative magnification of structures in the lung. When the beam direction is posteroanterior (PA), the heart is close to the film and is imaged accurately. When the beam direction is anteroposterior (AP), the heart is farther from the film and is magnified as a result of the divergence of the x-ray beam.

For different positions of the patient, gravity affects the radiographic appearance of the chest. The dependent pulmonary vessels are more distended with blood than are the nondependent ones and therefore appear larger. Large pulmonary vessels in the upper lung are, therefore, a normal finding in a supine chest but indicate some type of cardiac or fluid abnormality in an upright chest. In a decubitus view the dependent lung is partially collapsed, the nondependent lung is expanded, and the mediastinum is shifted to the dependent side. Rotation of the patient changes the contours of the heart and the mediastinum by rotating out laterally the structures that are directly anterior and posterior to the heart. When the patient is rotated to the left, the right hilum appears abnormally prominent, and the heart silhouette is large. When the patient is rotated to the right, the left hilum is prominent.

A low level of inspiration makes the heart appear wider and the pulmonary vessels appear large and crowded. The best indicator of the level of inspiration is the relationship of the lower portion of the heart to the diaphragm. Counting ribs is not recommended.

The film technique determines the absolute film exposure (blackness) and the relative density of structures. Low exposure produces a light film with good demonstration of pulmo-

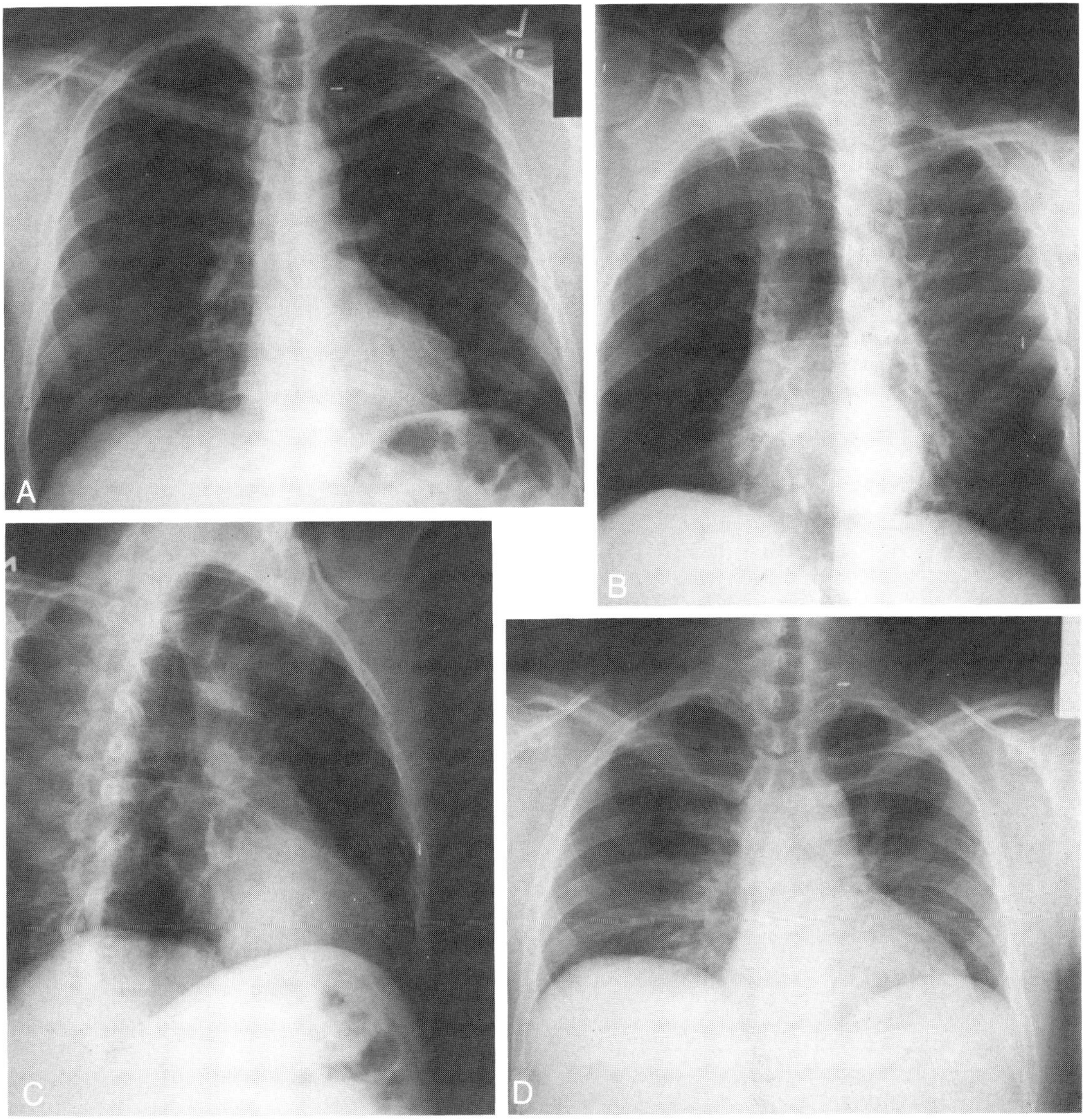

FIGURE 2–1. *A.* Upright posteroanterior (PA) chest radiograph taken at 6-feet (1.83 m) film distance. *B.* Upright left anterior oblique view. *C.* Normal upright right anterior oblique view. *D.* Normal supine, anteroposterior (AP) view at the end of expiration in the same patient. The shorter 40-inch focal distance, the lower level of inspiration, and the AP projection combine to make the heart look larger and the central vessels more prominent.

nary parenchyma but poor penetration of the mediastinum. A high kilovoltage technique gives good penetration of the patient but minimizes the density differences among structures.

Any orderly approach can then be undertaken to look at structures individually, beginning with foreign objects such as tubes, catheters, pacemakers, sutures, drains, prostheses, knives, or bullets. Identifying these objects and their exact location is often the most important part of the radiographic evaluation. The approach continues with a study of the bones, specifically the spine (in both frontal and lateral views), the clavicles, the scapulae, the humeri, the sternum, and the ribs. The most rapid and reliable way to assess the ribs is to look first at the posterior segments of the right ribs 1 to 12, then the right anterior segments, and finally the right lateral segments. The process is repeated for the left side. Scanning each rib continuously from back to front is impossible (the eye can follow a moving target, but it scans a stationary line in saccades) and frustrating.

Such a review of the bones in the PA view

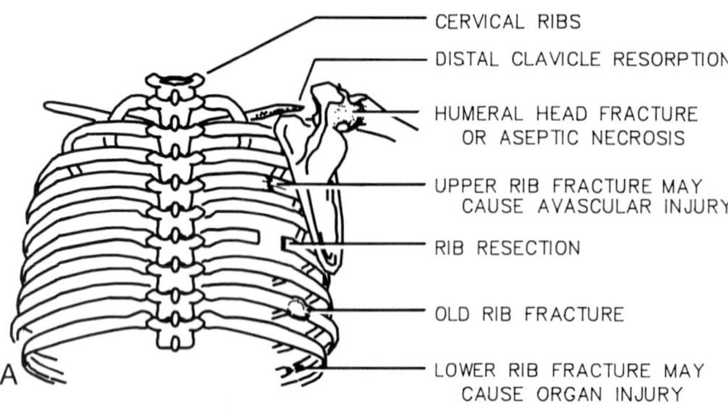

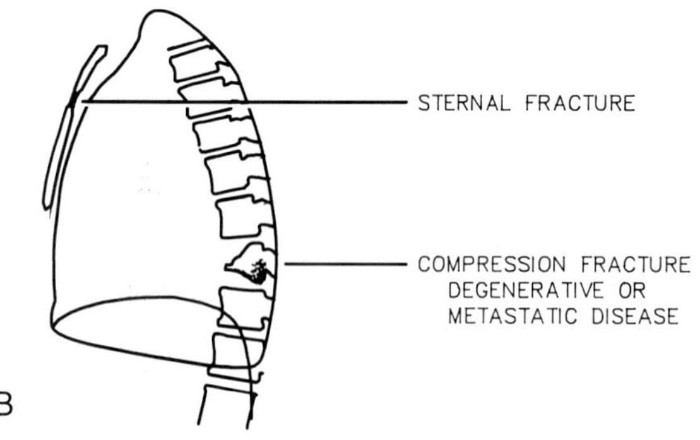

FIGURE 2–2. Location of important bone findings on chest radiograph. *A.* PA view. *B.* Lateral view.

(Fig. 2–2) can indicate such abnormalities as cervical ribs, which can cause nerve root compression; upper rib fractures, which can be associated with injury to the aorta or the brachiocephalic vessels; lower rib fractures, which can be associated with injury to abdominal organs; rib resection, which is indicative of previous surgery; old rib fractures, usually located laterally, which can indicate previous trauma, including child abuse; resorption of the distal clavicles, seen in rheumatoid arthritis; and fracture, dislocation, or necrosis of the proximal humerus. The lateral view can reveal sternum fracture, pectus excavatum, and ver-

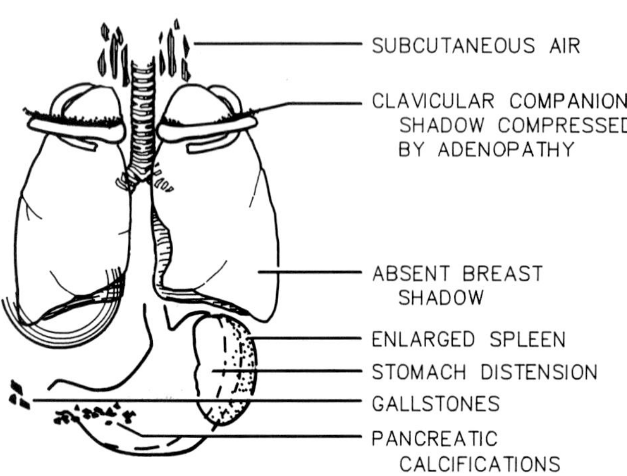

FIGURE 2–3. Soft tissue abnormalities on PA chest radiograph.

tebral body abnormalities, including degenerative disease, metastatic cancer, and compression fracture.

Next, the soft tissues are evaluated. An unusual contour of the soft tissues of the neck suggests a thyroid mass, adenopathy, or subcutaneous emphysema. Asymmetric breast shadows may indicate mastectomy. Abnormalities in the abdomen that are visible on the chest radiograph include hepatomegaly, splenomegaly, gallstones, abdominal calcifications, and gastric distention (Fig. 2–3).

The mediastinum appears as a series of bulges on the PA radiograph (Fig. 2–4*A*). Any deviation from the expected contours must be explained. The lateral radiograph can be particularly helpful in an evaluation of the anterior mediastinum and the hilar region for adenopathy, tumor, and other abnormalities. It also assists in locating structures spatially (Fig. 2–4*B*). The esophagus is not usually seen on the plain film, but an abnormality can be inferred when the right paratracheal stripe is widened (Fig. 2–4*C*). This widening is indirect evidence of a mass in the mediastinum. However, computed tomography (CT) can demonstrate large esophageal, paratracheal, and hilar masses in the mediastinum that are not evident on the plain chest film. Therefore, CT is indicated for any patient with clinical or radiographic findings that suggest a hilar or mediastinal mass.

Evaluation of the mediastinum is completed by assessment of the heart and then of the pulmonary vessels (Fig. 2–5). Heart contour and size (maximal diameter is half the width of the thorax), chamber position and size, valve position, presence of calcification (of valves, vessels, or aneurysm), and size of pulmonary vessels are evaluated. In addition to standard PA and lateral views, films obtained with the patient in the left and right anterior oblique position can be helpful.

The lungs are evaluated for symmetry, aeration, clarity of vessels, and the presence of focal or diffuse abnormal density. In a patient at risk for lung cancer, a careful search for pulmonary nodules must be made. Knowledge of the locations of segments of the lung in both PA and lateral projections allows the radiologist to determine the location of abnormalities and assess lung volume loss (Fig. 2–6). The right lung has three lobes (upper, middle, and lower) separated by pleural fissures; the right upper and the right middle lobes together have five segments, and the right lower lobe has five segments. The left lung has two lobes (upper and lower); the lingula, which is the left-sided counterpart of the right middle lobe, is part of the left upper lobe. The left upper and the left lower lobes each have four segments. Collapse of a lung segment results in loss of lung volume (manifested by shift of the mediastinum and elevation of the diaphragm), increased density of the collapsed segment, and obscuring of adjacent borders of the heart, the mediastinal structures, or the diaphragm.

Finally, the pleura is studied for the presence of fluid, scarring, apical thickening, plaques, and calcifications. A pleural effusion causes blunting of the costophrenic angles and loss of the border of the hemidiaphragm. On a decubitus view, this fluid can be seen to layer on the dependent side (Fig. 2–7).

Computed Tomography Interpretation

CT has greatly improved the diagnosis of chest disease. The broad range of density demonstrated by CT provides essential information about the predominantly air-filled lung, the soft tissues of the mediastinum, and the high-density bones. The scan can be photographed at level and window settings that optimize the density differences among these structures to best demonstrate them. Usually at least two settings are employed: one to show the lung parenchyma, the other to show the mediastinum and the bones (see Figure 1–5).

The lung setting demonstrates the lung parenchyma, the pulmonary vessels, and the major bronchial segments (Fig. 2–8*A*). Vessels normally taper toward the periphery. Consolidated areas and parenchymal masses are easily seen as high density against the low-density lung. Nodules are easily identified, and their CT numbers (density) can be determined. Nodules with a density similar to that of bone are always benign calcified lesions, usually granulomas. Nodules with CT numbers less than that of bone are indeterminate and must be evaluated by biopsy if clinical circumstances warrant.

The mediastinal setting demonstrates the vessels, the lymph nodes, the esophagus, the airway, and the heart (Fig. 2–8*B* to 2–8*F*). The lower slices show the heart. The pulmonary artery, the aorta, and the superior vena cava are visible more superiorly. The airway is anterior, and the esophagus is usually collapsed and positioned slightly to the left. Important lymph nodes are subcarinal, paratracheal, and hilar. The pulmonary hilum shows

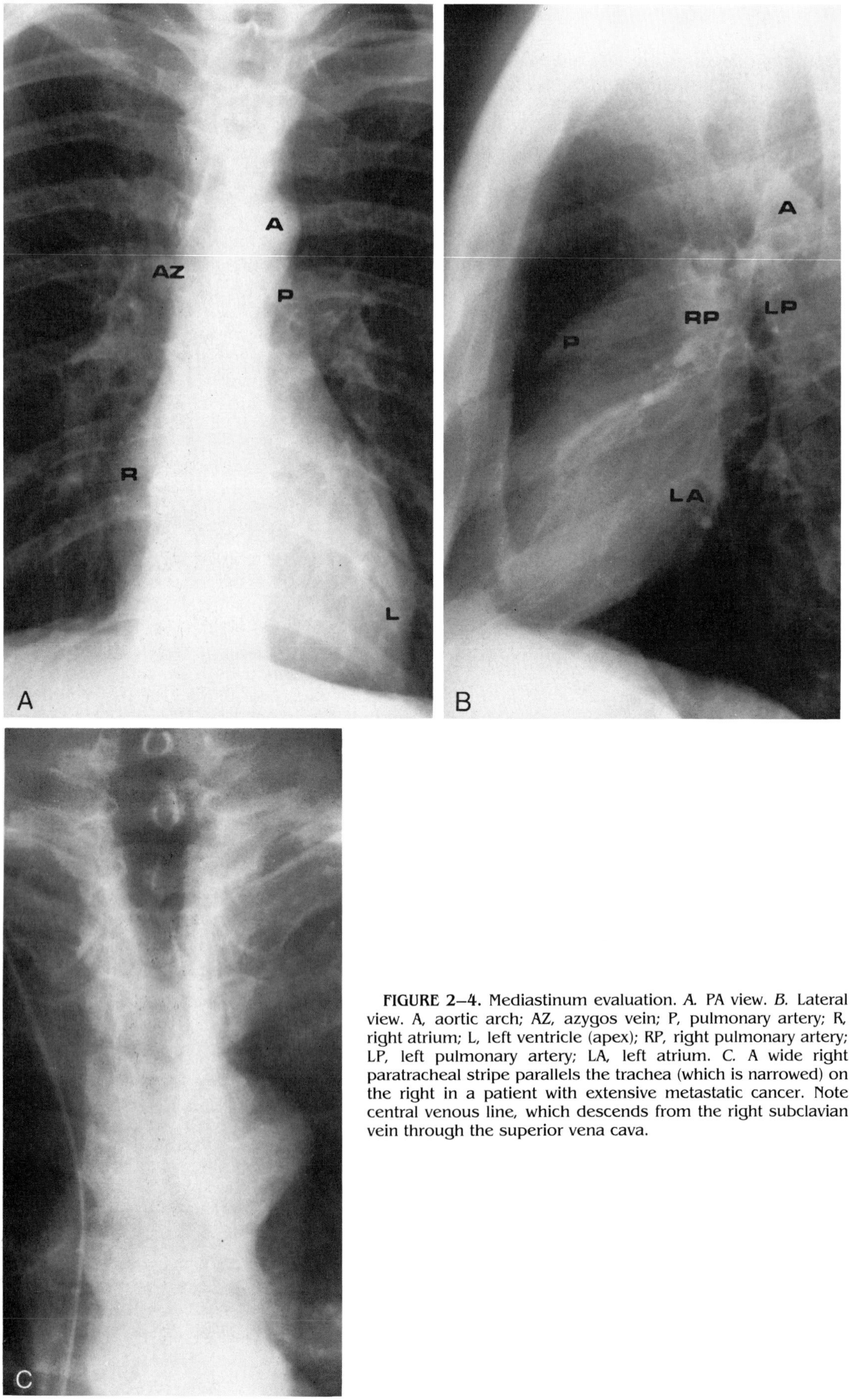

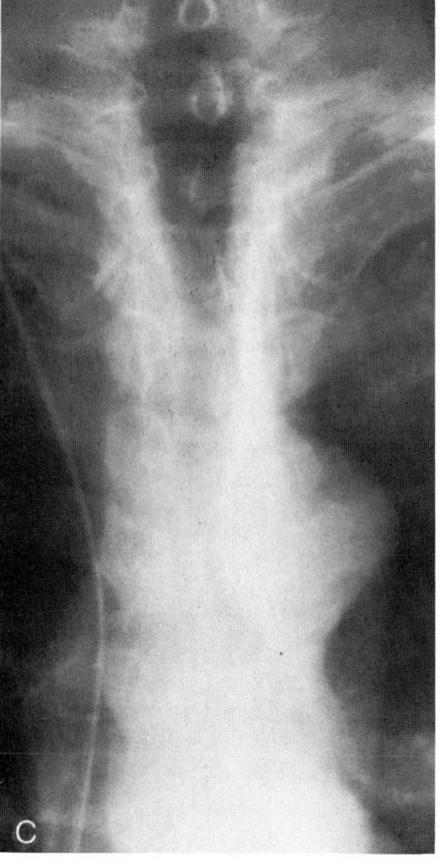

FIGURE 2–4. Mediastinum evaluation. *A.* PA view. *B.* Lateral view. A, aortic arch; AZ, azygos vein; P, pulmonary artery; R, right atrium; L, left ventricle (apex); RP, right pulmonary artery; LP, left pulmonary artery; LA, left atrium. C. A wide right paratracheal stripe parallels the trachea (which is narrowed) on the right in a patient with extensive metastatic cancer. Note central venous line, which descends from the right subclavian vein through the superior vena cava.

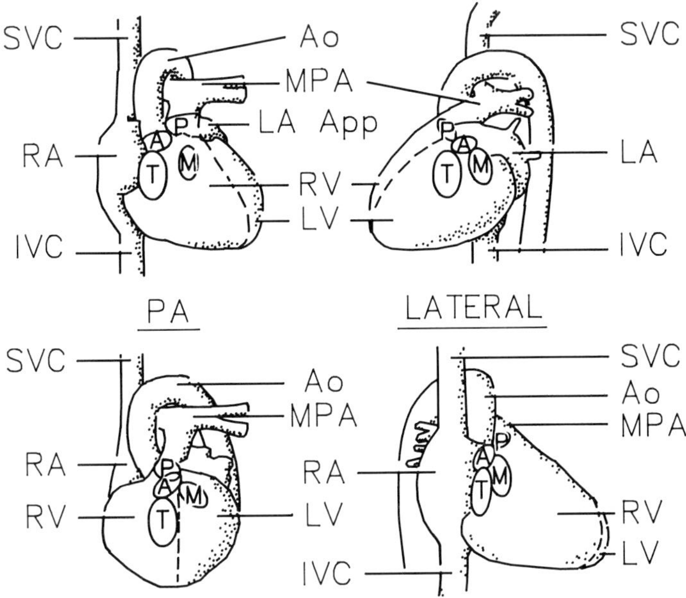

FIGURE 2–5. Positions of cardiac chambers and valves. Ao, aorta; SVC and IVC, superior and inferior vena cava; MPA, main pulmonary artery; RA and LA, right and left atria; RV and LV, right and left ventricles; LA App, left atrial appendage; A, P, T, and M, refer to the aortic, pulmonic, tricuspid, and mitral valves, respectively.

symmetrical tapering and branching of vessels and major bronchi. Contrast enhancement can usually demonstrate tumor or adenopathy in the hilum. The aortic arch and its three great vessels, the innominate vein, the esophagus, and the superior vena cava are visible more superiorly. The esophageal lumen is difficult to show even when oral contrast is given because it is often collapsed during the imaging.

Magnetic Resonance Imaging Interpretation

Magnetic resonance imaging (MRI) is most effective in evaluating mediastinal disease and chest wall abnormalities. Imaging in the coronal plane best shows tumor or adenopathy. Coronal chest anatomy is analogous to the frontal plain film of the chest. Advantages of MRI over CT include better vision of extension of the chest wall by tumor, separation of hilar adenopathy from the flow void in pulmonary vessels without the need for intravenous contrast, and detection of mediastinal adenopathy and vascular invasions (Fig. 2–9). Motion artifact is least severe at low-field strengths, and image contrast is best in short inversion time recovery (STIR) films (Fig. 2–10).

TRAUMATIC DISEASES

Traumatic injuries to the chest include injuries caused by penetration, blunt force, and toxic chemicals. The most common chest injuries are caused by motor vehicle accidents, which result in rib fractures, lung contusion, and aortic injury.

Penetrating Trauma

Penetrating trauma is usually produced by a knife or a bullet, but glass and other projectiles can also cause significant damage. A high-speed bullet causes a cone-shaped shock wave as it passes through the body, resulting in tissue disruption that is more extensive than the size of the bullet would suggest. Entrance and exit wounds indicate the path of the projectile, and injury to any structure in this path must be suspected. A penetrating wound to the lower chest can injure abdominal organs by passing through the high middle portion of the diaphragm (Fig. 2–11).

In any case of penetrating trauma, a careful search for fragments of the projectile or implement must be undertaken. Metallic projectiles and glass always appear relatively opaque on x-ray films and are easily detected. Other projectiles may be similar in radiographic density to body tissues and therefore are identified only by careful search. The geometric shapes of these nearly isodense objects are often an important clue to their presence. In any case of trauma, all foreign objects should be assumed to be within the patient until proved otherwise.

FIGURE 2–6. Lung segments. *A.* Right lung. *B.* Left lung.

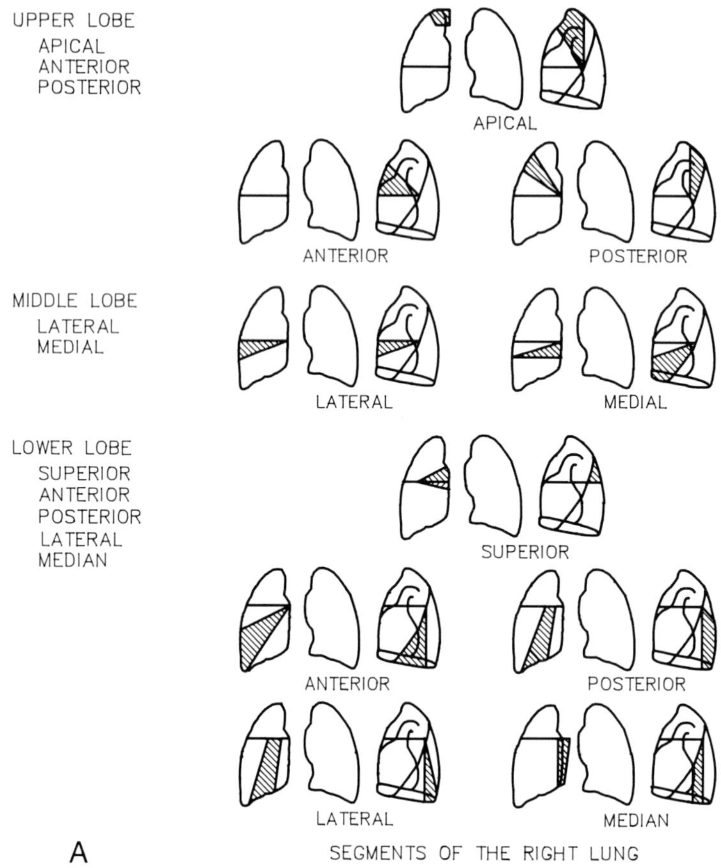

UPPER LOBE
APICAL
ANTERIOR
POSTERIOR

APICAL

ANTERIOR POSTERIOR

MIDDLE LOBE
LATERAL
MEDIAL

LATERAL MEDIAL

LOWER LOBE
SUPERIOR
ANTERIOR
POSTERIOR
LATERAL
MEDIAN

SUPERIOR

ANTERIOR POSTERIOR

LATERAL MEDIAN

A

SEGMENTS OF THE RIGHT LUNG

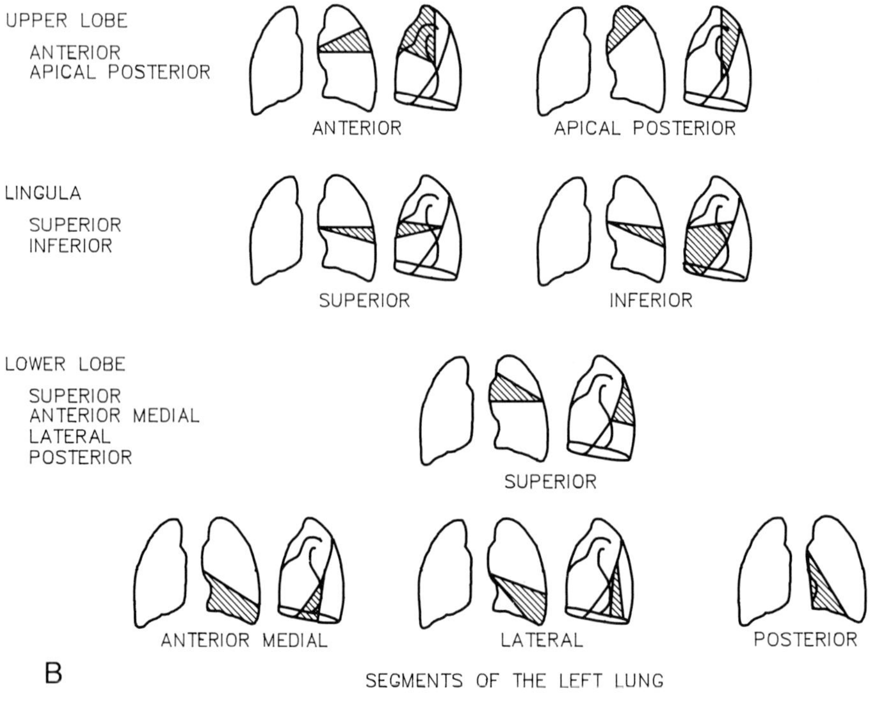

UPPER LOBE
ANTERIOR
APICAL POSTERIOR

ANTERIOR APICAL POSTERIOR

LINGULA
SUPERIOR
INFERIOR

SUPERIOR INFERIOR

LOWER LOBE
SUPERIOR
ANTERIOR MEDIAL
LATERAL
POSTERIOR

SUPERIOR

ANTERIOR MEDIAL LATERAL POSTERIOR

B

SEGMENTS OF THE LEFT LUNG

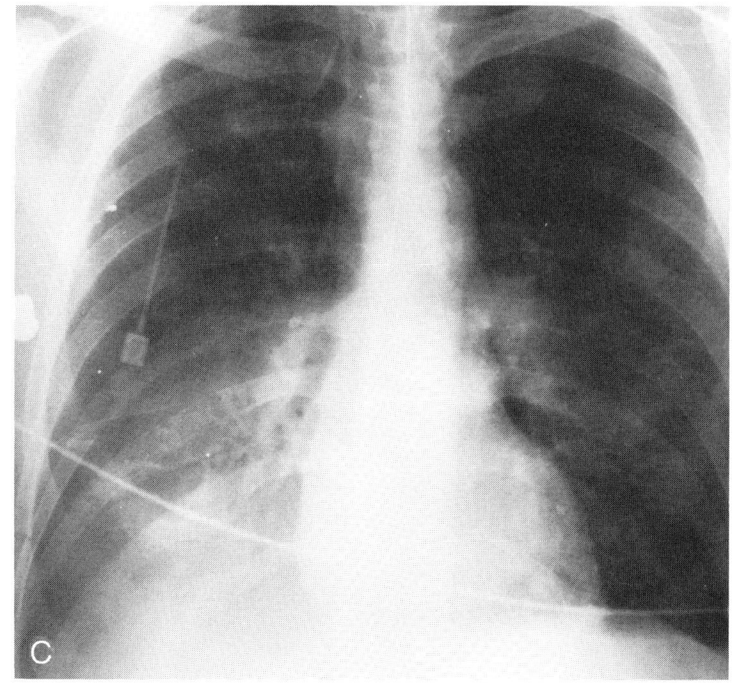

FIGURE 2–6 *Continued C.* Right lower-lobe collapse. An obstructing bronchogenic carcinoma (not seen) in the right lower-lobe bronchus caused lobe collapse. The collapsed segment is of increased density because it no longer contains air. Volume loss is evident from the shift of the heart to the right. The right diaphragm is obscured because the collapsed segment lies against it. The right heart border, being well anterior, is clearly seen.

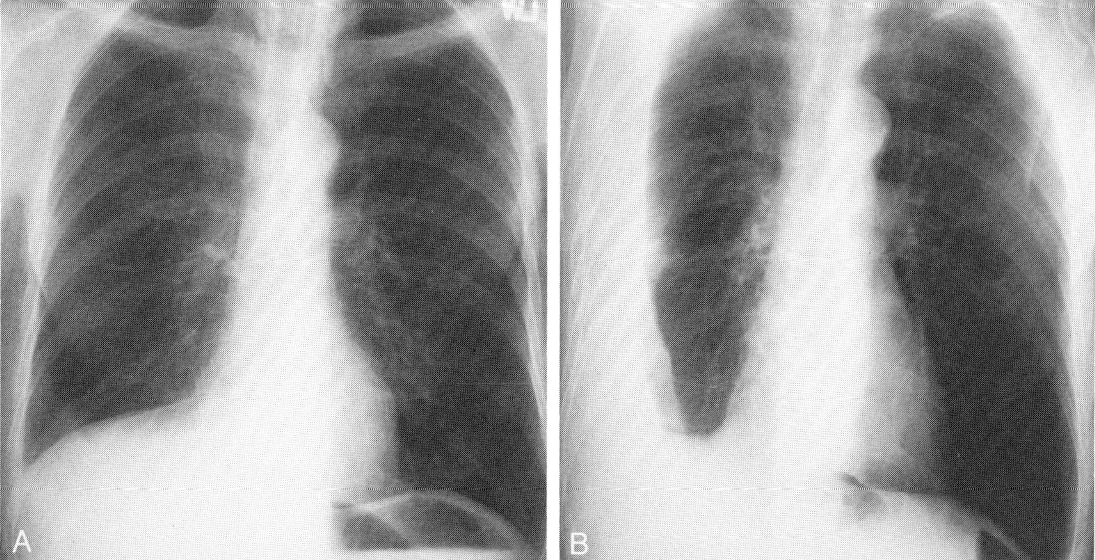

FIGURE 2–7. Pleural effusion. *A.* Upright PA chest film shows a right subpulmonic pleural effusion that elevates the right lung base. *B.* Right lateral decubitus view (right side down) clearly demonstrates the pleural fluid that flows along the right chest wall. The decubitus technique can also be used to show pneumothorax in the lung on top.

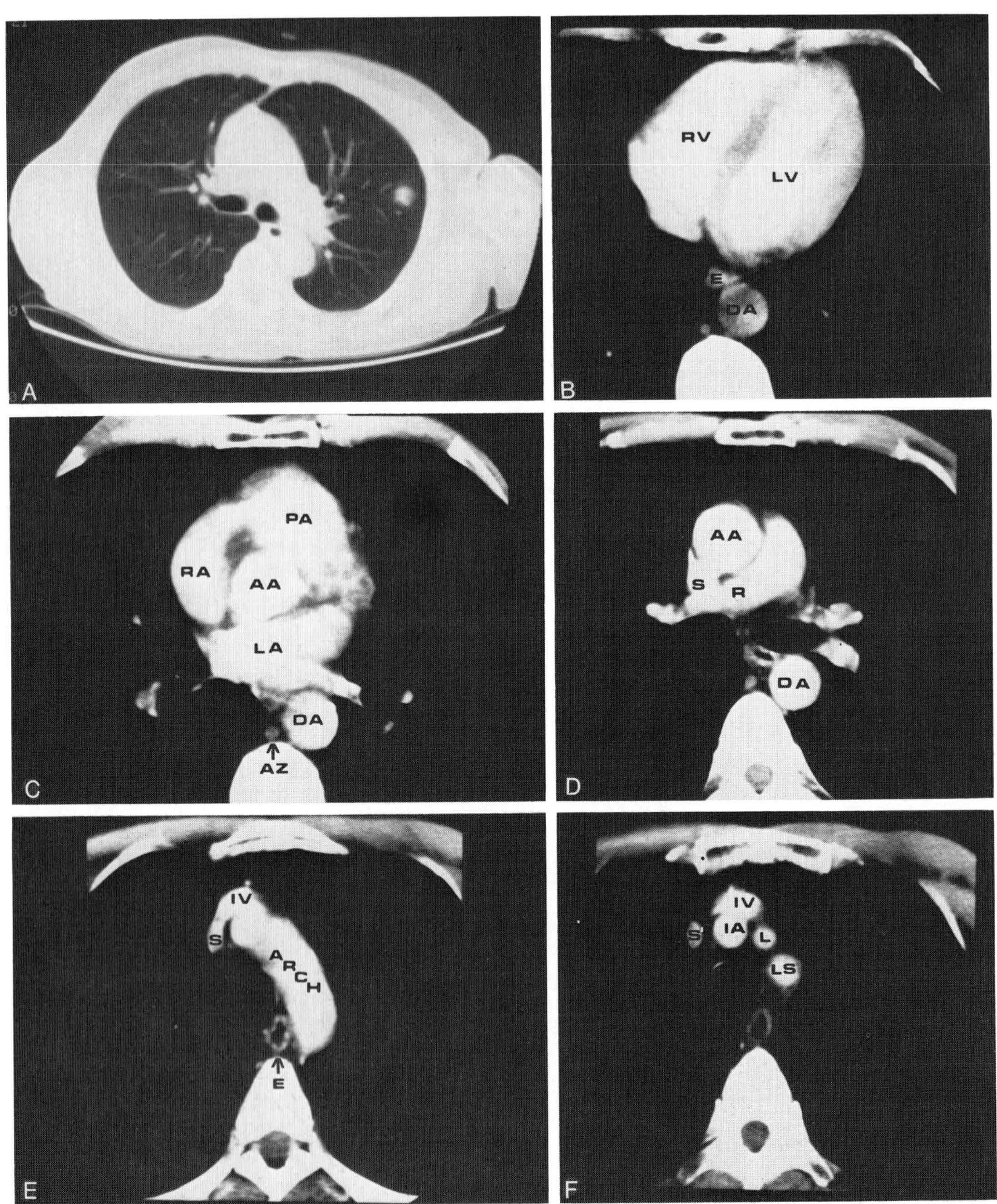

FIGURE 2–8. Chest computed tomographic (CT) evaluation. *A.* Lung window view reveals the right and left main bronchi in the mediastinum, branching pulmonary vessels, and a round, single nodule in the periphery of the left lung. This nodule was an adenocarcinoma of the lung. *B* to *F.* CT images of the mediastinum from inferior to superior. RV, right ventricle; LV, left ventricle; E, esophagus; DA, descending aorta; PA, pulmonary artery; RA, right atrium; AA, ascending aorta; LA, left atrium; AZ, azygous vein; S, superior vena cava; R, right pulmonary artery; IV, innominate vein; ARCH, aortic arch; IA, innominate artery (brachiocephalic); L, left common carotid artery; LS, left subclavian artery.

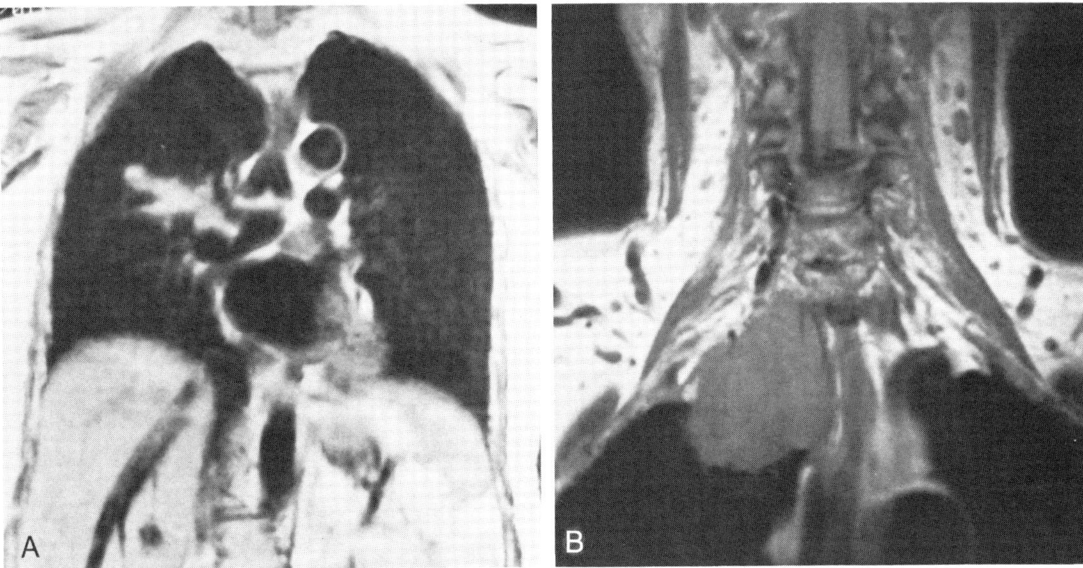

FIGURE 2–9. Magnetic resonance evaluation of lung carcinoma. *A.* Lung carcinoma. Coronal T1 spin echo image of the chest shows a right-lung mass that extends to the right hilum and associated adenopathy. *B.* Apical lung carcinoma in a different patient. T1 spin echo scan shows a large mass at the lung apex that invades the upper neck and spine and displaces the esophagus and trachea. The patient had right arm pain and numbness, as a result of brachial plexus involvement.

Blunt Trauma

Blunt trauma to the chest usually results from a motor vehicle accident or a blow by a fist. Fractures, especially of ribs, are common, and bone fragments often cause injury to nearby soft tissue and vessels (see Fig. 2–2). The most important results of blunt pulmonary and mediastinal injuries are pulmonary contusion, pneumothorax, pleural effusion, hemothorax, pneumomediastinum, esophageal rupture, and diaphragmatic rupture.

Blunt (or penetrating) chest injuries frequently cause blood, air, or other fluids to enter the pleural space, where they can cause compression of the adjacent lung. The most

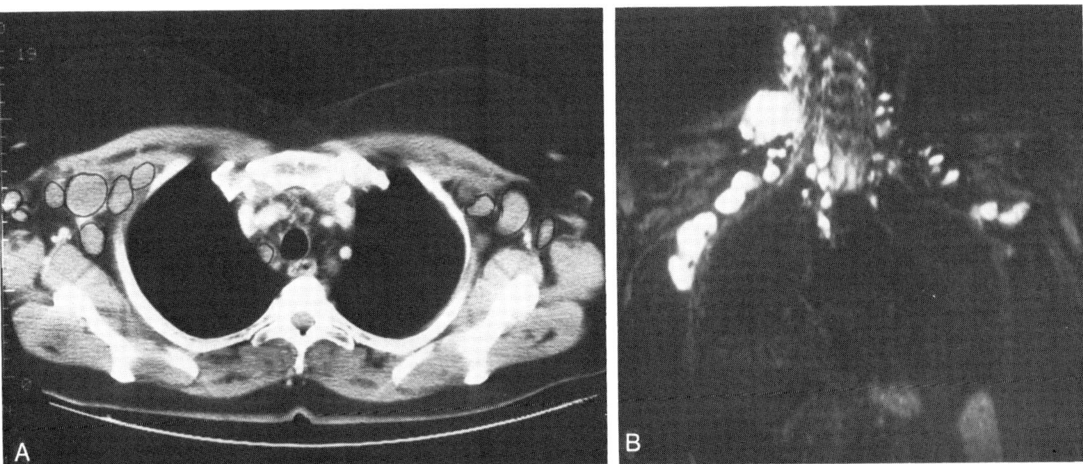

FIGURE 2–10. Non-Hodgkin's lymphoma. *A.* Contrast-enhanced CT scan shows numerous round masses in the upper mediastinum and in the anterior chest wall. These lesions also extended into the neck and throughout the chest, the abdomen, and the pelvis. The lesions here are enhanced graphically in order to distinguish them from normal muscle, which has a similar density on CT. *B.* Coronal short TI inversion recovery (STIR; see Chapter 1) magnetic resonance image shows bright abnormal signal in multiple areas of lymphomatous nodes in both axillae, in the neck, and in the upper mediastinum. Suppression of fat and low intensity of muscle tissue and air provide high contrast of tumor that is ideal for screening.

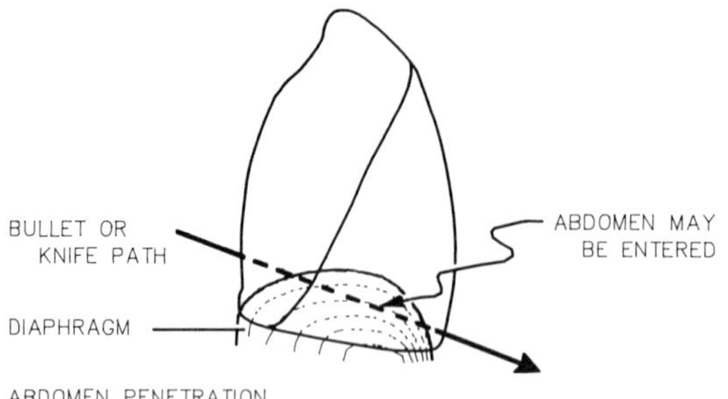

FIGURE 2–11. Abdominal penetration from a chest wound.

important results of these injuries are pneumothorax (air in the pleural space), hemothorax (blood in the pleural space), and pneumomediastinum (air in the mediastinum). In general, patients with these conditions are in severe respiratory distress.

Pulmonary Contusion. Pulmonary contusion is the most common blunt injury to the chest. The symptoms are chest pain and inspiratory discomfort. The contused lung appears as an area of increased radiographic density over the region of trauma (Fig. 2–12). It is evident immediately after the injury and resolves within 1 to 2 days. Effusion resulting from trauma indicates hemothorax, especially if adjacent lung contusion is evident. Occasionally, a cavity forms in the region of trauma and then fills with air or blood (hematoma). These traumatic cysts (pneumatoceles) may persist for months. A radiographic appearance similar to that of pulmonary contusion can occur in patients who have fractures that result in fat embolus to the lung. However, fat embolus does not cause symptoms or radiographic abnormalities until 24 to 48 hours after the injury.

Pneumothorax. Pneumothorax is best identified in the upright, expiration chest film by the presence of an air-filled pleural space, a collapsed lung, and a displaced pleural margin (Fig. 2–13*A*). The displacement of the pleural margin, identified as a thin, continuous line, best outlines the edge of the lung against the pneumothorax. However, a severely traumatized patient is usually examined supine, a position in which the appearance of pneumothorax may be subtle. On the supine radiograph, a deep costophrenic sulcus as a result of anteriorly loculated air is diagnostic of pneumothorax. Other findings such as areas of relative radiolucency, sharp heart margin, and apparently hyperlucent lung are less conclusive but helpful findings. When the supine film is inconclusive, a decubitus view with the abnormal side up shows the same findings as the upright view.

At times, a pneumothorax is simulated by the presence of a skin fold that can be mistaken for a displaced pleural margin. However, a skin fold can usually be distinguished by its course outside the lung, its discontinuous border, the absence of a thin pleural line, and the presence of lung parenchymal markings lateral to the fold (Fig. 2–13*B*).

Pleural Effusion, Hemothorax, and Chylothorax. Fluid, usually blood, in the pleural space (including the interlobar fissures) is frequently seen in thoracic trauma. Other types of effusion include chylous, serous, and malignant effusions and have the same appearance as hemothorax. Unless it is loculated or clotted, the fluid flows to the dependent parts of the pleural space. The appearance of the fluid depends on the position of the patient (Fig. 2–14). On a supine film, the fluid forms a smooth layer posteriorly and causes a diffuse increase in density of most of the lung without definite margins. On upright films, the upper level of the fluid has a meniscus easily seen on the lateral projection. The fluid causes a rounded blunting of the costophrenic angle on the AP

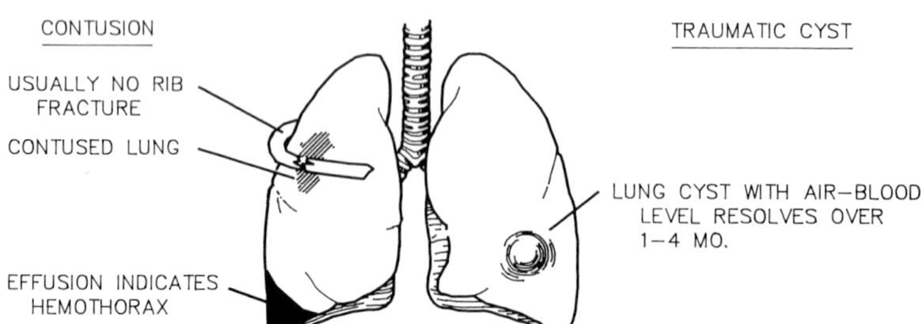

FIGURE 2–12. Pulmonary contusion and traumatic lung cyst.

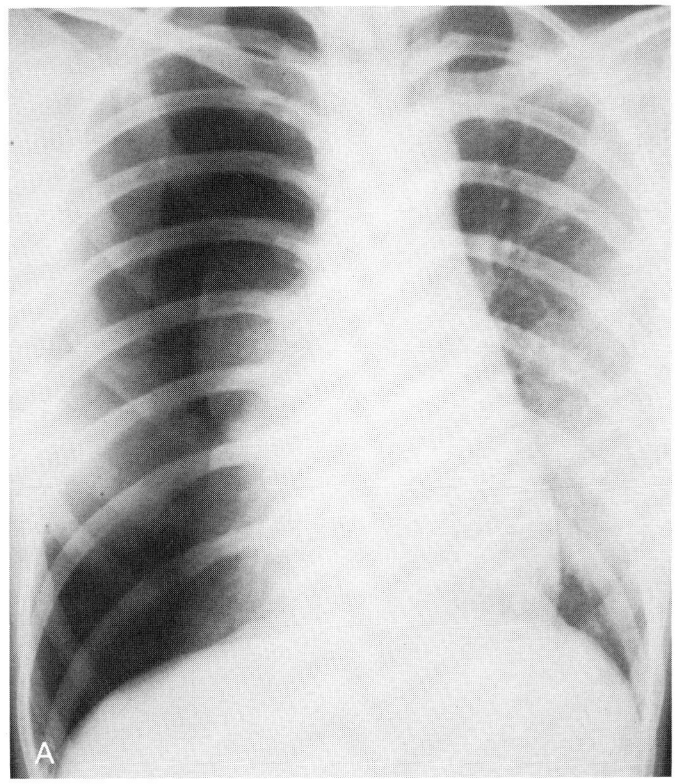

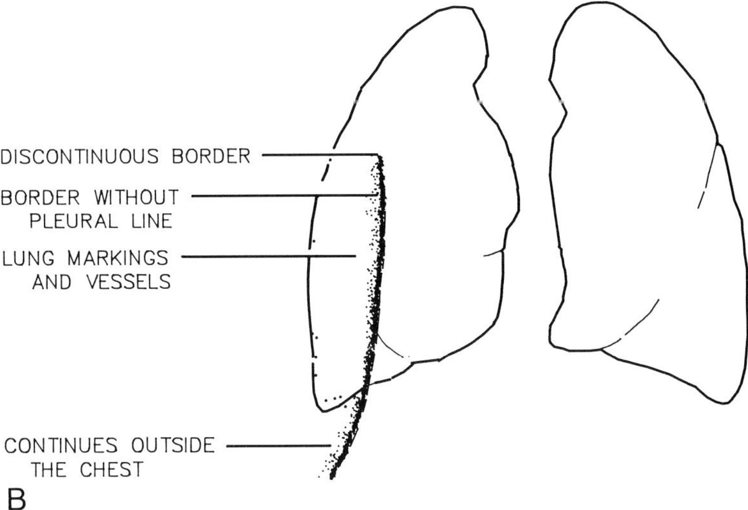

FIGURE 2–13. Pneumothorax. *A*. Right tension pneumothorax. Note the air-filled, right thorax and the collapse of right lung medially; the patient has been knifed in the chest. *B*. Skinfold simulating pneumothorax.

film if sufficient fluid (more than 400 mL) is present to fill the costophrenic sulcus posteriorly. The best plain film method for verification of a small amount of fluid is the decubitus view with the side of interest down; the fluid then layers out along the dependent margin (see Fig. 2–7*B*). Pleural effusions are seen easily on CT, which provides additional information regarding the adjacent lung and soft tissues. Ultrasonography is useful for locating small amounts of fluid for thoracentesis.

Hemopneumothorax occurs in penetrating injuries to the chest and appears as an air/fluid level in the pleural space (Fig. 2–15). Chylothorax results from interruption of the thoracic duct (which is right-sided in the lower chest and left-sided in the upper chest); it is usually caused by trauma or tumor.

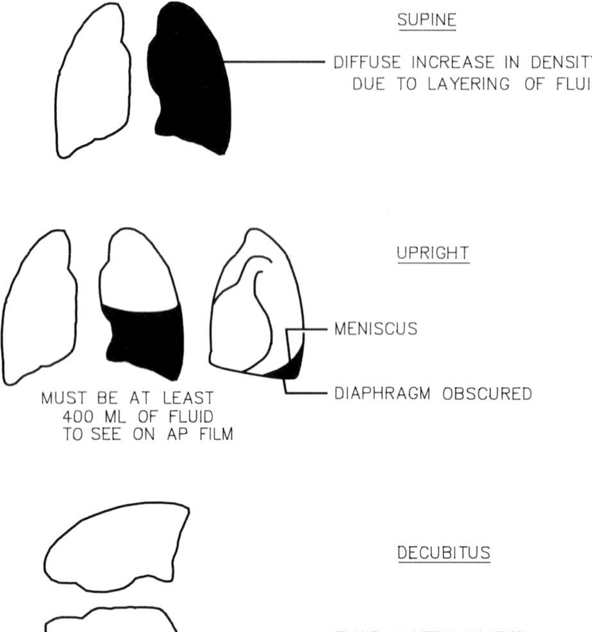

FIGURE 2–14. Various appearances of pleural effusion on plain film.

Pneumomediastinum. Air in the mediastinum may be the direct result of esophageal or tracheobronchial rupture, or it may occur in association with communicating pneumoperitoneum or pneumothorax. Air can be seen outlining vessels, mediastinal structures, and the medial part of the diaphragm. It can outline the medial pleural margin, best seen along the middle mediastinum on the left. On a supine film, an important finding is a continuous diaphragm, which is not normally seen in its midportion (Fig. 2–16). Subcutaneous emphysema occurs when the air dissects into the neck, often the most striking abnormality in pneumomediastinum. Pneumopericardium is

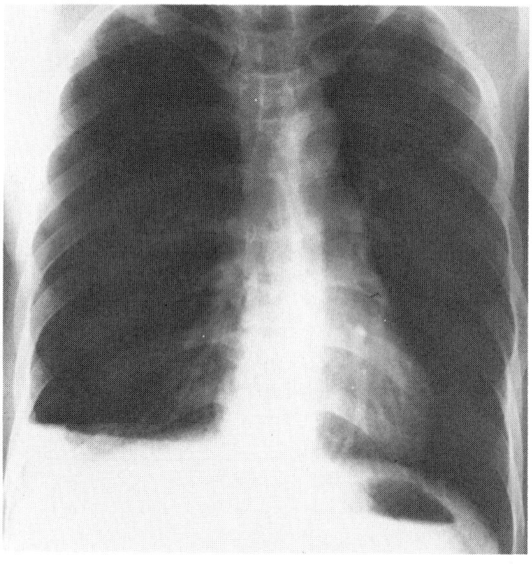

FIGURE 2–15. Hemopneumothorax. Upright PA chest film shows an air/fluid (blood) level above the right diaphragm in a young man stabbed in the chest.

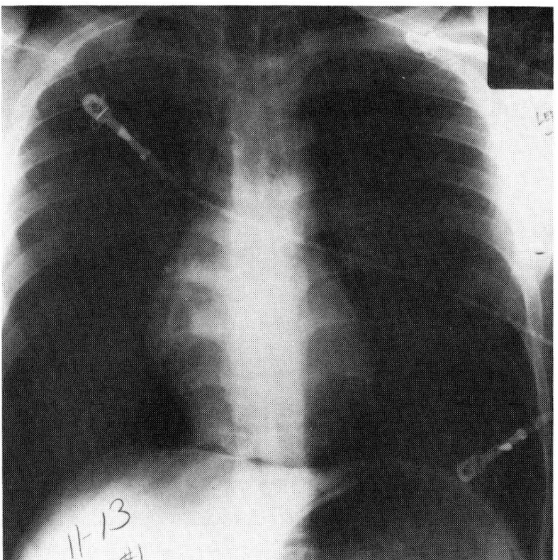

FIGURE 2–16. Pneumomediastinum. Upright PA chest film shows a continuous diaphragm across the midline and a diagonal line of air crossing the shadow of the superior vena cava, both of which indicate air in the mediastinum. Air also outlines the wall of the stomach. In this case, the air dissected along the esophagus after rupture during vomiting (Boerhaave's syndrome).

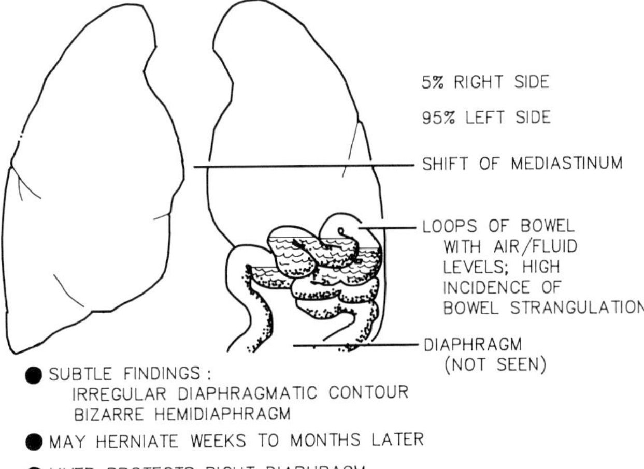

FIGURE 2–17. Characteristics of diaphragmatic rupture.

usually part of the spectrum of pneumomediastinum and is best evidenced by outline of the main pulmonary artery against air. Pneumothorax and pneumoperitoneum and signs of esophageal or tracheobronchial rupture should lead to suspicion of pneumomediastinum.

Esophageal Rupture. Esophageal rupture can be caused by blunt trauma but more frequently results from diagnostic endoscopy and therapeutic interventions (esophageal airway and esophagogastric tube placement and esophageal dilatation). Radiographic findings consist of pneumomediastinum (see Fig. 2–16), effusion, and lung consolidation. Severe, often fatal, mediastinitis can develop and requires immediate surgical intervention. Esophageal rupture is discussed further in Chapter 3.

Diaphragmatic Rupture. Severe, blunt trauma to the abdomen can cause the diaphragm to rupture, allowing the abdominal contents to herniate into the chest. Patients develop severe respiratory distress and bowel strangulation. Radiographs show opacification of one lung (usually the left), obscuring of the hemidiaphragm, and displacement of the mediastinum to the opposite side (Fig. 2–17). Diaphragmatic rupture must be suspected in any traumatized patient in whom the diaphragm is not well demonstrated. Minimal diaphragmatic injury can have a subtle appearance and lead to massive rupture weeks to months later.

Aortic Rupture and Dissection. Deceleration injuries, usually the result of motor vehicle accidents, cause shearing forces on fixed organs. Aortic rupture and dissection are discussed in Chapter 5.

Toxic Injury

Acute Inhalation Injury. Acute inhalation injury is most commonly caused by entry of noxious gases into the lungs. The most common inhalant is smoke, which contains carbon dioxide, carbon monoxide, and a multitude of other gases and suspended hot particles. The initial chest film may be normal despite ventilatory and biochemical abnormalities. The radiographic appearance may then progress to that of generalized interstitial lung disease. Inhaled toxins such as poison gas, fumes from volatile chemicals, and allergens produce a similar radiographic picture, although the cause may be hypersensitivity in addition to direct tissue injury.

Acute Aspiration. Aspirated fluids produce diffuse irritation of the lungs, usually as a result of a chemical pneumonitis. Supportive respiratory care is the primary therapy. Antibiotics are not generally indicated unless infection is demonstrated. The radiographic appearance varies from patchy areas of increased density to diffuse abnormality to pulmonary edema. The most commonly aspirated substances are hydrocarbons and gastric contents.

The most severe disease is caused by inhalation of hydrocarbons, including cleaning fluids, polishes, fuels, and lighter fluids. Direct aspiration or aspiration after ingestion results in an alveolar inflammation. Patients are short of breath, febrile, and hypoxemic. The chest film shows bilateral patchy areas of increased density or large areas of consolidation. Supportive respiratory care is the only therapy available, and patients generally recover in 1 to 2 weeks. As the consolidation clears, pneu-

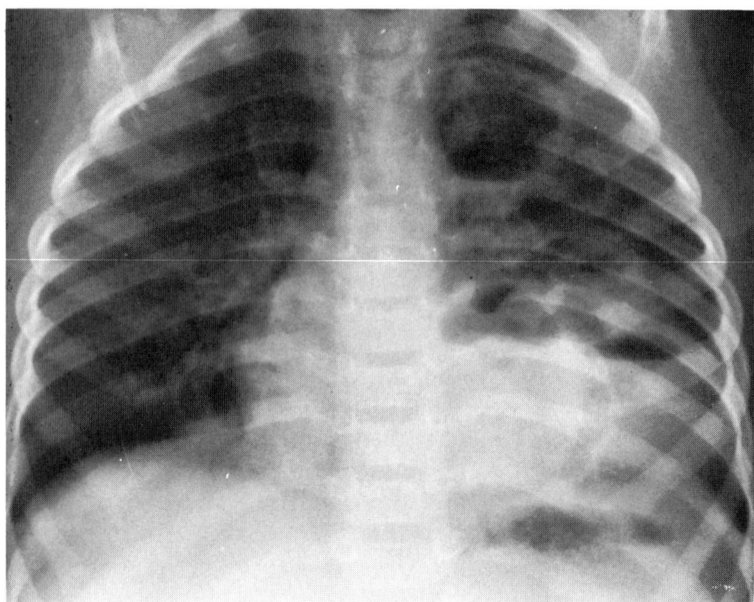

FIGURE 2–18. Hydrocarbon inhalation and ingestion. Chest film shows pulmonary consolidation and pneumatoceles in a child who had unsupervised access to furniture polish.

matoceles may form (Fig. 2–18). These pneumatoceles do not rupture, and they eventually resolve.

Foreign Body Aspiration. Foreign body aspiration is most common in children and can result in obstruction of a lung or a lung segment. Clinical symptoms in foreign body aspiration range from mild wheezing to severe hypoxia. The aspiration is often unnoticed by the parent and not remembered by the child. The radiographic appearance is a subtle difference in density between one lung and the other lung or between one segment and the remainder of the lung. When such a density difference is seen in a child suspected of foreign body aspiration, a decubitus film or an expiration film can demonstrate air trapping in the affected lung.

Radiation Injury. Most patients who develop radiation injury to the lungs have had radiation therapy for lung cancer. Such injury requires exposure to at least 20 Gy (2000 rad), and the severity of the injury depends on the total dose, the time course of therapy, and whether the radiation is from electromagnetic waves or from particles. Exposure to more than 60 Gy (6000 rad) always causes pneumonitis and fibrosis. During the first month after exposure, pneumonitis develops as capillary and alveolar cells are sloughed, but this is not usually evident radiographically. Radiographic abnormalities appear 1 to 2 months after treatment as areas of consolidation in the radiation field. These areas of abnormality progress to fibrosis and contraction in 6 to 12 months (Fig. 2–19). Injury to the lung can be amplified by chemotherapy or the withdrawal of steroids.

Drug Injury. Several chemotherapeutic agents may injure the lung. In 40% of patients treated with methotrexate, a granulomatous pneumonia develops and may progress to fibrosis (Fig. 2–20). Onset is anytime from 1 month to 5 years after initiation of therapy. Bleomycin sulfate causes alveolar or interstitial destruction and fibrosis in 2% to 6% of patients. The clinical and radiographic abnormalities usually become evident about the sixth week of therapy. Busulfan can cause destruction similar to that caused by bleomycin sulfate, but such injury is uncommon.

Cyclophosphamide (Cytoxan) causes temporary cardiac failure and pulmonary edema when it is administered in large doses for the treatment of resistant lymphoma. The process begins on the third or fourth day of treatment and persists for about 10 days. It resolves without therapy.

Nitrofurantoin macrocrystals (Macrodantin) can incite an allergic pneumonitis. Clinical and radiographic abnormalities usually develop after 4 days of exposure to the drug. The typical radiographic appearance is a basal reticular pattern of increased density, apparently caused by edema. Withdrawal of the drug usually results in prompt resolution, although some patients have symptoms for years.

Amiodarone hydrochloride, a drug used for prevention of recurrent ventricular arrhythmias, causes (in 5% of treated patients) a lipid storage abnormality in the lungs that incites

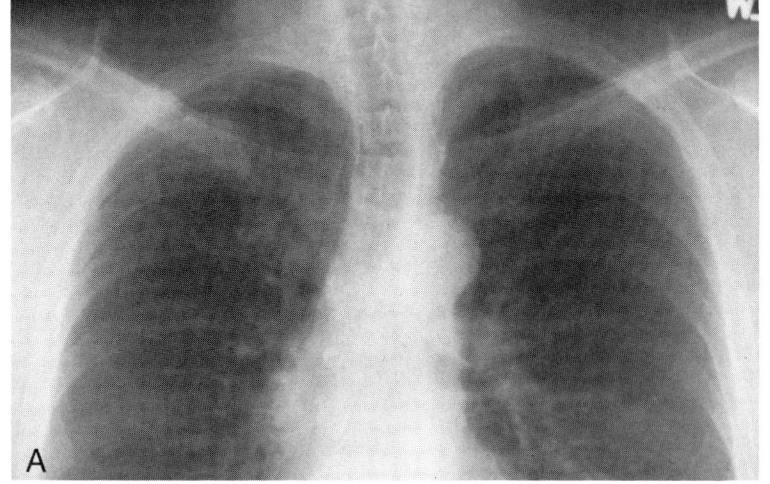

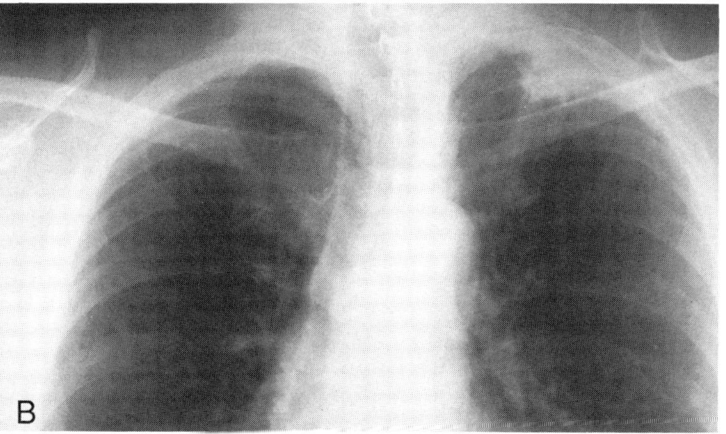

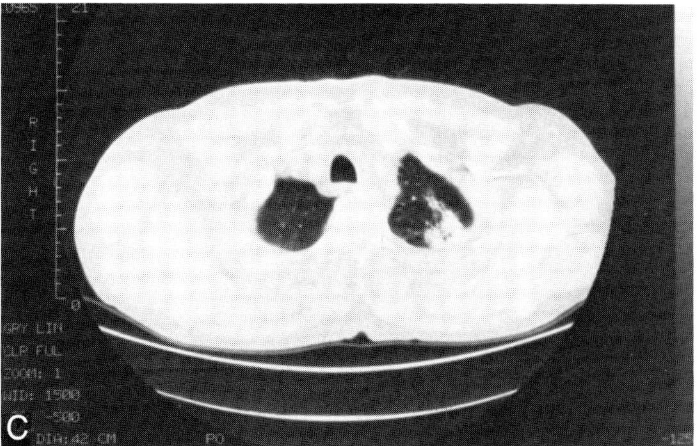

FIGURE 2–19. Lung injury after irradiation for cancer in the left neck and supraclavicular region. *A.* Preradiation chest radiograph shows no abnormality in the lung apexes. *B.* Six months after radiation, increased fibrotic density is seen in left apex. *C.* CT scan shows a pleura-based mass. Although the findings are consistent with recurrent or direct tumor spread, this abnormality did not change over 2 years.

an immunological response that can cause lung destruction. Symptoms, which usually begin after 6 months of continuous exposure to the drug, include dyspnea, weakness, and pleuritic chest pain. The radiographic appearance is highly variable and includes focal and diffuse interstitial consolidation. The abnormality disappears within 3 months after the drug is discontinued unless fibrosis has occurred.

CONGENITAL ABNORMALITIES

Bone and Soft Tissue Congenital Abnormalities

Congenital abnormalities of the bones and soft tissues in and near the chest are common. These abnormalities are usually not clinically

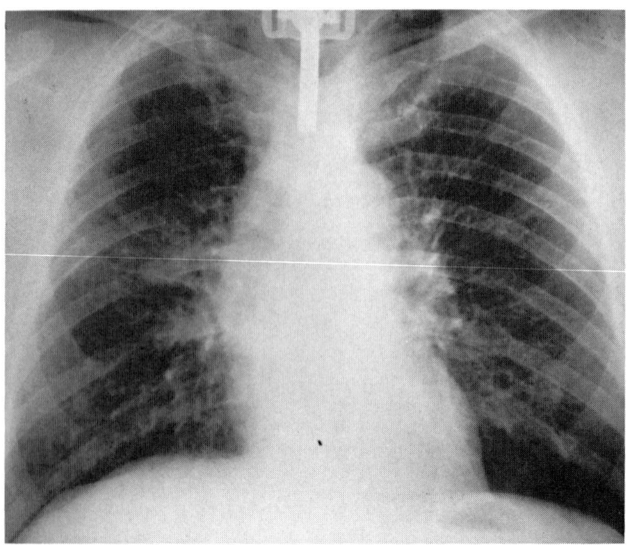

FIGURE 2–20. Methotrexate lung disease. PA chest film shows a predominantly lower lung interstitial process in a patient undergoing methotrexate therapy for cancer. The lower lung location is typical.

significant, but they may suggest an important diagnosis. Bone abnormalities include cervical ribs, bifid spinous processes, extra or fewer ribs (11 pairs of ribs is a common finding in Down's syndrome), and a double manubrial ossification center (also seen in Down's syndrome). A pectus deformity alters the appearance of the chest on the frontal radiograph (the anterior ribs have a vertical orientation, and the heart is displaced to the left). Important soft tissue findings on the chest radiograph are often seen in the upper abdomen. Malpositioned abdominal contents can be demonstrated. A mass seen in the lower chest may be a thoracic kidney.

Radiographs of the upper anterior mediastinum of neonates and young children show the thymus, which is not seen in adults. The thymus must not be mistaken for a mass, atelectasis, or pneumonia (Fig. 2–21). It is generally seen in patients up to age 6 years, but it can be visible as late as age 15. Under conditions of stress such as infection or cancer, the thymus atrophies. Thymus atrophy in a neonate or a young child is an important finding and indicates the need for further evaluation. The heart occupies a larger part of the chest in the child than in the adult and, in conjunction with the thymus, causes a different appearance of the frontal chest film. Lack of visualization of the thymus may also be caused by immune disease or by thymic aplasia. Cysts and tumors can arise in the thymus (Fig. 2–22).

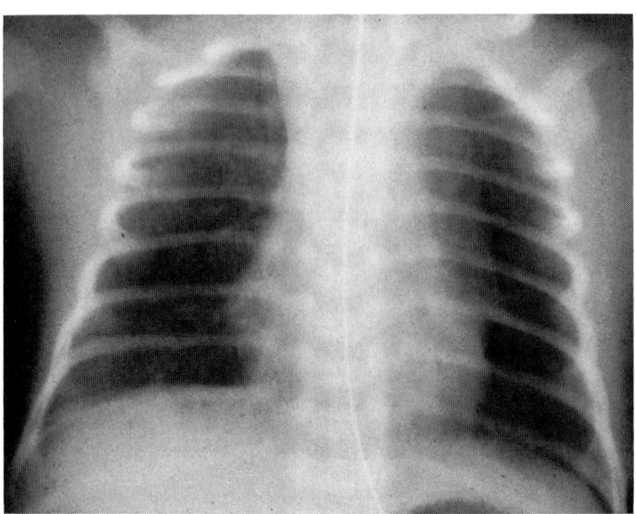

FIGURE 2–21. Thymus. Frontal chest film in a 1-month-old girl shows a large sail-shaped shadow that projects to the left of the mediastinum, the normal appearance of the thymus. Note also the large size of the heart in relation to the lungs. A nasogastric tube marks the path of the esophagus.

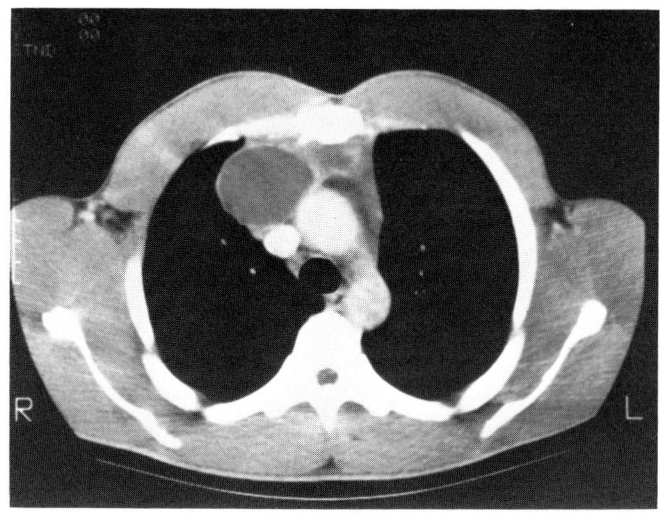

FIGURE 2–22. Thymus cyst. CT scan of upper mediastinum shows a round, circumscribed, low-density cyst in the mediastinum anterior to the densely opacified superior vena cava. This lesion was asymptomatic, a benign thymus cyst, and was removed surgically.

Intrathoracic Congenital Abnormalities

Most noncardiac congenital anomalies seen in the thorax are best classified as bronchopulmonary foregut abnormalities because all thoracic organs form simultaneously and the anomaly often involves several organs. The most important of these are diaphragmatic hernia, bronchogenic cyst, pulmonary agenesis, bronchial atresia, pulmonary sequestration, arteriovenous malformation, cystic adenomatoid malformation, and congenital lobar emphysema.

Diaphragmatic Hernia. Herniation of abdominal contents into the chest occurs as a result of the congenital absence or defect of the diaphragm. The appearance is similar to that of traumatic diaphragmatic rupture (Fig. 2–23; see also Fig. 2–17). These hernias commonly occur at openings for the esophagus, the aorta, and the inferior vena cava. Bochdalek's hernias result from incomplete closure of the pleuroperitoneal membrane posteriorly. Morgagni's hernias are rare, occur in adults, and are located at the mammary vessels. Eventration of the diaphragm is a benign condition caused by partial or complete failure of muscle development and results in a bulge in the otherwise smooth contour of the diaphragm.

Bronchogenic, Pericardial, and Neurenteric Cysts. Bronchogenic cysts are rare cystic lesions of the lung or the mediastinum and are lined with respiratory epithelium. They do not communicate with the bronchial tree. In the mediastinum, these cysts are always solitary and are usually subcarinal, but they can occur anywhere. In the lung, central lesions are usually solitary; peripheral lesions are multiple. Two thirds of lung lesions are found in the lower lobes (Fig. 2–24). The pericardial cyst is an extremely rare solitary lesion that arises in the pericardial membrane, usually in the anterolateral cardiophrenic region. Its radiographic appearance is similar to that of the bronchogenic cyst. Failure of the neural and gut elements to separate results in a cystic structure called a neurenteric cyst. It can be found anywhere along the spine and may communicate with the gastrointestinal tract or the subarachnoid space.

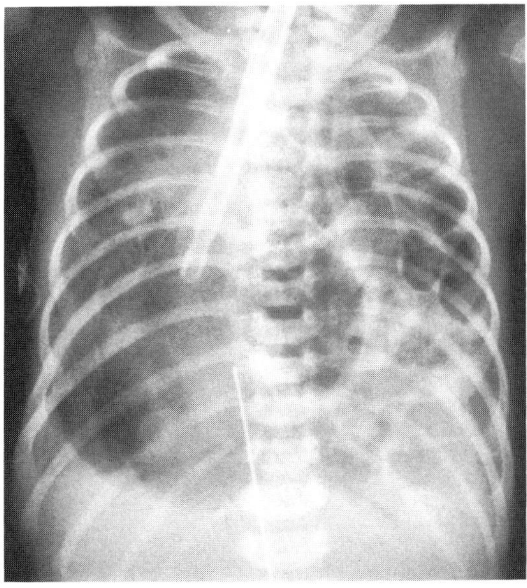

FIGURE 2–23. Congenital diaphragmatic hernia. The air-filled loops of bowel fill the left chest, compress the lungs, and shift the mediastinum to the right. The endotracheal tube shows the displacement of the trachea.

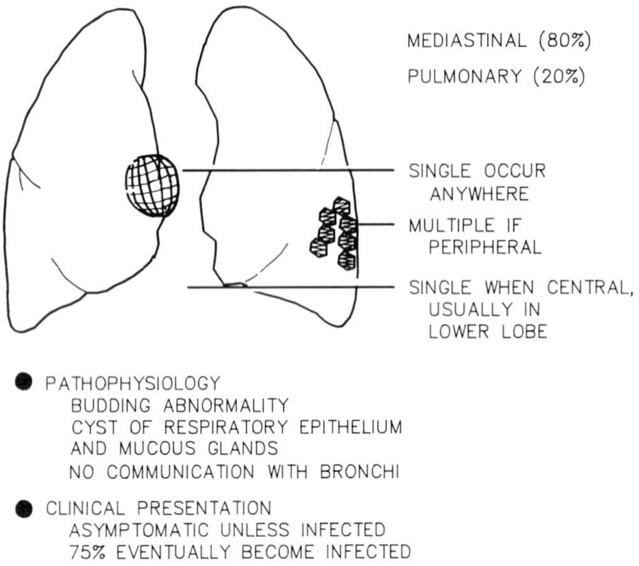

MEDIASTINAL (80%)
PULMONARY (20%)

SINGLE OCCUR ANYWHERE

MULTIPLE IF PERIPHERAL

SINGLE WHEN CENTRAL, USUALLY IN LOWER LOBE

- PATHOPHYSIOLOGY
  BUDDING ABNORMALITY
  CYST OF RESPIRATORY EPITHELIUM AND MUCOUS GLANDS
  NO COMMUNICATION WITH BRONCHI
- CLINICAL PRESENTATION
  ASYMPTOMATIC UNLESS INFECTED
  75% EVENTUALLY BECOME INFECTED

FIGURE 2–24. Development and characteristics of bronchogenic cysts.

Azygos Lobe. The azygos lobe is formed when early development of the azygos vein isolates a part of the right upper lobe during lung formation (Fig. 2–25). It occurs in 2% of the population and is of no clinical significance. In rare instances, isolated pneumonia or atelectasis causes a consolidated appearance.

Pulmonary Agenesis. Complete pulmonary agenesis is rare (1 in 10,000 infants) and results from failure of the lung bud to form. The normal opposite lung expands to fill the anatomical space and performs the function of the absent lung (Fig. 2–26). Cardiac and vertebral abnormalities are often present. A limited abnormality of lung development is termed pulmonary hypoplasia. This can be a result of an intrathoracic abnormality such as vascular insufficiency, thoracic cage deformity, or partial lung bud abnormality, or it can result from an extrathoracic event that prevents normal growth and expansion of the lung, such as diaphragmatic herniation, ectopic kidney, diaphragm eventration, or oligohydramnios.

Bronchial Atresia. Bronchial atresia results from interruption of a bronchial artery during lung formation. It is usually asymptomatic and is discovered in adulthood when the chest

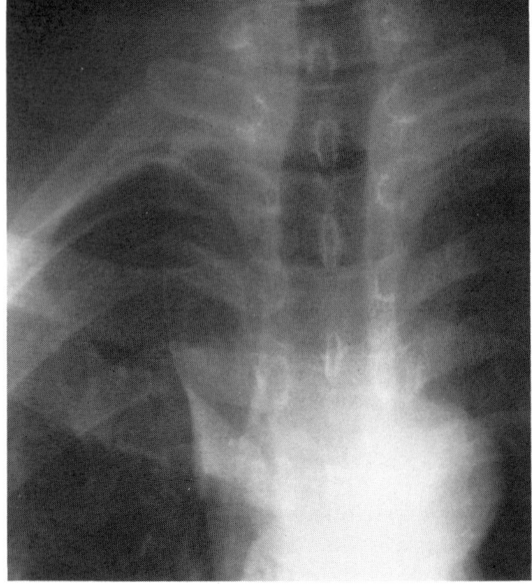

FIGURE 2–25. Azygos lobe. Detailed view of a frontal chest film shows an azygos lobe near the right apical midline. The thin pleural line ends in a triangular margin at the site of the azygos vein.

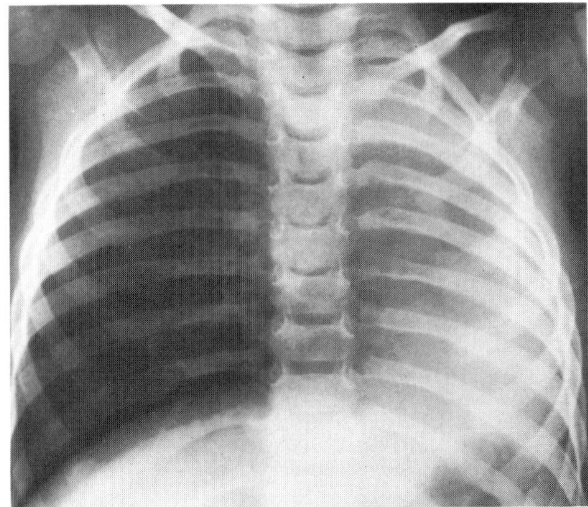

FIGURE 2–26. Left lung agenesis. Because of absence of the left lung, the heart fills the left thorax. The right lung shows hyperexpansion to provide compensatory pulmonary function. The mediastinum is consequently shifted to the left.

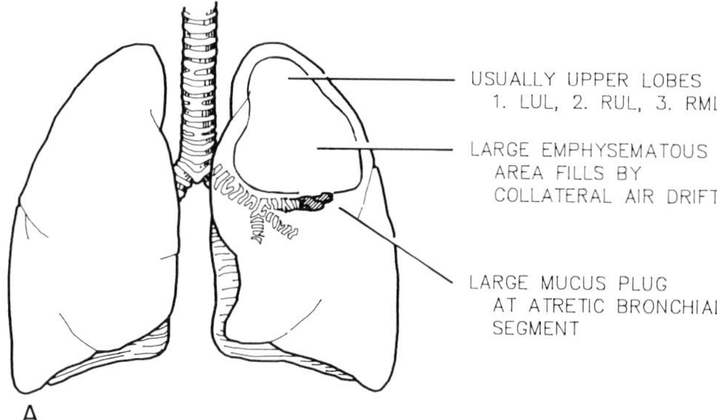

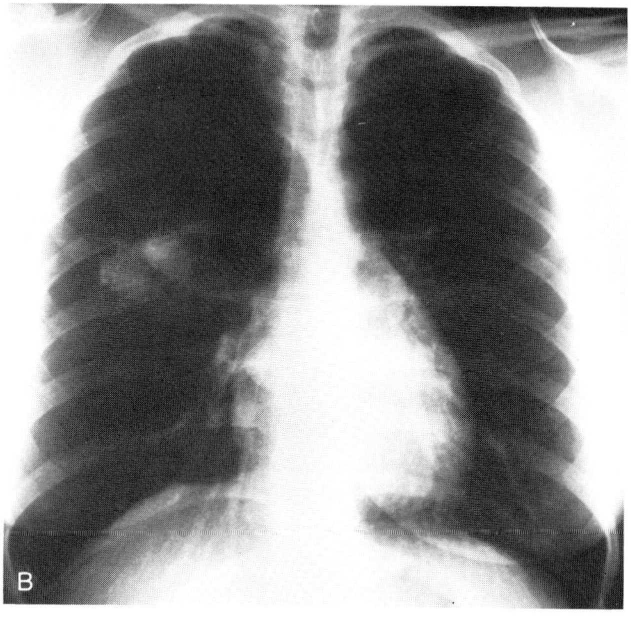

FIGURE 2–27. Bronchial atresia. *A.* Diagram. LUL, left upper lobe; RUL, right upper lobe; RML, right middle lobe. The three most common locations for this abnormality are (1) LUL, (2) RUL, and (3) RML. *B.* PA chest film shows a mass in the right upper lobe bronchus and a mucus plug in an atretic bronchus. Superiorly, a large, cystic lucency is visible without lung markings. This represents emphysematous lung distal to the atretic and plugged bronchial segment.

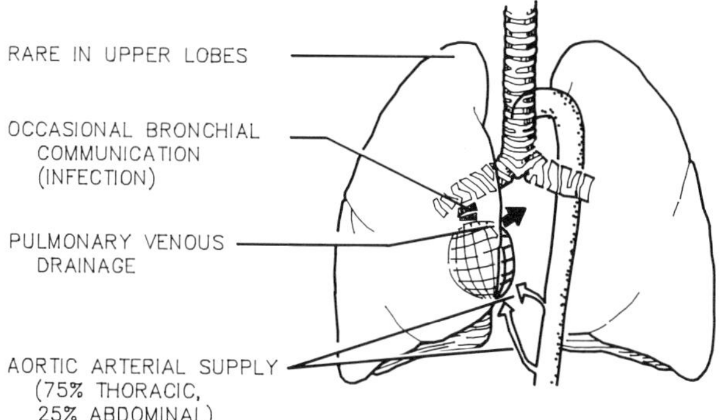

FIGURE 2–28. Characteristics of intralobar sequestration.

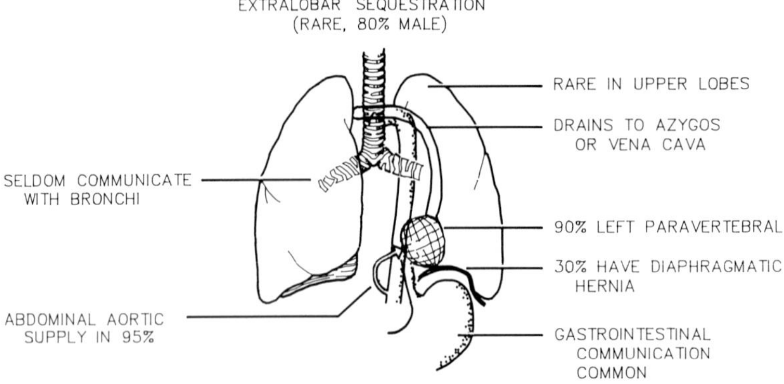

FIGURE 2–29. Characteristics of extralobar sequestration.

radiograph, obtained for other reasons, shows a hyperexpanded upper or middle lung segment, the result of obstruction by a central, massive mucus plug at the site of interruption. This radiographic appearance includes a central obstructing mass and peripheral hyperexpansion (Fig. 2–27) and is similar to that of an obstructing carcinoma of the lung.

Pulmonary Sequestration. Pulmonary sequestration is a localized collection of lung tissue that does not communicate with the tracheobronchial tree. Sequestrations are subclassified as intralobar and extralobar. Intralobar sequestration (Fig. 2–28) occurs within the visceral pleura; it typically receives systemic arterial blood (usually from the abdominal aorta) and drains via pulmonary veins. Extralobar sequestration (Figs. 2–29, 2–30) occurs outside the visceral pleura, receives systemic arterial blood, and usually drains via the azygos venous system. Extralobar sequestration is more likely to communicate with the gastrointestinal tract and to be associated with diaphragmatic defects.

Pulmonary sequestration manifests either as an asymptomatic mass on a chest radiograph obtained for other reasons or as a pulmonary infection caused by communication of the sequestered lung segment with the gastrointestinal tract or with a bronchus (Fig. 2–30).

Arteriovenous Malformation. An arteriovenous malformation (AVM) is a congenital collection of abnormal arterial to venous connections. The most important AVMs are in the brain and the lungs. Many patients who have pulmonary AVMs have hereditary telangiectasia. In the lungs, AVMs are usually asymptomatic, but some patients have hemoptysis and dyspnea. The diagnosis of AVM can often be suspected from the identification of a lung nodule that has an efferent vessel and an afferent vessel (Fig. 2–31) or by contrast enhancement on CT. Whenever there is suspicion that a pulmonary nodule is an AVM, arteriography should be performed before biopsy. Because AVMs are multiple in one third of patients, a careful search for additional lesions is indicated when one is identified.

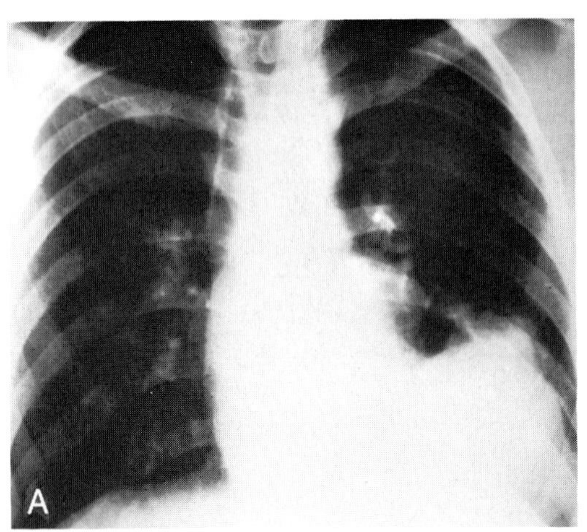

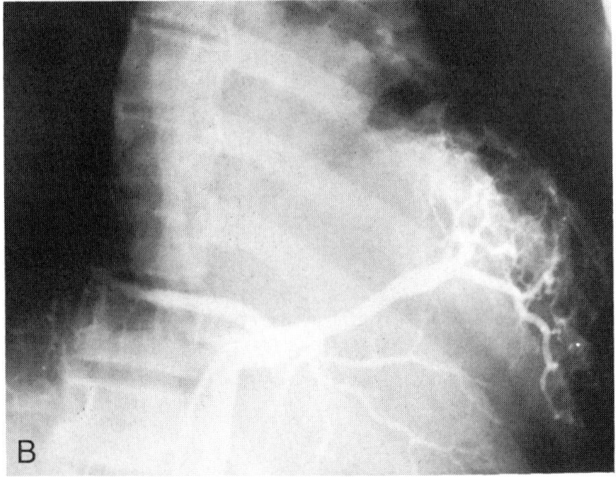

FIGURE 2–30. Extralobar sequestration. *A.* Chest film in a child with repeated pulmonary infections shows an opaque consolidated area in the left lower lobe. *B.* The blood supply to this lobe is shown by selective injection of an artery arising from the abdominal aorta.

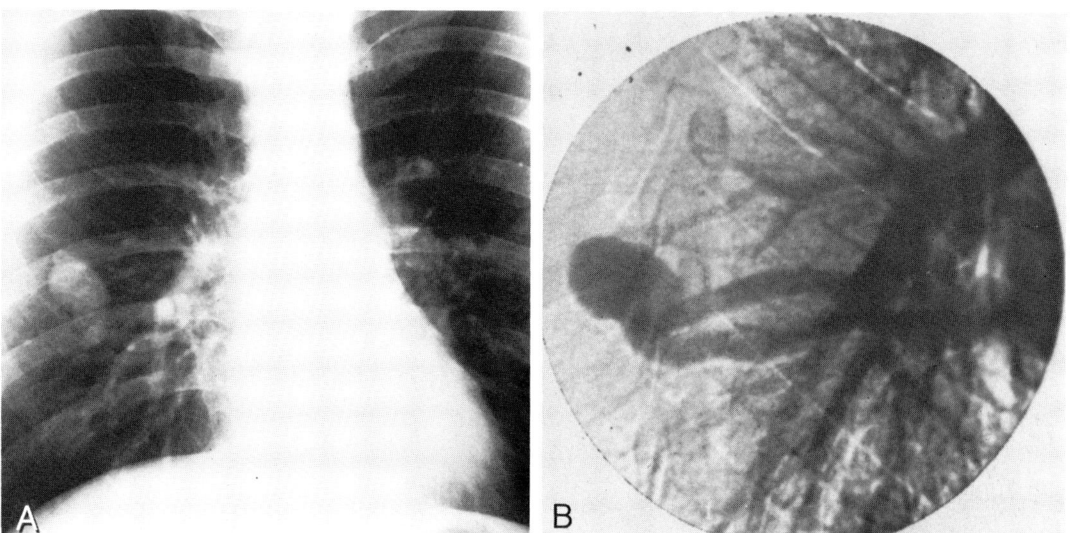

FIGURE 2–31. Arteriovenous malformation. *A.* Plain radiograph shows a smooth mass in the right lung. Close inspection suggests a linear density leading back toward the mediastinum. *B.* Arteriogram shows a large feeding vessel; early flow through a similar caliber vein returns to the left atrium.

Another vascular abnormality in the lung, which may have a similar radiographic appearance to an AVM, is a pulmonary varix, a congenital, locally dilated segment of the pulmonary vein. It is an asymptomatic lesion and is not associated with AVM.

Cystic Adenomatoid Malformation. A cystic adenomatoid malformation occurs when failure of mesenchymal formation of alveoli and terminal bronchioles results in the formation of multiple cystic structures in place of normal lung tissue. Usually an entire single lobe of the lung is involved. When it is detected in infants, the involved area of lung appears solid. When it is detected in children, the involved part appears cystic (Fig. 2–32).

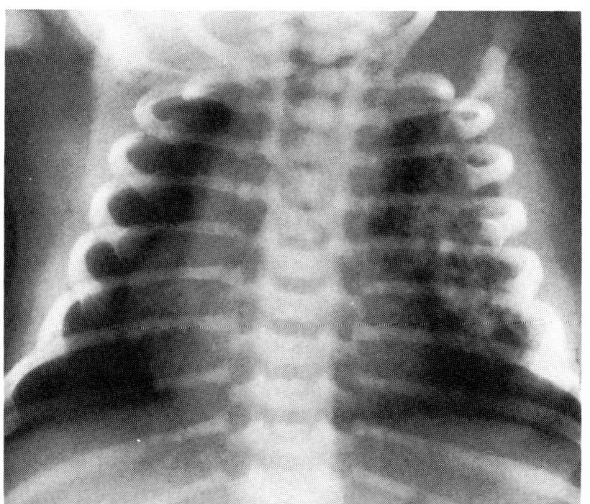

FIGURE 2–32. Cystic adenomatoid malformation. PA chest film shows mixed opacification in the left lung of an infant with mild respiratory distress.

Congenital Lobar Emphysema. Congenital lobar emphysema is probably caused either by failure of the alveoli to form normally or by congenital bronchial obstruction. Either of these results in a large, bullous lesion occupying an entire lobe, usually an upper lobe. Immediately after birth, the lesion is fluid filled and appears as a solid mass on chest radiographs (Fig. 2–33*A*). By the age of 3 days, the fluid is resorbed, and an air-filled emphysematous mass is evident (Fig. 2–33*B*). This appearance is nearly identical to that of bronchial atresia (see Fig. 2–27). Many patients (about 10%) have additional congenital abnormalities, such as hypoplasia of other lung segments and cardiac abnormalities.

Inherited Diseases

Neurofibromatosis. Neurofibromatosis comprises two inherited syndromes, discussed in detail in Chapter 8. The common manifestations are café au lait skin lesions, cutaneous fibromas, and neurofibromas of the central nervous system. Patients have increased incidence of most kinds of central nervous system tumors. A less common manifestation is upper-lobe, bullous lung disease and diffuse, lower-lobe interstitial lung disease (Fig. 2–34). The patient's clinical course is usually determined by the central nervous system disease, but those with lung disease can develop respiratory insufficiency.

Tuberous Sclerosis. Tuberous sclerosis is an autosomal dominant syndrome characterized

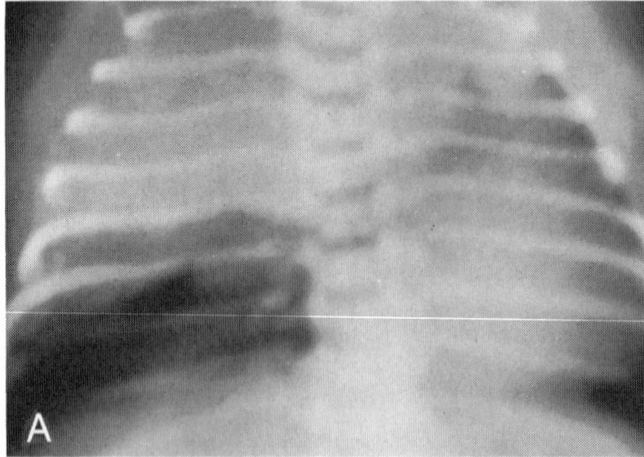

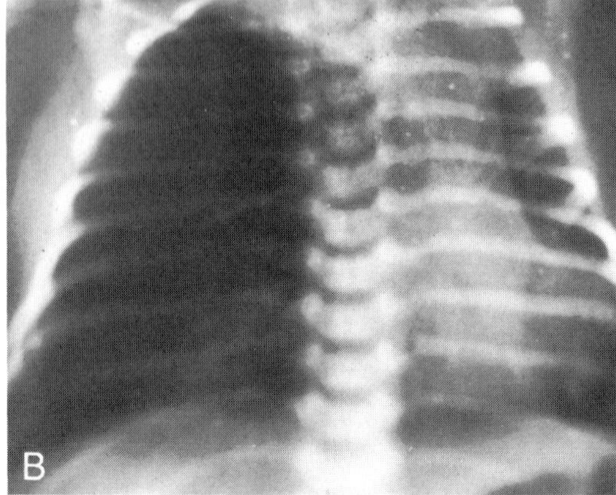

FIGURE 2–33. Congenital lobar emphysema. *A.* Shortly after birth, the right upper lobe is opaque. *B.* Later, the fluid has resolved, leaving hyperinflation and bullous changes. The overinflated right upper lobe displaces the mediastinum to the left.

clinically by mental retardation, seizures, and adenoma sebaceum. The most important lesions, hamartomas, occur in the brain (see Chapter 8); angiomyolipoma of the kidneys, rhabdomyoma of the heart, and subungual fibromas are less common manifestations. The lungs are involved in 0.1% of patients; in the lungs, smooth muscle proliferates and causes a reticulonodular appearance on the radiograph. These radiographic findings are similar to those of other types of interstitial fibrosis.

Sickle Cell Anemia. Sickle cell anemia is a hereditary abnormality that affects the beta chain of hemoglobin. This abnormality allows the red blood cells to assume a sickle shape under low oxygen tension, which results in hemodynamic and bone abnormalities that are visible on the chest radiograph (Fig. 2–35). The principal hemodynamic abnormality is cardiomegaly resulting from increased intravascular volume. Bone abnormalities are attributable to infarction and include necrosis of the humeral heads and biconcave appearance of the vertebral bodies.

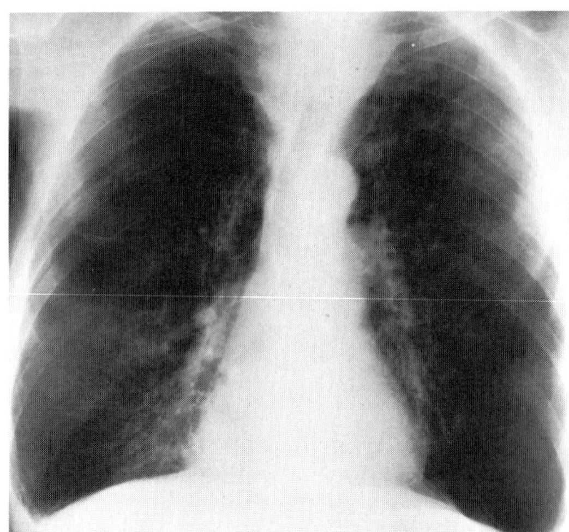

FIGURE 2–34. Neurofibromatosis. PA chest film shows hyperinflation, bullous abnormalities, and interstitial disease. Without clinical information, these findings would suggest the diagnosis of obstructive pulmonary disease.

Alpha$_1$-Antitrypsin Deficiency. Alpha$_1$-antitrypsin deficiency is a genetic defect in which the trypsin-inactivating enzyme is not made in sufficient quantities. The resultant elevation in serum trypsin, a proteolytic agent, causes digestion of the lungs. Patients usually become symptomatic early in adulthood as a result of development of respiratory difficulties. The lung destruction is characteristically most severe in the lower lobes (Fig. 2–36), resulting in a radiographic appearance of hyperlucency and vascular attenuation in the lower lobes and increased size of upper-lobe vessels. The reason for the lower-lobe destruction is not known.

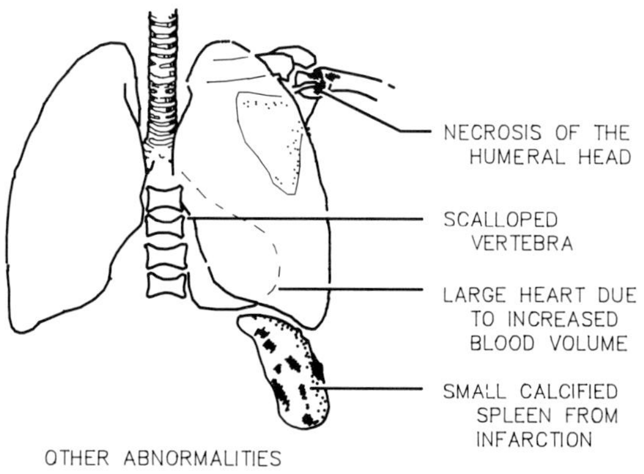

FIGURE 2–35. Characteristics of sickle cell anemia.

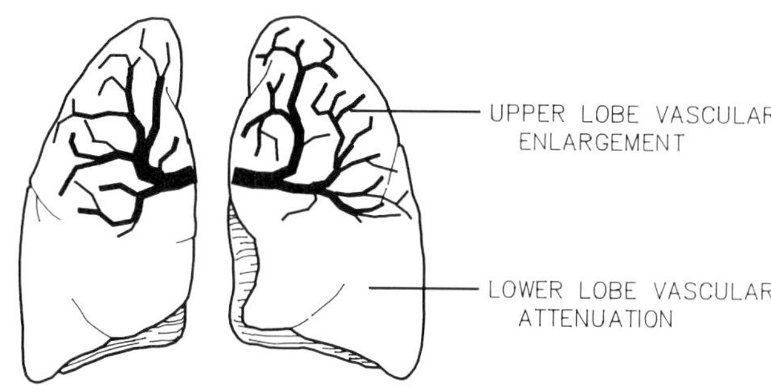

FIGURE 2–36. Characteristics of alpha$_1$-antitrypsin deficiency.

SYSTEMIC DISEASES

Endocrine Diseases

Most endocrine diseases manifest no abnormalities on chest radiographs. When the diseases do affect the chest, the abnormalities usually involve the bones as a result of changes in calcium metabolism (see Chapter 7). Other endocrine conditions that alter the appearance of chest radiographs are Cushing's syndrome and thyroid and parathyroid masses.

Cushing's Syndrome. The increase in soft tissue fat caused by corticosteroid excess either from Cushing's syndrome or from exogenous steroid therapy is manifested on chest radiographs as widening of the mediastinum and enlargement of the cardiac silhouette, both of which can be shown to be caused by increased fat on CT scans.

Thyroid Mass. The thyroid, normally small and not visible on chest radiographs, occasionally enlarges and appears as a mass in the lower neck. The enlarged thyroid (goiter) in the lower neck can cause asymmetry of soft tissue lines, loss of the clavicular companion shadow, and displacement of the trachea. Diagnosis is usually confirmed by nuclear medicine thyroid scan (see Chapter 9) or, occasionally, by ultrasonography. Infrequently, the thyroid extends below the clavicles and appears as a mass in the upper mediastinum. The diagnosis of intrathoracic thyroid gland is established by CT, MRI, or nuclear medicine thyroid scan.

Parathyroid Masses. Parathyroid glands can be found anywhere between the chin and the diaphragm, but most (96%) are in the neck near the posterior surface of the thyroid gland. Approximately 3% are found in the chest. The normal parathyroid gland is only 3 mm in diameter and is not detectable on plain radiographs. Ectopic parathyroid adenomas can be preoperatively detected in the neck by ultrasonography or in the neck and chest by CT, but their small size may make differentiation from adjacent structures such as lymph nodes, vessels, and muscle bundles difficult. Other radiological methods (for example, arteriography, venous blood sampling, MRI, and nuclear medicine scans) can be used to further evaluate a parathyroid adenoma.

Immunological Diseases

The immune responses to foreign material are classified into four types according to the mediator (Table 2–1). Types I (anaphylactoid) and III (Arthus) are the most important in lung disease. Immune disease in the chest can involve the mediastinum, the soft tissues, and

TABLE 2–1. TYPES OF IMMUNE RESPONSE

Type	Reaction	Mediator	Onset
I	Anaphylactoid	IgE	0 to 15 min
II	Humoral	IgG	Days
III	Arthus	IgG, IgM, immune complexes	Hours
IV	Cell-mediated	T lymphocytes	Weeks

IgE, IgG, and IgM, immunoglobulins E, G, and M.

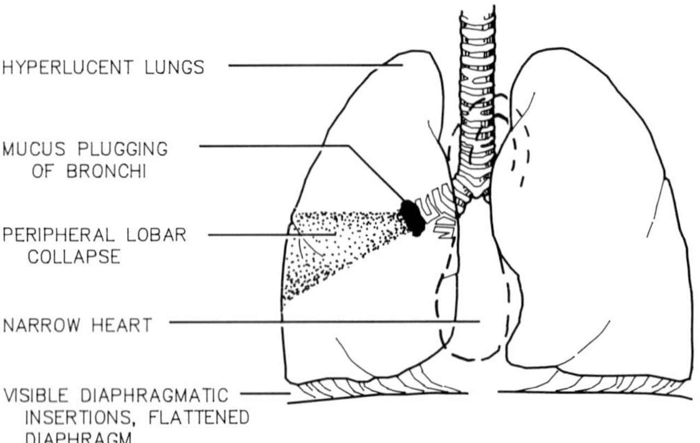

FIGURE 2–37. Characteristics of asthma.

the lungs. Mediastinal masses in immune disease can be the result of enlarged thymus, thymoma, or lymphoma. The lung nodules associated with rheumatoid arthritis or Wegener's granulomatosis most commonly involve the lung parenchyma but may involve the mediastinum. Enlargement of the cardiac silhouette in a patient with immune disease may indicate cardiomyopathy or pericardial effusion.

Lung Disease Caused by Extrinsic Agents

The most common chest abnormality in patients with immunological disorders is chronic inflammatory lung disease resulting from repeated infections. This type of disorder includes extrinsic allergic diseases such as asthma and extrinsic allergic alveolitis, deficiency of immunological response as a result of congenital cellular and biochemical abnormalities, and acquired deficiencies of immunological function, including cancer and the acquired immunodeficiency syndrome (AIDS). Iatrogenic immune suppression from steroid and cancer therapy is the most common cause of immunological disorders and requires the careful attention of the clinician and the radiologist.

Asthma. Asthma is a reversible, obstructive airway disease characterized by bronchospasm induced by an allergic response to environmental agents. It is most common in children. The chemical mediator is immunoglobulin E (IgE), but the slow-reacting substance of anaphylaxis (SRSA) has also been implicated. Radiographic abnormalities, when present, include hyperexpansion of the lungs, caused by air trapping, and mucus plugging of bronchi, which results in peripheral segmental atelectasis (Fig. 2–37).

Extrinsic Allergic Alveolitis. Extrinsic allergic alveolitis is alveolar hypersensitivity caused by inhalation of large quantities of particulate matter of up to 10 microns in diameter. A great variety of particles cause this condition, the most common being organic material, dusts, and feathers (Table 2–2). These particles cause a type III reaction in which antigen-antibody complexes form, and complement fixation and cell destruction by polymorphonuclear leukocytes occur about 6 hours after exposure. There is some evidence that a type IV (cell-mediated) response is also involved. Acute, subacute, and chronic radiographic changes occur in exposure to all types of offending agents, depending on the duration and intensity of exposure. Early granular appearance of the lungs may completely clear or may progress to reticulonodular abnormalities; this may clear or, with continued exposure, may progress to fibrosis and irreversible lung destruction (Fig. 2–38).

Lung Disease Associated With Collagen Vascular Diseases

The collagen vascular diseases are a group of diseases that involve collagen and vascular

TABLE 2–2. CAUSES OF EXTRINSIC ALLERGIC ALVEOLITIS

Disease	Cause
Farmer's lung	Actinomycetes (especially *Micropolyspora faeni*) from stored, moldy hay
Bird-fancier's lung	Bird serum, feces, feathers
Mushroom-worker's lung	Actinomycetes (grows during pasteurization)
Bagassosis	Bagasse fibers (from sugar cane), *Thermoactinomyces sachari*
Forced-air lung	*Thermoactinomycetes* species
Malt-worker's lung	*Aspergillus clavatus*
Maple-bark lung	*Cryptostroma corticale*
Pituitary snuff lung	Pig or ox pituitary extract
Suberosis	Cork dust
Sequoiosis	Redwood sawdust
Grain-weevil lung	Weevil
Byssinosis	Cotton dust
Cheese-washer's lung	Moldy cheese
Fish-meal lung	Fish meal
Coffee-worker's lung	Bean dust
Lycoperdonosis	Mushroom spores (from "puffball" inhaled to stop nosebleeds)
Detergent-worker's lung	*Bacillus subtilis* used in detergents to make proteolytic enzymes
Spray-starch lung	Starch
Wood-pulp lung	Mold *Alternaria*

tissues in the body. The specific cause of these diseases is unknown, but abnormalities in the patient's immune system are usually suggested by abnormal results of histological, biochemical, or immunological tests. All of these diseases can involve the lungs, in which they cause interstitial disease. Pleural or pericardial effusion, lung consolidation, or lung nodules may also be present. Advanced lung disease caused by collagen vascular diseases (and other interstitial lung diseases) is characterized by endstage lung destruction and interstitial fibrosis (called honeycomb lung). Pulmonary function studies can show severe restrictive impairment in excess of that suggested by radiographic findings. Biochemical and biopsy studies are needed to establish the diagnosis. Dramatic improvement in lung lesions often occurs when steroid therapy is instituted.

Despite similarities in the lung involvement associated with these collagen vascular diseases, each has certain distinguishing characteristics. Rheumatoid lung disease is often accompanied by parenchymal nodules and pleural effusion. Scleroderma is often associated with esophageal abnormalities. Both rheumatoid lung disease and scleroderma are common causes of severe lung destruction. Systemic lupus erythematosus (SLE) is associated with characteristic rash and immunological abnormalities. Although SLE is the most common of the collagen vascular diseases to involve the lungs, the findings of diffuse interstitial disease are nonspecific. The chest radiograph abnormalities of polymyositis and dermatomyositis, if they occur at all, are limited to reticulonodular interstitial density; the diagnosis is made on the basis of skin and muscle

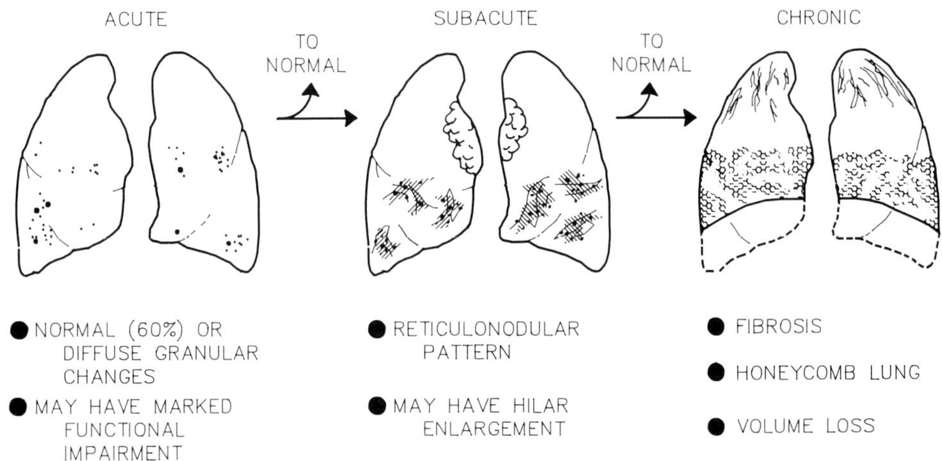

FIGURE 2–38. Characteristics of extrinsic allergic alveolitis.

involvement. Polyarteritis nodosa causes nonspecific alveolar densities in the lung; diagnosis depends on histological identification of necrotizing angitis.

Rheumatoid Lung Disease. Rheumatoid arthritis, a disease predominantly of middle-aged women, most commonly affects only the joint spaces. However, lung disease is common in men afflicted with rheumatoid arthritis, particularly those who have severe joint disease. Pulmonary radiographic findings are usually limited to diffuse interstitial fibrosis, but pleural effusion and lung nodules may also be present (Fig. 2–39). The interstitial disease usually has a fine basal reticular pattern, but in advanced disease, severe endstage lung destruction is seen. Pleural effusion, a sterile exudate, is usually unilateral (90%) and can be the only chest abnormality. Lung nodules are identical to the subcutaneous nodules seen elsewhere in the body. They are usually multiple and often cavitate. Arteritis of the pulmonary vessels can lead to pulmonary hypertension and cor pulmonale.

Scleroderma. Scleroderma is a systemic collagen vascular disease that affects the skin and smooth muscle of all organ systems. It usually affects women in the 30- to 60-year age group. The early chest radiographic abnormality is reticulonodular interstitial disease. This progresses to fibrosis, marked volume loss, and the development of microcysts. Esophageal

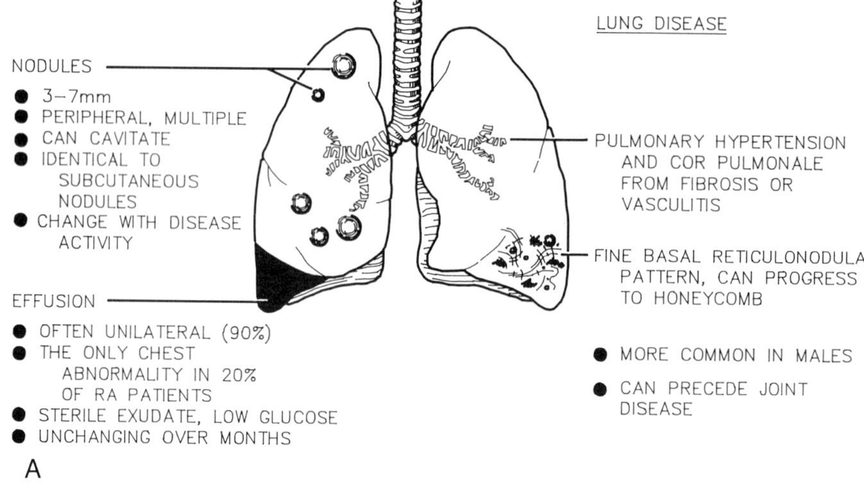

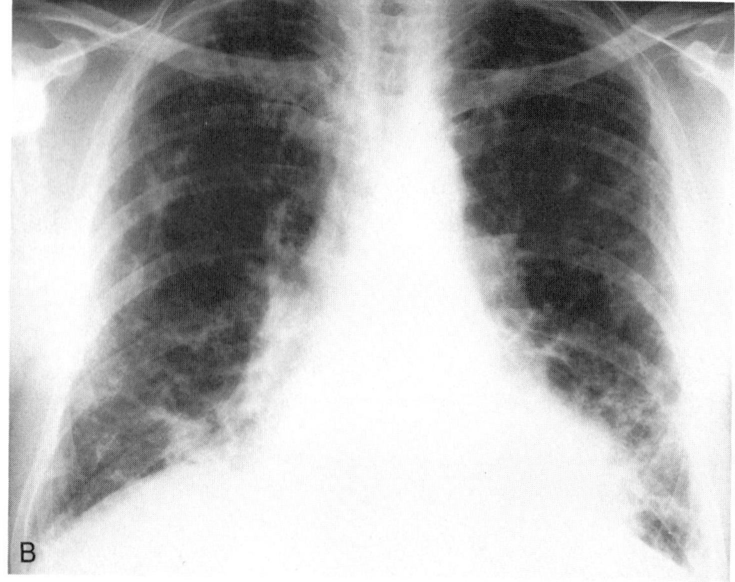

FIGURE 2–39. Rheumatoid lung disease. *A.* Diagram: rheumatoid arthritis. *B.* Chest film shows extensive interstitial opacification throughout the lungs in a patient with long-term rheumatoid arthritis.

involvement is common, resulting in esophageal dilatation and dysmotility, and leads to repeated aspiration pneumonitis.

Polymyositis and Dermatomyositis. Polymyositis and dermatomyositis are collagen vascular diseases that affect predominately the skin and striated muscle. Patients with polymyositis and dermatomyositis may have a normal chest, bibasilar reticulonodular lung abnormalities, or, if pharyngeal muscles are involved, evidence of repeated aspiration. The chest radiographic findings are nonspecific.

Lung Disease Associated With Immunological Disease

Other immunological diseases that affect the lungs are Wegener's granulomatosis, Goodpasture's syndrome, and ankylosing spondylitis. Wegener's granulomatosis results in a vasculitis and subsequent interstitial lung disease. Goodpasture's syndrome, an autoimmune reaction to the lungs and the kidneys, causes pulmonary hemorrhage and lung destruction. Ankylosing spondylitis, an arthritis of the spine associated with histocompatibility antigens, apparently causes lung disease as a result of consequent restriction of lung expansion.

Wegener's Granulomatosis. Wegener's granulomatosis is a disease of unknown cause, is probably attributable to autoimmunity, and manifests in adults as upper respiratory disease followed later by lung and kidney disease (Fig. 2–40). The upper respiratory disease leads to thickening of the sinus mucosa, which can eventually destroy bone. Lung involvement consists of interstitial fibrosis, multiple pulmonary nodules (granulomas), and associated vasculitis; it eventually leads to respiratory failure. Glomerulitis occurs later and results in renal failure. Patients often require dialysis or kidney transplantation. Some patients have a limited form of Wegener's granulomatosis that affects only the lungs. These patients have a slightly better prognosis. In many patients, response to steroids or cytotoxic agents is dramatic, including reversal of renal disease.

Goodpasture's Syndrome. Goodpasture's syndrome is an immune disease of young adults in which antibodies (immunoglobulin G) to the glomerular basement membrane and to the immunologically similar alveolar basement membrane cause renal failure and lung destruction. The manifesting sign is pulmonary hemorrhage or nephrotic syndrome. Repeated hemorrhage leads to diffuse interstitial fibrosis, hemosiderosis, and sclerosis of pulmonary vessels (Fig. 2–41). Vasculitis rarely occurs. Diagnosis can be made by means of lung or renal biopsy. Prognosis is poor (95% of patients die within 6 months); few patients survive 5 years. Corticosteroids and cytotoxic drugs are the only accepted treatment, although nephrectomy has reversed the pulmonary symptoms in some cases. Goodpasture's syndrome should not be confused with idiopathic pulmonary hemosiderosis, a disease of early childhood with similar lung changes; this latter disease is not an autoimmune disorder and does not affect the kidneys.

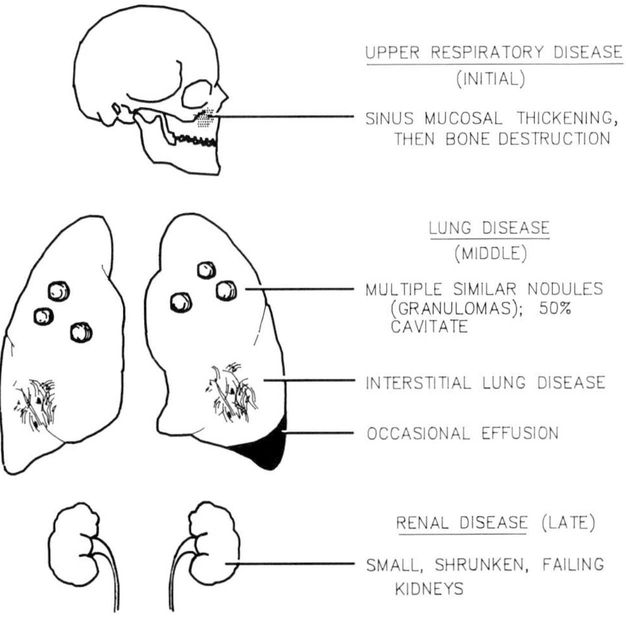

FIGURE 2–40. Characteristics of Wegener's granulomatosis.

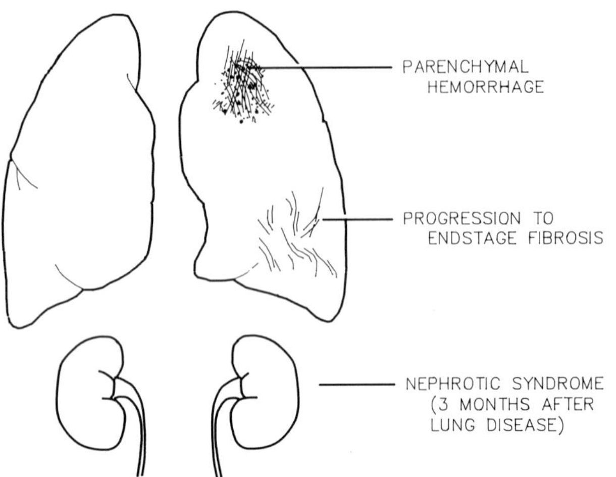

FIGURE 2–41. Characteristics of Goodpasture's syndrome.

Ankylosing Spondylitis. Ankylosing spondylitis is an arthritis of young men associated with the HLA-B27 histocompatibility antigen. It is characterized by sacroiliac and spinal ankylosis. When spine disease extends to the thoracic region, the upper thorax becomes fixed, and upper lung fibrosis develops. The radiographic appearance is similar to that of tuberculosis (Fig. 2–42).

Pulmonary Infiltrates With Eosinophilia

A variety of lung diseases are associated with eosinophilia, either within the lesions or in the peripheral blood. These diseases manifest radiographically by peripheral infiltrates and are called the PIE (*p*eripheral *i*nfiltrates with *e*osinophilia) syndrome. The most common of these diseases are Löffler's syndrome, acute or chronic eosinophilic pneumonia, tropical eosinophilic pneumonia (filariasis), allergic bronchopulmonary aspergillosis, and polyarteritis nodosa. The eosinophilia may be attributable to hypersensitivity or parasitic infestation, or it may be idiopathic.

Löffler's Syndrome. Löffler's syndrome is characterized radiographically by transient migratory interstitial or alveolar density in the lung (fleeting pneumonia) caused by eosino-

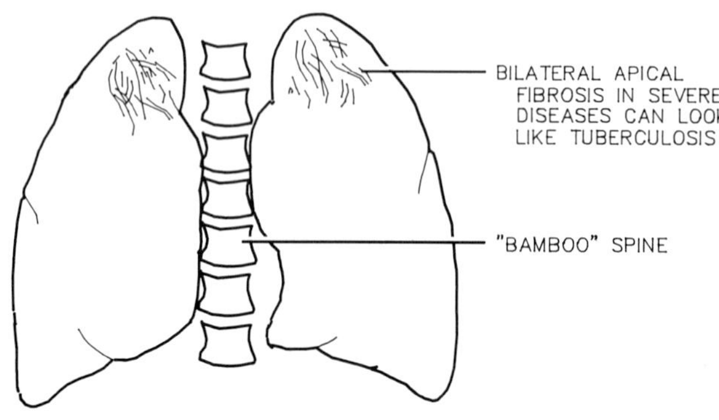

FIGURE 2–42. Characteristics of ankylosing spondylitis.

philic infiltration. The patient may be asymptomatic or may have a cough or general malaise. The blood eosinophil count is elevated. Most patients have a history of atopy. The disease can be caused by allergic reaction to either worms (*Ascaris, Trichuris, Strongyloides,* and *Ancylostoma*) or drugs or hypersensitivity to fungal organisms (bronchopulmonary aspergillosis). It is self-limiting and usually resolves within 1 month if the offending organism or agent is removed.

Chronic Eosinophilic Pneumonia. Chronic eosinophilic pneumonia is similar in cause and presentation to Löffler's syndrome except that the course is more prolonged. Increased density is seen on radiographs, predominantly in the periphery of the lung, as a "reverse batwing" pattern (i.e., a photographic negative of pulmonary edema). The interstitial or alveolar density is caused by infiltration by histiocytes and eosinophils. The known causes are drugs (sulfa and nitrofurantoin), allergens, and parasites. Patients who have an allergic cause of chronic eosinophilic pneumonia have often received desensitization treatments to the offending agent. Various parasites, notably *Ascaris, Strongyloides, Ancylostoma, Necator, Toxocara,* and *Schistosoma,* pass through the lungs during their cycle, and there they incite an allergic reaction. In 5% of cases of schistosomiasis, the ova become lodged in the pulmonary vessels and cause an obliterative alveolitis and resultant pulmonary hypertension.

Usually, patients with chronic eosinophilic pneumonia are middle-aged, atopic women who are moderately ill with symptoms similar to those of tuberculosis (i.e., fever, weight loss, sweats, and cough). Sixty-five percent of patients have an elevated blood eosinophil count; rapid improvement follows steroid therapy, but the disease tends to recur. A less common eosinophilic pneumonia has an abrupt, rapid presentation that results in respiratory failure in a few days. Therapy with a brief course of steroids (several weeks) is curative.

Tropical Eosinophilic Pneumonia (Filariasis). Tropical eosinophilic pneumonia (filariasis) is caused by infestation by filariae (primarily *Wuchereria bancrofti*), which lodge in the pulmonary capillaries and induce an allergic alveolitis that causes fibrosis and eosinophilic infiltration. The disease is most common in 20- to 40-year-old inhabitants of India and Malaysia. Symptoms are similar to those of asthma, and the blood eosinophil count is elevated. If fibrosis is not extensive, the chest abnormalities may resolve after treatment with diethylcarbamazine. If fibrosis is advanced, the patient has persistent restrictive lung disease.

Allergic Bronchopulmonary Aspergillosis. Allergic bronchopulmonary aspergillosis is a complex immunologic reaction to *Aspergillus fumigatus*. The disease affects asthmatics, occurs most commonly in winter, and causes cough, fever, wheezing, and sputum production. The sputum and the peripheral blood contain eosinophils. The spores are inhaled and cause a type I reaction in the bronchi. A later type III reaction causes bronchial necrosis and eosinophilic consolidation. Hyphae and eosinophils collect in the bronchi to form obstructing plugs. Radiographs show that lobar or segmental consolidation results distal to the obstructing plugs. These mucus plugs, composed of eosinophils and hyphae, produce smooth dilatation of the central bronchi, described as a toothpaste or gloved-finger appearance. Treatment of allergic bronchopulmonary aspergillosis is directed toward therapy for asthma. The pulmonary disease clears in days to weeks after institution of bronchodilator and steroid therapy.

Polyarteritis Nodosa. Polyarteritis nodosa is the prototype necrotizing angiitis of small and medium-sized vessels; it is caused by an autoimmune hypersensitivity reaction. The disease affects middle-aged adults, primarily women, and manifests as fever, weight loss, and anorexia. Vessels in all parts of the body can be affected; the lungs are involved in about 20% of patients. The kidneys are involved in 80% of patients, with resultant renal failure and hypertension. Unfortunately, even with steroid and cytotoxic drug therapy, the 5-year survival rate is only 50%. The cause is unknown, although some cases have resulted from acute drug reaction, and patients usually have positive reactions to the hepatitis-B surface antigen. Vascular necrosis, inflammation, and, later, fibrosis are seen in histological examination. Although the cause is unknown, the radiographic findings are similar to the fleeting abnormalities of Löffler's syndrome (Fig. 2–43). In addition, miliary nodules, effusion, and cavitating nodules may be present.

INFECTIOUS DISEASES

Infection in the lung is caused by bacteria (pyogenic, enteric, and atypical), fungi and mycobacteria, viruses, protozoans, and worms (Table 2–3). The radiographic appearances of

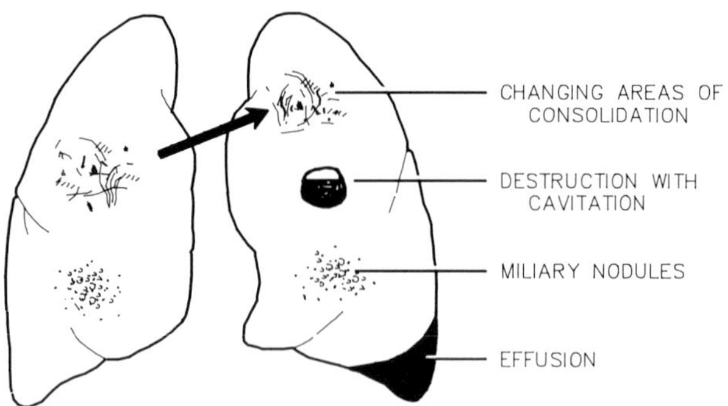

- NECROTIZING ANGIITIS OF SMALL/MEDIUM VESSELS
- MIDDLE AGE
- 20% HAVE LUNG DISEASE
- 50% – 5 YEAR SURVIVAL

FIGURE 2–43. Characteristics of polyarteritis nodosa.

many pneumonias are similar, and although it is often not possible to differentiate pneumonia from other lung diseases, certain characteristic radiographic patterns may facilitate the correct diagnosis. Often the radiologist can suggest the diagnosis on the basis of clinical history even with a paucity of radiographic findings. It is therefore important for the radiologist to be aware of clinical aspects of pneumonia and to obtain a thorough clinical history in evaluating chest infection. The most common infections are caused by pyogenic bacteria.

Most infections that occur in adults can occur in children, and the radiographic appearances are usually identical; however, pneumonia in children often has a subtle appearance on radiographs and several radiographic abnormalities are not found in adults with pneumonia. Peribronchial thickening is often the earliest finding in childhood pneumonia. Atrophy of the thymus, if the patient is young, can also suggest early disease. Recurrent pneumonia in children, radiographically evident from chronic lung disease, can be attributable to a variety of causes.

Bacterial Pneumonia Caused by Gram-Positive Organisms

Pneumococcal Pneumonia. *Streptococcus pneumoniae* causes 40% of all cases of pneumonia. Of the more than 88 serotypes of *S. pneumoniae,* only a few are common. Infection occurs by aspiration, often from the patient's own normal oral flora. Patients exhibit leukocytosis, fever, and usually a single, shaking chill, and they produce bloody sputum loaded with leukocytes and organisms. Patients with sickle cell disease and those who have undergone splenectomy have a higher incidence of episodes of pneumococcal pneumonia than do people in the general population.

Infection in the lung causes airspace, usually lower-lobe, consolidation that spreads to adjacent lung segments through Kohn's pores. Thus the disease is not segmental but is usually confined to one lobe. Radiographs show nonsegmental consolidation limited to a single lobe (Fig. 2–44). Air bronchograms can usually be identified, and pleural effusion is common. Cavitation is rare. All serotypes are sensitive

TABLE 2–3. IMPORTANT CAUSES OF PNEUMONIA

Gram-Positive Bacteria	Gram-Negative Bacteria	Other	Fungi	Atypical Organisms
Pneumococcus	*Escherichia coli*	*Mycobacterium*	*Aspergillus*	*Mycoplasma*
Streptococcus	*Klebsiella*	*Actinomyces*	*Histoplasma*	*Chlamydia*
Staphylococcus	*Enterobacter*	*Nocardia*	*Coccidioides*	*Rickettsia*
Bacillus	*Pseudomonas*		*Candida*	
Listeria	*Haemophilus influenzae*		*Blastomyces*	
			Cryptococcus	

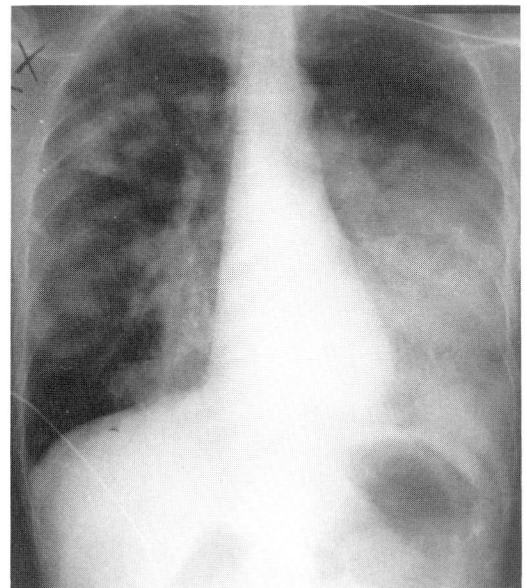

FIGURE 2–44. Pneumococcal pneumonia. PA chest film shows nearly complete left lower-lobe opacification and additional patchy areas in the right lung in a man with extremely high fever.

to penicillin. Clinical symptoms usually resolve in 24 to 48 hours after therapy is begun. However, radiographic abnormalities clear more slowly, returning to normal within about 2 weeks.

Beta-Hemolytic Streptococcal Pneumonia. Of the beta-hemolytic streptococci, the Lancefield group A is the most common cause of pneumonia; 20% of the population carry these organisms as normal oral flora. Infection by streptococci results in patchy or homogeneous consolidation limited to one lung segment. In severe or untreated cases, empyema and, later, pleural scarring develops. The organism is always sensitive to penicillin. Diseases caused by streptococci outside the chest include strep throat, scarlet fever, rheumatic heart disease, acute glomerulonephritis, and impetigo.

Group B beta-hemolytic streptococcus causes a usually fatal pneumonia in neonates that is characterized by diffuse patchy consolidation associated with bacteremia (Fig. 2–45). Additional radiographic abnormalities include hyperexpansion of the lungs, pleural effusion, and thymic atrophy.

Staphylococcal Pneumonia. *Staphylococcus aureus,* a gram-positive, coagulase-producing bacterium, causes pneumonia increasingly commonly because of its presence as normal oral flora and its ability to develop antibiotic resistance. It usually affects hospitalized or debilitated patients. Radiographs show segmental consolidation, which often involves more than one lobe. The infection is often progressive, resulting in severe lung destruction, the formation of abscesses, and cavitation. Extension of infection to the pleural space (empyema) often occurs. In children the cavity often develops into a pneumatocele and can cause pneumothorax. Staphylococcal pneumonia is difficult to treat because of its resistance to drugs.

Pneumonia Caused by Unusual Gram-Positive Bacteria

***Bacillus anthracis* Pneumonia.** *Bacillus anthracis* is a gram-positive rod that forms spores. It causes disease in cattle, sheep, and goats and is transferred to humans from the fur and the hides of these animals. After the spores are inhaled, they enter the lymphatics and the blood stream. Chest films show patchy areas of increased density that are attributable to hemorrhagic pneumonitis. Pleural effusion and hilar enlargement are often present. The clinical symptoms of fever and bloody sputum and the radiographic appearance of pneumonia caused by *B. anthracis* are nonspecific. Unless the disease is suspected and treated, the pa-

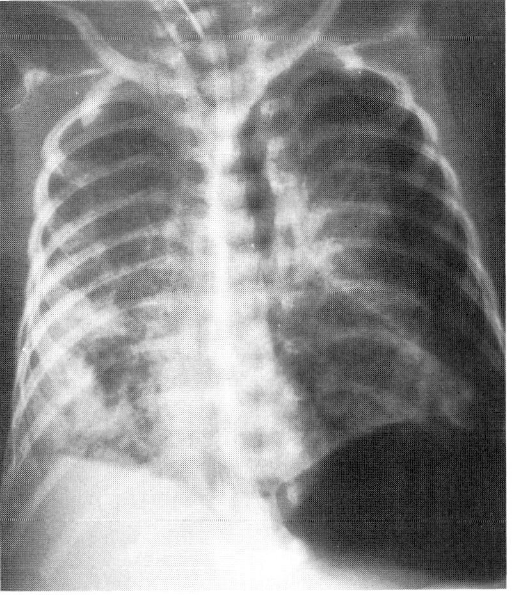

FIGURE 2–45. Streptococcal pneumonia. Chest film shows extensive, patchy areas of lung opacification caused by a group B beta-hemolytic *Streptococcus* infection in an infant. Treatment of this infection was complicated by a pneumothorax that resulted from high-pressure mechanical ventilation. (Note endotracheal tube.)

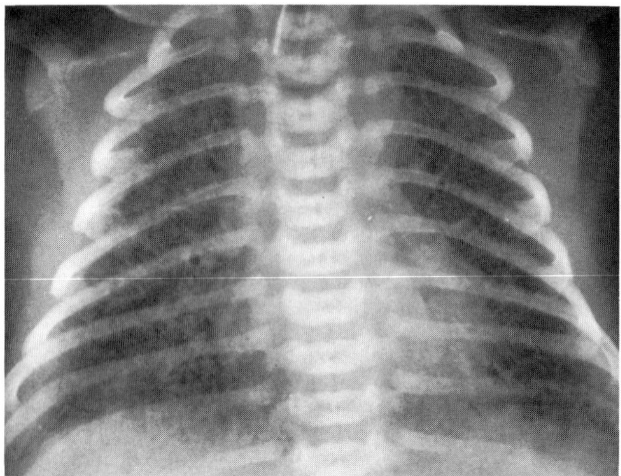

FIGURE 2–46. *Listeria* pneumonia. Chest film in a newborn with respiratory distress shows patchy areas of consolidation. The infant required endotracheal intubation and assisted ventilation. Note thymic atrophy, indicative of stress.

tient dies within a few days after development of pneumonia.

***Listeria* Pneumonia.** *Listeria monocytogenes,* also a gram-positive rod, affects immunodeficient patients (infants or immunosuppressed adults). Infants acquire the infection during passage through the birth canal and develop a severe, often fatal, pneumonia. Radiographs show coarse and patchy areas of increased density (Fig. 2–46). Hyperexpansion of the lungs differentiates *Listeria* pneumonia from restrictive lung disease. Thymic atrophy indicates stress.

Pneumonia Caused by Gram-Negative Organisms

The gram-negative bacteria are increasingly common causes of pneumonia, particularly in immunosuppressed or debilitated patients. Gram-negative infections are more serious than gram-positive infections because of their resistance to drugs, the production of endotoxin, and their tendency to cause septicemia.

***Escherichia coli* Pneumonia.** *Escherichia coli* has become a common cause of pneumonia. It primarily affects debilitated hospitalized patients who are receiving multiple antibiotic therapy. Chest radiographs show multilobar consolidation often with pleural effusion. *E. coli* pneumonia rarely causes cavitation.

***Klebsiella* Pneumonia.** *Klebsiella* species cause 5% of all cases of pneumonia. The organism produces an acute, fulminating, airspace consolidation, usually in debilitated hospitalized patients or in alcoholics. The radiographic appearance is the same as that of pneumococcal pneumonia except that (1) the inflammatory exudate expands the affected part of the lung, (2) abscess cavitation is common, and (3) effusion and empyema are usually present (Fig. 2–47). In 50% of patients, the disease is fatal within the first 48 hours, and so treatment must be started early.

***Enterobacter* and *Serratia* Pneumonia.** *Enterobacter* and *Serratia* pneumonias also occur

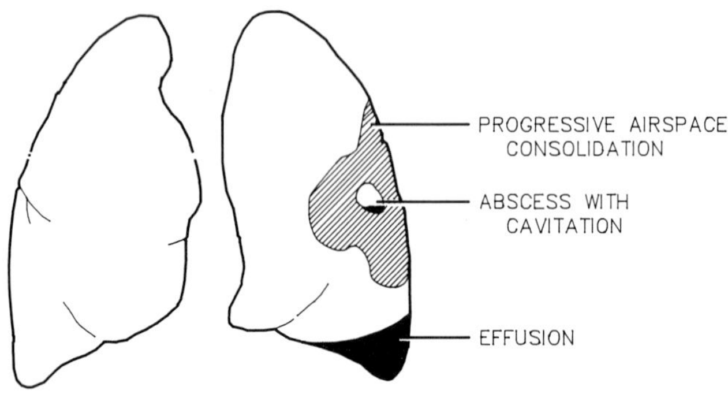

FIGURE 2–47. Characteristics of *Klebsiella* pneumonia.

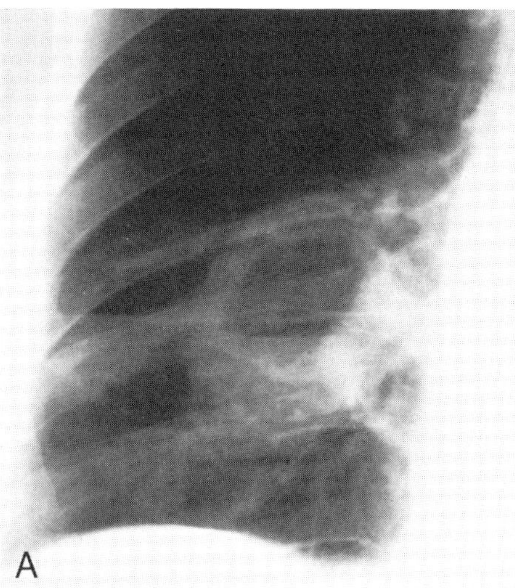

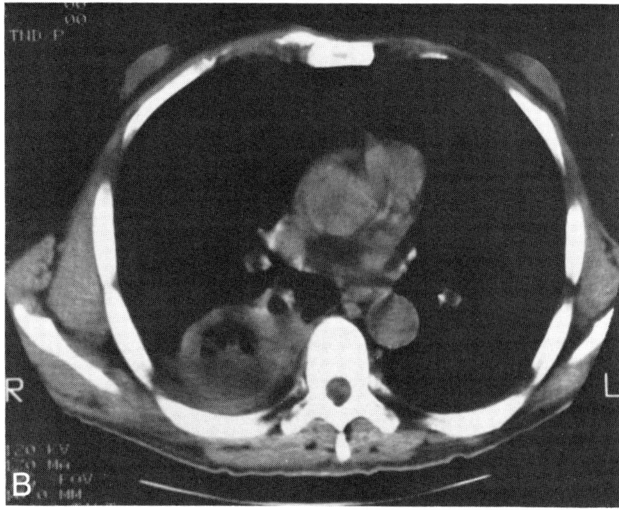

FIGURE 2–48. Anaerobic pneumonia. *A.* PA view. Chest radiograph shows an air-fluid level inside a right lower-lobe cavity lesion. *B.* CT scan shows a large, round mass lesion with central cavitation. A smaller cavity is seen in a second mass anterior and medial to it. The patient, an alcoholic, first developed an aspiration pneumonia, which was then complicated by a mixed, anaerobic infection and cavitation.

in debilitated patients and exhibit a radiographic picture similar to that of *Klebsiella* pneumonia but without abscess formation. *Serratia* pneumonia in particular has become a common nosocomial disease. Both *Enterobacter* and *Serratia* produce cephalosporinase and are difficult to treat.

***Pseudomonas* Pneumonia.** *Pseudomonas aeruginosa* is an opportunistic, gram-negative bacillus that causes a usually fatal pneumonia in debilitated patients. The organism grows easily and colonizes virtually all hospital materials, including respirators. It is resistant to nearly all antibiotics. The radiographic appearance of the pneumonia is the same as that of staphylococcal pneumonia, although patchy consolidative forms also are seen.

Pseudomonas pseudomallei causes a disease (melioidosis) endemic in Southeast Asia. On radiographs, it produces a nodular pattern in the lungs (and other organs) because of microabscesses, which may coalesce and cavitate. The acute form of the disease is rapidly fatal if untreated. The chronic form is that of unresolved pneumonia, which mimics tuberculosis clinically and radiographically. The organism grows easily on all types of media, and the diagnosis is often easy to make.

***Haemophilus influenzae* Pneumonia.** *Haemophilus influenzae* typically causes disease in children aged 2 months to 3 years, although immunocompromised adults may also be afflicted. The radiographic appearance is the same as that of *Streptococcus pneumoniae* pneumonia.

Pneumonia Caused by Anaerobes. Anaerobic pulmonary infections are caused by aspiration of oral flora or by septicemia and commonly occur in alcoholics, epileptics, and debilitated patients (especially those with dysphagia). Aspiration is usually into the lowest (most dependent) portions of the lung and produces a homogeneous, segmental consolidation (Fig. 2–48). Cavitation is common and extensive. The infections are usually clinically insidious.

Pneumonia Caused by Bacteria-Like Organisms

Tuberculosis. Mycobacterial disease is most commonly caused by *Mycobacterium tuberculosis,* and in the United States, it affects alcoholics, members of low socioeconomic groups, immunocompromised patients, and immigrants from Asia and Central and South America. The clinical symptoms and the radiographic appearance depend on the stage of disease and the type of involvement. Primary tuberculosis, the initial infection, is usually asymptomatic. A hypersensitivity reaction occurs 4 to 8 weeks after the initial infection and leads to caseation. The lesion later becomes walled off by scar tissue but still contains viable organisms. The radiographic features of primary tuberculosis include a focal area of consolidation, often with cavitation, asymmetrical adenopathy, and, in up to 40% of patients,

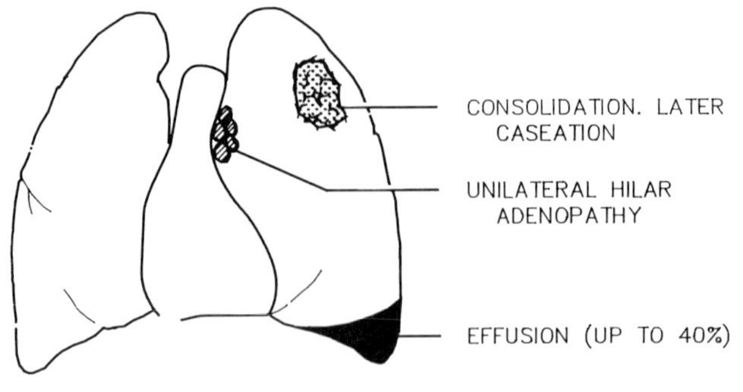

FIGURE 2–49. Characteristics of primary tuberculosis.

pleural effusion (Fig. 2–49). Calcification of the parenchymal scar, called Ghon's lesion, occurs in 25% of patients. The combination of Ghon's lesion and calcified lymph nodes is called a Ranke complex.

Reactivation tuberculosis occurs when viable organisms are released into the blood stream from primary lesions. A pulmonary reinfection occurs, primarily in the better aerated upper lobes, and causes clinical signs of fever, night sweats, and general malaise. The radiographic appearance is apical consolidation with pleural thickening and bronchiectasis. The hila are elevated as a result of the apical scarring and retraction (Figs. 2–50, 2–51). In most cases the activity of the disease cannot be determined from the chest film. Cavitation usually indicates active disease. When no change in the radiographic abnormality is seen over months, it may be assumed that the disease is inactive.

Miliary tuberculosis, a severe disseminated form, occurs when hematogenous spread of organisms causes septicemia, usually in a debilitated person. Multiple 1-mm (millet seed–sized) densities are seen uniformly spread throughout the lungs (Fig. 2–52). Patients are severely ill. The disease is fatal unless treated early and vigorously.

Atypical mycobacteria, most commonly *Mycobacterium kansasii* and *M. intracellulare,* cause 1% of cases of pulmonary tuberculosis. Most cases are in immunocompromised patients. *M. fortuitum* and *M. scrofulaceum* rarely cause lung disease. The clinical symptoms in atypical tuberculosis are similar to but milder than those of the more common form. The radiographic pattern is indistinguishable from that of *M. tuberculosis* infections.

Actinomycetes: Actinomycosis and Nocardiosis. The actinomycetes include *Actinomyces* species (*israelii* and *bovis*), *Nocardia (asteroides),* and *Streptomyces* species; they were originally classified as fungi because of their mycelial tissue forms. They are now grouped with the bacteria because they also have a bacterial form and respond to antibiotics. In the bacterial form, they appear as gram-positive rods. Acid-fast staining is highly dependent on decolorization strength and leads to much confusion: *Actinomyces* is not acid-fast, whereas *Nocardia* is. *Actinomyces* and *Nocardia* organisms do not respond to antifungal agents.

Actinomyces israelii is a constituent of the anaerobic flora of the normal mouth. The most common form of infection (60%) is caused by direct extension from the mouth into the cervicofacial region (called lumpy jaw). In 20% of patients, actinomycosis affects the abdomen, usually the appendix, and can extend to involve the liver and pelvic organs. Fifteen percent of cases are thoracic as a result of aspiration of the organism, which causes a nonsegmental cavitary pneumonia (Fig. 2–53). Untreated, the disease can penetrate the chest wall by means of proteolytic enzymes. The diagnosis of actinomycosis is confirmed by the presence of yellow (sulfur) granules in the sputum or in biopsy material or by growth of the organism. The infection is treated by long-term, low-dose penicillin.

Nocardia asteroides is an anaerobe found in the soil. It can cause disease when it is inhaled, particularly in immunosuppressed patients. Clinical features, results of acid-fast staining, and radiographic findings are similar to those of tuberculosis. Unlike *Actinomyces,*

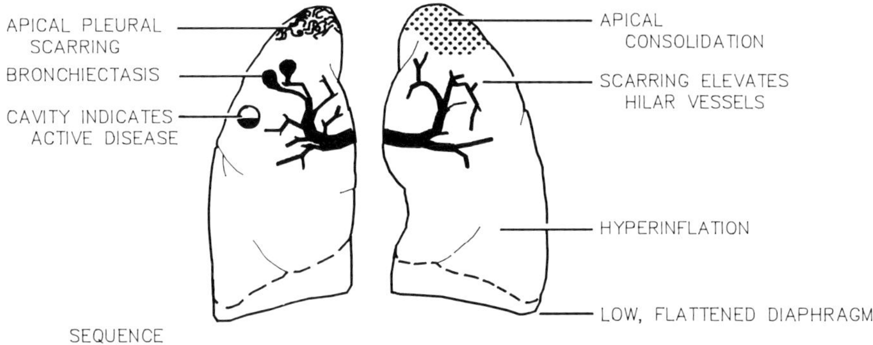

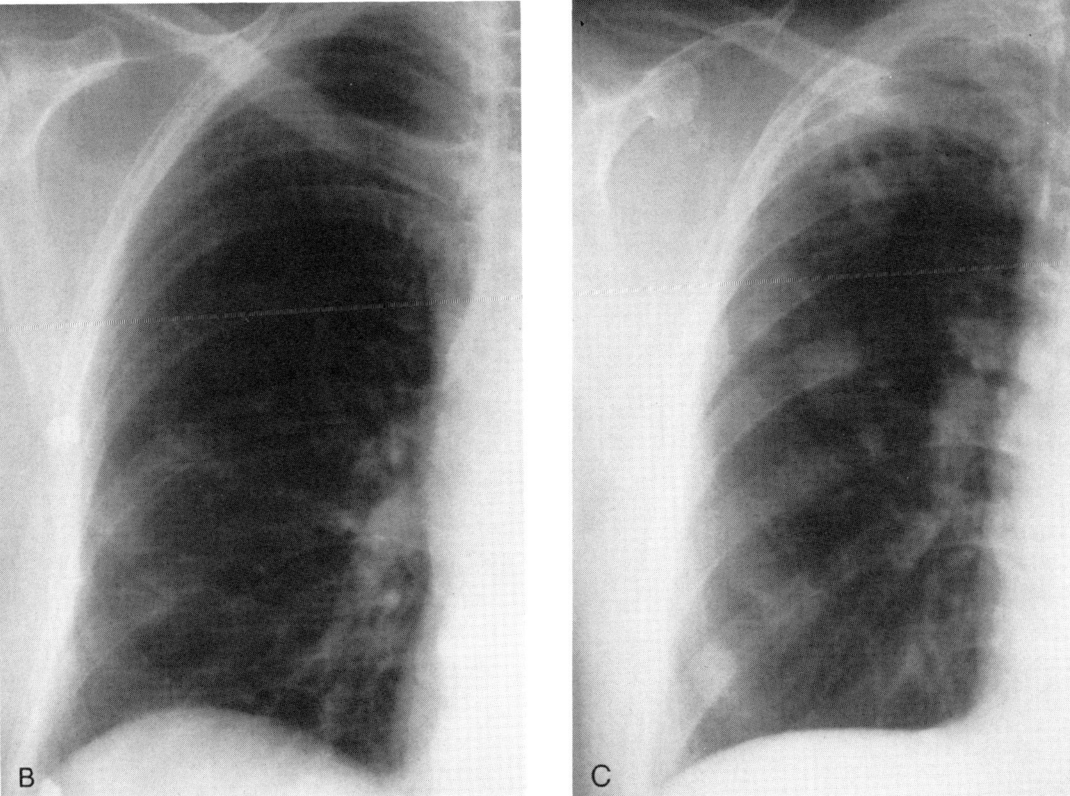

FIGURE 2–50. Reactivation tuberculosis. *A.* Diagram. *B.* Chest film in a man who had had a previous tuberculosis infection and had developed a fever and another infection shows minimal opacification in the right lung. *C.* In a radiograph taken 4 weeks later, scattered alveolar densities had become obvious throughout the lung. The prominent involvement is in the right apex.

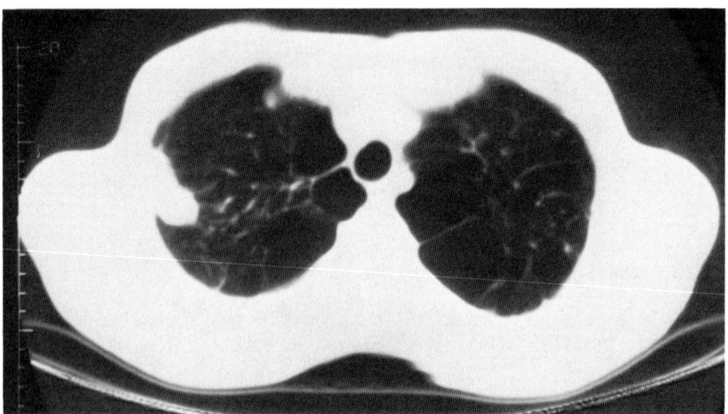

FIGURE 2–51. Chronic, inactive tuberculosis. CT scan of the upper lung photographed at lung windows demonstrates large bullae. In addition, a large scar is present in the lateral right lung. This abnormality was stable, which indicates that active disease was not present in the patient, a 65-year-old man with a history of tuberculosis.

Nocardia does not penetrate the chest wall (Fig. 2–54). The organism is responsive to the sulfonamides and the tetracyclines, but not to penicillin.

Fungal Pneumonias

Aspergillosis. The fungus *Aspergillus fumigatus,* widespread in nature, is commonly found as a nonpathogen in the respiratory tract. It causes four types of lung disease: primary pneumonia, allergic bronchopulmonary aspergillosis, mycetoma, and diffuse pneumonia. Primary pneumonia is exceedingly rare, and its radiographic appearance is like that of pneumococcal pneumonia. Its clinical manifestation is as a chronic infection. Allergic bronchopulmonary aspergillosis is a complex, allergic reaction to *A. fumigatus* characterized by plugging of bronchi by hyphae and inflammatory cells (see the Immunological Diseases section). Mycetoma (fungus ball) is a collection of hyphae and mucus that forms in a cavity in the lung (Fig. 2–55). The cavity may be caused by a previous or concomitant infection from another organism (especially tuberculosis), or it may be caused by carcinoma, bronchiectasis, sarcoidosis, or lung destruction. No invasion of lung tissue occurs in mycetoma. In debilitated or immunosuppressed patients, a fulminant diffuse pneumonia can occur.

Histoplasmosis. *Histoplasma capsulatum* is found in the soil, particularly in river valleys

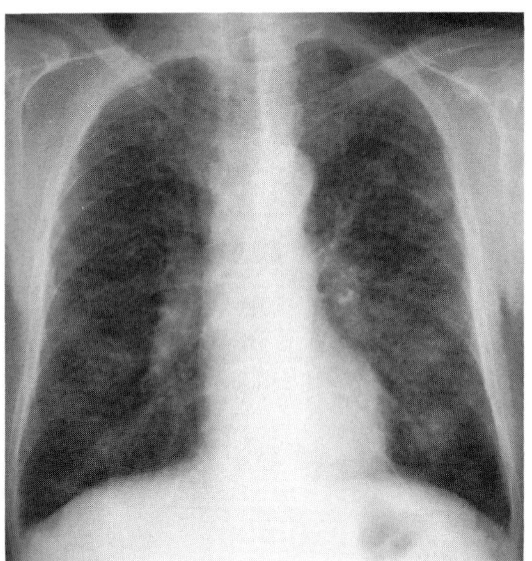

FIGURE 2–52. Miliary tuberculosis. PA chest film shows a diffuse pattern of small densities throughout both lungs. The patient, who was immunocompromised as a result of chemotherapy treatment for lymphoma, has disseminated (miliary) tuberculosis.

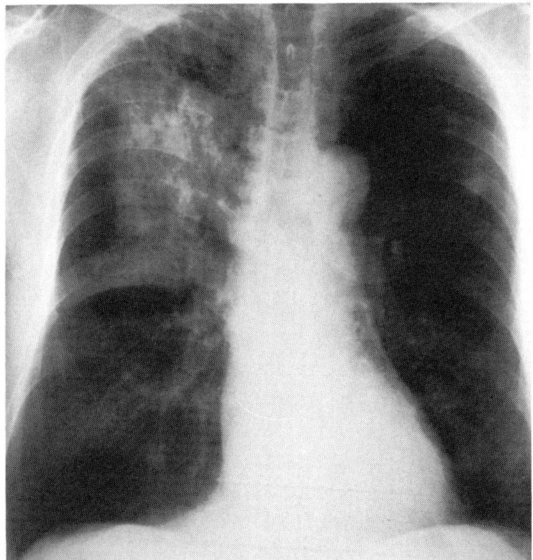

FIGURE 2–53. Actinomycosis. PA chest film shows right upper-lobe consolidation in a 35-year-old man with productive cough. Sputum analysis showed yellow "sulfur" granules, and the patient responded to long-term, low-dose penicillin.

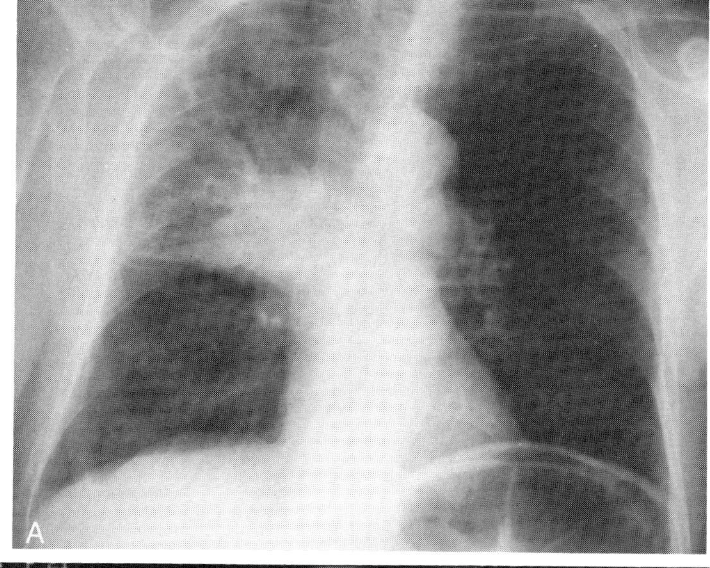

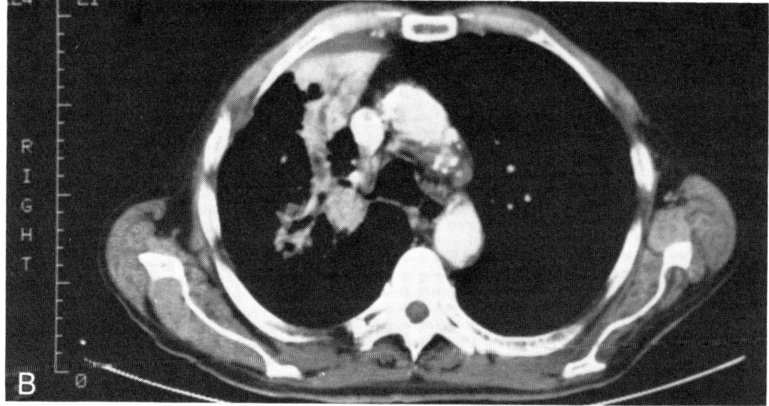

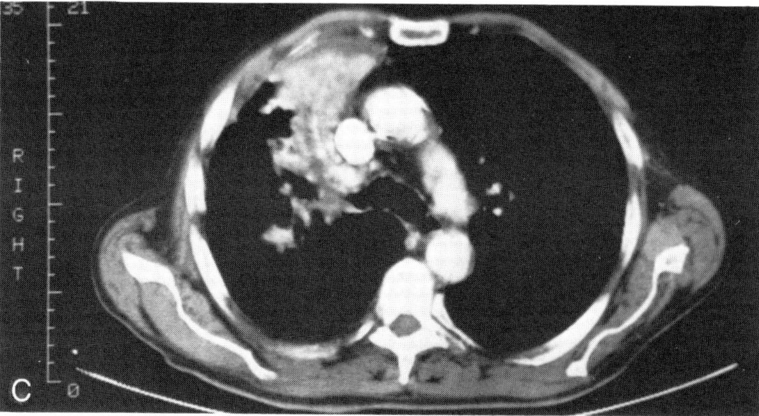

FIGURE 2–54. Nocardia pneumonia. Chest film *(A)* shows a mass lesion near the right hilum. CT sections *(B* and *C)* below the aortic arch show that this mass obstructs the right upper-lobe bronchus, causing collapse. The mass represented a focal *Nocardia* infection.

(Ohio, Mississippi, and Saint Lawrence), where it thrives on bird and bat feces and sporulates; it is inhaled into the lungs and phagocytosed by the cells of the reticuloendothelial system and then enters the blood stream. Hematogenous infection always occurs but may not be evident on clinical examination. The primary form of infection is usually a benign flu-like illness that is associated radiographically with patchy areas of pneumonia and lung nodules (Fig. 2–56). Lymph node enlargement can occur either in conjunction with the pneumonia or as the only abnormality. The infection can cause obstruction of nearby vessels, bronchi, or the esophagus. In an endemic area, the combination of pneu-

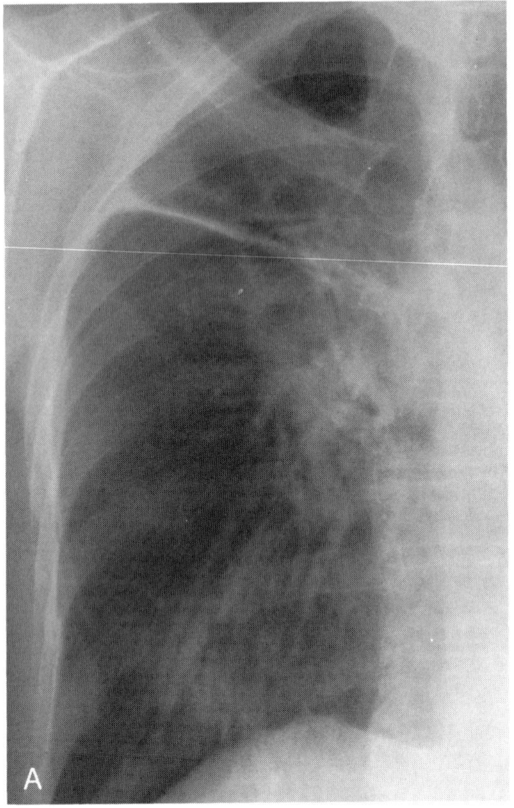

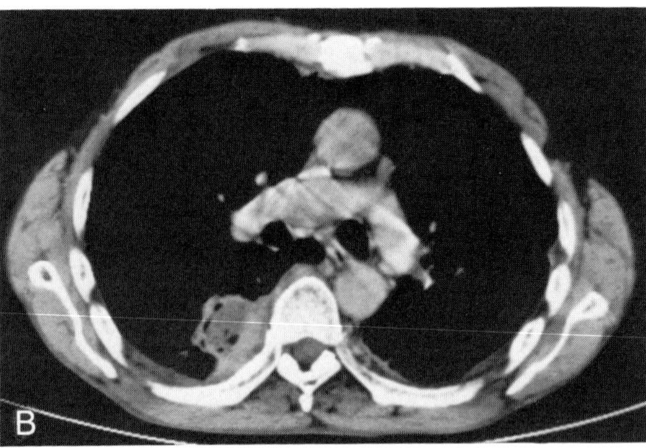

FIGURE 2–55. Mycetoma. *A.* Chest film shows an *Aspergillus* fungus ball complicating a case of extensive bullous emphysema. Note the elevation of the hilum and the minor fissure. A few cavities in the right upper lobe remain. The mass projects along the vertebral column and obscures its right border. *B.* CT scan shows a thick-walled cavity containing the mycetoma and air bubbles adjacent to the vertebral body.

monia and lymph node enlargement is highly suggestive of histoplasmosis.

A reinfection form of histoplasmosis is characterized radiographically by parenchymal consolidation, usually in the upper lobes. It may be diffuse and severe, often occurring in debilitated patients. Multiple calcified granulomas are seen as evidence of old, diffuse disease. In some cases the calcified granulomas can erode into the peripheral airways and be coughed up as broncholiths.

Coccidioidomycosis. *Coccidioides immitis* is found as spherules in the soil, particularly in the southwestern United States. These spherules release spores that are inhaled into the lungs, in which they incite a granulomatous reaction. Lung disease is usually mild; 60% of the patients are asymptomatic. The rest have a flu-like illness. Only 1% have a prolonged illness, and 0.02% have disseminated disease. The radiographic findings depend on the severity and the time course of the disease.

Four radiographic forms are seen. A fleeting pneumonia generally affecting the upper lobes is the most common form (60%). A focal consolidative infection, usually in the lower lobes, occurs in 20%; one fifth of patients with these infections have hilar adenopathy, and most recover without treatment. The nodular form, characterized by single or multiple thin-walled cavities in the upper lobes, occurs in 10% of patients (Fig. 2–57). The disseminated form, characterized by diffuse micronodules, is rare. Coccidioidomycosis is commonly associated with tuberculosis (10% of patients) and erythema nodosum in women (20%).

Candidiasis. *Candida albicans,* a fungus that rarely causes disease in the chest, is a common inhabitant of the mouth and perineum. However, this fungus can cause lung disease in debilitated adults or in infants contaminated via the birth canal. Drug addicts are particularly prone to *Candida* endocarditis, and septicemia from *Candida* occurs in severely debilitated or immunosuppressed patients, especially those treated with several antibiotics. There is no distinctive pulmonary radiographic pattern, and biopsy is usually required in order to establish the diagnosis.

Blastomycosis. *Blastomyces dermatitidis* causes a granulomatous infection of the skin and lungs (North American blastomycosis). The organism is found in the soil and infects inhabitants of the central and southeastern United States and, more recently, Africa. Lung disease is extremely rare and affects only

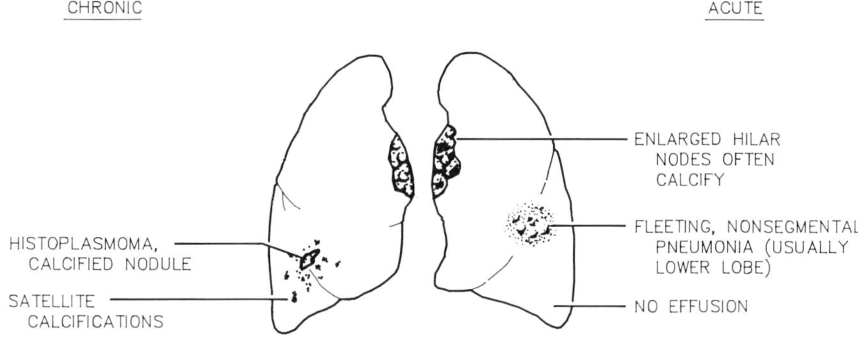

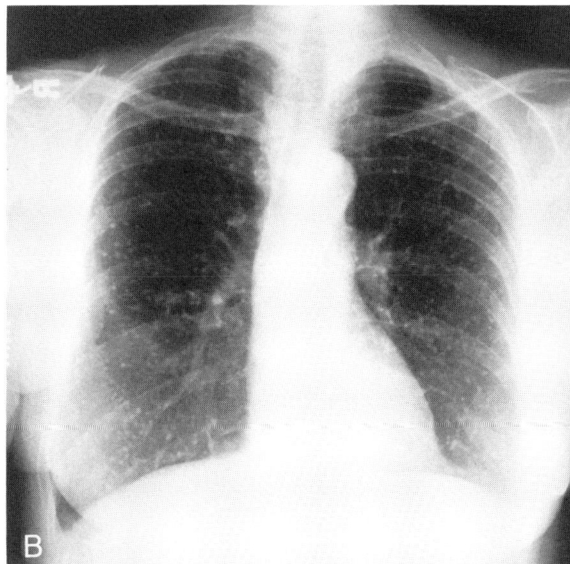

FIGURE 2–56. Histoplasmosis. *A.* Diagram. *B.* Old histoplasmosis. Chest film shows multiple calcifications in an absolutely asymptomatic man from Mississippi.

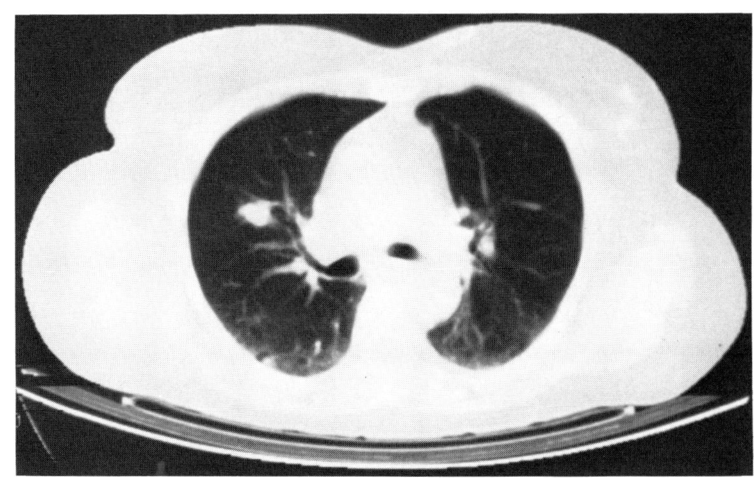

FIGURE 2–57. Coccidioma. CT scan viewed at lung windows shows a nodular density in the right upper lung. This was a healed granulomatous lesion from coccidiodomycoisis but looks similar to a malignant pulmonary nodule (see Fig. 2–8*A*).

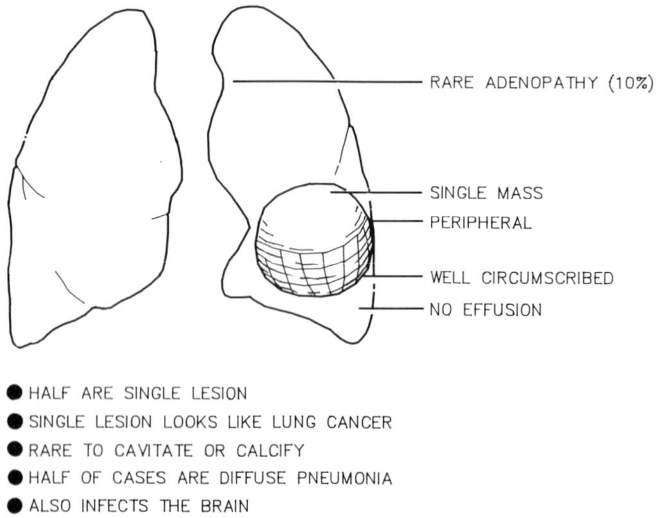

RARE ADENOPATHY (10%)
SINGLE MASS
PERIPHERAL
WELL CIRCUMSCRIBED
NO EFFUSION

- HALF ARE SINGLE LESION
- SINGLE LESION LOOKS LIKE LUNG CANCER
- RARE TO CAVITATE OR CALCIFY
- HALF OF CASES ARE DIFFUSE PNEUMONIA
- ALSO INFECTS THE BRAIN

FIGURE 2–58. Characteristics of cryptococcosis.

immunocompromised patients. Chest radiographic findings are nonspecific and usually reveal acute, nonsegmental airspace consolidation. Pleural effusion, hilar adenopathy, and calcification do not occur. Skin granulomas are common and may become ulcerative and purulent.

Cryptococcosis. *Cryptococcus neoformans* is an increasingly common cause of lung disease in immunosuppressed patients, especially those with lymphoma, leukemia, SLE, renal transplants, and chronic lung disease. It most often involves the central nervous system of debilitated and immunocompromised patients (see Chapter 8). The organism, found in pigeon feces, can be inhaled, enter the blood, and then cause pulmonary or central nervous system infection. The most common radiographic appearance is either a single, well-circumscribed mass lesion in the lung periphery or a diffuse consolidative pattern (Fig. 2–58).

Pneumonias Caused by Atypical Organisms

***Mycoplasma* Pneumonia.** *Mycoplasma* is a primitive bacterial type of organism that is inhaled and causes an atypical pneumonia. The disease generally affects children and young adults and is usually clinically mild despite considerable radiographic abnormalities. Radiographic differentiation from viral pneumonia or other bacterial pneumonia is usually impossible (Fig. 2–59).

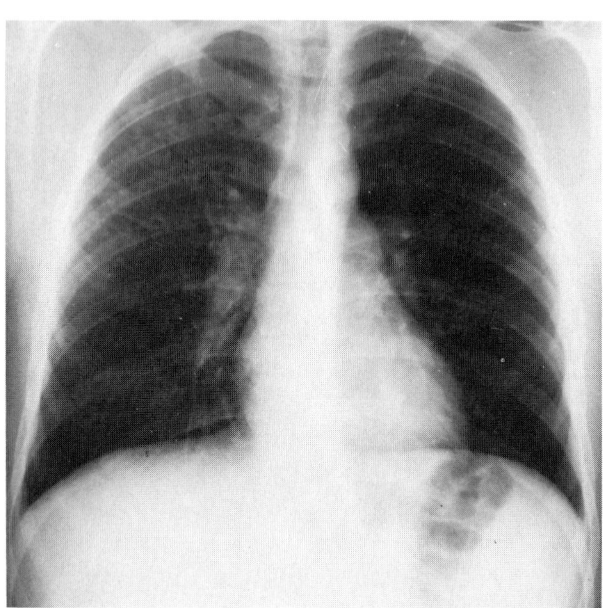

FIGURE 2–59. Mycoplasma pneumonia. Chest film shows areas of right upper-lobe opacification in a 16-year-old with a mild fever. The opacifications are interstitial.

Psittacosis and Ornithosis. *Chlamydia psittaci* is a virus-like organism present in bird excretions. When it is inhaled, usually by bird handlers, it causes a diffuse, interstitial pneumonia similar to that caused by the viruses. Disease acquired from parrots is called psittacosis; ornithosis refers to disease acquired from all types of birds. The chest radiograph shows nonspecific interstitial abnormalities.

Rickettsial Pneumonia. Some rickettsiae occasionally cause pneumonia. In Q fever (Queensland fever, caused by *Coxiella burnetii*), chest radiographs show discrete areas of homogeneous segmental consolidation, usually in the lower lobes, and occasionally pleural effusion. The disease is self-limiting. Epidemic typhus and Rocky Mountain spotted fever do not cause pneumonia. Scrub typhus (due to *Rickettsia tsutsugamushi*) rarely causes an interstitial or consolidative pneumonia.

Viral Lung Disease

Upper respiratory viral disease is common but does not usually cause pneumonia. A large variety of viruses can cause respiratory problems (Table 2–4). Symptoms are nonspecific, and radiographic findings are highly variable. The radiographic viral patterns of varicella pneumonia, Swyer-James syndrome, and laryngeal papillomatosis are distinctive.

***Varicella* Pneumonia.** The herpes virus, *Varicella zoster,* is the causative agent of chickenpox and the segmental skin disease known as shingles. It causes pneumonia in a small percentage of children and in half the adults who develop chickenpox. This pneumonia is of no consequence in children, but it can be fatal in adults. Radiographs in acute varicella pneumonia show diffuse consolidation. Residual changes in 1% of patients are multiple, punctate calcifications scattered throughout the lung and similar to those seen after the diffuse form of histoplasmosis (see Fig. 2–56).

Swyer-James Syndrome. Swyer-James syndrome is a group of radiographic findings that reflect diffuse postinfectious pulmonary injury, usually involving a lobe or an entire lung. It is caused by infection by Coxsackie virus B (and probably other viruses) at an early age, resulting in bronchiolitis and obliteration of small airways. Airtrapping, parenchymal destruction, and decreased growth occur in the af-

TABLE 2–4. VIRUSES THAT CAUSE RESPIRATORY INFECTION

Group Type	Entry	Respiratory Involvement
Ribonucleic Acid Viruses		
Myxoviruses		
Influenza (A and B)	Inhaled	Trachea and bronchi; severe pneumonia in ill or aged; predisposition to bacterial superinfection
Parainfluenza (four types)	Inhaled	Croup in children; pharyngitis in older patients
Respiratory syncytial (one type)	Inhaled	Bronchopneumonia in children less than 2 years old
Rubeola (one type)	Inhaled	Measles; pneumonia in 20%
Picornaviruses		
Coxsackie (30 types)	Alimentary	Very rarely pneumonia; type B causes Swyer-James syndrome
Rhinovirus (89 types)	Inhaled	Causes 50% of upper respiratory infections; rarely causes lower respiratory infection
Deoxyribonucleic Acid Viruses		
Adenovirus (33 types)	Oral	Common cold to severe pneumonia
Herpes		
Varicella	Inhaled	*V. zoster* causes chickenpox and shingles; diffuse pneumonia in adults
Simplex (I and II)	Contact	Fulminant infection in the neonate
Cytomegalovirus	Contact	Pneumonia in immunodeficient patients
Papovavirus	Contact	Laryngeal papillomatosis

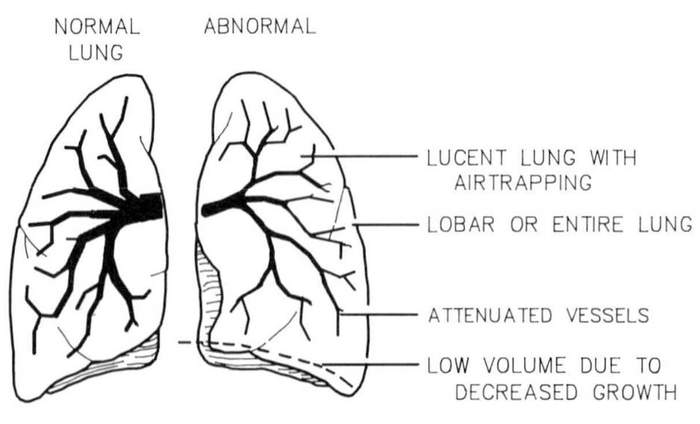

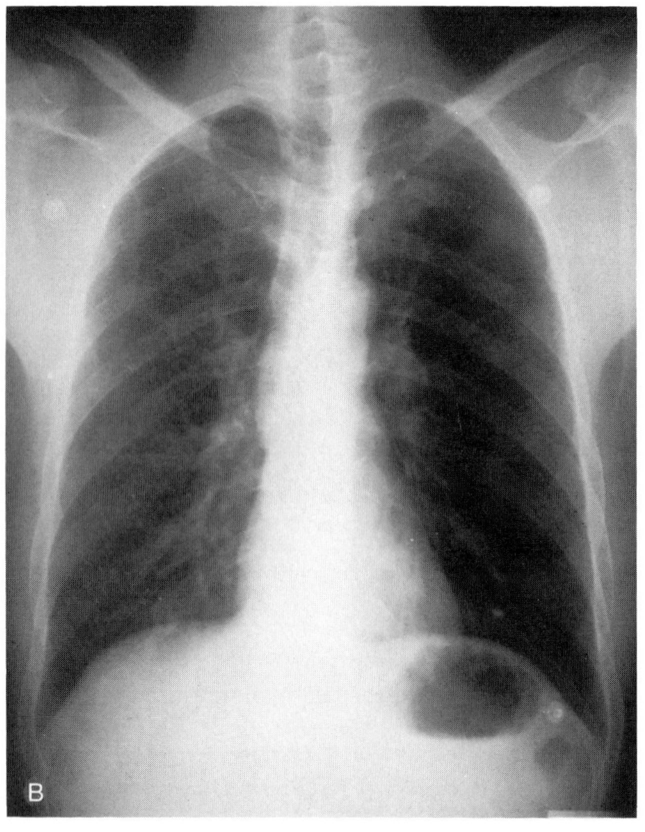

FIGURE 2–60. Swyer-James syndrome. *A.* Diagram. *B.* Chest radiograph shows a hyperlucent left lung in a 20-year-old man who claimed to be a long-distance runner and who had suddenly developed shortness of breath. Actually, he was psychotic, had never been a runner, and had no pulmonary symptoms.

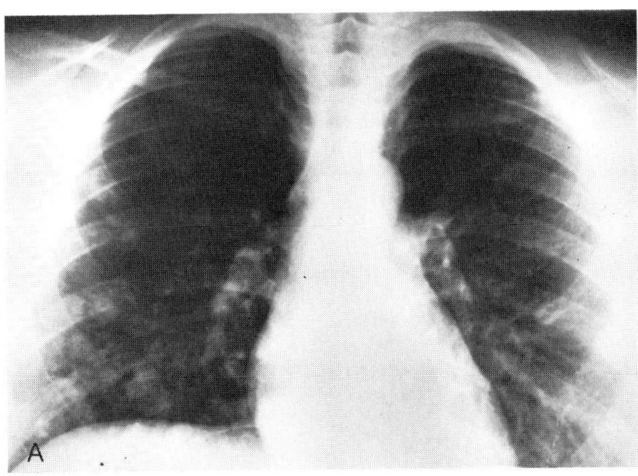

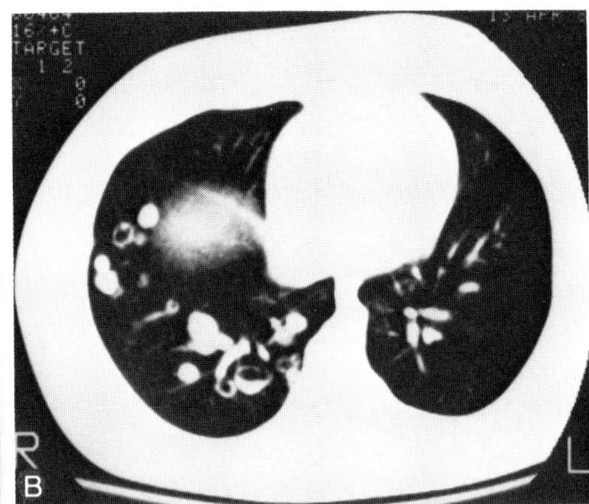

FIGURE 2–61. Laryngeal papillomatosis. *A.* A chest radiograph shows multiple round densities in the lungs, especially on the right. The patient had extensive laryngeal papillomatosis with lung involvement. *B.* The chest CT scan shows several of these densities to be cavitary lesions.

fected portion of the lung. Chest radiographs show a hyperlucent lung or lobe and attenuated vessels (Fig. 2–60). Clinical circumstances usually allow distinction between the Swyer-James syndrome and other causes of unilateral lucent lung (see the Radiographic Differential Diagnosis section).

Laryngeal Papillomatosis. The papovavirus that causes warts occasionally causes papillomatous lesions on the mucosal surface of the larynx. If these lesions spread to the bronchi and bronchioles, they cause subsegmental obstruction and form cysts. Cavitation of these cysts can occur. Occasionally the papillomas are visible in profile within the airway on chest radiographs (Fig. 2–61).

Protozoan Lung Diseases

Amebiasis. Amebiasis usually affects the gastrointestinal tract but may involve the lungs by direct extension of liver abscess or by hematogenous spread. Of the patients who have gastrointestinal tract involvement, 10% also have liver involvement, and 2% have lung involvement. When infection occurs in the lungs, it is usually in the right lower lobe as a result of direct spread through the diaphragm from the liver. Radiographic findings are consolidation with cavitation and pleural effusion (Fig. 2–62).

***Pneumocystis* Pneumonia.** *Pneumocystis carinii,* a protozoan, probably exists as a nonpathogen in the lungs of normal individuals. However, the organism can cause pneumonia in immunocompromised patients, particularly in premature infants (because of immature immune systems), immunodeficient children, patients with acquired immune disorders (leukemia and lymphoma), patients taking immunosuppressive drugs (chemotherapy or steroids; transplant patients), and patients who have AIDS. The pattern of pulmonary involvement varies from reticular interstitial disease to diffuse hilar consolidation resembling pulmonary edema. No effusion is associated with pneumocystis pneumonia (Fig. 2–63). Infection often is concomitant with cytomegalovirus (in up to 70% of patients).

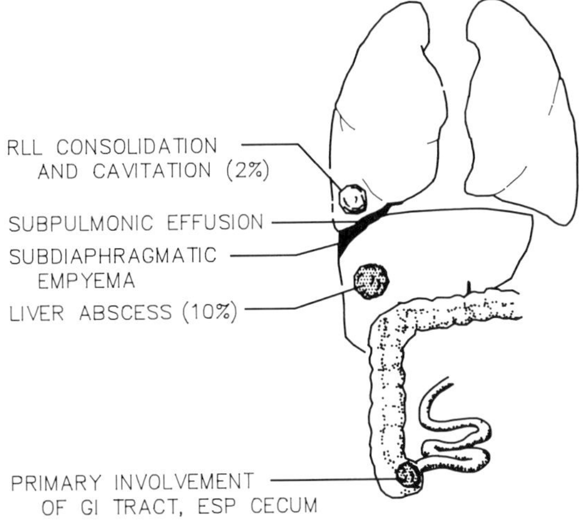

FIGURE 2–62. Characteristics of amebiasis.

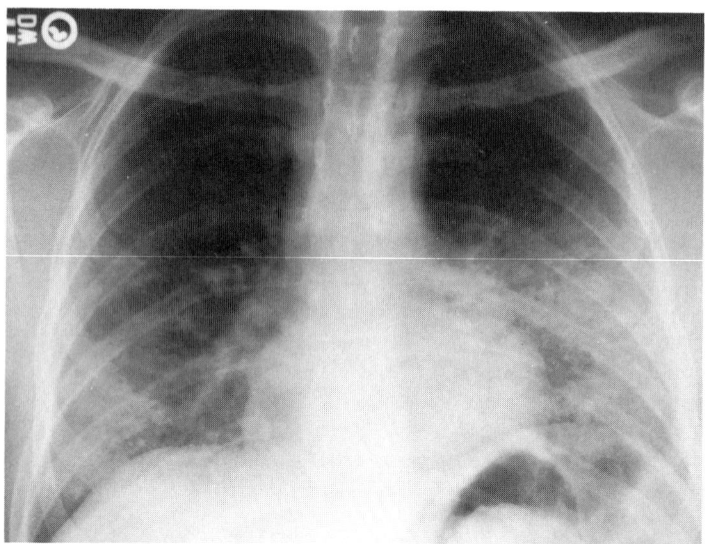

FIGURE 2–63. *Pneumocystis* pneumonia. The patient, a 35-year-old man with acquired immunodeficiency syndrome (AIDS), came to the emergency room with rapidly progressing respiratory distress. Chest film shows interstitial pulmonary opacification on the right and alveolar consolidation on the left.

Diseases Caused by Worms

Echinococcosis. *Echinococcus granulosis* is a small tapeworm, 3 to 6 mm long, that is transmitted from dogs and wolves to humans by way of two types of intermediaries: sheep and cows are the link in the pastoral form (common in the Mediterranean, Asia, and southern South America), and deer and mice are the link in the sylvian form (Alaska and northern Canada). In humans, the ingested larvae are usually trapped and encapsulated in the liver and lungs, where they produce echinococcal (hydatid) cysts. The cyst in the lungs is typically a single, spherical, fluid-filled mass that contains numerous daughter cysts of the inner wall (Fig. 2–64). The organism occasionally spreads beyond these organs to cause disease in the brain, bones, kidneys, and spleen.

Cysticercosis. Cysticercosis is caused by various tapeworms, most commonly *Taenia solium.* Disease occurs when the eggs are ingested and disseminated via the blood to the muscles, the brain, and the eyes, where mature organisms form and calcify into 3 × 10 mm oval lesions. On chest radiographs, these lesions appear as multiple calcified densities in the muscles of the chest wall. Cysticercosis is discussed in detail in Chapter 8.

Paragonimiasis. Paragonimiasis is a mild pulmonary infection caused by the fluke *Par-*

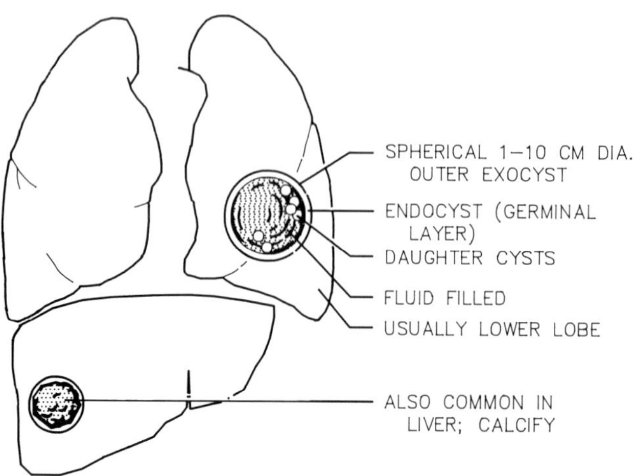

FIGURE 2–64. Characteristics of echinococcosis. DIA, diameter.

agonimus westermani (a trematode) and occurs predominantly in the Far East. The life cycle of the fluke is complicated. Infection results when humans eat infected crabs or crayfish. The metacercarial forms pass from the intestines to the lungs by direct penetration. In the lungs, they develop into mature flukes and discharge their eggs into the bronchioles. Chest radiographs can show a variety of abnormalities, including hazy and inhomogeneous shadows, homogeneous shadows, cystic areas within shadows, ring shadows, and thin-walled cysts. Patients may have hemoptysis, fever, and weight loss, but most are asymptomatic. Spread to the brain causes an encephalitis, which can be fatal.

NEOPLASTIC DISEASES

Benign Tumors of the Lung and Respiratory Tract

Primary benign tumors of the lung are rare, constituting fewer than 5% of all lung tumors. The most common of these are bronchial adenomas, hamartomas, smooth-muscle tumors, and lipomas.

Bronchial Adenoma. Bronchial adenomas, which constitute half of all benign lung tumors, arise from ductal epithelium of bronchial mucous glands. Most bronchial adenomas are of the carcinoid histological type, but they rarely cause the clinical carcinoid syndrome. They are low-grade malignancies that can metastasize late in their natural history. The rest are benign salivary types. The central adenomas most often cause obstruction, which result in distal atelectasis and consolidation. The peripheral adenomas usually appear on radiographs as nodules and do not cause symptoms, but they have a higher incidence of cellular atypia. Simple resection is adequate therapy for all these lesions (Fig. 2–65).

Pulmonary Hamartoma. A pulmonary hamartoma is a mass of benign pulmonary tissue that is structurally disorganized. Although present at birth, it causes no symptoms and is usually detected incidentally when the patient is about 50 years old. On radiographs, it appears as a solitary, peripheral, well-circumscribed, lobulated mass. It is often irregularly calcified, which causes a popcorn appearance. The lesion has no malignant potential.

Smooth Muscle and Connective Tissue Tumors. The leiomyoma is a rare, benign tumor of the lung, usually appearing as a solitary, peripheral, nodular lesion. It can become very large (up to 13 cm) and can calcify. Most leiomyomas, however, are small and do not produce symptoms. When multiple leiomyomas are present, they are of various sizes and are located in all areas of the lung. This condition is called leiomyomatosis and is thought to be caused by metastases from a low-grade leiomyosarcoma.

The fibroma (and fibrosarcoma) can occur centrally, causing obstruction, or peripherally as a solitary nodule. A fibroma arising from the pleura is called a local benign mesothelioma; the tissue of origin is often indeterminate. In contrast to malignant mesothelioma, local benign mesothelioma is not related to exposure to asbestos or cigarette smoke.

The lipoma usually arises from the wall of the trachea or the large bronchi (80%). It is more common in men than in women (5:1) and is usually solitary. It appears on radiographs as a smooth elevation of the mucosal surface, and its appearance occasionally changes when the patient changes position. Lipomas can also arise from the pleura.

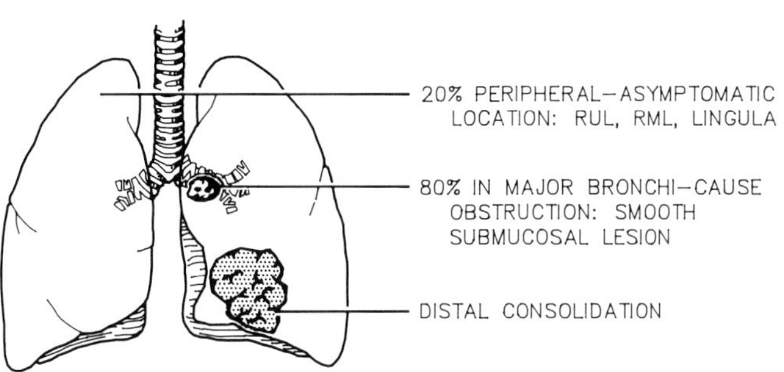

FIGURE 2–65. Characteristics of bronchial adenoma. RUL, right upper lobe; RML, right middle lobe.

Malignant Tumors of the Lung and the Respiratory Tract

A variety of malignancies affect the lung, but the most common is bronchogenic carcinoma. Most of these are of the squamous cell type. Many tumors metastasize to the lungs because malignant cells are trapped by the pulmonary capillaries.

Primary Lung Cancer. Primary lung cancer, which is composed of five cell types (Table 2–5), is the most common malignancy in men and, in some series, in women as well. The average age of onset is 45 to 55 years. Of these tumor types, all except alveolar cell (bronchoalveolar) carcinoma are related to cigarette smoking. Other factors associated with the development of lung cancer are exposure to asbestos (the incidence is 10 times that of persons not exposed and 100 times among exposed persons who are also smokers), radioactivity, nickel, ether, silica, coal dust, and toxic gas. Tuberculosis does not predispose patients to lung cancer, but it makes identification of a lung tumor difficult. Presenting symptoms of bronchogenic carcinoma are caused by impaired drainage of the airway and include severe suppurative or ulcerative bronchitis and bronchiectasis. Atelectasis is the most common radiographic manifestation with or without identification of the tumor mass.

Primary lung tumors can occur anywhere in the tracheobronchial tree, but most (70%) are in the segmental or subsegmental bronchi; fewer than 1% arise in the trachea. Medially located tumors are most often of the squamous cell or oat-cell types. Laterally located tumors are of all types. When primary lung tumors occur in the superior pulmonary sulcus (4% of all lung carcinomas), they are called superior sulcus, or Pancoast's, tumors (see Fig. 2–9*B*). This designation is not specific for any particular cell type; in fact, the relative incidence of the various cell types is the same as that elsewhere in the lung. Superior pulmonary sulcus tumors classically produce arm weakness, caused by involvement of the brachial plexus, and Horner's syndrome (ptosis, miosis, and anhidrosis), caused by involvement of the superior cervical ganglion. Any tumor that invades the structures of the thoracic inlet could produce such symptoms. Superior sulcus tumors are more accessible for biopsy or resection than are most lung carcinomas.

The radiographic abnormalities of primary lung cancer are the mass itself, the obstruction caused by the tumor mass, mediastinal spread, and distant metastasis. The most common manifestation is an obstructing endobronchial lesion, with secondary atelectases, oligemia, or infection (Figs. 2–66 and 2–67; see also Figs. 1–5, 2–9). Cavitation may be present, especially with squamous cell carcinoma, because of central tumor necrosis or the development of lung abscess. The second most common manifestation of lung cancer is infection in the obstructed lung segment; therefore pneumonia in the age group at risk must be observed until the abnormality completely resolves.

Hilar enlargement (usually unilateral) may indicate local spread of tumor or lymph node involvement (particularly with oat-cell carcinoma). Mediastinal widening can be caused by tumor, infiltration of lymph nodes, or obstruction of the superior vena cava (SVC). Lymphangitic spread of tumor is uncommon, but it is an important consideration because the appearance is similar to that of congestive heart failure (Fig. 2–68). Effusion occurs in 10% of patients and indicates pleural involvement. Distant metastases to bones, the brain, or the liver may be detected clinically before the primary lung tumor is discovered. Bone

TABLE 2–5. CHARACTERISTICS OF PRIMARY LUNG CANCER

Tumor Type	Percentage	Location: *Central*	Location: *Peripheral*	Metastatic Spread
Squamous cell (epidermoid)	60	Yes	Yes	Contiguous, lymphatic, hematogenous
Adenocarcinoma	15	No	Yes	Hematogenous, contiguous, lymphatic
Large cell (giant cell)	10	Yes	Yes	Contiguous, hematogenous, lymphatic
Small cell (oat cell)	10	Yes	Yes	Hematogenous to bone, marrow, and mediastinum
Alveolar cell (bronchoalveolar)	2	No	Yes	Contiguous to lymph and blood

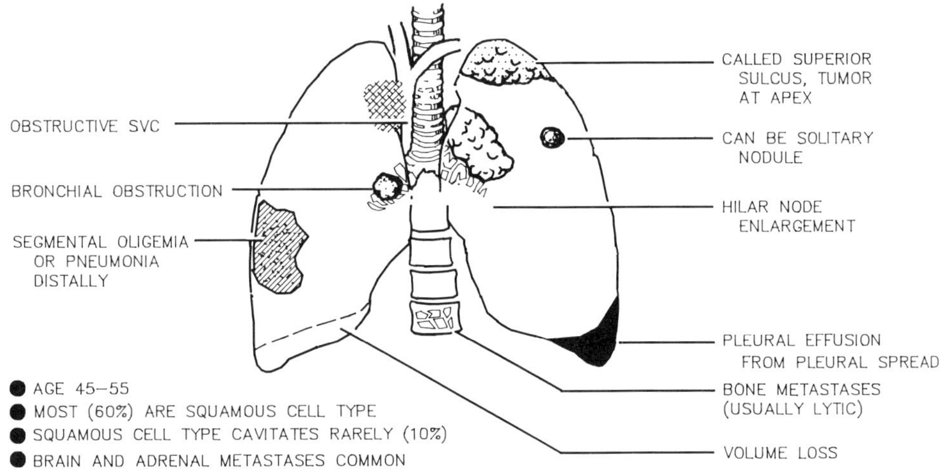

FIGURE 2–66. Characteristics of lung cancer. *SVC,* superior vena cava.

metastases are invariably "hot" (show dense uptake) on bone scans and, if visible on radiographs, are usually lytic. If they involve the spine, they can cause neurologic deficit as a result of cord or nerve root compression. Lung tumors commonly spread to the adrenal gland, and so the metastatic work-up should include evaluation of this area.

Although the diagnosis of lung cancer is usually suggested by results of clinical examination and chest radiograph, tissue diagnosis by aspiration or biopsy is required. Bronchoscopy washing or biopsy, open biopsy, and radiographically guided needle biopsy are the usual methods of obtaining tissue for diagnosis. Before therapy, such factors as mediastinal spread, local bone or chest wall involvement, metastasis to other parts of the lung or to distal locations (especially to the adrenal glands and the brain), and involvement of the opposite lung must be evaluated to determine the type of treatment. In most patients, any of these additional abnormalities precludes surgery as a treatment alternative. CT and MRI are particularly effective in evaluating lung tumors because they demonstrate the anatomical structure and the tumor and because they are highly sensitive to the presence of metastases and tumor-related abnormalities.

Some patients with lung cancer have unusual symptoms. Patients with alveolar cell carcinoma often complain of cough and abundant mucoid sputum production. Although in 80% of patients the radiographs show a solitary

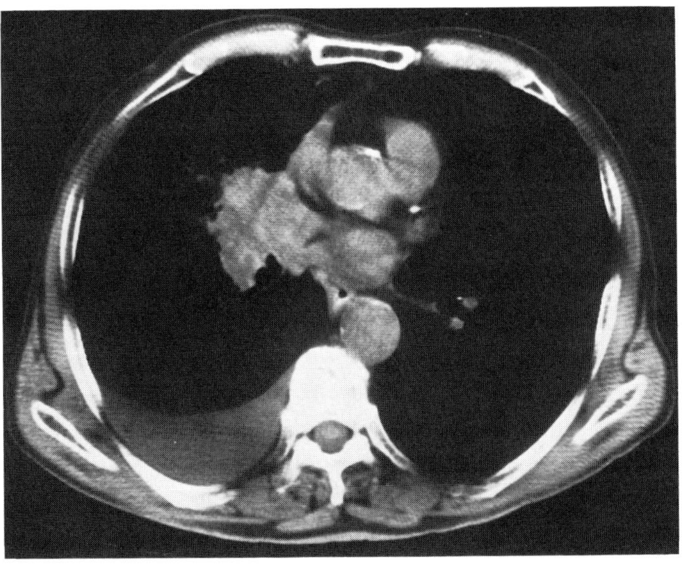

FIGURE 2–67. Bronchogenic carcinoma. CT scan shows a mass in the right hilum in a 50-year-old man with cachexia. Note also a right-sided malignant pleural effusion.

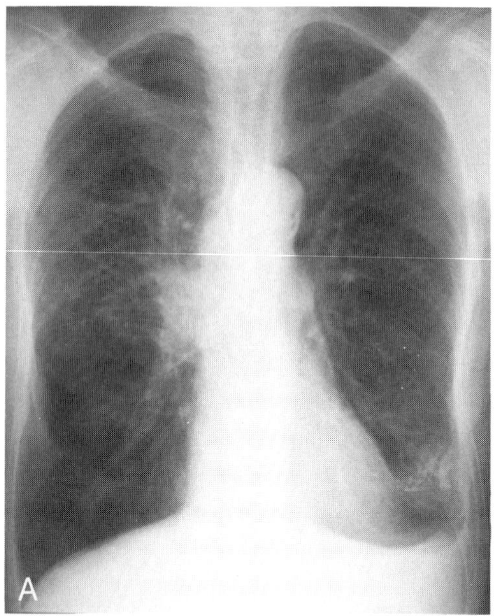

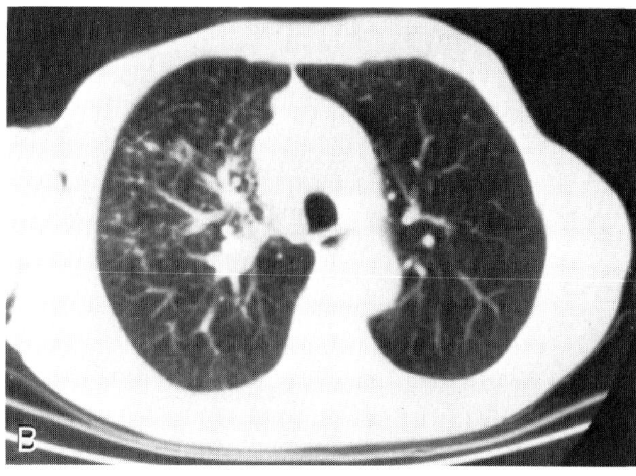

FIGURE 2–68. Lymphangitic spread of lung cancer. *A.* Plain film shows abnormal density in the right hilar region, indicating primary lung carcinoma. The peripheral interstitial areas of the lung show linear abnormalities, indicating lymphangitic spread of the tumor. This appearance is often indistinguishable from that of congestive heart failure. *B.* CT scan confirms the tumor mass and interstitial abnormalities.

peripheral mass, 20% have a diffuse form of tumor involvement, which appears on radiographs as a generalized airspace consolidation with lymphatic infiltration (Fig. 2–69).

Prognosis is poor for all types of primary lung cancer. Despite some response of these tumors to radiation and chemotherapy, the average patient survives less than 1 year after detection of the tumor. In most long-term survivors, the tumor was detected when it was small and was treated aggressively with surgery, radiation, and chemotherapy.

Some patients develop symptoms that are not directly related to the tumor. These extrathoracic paraneoplastic syndromes are distinct from tumor involvement and cause symptoms in the neuromuscular system, the connective tissues, the vascular/hematopoietic system, and the endocrine glands (Table 2–6). Oat-cell tumors are especially likely to cause paraneoplastic syndromes (20% of patients).

Metastases. Metastases to the lung are most commonly from primary tumors of the lungs, the breasts, the kidneys, the bones, the gastrointestinal tract, and the trophoblastic tissue. Involvement is usually the result of hematogenous dissemination but can also be by means of direct local extension or lymphangitic spread. The appearance of the metastatic lesion may be that of a solitary pulmonary nodule, diffuse consolidation, or multiple round masses (Fig. 2–70).

Two percent of all solitary nodules in the lung are metastases. These nodules usually appear as smooth, lobulated, noncalcified masses in the lower lobes. Most solitary nodular metastases (30%) are from colon carci-

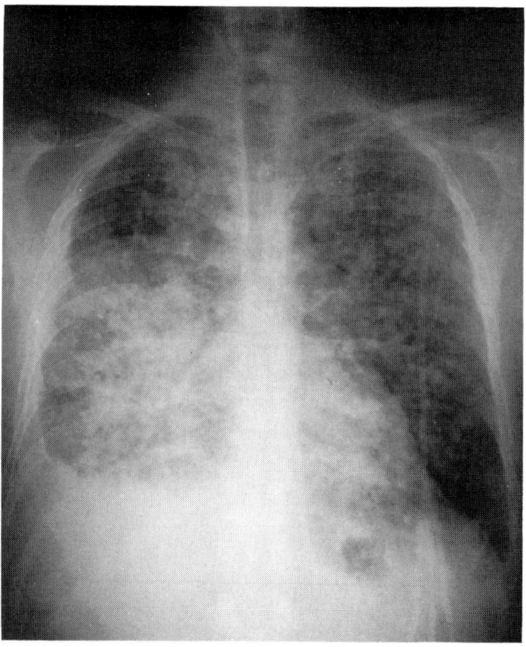

FIGURE 2–69. Alveolar cell carcinoma. Frontal radiograph in a 40-year-old man shows bilateral alveolar infiltrates, which are most severe in the right lung base, and associated pleural effusion that represents diffuse spread of alveolar cell carcinoma. This appearance can easily be confused with that of congestive heart failure or pneumonia.

TABLE 2–6. EXTRATHORACIC PARANEOPLASTIC SYNDROMES

System Affected	Syndrome	Cause
Neuromuscular	Myasthenia, peripheral neuropathy, and cerebellar degeneration	60% oat cell, 20% squamous cell, 15% large cell, and 5% adenocarcinoma
Connective tissues	Hypertrophic osteoarthropathy, clubbing, dermatomyositis, and acanthosis nigricans	Squamous cell
Vascular/hematopoietic	Thrombophlebitis and thrombocytopenia	All types
Endocrine	Gynecomastia	All types
	Inappropriate antidiuretic hormone	Oat cell
	Cushing's syndrome	Oat cell and others
	Hyperparathyroidism	70% squamous cell and 30% large cell

nomas; others are from osteogenic sarcoma, renal cell carcinoma, and testicular carcinoma. Tumors hematogenously spread to the lung can cause diffuse consolidation or multiple round lesions (called cannonball lesions). These tumors are generally vascular and include renal cell carcinoma, osteogenic sarcoma, thyroid carcinoma, choriocarcinoma, melanoma, and testicular carcinoma.

Lymphangitic lung metastases occur when tumor spreads hematogenously to the lung periphery, where it invades the lymphatic system and infiltrates centrally. The diffuse reticular peripheral density is radiographically indistinguishable from interstitial edema and interstitial lung disease. Hilar enlargement and bronchial wall thickening are often present. The tumors that most commonly spread to the lymphatic system are breast, stomach, and thyroid carcinomas. In contrast to primary lung tumors, lung metastases seldom cavitate (fewer than 4%).

Lymphoma, Leukemia, and Myeloma

Hodgkin's Disease. Hodgkin's disease is a malignant lymphomatous process characterized histologically as a proliferation of abnormal T lymphocytes (and identified histologically by the presence of histiocytic giant cells called Reed-Sternberg cells). The disease primarily affects young adults (it is slightly more common in men) and is localized to the axial lymph nodes, particularly in the neck and chest. This nodal involvement is generally continuous along the axial skeleton from the cervical nodes down to the most inferior extent of disease. It can extend into the abdomen.

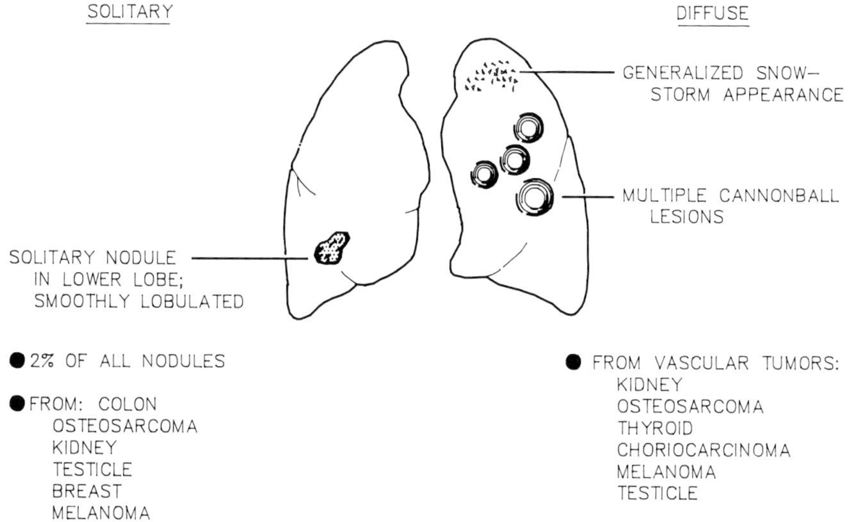

FIGURE 2–70. Characteristics of metastases to the lung.

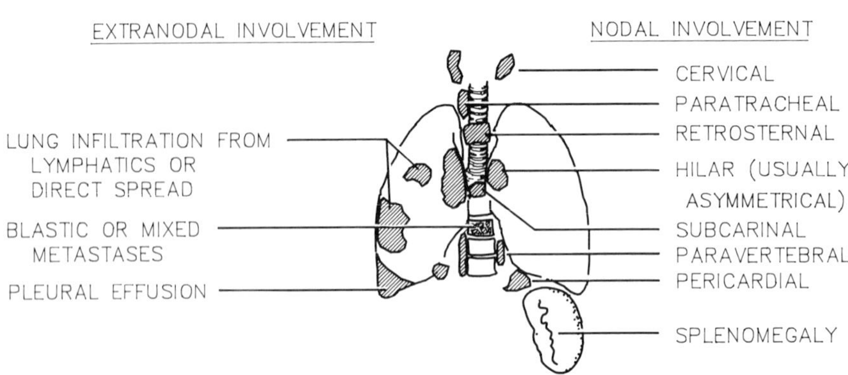

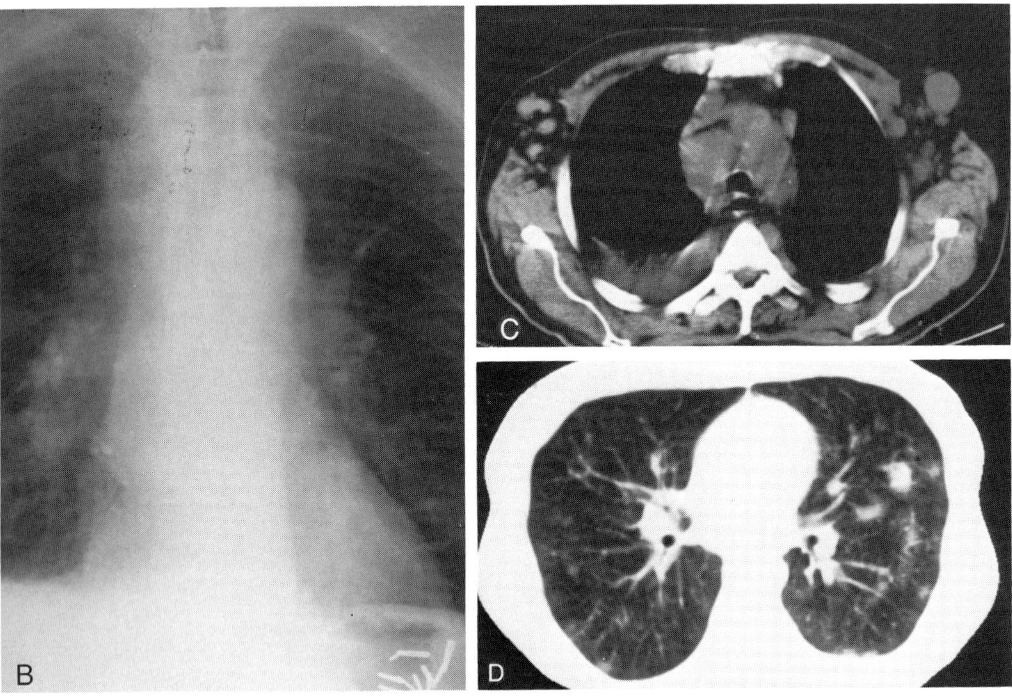

FIGURE 2–71. Lymphoma in the chest. *A.* Characteristics of lung abnormalities in Hodgkin's disease. *B.* Chest film in a middle-aged man with non-Hodgkin's lymphoma shows a mass in the mediastinum, predominantly to the right of the trachea. The right hemidiaphragm is not well-delineated. The patient had had a splenectomy, and surgical clips are visible below the diaphragm. *C.* CT scan through this level shows a right mediastinal mass that represented non-Hodgkin's lymphoma. Right pleural effusion and axillary adenopathy are also demonstrated. *D.* CT scan of the midchest viewed at lung windows demonstrates widening of the mediastinum as a result of extensive adenopathy. A pleural effusion is present in the left base, which was better shown at mediastinal windows. Diffuse opacification throughout the lung is in a somewhat nodular pattern as a result of lymphomatous involvement of the lung parenchyma. The patient, a 41-year-old woman, had lymphomatous involvement throughout the chest, abdomen, and pelvis, including focal liver lesions.

The most common clinical manifestation is an asymptomatic neck mass, but some patients have cachexia, fever, and anemia. At the time of diagnosis, two thirds of patients have lymph node involvement in the chest, and 10% have lung infiltration. The predominant radiographic finding is asymmetrical mediastinal adenopathy (Fig. 2–71*A*), best seen on CT scan or MRI. Other abnormalities visible on the chest radiograph or the CT scan include lung parenchymal masses, pleural effusion, blastic metastases, and splenomegaly. Hodgkin's disease responds well to radiation therapy, which results in complete cures in patients with limited disease.

Non-Hodgkin's Lymphoma. Non-Hodgkin's lymphoma arises from B lymphocytes, stem cells, or histiocytes. It afflicts men and women in the 30- to 70-year age group and usually involves the abdomen. Thoracic involvement, primarily mediastinal and peribronchial lymphadenopathy, occurs mainly as a result of diffuse or advanced disease (Fig. 2–71*B;* see also Fig. 2–10). The radiographic abnormalities of non-Hodgkin's lymphoma in the chest include adenopathy, localized mass, diffuse nodules, pleural effusion, and splenomegaly.

Leukemia. Leukemia frequently infiltrates the lungs but seldom is apparent on radiographs. Chest abnormalities are usually the results of infection or congestive heart failure. Initial leukemic marrow involvement is usually focal but becomes generalized to all normal erythropoietic (red) marrow; even areas of fatty (yellow) marrow may be occupied by abnormal masses of white cells.

Myeloma. Myeloma occurs in two forms in the chest: either as a soft tissue mass that spreads directly from a rib lesion or as a solitary plasmocytoma in the upper respiratory tracts of lung. The former is easily recognized by its bone origin and soft tissue mass (Fig. 2–72). The latter appears as a solid mass in the chest and requires biopsy for diagnosis. Solitary plasmocytoma is extremely rare. In rare cases, patients with hypercalcemia and hyperphosphatemia caused by myeloma have metastatic calcification in the lung parenchyma.

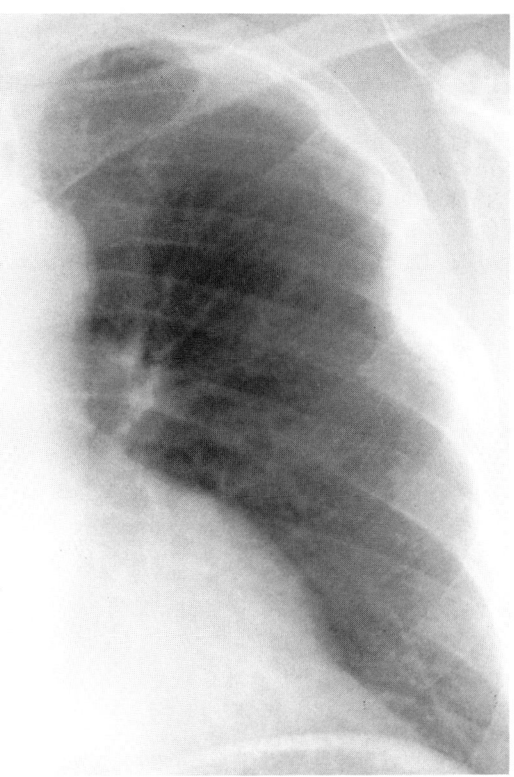

FIGURE 2–72. Myeloma. Involvement of the lateral aspect of the fourth rib in a patient with myeloma, shown on this detailed view of the left chest, causes enlargement, loss of normal rib definition, and a soft tissue mass.

Mediastinal Tumors

The mediastinum is divided into three parts. The anterior part is bordered anteriorly by the sternum and posteriorly by the trachea. It includes the retrosternal space, the thymus, intrathoracic thyroid tissue, and lymph nodes anterior to both the trachea and the major bronchi. The middle mediastinum extends from the trachea to the spine and includes the trachea, the esophagus, deep mediastinal lymph nodes, the heart, and the vessels. The posterior mediastinum includes the spine, nerves, and the descending aorta. Mediastinal tumors are diagnosed radiographically by their position in the mediastinum and by their appearance. The most important anterior mediastinal tumors are thymoma, thyroid tumor, germ-cell tumor, and lymphoma (discussed earlier). Other anterior mediastinal tumors are lipoma, fibroma, hemangioma, and lymphangioma.

Thymoma. Thymoma is the most common tumor in the anterior mediastinum (it occurs less commonly in the middle mediastinum) and constitutes 10% to 15% of all mediastinal tumors. The tumor develops at any age, but most patients are over 20 years old at the time of detection. Ninety percent of thymomas are benign, as indicated by calcification and encapsulation of the mass. Most (95%) are solid, and the rest are cystic (see Fig. 2–22). On radiographs, a thymoma appears as a large anterior mediastinal mass that displaces but does not compress adjacent structures. Because they do not immediately produce symptoms when they compress vital structures, they can become very large. There is a definite association between thymoma and myasthenia gravis: 15% of patients with myasthenia gravis have thymomas, and 25% to 50% of patients with thymomas have myasthenia gravis. The tumor spreads by local invasion; metastasis is rare.

Thyroid Tumor. A thyroid mass in the anterior mediastinum is usually an asymptomatic goiter (thyroid carcinoma is uncommon in the thorax). The goiter is usually encapsulated and can be cystic and calcified. It can be located either in the anterior or in the posterior mediastinum. The diagnosis of thyroid masses is discussed earlier in the Systemic Diseases section and in Chapter 9.

Germ-Cell Tumors. Germ-cell tumors constitute 10% to 15% of all mediastinal tumors. They arise from midline cell rests and become evident when the patient is about 20 years old. Eighty percent are benign. Most are in the anterior mediastinum and are teratomas. The radiographic appearance depends on the cell types present. Radiographs show a mass, often with calcification, that compresses adjacent structures.

Other Mediastinal Masses. Causes of middle mediastinal masses are lymphoma, leukemia, metastatic tumor (primarily from the lungs, the upper gastrointestinal tract, the prostate, or the kidneys), cysts (see the Congenital Diseases section), diaphragmatic hernias, abnormal cardiovascular structures, and esophageal tumors (see Chapter 3).

Posterior mediastinal masses are primarily neurogenic (see Chapter 8). The most common are (in order of decreasing frequency) neurofibroma, neuroblastoma, pheochromocytoma, and chemodectoma. Many of these tumors are malignant.

Pleural Tumor

Malignant Mesothelioma. Malignant mesothelioma is a tumor of the pleura that has a high association (80%) with long-term exposure to asbestos. Patients are usually 40 to 60 years old and have severe respiratory difficulty and cachexia. The tumor is generally a large, irregular mass that covers and invades the surface of the lung. Chest radiographs or CT scans demonstrate a predominantly pleura-based lesion. Pleural effusion is common. Most patients die within 1 year of diagnosis.

VASCULAR DISEASES

Vascular diseases of the lungs include embolism and processes that affect fluid balance and blood pressure. The most important cause of embolism is thrombus formation, but other types of emboli must be considered in some clinical circumstances.

Pulmonary Thromboembolism. Pulmonary thromboembolism, with or without infarction, is one of the most common lung diseases. It usually does not produce symptoms, but it is the immediate cause of death in a large proportion of hospitalized and immobilized patients. Diagnosis is especially important because it often occurs in young, healthy people, is potentially fatal, and is treatable.

The usual sources of emboli are the veins of the pelvis and thigh, but for half of documented emboli, no source is identified. Because chest radiographs often show no abnormality, the diagnosis is difficult. Most chest film abnormalities, such as pleural effusion and elevated hemidiaphragm, are nonspecific. The most helpful findings of hyperlucency in the obstructed lung caused by shunting of blood away from the abnormal area (Westermark's sign), wedge-shaped peripheral infarct (Hampton's hump), and enlargement of the pulmonary artery (caused by the presence of a large clot) are present in fewer than 5% of patients (Figs. 2–73, 2–74). Sometimes the radiographic appearance is of pulmonary hypertension with proximal enlargement and peripheral attenuation of pulmonary arteries.

When pulmonary embolus is suspected, an orderly evaluation requires measurement of arterial blood gases, chest radiography, ventilation perfusion scanning (see Chapter 9), and consultation with a pulmonary specialist. If the results of this evaluation are equivocal, pulmonary angiography should be performed. Therapy includes anticoagulation, prevention of further emboli, and, occasionally, surgical removal of clot. In some cases, mechanical barriers to the advance of further emboli, such as Kimray-Greenfield filters or vena cava plication, are required. The hyperlucency caused by pulmonary embolus can resolve within 24 hours after therapy is begun. The wedge-

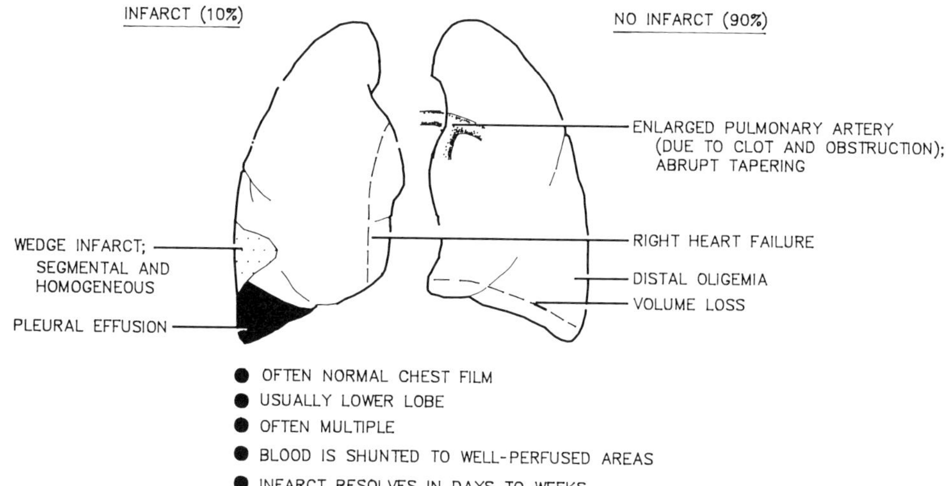

FIGURE 2–73. Characteristics of pulmonary embolism and infarction.

shaped infarct gradually becomes resorbed over 1 week or more; it does not cavitate.

Fat Embolism. Fat embolism usually results from the entrance of bone marrow fat into the veins after a fracture. The fat can be deposited in the lungs, the kidneys, the brain, and the skin. Respiratory and cardiac impairment typically develop 24 to 72 hours after the fracture. Hypoxemia and decreased oxygen-diffusing capacity occur regardless of whether abnormalities are visible on the chest radiograph, and they probably represent a diffuse alveolitis rather than an obstructive phenomenon. The diagnosis can be suspected clinically by the presence of a petechial skin rash (caused by fat in the dermis), fat in the urine, and onset of respiratory symptoms 1 to 2 days after the fracture.

Chest radiographs show peripheral airspace consolidation that is similar to that of pulmonary contusion or noncardiogenic pulmonary edema. In fact, the clinical and radiographic findings may be compatible with all three of these processes in a patient who has multiple traumatic injuries. Treatment is directed toward supportive respiratory care. It is not known how many patients survive mild fat embolism. The mortality rate among patients

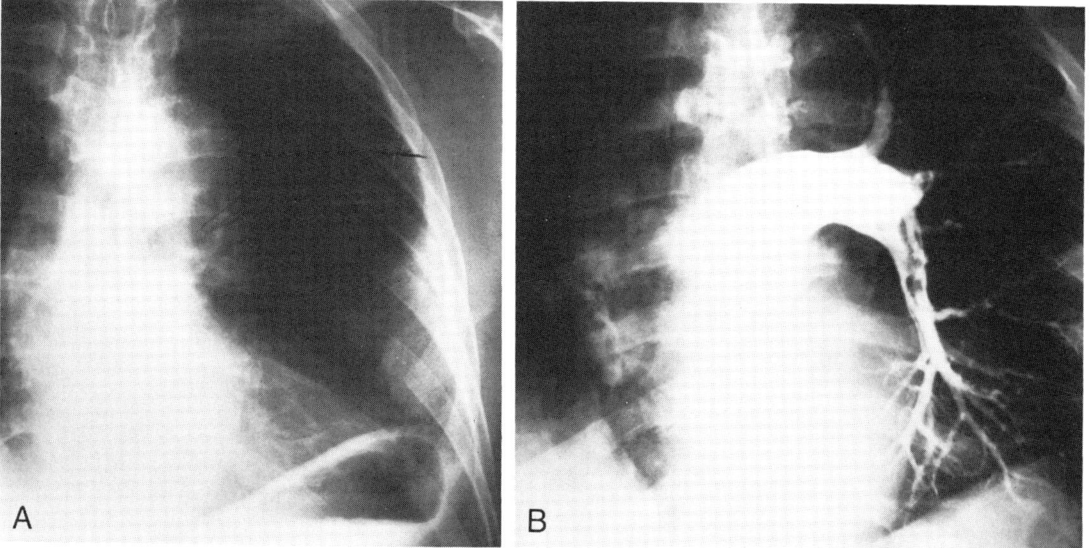

FIGURE 2–74. Peripheral infarction. *A.* Chest film shows a peripheral opacification in the left lower lobe. This mound-shaped abnormality (called Hampton's hump) suggests a wedge-shaped infarct peripherally. *B.* Arteriogram shows a large embolus in the artery to this area of the lung.

who have severe respiratory symptoms, cardiac decompensation, and petechial skin rash is high (10% to 15%).

Embolism of oil-based contrast material may occur after lymphangiography. It is most severe when lymphatic obstruction diverts the contrast material directly to the venous system. Chest radiographs appear abnormal in half of the patients, showing a fine reticular pattern that clears in about 7 days. Oxygen-diffusing capacity decreases by 20% during the first 24 hours after the procedure and returns to normal within 1 month.

Amniotic Fluid Embolism. Amniotic fluid embolism accounts for about 5% of maternal deaths and is the most common cause of immediate postpartum maternal death. Normally, no amniotic fluid enters the maternal circulation, but precipitous labor, oxytocin-induced labor, older age of the mother, multiparity, and intrauterine death are conditions that predispose the mother to rupture of pelvic veins and entrance of amniotic fluid into the venous system. The amniotic fluid, which contains fetal material (notably, meconium and cellular debris), can then pass to the lungs, causing obstruction of pulmonary arterioles and capillaries. The result is pulmonary hypertension and vascular collapse. Anaphylactoid reaction, caused by the meconium, and disseminated intravascular coagulation (amniotic fluid contains large amounts of coagulation factors) also occur. The patient's symptoms suggest massive pulmonary embolism or aspiration. Airspace consolidation indistinguishable from that of pulmonary edema is the radiographic picture, but a chest film is not usually obtained. Amniotic fluid embolism is usually fatal to the mother within 6 hours after giving birth, because of respiratory insufficiency or uterine hemorrhage.

Parasitic Emboli. Parasitic emboli are primarily schistosomal (*Schistosoma haematobium, S. mansoni,* and *S. japonicum*) eggs that enter the blood and lodge in the pulmonary arteries. These emboli cause an obliterative alveolitis and resultant pulmonary hypertension in about 5% of infected patients. Other parasites that affect the lungs do not obstruct vessels enough to cause symptoms.

Tumor Embolism. Embolism commonly occurs in tumors that invade the inferior vena cava, such as renal cell carcinoma and hepatocellular carcinoma. Otherwise, although hematogenous spread of tumor is common (occurring in 30% of patients with cancer), embolism of particles large enough to cause respiratory signs and symptoms is rare. Radiographic findings depend on the location and the size of the tumor embolus.

Air Embolism. Air can be introduced into the venous circulation by intravenous catheter or during surgery and can occlude the pulmonary vessels. The onset of ventilatory insufficiency is usually abrupt. A large air collection obstructing a major vessel can be seen as low density on radiographs. Venous air can enter the arterial side by crossing an atrial or a ventricular septal defect and cause cerebral infarction.

Foreign Body Embolism. Intravenous drug users often inject microorganisms and other materials, which results in both septic and aseptic embolism. Septic emboli to the lungs and other organs are usually composed of tissue infected by *Staphylococcus aureus.* The sites of origin of this tissue include septic heart valves (common among drug users) and infected clot in the veins caused by nonsterile injection or indwelling catheters. The lesions are usually multiple, round or wedge-shaped areas of increased density, often with cavitation. Talc (magnesium silicate, a component of methylphenidate hydrochloride), tripelennamine tablets (an antihistamine), cornstarch (used in dilution of heroin), and cotton fibers (used in filters) all cause interstitial fibrosis. The early chest film findings are diffuse micronodules; these progress to fibrosis and pulmonary hypertension (Fig. 2–75). The findings are similar to those of interstitial lung disease of any cause (see the Diseases of the Airways section). The condition is progressive even when injections are stopped.

Venous catheters can embolize to the lungs if they break or are inadvertently sheared off. The catheter is easily identified radiographically if it is radiopaque.

Pulmonary Edema

Pulmonary edema is the result of increased fluid within the interstitium and, if severe, within the airspaces of the lungs. The normal fluid balance in the lungs can be upset by abnormalities of pressure, osmolarity, and capillary permeability. The radiographic appearance of pulmonary edema depends on the amount of interstitial fluid and varies from mild interstitial haziness to confluent alveolar edema. Cardiac failure and fluid overload are the most common causes of pulmonary edema and are usually easy to diagnose because of

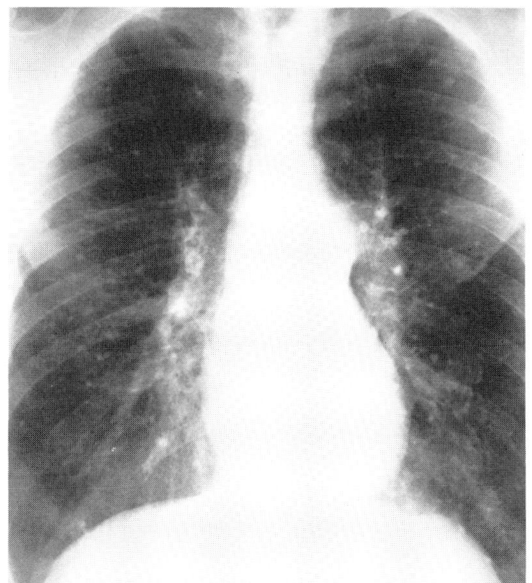

FIGURE 2–75. Lung disease in a drug user. Chest film shows diffuse micronodules in both lungs of a young adult male who was an intravenous heroin user. These are early findings of interstitial fibrosis caused by foreign body emboli.

TABLE 2–7. CARDIAC CAUSES OF PULMONARY EDEMA

Enlarged Cardiac Silhouette
Congestive heart failure
Mitral stenosis
Fluid overload
Renal failure
Glomerulonephritis
Cor triatriatum
Left atrial myxoma
Obstructed pulmonary veins
Normal Cardiac Silhouette
Acute myocardial infarction
Arrhythmia
Constrictive pericarditis
Cardiotoxic drugs

enlargement of the heart. Many other diseases also result in pulmonary edema. It is difficult to distinguish these diseases from lung diseases characterized by alveolar or interstitial consolidation. The adult respiratory distress syndrome and pulmonary alveolar proteinosis are two important lung diseases that have the appearance of pulmonary edema.

Cardiogenic Pulmonary Edema. There are many cardiac causes of pulmonary edema (Table 2–7), but the most common is congestive heart failure. When the failing heart is unable to pump blood efficiently, the pulmonary venous pressure increases and causes interstitial fluid and, if severe, alveolar fluid to accumulate. Patients with severe congestion have shortness of breath and orthopnea and, in severe cases, produce pink, frothy sputum. The radiographic appearance depends on the severity of the edema (Fig 2–76, 2–77). The earliest radiographic change is a diversion of blood flow to the upper lobes. If the cardiac failure persists, perivascular transudation of fluid occurs and the pulmonary vessels become indistinct. Kerley's lines (the most common are Kerley's B lines) appear visible when fluid fills the interlobular septa of the lung. These lines are seen in instances of acute and chronic heart failure, long-standing mitral valve disease, cardiac shunts, and pneumoconiosis (Fig. 2–78). In the most severe cases of pulmonary edema, fluid fills the alveoli and appears as patchy areas of increased density on the chest

FIGURE 2–76. Characteristics of pulmonary edema.

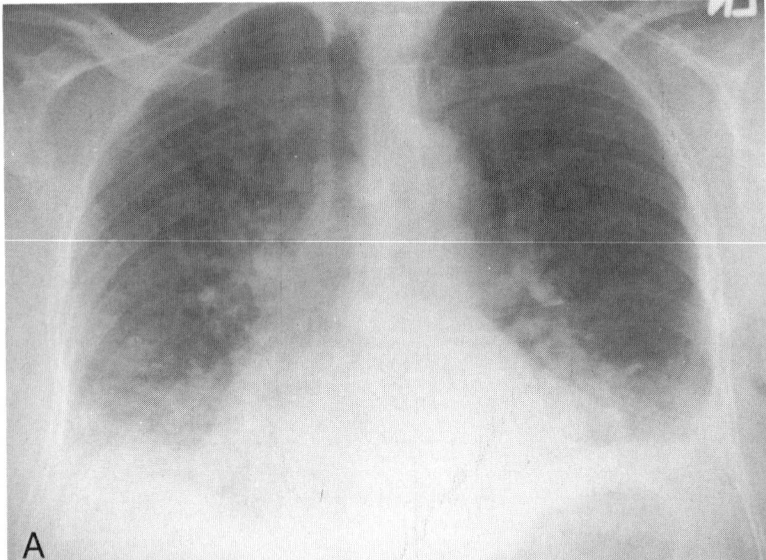

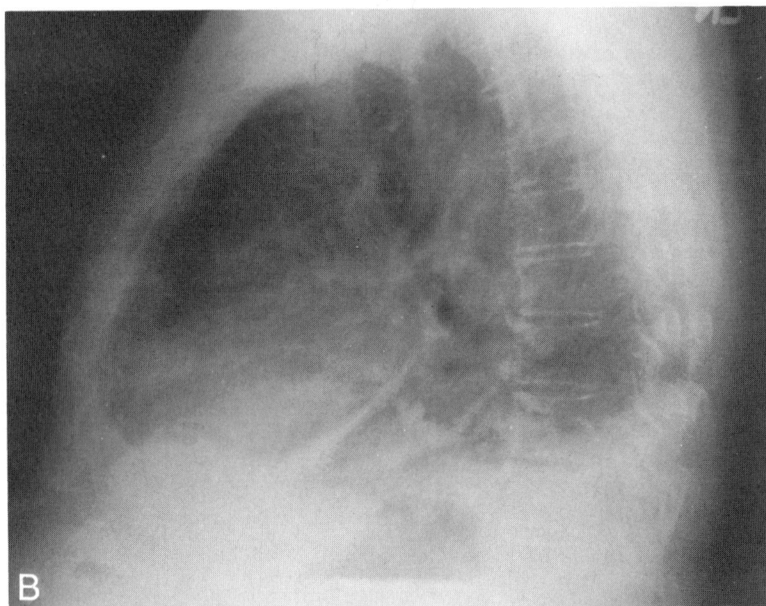

FIGURE 2–77. Pulmonary edema. *A.* Frontal chest film shows a poor inspiratory effort, bilateral pleural effusions, and diffuse increase in size of vessels and indistinctness of their contours, all of which are indicative of pulmonary edema. The heart size is indeterminate because of the insufficient inspiration. The patient had suffered acute left ventricular failure after myocardial infarction. *B.* Lateral view shows fluid in the major fissures, pleural effusions, and an end-on appearance of the engorged indistinct vessels.

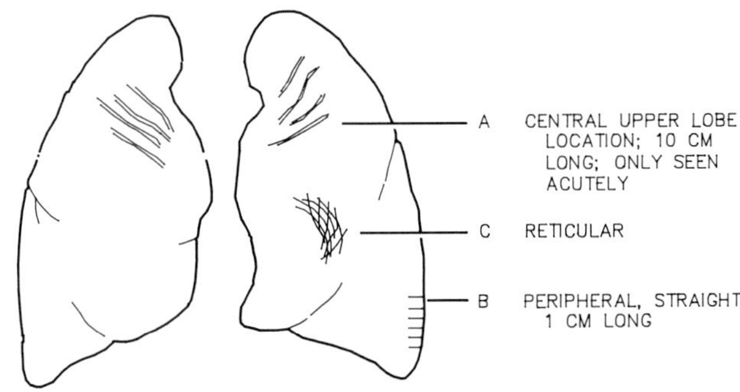

FIGURE 2–78. Characteristics of Kerley's lines.

film. Although most causes of cardiogenic pulmonary edema are associated with cardiac enlargement, several important causes, including myocardial infarction, are often associated with a normal heart size.

Noncardiogenic Pulmonary Edema. Many toxic and traumatic injuries to the lung cause pulmonary edema by increasing the permeability of the vascular wall (Table 2–8). The radiographic appearance is that of perivascular or alveolar edema and a normal heart.

Adult Respiratory Distress Syndrome. A severe form of lung disease that can cause pulmonary edema is the adult respiratory distress syndrome (ARDS). In this disease, hypoxia, hemorrhage, or a toxic injury from inhalation causes injury to the respiratory epithelium that results in structural abnormalities, which can be seen on radiographs, and functional abnormalities. The diagnosis is based on clinical and laboratory findings and on the time course of the disease. The most important abnormalities in ARDS are alveolar consolidation and thickening of the interstitium, which result in reduced oxygen diffusion, restriction of lung expansion, and shunting of blood to poorly aerated parts of the lung (Table 2–9).

The radiographic appearance is patchy consolidation similar to that of pulmonary edema. The development of radiographic abnormalities occurs over a period of days to weeks (Table 2–10). Both functional and radiographic findings must be present and other causes of disease ruled out before a diagnosis of ARDS can be made. Depending on the severity of the process, ARDS may clear completely in 7 days or may progress to interstitial fibrosis.

Alveolar Proteinosis. Alveolar proteinosis is a rare process caused by protein and lipid deposition in the airspaces. It occurs in patients 20 to 50 years old. The cause is unknown. One third of the patients are asymptomatic. Those with severe disease develop respiratory distress, infection, or both. Chest radiographs show bilateral alveolar consolidation similar in appearance to that of pulmonary edema, but the heart size is normal and interstitial edema is absent (Fig. 2–79). One third of all afflicted patients die despite intensive bronchial lavage.

TABLE 2–8. NONCARDIAC CAUSES OF PULMONARY EDEMA

Acute radiation pneumonitis
Inhalation (CO, NO_2, SO_2, NH_3, smoke, hydrocarbons)
Aspiration (near drowning, acidic gastric secretions, radiographic contrast)
Neurogenic (trauma, seizure, hydrocephalus)
High altitude
Heroin overdose
Rapid re-expansion of a collapsed lung
Reaction to blood transfusion
Fat embolism
Adult respiratory distress syndrome (ARDS)
High-dose cytoxan therapy
Pulmonary alveolar proteinosis

TABLE 2–9. ABNORMALITIES IN ADULT RESPIRATORY DISTRESS SYNDROME (ARDS)

Abnormality	Findings
Alveolar	Proteinaceous material in the alveoli; increased capillary permeability
Radiographic	Patchy interstitial consolidation appearing as pulmonary edema
Diffusion	Thickened interstitium causes poor diffusion and decreased lung compliance
Shunting	Shunting of blood to poorly aerated areas of the lung results in low arterial oxygenation

DISEASES AFFECTING THE AIRWAYS

Tracheal and Bronchial Diseases

Important diseases of the trachea and bronchi include tumors (50% squamous cell carcinoma and 45% cylindroma, both of which are rare), saber-sheath trachea (narrowed lateral diameter of the extrathoracic trachea, seen in chronic smokers), tracheobronchomegaly (dil-

TABLE 2–10. TIME COURSE OF ADULT RESPIRATORY DISTRESS SYNDROME

Time After Onset of Symptoms	Radiographic Findings
0 to 12 hr	Normal
12 to 24 hr	Patchy interstitial consolidation; normal heart size
24 to 48 hr	Marked consolidation; no effusion unless pneumonia is also present
5 to 7 days	Clearing of edema
Beyond 7 days	Interstitial fibrosis

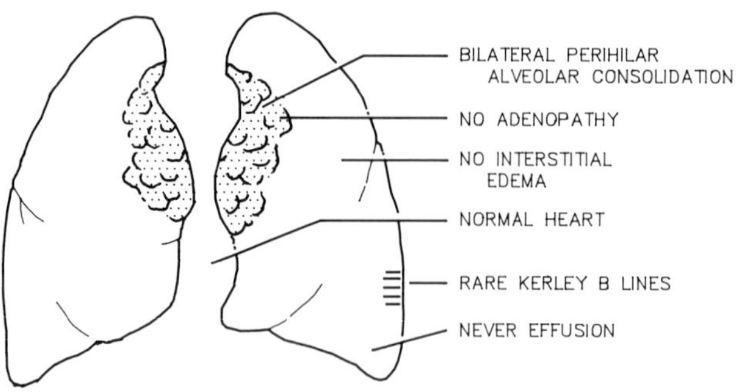

FIGURE 2–79. Characteristics of alveolar proteinosis.

atation of the bronchial tree to more than 3 cm as a result of increased elasticity), tracheopathia osteoplastica (bone and cartilage spicules in the tracheal and bronchial submucosa), and tracheomalacia (weakness and loss of cartilage in the tracheal wall). Iatrogenic tracheal stenosis can occur after prolonged endotracheal intubation.

Many tracheal or bronchial abnormalities can be suspected from thickening of the walls, evidence of obstruction, or from displacement seen on chest films. CT can best demonstrate the large airways and show calcification and soft tissue masses if they are present. Endoscopy is necessary to confirm intraluminal abnormalities.

Diseases of the Small Airways

The small airways are affected by a variety of toxic, infectious, and obstructive processes. The most important of these are chronic obstructive lung disease and bronchiectasis.

Chronic Obstructive Lung Disease. Chronic obstructive lung disease comprises the entire spectrum of chronic bronchitis, emphysema, restrictive disease, and obstructive disease. It occurs predominantly in middle-aged and elderly men and is caused by smoking, air pollution, and occupational exposure, often with infection as an aggravating factor. Patients develop progressive shortness of breath, intolerance of exercise, and respiratory embarrassment. They have obstructive and often restrictive disease. To maintain positive pressure in the airways in order to keep them open, they breathe in at large lung volumes and expire against pursed lips. Interstitial fibrosis leads to pulmonary hypertension and, later, cor pulmonale.

Radiographs show lucent, overexpanded lungs and increased interstitial markings. If the disease is severe, there are signs of pulmonary hypertension (Fig. 2–80; see also Chapter 5). Patients have progressive respiratory impairment, which is eventually fatal. Many patients develop lung cancer. If lung disease is detected early and ingestion of the offending agent is stopped, the lung disease may disappear.

Bronchiectasis. Bronchiectasis, an irreversible, localized dilatation of the bronchial tree, is usually caused by chronic inflammation or obstruction. Trauma, chronic infection, and immunodeficiency are the important predisposing factors (Table 2–11). It is becoming less common because of antibiotic therapy. Patients who have bronchiectasis develop pneumonia, sputum production, or hemoptysis. Chest radiographs show signs of interstitial lung disease and can show the dilated bronchi. Often, the thickened walls have a tram-track appearance. Air/fluid levels can be seen within the cylindrical or saccular bronchial dilatations. Most patients are treated conservatively. Saccular bronchiectasis, however, is treated surgically because of the risk of rupture. Cystic fibrosis is a syndrome that causes bronchiectasis.

Cystic Fibrosis. Cystic fibrosis (mucoviscidosis) is an inherited autosomal recessive disease of children in which abnormally viscous mucus is produced by all glandular secreting tissue, including the pancreas, the intestines, and the lungs. In the lungs, these secretions obstruct the airway and cause bronchiectasis, recurrent pneumonia, and fibrosis. Chest radiographs show hyperexpanded lungs with bronchiectasis and interstitial disease (Fig. 2–81). Cystic fibrosis is eventually fatal, usu-

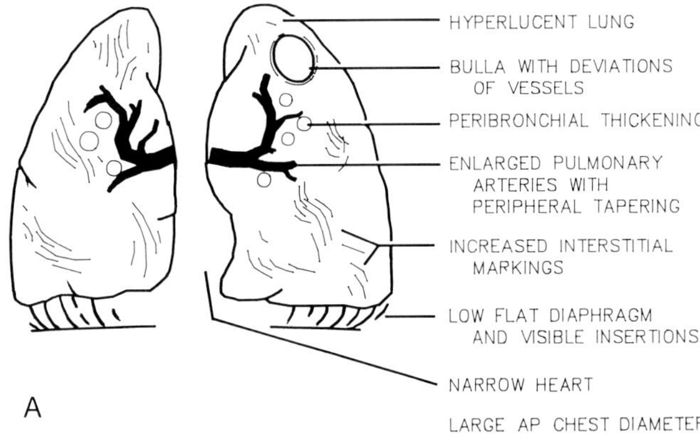

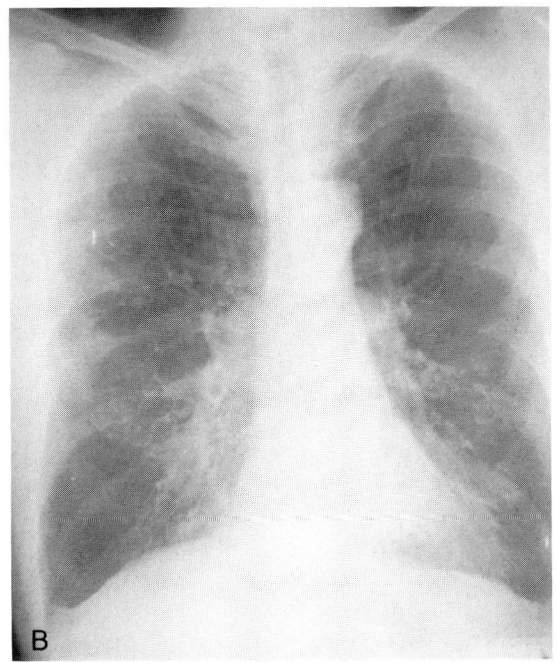

FIGURE 2–80. Chronic obstructive lung disease. *A.* Diagram. AP, anteroposterior. *B.* Chest film shows hyperinflated lungs in a patient with emphysema. Although the radiographic findings are not always correlated with the severity of the clinical disease, they are valuable for detecting such complications as infection, tumor, pneumothorax, pulmonary artery hypertension, and congestive heart failure.

ally by the late teen years, but some patients live to age 30 years. The gastrointestinal abnormalities of this disease are discussed in Chapter 3.

TABLE 2–11. CAUSES OF BRONCHIECTASIS

Traumatic
- Bronchial obstruction by foreign body or trauma

Congenital
- Immunoglobulin deficiency
- Tracheoesophageal fistula
- Cystic fibrosis

Inflammatory
- Chronic aspiration (alcoholism, esophageal dysfunction, scleroderma)
- Infection (tuberculosis, aspergillosis, measles, whooping cough)

Inhalation Diseases

Silicosis. Silicosis occurs in miners, sandblasters, potters, and other workers exposed for long periods to high concentrations of silica dust. The particles are trapped in alveoli, in which a mononuclear response destroys the lung parenchyma. Patients develop respiratory difficulty as pulmonary fibrosis progresses. Many develop lung cancer. On radiographs, a small nodular pattern progresses to larger coalescent masses, predominantly in the upper lobes (Figs. 2–82, 2–83). Hilar adenopathy can develop at any time, and eggshell calcification of lymph nodes occurs in about 5% of patients. Such calcification is virtually pathognomonic of silicosis (rarely is eggshell calcification present in sarcoid and coccidioidomycosis), as is

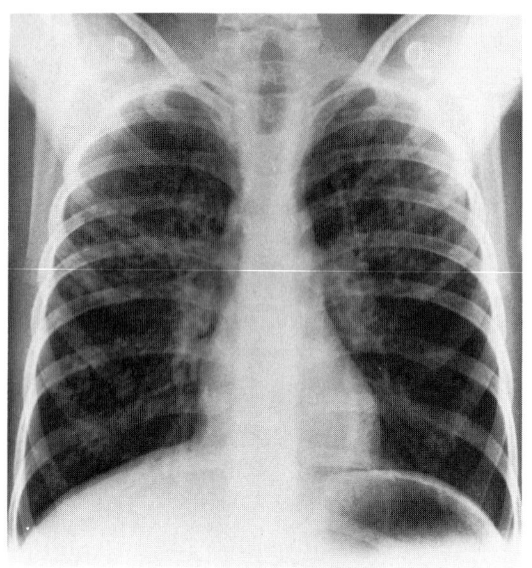

FIGURE 2–81. Cystic fibrosis. Chest film shows characteristic hyperinflation and diffuse, coarse, interstitial markings in a teenage male with cystic fibrosis.

the finding of coalescent upper-lobe masses. The disease is progressive even if exposure to silica is stopped.

Asbestos Lung Disease. Miners, processors of asbestos, and workers in the insulation, textile, construction, shipbuilding, and automobile manufacture industries are exposed to asbestos. Long-term inhalation (over 10 to 20 years) of the asbestos fibers results in a mononuclear response in the respiratory bronchioles and alveoli and, consequently, pulmonary hemorrhage and edema. Patients have gradual and progressive respiratory impairment. Pleural thickening and generalized fibrosis occur, predominantly in the lower lobes. The most common radiographic findings are pleural thickening and calcification (Fig. 2–84). The incidence of squamous cell carcinoma of the lung is 10 times higher among patients with long-term asbestos exposure (100 times if they are also smokers) than among persons not exposed to asbestos. A large proportion of patients with malignant mesothelioma have been exposed to asbestos. Extrathoracic malignancies are also common in patients exposed to asbestos; these malignancies include carcinomas of the pancreas, the esophagus, and the larynx.

Coal Worker's Pneumoconiosis. Coal miners acquire pulmonary fibrosis from inhaling coal dust, which causes a local tissue reaction. Aside from the insult caused by coal dust particles, some coals have associated silica particles. Coal particles less than 5 microns in diameter overwhelm the mucous transport system and remain in the respiratory bronchioles and alveoli. Fibroblasts, macrophages, and coal dust particles form small nodules that are uniformly distributed. A reticulonodular pattern is the only radiographic finding in most patients. Such patients usually have no functional impairment. In about 30% of patients, the small nodules become larger (1 cm or more), usually in the upper lobes; this condi-

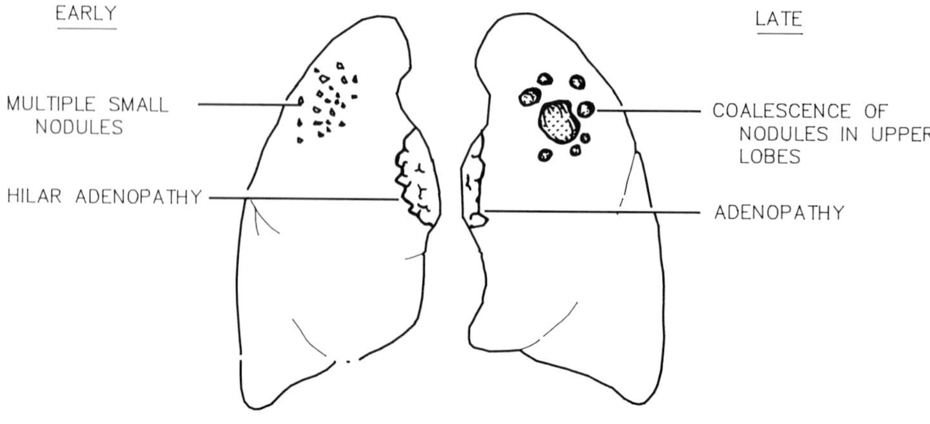

FIGURE 2–82. Characteristics of silicosis.

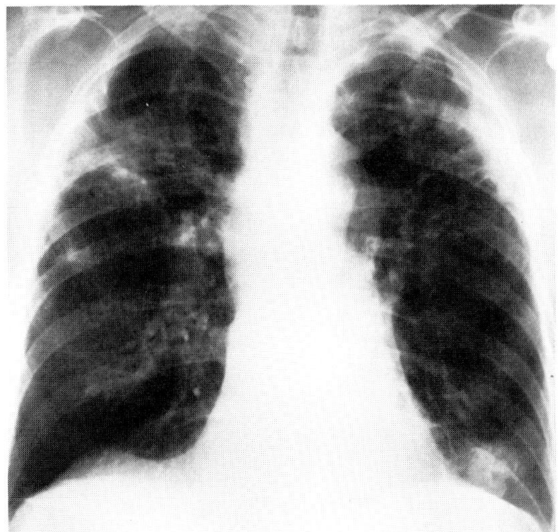

FIGURE 2–83. Silicosis. Chest radiograph of a miner shows coalescent lung masses that accumulated slowly over years. Areas of pleural thickening are also evident.

tion is called progressive massive fibrosis. The cause of this condition is not clear. Rheumatoid, antinuclear, and antilung antibodies are commonly present and suggest an immunological mechanism.

IDIOPATHIC DISEASES

Sarcoidosis. Sarcoidosis is a disease of unknown cause, most common in young American blacks, characterized by noncaseating granulomas in several organs. In the lung, hilar adenopathy is an early finding, fibrosis a late one. Patients develop symptoms of interstitial lung disease and, in severe cases, pulmonary hypertension. The usual radiographic course is bilateral hilar and paratracheal adenopathy followed by interstitial lung disease (Fig. 2–85). Some patients develop only adenopathy, and they are usually asymptomatic. Others develop only lung disease. Frequently, the adenopathy disappears and the lung disease progresses, often (in 20% of patients) to severe fibrosis. The liver, the spleen, the heart, the bone marrow, the skin, and the lymph nodes are also involved. Patients with severe disease die of endstage interstitial lung disease and pulmonary hypertension.

Interstitial Lung Disease. Because the response to lung injury is limited, the cause often is not determined. A histological classification of interstitial lung disease (Table 2–12) is useful for categorizing such diseases, but the

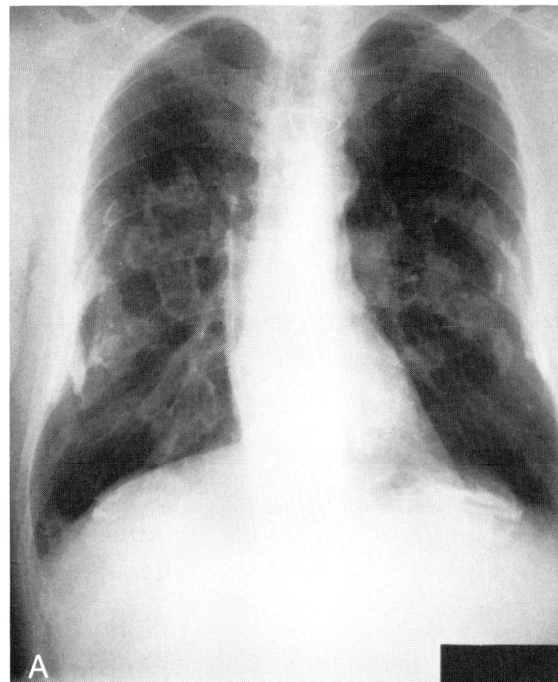

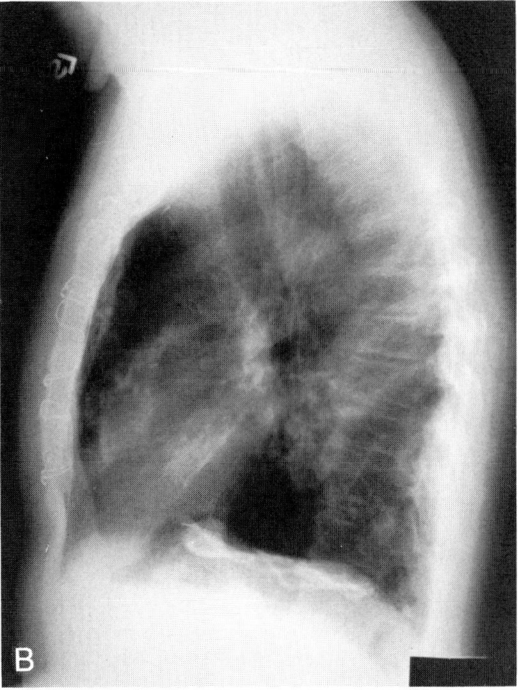

FIGURE 2–84. Asbestos-related lung disease. *A.* Frontal chest film shows multiple calcified, mass-like densities overlying the lungs. From the frontal film it is not possible to determine whether these densities are within the lung, although their clear margination and the presence of lesions along the diaphragm and the lateral margins suggest that they are outside the lung parenchyma. *B.* Lateral view shows that the calcified abnormalities are along the anterior chest wall and pleural margins inferiorly.

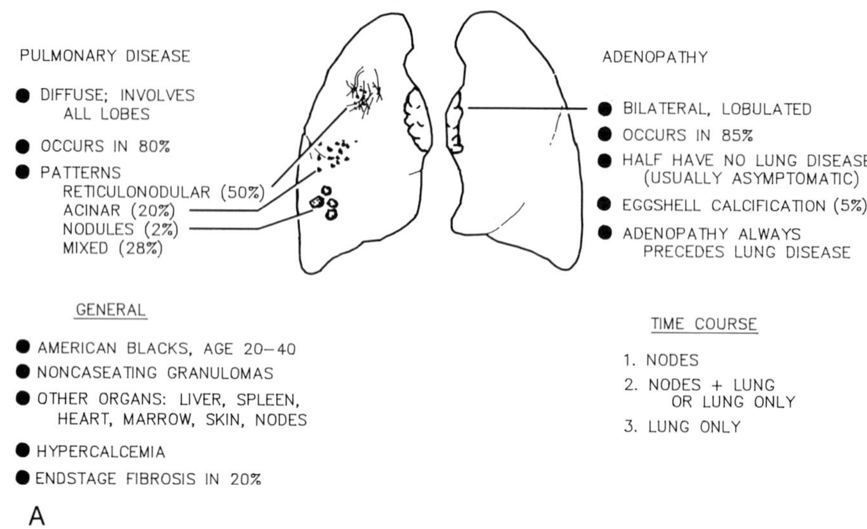

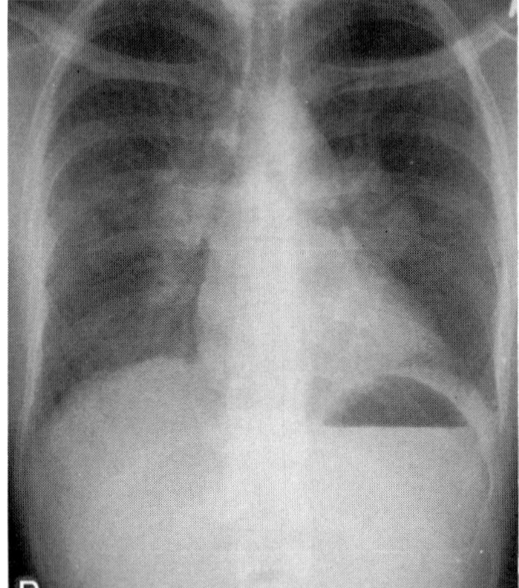

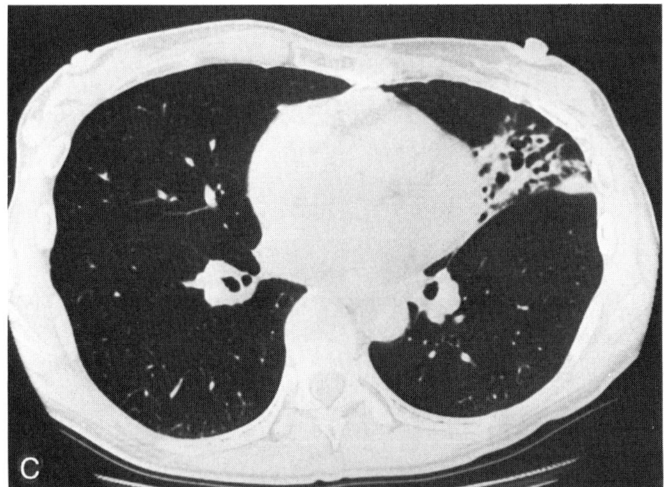

FIGURE 2–85. Sarcoidosis. *A.* Diagram. *B.* Chest film in a patient with early sarcoidosis shows mild right paratracheal and massive bilateral hilar adenopathy. *C.* High-resolution CT scan of the chest of a 59-year-old black woman with late-stage disease shows a confluent area of increased density in the lingula, with a coarse honeycomb appearance. Pneumatoceles are also evident within the abnormality. High-resolution CT imaging can demonstrate the interstitial pattern and help in the assessment of other abnormalities such as lymphadenopathy, pleural disease, and superinfection.

TABLE 2–12. CLASSIFICATION OF INTERSTITIAL PNEUMONIAS

Type	Abnormalities
Usual	Interstitial pneumonia
Bronchiolar	Bronchiolitis obliterans plus usual interstitial pneumonitis
Desquamative	Desquamation of lung tissue with mononuclear infiltration
Lymphoid	Lymphoid infiltration of the lung
Giant cell	Giant cell infiltration

radiographic appearances of the five categories are indistinguishable: all show diffuse interstitial changes progressing to fibrosis, honeycombing, and endstage lung disease. The radiographic finding common to all of the categories is a reticulonodular pattern with a hazy ground-glass appearance of the lungs. The prognosis of such patients is variable. Many live for many years with worsening respiratory function, and others, such as those with the Hamman-Rich syndrome (Fig. 2–86), have a rapid, progressive, diffuse, interstitial

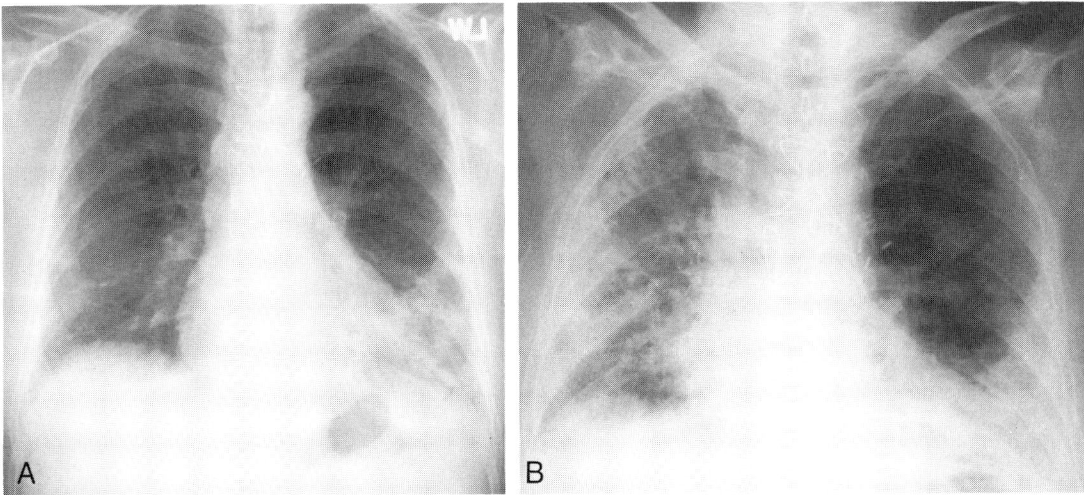

FIGURE 2–86. Hamman-Rich syndrome. *A.* Frontal chest film shows bilateral interstitial abnormalities in a middle-aged man. These developed rapidly over 1 month. *B.* Chest film 1 month later revealed extensive progression in disease of interstitial fibrosis. The patient died shortly after this film was obtained.

fibrosis leading to death in less than 1 year after diagnosis.

Histiocytosis X. Most forms of histiocytosis X affect young people (see Chapters 7 and 8). A rare form is limited to lung involvement and occurs in adult males. The disease is characterized by infiltration of alveolar septa and bronchial walls by histiocytes. This infiltration produces the radiographic picture of diffuse, primarily middle- and upper-lobe nodular abnormalities (Fig. 2–87). The interstitial lung disease usually progresses to fibrosis and honeycombing. Most patients die of respiratory insufficiency.

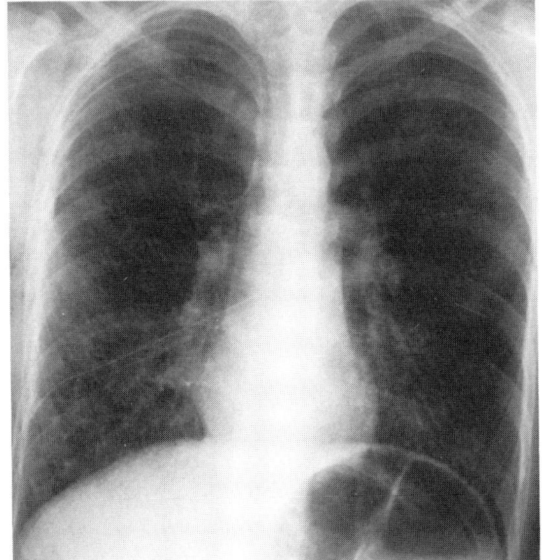

FIGURE 2–87. Histiocytosis X lung disease in a 17-year-old male. Frontal chest film shows hyperinflated lungs with coarse interstitial markings. A chest tube was required after open lung biopsy, which established the diagnosis of histiocytosis X lung disease.

PEDIATRIC LUNG DISEASE

Lung Disease in the Neonate

Lung disease in the neonate can be difficult to diagnose and can be easily confused with heart disease manifested by pulmonary edema or vascular engorgement. The list of lung diseases of neonates is limited. The clinical information (i.e., time of onset, progression, and birth history) and radiographic findings (the size of the heart, the pulmonary vessels, and the liver; the degree of lung aeration; and the pattern of consolidation) usually allow the diagnosis to be made. The most important conditions are retained fetal lung fluid, hyaline membrane disease, pneumonia, meconium aspiration, and pulmonary hemorrhage (Table 2–13). Less common causes of lung disease in newborns include pulmonary hemorrhage; Wilson-Mikity syndrome; pulmonary congestion as seen with hypoglycemia, erythroblastosis fetalis, and polycythemia; pulmonary lymphangiectasis; and pulmonary hypoplasia.

Retained Fetal Lung Fluid. The most common cause of lung consolidation in the newborn is retained fetal lung fluid. In utero, the lungs are filled with fluid, which must be removed so that the lungs can be aerated. Most likely, the fluid is cleared by peribronchial lymphatics and veins. Much of this fluid is

TABLE 2–13. LUNG DISEASES OF NEWBORNS

Disease	Lung Expansion	Pulmonary Consolidation	Onset	Progression	Clinical Factors
Retained fetal lung fluid	Increased	Diffuse increased density; often with effusion	Birth to 6 hr	Clears by 72 hr	Failure to expel fetal lung fluid; common in cesarean section or rapid delivery
Hyaline membrane disease	Decreased	Diffuse bilateral granular lungs; low lung volumes; can develop pneumothorax	Birth	Often fatal; otherwise, clears over 2 to 3 weeks	Immature lung has insufficient surfactant to allow lung expansion; common in premature infants
Pneumonia	Increased	Asymmetrical patches of increased density, often with effusion	Birth	Improvement on antibiotics, unless caused by beta streptococci (fatal in 12 hr)	Prolonged ruptured membranes, maternal infection; caused by group B beta streptococci, *Listeria*, *Escherichia coli*
Meconium aspiration	Increased	Coarse patches of density; asymmetrical and bilateral; usually no effusion	Birth	Some infants die rapidly; most cases clear over 1 week	Born through meconium, not septic; occurs in full-term infants
Pulmonary vascular congestion, hypoglycemia, and IDM	Moderate	Homogeneous consolidation	1 to 3 days	Clears in hours with therapy	Occurs in complicated pregnancy, postmaturity, hypoxia, and hypothermia
Hypervolemia and polycythemia	None	Pulmonary edema	Birth	Clears over a few days	Increased vascular volume causes interstitial edema; causes: late clamping of cord, overtransfusion, placental dysfunction, polycythemia
Erythroblastosis fetalis	None	Hemorrhage or edema	6 to 72 hr	Clears in 24 hr with therapy	Antibodies from sensitized mother destroys Rh+ fetal red blood cells; yellow umbilical cord, jaundiced fetus
Pulmonary dysmaturity (Wilson-Mikity syndrome)	Moderate	Bubbly-appearing lungs	1 week	2- to 5-week bihilar haze, 5-week to 5-month microcysts, then returns to normal	Normal in first week; occurs in premature infants weighing less than 1500 g due to immature lungs; self-limited
Congenital pulmonary lymphangiectasis	Moderate	Diffuse reticular bilateral disease	Birth	Death within hours	Dyspnea and cyanosis

IDM, infant of a diabetic mother.

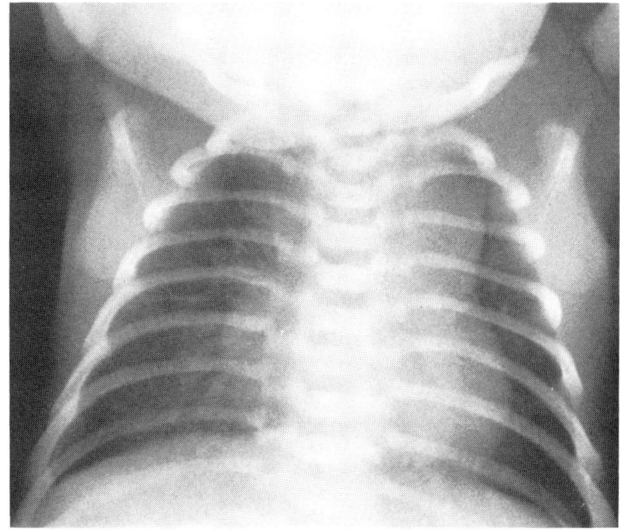

FIGURE 2–88. Retained fetal lung fluid (transient tachypnea of the newborn). AP view of thorax shows hyperinflation, fluid in the fissures, vascular prominence and poor vascular definition, and slight enlargement of the cardiac silhouette. The fluid resolved shortly after birth in the infant, who had been delivered by cesarean section.

expelled during vaginal delivery by compression of the infant's thorax. When the fluid is incompletely removed at birth, respiratory embarrassment occurs, and the infant develops tachypnea. Newborns delivered by cesarean section and those delivered rapidly are especially likely to have retained lung fluid. The radiographic appearance is that of hyperexpanded lungs with perihilar streaking, mild enlargement of the cardiac silhouette, and, frequently, pleural effusions that are most prominent in the fissures (Fig. 2–88). The disease is self-limited. The fluid is absorbed in 1 to 3 days, and the radiographic and clinical abnormalities disappear.

Hyaline Membrane Disease. Hyaline membrane disease is a respiratory distress syndrome of premature infants that is characterized clinically by hypoxia and acidosis, radiographically by poorly expanded, granular-appearing lungs with air bronchograms (Fig. 2–89), and histologically by collapsed alveoli and by hyaline membranes deposited on the terminal bronchioles. It occurs because immature lungs lack sufficient surfactant to allow expansion of the alveoli after birth. Initially, radiographs appear normal. Later (about 5 to 12 days of age) the lungs develop a hazy appearance that gradually returns to normal after 2 to 3 weeks.

Infants with mild disease are typically extubated within 7 to 10 days. In most infants with hyaline membrane disease, the lungs are noncompliant and require assisted ventilation for adequate oxygenation. When high ventilation pressures are required, interstitial emphysema and pneumothorax can develop. Prolonged, artificial ventilation can cause pulmonary fibrosis, bronchiolar damage, and uneven aeration of the lungs, called bronchopulmonary dysplasia (Fig. 2–90). Prenatal administration of corticosteroids can accelerate lung maturity, enhancing surfactant production and thereby preventing hyaline membrane disease.

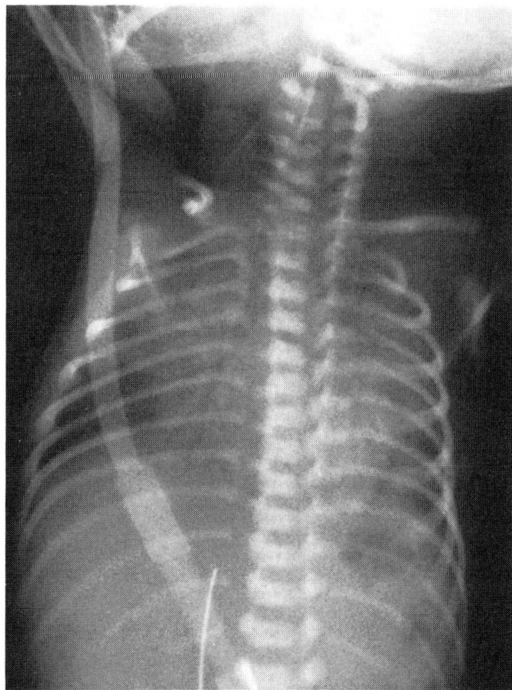

FIGURE 2–89. Hyaline membrane disease. Slightly rotated frontal view of the thorax shows underinflated lungs with a granular appearance. Air bronchograms are also evident.

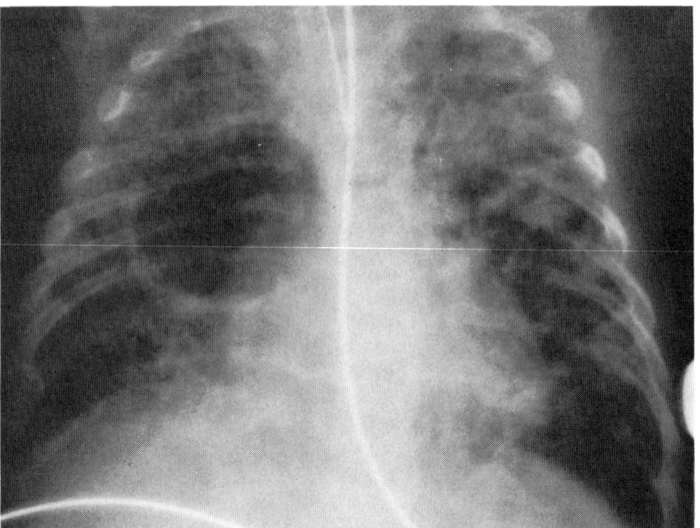

FIGURE 2–90. Bronchopulmonary dysplasia. AP view of thorax shows an area of hyperinflation surrounded by areas of scarring in a premature infant who required prolonged ventilator support.

Pneumonia. Pneumonia in the neonate is usually caused by the Lancefield group B, beta-hemolytic streptococci. Other organisms that cause pneumonia include *Listeria monocytogenes, Staphylococcus aureus,* and the enteric gram-negative bacteria, especially *Escherichia coli.* Causes of pneumonia include maternal infection and premature membrane rupture with amnionitis. Infants are severely ill with fever, respiratory difficulty, and hypoglycemia. The most common radiographic appearance is of hyperexpanded lungs containing patches of increased density in an asymmetrical distribution (Fig. 2–91). However, neonatal pneumonia can mimic any process, particularly transient tachypnea of the newborn and hyaline membrane disease. The prognosis for streptococcal pneumonia is, in general, poor. The mortality rate is high among infants who develop fulminant sepsis and shock.

Meconium Aspiration. Meconium, the first neonatal intestinal excretion, is usually passed after birth; it is occasionally passed before birth as a result of hypoxia. If this meconium is aspirated by the neonate, the particles can lodge in the small peripheral bronchi, causing overexpansion of the lungs and subsequent pneumothorax and pneumomediastinum. A chemical pneumonitis can also develop. Radiographs show hyperexpanded lungs with bilateral and asymmetrical patches of increased density (Fig. 2–92); this appearance is similar

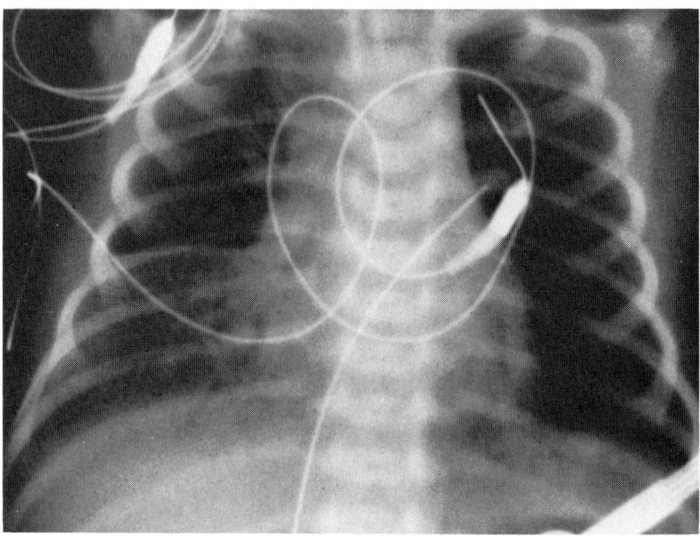

FIGURE 2–91. Neonatal pneumonia. AP view of chest shows pleural fluid in the minor fissure and patchy opacification in the right lower lung. The infant had been born after prolonged membrane rupture when a maternal infection developed.

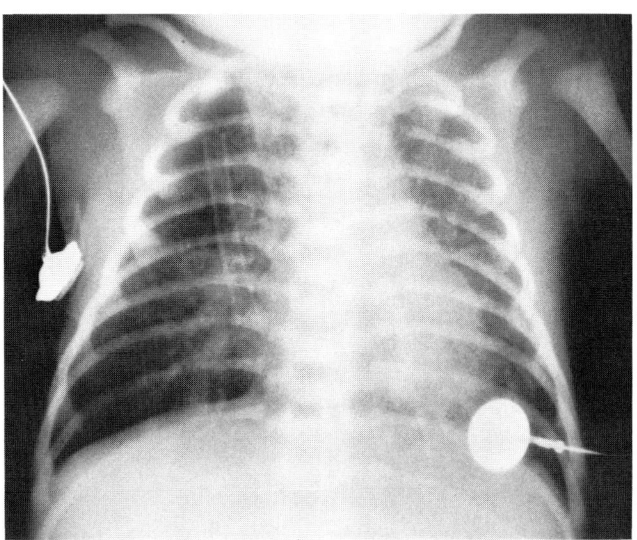

FIGURE 2–92. Meconium aspiration. AP view of the thorax shows hyperinflation of the lungs with coarse, streaky densities throughout. These findings resulted from meconium aspiration and are indistinguishable from those of pneumonia. The infant was born through meconium and had no fever, and there was no evidence of maternal sepsis.

to that of pneumonia. Associated evidence of airway rupture is frequently present (i.e., pneumothorax and pneumomediastinum).

Pneumonia and meconium aspiration are difficult to distinguish radiographically. Meconium aspiration can be distinguished clinically from hyaline membrane disease by gestational age. Hyaline membrane disease occurs in premature infants; meconium aspiration usually occurs in postmature infants. Infants suffering from meconium aspiration are routinely treated with antibiotics until results of cultures prove negative. Suctioning of the trachea in the delivery room is the most important treatment to prevent aspiration below the vocal cords. Infants with aspiration into the tracheobronchial tree frequently require assisted ventilation. The mortality rate is high among these infants. Many infants who recover have radiographic abnormalities for days or weeks (Fig. 2–92).

Pulmonary Hemorrhage. Pulmonary hemorrhage is usually secondary to severe hypoxia and capillary damage, as seen in hyaline membrane disease, meconium aspiration, or neonatal pneumonia. The radiographic findings are usually that of the underlying process, unless the hemorrhage is massive. In the latter case, the radiograph shows homogeneously opaque lungs.

Pulmonary Congestion. Hypoglycemia occasionally occurs in neonates, particularly in infants of diabetic mothers. Radiographs frequently show pulmonary congestion and an enlarged cardiac silhouette, which clears on correction of the hypoglycemia. Infants of diabetic mothers frequently show liver and spleen enlargement and increased fat thickness on radiographs.

Polycythemia. Polycythemia can result from excessive umbilical cord milking or twin transfusion, but it can also occur as a primary phenomenon. Radiographs show an enlarged cardiac silhouette and vascular congestion that simulates retained fetal lung fluid or cardiac disease.

Erythroblastosis Fetalis. Erythroblastosis fetalis occurs when a mother with Rh-negative factor develops antibodies to a fetus with Rh-positive factor. The antibodies cross the placenta and enter the fetus, causing hemolysis and anemia in the fetus. Chest radiographs of the fetus frequently show pulmonary vascular congestion caused by high-output cardiac failure. Additional findings are ascites, hydrothorax, and an enlarged cardiac silhouette.

Pulmonary Dysmaturity. Pulmonary dysmaturity (Wilson-Mikity syndrome) primarily affects premature infants weighing less than 1500 g. Usually these infants do not have respiratory difficulties until after the first few days of life. Initial chest radiographs are usually normal. Over the next few days the radiographs show nodular, coarse densities alternating with areas of hyperaeration. The abnormalities progress to a bubbly appearance of the lungs. The radiographic changes resemble those seen in bronchopulmonary dysplasia, but pathological examination reveals no fibrosis in Wilson-Mikity syndrome, as there is in bronchopulmonary dysplasia. The radiographic abnormality in Wilson-Mikity syndrome gradually clears over 2 years.

Congenital Pulmonary Lymphangiectasis. Congenital pulmonary lymphangiectasis is an isolated disease that manifests at birth and is rapidly fatal. The cause is considered to be an early arrest of pulmonary lymphatic development and persistence of large dilated and obstructed lymphatic channels. Radiographs show a reticular or coarsely nodular pattern in the lungs with generalized hyperaeration.

Pulmonary Hypoplasia. Bilateral pulmonary hypoplasia is usually the result of intrauterine compression of the fetal thorax. The best known cause of pulmonary hypoplasia is extrathoracic compression in the oligohydramnios syndrome, which in turn is caused by fetal renal agenesis and resultant fetal anuria. Maternal oligohydramnios develops as a result of anuria, which leads to compression of the fetal thorax and lungs by the uterus. Radiographs of infants with bilateral pulmonary hypoplasia as a result of maternal oligohydramnios show a bell-shaped thorax and, frequently, pneumothorax or pneumomediastinum. Any fetal renal anomaly resulting in decreased urine output and maternal oligohydramnios can cause similar findings.

Other causes of bilateral lung hypoplasia include large abdominal masses that elevate the hemidiaphragms and compression of the lungs by the fetal bony thorax, by diaphragmatic hernia, and by chylothorax. Primary pulmonary hypoplasia (discussed in the Congenital Diseases section) also results in small lungs.

RADIOGRAPHIC DIFFERENTIAL DIAGNOSIS

A single radiographic finding or pattern frequently suggests a limited list of diagnoses. Additional findings and clinical history can then assist in further limiting the list or in making a firm diagnosis. The following approaches to evaluation of radiographic findings can provide assistance in differential diagnosis.

PATTERNS OF LUNG DISEASE

Abnormal density in the lung is caused by the presence of air, fluid, or cells; the pattern of distribution of this abnormal density suggests a specific differential diagnostic list. The four basic patterns of lung disease are disseminated airspace consolidation, localized airspace consolidation, lobar consolidation, and interstitial lung density.

1. Disseminated Airspace Consolidation
   A. Acute
      - Pneumonia (viral and atypical)
      - Pulmonary edema
      - Hemorrhage
      - Adult respiratory distress syndrome (ARDS)

   B. Chronic
      - Sarcoidosis
      - Lymphoma
      - Alveolar cell carcinoma
      - Alveolar proteinosis
      - Pneumoconiosis
2. Localized Airspace Consolidation
   - Pneumonia (bacterial)
   - Tumor
   - Infarction
   - Tuberculosis
   - Fungal infection
   - Contusion
   - Radiation injury
3. Lobar Airspace Consolidation
   - Pneumonia (bacterial)
   - Bronchial obstruction
   - Tuberculosis
   - Lymphoma
   - Aspiration
   - Infarction
4. Interstitial Pattern
   A. Linear pattern (Kerley's B lines)
      - Pulmonary edema
      - Chronic congestive heart failure
      - Pneumoconiosis
      - Lymphangitic metastases
      - Lymphoma
      - Pneumonia

   B. Nodular (Miliary) Pattern
      - Granulomatous diseases: tuberculosis, histiocytosis X, sarcoidosis, and pneumonoconiosis
      - Metastatic disease

   C. Destructive Pattern (Honeycomb Lung)
      - Chronic lung disease
      - Collagen vascular diseases

APPROACH TO THE EVALUATION OF INTERSTITIAL LUNG DISEASE

Although the causes of interstitial lung disease are numerous, a direct approach can limit the possibilities and identify treatable diseases. The first step is to suggest two treatable causes: congestive heart failure and pneumonia (especially the types caused by viruses and atypical organisms). Next, obtaining four elements of the clinical history assists in identifying most other causes of interstitial lung disease: (1) work and exposure, (2) underlying disease (especially cancer and collagen vascular disease), (3) drug therapy, and (4) immunosuppression. If this direct method is inconclusive, the following causes must be systematically investigated:

Congenital (neurofibromatosis, tuberous sclerosis, cystic fibrosis)
Systemic (collagen vascular diseases, immune deficiency, eosinophilic lung disease, extrinsic allergic alveolitis, Goodpasture's syndrome, Wegener's granulomatosis)
Infectious (viral, atypical, opportunistic, protozoan)
Neoplastic (metastases: hematogenous and lymphangitic)
Vascular (embolism, *Strongyloides* infestation)
Airway (chronic lung disease, pneumoconiosis)
Idiopathic (sarcoidosis, histiocytosis X)

UPPER-LOBE LUNG DISEASES

Only a few diseases are limited to the upper lobes of the lungs. They have characteristic radiographic appearances and can usually be distinguished from one another.

Tuberculosis
Sarcoidosis
Fungal pneumonia
Silicosis
Histiocytosis X
Ankylosing spondylitis

INTERPRETATION OF A SOLITARY PULMONARY NODULE

A solitary, pulmonary nodule is a single lesion in the lung, ranging in size from a few millimeters to a few centimeters. Such a lesion is benign if it shows central calcification, high CT density (similar to that of bone), and no change in 3 years. Otherwise, such a lesion should be considered an early carcinoma. It is important to verify that the nodule is in the lung rather than on the chest wall or even outside the patient.

Lesion	*Prevalence*
Granuloma	60%
Lung carcinoma	30%
Hamartoma	7%
Tumor metastases	2%
Bronchial adenoma	Rare
Arteriovenous malformation	Rare
Benign mesothelioma	Rare

CAUSES OF CAVITATING LUNG LESIONS

Cavitating lung lesions are single or multiple lung nodules that have a central cavity filled with fluid. Any type of lesion can become infected or have a necrotic center. The appearance of the cavity or the thickness of the wall (indicated in parentheses) is helpful but never conclusive in establishing a diagnosis.

1. Trauma

   Traumatic cyst
   Traumatic diaphragmatic hernia

2. Congenital

   Bronchogenic cyst (smooth, thin wall)
   Sequestration (lung bases, usually left)

3. Systemic

   Wegener's granulomatosis (multiple, round, circumscribed nodules; half cavitate, with shaggy inner walls)
   Rheumatoid (multiple nodules)

4. Infection

   Tuberculosis (upper lobe, thick wall)
   Histoplasmosis (thick wall)
   Coccidioidomycosis (thin or thick wall)
   Staphylococcus aureus (shaggy, multiple; in adults, abscess; in children, pneumatoceles, often with air/fluid levels)
   Aspergillus fungus ball (moves on decubitus view)
   Echinococcal cyst (contains daughter cysts)

5. Neoplasms

   Primary lung cancer (especially squamous cell)
   Hodgkin's disease
   Metastases

6. Vascular

   Infarct
   Septic embolism

7. Idiopathic

   Not sarcoidosis (nodules are rare)
   Not histiocytosis X (nodules are rare)

CAUSES OF BILATERAL HILAR ADENOPATHY

Bilateral hilar adenopathy has few causes. The pattern is often helpful in arriving at the correct diagnosis. The hilar adenopathy of tuberculosis is usually unilateral.

Sarcoidosis (symmetrical)
Lymphoma (asymmetrical)
Viral infection (infectious mononucleosis)
Metastases (testicular, bone, gastrointestinal tract)

CAUSES OF HONEYCOMB LUNG

Endstage lung destruction results in a honeycomb pattern of interstitial fibrosis. Although there are many causes of interstitial lung disease (see the Approach to the Evaluation of Interstitial Lung Disease), six are common.

Pneumoconiosis
Sarcoidosis

Scleroderma
Rheumatoid lung disease
Histiocytosis X
Hamman-Rich fibrosis

CAUSES OF LUNG CALCIFICATION

Disseminated calcification in the lung has a characteristic appearance and can be caused by several important diseases. In all cases, the calcium is deposited after diffuse parenchymal injury.

Metastases (from bone, cartilage, gastrointestinal tract)
Histoplasmosis
Varicella pneumonia
Coccidioidomycosis
Mitral stenosis (hemosiderin deposits calcify)
Metastatic calcification (from calcium disorders)

CAUSES OF KERLEY'S B LINES

Prominent intralobular septa in the lungs, when seen as short, thin, horizontal lines terminating at the lateral edge of the pleura, are called Kerley's B lines. The cause of these prominences can be fluid or interstitial fibrosis. The most common cause is congestive heart failure.

Congestive heart failure
Mitral stenosis
Cardiac shunt (especially atrial septal defect)
Pneumoconiosis

CAUSES OF UNILATERAL LUCENT LUNG

When lucency is seen in only one lung, the cause is usually a chronic disease. Because it is treatable and potentially fatal, pulmonary embolus should be considered if clinical circumstances warrant.

Pulmonary embolus
Bullous emphysema
Pulmonary artery hypoplasia
Swyer-James syndrome
Alpha$_1$-antitrypsin deficiency
Unilateral absence of pectoralis muscles
Mastectomy

Suggested Readings

Fraser RG, Paré JA: Diagnosis of Diseases of the Chest, 3rd ed. Philadelphia: WB Saunders, 1990.

Nadich DP, Zerhouni EA, Siegelman SS: Computed Tomography and Magnetic Resonance of the Thorax, 2nd ed. New York: Raven Press, 1991.

Reed JC: Chest Radiology: Plain Film Patterns and Differential Diagnoses, 2nd ed. Chicago: Year Book Medical, 1987.

3

Alimentary Tract and Abdominal Radiology

Michael Davis
Michael R. Williamson
Susan L. Williamson
Gary K. Stimac

Abdominal imaging is complex because the several organ systems contained require special expertise in many imaging modalities. This chapter is therefore organized in three parts. Part I covers the tubular gastrointestinal (GI) tract and features plain film and contrast examinations as the predominant methods of evaluation. Part II covers imaging of the solid organs of the abdomen. Part III deals with imaging of the abdomen for conditions caused by trauma, infection, or tumor that can involve multiple organs, abdominal spaces, and mesenteric planes, including the peritoneal cavity and the retroperitoneum. This latter section demonstrates the use of computed tomography (CT), ultrasonography, and magnetic resonance imaging (MRI) in the evaluation of complex masses, abscesses, and benign and malignant tumors. The "Basic Evaluation," "Topics in Pediatric Radiology," and "Radiographic Differential Diagnosis" sections are in their usual places within the chapter. Pelvic disease and the genitourinary system are covered in Chapter 4 in a similar format.

BASIC EVALUATION

Plain Film Interpretation

The evaluation of the abdomen is complex and often requires several complementary examinations for diagnosis. The first imaging examination is usually plain film radiography, which is especially helpful in the assessment of specific abdominal complaints and localizing signs. Both supine and upright views should be obtained (Fig. 3–1) in order to identify abnormal patterns of fluid and air. Attention should be directed to the bones, the soft tissues, the abdominal organs, and the bowel gas pattern. The lung bases are usually included on the abdominal film, and because this film employs different radiographic techniques, it may reveal pulmonary lesions not shown on the routine posteroanterior (PA) chest radiograph.

The bones are first examined for fractures, metastases, arthritis, and abnormal calcifications (Fig. 3–2). Fractures of the lower ribs are often associated with injuries to adjacent organs. Metastases to the spine and the pelvis can be lytic (of low density), sclerotic (blastic or of high density), or of mixed density. Many types of arthritis involve the hips, the sacroiliac joints, and the spine and are detectable on abdominal films. Pathological calcifications in

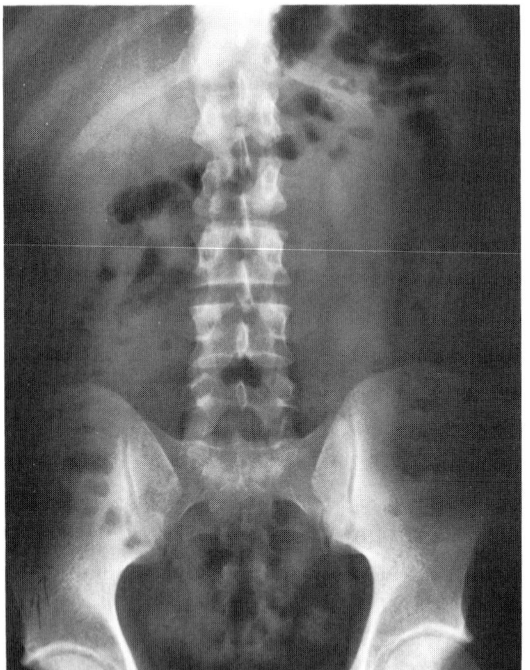

FIGURE 3–1. Upright plain film of the abdomen. The abdominal plain film is capable of demonstrating organ size, calcifications, fluid, and air. The presence of mass lesions can be inferred from displacement of normal structures. Air and fluid change appearance when the patient assumes an upright position.

the abdomen may indicate acute disease such as ureteral obstruction by a calculus, or they can suggest a chronic process such as tumor, inflammation, or infection. Although calcifications in the gallbladder (gallstones), the pancreas, or the appendix (appendicoliths) are the result of chronic processes, they may also be associated with acute inflammation in patients with symptoms of cholecystitis, pancreatitis, or appendicitis, respectively.

The soft tissues and abdominal organs are evaluated next (Fig. 3–3). The liver appears on plain films as a homogeneous density in the right upper quadrant; effacement of its lower edge on the supine film suggests free intraperitoneal fluid. Because of its pyramidal shape, the size (and volume) of the liver cannot be accurately determined from plain films. The spleen is often not seen on abdominal films because it is small and overlaps the stomach and splenic flexure of the colon. Splenomegaly is associated with many diseases, most commonly portal hypertension, hemorrhage (spontaneous or traumatic), leukemia, and lymphoma. The pancreas is not seen on plain films unless it contains calcification, a common finding in patients with chronic pancreatitis. Renal outlines are often visible, allowing kidney size to be estimated, but they are seldom seen well enough to reliably diagnose perinephric abscess or hematoma. The full bladder appears as a round homogeneous mass in the pelvis and is occasionally mistaken for a tumor. Poor visualization of the psoas muscle margin suggests the presence of retroperitoneal fluid, an abscess, or a mass. Often, this margin is poorly seen in normal patients who have no pathological process in the retroperitoneum.

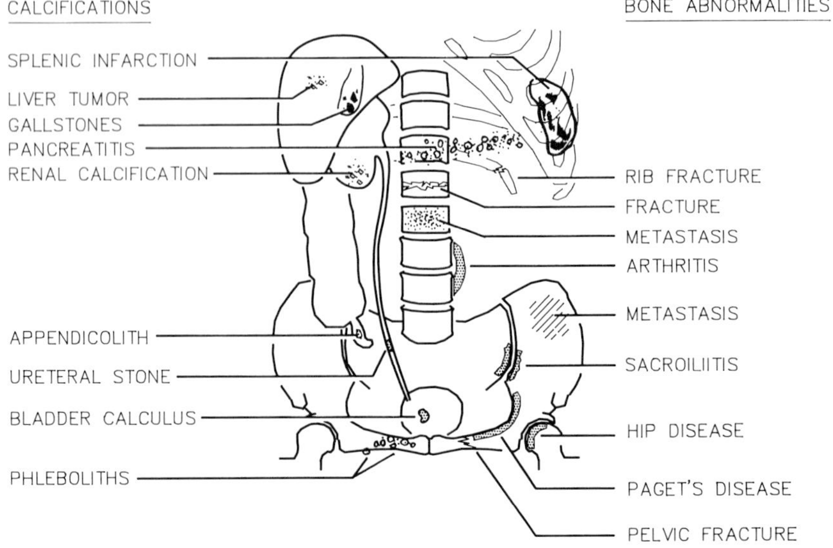

FIGURE 3–2. Bone lesions and abnormal calcifications seen on abdominal films.

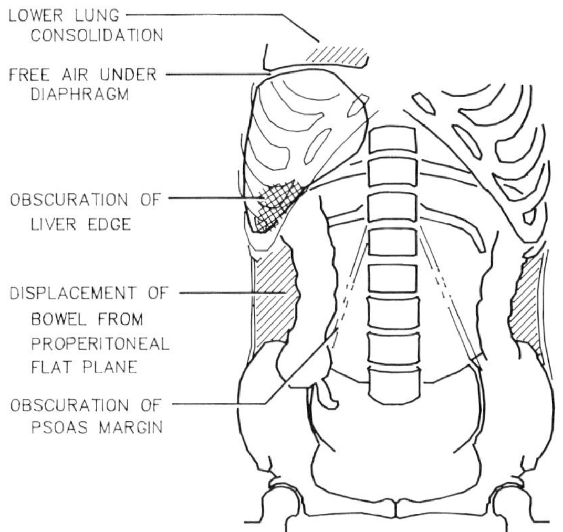

FIGURE 3–3. Soft-tissue abnormalities seen on abdominal films.

Abnormal Bowel Gas Pattern. The bowel gas pattern is usually nonspecific, but its appearance may suggest abnormalities that can be confirmed by other examinations (Fig. 3–4*A*). Displacement of the colon medially from the properitoneal fat planes occurs when free intraperitoneal fluid or blood lies in the paracolic gutters. Obstruction is suggested by the presence of dilated segments and air/fluid levels in the bowel proximal to the obstruction and by the absence of gas distal to the obstruction. When all segments of the bowel are distended with gas, the patient is more likely to have a paralytic ileus, also referred to as adynamic ileus (or, simply, ileus). Such a nonobstructed, atonic bowel gas pattern may be associated with ischemia, acute inflammation, drugs, surgery, trauma, neuromuscular disorders, and various other diseases such as heart failure, pneumonia, shock, diabetes, and uremia. Early or partial bowel obstruction can be difficult to detect in the absence of sufficient fluid, gas, and distention proximal to the obstruction.

Pneumoperitoneum. Pneumoperitoneum, the presence of free air in the peritoneal cavity, is usually caused by the disruption of the bowel wall. Causes include ulcerations, blunt traumatic ruptures, iatrogenic perforation from instrumentation, perforation of a hollow viscus by a foreign body, inflammatory bowel disease, diverticulitis, peptic ulcer or obstruction of Meckel's diverticulum, neoplasm, and infection. Other less common causes include penetration injury, air from the female genital tract, or gas from intra-abdominal abscess. The most common cause of free intraperitoneal air is

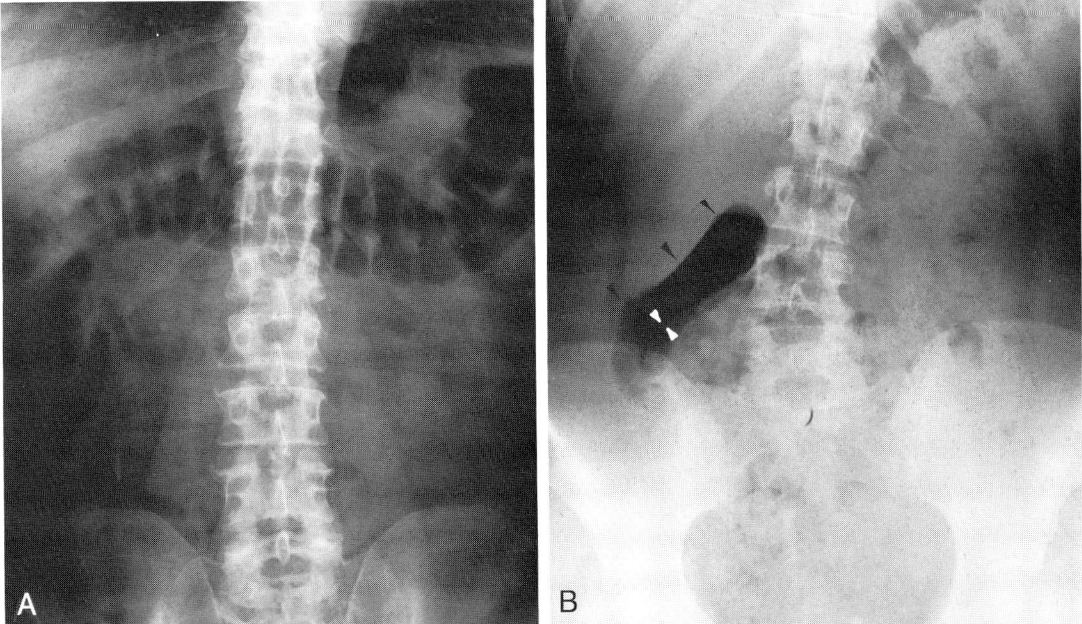

FIGURE 3–4. Abdominal gas pattern. *A.* Bowel air. Abdominal plain film shows air throughout the transverse colon. The bowel is not dilated, and there are no signs of obstruction. The patient is an older woman with epigastric discomfort. *B.* Free abdominal air. Supine abdominal film shows elliptical collection of free air that clearly outlines the inferior margin of the liver. Air also outlines both the inner and outer walls of the bowel *(arrowheads),* which is called the double-wall sign.

recent abdominal surgery, the air normally being visible for 3 to 5 days. In the absence of surgery, bowel rupture is usually the cause. Free air can be seen beneath the diaphragm on upright views or outlining the falciform ligament, the liver edge, or the bowel wall on supine views (Fig. 3–4*B*). Sometimes the bowel ruptures into the retroperitoneal space, where the air is difficult to detect on plain films, but it occasionally outlines the kidneys or the psoas margins.

Intraperitoneal Fluid. Excess, free intra-abdominal (peritoneal) fluid can be composed of ascites, blood, pus, chyle, urine, bile, and intestinal contents. None have any distinguishing characteristics on abdominal plain films. Fluid can be seen to obscure the liver edge or displace the colon medially. Diagnosis can be made manually by percussion and demonstration of shifting dullness, but ultrasonography and CT are far superior for detecting fluid collections and greatly assist in determining their causes.

Contrast Examination of the Gastrointestinal Tract

Contrast examinations (upper GI series, small-bowel series, enteroclysis, and barium enema studies) are the best radiological methods for evaluating the lumen of the GI tract. These examinations provide excellent detail of the lumen and the mucosal surface of most of the GI tract. Barium suspensions, modern filming techniques, and the simultaneous use of air as a second contrast agent (double-contrast examinations) greatly increase the diagnostic value of these examinations. Fluoroscopic images can be recorded on videotape, by spot film cameras, by film cassette devices, on large films, and by digital computers.

The proximal GI tract (the mouth, the pharynx, the esophagus, the stomach, and the small bowel) is studied by upper GI series through the use of single- or double-contrast examination techniques. On single-contrast examination, medium-density barium (50% to 60%, weight per volume) is used to outline the lumen in the distended and collapsed states. The double-contrast examination entails the use of high-density barium (200%, weight per volume), which adheres to the bowel wall and provides a smooth uniform coating. This coating of the mucosal surface in combination with distension of the lumen by air provides a see-through view of the lumen and the mucosal surface. The most complete examination of the upper GI tract, the biphasic examination, entails the use of both single- and double-contrast techniques. The single-contrast esophagram can show strictures, masses (intrinsic and extrinsic), dysmotility, diffuse spasm, moderate to high grades of inflammation and infection, aberrant vascular structures, diverticula, and varices. With the double-contrast technique, the normal esophagus is seen as a tube with a satin-smooth surface (Fig. 3–5). When the esophagus is partially collapsed, smooth, longitudinal folds are evident. Occasionally, small, transverse folds are identified during contractions. The double-contrast esophagram can show most of the same abnormalities as the single-contrast examination can but can also demonstrate very early stages of mu-

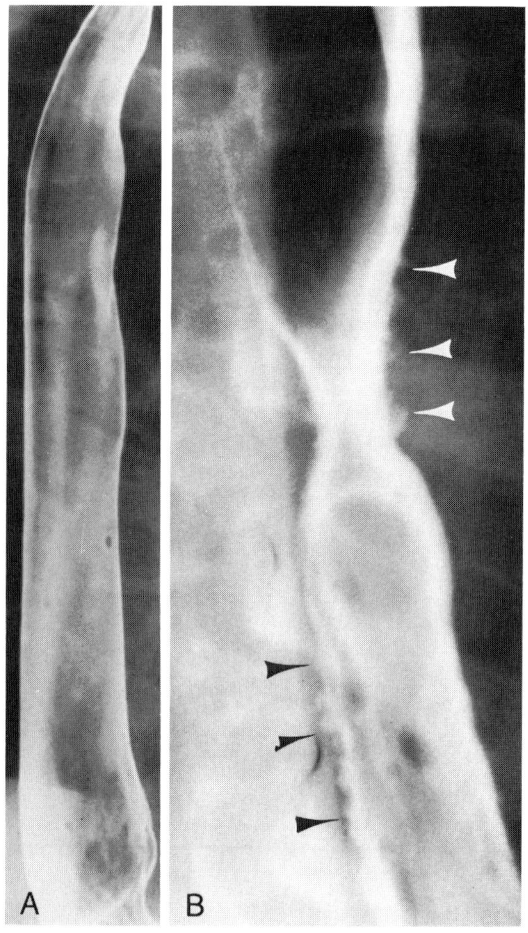

FIGURE 3–5. Esophagus examination. *A.* Normal double-contrast esophagram shows a satin-smooth texture of the mucosa. *B.* Esophagram in a patient with herpes simplex esophagitis shows narrowing in the mid esophagus associated with multiple, spiculated ulcers along both margins *(arrows).*

cosal disease, including inflammation, ulceration, infection, and tumor.

Esophageal motility is assessed fluoroscopically for primary (swallow-induced) and secondary (locally induced) stripping waves. Barium in the stomach usually does not flow back into the esophagus, but, if reflux of small amounts into the lower esophagus is seen and is rapidly cleared, it is unlikely to be clinically significant. The stomach and the duodenum are systematically evaluated for thickened or nodular folds, the presence of mucosal lesions (including erosions, ulcers, and masses), and restricted distensibility, especially in the region of the gastric antrum. A benign ulcer (Fig. 3–6) appears as a rounded pool of barium surrounded by a lucent rim of edema. Extrinsic masses may be seen displacing the stomach and duodenum.

The small bowel, which measures approximately 20 feet (6.1 m) from gastric pylorus to ileocecal valve, is most easily examined by small-bowel series (small-bowel follow-through). This examination comprises a series of radiographs that follow the barium as it passes through the bowel to the colon. The most important findings are abnormal distention or narrowing of the bowel lumen; thickening or nodularity, or both, of the small intestinal mucosal folds; the presence of intraluminal masses; and compression or tethering of the bowel by extraluminal masses (Fig. 3–7). A small-bowel study is indicated when clinical signs and symptoms indicate disease in the small bowel or when a source of bleeding has not been found in the esophagus, the stomach, or the colon after they have been examined by contrast studies or endoscopy. It is too time consuming and expensive to be considered a general screening examination.

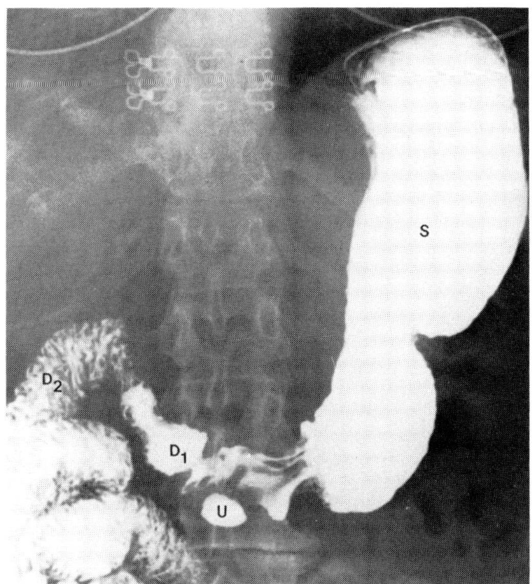

FIGURE 3–6. Benign gastric ulcer and normal duodenum. Isolated oval collection of barium projects outside the antrum of the stomach (S). The benign ulcer mound and radiating folds are diagnostic of peptic ulcer (U). Note the normal duodenal bulb (D1) and the normal descending duodenum (D2). Also, the small bowel is malrotated with several loops of barium-filled bowel in the right abdomen.

The colon is studied through the use of either single- or double-contrast barium enema. Both examinations can reveal small polyps and other intraluminal defects (including benign and malignant mucosal abnormalities), as well as strictures, malrotation, and extrinsic masses; however, the double-contrast examination is superior for evaluation of the mucosal surface (Fig. 3–8), enabling detection of small polyps, superficial erosions, and ulcers. In general, the double-contrast barium enema study can reveal subtle or very early colon disease. The most important abnormalities detectable by means of barium enema are benign and malignant tumors, diverticula, ischemic disease, inflammatory bowel disease, and infectious bowel disease.

Other contrast studies are used when circumstances warrant, which is usually after a standard examination is inconclusive. These include video fluoroscopic esophagram (a video recording of the barium swallow to demonstrate esophageal motility), enteroclysis (a single- or a double-contrast examination of the small bowel after duodenal or jejunal intubation), and peroral pneumocolon (a small-bowel follow-through examination with barium) followed by rectal insufflation of air when barium reaches the right colon. This latter study allows visualization of the proximal right colon and the terminal ileum. Although the liver and the gallbladder can be evaluated with the use of injected or ingested contrast materials (intravenous cholangiogram for the biliary system and oral cholecystogram for the gallbladder), these studies are less commonly performed because CT, ultrasonography, and MRI provide more specific information. The intrahepatic biliary system can be examined through percutaneous needle injection or through endoscopic retrograde injection of the common bile duct and the pancreatic duct (also called endoscopic retrograde cholangiopancreatography) (Fig. 3–9).

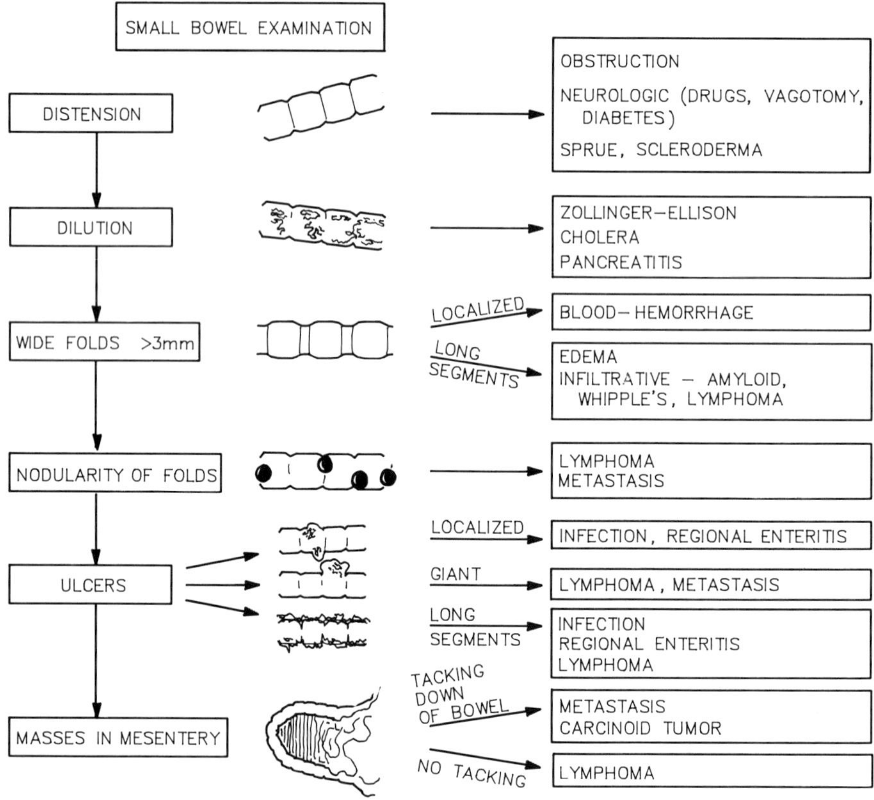

FIGURE 3–7. Small bowel evaluation.

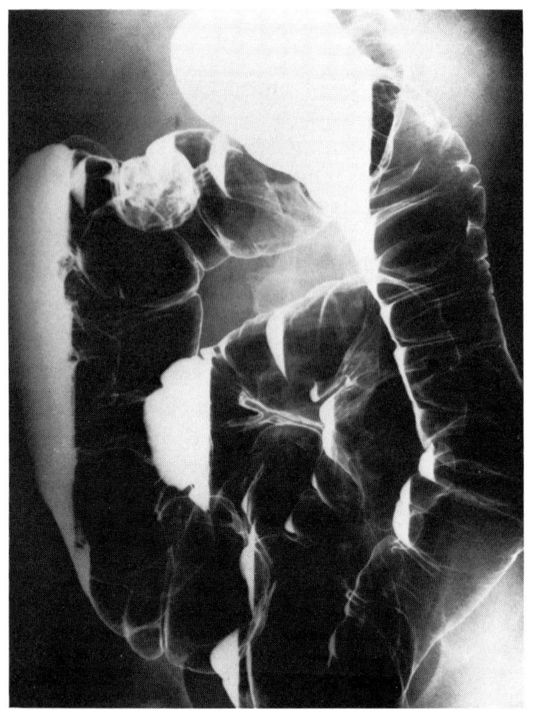

FIGURE 3–8. Full-sized decubitus film of a double-contrast barium enema shows detail of the mucosa of the nondependent side of the bowel. The opposite decubitus view showed the other side of the bowel. The technique can demonstrate polyps, tumors, and other intraluminal masses. In this case, a villous adenoma is demonstrated near the hepatic flexure.

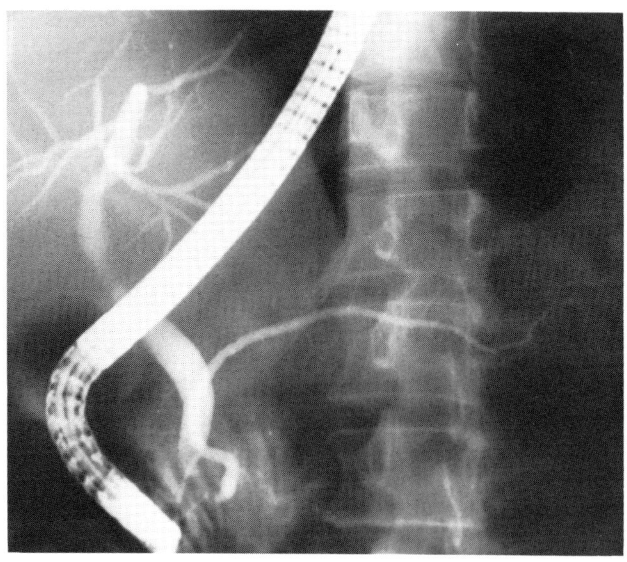

FIGURE 3–9. Biliary and pancreatic ducts. Fluoroscopic spot film, obtained after injection of contrast material into the pancreatic and common bile ducts, shows normal branching and contour of the intra- and extrahepatic biliary system. The pancreatic duct has a mildly irregular contour as a result of senescent changes. The contrast was injected through an endoscope during a retrograde cholangiopancreatic procedure.

Computed Tomography

CT of the abdomen is the standard method for evaluation of the solid abdominal organs, the mesentery, and the retroperitoneum. It is therefore especially valuable in the study of trauma for detecting and assessing multiple injuries, in the study of cancer for evaluating the extent of cancer and metastases, in surgery for planning and follow-up, and for assistance in difficult diagnostic situations. Evaluation includes assessment of organ size and location and the presence of masses and hemorrhage (Fig. 3–10). Upper abdominal transverse images show the lung bases, the liver, the spleen, the stomach, the aorta, and the spine. These structures are evaluated for evidence of pleural effusion, spleen or liver enlargement, gastric distension, and ascites. The liver should have a homogeneous appearance without focal defects. Defects of low or high density are generally attributable to tumor or abscess. Regularly spaced, enlarged, tubular structures of low density usually represent dilated bile ducts and may indicate pancreatic or bile duct tumor, stones, or biliary stricture. Generalized decrease in liver density, revealing the enhancing vessels, indicates fatty liver infiltration. The anterior margin of the spleen should extend to about midabdomen. Midabdominal CT sections show the midliver, the pancreas, the vessels, the adrenal glands, and the left kidney. Important findings include pancreatic calcifications, aortic aneurysm, and renal and adrenal masses. Cystic collections may represent tumors, cysts, or a fluid-filled bowel. The lower CT sections show the inferior liver, both kidneys, the aorta, the vena cava, and the bowel.

Knowledge of anatomical compartments and potential spaces allows precise determination of the locations and the probable causes of many abdominal abnormalities (including blood, pus, and free intraperitoneal fluid). These determinations greatly assist in diagnosis of abdominal disease (Fig. 3–11). The compartments are complex and difficult to visualize in three dimensions; however, an understanding of them is necessary for interpretation of plain film and cross-sectional imaging examinations. The peritoneal cavity is the primary space in the abdomen and contains most of the bowel, the liver, and the spleen. Most of the liver is within the superior right side of the peritoneal cavity. The posterior subhepatic space (Morison's pouch) is the extension of the peritoneal cavity behind the liver. In the supine patient, this space is the most dependent part of the peritoneal cavity and can be a site of collections of pus or blood. The duodenum and transverse colon abut the peritoneal cavity and form the posteroinferior boundary of the anterior subhepatic space. Because the posterior walls of these organs are contiguous with the retroperitoneum, rupture of these segments of bowel can result in intraperitoneal or retroperitoneal extravasation (shown later in Fig. 3–29).

On the left side of the abdomen, the peritoneal cavity surrounds the spleen and the left lobe of the liver. This large space communi-

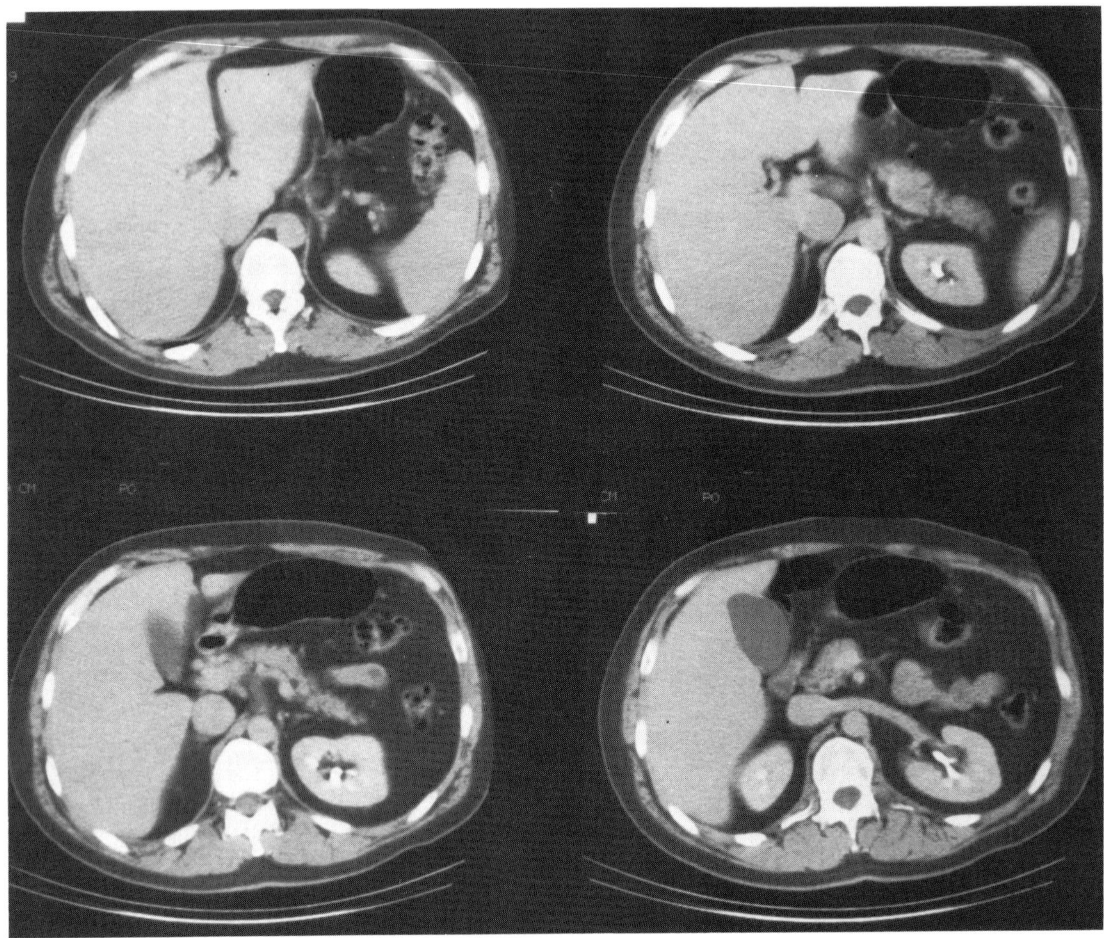

FIGURE 3–10. CT evaluation of the abdomen. Four slices from an abdominal CT demonstrate the normal locations and relationships of structures. In the patient, who had a large amount of abdominal fat, delineation of anatomical structures was excellent. The highest slice (top left) shows the fissure for the falciform ligament separating lateral and medial segments of the left lobe of the liver. The aorta is of normal size; the inferior vena cava (IVC) is intrahepatic. The spleen is seen on the patient's left and the top of the left kidney is visible. The next slice (top right) shows the IVC and more of the left kidney. The right adrenal gland lies behind the IVC; the left adrenal gland has a triangular shape and is anterior and medial to the left kidney. A lower slice (bottom left) shows the pancreas and, dorsal to it, the mesenteric vessels. The bowel is outlined by fat. The lowest slice shows the gallbladder, both kidneys, and the bowel. The left renal vein passes between the aorta and superior mesenteric artery as it enters the IVC. Directly anterior to the IVC is the head of the pancreas. The duodenum lies between the gallbladder and the IVC.

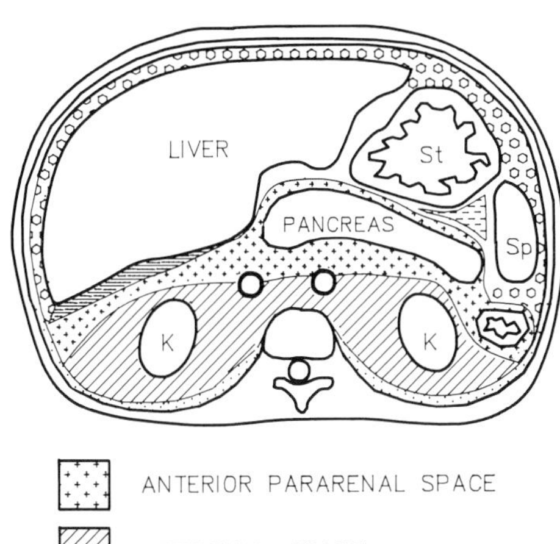

ANTERIOR PARARENAL SPACE

PERIRENAL SPACE

POSTERIOR PARARENAL SPACE

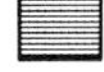

SUBHEPATIC PERITONEAL SPACE (MORISON'S POUCH)

PERITONEAL CAVITY

LESSER SAC

A

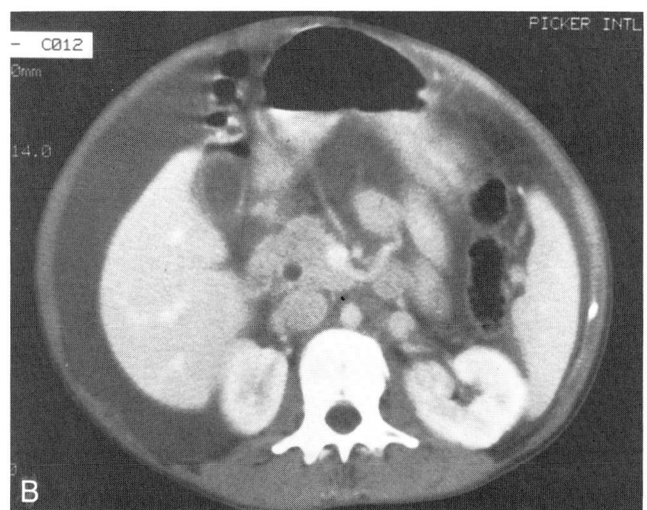

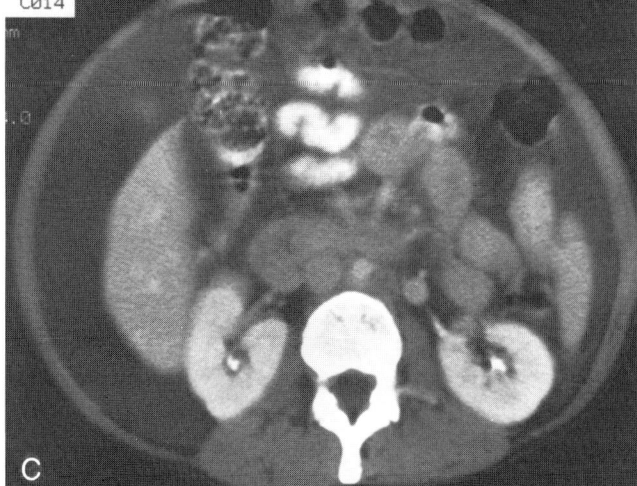

FIGURE 3–11. Anatomical compartments and potential spaces in the abdomen. *A.* Diagram. St, stomach; Sp, spleen; K, kidney. *B.* CT shows a large amount of intraperitoneal fluid; the patient had ascites as a result of portal venous occlusion. The fluid clearly outlines the liver, the spleen, and the bowel. The gallbladder wall is thickened, and fluid is seen within the lesser sac. *C.* Lower slice shows loops of bowel floating in the fluid. The kidneys and vessels are retroperitoneal. (Courtesy of J. Borrow, First Hill Diagnostic Imaging Center, Seattle.)

cates freely with the remainder of the peritoneal cavity, and so abscesses can spread easily. A portion of the peritoneal cavity, called the lesser sac, becomes isolated behind the stomach during development. The lesser sac communicates with the main peritoneal cavity via the foramen of Winslow. It lies behind the stomach, the duodenal bulb, and the lesser omentum and is limited inferiorly by the transverse mesocolon. The lesser sac is an important and frequent site of infection. Inferiorly, the peritoneal cavity contains the small bowel and loops of the sigmoid colon. A central space between the bladder and the rectum, the pouch of Douglas, is often filled with fluid, pus, or blood when the patient is either supine or upright. The peritoneal cavity extends beyond (lateral to) the ascending and descending portions of the colon (which are retroperitoneal), allowing fluid to displace these segments of bowel medially.

The retroperitoneum is divided into the anterior pararenal, the posterior pararenal, and the perirenal spaces. The anterior pararenal space is a thin plane of fat separating the pancreas and the ascending and descending portions of the colon from the peritoneal cavity. It extends vertically down to the pelvis. The posterior pararenal space is a thin rim of fat posteriorly that contains no organs. It extends laterally to form the properitoneal fat seen on plain films. Medially, it follows the psoas muscle. The perirenal space is nearest to the kidney and contains abundant fat surrounding the kidneys and adrenal glands. It extends inferiorly to the level of the iliac crest. These three spaces are important for the diagnosis of effusions, hemorrhage, and abscesses.

The anatomical relationships of the structures in the upper abdomen are constant and are helpful in CT and ultrasonographic studies (Fig. 3–12; see also Figs. 3–10, 3–11). In general, the organs are anterior and the vessels posterior in the abdomen. The relationship of the pancreas to the superior mesenteric artery and vein enables identification of pancreatic masses, adenopathy, and periportal lesions, even when pancreatic tissue is not optimally seen. Distortion of the close relationship of the tail of the pancreas to the splenic vein is indicative of pancreatic tail masses and splenic or perisplenic hemorrhage. Familiarity with the structures that pass between the aorta and the superior mesenteric artery enables differentiation of the duodenum, the lymph nodes, and tumors. Fluid collections, abscesses, and cystic tumors are also detectable from these anatomical relationships in both CT and ultrasonography.

CT best depicts abdominal tissues and other contents of widely differing density, such as fat, air, and calcium. The radiographic contrast of CT is best in patients with an abundance of body fat. Interfaces between tissues or fluids of similar density are not well-delineated by CT. Difficulties that arise in differentiating normal loops of bowel, ureters, and vessels from abnormalities are eliminated in most cases by the use of orally and intravenously administered contrast material. Rectally administered contrast material can assist in pelvic evaluations for tumor or infection.

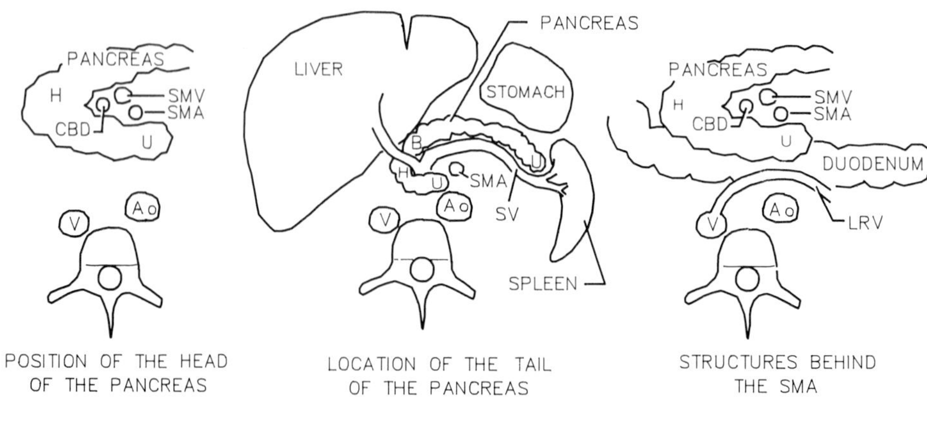

FIGURE 3–12. Anatomy of the upper abdomen. Diagram shows the relationship of the head (H), the body (B), the tail, and the uncinate process (U) of the pancreas. SMA and SMV, superior mesenteric artery and vein; CBD, common bile duct; V, vena cava; Ao, aorta; SV, splenic vein; LRV, left renal vein.

Ultrasonography

Ultrasonography is applied to evaluation of the liver, the biliary system (including the gallbladder), and the pancreas. It is one of two methods used for the diagnosis of acute cholecystitis (the other is the technetium iminodiacetate scan; see Chapter 9) and is the most informative noninvasive technique for evaluating the biliary system (Fig. 3–13). Ultrasonography readily demonstrates dilated ducts and cysts in the pancreas and can assist in the evaluation of liver masses, biliary obstruction, and abdominal infection. As with CT, familiarity with the predictable, normal anatomical relationships enables the ultrasonographer to describe the abnormalities accurately.

Loculated collections of fluid and interfaces between structures are depicted well on ultrasonograms because the sound easily passes through simple fluid collections and is reflected from any tissue interface. Because only a small portion of any large organ (such as the liver or the spleen) is seen at one time and because it is difficult to be sure of surveying an entire organ, ultrasonography is not as reliable as CT in assessing liver metastases or multiple abscesses. CT and ultrasonography are therefore complementary: often both are needed in order to establish a diagnosis. Ultrasonography is most effective for examining a thin patient who has no gaseous distension or extensive calcification. Because the equipment is portable and the examination is easy to perform, ultrasonography is effectively used to direct biopsies, aspirations, and placement of drainage tubes.

Magnetic Resonance Imaging

MRI is applied primarily to the solid organs of the abdomen. As with CT, its greatest value in GI tract evaluation is in evaluating large masses, adenopathy, and metastases. Also, as with CT, MRI of the abdomen is more difficult than imaging of other areas (such as the brain) because of the large size of the abdomen, the variability of appearance of structures, and motion caused by respiration and peristalsis. The tubular GI tract is difficult to image because of peristalsis, lack of adequate spatial resolution, and lack of sufficient difference in tissue contrast between it and surrounding structures. Rapid imaging sequences, motion suppression algorithms, and the capability of showing high tissue contrast allow diagnosis of some tumors and metabolic conditions.

MRI evaluation is similar to CT evaluation. The transverse (axial) views are interpreted in a manner similar to that in CT by identification of the size, the shape, and the intensity of each organ. Coronal views are best for general screening of the abdomen and the initial identification of adenopathy. These views can be evaluated through an approach analogous to the evaluation of the AP abdominal plain film. High-contrast images, especially short TI (inversion time) inversion recovery (STIR) images, show fluid, blood, tumor, pus, and adenopathy as high intensity (Fig. 3–14). An understanding of signal intensity characteristics of various tissues and normal anatomical structures in sagittal, coronal, and transverse planes is the basic requirement for MRI interpretation.

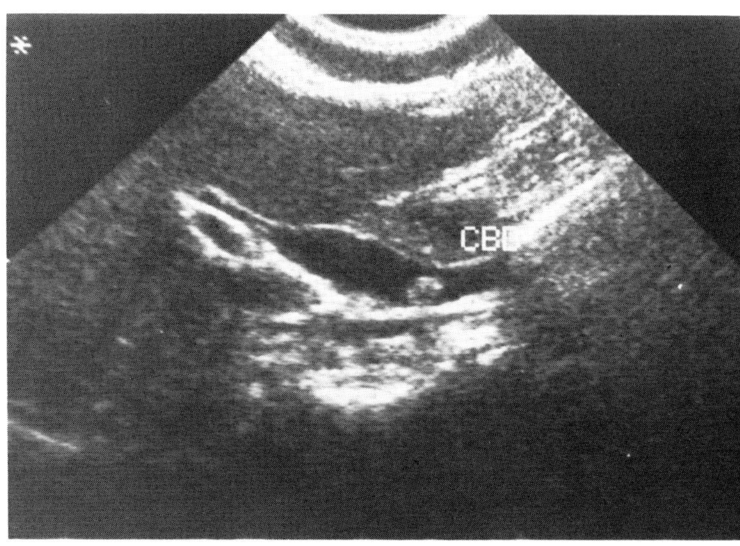

FIGURE 3–13. Common bile duct stone. A longitudinal ultrasonogram shows a stone within the common bile duct. Note the shadowing behind the stone. Proximal to the stone, the common bile duct measures 9 mm.

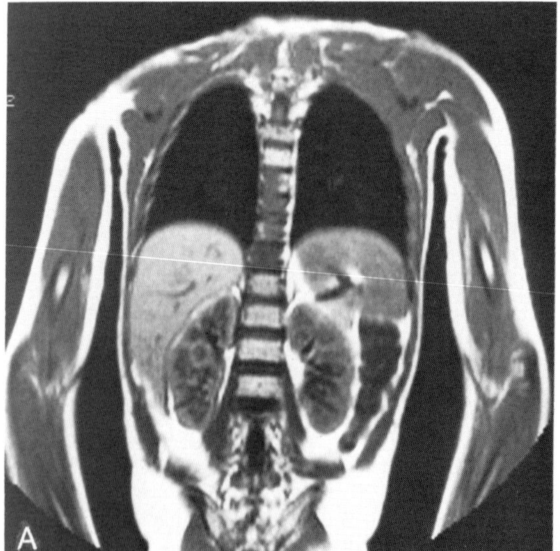

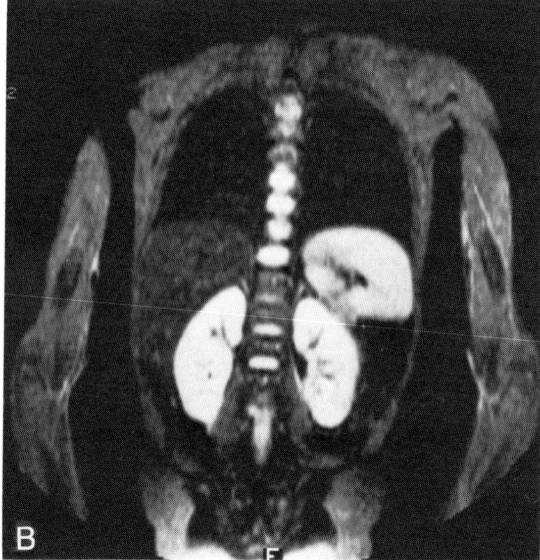

FIGURE 3–14. Coronal abdomen. *A.* Coronal T1 spin echo scan of the posterior abdomen shows the normal appearance of the liver, the kidneys, the spleen, and the descending colon. Because the patient was a 9-year-old child, a large field of view permitted examination of the lungs and the majority of the abdomen. The gray-appearing marrow is normal. The midthoracic vertebral bodies show low intensity because of diffuse involvement by metastatic rhabdomyosarcoma. *B.* Matching short TI inversion recovery (STIR) sequence shows the normal appearance of the liver and normal bone marrow as dark. Fat and muscle also appear dark. The spleen, the gastric contents, and the kidneys have a high-intensity appearance on STIR images. Tumor involving the midthoracic vertebrae is hyperintense (white) on STIR images. Bowel fluid can also be of high intensity; however, in this case, the bowel is filled with air. (Courtesy of J. Smith, First Hill Diagnostic Imaging Center, Seattle.)

The solid portions of the liver and the spleen provide homogeneous MRI signals. The vessels within these organs are well seen because they contribute little or no signal. Because tumors and metabolic diseases are usually characterized by prolonged T1 or T2 relaxation times, the two imaging techniques that have been most successful for liver imaging are the spin echo and inversion recovery techniques. Spin echo technique with a long repetition time (2.0 seconds or longer) and late echo delay (echo time of 80 milliseconds or longer) demonstrates most tumors and focal abnormalities as high-intensity areas that are well-delineated from normal liver and splenic tissue. Vascular displacement and bile duct dilatation can be easily evaluated.

Inversion recovery techniques demonstrate the prolonged T1 of tumor, adenopathy, and fluid collections if repetition and inversion times are chosen properly. For intermediate repetition times (1 to 2 seconds), inversion time can be chosen so that the signal from fat is nearly zero at the time of detection (about 100 to 150 milliseconds). In this technique (called STIR), the signal from muscle is low, that of fat is markedly suppressed, and most abnormalities are of high intensity (Fig. 3–15). The normal liver and pancreas are also of low intensity on STIR images. Fatty liver infiltration gives an appearance similar to that of suppressed fat (very dark). The spleen, the kidneys, and fluid-filled loops of bowel have high intensity (see Fig. 3–14). Normal anatomical relationships and pathological processes in the pancreas can be demonstrated in spin echo and inversion recovery techniques.

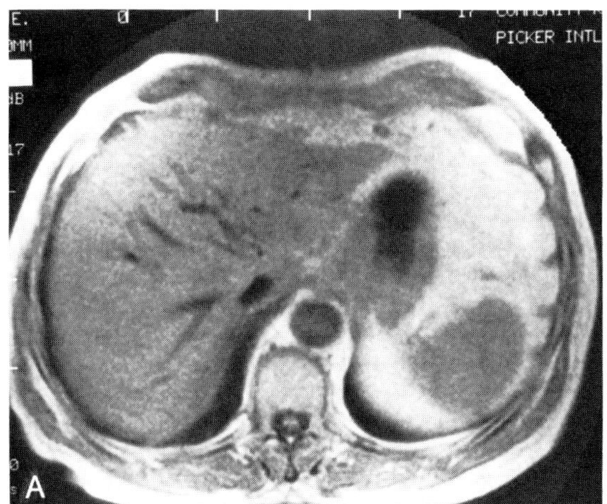

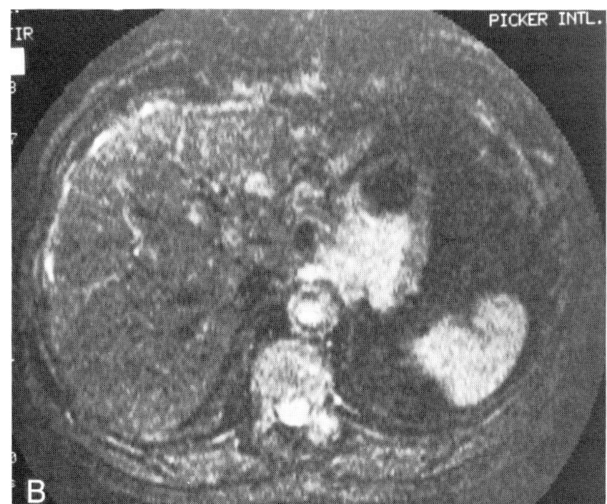

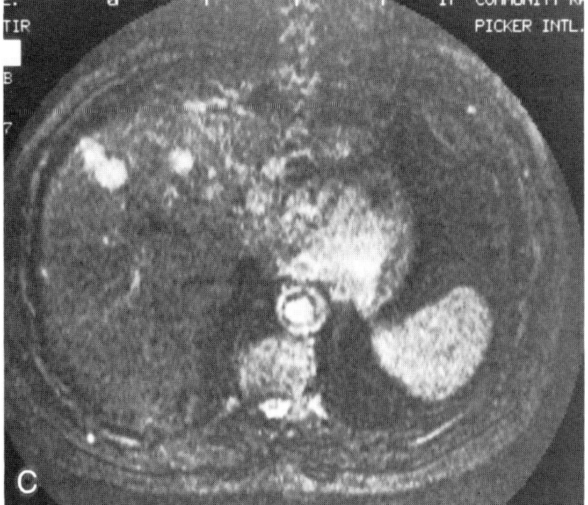

FIGURE 3–15. Adenocarcinoma involving the stomach and esophagus. *A.* T1 spin echo image shows normal appearance of the liver, the spleen, and upper abdominal fat. Thick soft tissue around the posterior stomach is abnormal. *B.* STIR image shows high intensity of abnormal tissue, which represented adenocarcinoma involving the esophagus and the stomach, that was not detected on computed tomography (CT) or radionuclide scan. *C.* STIR image at a lower level shows several peripheral metastatic liver lesions. Note on the STIR image the suppression of the abdominal fat and the high intensity of the tumor, the spleen, the metastatic lesions, cerebrospinal fluid, and blood flow in the aorta. (Courtesy of D. Olson, Bluefield, West Virginia.)

Part I
Alimentary Tract

OVERVIEW

Diseases of the alimentary or tubular GI tract share many similarities despite the different functions of each part of the tract. The presence of a tubular lumen and the sensitivity of the mucosa cause similar appearances of trauma, inflammation, and neoplasms. These general characteristics are described in this section, before discussions of individual alimentary tract organs.

Trauma

Trauma to the GI tract can be caused by either penetration or blunt injury. Penetration trauma, from a knife, a bullet, another projectile, or a surgical instrument, causes laceration of the bowel wall or of the abdominal organs and retroperitoneal structures and may result in hemorrhage. Later, peritonitis or fistula formation may occur. Penetration injuries that appear to be entirely above the diaphragm may injure subdiaphragmatic organs (see Fig. 2–11). Upper GI series or enemas with water-soluble contrast material are indicated when penetration injury to the tubular GI tract is suspected. Iodinated, water-soluble contrast is used because barium leaking into the mediastinal, intraperitoneal, or extraperitoneal cavities causes a granulomatous inflammatory reaction, whereas iodine solutions do not. Such examinations can demonstrate extravasation of contrast material caused by bowel laceration or obstruction caused by submucosal hemorrhage or bowel-wall edema.

Blunt injury to the abdomen may involve fixed portions of the tubular GI tract, such as the esophagus as it crosses the diaphragm, the retroperitoneal portion of the duodenum, the ascending and descending portions of the colon, and the rectum. The movable intraperitoneal loops of small intestine, the sigmoid colon, and the stomach are able to move away from the blunt force and are usually not damaged. The most common blunt injuries result in intramural or mesenteric hematoma. As with penetration injuries, contrast examinations with water-soluble material are most informative in evaluation of injury to the tubular GI tract, but contrast CT (including diluted oral contrast) is most informative in evaluation of blunt abdominal injury because it can demonstrate injuries to adjacent organs and the mesentery.

Congenital Abnormalities

Most congenital abnormalities of the alimentary tract are caused by in utero vascular accidents or by failure of recanalization of the gut or are related to abnormal positions of the gut that result from incomplete in utero rotation and subsequent abnormal attachments and bands.

Inflammation and Infection

Inflammatory disease may affect any part of the alimentary tract. Whereas peptic inflammatory disease is most common in the esophagus, the stomach, and the duodenum, regional enteritis (Crohn's disease) involves predominantly the small bowel and the colon. Regional enteritis often involves several segments of these portions of the GI tract, and the terminal ileum is the most common site. Ulcerative colitis affects predominantly the colon, usually the distal portion, and is characterized by involvement of a continuous portion of the colon. It may involve the entire colon.

Infectious involvement of the alimentary tract depends on the effectiveness of protective mechanisms, types of irritants, and the ability of the normal flora of the gut to suppress opportunistic infection. Different infections therefore occur in typical locations (Fig. 3–16). Many infections of the esophagus and the stomach are viral because these organs are protected from bacterial and parasitic agents by oral and gastric secretions. In the middle and distal portions of the bowel, normal flora and the composition of bowel contents facilitate infection of the alimentary tract by a wider variety of organisms.

Neoplasms

Tumors of the alimentary tract are most common in the proximal and distal portions, probably because they are most frequently

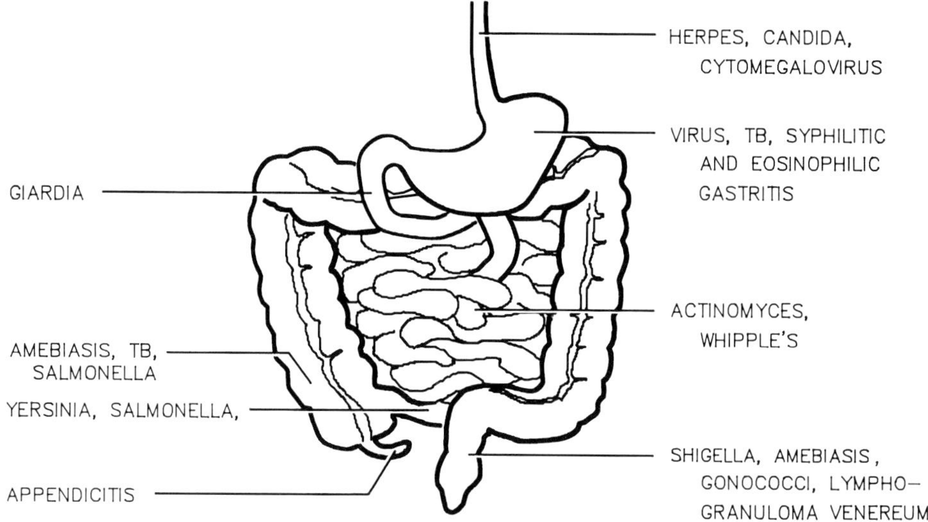

FIGURE 3–16. Locations of infection in the alimentary tract. TB, tuberculosis.

exposed to carcinogens and because of the propensity of these tissues to undergo malignant transformation as a result of chronic irritation. Tumors of the small bowel are rare. Metastatic tumor to the bowel can occur from any source, but hematogenous spread of most tumors, notably those of the lung and the breast and melanoma, are most common. They produce ulcerating, submucosal lesions, often described as having a bull's-eye appearance on barium examinations. Primary abdominal and pelvic tumors also spread to the alimentary tract by direct extension. Ovarian carcinoma is noted for seeding of the mesentery, the omentum, and the serosal surfaces of the bowel. Lymphoma, usually the non-Hodgkin's type, involves the bowel or the mesentery in many patients. Various premalignant lesions, including polyps, are found throughout the alimentary tract, especially in association with certain polyposis syndromes, with inflammatory bowel disease, and with chronic irritation.

Vascular Disease

Vascular diseases occur in all parts of the alimentary tract. In the proximal and distal ends, in which the blood supply is rich, the usual manifestation is hemorrhage. The cause of hemorrhage may be ulceration, inflammation, obstruction, or necrosis resulting from tumor or ischemia. In the middle portions of the bowel, in which arterial blood supply is tenuous, ischemic necrosis is more common.

Motility Disorders

The peristalsis that propels food through the gut depends on a complex pattern of neuromuscular coordination. It can be disturbed by neuromuscular abnormalities as well as local factors such as obstruction, stricture, inflammation, and tumor. Such disorders are most important in the proximal portion of the alimentary tube, in which function and coordination is most complex. Evaluation of motility disorders requires real-time fluoroscopic examination to demonstrate the abnormal esophageal or bowel peristalsis.

Diverticular Disease

Diverticula of the GI tract are outpouchings of the mucosa either acquired through weakened muscularis or caused by traction on the outer wall. They occur throughout the GI tract. Esophageal diverticula produce symptoms of dysphagia and obstruction. In the colon, inflamed diverticula result in infection, hemorrhage, and bowel rupture. Elsewhere, they are usually asymptomatic. A diverticulum can be distinguished from a polyp on a barium contrast study because it projects outside the

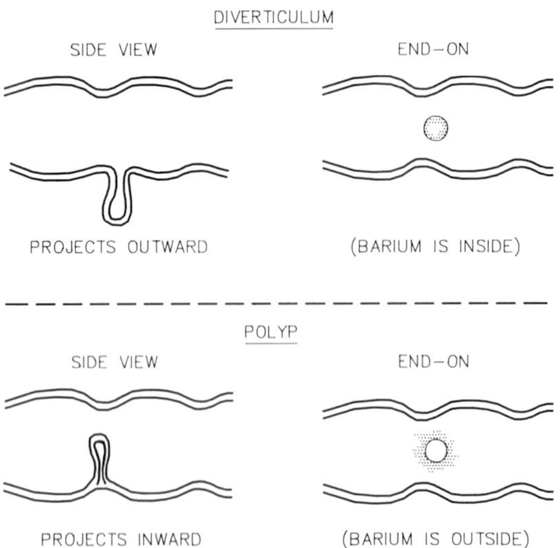

FIGURE 3–17. Appearance of polyp and diverticulum on contrast gastrointestinal (GI) examination.

lumen and because it fills with barium (Fig. 3–17; see also Fig. 3–52).

ESOPHAGUS

Trauma

Penetration injuries to the esophagus from a knife or a bullet can cause esophageal rupture and communication with the mediastinum. Leakage of esophageal contents into the mediastinum causes mediastinitis, a serious and often fatal inflammatory response. Entrance of such material into the tracheobronchial tree results in chronic aspiration and lung disease. Blunt or deceleration trauma can sever the esophagus at its distal site of fixation at the diaphragm. The most common causes of lower esophageal ruptures are iatrogenic and include the placement of esophageal and gastric tubes used to drain the stomach, tamponade bleeding esophageal varices, or dilate esophageal strictures. Diagnostic endoscopy can cause esophageal rupture, but this is rare. Evaluation of acute esophageal injury is by single-contrast, water-soluble esophagram. It can show extravasation or mucosal injury. CT accurately shows contrast extravasation, pneumomediastinum, and pleural effusion.

Spontaneous Esophageal Rupture. Spontaneous esophageal rupture (Boerhaave's syndrome) occurs when the esophageal pressure is raised abruptly. Common precipitating factors include severe vomiting, blunt trauma, and, in rare instances, childbirth. The tear is usually at the left posterolateral part of the lower third of the esophagus and causes rapidly developing pleural effusion and pneumomediastinum, well demonstrated on plain films (see Fig. 2–16). The air from pneumomediastinum may dissect into the soft tissues of the neck. Immediate surgical drainage is indicated because empyema and mediastinitis develop within 24 hours of the injury.

Mallory-Weiss Tear. The Mallory-Weiss tear is a linear perforation of the esophageal mucosa and submucosa. Such perforations (which are often multiple) occur in alcoholics as a result of violent retching or vomiting after a drinking binge. Other causes of severe vomiting, such as gastritis or brainstem tumor, can also result in Mallory-Weiss tears. Patients commonly have hematemesis but, because actual esophageal rupture does not occur, do not have symptoms of mediastinitis or pleural irritation. Nearly all Mallory-Weiss tears (95%) are evident on endoscopy, but they are difficult to diagnose on radiographs because (1) it is difficult to fully distend the esophageal lumen and (2) the vertical linear tears have an appearance similar to that of mucosal folds. Mallory-Weiss tears may require surgical intervention but usually heal spontaneously in 48 to 72 hours.

Congenital Abnormalities

Because the esophagus develops embryologically from the foregut at the same time as the lung, some abnormalities associated with the esophagus also involve the tracheobronchial tree. The most important congenital abnormalities of the esophagus are atresia (often with associated communication between the esophagus and the trachea), duplication, and obstructing webs. Compression of the esophagus by vascular rings, pulmonary slings, and brachiocephalic vessels is uncommon and usually does not cause high-grade obstruction.

Esophageal Atresia and Tracheoesophageal Fistula. Congenital absence of a segment of the esophagus (esophageal atresia) is a rare failure of formation at the time of separation of the respiratory diverticulum from the foregut. It is often accompanied by tracheoesophageal fistula. Esophageal atresia is evident shortly after birth because the infant is unable to retain food. If the esophagus communicates with the trachea, food or secretions are aspirated into the lungs, which causes respiratory distress or pneumonia. The most common form of esophageal atresia occurs at the mid-esophageal level and is associated with communication between the trachea and lower esophagus (Fig. 3–18). The barium esophagram is used for both diagnosis and follow-up after surgical repair. Vertebral, cardiac, and renal anomalies are often also present and should be sought on radiographs. The esophageal portion that is absent and the type of communication with the trachea determine the seriousness of symptoms and the type of surgical treatment available. Surgical repair is usually successful, but stenosis and absent lower esophageal peristalsis can limit function.

Esophageal Duplication. Esophageal duplication is a rare error of foregut development. The duplicated segment is usually a hollow intramural mass; its lumen does not communicate with the true esophageal lumen.

Esophageal Webs, Rings, and Vascular Slings. Congenital esophageal webs and rings are rare but can obstruct the esophageal lumen. Esophageal webs are infrequently found incidentally (4%) in patients examined with upper GI series for other GI complaints and are usually located in the cervical esophagus. Congenital external restrictive bands or rings can occur anywhere in the esophagus. Occasionally, these rings are cartilaginous (predominantly in the lower third of the esophagus).

External compression of the esophagus by aberrant vessels (vascular rings and pulmonary slings) causes indentation of the esophagus and is easily shown on barium esophagram. The most common vessels to compress the esophagus are an isolated, aberrant subclavian artery (which passes behind the esophagus and causes an oblique posterior indentation), an aberrant left pulmonary artery (which passes in front of the esophagus, compressing it anteriorly), and variations of the double aortic arch. When an aberrant subclavian artery or a double aortic arch is associated with a vascular ring, circumferential impression of the esophagus results. Because these patients also have tracheal compression, wheezing and other respiratory symptoms occur. When the esophagram suggests a vascular ring, MRI or angiography can confirm the anatomical variant before surgery.

Inflammation

Toxic Injury. The esophagus can be injured by endogenous and exogenous agents. The

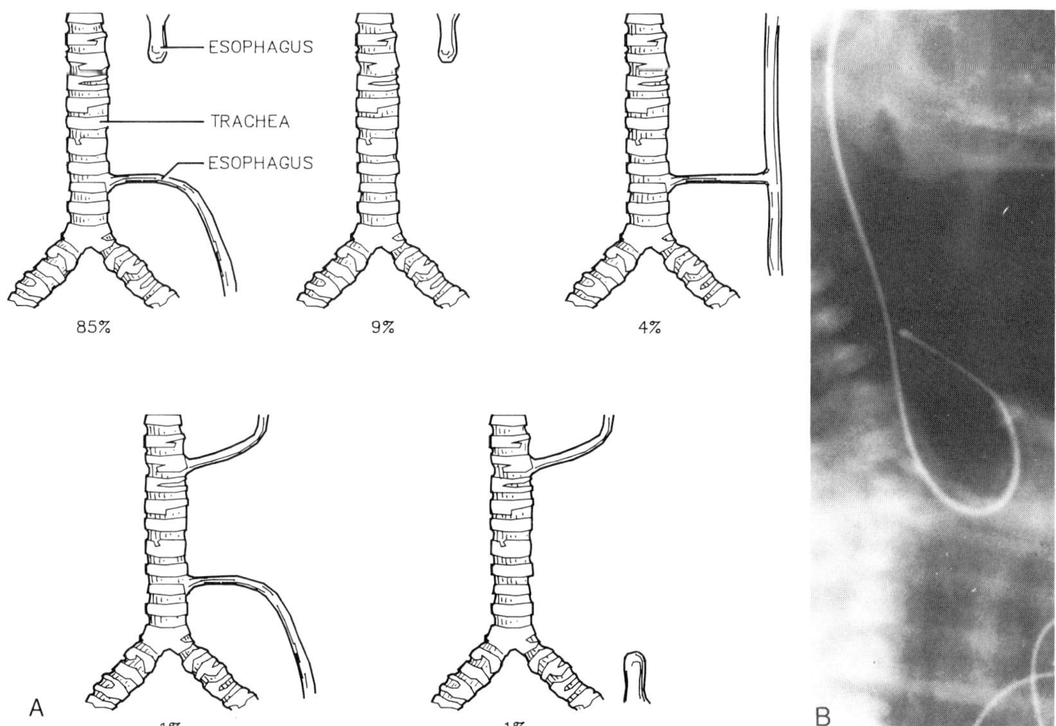

FIGURE 3–18. Tracheoesophageal fistula and atresia. *A.* Diagram. *B.* Plain film shows nasogastric tube in a blind pouch at the termination of the esophagus in a patient with the most common type of tracheoesophageal fistula.

most common exogenous agents are lye, drain cleaners, dishwasher detergent, and acids. Alkaline substances penetrate deep into the esophageal mucosa and cause more serious injuries than do acids. The radiographic appearance of caustic injuries varies, depending on how long after injury the film is made. Initially, contrast can be demonstrated within submucosal irregularities. Altered motility develops later as a result of interruption of the normal peristalsis. Strictures and ulceration develop within 2 weeks after a severe injury (Fig. 3–19). Long-term complications of such injuries include chronic aspiration, gastroesophageal reflux, mediastinal fibrosis, and the development of carcinoma of the esophagus.

Reflux Esophagitis. Esophagitis caused by endogenous acid occurs when gastric acid flows back into the lower esophagus through an incompetent lower esophageal sphincter or a hiatal hernia. Patients develop burning epigastric pain (heartburn) shortly after eating. The pain is worst when the patient lies supine and improves when the patient sits or stands upright. It may mimic chest pain from cardiac disease. Nearly all patients with chronic reflux esophagitis have hiatal hernia or Barrett's esophagus (to be discussed). Other conditions associated with reflux esophagitis include obesity, scleroderma (caused by incompetence of the lower esophageal sphincter and absence of peristalsis in the esophagus), indwelling nasogastric tubes, and gastric surgery.

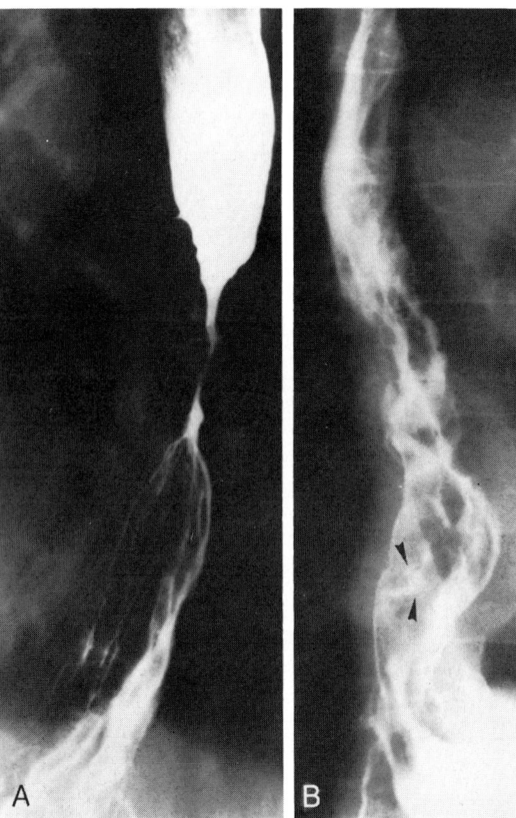

FIGURE 3–19. Esophageal inflammation. *A.* Stricture. Esophagram shows extensive stricture caused by long-term gastroesophageal reflux. *B.* Ulceration is present throughout Barrett's-type mucosa of the lower esophagus. A persistent deformity *(arrowheads)* represented esophageal carcinoma.

The biphasic esophagram is most effective in evaluating esophagitis by showing mucosal thickening, nodularity, erosions, ulcerations, stricture, spasm, and spiculated margins. Associated findings include reflux, hiatal hernia, and stricture formation. Mild reflux esophagitis produces mucosal erythema without demonstrable radiological abnormalities. More advanced disease causes inflammation of the esophageal mucosa, which results in a granular appearance and thickening or slight irregularity of folds. More severe esophagitis produces more fold thickening and ulcerations, usually just proximal to the esophagogastric junction.

Superficial ulcerations often have a linear appearance, with fine radiating folds and slight retraction of the wall. The ulcerations are usually longitudinal and must be distinguished from barium collections between normal folds. Stricture is identified by fixed deformity and lack of distensibility. Ulcers similar to those seen in the stomach and the duodenum can also be seen in the esophagus and appear as deeper focal lesions. These ulcers are usually near the esophagogastric junction and are always associated with hiatal hernia. They may also occur in the midesophagus in patients with Barrett's esophagus.

The radiological findings of inflammation and ulceration are not specific for reflux esophagitis and can also be seen in caustic esophagitis and esophageal infection. The enlarged, serpiginous, irregular folds seen in reflux esophagitis can simulate esophageal varices or varicoid carcinoma of the esophagus. In reflux esophagitis, the response to treatment on follow-up examinations indicates the correct diagnosis. Varices change in size or shape or may disappear during esophageal contraction or distension, whereas the changes associated with carcinoma and esophagitis remain constant. In indeterminate cases, biopsy or close follow-up is required.

Treatment of reflux esophagitis requires elimination or neutralization of gastric acid secretions and the prevention of reflux. Antacids and histamine blockers, as well as dietary changes, reduce the acid content and secretions in the stomach. Slight elevation of the head and thorax reduces reflux. Hiatal hernia and an incompetent esophageal sphincter can be repaired surgically.

Barrett's Esophagus. The presence of columnar gastric mucosa in the lower esophagus (Barrett's esophagus) is associated with excessive acid in the lower esophagus. This displacement of gastric mucosa may be either congenital or the result of changes caused by chronic reflux esophageal irritation. Barrett's esophagus is associated with an increased incidence of adenocarcinoma of the columnar epithelium of the distal esophagus. In contrast, squamous cell tumors occur throughout the esophagus (see Fig. 3–19*B*).

Hiatal Hernia. Hiatal hernia, the herniation of a portion of the stomach through the diaphragm, is a common abnormality that often results in reflux of gastric contents and digestive juices into the lower esophagus. The abnormality can be either an elevation of the cardia of the stomach through the esophageal hiatus in the diaphragm (sliding hernia) (Fig. 3–20) or a true hernia of the stomach through a separate defect in the diaphragm, which is usually caused by traumatic diaphragmatic rupture. Patients with symptomatic hiatal hernias experience the burning epigastric pain of reflux esophagitis. Most hiatal hernias do not cause symptoms. However, most patients with symptoms of esophagitis have hiatal hernia.

The radiographic diagnosis of hiatal hernia requires both physiological and radiological evaluation, both of which can be conducted during an upper GI examination. Demonstration of reflux of barium from the stomach into the esophagus can be shown during fluoroscopy by use of various maneuvers, including placement of the examination table in the head-lowered position, having the patient perform the Valsalva maneuver, or application of pressure to the stomach. Hiatal hernia is easily diagnosed when the hernia is large, but the demonstration of small or intermittent herniations requires careful attention to technique. Patients with symptomatic hiatal hernia are first treated with antacids. If this therapy is unsuccessful, surgical repair is curative.

Radiation Injury. Radiation to the mediastinum for the treatment of Hodgkin's disease, esophageal carcinoma, metastatic disease to the mediastinum, and lung cancer can cause motility disturbances, acute esophagitis, or the later development of esophageal strictures. The severity of the injury depends on the amount of radiation and the duration of therapy. Most symptomatic patients have received more than 4500 rad over a period of less than 8 weeks. The appearance is similar to that

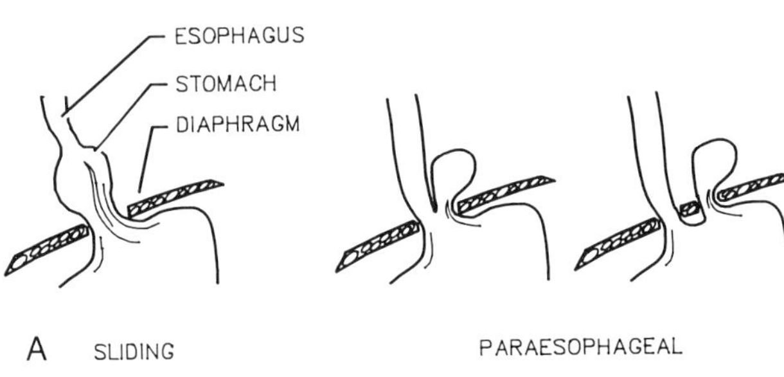

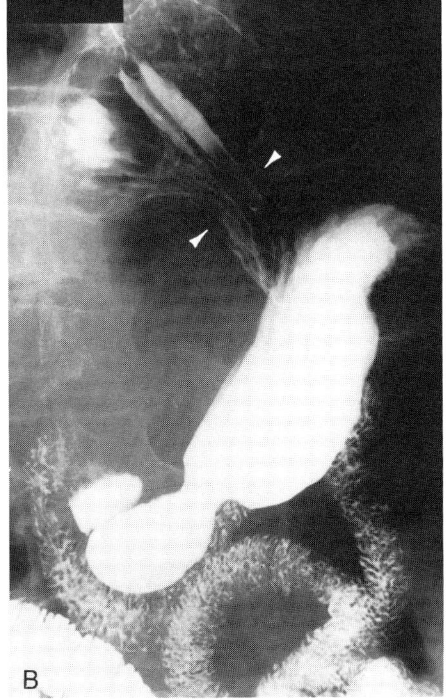

FIGURE 3–20. Hiatal hernia. *A.* Diagram. *B.* Sliding hiatal hernia. Upper GI series shows a large herniation of stomach above the diaphragm *(arrowheads).*

caused by esophagitis. The disease is confined to the irradiated portion.

Inflammatory Disease. Nonspecific inflammatory diseases can affect the esophagus but are uncommon. Regional enteritis (Crohn's disease) seldom involves the esophagus, but when it does, other parts of the GI tract are almost always involved as well. Esophageal lesions seen in regional enteritis include longitudinal and transverse ulcerations and aphthous lesions similar to those seen elsewhere in the GI tract (to be discussed). Less common inflammatory diseases of the esophagus include bullous pemphigoid, Behçet's disease, and dermatomyositis.

Infection

Infectious lesions of the esophagus usually occur in debilitated or immunosuppressed patients. The most important infections of the esophagus are viral (herpes simplex and cytomegalovirus) and fungal, mainly *Candida albicans* (the most common cause of infection of the esophagus) and *Candida tropicalis* (a more virulent fungus that invades the gut).

Viral Infection. Viral infections of the esophagus are usually caused by herpes simplex or cytomegalovirus. They occur in debilitated or immunosuppressed patients such as those with cancer, those receiving immunosuppressive chemotherapy, and those with primary diseases of the immune system, including acquired immunodeficiency syndrome (AIDS). The primary symptom of viral esophagitis is severe odynophagia. Barium esophagram shows ulcers and linear irregular, nondistensible defects in the lower two thirds of the esophagus (Fig. 3–21; see also Fig. 3–5). The distinction between herpes and cytomegalovirus cannot always be made on radiographs, although cytomegalovirus ulcers are often very large. Viral esophagitis is usually self-limiting.

Candidiasis. *Candida albicans* and *C. tropicalis* affect the oropharynx and the esophagus of patients with immunosuppression or with advanced cancer or when antibiotic therapy has suppressed the normal oral flora and allowed overgrowth of other organisms. The usual symptom is odynophagia (painful swallowing); about half of patients with esophageal candidiasis also have oral infection (thrush). Barium esophagram shows abnormal peristalsis and varying degrees of ulceration and exudate, which cause a shaggy appearance of the mucosa that may involve long segments of the esophagus (Fig. 3–22). The identification of a cobblestone appearance caused by a combination of ulcers and plaques is helpful for establishing the diagnosis. In some patients, the entire esophagus is involved. The infection responds well to oral antifungal agents.

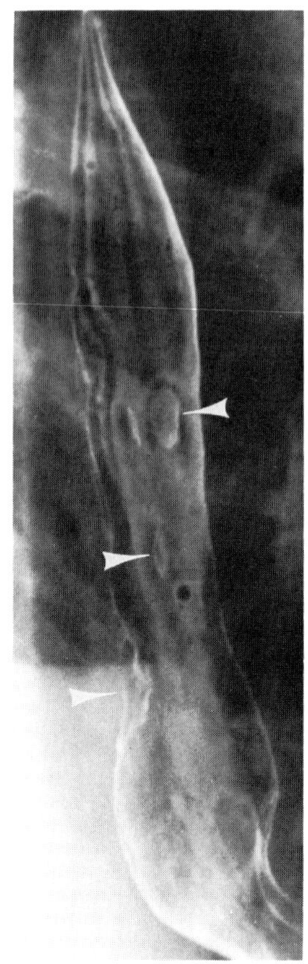

FIGURE 3–21. Cytomegalovirus infection. Esophagram in a patient with cytomegalovirus esophagitis shows several oval ulcerations of varying size scattered throughout the lower esophagus *(arrowheads)*.

Neoplasms

Benign tumors of the esophagus are rare and seldom symptomatic until they become large. The most common is the leiomyoma, a tumor of smooth muscle that arises in the wall of the lower two thirds of the esophagus. The usual radiographic appearance is a smooth, submucosal mass without associated obstruction. Other, less common benign tumors of the esophagus include squamous papilloma, lipoma, neurofibroma, and inflammatory polyp. Malignancy of the esophagus depends on the transformation of squamous cell epithe-

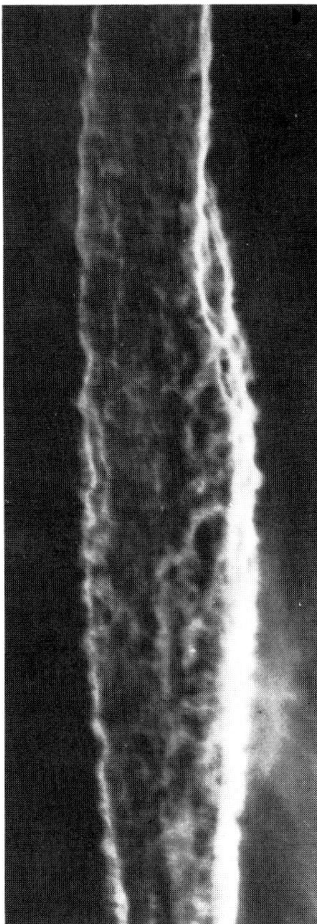

FIGURE 3–22. *Candida* esophagitis. Esophagram shows irregular and ragged esophageal mucosa in an immunosuppressed patient. *Candida* infection is primarily exudative rather than ulcerative.

lium to squamous cell carcinoma. Adenocarcinoma can develop from columnar epithelium in Barrett's esophagus as a result of changes caused by reflux esophagitis. Other tumors of the esophagus include metastases (especially bronchogenic carcinoma and melanoma), lymphoma, and leiomyosarcoma. Gastric carcinoma sometimes spreads to the esophagus by direct invasion.

Esophageal Carcinoma. Primary squamous cell carcinoma is the most common malignant tumor of the esophagus. It may occur anywhere in the esophagus and is most common in men aged 60 to 70 years. The tumor is associated with chronic irritation, such as that caused by long-term alcohol abuse and cigarette smoking. Other predisposing conditions include head and neck tumors, achalasia, and lye stricture. Adenocarcinoma is almost always associated with Barrett's esophagus. Patients with esophageal carcinoma generally have symptoms of increasing dysphagia and weight loss.

Nearly all primary esophageal carcinomas are of the squamous cell type. In very rare instances, a primary adenocarcinoma arises in the esophagus. Adenocarcinoma found in the lower esophagus is usually the result of spread of a gastric carcinoma or has developed from Barrett's-type epithelium (see Figs. 3–15 and 3–19*B*). Patients with esophageal carcinoma develop dysphagia and initially have difficulty swallowing solid foods. As the disease progresses, obstruction of liquids develops. Weight loss may result from lack of food intake and the generalized cachexia of cancer. Chest pain can develop when the tumor invades the mediastinum, and exsanguination may occur when major vessels are eroded.

The radiographic diagnosis of esophageal carcinoma is best made by barium esophagram, which can show several patterns (Fig. 3–23). Early lesions are broad-based, slightly elevated, 2 × 4 mm mucosal plaques. Shallow ulceration may be present on the surface of the plaque. Late findings are mural infiltration, constriction, ulceration, and fistula formation. The infiltrative malignant lesions cause an irregular, tapered stricture and, often, an abrupt, shelf-like margin. The stricture may appear similar to that seen in esophagitis. Therefore, patients with benign-appearing strictures should receive follow-up examinations in order to determine whether healing occurs. Biopsy is usually necessary to distinguish between postinflammatory strictures and carcinoma.

Some esophageal tumors are multifocal because of the spread of tumors to other parts of the esophagus (and to other organs) by the lymphatics. Some esophageal carcinomas are polypoid masses (usually adenocarcinomas) that cause luminal narrowing and irregularity. When these lesions are elongated and irregular or nodular, they may simulate esophageal varices. This type of tumor, called a varicoid carcinoma of the esophagus, does not change in appearance from film to film or during fluoroscopic maneuvers, whereas varices change configuration with changes in the patient's position, with changes in degree of distention of the esophagus, and during the Valsalva maneuver. Varicoid carcinoma is a more invasive type of tumor and spreads quickly into the trachea and the paraesophageal mediastinum.

CT or MRI is required in order to fully define the extent of tumor and to stage the disease. The most important findings are invasion of the mediastinum and adenopathy.

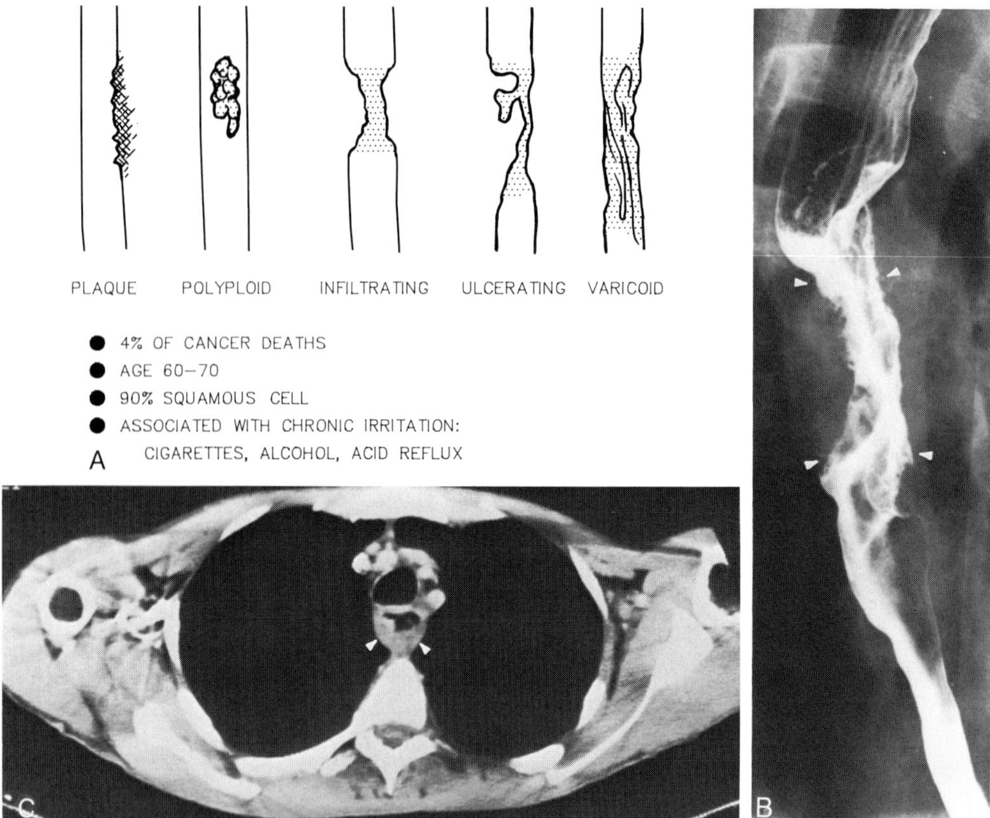

FIGURE 3–23. Esophageal carcinoma. *A.* Diagram. *B.* Esophagram shows a circumferentially infiltrating lesion of the midesophagus *(arrowheads)* in a patient with severe dysphagia. The irregular surface pattern is caused by mucosal destruction. *C.* CT in a different patient shows involvement of the posterior and right lateral wall of the esophagus by an infiltrative squamous cell carcinoma. Note the irregular wall thickening and deformation of the lumen *(arrowheads).*

Vascular encasement, lung or airway invasion, and liver involvement are indications of advanced, inoperable disease.

Esophageal carcinoma is both destructive and invasive. Adjacent spread via the lymphatics involves other areas of the esophagus and the mediastinum. Direct extension into the mediastinum can involve the airway, the vessels, and the nerves, including the vagus and the recurrent laryngeal nerves. Although gastric carcinoma can cross the diaphragm to involve the esophagus, it is less common for esophageal carcinoma to spread to the stomach. Liver metastases indicate disseminated disease (see Fig. 3–15).

Because the tumor is usually detected late in its development, the prognosis for patients with esophageal carcinoma is poor. Tumors in the upper half are treated by radiation. Limited tumors in the lower half can be treated surgically. However, therapy seldom results in cure. Most patients die within 6 to 12 months after diagnosis. Resection is unsuccessful when the tumor has penetrated into the mediastinum.

Other Esophageal Malignancies. Other malignancies of the esophagus are caused by extension from gastric tumors and gastric lymphoma. Direct spread from lung carcinoma occasionally involves the esophagus. The distinction is best made with CT, which can show the primary lesion, local invasion, and adenopathy (Fig. 3–24).

Vascular Diseases

Esophageal Varices. Vascular abnormalities of the esophagus are almost always acquired. The most important is esophageal varices, which are submucosal esophageal veins that become dilated when venous blood flow is obstructed. The obstruction can affect the veins of the lower esophagus, which join the

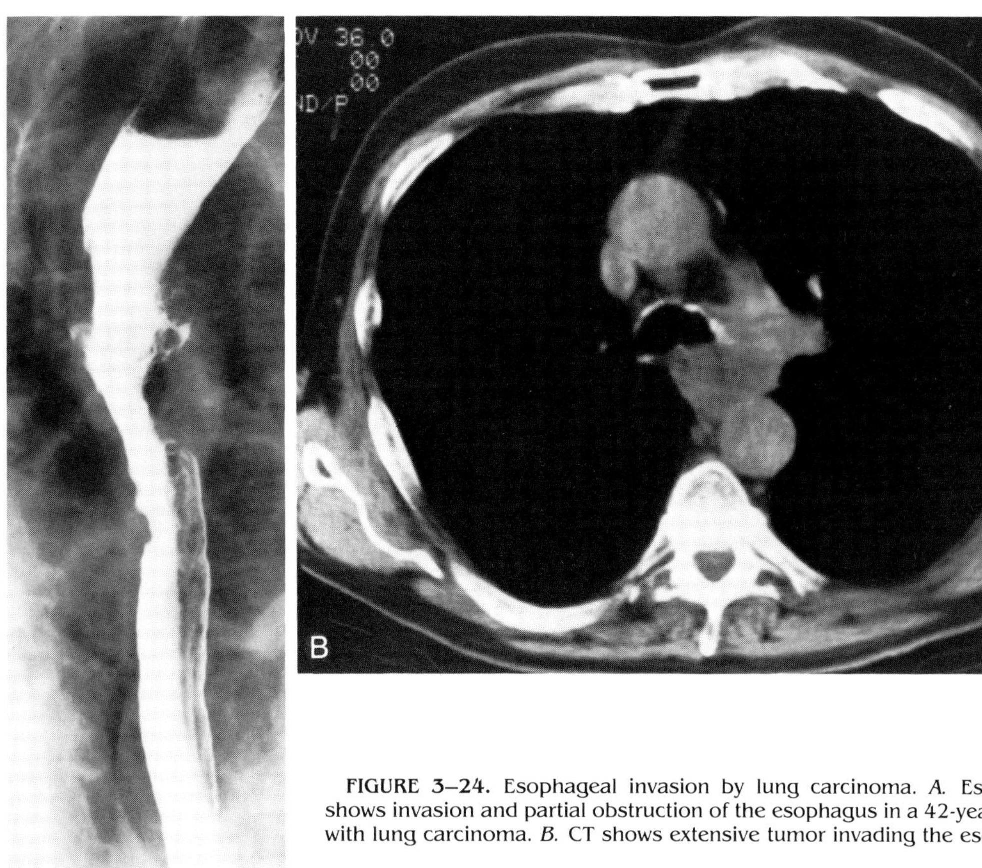

FIGURE 3–24. Esophageal invasion by lung carcinoma. *A.* Esophagram shows invasion and partial obstruction of the esophagus in a 42-year-old man with lung carcinoma. *B.* CT shows extensive tumor invading the esophagus.

portal venous system, or the veins of the upper esophagus, which drain into the azygos vein and the superior vena cava. Alcoholic cirrhosis of the liver is the most common cause of lower esophageal varices, but other causes of portal venous obstruction such as splenic vein thrombosis, obstruction of the inferior vena cava at the level of the right atrium, congestive heart failure, and congenital hepatic fibrosis can also cause varices. Obstruction of the cephalic venous drainage of the esophagus is usually associated with the superior mediastinal syndrome caused by lung cancer or by metastatic or chronic mediastinal inflammatory disease, such as histoplasmosis. Trauma and surgery may also cause obstruction of the azygos vein or the superior vena cava.

When these dilated veins rupture into the esophageal lumen, the patient vomits bright red blood and develops signs of acute blood loss (i.e., hypotension with tachycardia). The diagnosis of variceal bleeding is made clinically by the presence of hematemesis, and the varices are best identified by endoscopy. Occasionally, the radiologist is asked to identify varices in a patient who is not actively bleeding. They can sometimes be shown as serpentine filling defects that change in size with a Valsalva maneuver during barium esophagram (Fig. 3–25). However, in many cases, the barium examination fails to demonstrate them. When varices are actively bleeding, angiography can identify the source.

Acute treatment includes management of blood pressure and control of bleeding. The bleeding varices can be tamponaded with the use of an esophageal tube fitted with a balloon that can be inflated to compress the varices. Other therapy can be administered by the radiologist. Sometimes the bleeding can be controlled by the infusion of intra-arterial pressor agents to cause spasm of the feeding arteries. Embolization of the blood supply (usually the left gastric artery) can decrease the inflow to the varices. Ultimately, most patients require a splenorenal or portocaval shunt to bypass the liver and thus relieve the pressure on the bleeding vessels.

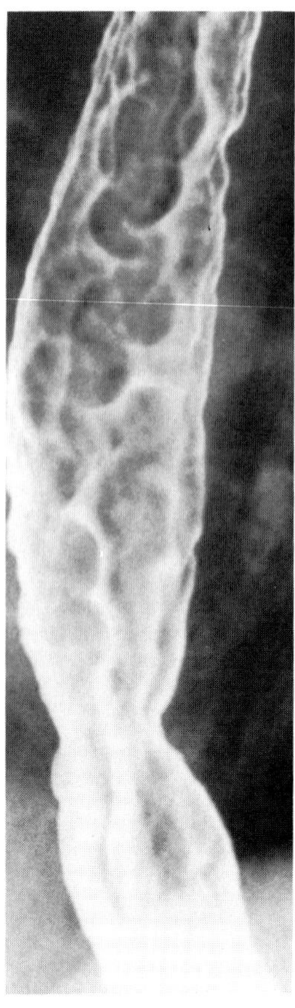

FIGURE 3–25. Esophageal varices. Esophagram shows large serpiginous folds in the distal esophagus of an alcoholic patient with liver disease. These varices changed shape during the examination, which ruled out a varicoid carcinoma of the esophagus.

Motility Disorders

Normal esophageal peristalsis consists of primary and secondary stripping waves. The primary wave is initiated by swallowing and progresses by sequential activation of successively lower nerve fibers in the esophagus. Any material not cleared by this primary stripping wave is cleared by a secondary wave initiated by a stretch at the location of this material and progressing to the gastroesophageal junction. Both the primary and secondary waves initiate relaxation of the lower esophageal sphincter. This complex function of swallowing involves the brainstem, the vagus nerve, the muscles of the esophagus, and the lower esophageal sphincter. When these processes are disturbed, motility becomes disordered, as characterized by tertiary (ineffective, random) contractions and failure of function of the lower esophageal sphincter. Disease at any level of the control of peristalsis can result in esophageal dysmotility (Fig. 3–26). Complications of these diseases include obstruction, reflux esophagitis, candidiasis, and the development of carcinoma.

Brainstem and Vagus Nerve Abnormalities. Brainstem tumors, multiple sclerosis, amyotrophic lateral sclerosis, and poliomyelitis can affect the nucleus of the vagus nerve, resulting

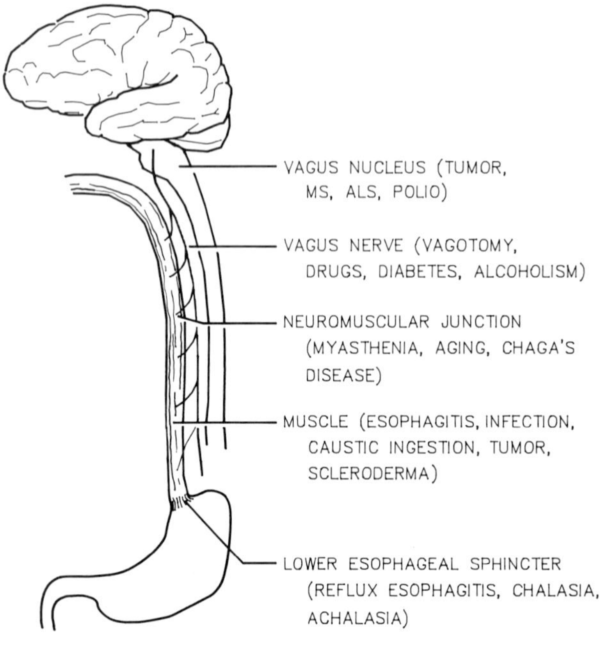

VAGUS NUCLEUS (TUMOR, MS, ALS, POLIO)
VAGUS NERVE (VAGOTOMY, DRUGS, DIABETES, ALCOHOLISM)
NEUROMUSCULAR JUNCTION (MYASTHENIA, AGING, CHAGA'S DISEASE)
MUSCLE (ESOPHAGITIS, INFECTION, CAUSTIC INGESTION, TUMOR, SCLERODERMA)
LOWER ESOPHAGEAL SPHINCTER (REFLUX ESOPHAGITIS, CHALASIA, ACHALASIA)

FIGURE 3–26. Causes of motility disturbance in the esophagus. MS, multiple sclerosis; ALS, amyotrophic lateral sclerosis.

in loss of initiation of swallowing. Drugs or surgical procedures that affect the vagus nerve and the neuropathy that occurs in alcoholism or diabetes can also result in interruption of the sequential activation of the esophageal nerve branches.

Neuromuscular Junction Dysfunction. Myasthenia gravis, aging, parasitic infestation, and muscular dystrophy can cause dysfunction at the neuromuscular junction and result in loss of the swallowing reflex. In myasthenia gravis, the acetylcholine receptors are blocked by the attachment of antibodies. The disease is limited to the upper third of the esophagus, in which striated muscle is present. Progressive loss of ganglion cells in elderly patients results in a condition of impaired swallowing (presbyesophagus). Infestation by the parasite *Trypanosoma cruzi* destroys the ganglion cells of the smooth muscle, resulting in poor function of the lower esophagus and the lower esophageal sphincter. Patients have signs and symptoms of obstruction of the lower esophagus and their radiographs are indistinguishable from those of patients with achalasia (to be discussed). The parasitic infestation (called Chagas's disease) also causes cardiac arrhythmias.

Diseases Affecting the Muscle. Any injury to the muscles of the esophagus can result in altered motility. The most common causes are reflux esophagitis, infection, caustic ingestion, tumor, and scleroderma. The abnormal portion of the esophagus in tracheoesophageal fistula generally has no peristaltic activity; this abnormality persists after surgical repair. Muscular dystrophy is an inherited disease of muscle characterized by progressive muscle weakness and wasting; the diseased esophageal striated muscle has ineffective peristalsis.

Diseases Affecting the Lower Esophageal Sphincter. Diseases that affect the lower esophageal sphincter delay emptying or cause obstruction, which results in altered motility. Reflux esophagitis is the most common cause. Achalasia is the intermittent failure of the lower esophageal sphincter to relax as a result of a lack of ganglion cells at this location. It usually occurs in the 30- to 50-year age group and becomes evident when dysphagia develops. Eventually, the patient develops a large, dilated esophagus without peristalsis (Fig. 3–27). The esophagram shows an air/fluid level in the midesophagus and barium mixed with retained food particles. A symmetrically tapered, severely narrowed lower segment is seen at the gastroesophageal junction, through which intermittent spurts of barium pass.

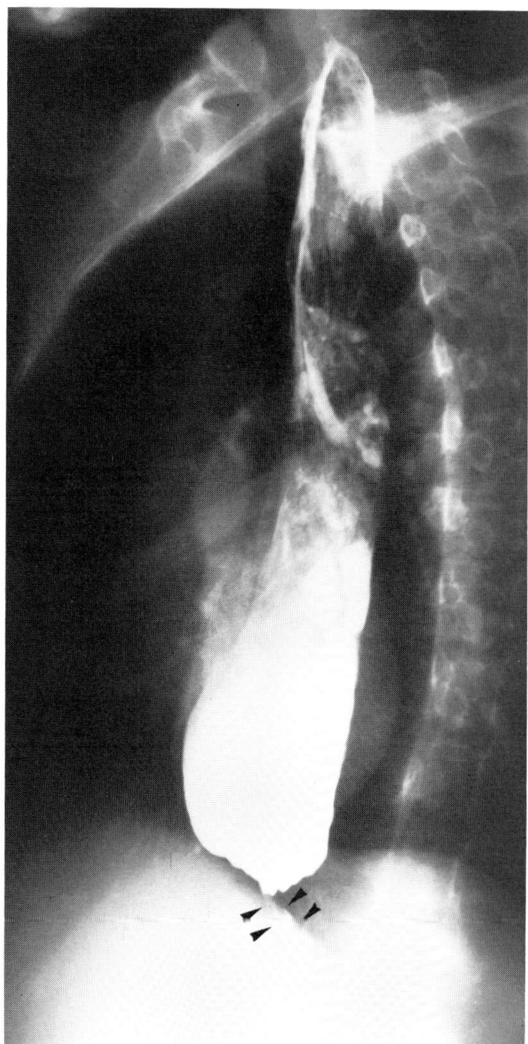

FIGURE 3–27. Achalasia. Left anterior oblique view after barium swallow shows marked distention of the esophagus with retained food particles and fluid diluting the barium. Marked narrowing is present at the gastroesophageal junction *(arrowheads)*. The patient, a 36-year-old woman from Central America, complained of difficulty swallowing.

There is no peristalsis in the distal two thirds of the esophagus (composed of smooth muscle). Patients with severe obstruction require balloon dilatation or surgery.

Diverticular Disease

Diverticula occur at three locations in the esophagus: (1) just above the upper esophageal sphincter, (2) at the level of the pulmonary hilum, and (3) in the lower esophagus (Fig. 3–28). Most esophageal diverticula are

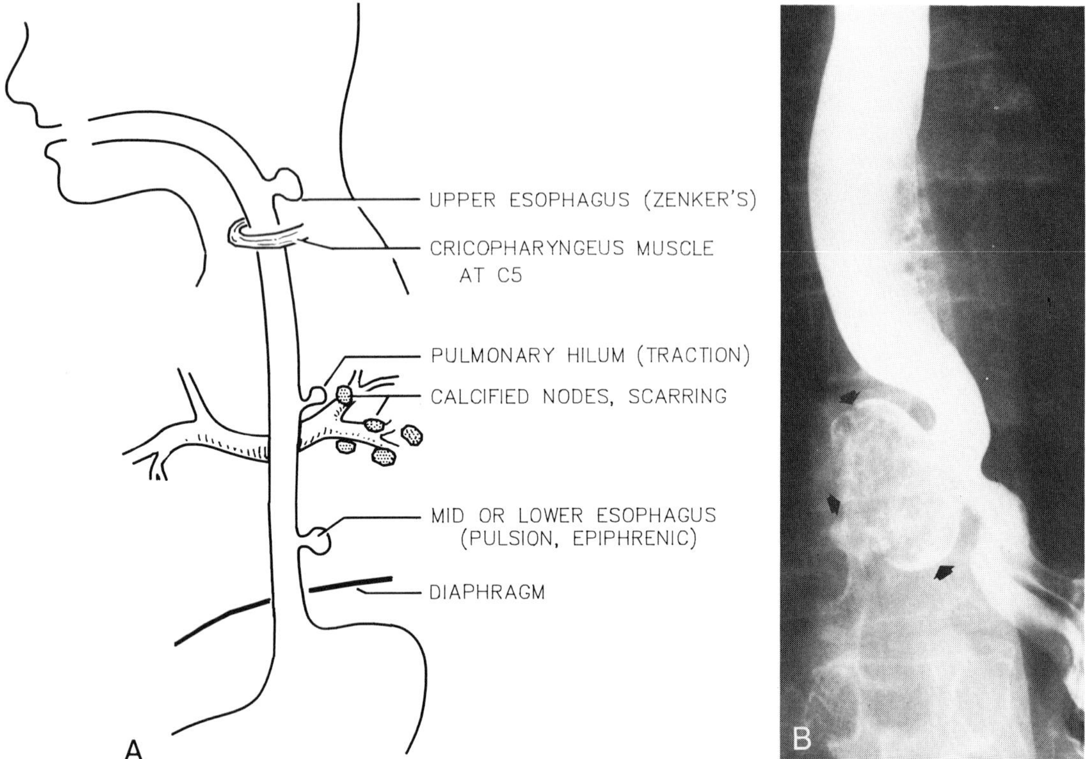

FIGURE 3–28. Esophageal diverticula. *A.* Diagram. *B.* Esophageal epiphrenic diverticulum. Esophagram shows outpouching in distal esophagus containing food particles *(arrowheads)* in a middle-aged woman with symptoms of gastroesophageal reflux.

single, are acquired in middle age, and do not cause symptoms. They are easily diagnosed on barium esophagram.

A pharyngeal diverticulum, called Zenker's diverticulum, occurs just above the upper esophageal sphincter (the cricopharyngeus muscle) and is located posteriorly or posterolaterally. It can trap food passing into the esophagus during swallowing and result in discomfort, dysphagia, and regurgitation. When a large Zenker's diverticulum is distended with food, it can obstruct the esophageal lumen and cause aspiration into the trachea.

A traction diverticulum occurs when scarring at the pulmonary hilum, usually from tuberculosis or tumor (or x-ray therapy of tumor), places traction on the esophagus as it passes through the mediastinum. Symptoms depend on the underlying disease and the degree of traction.

A pulsion diverticulum is an acquired outpouching of a weakened esophageal wall caused by repeated increases in intraluminal pressure. Such a diverticulum is usually seen near the carina. Epiphrenic diverticula are found in the middle and lower thirds of the esophagus. Often they are just above the diaphragm and are larger than the traction and the pulsion diverticula. They are usually associated with esophageal stricture, hiatal hernia, or gastroesophageal reflux.

STOMACH AND DUODENUM

Trauma

The stomach is rarely injured by trauma because of its relatively unrestricted and protected position in the upper abdomen. Penetration injuries usually also involve adjacent organs and thus are of more serious immediate consequence. Blunt injury can cause rupture of the stomach and expulsion of the contents into the peritoneal cavity or cause an intramural hematoma. Diaphragmatic rupture can cause herniation of the stomach and the bowel into the chest (see Chapter 2).

The duodenum and the proximal jejunum are fixed by their retroperitoneal attachments and the ligament of Treitz. The most common GI tract injuries are at these sites where they are sheared from these attachments or where the bowel is compressed against the spine. The injuries range from intramural hematoma, which can cause duodenal obstruction, to rupture and expulsion of duodenal contents into either the peritoneal cavity or the retroperitoneum. Intraperitoneal rupture results in acute peritonitis, and retroperitoneal rupture results in hemorrhage or abscess formation.

The diagnosis of intraperitoneal rupture can often be made by the detection of subdiaphragmatic air and intraperitoneal fluid on abdominal films. Rupture into the retroperitoneum results in extravasation of air, food, and digestive juices into the anterior pararenal space, almost always on the right side. Plain films often appear normal. A limited upper GI examination can be performed by administration of a small amount of dilute water-soluble contrast to the patient, who lies prone on the fluoroscopy table in a slightly right-side-down position (the GI position). With the patient in this position, the contrast material passes quickly into the duodenum, and extravasation can be demonstrated.

CT can show air, contrast extravasation, and bowel wall thickening caused by hematoma (Fig. 3–29). Hematoma may also be present in the mesentery. Air may be in the anterior pararenal space if the rupture is retroperitoneal, or it may be seen as pneumoperitoneum if the rupture is anterior. Because of its proximity to the duodenum, the head of the pancreas may also be injured and may show hemorrhage or enlargement. CT is most informative in the evaluation of such injuries, showing hemoperitoneum and injuries to solid organs in addition to the aforementioned injuries related to the bowel trauma.

Congenital Abnormalities

Congenital lesions of the stomach are usually discovered because of obstruction or the development of acid peptic disease. The most important of these diseases are duplication, antral web, pyloric stenosis, and heterotopic pancreatic tissue. Although not congenital, pyloric stenosis is detected in the first or second month after birth and is discussed in this section. The most important congenital abnormalities of the duodenum are duplication, atresia, and compression by external congenital bands associated with incomplete rotation of the small bowel and the colon and with structures such as annular pancreas (discussed later in sections on pancreatic abnormalities).

Pyloric Stenosis. Pyloric stenosis, a narrowing of the pyloric channel, is caused by circumferential hypertrophy of the pyloric muscle at the junction of the stomach and duodenum. Eighty percent of patients are male and are usually firstborn children, and there is a familial tendency for the disorder to occur. The hypertrophied muscle causes gastric outlet obstruction, usually between the ages of 2 and 8 weeks, manifested by postprandial, projectile vomiting. The diagnosis can often be made from the presence of a palpable mass in the region of the pylorus and from the clinical symptoms. If no mass is palpated, the diagnosis can be confirmed by ultrasonography or upper GI series.

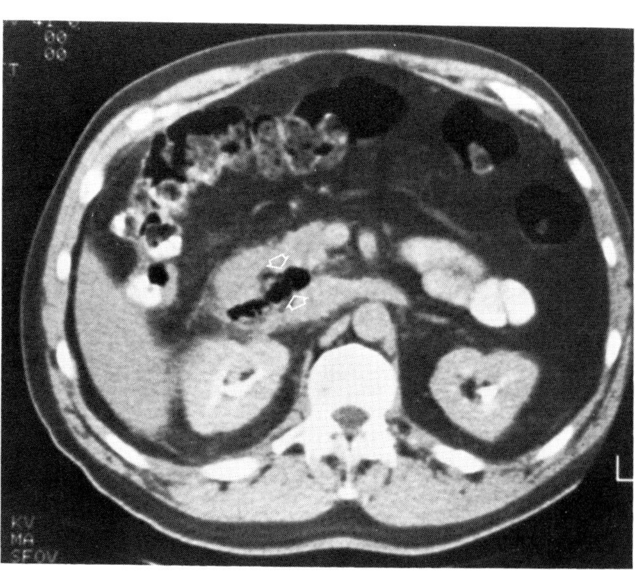

FIGURE 3–29. Rupture of duodenal diverticulum from foreign body perforation. A mass to the right of the midline contains irregular retroperitoneal gas collections *(arrowheads)* caused by rupture and leakage of air as a result of perforation. A secondary response has resulted in an inflammatory mass.

Ultrasonography is the preferred examination because it can show the hypertrophied and elongated pyloric muscle and the failure of the pyloric channel to open (Fig. 3–30). Enlargement of the pyloric muscle to more than 4 mm is considered diagnostic. The upper GI series is best performed by placement of a nasogastric tube into the antrum of the stomach and injection of a small amount of barium to document the obstructed, narrowed, and elongated pylorus. Myotomy of the long axis of the hypertrophied (but otherwise normal) muscle is curative.

A mild form of pyloric stenosis, called pyloric hypertrophy, is usually diagnosed in infants but can be seen in adults. This hypertrophy of the pyloric muscle causes a partial gastric outlet obstruction. Radiographs show elongation of the antrum and narrowing in the pyloric region. This appearance can be similar to that of other diseases, such as scarring from peptic ulcer or caustic ingestion.

Heterotopic Pancreatic Tissue. Heterotopic or aberrant pancreatic tissue can be found in many sites, but the most common are the antrum and the pylorus of the stomach. It is characteristically seen as a round or ovoid mass, usually not larger than 2 cm in diameter, with a central dimple or depression that represents the orifice of a pancreatic duct. Such tissue is seen in 2% of autopsy specimens and is usually an incidental finding. In rare cases, patients have symptoms of obstruction by the mass, or the lesion may be seen incidentally on upper GI examination and require explanation. The appearance may simulate tumor or ulcer. When the mass is large, an upper GI series shows an intramural mass compressing the gastric lumen.

Antral Web. An antral web, a circumferential enfolding of gastric mucosa with a small central orifice, is a rare abnormality that causes obstruction 1 to 2 cm proximal to the pylorus. Although the lesion is present from birth, the patient can develop obstruction, usually partial, at any age. Many patients also develop ulcers. The web can be missed on endoscopy if the endoscope passes easily through the opening.

Volvulus: Gastric Rotation. Gastric rotation can occur in a patient who lacks normal fixation of the stomach by the hepatogastric, splenogastric, cologastric, and phrenogastric ligaments or when diaphragmatic abnormalities allow increased mobility of the stomach. The abnormality is of two types: (1) torsion (or organoaxial rotation), in which the stomach, the esophagus, and the duodenum all rotate about a common axis, and (2) mesenteroaxial (or true volvulus), in which the stomach rotates upon itself and becomes obstructed. This rotation can occur at any age. Such patients have

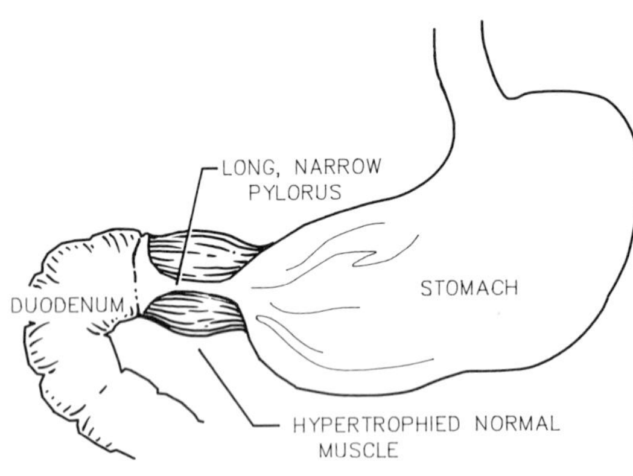

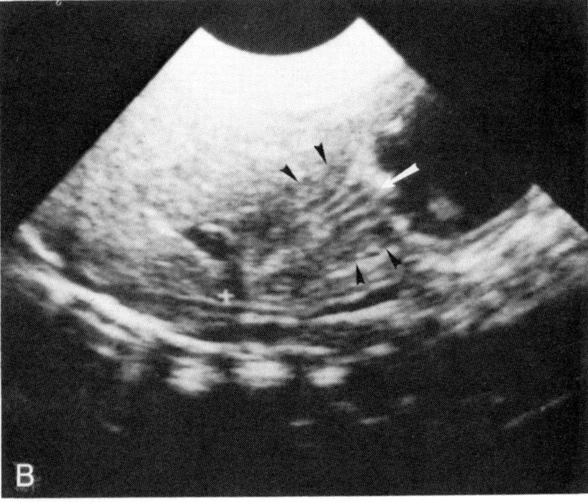

FIGURE 3–30. Pyloric stenosis. *A.* Diagram. *B.* Longitudinal ultrasonogram shows thickening of the muscle *(arrowheads)* and elongation of the pyloric channel (arrow) of a 4-week-old boy with projectile vomiting. The muscle wall thickness measured 6 mm.

signs of acute gastric obstruction that may be at the cardia, where it causes a beak-shaped narrowing of the distal esophagus, or at the pylorus of the stomach. The diagnosis is best made through upper GI examination, which shows the obstruction and the abnormal position of the stomach. In some cases, CT may be helpful for determining the locations of the abdominal organs.

Duodenal Duplication and Atresia. Duodenal duplication is rare and results in a second lumen that does not usually communicate with the primary lumen. Duodenal atresia results from an unknown in utero mechanism. Other anomalies are often present; for example, duodenal atresia is seen in 25% of patients with Down's syndrome. The diagnosis of duodenal atresia is suggested when the obstruction produces two collections of air in the stomach and the proximal duodenum seen on plain radiographs (called the double bubble). This double bubble can also be seen with congenital bands, annular pancreas, and duodenal diaphragm.

External Compression. Three uncommon causes of duodenal compression are annular pancreas, peritoneal bands, and the superior mesenteric artery syndrome. When the pancreas fails to form properly, it can encircle and obstruct the duodenum. When the colon fails to rotate properly as it returns to the abdomen, the fibrous bands of the mesentery of the ascending colon (called Ladd's bands) cross over the duodenum and compress it.

The superior mesenteric artery occasionally compresses the third portion of the duodenum passing between it and the aorta. Patients are usually teenagers or young adults and underweight. They develop vomiting and, as a result, are poorly nourished.

Inflammation and Infection

The most common diseases of the stomach and the duodenum are those caused by acid secretion. Inflammatory diseases that involve the stomach and duodenum include regional enteritis and eosinophilic gastroenteritis.

Gastritis, Duodenitis, and Peptic Ulcer Disease

Gastritis, duodenitis, and peptic ulcer disease are among the most common upper gastrointestinal diseases, all of which are caused by or exacerbated by acid. Peptic ulcer disease is the best known of these injuries to the gastric and duodenal mucosa and affects a quarter of the population of the United States at some point in their lives. Gastritis and duodenitis, which are much more common, are the result of less severe inflammation without ulceration. Patients with gastritis and duodenitis have symptoms related to mucosal irritation, including epigastric fullness, early satiety, nausea and vomiting, and anorexia. Inflammatory cells in the mucosa can be detected through endoscopic biopsy. The injury in all forms of acid-related disease is usually most severe in the gastric antrum and the duodenal bulb. The inflammatory response renders the folds edematous and poorly distensible and, if severe enough, causes the development of ulcers (Fig. 3–31).

Gastric Ulcer. A gastric ulcer is a local excavation of the mucosal surface that is produced by sloughing of inflammatory tissue. Ulcer configurations can be round or oval, linear, rectangular, or flame-shaped. Multiple ulcerations are common. Eighty-five percent of benign gastric ulcers are on the lesser curvature and are more likely to be found on the posterior wall. However, the location of a gastric ulcer is not a reliable indicator of benign disease. Gastric ulcers may vary in size from 1 mm to several centimeters. The size of a gastric ulcer is also of no value with regard to the likelihood of malignant disease. A gastric ulcer larger than 4 cm in diameter (giant ulcer) carries an increased risk of penetration and perforation.

In addition to peptic disease (the most common cause of gastric ulcer), gastric ulcers are caused by aspirin ingestion, corticosteroids, phenylbutazone, and nonsteroidal anti-inflammatory medications. Bile acid reflux from the duodenum, stress ulcers (often seen in burn patients), and debilitating diseases such as chronic obstructive pulmonary disease, chronic renal failure, and liver disease are also associated with gastric ulcers. Patients with gastric ulcers have epigastric pain on an empty stomach; the pain is relieved by food, antacids, or vomiting. They may be anemic and have occult fecal blood. Many patients have a history of aspirin use.

Radiographic features of benign gastric ulceration are varied. The more definite appearance with barium contrast is a fixed collection of barium that protrudes beyond the profile of the stomach. When seen end-on, the ulcer contains a central, rounded collection of barium with evenly distributed radiating gastric mucosal folds that stop abruptly at the ulcer

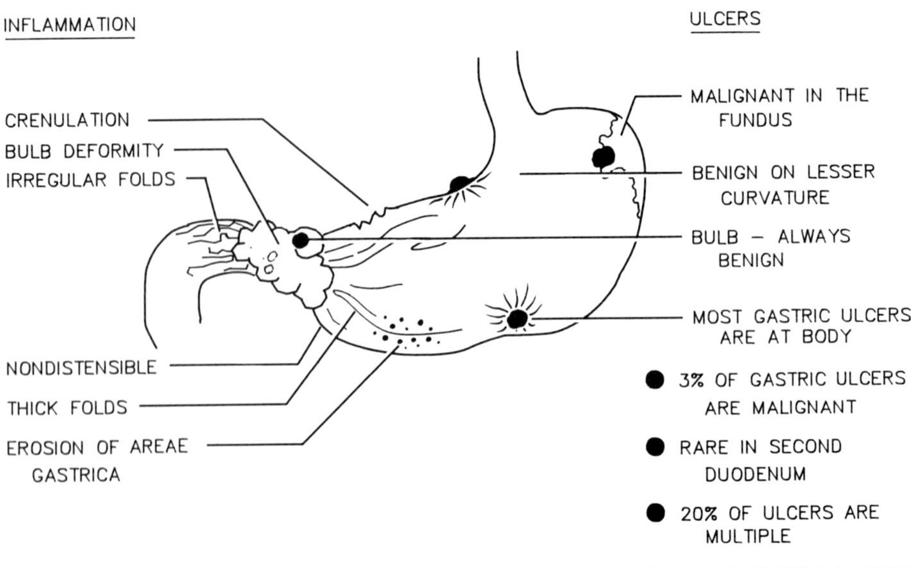

FIGURE 3–31. Characteristics of gastric and duodenal inflammation and ulcer disease.

margin (see Fig. 3–6). Hampton's line, a thin (1-mm), sharply demarcated, and lucent line, represents undermined gastric mucosa at the orifice of the ulcer niche. When more extensive edema and inflammation occur at the margin of the ulcer, a thicker band of mucosa is interposed between the ulcer crater and the lumen of the stomach. This band is called an ulcer collar when seen in profile (Fig. 3–32). With more severe edema and inflammation, this area becomes an ulcer mound.

The most important aspect of gastric ulcer diagnosis is determining whether the lesion is benign or malignant. The vast majority of gastric ulcers are benign. In profile views, a benign gastric ulcer crater appears to project beyond the lumen of the stomach. The margin of the ulcer crater is sharply defined and smooth with regular borders. Hampton's line is never seen in malignant ulceration. When the radiographic findings do not clearly establish benign disease, the ulcer is considered indeterminate, and biopsy is required in order to exclude the possibility of malignancy.

Benign gastric ulcers are treated conservatively with diet, antacid therapy, and anticholinergic drugs. When a benign gastric ulcer heals, a small, round residual radiographic deformity (scar) may persist. The most common radiographic findings of a gastric ulcer scar are mucosal folds that merge into a flat area at the previous ulcer site. Infrequently, a linear ulcer scar appears at the center of the converging folds. An ulcer that persists for more than 8 weeks without evidence of healing must be considered malignant.

Erosive Gastritis. Gastric erosions are seen frequently in patients who consume alcohol heavily or use aspirin frequently. Erosions are seen on radiographs as one or more, and sometimes many, tiny defects (aphthae) in the antral mucosa. They are best seen with the double-contrast technique but can be seen with single-contrast compression technique as barium is pushed into the small erosions. The erosions are superficial and generally heal if the cause of irritation is eliminated.

Duodenal Ulcer. Duodenal ulcers result from the combined actions of acid and pepsin. They are usually seen in young adults and are three times as common as benign gastric ulcers. Nearly all duodenal ulcers (95%) are found in the duodenal bulb, and thus they are relatively easy to identify. They range in size from a few millimeters to 2 cm in diameter.

Patients usually have a burning sensation (heartburn) near the midline epigastrium that develops about 45 to 60 minutes after meals. This burning pain can radiate to the back, the right shoulder, or the costal margins. Relief occurs quickly after ingestion of food or antacids or after vomiting because the acid is neutralized or eliminated.

The upper GI examination shows a round or oval collection of barium surrounded by a lucent halo of edema. Single-contrast technique often reveals an indentation of the duodenal wall opposite to the ulcer (called an

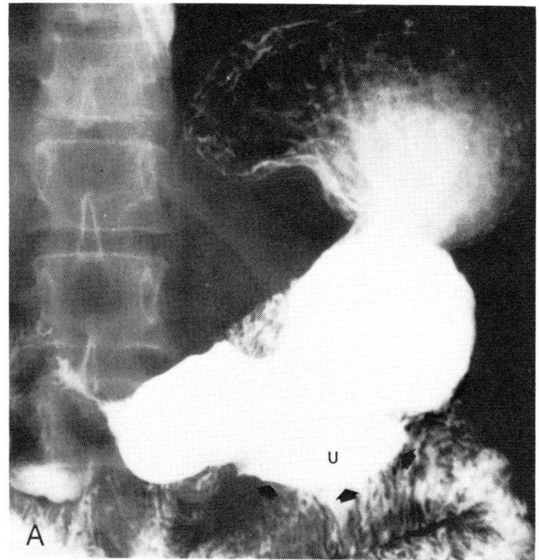

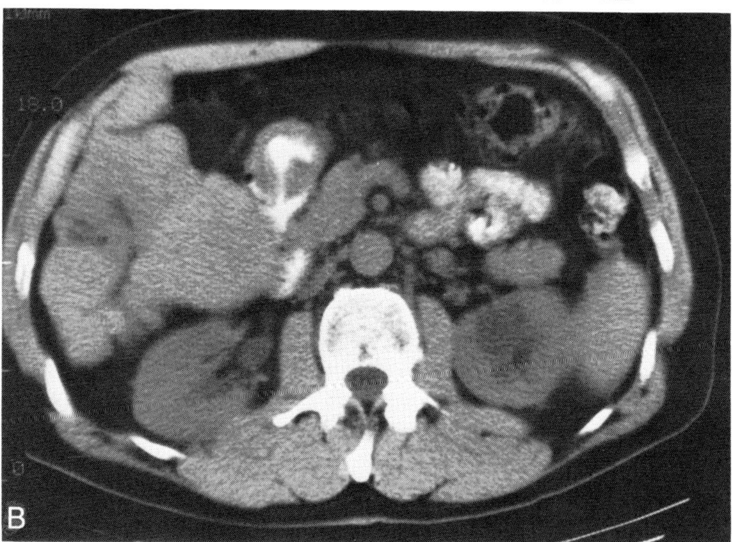

FIGURE 3–32. Gastric ulcer. *A.* Upper GI study shows a giant, excavating gastric ulcer along the greater curvature of the stomach *(arrowheads).* The projection of the ulcer crater beyond the gastric lumen, the sharp margination, and the smooth borders indicate a benign ulcer in a man with acid peptic disease. The thick margin of indentation is called the ulcer collar. *B.* In a different patient, CT after administration of oral contrast shows a rounded collection in the distal antrum that thins in the pylorus. Inferior to the pylorus is the arrowhead-shaped collection in the duodenal bulb. The left lateral outpouching of the contrast in the distal antrum represented a duodenal ulcer in a patient who had a history of gastric ulcers.

incisura) that represents contraction from scarring and inflammation (Fig. 3–33). The incisura therefore almost always points to the center of the ulceration.

Multiple ulcers may occur, causing extensive deformity from inflammation and edema. Healing of large ulcers or multiple ulcers results in pseudodiverticula formation, a cloverleaf deformity. When ulcers are seen in the postbulbar duodenum, causes other than simple peptic ulcer disease should be considered. Ulcerations in the postbulbar duodenum heal with excessive scarring and stricture formation.

Hypertrophic Gastritis. Hypertrophic gastritis is a poorly understood disease of the stomach characterized by enlargement of folds and increased secretions. The process shows hyperplasia (not hypertrophy) of gastric epithelium, which results in widened gastric folds. The proliferation of epithelial cells can result in fluid and protein exudation, mainly albumin.

An uncommon manifestation of hypertrophic gastritis is Ménétrier's disease. The disease involves predominantly the body of the stomach. Most patients are men and manifest hypoproteinemia (hypoalbuminemia) and decreased acid secretion in conjunction with large gastric folds. An upper GI series reveals giant rugal folds and dilution of the barium as a result of increased gastric secretions (Fig. 3–34). The disease is generally irreversible, and gastrectomy is required. In rare instances, patients develop gastric carcinoma.

Zollinger-Ellison Syndrome. Rare, gastrin-secreting tumors, usually of the pancreas (to be discussed) can result in a 500-fold increase

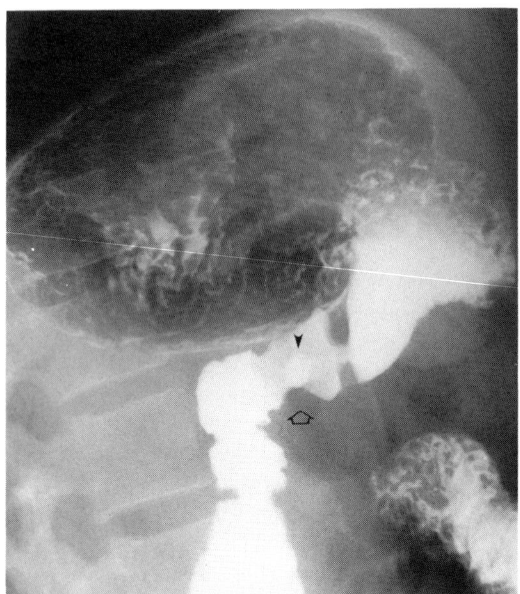

FIGURE 3–33. Duodenal ulcer. Upper GI study shows a benign duodenal ulcer *(arrowhead)* in central portion of duodenal bulb. The enfolding of the duodenal lumen just beneath the ulcer *(open arrow)* represents a scarring response called an incisura, a common finding in peptic ulcer disease.

in gastric acid production, the Zollinger-Ellison syndrome. The acid produces peptic ulcers predominantly in the duodenal bulb but also the stomach, the postbulbar duodenum (15% of patients), and the jejunum (10%). The ulcers characteristically are multiple.

The radiographic appearance of the Zollinger-Ellison syndrome is variable. The syndrome may initially take the form of a simple peptic ulcer, but the radiograph often reveals one or more ulcers in the stomach and duodenum. The presence of ulcers in unusual locations, such as the second and third portions of the duodenum and the proximal jejunum, is highly suggestive of the diagnosis. Additional important findings are the dilution of barium and rapid transit due to increase in secretions during barium contrast studies (see Fig. 3–7) and thickening of gastric, duodenal, and jejunal folds.

Eosinophilic Gastroenteritis. Eosinophilic gastroenteritis is a rare inflammatory disease of the stomach and the small bowel that is associated with an elevated blood eosinophil count. The disease is most common in children, and half of patients have a history of allergy. Sixty percent have an elevated blood eosinophil count, and the serum protein level is often decreased. An upper GI series shows contraction and nondistensibility of the gastric antrum and thickened folds. The entire stomach is usually involved, often with extension to the proximal small bowel. The lesions contain a predominance of eosinophils. Spontaneous remission is the usual course.

Atrophic Gastritis. Atrophic gastritis is a common finding in elderly patients with achlorhydria. Biopsy reveals thinning of the mucosa and a decrease in glandular elements. Symptoms of pain and early satiety are common. Upper GI shows smaller and less numerous gastric folds. Atrophic gastritis is also associated with increased incidence of adenomatous polyps and gastric carcinoma.

Regional Enteritis. Regional enteritis (Crohn's disease, granulomatous gastritis) involves the stomach in 20% to 40% of patients, almost always in conjunction with disease elsewhere in the GI tract. It involves the duodenum in 3% of patients. Symptoms are usually caused by more severe disease in the colon or the terminal ileum (to be discussed). An upper GI examination reveals aphthous lesions (small excavations with a surrounding halo of edema) in the antrum of the stomach. In advanced disease, granulomatous transmural involvement is present and is similar to that

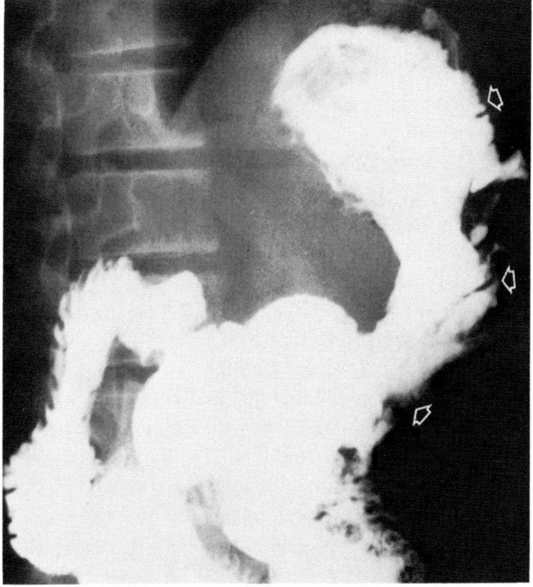

FIGURE 3–34. Hypertrophic gastritis. Upper GI study shows large irregular gastric folds throughout the greater curvature of the stomach *(open arrowheads)*. Although other gastric diseases may have a similar appearance, the patient, a middle-aged man, had hypoalbuminemia and decreased acid secretions, which indicated Ménétrier's disease.

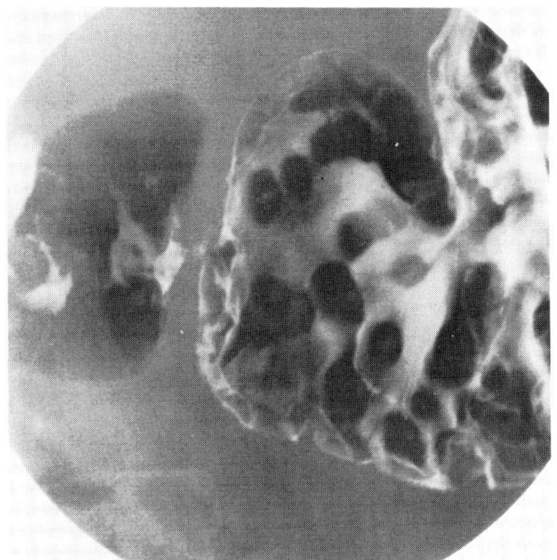

FIGURE 3–35. Regional enteritis of the stomach. Upper GI study shows numerous aphthous lesions in the gastric antrum in a young woman with regional enteritis. She also had advanced involvement of the terminal ileum and the stomach. The large defects are the result of halos of edema surrounding the small, barium-filled aphthous lesions. Aphthous lesions are consistent with, but not pathognomonic of, regional enteritis.

seen in the distal GI tract (Fig. 3–35). In the duodenum, the findings of thickened folds and ulceronodular changes are nonspecific.

Corrosive Gastritis. Ingestion of corrosive agents, whether acid or alkaline, produces a severe gastritis that may lead to necrosis and perforation. Ingestion of household bleach in liquid or tablet form is a common cause of corrosive gastritis. An upper GI examination reveals a variable appearance depending on the amount and the type of corrosive agent ingested. The esophagus is more severely involved by liquid corrosives. The most severe gastric involvement is usually seen in the dependent portion of the stomach along the greater curvature and the antrum. Varying degrees of mucosal destruction and excavation can occur. Mucosal thickening from hemorrhage and edema narrows the affected area. Stricture occurs within a few weeks after injury. Prompt treatment can prevent or reduce residual deformity.

Gastric Infections. Infection of the stomach is rare because of the protective function of gastric acid. When it does occur, it is usually a nonspecific viral gastritis. Viral gastritis causes generalized stomach upset, nausea, and vomiting. A diagnosis is usually made without radiographic examination, and the disease is self-limiting. An upper GI examination is obtained only for ruling out a more serious disease. The radiographic findings are nonspecific.

Tuberculosis and syphilis are rare infections of the stomach that usually involve the gastric antrum. In many patients with tuberculosis, lung disease is not evident on chest radiographs, and so the diagnosis is not always suspected. The upper GI examination in gastric tuberculosis and syphilis shows deep mucosal ulcerations, narrowing of the gastric lumen, and thickened folds primarily in the body and the antrum of the stomach. Although these findings are not specific, they usually lead to endoscopic biopsy and the correct diagnosis.

Giardiasis involves the duodenum and jejunum and produces nonspecific symptoms of epigastric discomfort. It is usually caused by ingestion of *Giardia lamblia*–infected water, frequently by hikers who drink from mountain streams. Results of an upper GI examination are usually normal, but edema of the mucosal folds in the duodenum and the jejunum often occurs and is suggestive of the diagnosis. Diagnosis is confirmed by duodenal aspirate or by a trial of antiparasitic therapy.

Neoplasms

Gastric Polyps and Polyposis. Gastric polyps are classified histologically as hyperplastic or adenomatous. Most (95%) are hyperplastic. Hyperplastic polyps result from chronic irritation and are the result of overgrowth and heaping up of the mucosa. They have no malignant potential. Adenomatous polyps, on the other hand, have considerable malignant potential, although they are uncommon in the stomach. The two types of polyps are indistinguishable on radiographs. They may be single or multiple, are usually smooth, and vary in size from 5 mm to more than 2 cm in diameter. Some gastric polyps have a pedicle, but most are sessile. Villous adenomatous polyps are intraluminal, trabeculated, and slightly irregular. When polyps become irregular or ulcerated, malignancy should be suspected.

Gastric polyps occur in several syndromes, including familial polyposis, Peutz-Jeghers syndrome, and Cronkhite-Canada syndrome (Table 3–1). Identification of these syndromes is important because the polyps of familial polyposis and Peutz-Jeghers syndrome have malignant potential. They are therefore considered premalignant lesions.

TABLE 3–1. INTESTINAL POLYPOSIS SYNDROMES

Syndrome	Transmission	Age (Years)	Incidence	Malignant Potential	Location	Symptoms	Description of Polyps	Associated Lesions
Familial polyposis	Autosomal dominant	15 to 30	Uncommon	Yes: in 15 years	Colon (100%); Less in small bowel and stomach	Vague	Hundreds of polyps of variable size	All patients develop colon carcinoma after about 15 years
Gardner's syndrome	Autosomal dominant	15 to 30	Rare	Yes: in 15 years	Colon (100%); less in small bowel and stomach	Vague	Multiple adenomas	Multiple osteomas (sinuses), soft-tissue fibromas, sebaceous cysts
Peutz-Jeghers syndrome	Autosomal dominant	10 to 30	Rare	Yes: in 2%	Small bowel (95%), colon (30%), stomach (5%)	Pain, bleeding, intussusception	Pedunculated hamartomas of the muscularis	Mucocutaneous pigmentation of the lips and buccal mucosa
Multiple juvenile polyposis	Autosomal dominant, sporadic	5 to 15	Rare	Possible	Colon (100%), small bowel (5%), stomach (5%)	Diarrhea, anemia	Multiple juvenile polyps	Protein-losing enteropathy
Cronkhite-Canada syndrome	None	40 to 70	Very rare	No	Colon (100%), stomach (100%), small bowel (50%)	Diarrhea	Inflammatory polyps	Ectodermal abnormalities: alopecia, nail pitting, and hyperpigmentation
Turcot's syndrome	Autosomal recessive	10 to 20	Very rare	Yes: in 25%	Colon (100%)	Diarrhea	Adenomatous polyps	Central nervous system tumors

Carcinoid Tumor. The carcinoid tumor is an uncommon, benign tumor that usually occurs in the ileum. It has a nonspecific appearance but is usually polypoid or sessile. It ranges in size from 1 to 6 cm in diameter. In the stomach, it may be malignant and, in such cases, metastasizes early in its development. It does not cause the carcinoid syndrome unless it has metastasized to the liver.

Mesenchymal Tumors. Mesenchymal tumors occur in the stomach as well as elsewhere. The most frequent benign mesenchymal tumor is the leiomyoma. It is usually asymptomatic, but it may cause hemorrhage if it is ulcerated or, occasionally, obstruction if located in the antrum. On upper GI series, the leiomyoma appears as a smooth mass protruding into the lumen (Fig. 3–36). It is usually located in the fundus, but it may be seen elsewhere in the stomach. Other mesenchymal tumors include fibromas, neurogenic tumors, leiomyosarcoma, lipoma, vascular tumors, and glomus tumors. These submucosal tumors of the stomach are variable in size and usually indistinguishable from one another radiographically, except for the lipoma, which shows fat density on CT and MRI.

Gastric Adenocarcinoma. Adenocarcinoma is the most common malignant gastric tumor. The incidence varies markedly in different parts of the world; it is particularly common in Japan, Finland, Chile, and Iceland. It affects men twice as often as women, and most patients are 30 to 45 years of age. The tumor is most common in the antrum, usually along the lesser curvature, but may be located anywhere in the stomach. It almost never crosses the pylorus. When it occurs in the gastric fundus, it may extend into the esophagus.

Adenocarcinoma is associated with abnormal gastric acid secretion (achlorhydria), pernicious anemia, atrophic gastritis, gastric ulcer disease, and previous gastric surgery. It is also associated with adenomatous polyps and intestinal metaplasia. The pathological appearance of the tumor may be of four types: polypoid and intraluminal (I), noninfiltrative with ulceration (II), infiltrative with ulceration (III), and

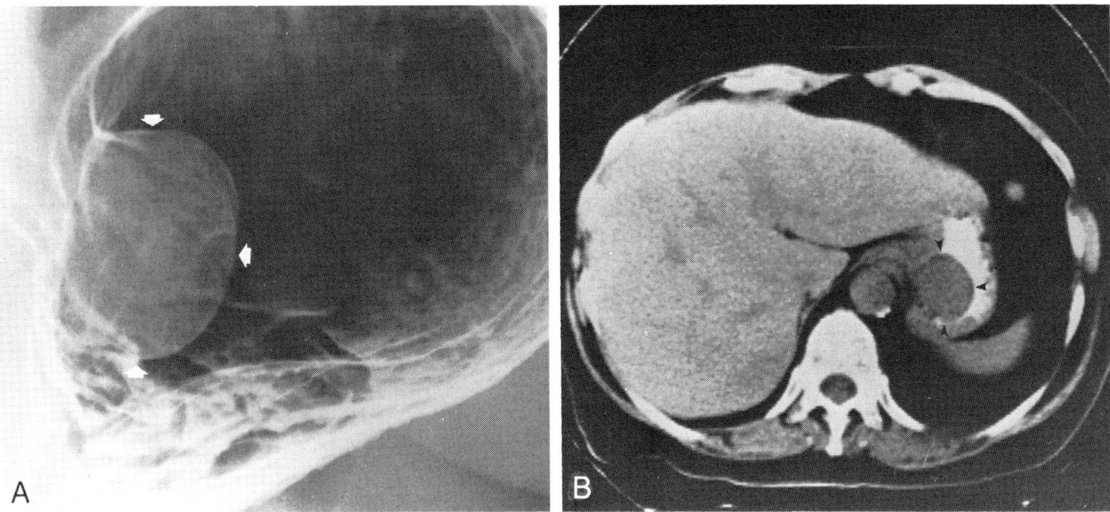

FIGURE 3–36. Intramural gastric leiomyoma. *A.* Double-contrast, upper GI study shows a large, smooth mass protruding into the lumen of the stomach *(arrowheads). B.* CT through the tumor shows a homogeneous mass originating from the posterior wall of the stomach *(arrowheads),* smoothly deforming the lumen.

diffusely infiltrative (IV). Prognosis is best for type I and worst for type IV.

Symptoms of early gastric carcinoma may be nonspecific or absent. The most common are abdominal pain, weight loss, anemia, weakness, anorexia, early satiety, nausea, and vomiting. These symptoms reflect both gastric dysfunction and the systemic effects of carcinoma. Some symptoms reflect obstruction at the pylorus or the gastroesophageal junction. When ulceration is present, patients may experience temporary relief with antacid therapy, and the diagnosis is delayed.

Several radiographic manifestations of gastric carcinoma are seen. The tumor may be superficial, polypoid, scirrhous, ulcerating with a mass, and ulcerating without a mass. Ulcerations are frequently irregular with irregularly thickened, often nodular folds of varying sizes. These folds do not approach the ulcer crater because of infiltrating submucosal tumor, a feature indicating the malignant nature of the lesion. The ulcer is within the mound of tumor and is therefore *inside* the profile of the gastric wall, in contrast to a benign ulcer, which projects *outside* the wall.

The diagnosis of gastric adenocarcinoma can often be suspected from the appearance on an upper GI series, but biopsy is necessary for confirming it. The examination reveals a mucosal mass (with or without an ulcer) and nondistensibility of the involved portion of the stomach (Fig. 3–37). Further evaluation and staging are performed through CT, which, in addition to demonstrating the mass, can show thickening of the gastric wall, infiltration of adjacent organs and of anatomical spaces, lymphadenopathy, and hepatic metastases.

Superficial or early gastric carcinomas are best diagnosed by double-contrast technique, which reveals subtle mucosal irregularity, slightly thickened folds in a focal area, or focal rigidity of the gastric wall. The polypoid carcinoma is less common and appears as a regular protruding mass of varying size with or without ulceration. Carcinoma with ulceration is more common and appears as an irregular mass containing an irregular ulcer.

The scirrhous form of adenocarcinoma (linitis plastica) is a primarily submucosal infiltration of a tumor that initially causes gastric fold flattening and rigidity and progresses to rigidity of long segments of the stomach and narrowing of the lumen.

Gastric carcinoma spreads locally to regional lymph nodes, the liver, and the esophagus, but it seldom crosses the pylorus. It can also result in general seeding (carcinomatosis) of the abdomen. The prognosis is dismal; the 5-year survival rate after surgery is about 10%. However, patients with superficial lesions that are detected early can be cured by surgery.

Gastric Lymphoma. Non-Hodgkin's lymphoma represents about 10% of all gastric malignancies and is becoming more common as the incidence of gastric adenocarcinoma decreases. It may be a primary lymphoma, or it may be part of more generalized involve-

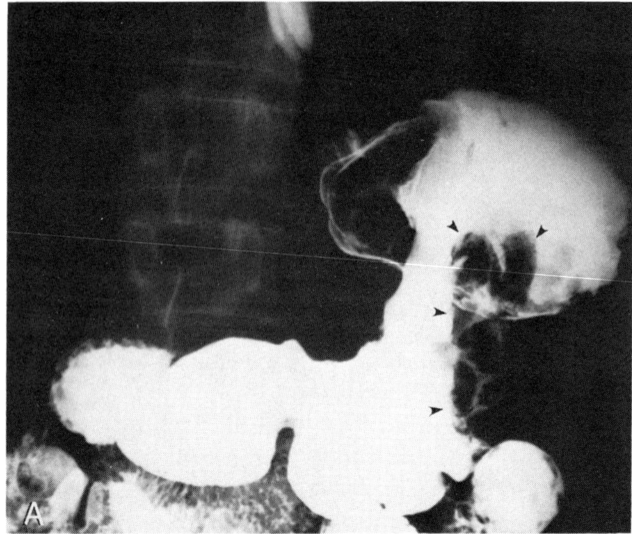

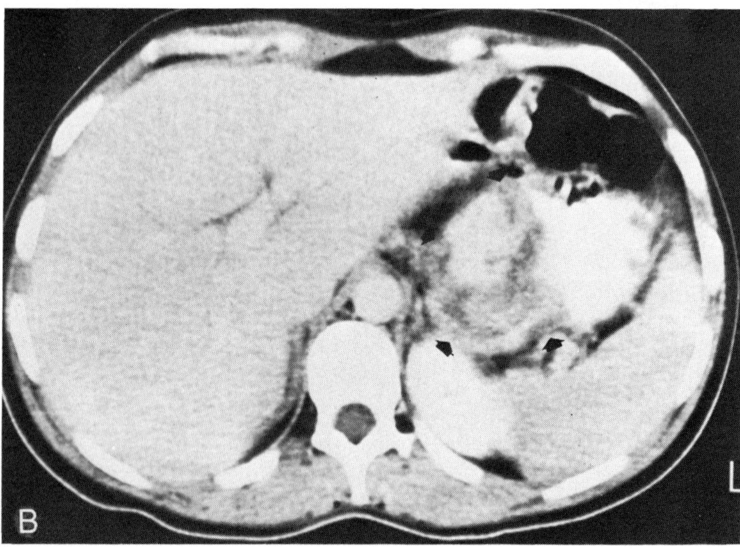

FIGURE 3–37. Gastric adenocarcinoma. *A.* Upper GI examination shows a large, irregular gastric mass along the greater curvature *(arrows),* which projects into the lumen of the stomach; this is indicative of malignancy in a 45-year-old man who experienced early satiety and weight loss. *B.* CT through the lesion shows deformity of the gastric wall and a large intramural mass posteriorly *(arrowheads)* but no hepatic metastases or adjacent adenopathy.

ment. Gastric lymphoma generally occurs in adults and can affect any portion of the stomach. The submucosa is infiltrated and occasionally contains superficial mucosal abnormalities, ulceration, and large gastric folds. The lesion can extend through the pylorus into the duodenum (unlike gastric adenocarcinoma) and may also extend superiorly to the esophagus. As in adenocarcinoma, the presenting symptoms include abdominal pain, anorexia, weight loss, nausea, and vomiting. Endoscopic biopsies, which are often superficial, may miss the submucosal infiltration, and so persistent symptoms or radiographic abnormalities should be further investigated.

The radiological findings of non-Hodgkin's gastric lymphoma include infiltration that may be focal, diffuse, or polypoid. Large gastric folds and one or more ulcerations may be associated with a mass. Lymphoma and adenocarcinoma are often indistinguishable; however, lymphomatous gastric folds are usually more pliable to palpation during fluoroscopic examination than is carcinoma. CT and MRI may reveal a mass in the gastric wall with local invasion. If gastric involvement is secondary to abdominal lymphoma, these examinations usually reveal lymphadenopathy (discussed later in Part III). Survival depends on the stage of the tumor. Gastric lymphoma carries a better prognosis than does adenocarcinoma: the 5-year survival rate is as high as 60% (Fig. 3–38).

Other, less common gastric malignancies include leiomyosarcoma, carcinoid tumor, and metastases, generally from melanoma, lung,

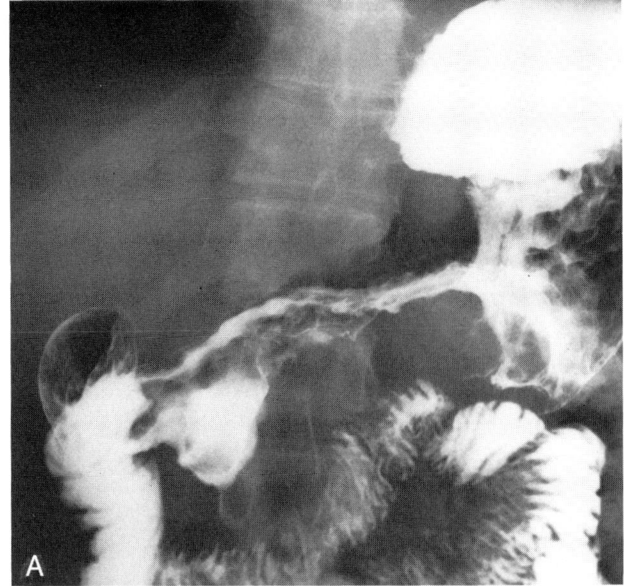

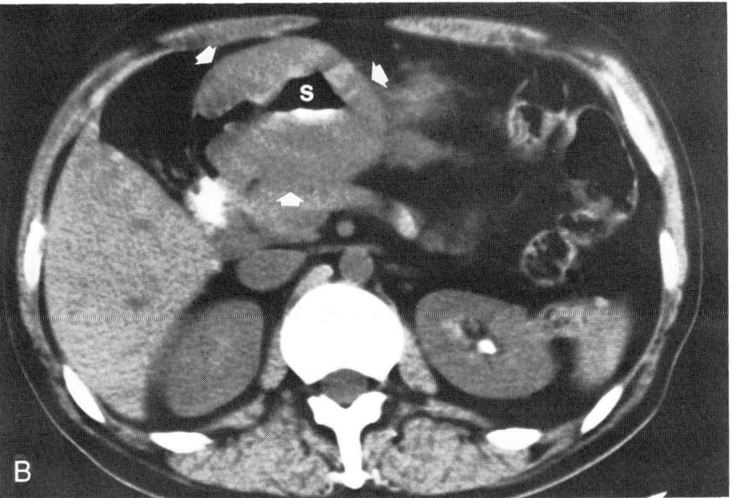

FIGURE 3–38. Gastric lymphoma. *A.* Upper GI study shows a huge, infiltrating mass involving primarily the greater curvature of the stomach. Note the irregular margins. *B.* CT through the lesion shows a greatly thickened gastric wall with deformity of the lumen *(arrowheads).*

and breast tumors. Leiomyosarcomas are typically large, lobulated, and irregular and contain large central ulcerations. Leiomyosarcoma and leiomyoma may be indistinguishable. Gastric carcinoid is usually not associated with the carcinoid syndrome. Metastases to the stomach are usually multiple, and some may have a bull's-eye appearance—that is, a nodule with central ulceration.

Malignant duodenal tumors are rare. The most common are adenocarcinoma, lymphoma, leiomyosarcoma, and metastatic lesions. Such tumors are usually identified when patients have atypical symptoms or respond poorly to therapy for presumed duodenal ulcer disease.

Vascular Disease

Gastric Varices. The gastric veins drain into the portal venous system; they can become dilated and can hemorrhage when the portal vein pressure increases as a result of liver disease or portal vein thrombosis. The signs and symptoms are similar to those of esophageal varices, which frequently coexist. The diagnosis is confirmed by clinical presentation and endoscopy. On an upper GI series, gastric varices, usually located near the gastroesophageal junction, can be confused with inflammation or an infiltrating tumor. In splenic vein thrombosis, the obstruction is proximal to the drainage of the esophageal veins, and only gastric varices result. Angiographic infusion of pressor agents into the left gastric artery or embolization of this vessel is often required to control active bleeding. Long-term therapy requires a portal-systemic bypass to relieve the elevated portal venous pressure.

Diverticular Disease

Gastric diverticula are commonly seen in the fundus of the stomach along the lesser curvature and are asymptomatic. Duodenal diverticula are more common, may be multiple, and are asymptomatic.

SMALL BOWEL (JEJUNUM AND ILEUM)

Trauma

Injury to the small bowel is usually at the proximal end because of the retroperitoneal fixation of both the duodenum and the ligament of Treitz. The remainder of the small bowel is freely movable within the peritoneum. Blunt or penetration injuries can cause extravasation of bowel contents into the peritoneal cavity and result in life-threatening peritonitis. In addition, such injuries can predispose a patient to the development of fistulas from one loop of bowel to another or sinus tracts to the skin surface. The most common small-bowel injuries are lacerations and intramural hematomas. Mesenteric hematomas, pneumoperitoneum, and hemoperitoneum also occur with bowel trauma. Radiographic examinations may reveal extravasation of contrast material, a thickened bowel wall with or without luminal narrowing, or intraperitoneal air, fluid, or blood. Most patients with penetration injuries require immediate surgical exploration, removal of the injured bowel, and extensive peritoneal irrigation and antibiotic therapy. Patients who develop fistulas require radiographic examinations in which the fistulas and any drainage tubes are injected in order to identify the locations of communications.

Congenital Abnormalities

The most important congenital abnormalities of the small bowel are abnormalities of development, including atresia, duplication, Meckel's diverticulum, malrotation, and cystic fibrosis, a hereditary disease characterized by viscous secretions that significantly affect the small bowel. Atresias and duplications are rare and can occur anywhere in the small bowel. Their characteristics are similar to those of atresias and duplications in the duodenum. Other anomalies are often associated with and may be the cause of atresia (such as acquired volvulus secondary to meconium ileus and malrotation).

Meckel's Diverticulum. Meckel's diverticulum is a local persistence of the omphalomesenteric duct at its junction with the ileum. It occurs 15 to 90 cm from the ileocecal valve and may contain gastric mucosa (in 15% of patients) and pancreatic mucosa (5%). Patients usually become symptomatic by 2 years of age when ulceration results from acid secretion from the aberrant gastric mucosa. Intestinal obstruction and inflammation occur less frequently. The diagnosis can be made through the demonstration of gastric mucosa on a nuclear medicine scan (Chapter 9). Contrast radiographic examinations are only sometimes helpful, but they can also rule out alternative diagnoses (Fig. 3–39).

Malrotation. Malrotation is abnormal intestinal positioning resulting from the failure of normal return of the bowel from the embryonic hernial sac. The malrotation can cause obstruction from fibrous bands or from twisting of the bowel on its mesenteric axis (volvulus). Important diagnostic considerations are the location and mobility of the cecum, the position of the small bowel, and the presence of obstruction. Duodenal bands (Ladd's bands) can be associated with malrotation; they cause proximal obstruction. Both upper GI and barium enema examinations can assist in the diagnosis of malrotation.

Cystic Fibrosis. Cystic fibrosis is an inherited autosomal recessive disease characterized by thick mucous secretions (therefore it is also called mucoviscidosis) by all glandular secreting tissue, including the lungs, the pancreas, and the intestines. These thick secretions in the small bowel result in intestinal obstruction and intussusception.

In 10% to 15% of neonates with cystic fibrosis, bowel obstruction results from abnormally viscous meconium in the distal ileum, a condition called meconium ileus. Bowel obstruction also occurs in adults with what appears to be a mild form of cystic fibrosis. The obstruction, called meconium ileus equivalent, causes less severe symptoms. The pulmonary complications of cystic fibrosis (see Chapter 2)

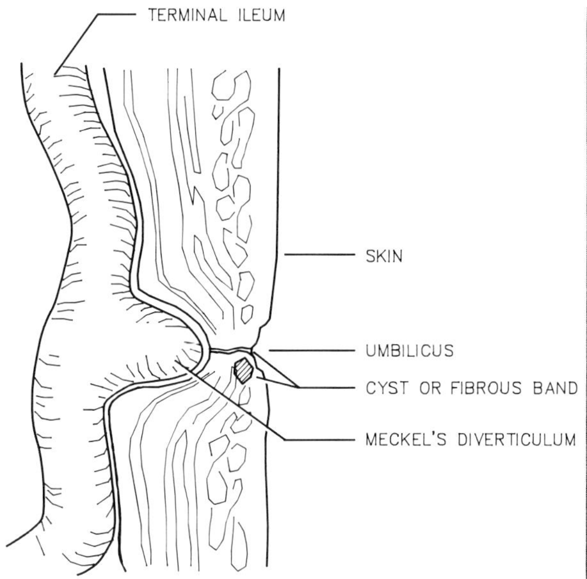

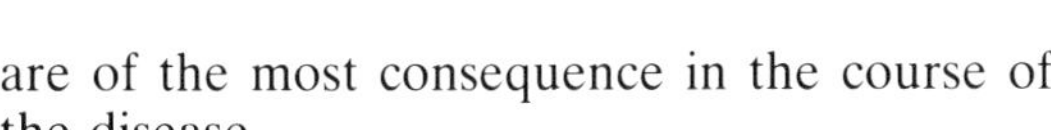

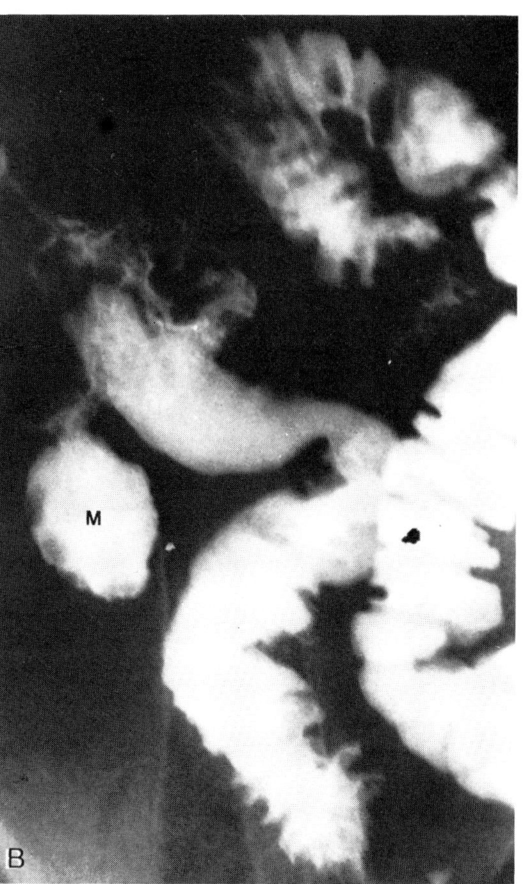

FIGURE 3–39. Meckel's diverticulum. *A.* Diagram. *B.* Small-bowel study shows a small outpouching (M) from the terminal ileum. This diverticulum caused abdominal pain in a young boy.

are of the most consequence in the course of the disease.

Scleroderma. Scleroderma, also called progressive systemic sclerosis, affects the entire GI tract by proliferation of fibrous connective tissue and vasculitis. The small bowel is affected much less commonly than is the esophagus. The submucosal muscular layer becomes fibrotic, which results in weakening, loss of tone, and impaired peristalsis. The mucosa is not affected. Decreased motility results in delayed transit time, which not only interferes with digestion but also facilitates bacterial overgrowth. The predominant radiographic finding in the small bowel is dilatation (see Fig. 3–7). Scattered areas show pseudosacculations caused by weakness of the wall. These pseudodiverticula have wide necks and are thus differentiated from true diverticula, which have narrow necks.

Nontropical Sprue. Nontropical sprue is caused by an allergy or sensitivity to gluten that is found in harvest grains, notably wheat. The sensitivity manifests clinically as malabsorption of many substances, including fat. The small intestine shows a diminished number and decreased height of mucosal folds and dilatation of long segments. Increased amounts of fluid within the intestinal lumen dilute the barium. Nontropical sprue is a premalignant condition of the small intestine that predisposes the patient to the development of lymphoma after decades. Because the radiographic appearances of nontropical sprue and lymphoma are similar, a sudden change in clinical condition, such as fever, must be suspected as indicating the development of lymphoma.

Intestinal Lymphangiectasia. Intestinal lymphangiectasia is a rare disorder of the small intestine that results in a protein-losing enteropathy. The mucosal folds become thickened as a result of dilatation of submucosal lymphatics, loss of protein, and resulting edema.

Inflammation

Regional Enteritis. Regional enteritis (Crohn's disease) is a chronic granulomatous

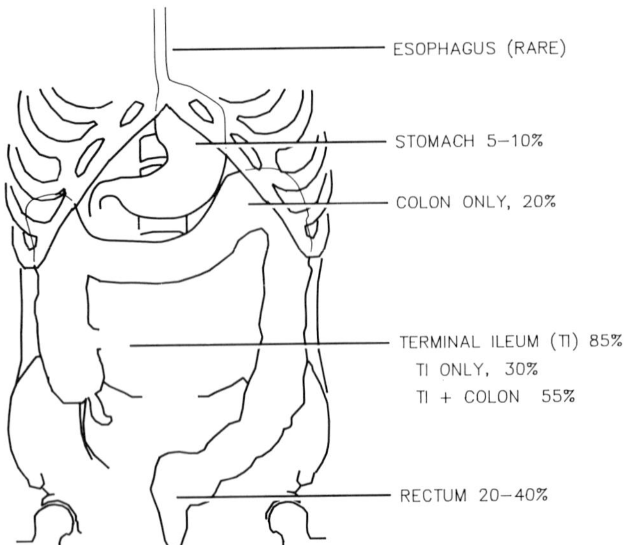

FIGURE 3–40. Locations and frequencies of involvement of regional enteritis.

disease of unknown cause that primarily involves the terminal ileum. Other areas include the colon, the rectum, and the proximal GI tract (Fig. 3–40). Patients develop diarrhea, abdominal pain, and varying degrees of obstruction. Many patients have additional diseases associated with but not directly related to the bowel disease. These include arthritis, ankylosing spondylitis, skin lesions, and uveitis.

Small-bowel involvement by regional enteritis is best diagnosed by small-bowel follow-through or enteroclysis with particular attention directed to the terminal ileum. Barium enema is usually obtained to evaluate the colon and can also demonstrate the terminal ileum if the ileocecal valve is incompetent. The radiographic findings are attributable to the transmural inflammatory involvement of the bowel wall. Abscess, ulceration, stricture, and the formation of fistulas are the most common complications (Fig. 3–41).

Initially, the small-bowel mucosa shows nodularity from apparent enlargement of the lymphoid follicles. Later, there is segmental, often asymmetrical, thickening of the valvulae conniventes (the small-bowel folds) from edema and aphthoid ulcerations. As the disease progresses, transmural involvement of the bowel wall occurs. Ulcers may penetrate through the bowel wall and form fistulas with other segments of the small bowel, the colon, the mesentery, and other organs. When transmural disease is severe, the bowel wall becomes markedly thickened and the lumen becomes narrow. Upper GI examination reveals abnormal separation of the bowel loops caused by the thickened walls. In advanced disease, marked thickening of the wall of the terminal ileum together with spasm causes severe narrowing (the string sign). Premature filling of adjacent loops of small-bowel or colon segments indicates fistula formation.

The clinical course of regional enteritis is one of intermittent exacerbation and remission. A barium contrast examination is important in establishing the diagnosis of regional enteritis and can be used to monitor changes during the course of the disease. Surgical resection of a diseased area is often curative when disease is limited to the colon, but in most patients with involvement of the terminal ileum, the disease recurs at that site after surgical resection.

Patients generally have continued and progressive disability as a result of their disease. Associated arthritis and ankylosing spondylitis can also be assessed radiographically but generally do not respond to therapy. Approximately 10% of patients with ulcerative colitis (to be discussed) develop retrograde involvement of the terminal ileum, called back-wash ileitis, that can be confused with regional enteritis. However, back-wash ileitis is characterized by a normal or dilated lumen, as opposed to the narrowed, irregular lumen of regional enteritis.

Eosinophilic Gastroenteritis. Eosinophilic gastroenteritis is a condition of unknown origin characterized by focal or diffuse lesions of the stomach and the small intestine. Biopsy of the intestinal mucosa shows increased numbers of

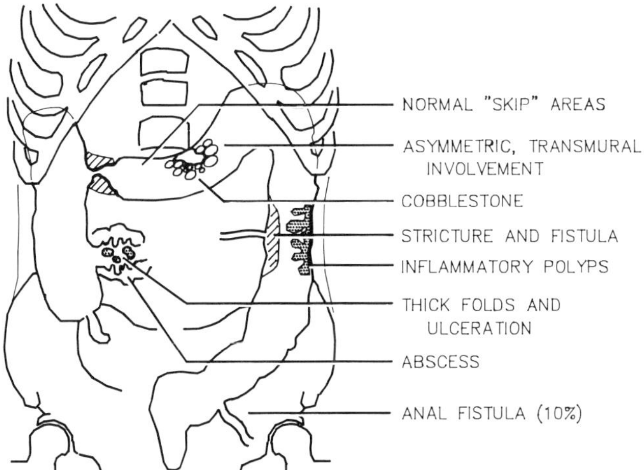

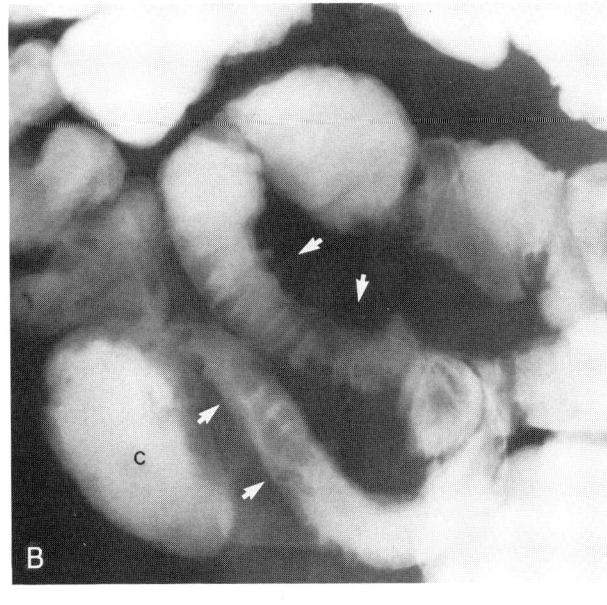

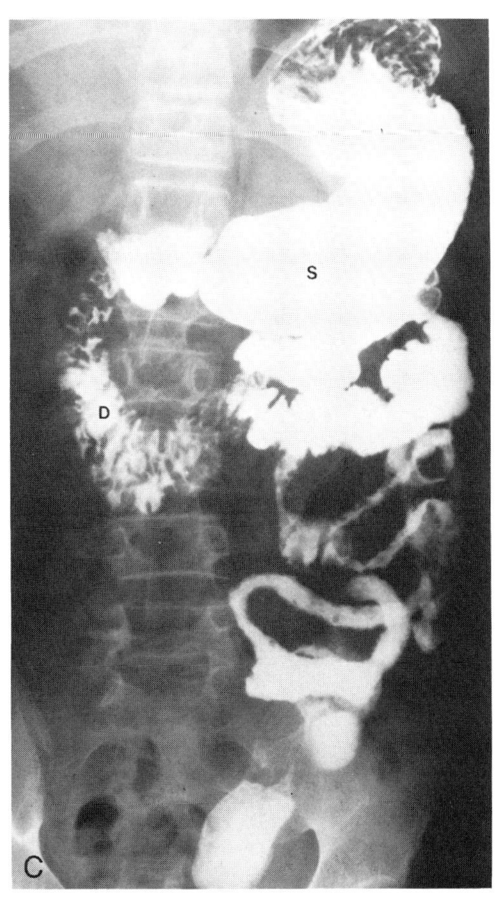

FIGURE 3–41. Regional enteritis. *A.* Diagram. *B.* Small-bowel study shows marked segmental thickening of the mucosal folds of the terminal ileum with spiculations along the margins *(arrows).* Nodularity is also evident, as are areas of normal mucosa. C, cecum. *C.* Small-bowel series in advanced and diffuse regional enteritis shows multiple loops of markedly narrowed, irregular, and ulcerated small bowel. The wide separation of loops is caused by transmural involvement that has caused thickening of the bowel wall. S, stomach; D, duodenum.

eosinophils. Varying degrees of bowel-wall thickening, nodularity, and ulceration are seen on upper GI series. Occasionally, strictures form.

Radiation Enteritis Injury. Because the cells of the small bowel divide rapidly, they are especially prone to injury by radiation, which results in inflammation, edema, ulceration, and stenosis. Patients who receive abdominal radiation for cancer may develop obstruction or bowel necrosis. In the acute stage, the mucosa is sloughed. Later, the bowel may become fibrotic with consequent stricture. The mesentery can become thickened and restrict the movement of the bowel, causing varying degrees of obstruction.

Infection

Infections of the small bowel are uncommon. When they occur, they are usually associated with medical or surgical therapy. Surgical creation of a blind loop in the bowel as a result of resection or gastric bypass can result in areas of stasis of food and overgrowth of enteric organisms. Chronic antibiotic suppression of normal flora can also allow overgrowth of organisms that are normally few in number. As a result, most infections of the small bowel are caused by unusual organisms, and nonspecific abnormalities are present on radiographic examinations.

Bacterial Infection. *Yersinia enterocolitica,* a gram-negative bacterium, causes an acute infection of the terminal ileum, usually of the distal 20 cm. In rare instances, it extends into the colon. Patients have symptoms of hypermotility, manifested by cramping and diarrhea. A small-bowel follow-through or reflux from a barium enema shows aphthoid or larger ulcers, nodularity, and thickened folds. These findings are indistinguishable from those of regional enteritis. However, with therapy, the process resolves completely in about 8 weeks.

Both *Salmonella* species and *Campylobacter fetus* can involve the terminal ileum, the ileocecal valve, and the proximal colon. *Salmonella* is rarely seen in the proximal small bowel. Both cause nonspecific symptoms and radiographic findings of nodularity and wall thickening.

Whipple's disease is an infection of the small bowel by a gram-positive, rod-shaped bacillus. Patients have malabsorption, diarrhea and steatorrhea, and fever. The bowel wall, predominantly the jejunum, is infiltrated by fat, inflammatory cells, and bacteria. Small-bowel examination reveals irregularly thickened folds as a result of infiltration, but these findings are not diagnostic. Small-bowel biopsy from which periodic acid–Schiff (PAS) positive macrophages can be demonstrated is required for diagnosis. The diagnosis is important because patients respond to antibiotics.

Unusual Infections. Tuberculosis of the small intestine usually involves the ileum and the cecum and results from the swallowing of infected sputum by patients with pulmonary tuberculosis. Many such patients have a normal chest radiograph. Early disease shows thickened, nodular folds with irregular ulceration. With progression, more extensive ulcerations and fistula formation may be seen. Tuberculosis of the terminal ileum may simulate regional enteritis. The terminal ileum may also be involved by granulomas from histoplasmosis as a result of ingestion of the organism. Colonization of the terminal ileum results in an irregular mucosal pattern and multiple ulcerations. Actinomycosis involves the small bowel and is also limited to the ileocecal region. A mass and fistulas to other parts of the bowel or sinus tracts to the skin are often present and help establish the diagnosis.

Neoplasms

Benign Tumors

Tumors of the small bowel constitute fewer than 3% of all alimentary tract tumors. The most common benign tumors are leiomyomas, lipomas, hemangiomas, adenomas, and neurogenic tumors. Two polyposis syndromes, Peutz-Jeghers and Cronkhite-Canada, substantially involve the small bowel (see Table 3–1). The multiple polyps are easily identified, and the clinical history and associated findings help establish the diagnosis in both of these syndromes. Peutz-Jeghers syndrome is an inherited autosomal dominant syndrome characterized by multiple, hamartomatous polyps of the small intestine (the small intestine is involved in 95% of patients), the colon (30%), and the stomach (25%). Associated pigmented mucocutaneous skin lesions are present from birth. In 2% of patients, these lesions are premalignant. There is an increased incidence of carcinoma in the stomach, duodenum, and colon in patients with this syndrome. There is also a high incidence of extraintestinal malignancy.

Cronkhite-Canada syndrome is a rare, noninherited syndrome characterized by multiple inflammatory polyps of the small bowel (in 50% of patients), the colon (100%), and the stomach (100%). Associated ectodermal abnormalities include alopecia, nail pitting, and hyperpigmentation. These polyps have no malignant potential. The average age of onset is 60 years. Patients develop watery diarrhea and protein loss that can eventually become life-threatening.

Carcinoid Tumor. One third of carcinoid tumors occur in the small bowel (most others occur in the appendix; to be discussed). Carcinoid tumors constitute 25% of all small-bowel tumors. Most of these are in the ileum, where they are more invasive. One third of small-bowel carcinoid tumors are malignant, one third are associated with a second endocrine tumor, and one third metastasize (usually to lymph nodes, liver, or lungs). The tumor grows slowly, and so symptoms are often insidious. Patients are generally 25 to 45 years of age. Serotonin and other substances produced by these tumors can cause the carcinoid syndrome of cutaneous flushing, hypotension, diarrhea, telangiectasis, and bronchial constriction. This syndrome usually indicates that spread to the liver has occurred.

Small-bowel examination or CT can reveal a mass that fixes the bowel and mesentery (see Fig. 3–7). The adjacent bowel wall is thickened. The prognosis depends on the malig nant potential of the tumor. Because most grow slowly, resection or palliative therapy is possible.

Malignant Tumors

Malignant tumors of the small bowel are rare, accounting for only 3% of malignant alimentary tract tumors. The majority are metastases from breast carcinoma, melanoma, and lung carcinoma. Primary tumors include adenocarcinoma, lymphoma, malignant carcinoid, and leiomyosarcoma.

Adenocarcinoma. Adenocarcinoma of the small bowel accounts for 25% of small-bowel malignancies. The tumor usually occurs in the proximal jejunum and the duodenum (lymphoma more often involves the ileum). Only 10% occur in the ileum. Small-bowel evaluation can reveal a polypoid or infiltrating mass and narrowing of the lumen. Ulceration, hemorrhage, and obstruction may occur.

Lymphoma. Lymphomatous involvement of the small bowel is usually of the non-Hodgkin's type and can be primary or part of a generalized process. Patients develop signs and symptoms of obstruction, perforation, or intussusception or the constitutional symptoms associated with lymphoma. The lesions are usually multifocal but may be solitary or diffuse. The ileum is more commonly involved than is the jejunum.

When Hodgkin's lymphoma involves the abdomen, it is usually by progressive, continuous nodal spread, first affecting the spleen, then the celiac lymph nodes, and then the mesenteric and periaortic nodes. Knowledge of such a progression is valuable in the differentiation of Hodgkin's from non-Hodgkin's lymphoma and, more important, differentiation of tumor from other processes (such as abscess in a patient with known Hodgkin's disease).

Radiographic findings include the presence of multiple nodules or a diffuse mass, infiltration of the bowel wall, ulceration, mesenteric invasion, and the development of a fistula (Fig. 3–42; see also Fig. 3–7). As the tumor infiltrates submucosally, the myenteric plexus is destroyed and bowel tone is diminished. The resultant aneurysmal dilatation, if present, can help differentiate lymphoma from adenocarcinoma. Bulky lesions may also appear to expand the lumen because of necrosis of the luminal portions of the mass.

Metastatic Tumors. Metastatic tumors most often involve the small bowel by hematogenous or intraperitoneal spread and less often by direct extension and lymphatic spread. The tumors that most frequently spread to the small bowel by intraperitoneal spread are pancreatic, stomach, colon, ovarian, and endometrial carcinoma. Breast carcinoma, bronchogenic carcinoma, and melanoma spread to the small bowel hematogenously.

Early metastatic lesions seen on small-bowel examination manifest as submucosal and intramural masses. With further growth, the overlying mucosa becomes altered and eventually destroyed as the tumor progresses and ulcerates. The lesions may be round, polypoid, or primarily ulcerative and may be pedunculated. A bulky mass may enlarge and obstruct the lumen. Long segments of mucosal destruction with ulceration occur in advanced disease. Melanoma often causes multiple masses, ulceration, and intussusception.

Vascular Disease

Ischemia. Vascular lesions are uncommon in the small bowel. The most common are

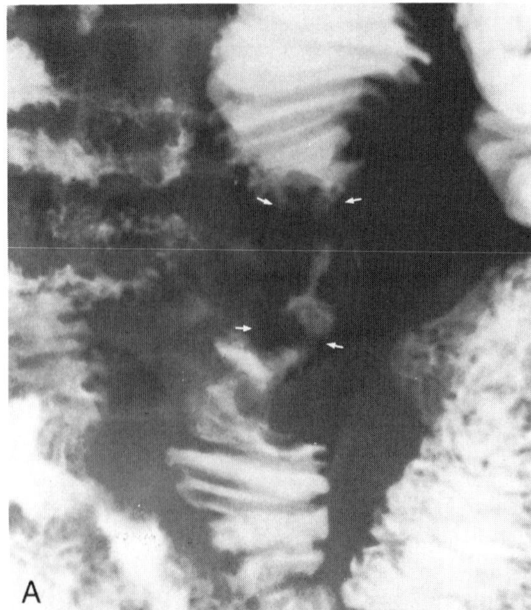

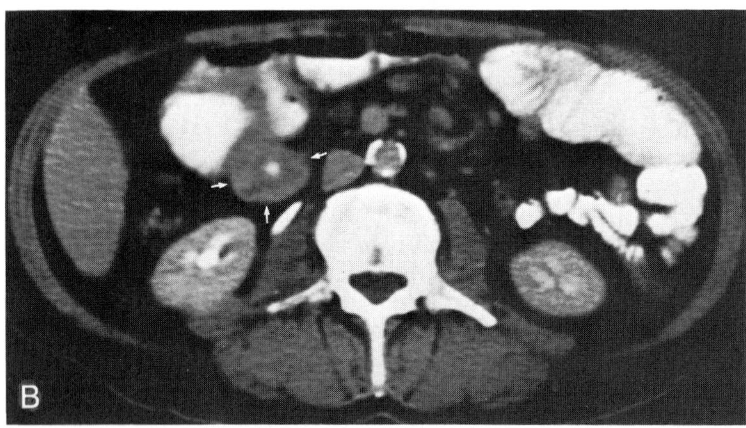

FIGURE 3–42. Small-bowel lymphoma. *A.* Small-bowel study shows a segment with markedly narrowed lumen and irregular mucosal pattern *(arrows)* in a young man with intermittent abdominal pain. *B.* CT in another patient with lymphoma shows circumferential involvement of the duodenal wall and narrowing of the barium-filled lumen *(arrows).*

acute and chronic intestinal ischemia, focal ischemia, vasculitis, and venous thrombosis. The primary radiographic finding of ischemia is mucosal and submucosal hemorrhage, which results in thickened folds. Mural and portal venous air are signs of associated mucosal destruction and infection with gas-forming bacteria, but they may be seen in several other diseases. Angiography (and, in rare instances, CT) can reveal thrombus, embolus, or atherosclerotic narrowing in the superior mesenteric artery or vein.

Hemorrhage. Hemorrhage is usually the result of anticoagulation, trauma from blunt injury, or a coagulopathy. Hemorrhage in the mesentery causes extramural indentations of the bowel lumen, called thumbprinting. These indentations, however, may also be seen with extramural masses. Necrotizing enterocolitis, which involves the large bowel and the small bowel, is discussed later in the section on vascular diseases of the colon.

Diverticular Disease

Diverticula of the small bowel (except for Meckel's diverticulum, discussed earlier) are acquired, asymptomatic, and discovered incidentally on contrast examinations. A diverticulum can occasionally be mistaken for a giant ulcer, but the presence of normal mucosa and the lack of edema and inflammatory changes are usually conducive to a correct interpretation. Jejunal diverticulosis is the development of multiple diverticula of the jejunum. These diverticula, which are uncommon, occur in elderly patients and are usually asymptomatic. However, they can cause a blind-loop syndrome, anemia, inflammation, or hemorrhage.

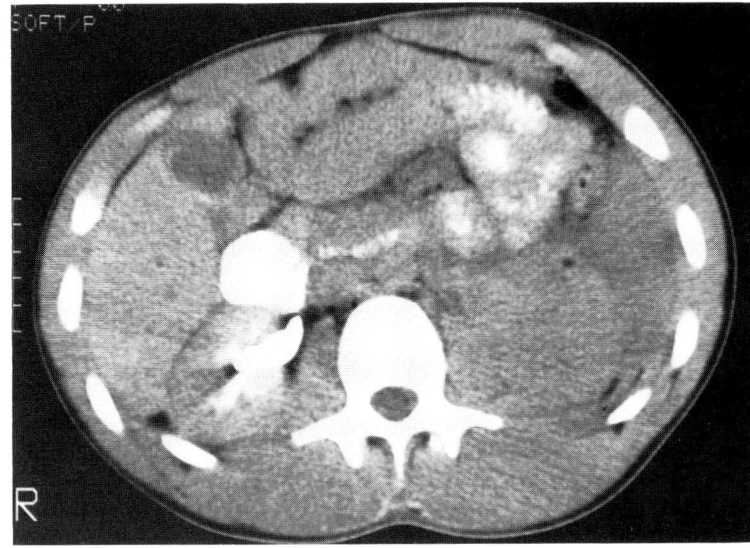

FIGURE 3–43. Bowel injury. CT shows thickening of the duodenal wall resulting from hematoma in a young man injured in an automobile accident. The wall thickening causes narrowing of the lumen of the transverse portion of the duodenum. The left kidney is enlarged and nonfunctioning as a result of severe injury.

COLON

Trauma

The colon is injured in 5% to 10% of cases of abdominal trauma. The sigmoid colon, the transverse colon, and the cecum are the most common sites, and the causes include blunt impact, penetration injury, and colonoscopy. Penetration injuries with extravasation of colonic contents lead to the development of fistulas and sinus tracts similar to those caused elsewhere in the GI tract. Plain films show intraperitoneal air, fluid, or blood. An abnormal bowel gas pattern can suggest bowel obstruction or adynamic ileus. CT may reveal bowel-wall thickening, mesenteric hematoma, hemoperitoneum, or pneumoperitoneum (Fig. 3–43).

Blunt or decelerating injuries damage the fixed portions of the bowel (the ascending and descending portions of the colon and the rectum). Such injuries usually result in retroperitoneal extravasation of fecal material. Traumatic injuries to the rectum are most commonly caused by insertion of foreign objects and by unconventional sexual techniques. Ingested foreign objects (even long, sharp ones) are usually passed through the colon without injury, although obstruction and perforation can occur. Such ingestions are common among prisoners as a method for admission to a hospital and are also seen in mental patients. Serial, abdominal films can document the usually uneventful passage of the objects through the GI tract.

Congenital Abnormalities

Congenital abnormalities of the colon include aberrant anatomical formation, such as atresia and duplication, and abnormalities characterized by dysfunction. Colonic atresia and duplication are rare and have the same characteristics in the colon as elsewhere in the GI tract. The most important dysfunctional disease of the colon is aganglionosis (Hirschsprung's disease).

Imperforate Anus. Imperforate anus, the lack of an opening between the skin and the rectum, indicates abnormalities in the anal canal, the rectum, or the lower urogenital system. A urogenital fistula is often present, and half of infants with imperforate anus have other anomalies. Full evaluation requires examination of both the genitourinary and lower GI tracts. Radiographs with the pelvis elevated to allow bowel gas to rise to the most distal part of the rectum document the length of the rectal pouch. However, ultrasonography enables a more accurate determination of the length of the atretic segment. A short segment is easily opened and repaired. A long, atretic segment requires complicated reconstructive surgery, particularly when other anomalies are present.

Aganglionosis. Aganglionosis (Hirschsprung's disease)—the congenital absence of parasympathetic ganglion cells in the submucosa of the colon, usually that of the rectum and the distal colon—results in constriction of the rectum and the distal colon and dilatation of the proximal bowel. The disease is most common in male infants and usually manifests as neonatal obstruction. It is not detected in some patients until late childhood or even early adulthood. These patients have constipation and vomiting or signs of bowel obstruction. The presumptive diagnosis is made through the use of barium enema without the use of cleansing enemas. The study must be performed by a skilled pediatric radiologist because of the difficulty of demonstrating the transition zone between the normal and abnormal bowel and because of the risk of perforation. The examination reveals a large, dilated proximal colon and a narrow, irregular rectosigmoid (Fig. 3–44). A delayed (24-hour) film shows stasis of the barium. The conclusive diagnosis is usually made by biopsy.

Surgical resection of the aganglionic segment and pull-through of the remaining colon is curative, especially when disease is limited to the rectosigmoid (80% of patients). Complications of aganglionosis other than bowel obstruction include the development of enterocolitis.

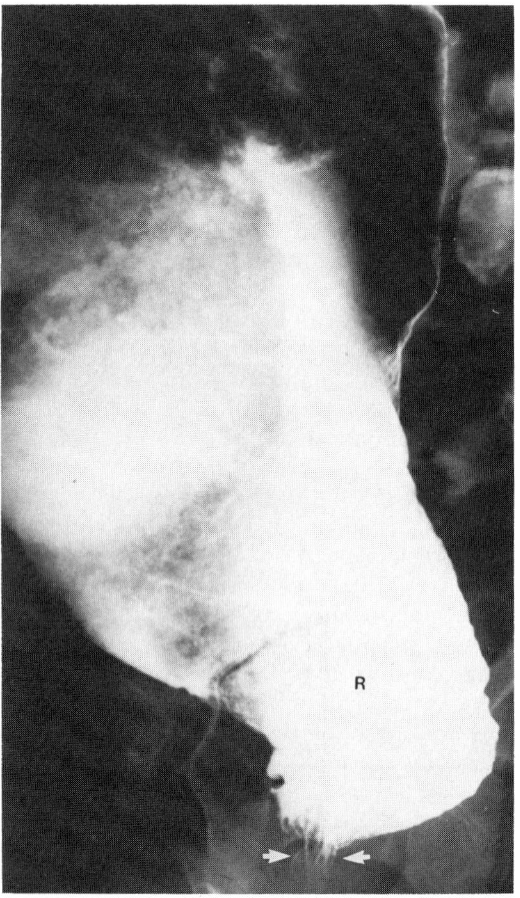

FIGURE 3–44. Aganglionosis. Barium enema study shows a greatly dilated sigmoid colon in an infant with distal large-bowel obstruction. The rectum (R) is markedly narrowed over a short distance *(arrows)*.

Inflammation

Toxic injury to the colon is usually the result of abuse of cathartic agents. High doses of over-the-counter cathartics produce chronic mucosal inflammation, primarily in the cecum and the ascending colon. Barium enema initially shows a large hypotonic colon and, later, an ahaustral, contracted colon. These changes occur as a result of decades of laxative abuse. Contrast studies show nonspecific mucosal inflammation, usually without ulceration.

Radiation colitis of variable degree and duration is common in patients being treated for abdominal or pelvic cancer. Edema and ulceration occur initially, followed by fibrosis and stenosis. The barium enema findings are indistinguishable from those of other forms of colitis. The effects of radiation colitis mimic those of ischemia.

Inflammatory bowel disease can involve any portion of the colon. The most important diseases are ulcerative colitis and regional enterocolitis (Crohn's colitis). Whereas ulcerative colitis involves the rectum and extends proximally, regional enteritis is most severe in the terminal ileum. The asymmetry of involvement and the presence of normal areas (skip areas) between inflamed segments are helpful in establishing the diagnosis of regional enteritis.

Ulcerative Colitis. Ulcerative colitis is an inflammatory bowel disease of unknown cause characterized by symmetrical (i.e., circumferential) mucosal inflammation beginning at the rectum and extending proximally. The disease is most common in girls and young women, usually Caucasian. The usual symptoms are rectal and abdominal pain, bleeding, and diarrhea. The usual clinical course is intermittent exacerbations followed by quiescent periods. Disease limited to the rectum and the sigmoid colon, called ulcerative proctitis, is usually less severe. More commonly, ulcerative colitis involves the rectum, the sigmoid colon, and the descending colon. The inflammatory process can extend into the ascending colon and even into the terminal ileum, where it is called backwash ileitis.

The most important radiographic features of ulcerative colitis are demonstrated on barium enema examination, which reveals continuous mucosal involvement beginning at the distal rectum and extending proximally (Fig. 3–45). Early disease causes granularity of the mucosa. More advanced disease is characterized by ulcerations (Fig. 3–46). Other findings include the development of inflammatory polyps (pseudopolyps) and, in advanced disease, shortening and narrowing of the colon (which give it the appearance of a pipe). In most cases, it is possible to distinguish ulcerative colitis from regional enteritis (Crohn's colitis) by the locations, the symmetry, and the characteristics of the inflammatory involvement.

Patients experience intermittent flare-ups of the disease, which often respond to steroid enemas, systemic steroid therapy, or antibiotics. Many patients have extracolonic diseases similar to those associated with granulomatous colitis. Colon carcinoma can develop as early as 10 years after onset of the disease, and the risk increases incrementally by about 1% per year beginning 10 years after onset of the disease. Severe disease also predisposes a patient to the development of toxic megacolon, a severe form of adynamic ileus, which can result in bowel rupture because of the extreme friability of the bowel wall.

Regional Enterocolitis. Regional enterocolitis (also called Crohn's disease, Crohn's colitis, and granulomatous enterocolitis) is characterized by asymmetrical, segmental inflammation affecting the full thickness of the bowel wall. The disease almost always involves the terminal ileum (see Figs. 3–40 and 3–41). Segments of the colon are involved in more than half of cases. Fistulas between bowel segments, sinus tracts to the skin, and abscesses are common, especially in the anus and the rectum. Barium enema studies can demonstrate eccentric (asymmetrical) colonic inflammation, including stricture, inflammatory polyps, cobblestone ulceration, and fistulas. It also can identify disease that recurs after surgical resection, which is often at the site of anastomosis at the terminal ileum. CT is most effective in identifying abscesses, which occur in 25% of patients.

Regional enterocolitis can usually be distinguished from ulcerative colitis by the asymmetrical, transmural involvement and by the presence of normal areas (skip areas) between diseased segments (Fig. 3–47). When disease is limited to the colon, surgical resection of the abnormal segment is often curative. The development of toxic megacolon and carcinoma in patients with regional enteritis is much less common than in patients with ulcerative colitis.

Infection

Infectious diseases of the colon are usually bacterial and generally result in a superficial mucosal inflammation. Radiographic examination is not performed unless unusual features or severe symptoms cause consideration of other diseases. Barium enema studies may yield normal results or may demonstrate the mucosal inflammation with or without ulceration. The location of infection can suggest the organism (see Fig. 3–16). Diverticulitis with abscess is discussed later in the "Diverticular Disease" section.

Bacillary Infection. *Shigella* species usually involve the rectum and the sigmoid colon and, in rare instances, the descending colon. *Salmonella* species usually involve the right portion of the colon and the distal small bowel. *Yersinia* infections, although usually limited to the terminal ileum, can extend into the colon. *Campylobacter fetus* infections affect all portions of the colon. Appendicitis, infection of the obstructed appendix, is a common, acute disease that usually occurs in children.

Acute Appendicitis. The appendix, a blind tubular bowel segment attached to the cecum, can become obstructed and trap bacteria and digestive residues, which form an infected mass. The inflamed appendix may rupture, causing life-threatening peritonitis. Such obstruction and infection, called appendicitis, can occur at any age but is most common in young children. The usual early clinical symptoms are fever and periumbilical abdominal pain (caused by inflammation of the visceral peritoneum). When rupture occurs, the fever intensifies, the white blood cell count becomes elevated, and the pain becomes localized over the appendix in the right lower quadrant (because of inflammation of the parietal peritoneum).

Usually the clinical manifestation of appendicitis leads to the correct diagnosis, and radiographs are not obtained. When the signs and symptoms are not typical or in older patients when other diseases are considered, plain films, barium enema studies, ultrasonography, and CT may complement the physical diagnosis. Plain films can show air or a stone (appendicolith) in the appendix, evidence of a mass or an abnormal fluid collection adjacent to the

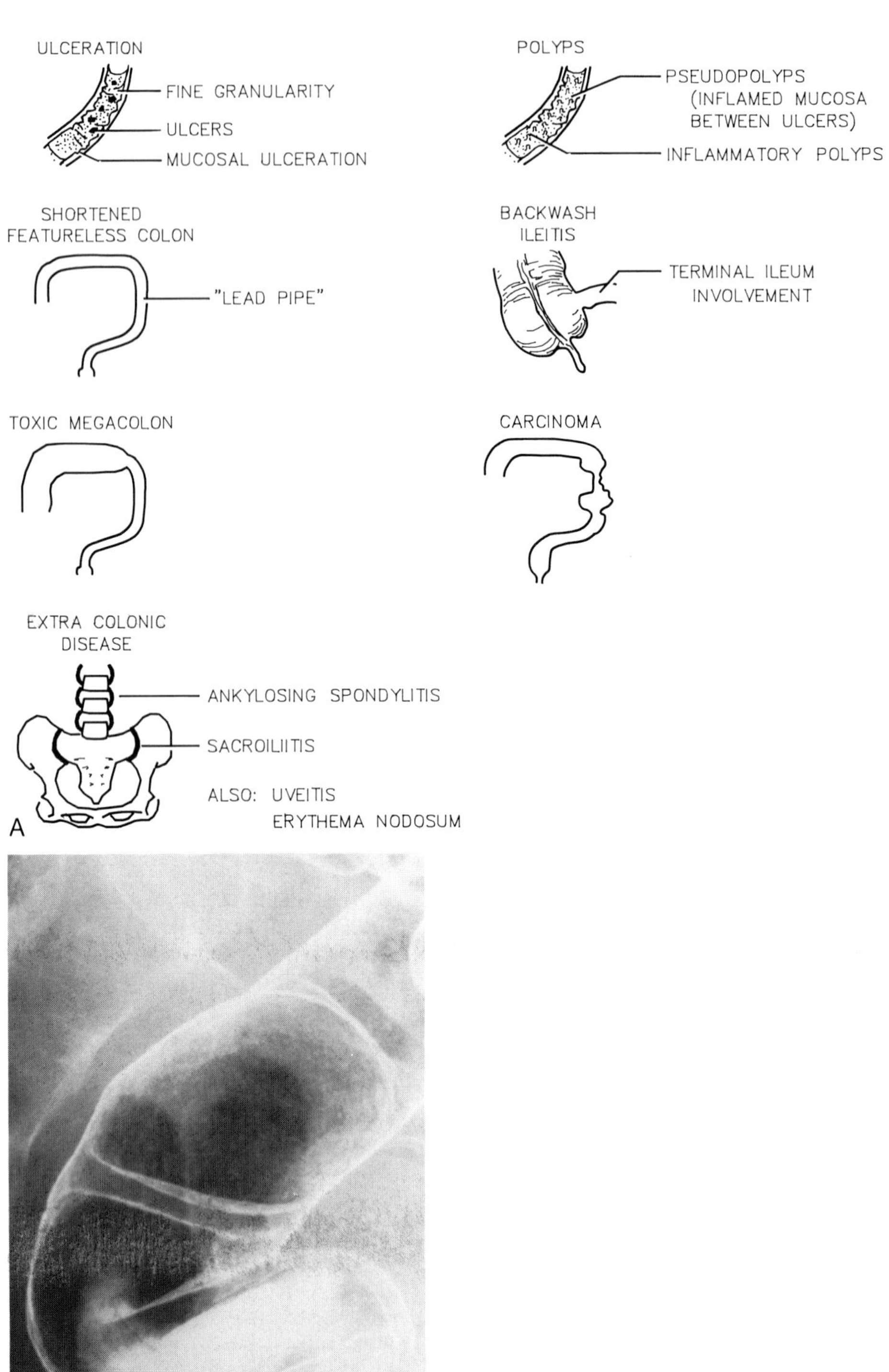

FIGURE 3–45. Ulcerative colitis. *A.* Diagram. *B.* Lateral view from double-contrast barium enema study shows multiple superficial ulcerations scattered throughout the mucosal surface of the rectum.

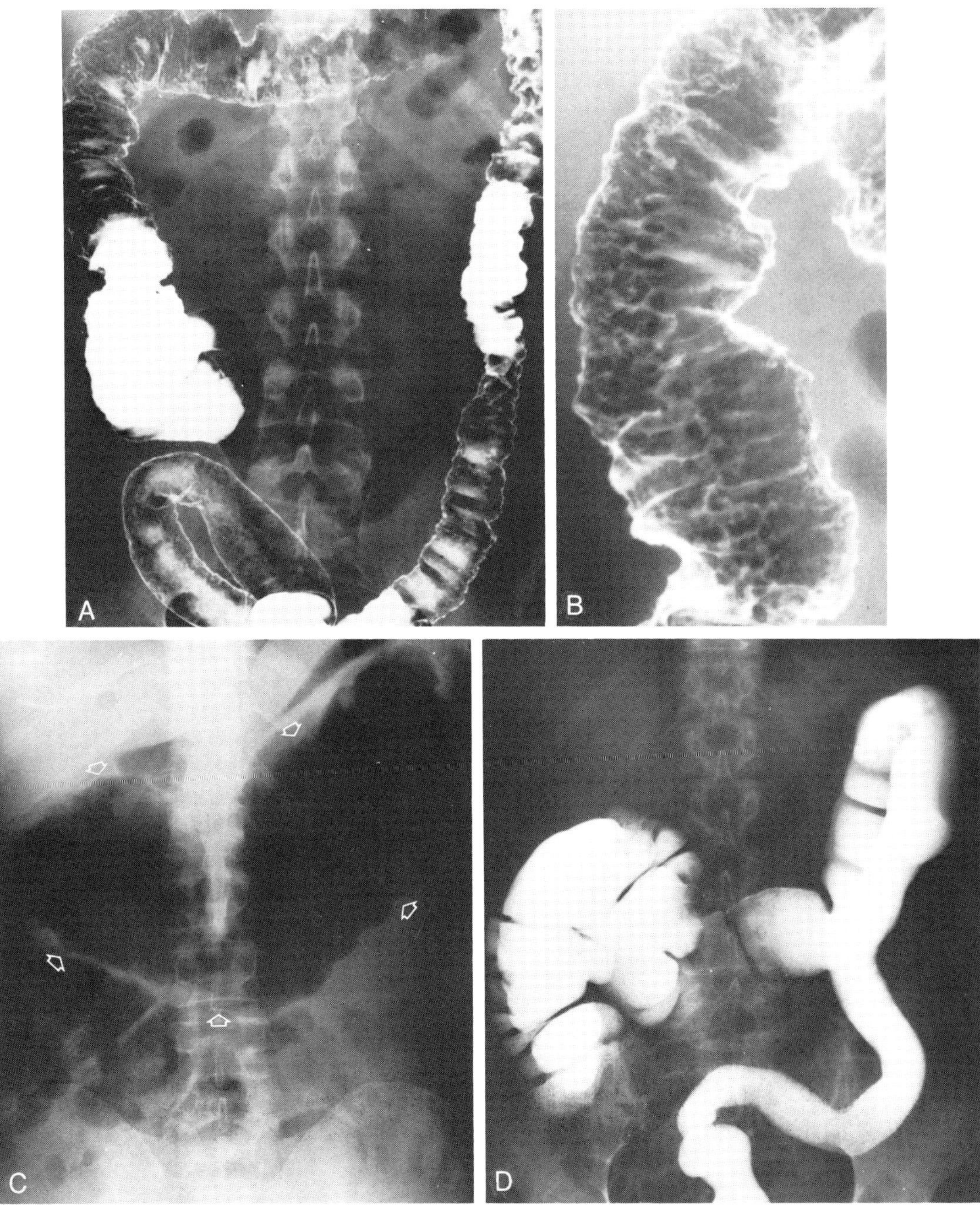

FIGURE 3–46. Advanced ulcerative colitis. *A.* Double-contrast barium enema study shows diffuse involvement of the entire mucosal surface pattern of the colon. Note loss of normal haustral folds of the colon and narrowing of the lumen. *B.* Magnified view of a segment of descending colon. *C.* Dilated transverse colon *(open arrowheads)* in a different patient with ulcerative colitis who developed toxic megacolon. *D.* Single-contrast barium enema shows featureless descending and sigmoid portions of the colon in a young woman with long-standing ulcerative colitis. This appearance, caused by destruction of mucosa, is likened to that of a pipe.

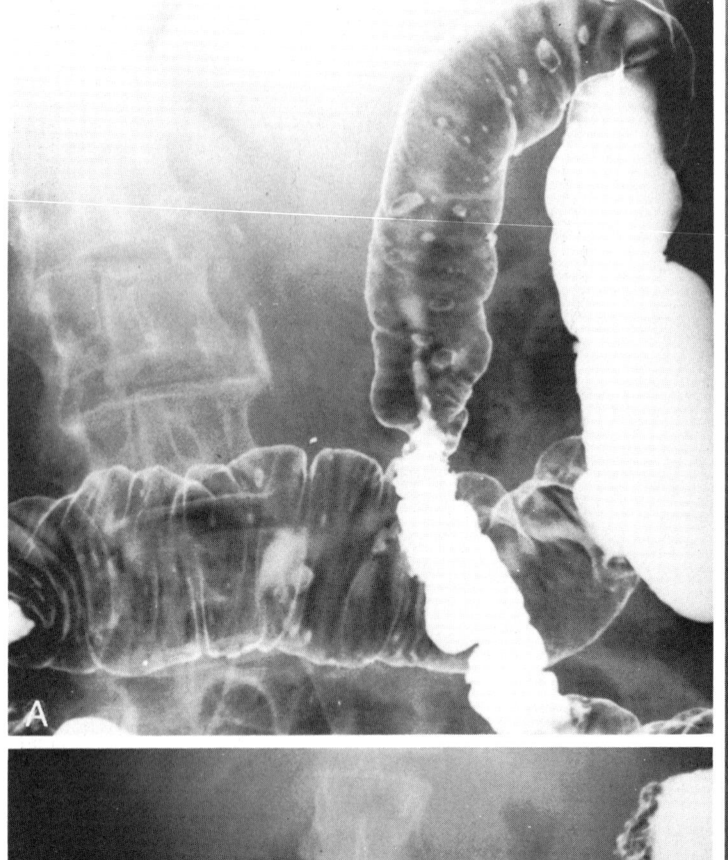

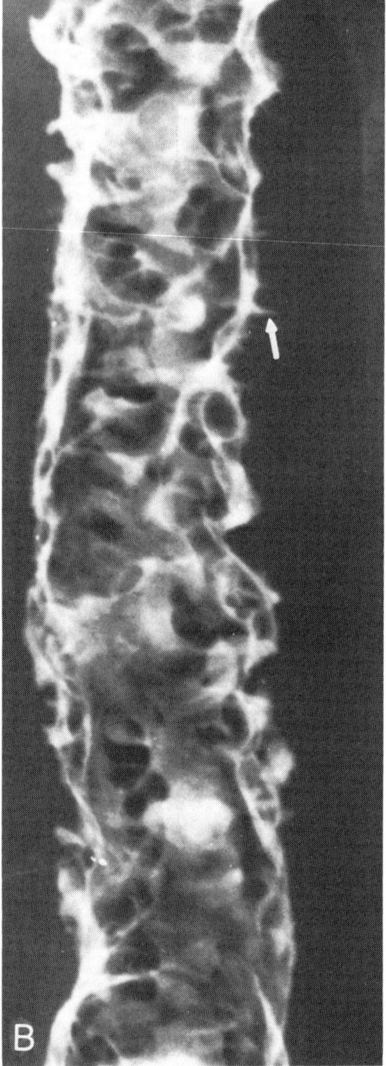

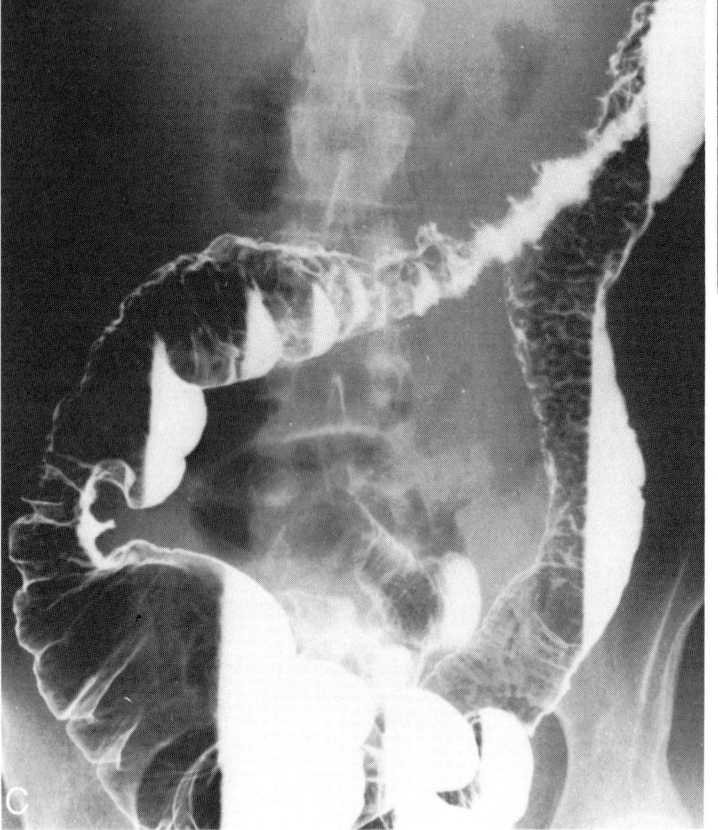

FIGURE 3–47. Regional enteritis with colon involvement. *A.* Double-contrast barium enema study shows numerous, shallow ulcerations of varying size that represent the aphthous lesions of a midstage regional enteritis. *B.* Double-contrast barium enema study, magnified view of a segment of the descending colon shows multiple mucosal irregularities that represent acute and chronic stages of regional enteritis. Ulcerations project from the lumen, best seen in profile. The curved spiculations (*arrow*) have a rose-thorn appearance and are commonly seen in regional enteritis. *C.* A double-contrast barium enema shows diffuse involvement of the left transverse colon and proximal half of the descending colon.

cecum, and evidence of bowel obstruction or localized adynamic ileus (Fig. 3–48). Barium enema studies can demonstrate extravasation or nonfilling of the appendix, effects of a mass (abscess) displacing the colon or the terminal ileum, and spasm or obstruction in the terminal ileum or cecum.

Ultrasonograms and CT scans can show masses and calcification. Ultrasonography can be used (1) to demonstrate the enlarged appendix and mural thickening and (2) to demonstrate that it does not collapse when compressed by the transducer. If the appendix measures 7 mm or more in diameter and cannot be compressed in a patient without causing right lower quadrant pain, the diagnosis of appendicitis is likely correct. Any patient who has acute, right lower quadrant pain and in whom an appendicolith is seen is also considered to have appendicitis. CT is most effective in demonstrating an abscess or an inflammatory mass associated with a ruptured appendix. Also, because most patients with right lower quadrant pain do not have appendicitis, CT and ultrasonography can show abnormalities related to other diseases.

Patients with acute appendicitis require surgery. A chronic appendiceal abscess can be treated initially with antibiotics. A patient with a well-defined abscess can often be treated by percutaneous drainage under CT or ultrasonographic guidance.

Tuberculosis. Tuberculosis of the colon is rare in the United States but is the second most common cause of infectious bowel disease worldwide. The infection usually is at the ileocecal valve, where it causes obstruction or abscess formation. In many patients, the result of a fecal smear for acid-fast bacilli is negative. The barium study reveals thickened and ulcerated mucosa in the region of the ileocecal valve, effects of the abscess, and narrowing of the bowel lumen (Fig. 3–49).

Amebiasis. Amebiasis is the commonest cause of infectious bowel disease worldwide, but it is relatively rare in the United States. Many patients are immunosuppressed or have poor sanitary habits. The infection usually involves the ascending colon, the rectum, and, in rare instances, the terminal ileum, in which it causes a transmural ulcerative inflammatory process. The clinical symptoms and the radiographic appearance of amebiasis are usually indistinguishable from those of granulomatous colitis (Crohn's disease). Barium enema studies reveal mucosa that is ragged as a result of inflammation, as well as edema and the formation of a pseudomembrane (Fig. 3–50). Patients with amebiasis also develop liver abscesses (to be described) and lung disease (see Chapter 2).

Pseudomembranous Colitis. Colitis associated with antibiotics is known as pseudomembranous colitis. The normal flora of the mucosal surface of the colon are altered because of the antibiotic therapy, allowing for colonization by *Clostridium difficile.* This bacterium produces a toxin that breaks down the substructure of the colonic mucosa and produces an extensive fibrin exudate. Patients develop fever and leukocytosis, which are suggestive of abdominal abscess.

Barium enema studies reveal local patches or large segments of irregular mucosa, often covered with a pseudomembrane. Edema causes effacement of the normal haustral colonic folds and separation of bowel loops. The most constant radiographic findings are a dilated intestinal lumen, thickened folds, and a shaggy appearance of the mucosa (Fig. 3–51). CT scans can show thickened colon wall. The findings on barium enema and CT studies are generally nonspecific and may simulate other diseases such as colitis caused by *Campylobacter* species, ulcerative colitis, and regional enterocolitis.

Neoplasms

Most benign tumors of the colon are adenomatous or hyperplastic polyps (Table 3–2). These are often detected incidentally when patients are evaluated for unrelated bowel symptoms. Because of the ease of removal of polyps through the colonoscope, all should be removed or evaluated in biopsy; further therapy is directed by the results.

The congenital polyposis syndromes (see Table 3–1) all involve the colon with multiple polyps. These syndromes are uncommon, but they are noteworthy because of their mode of genetic transmission, associated lesions, and malignant potential.

Hyperplastic Polyps. Hyperplastic polyps are small, nonneoplastic masses, usually about 5 mm in size. They appear identical to adenomatous polyps of the same size. They have no malignant potential.

Adenomatous Polyps. Adenomatous polyps are the most common colonic tumors. They occur in all age groups and may be single or multiple. These tumors arise from the colonic epithelium and are usually asymptomatic.

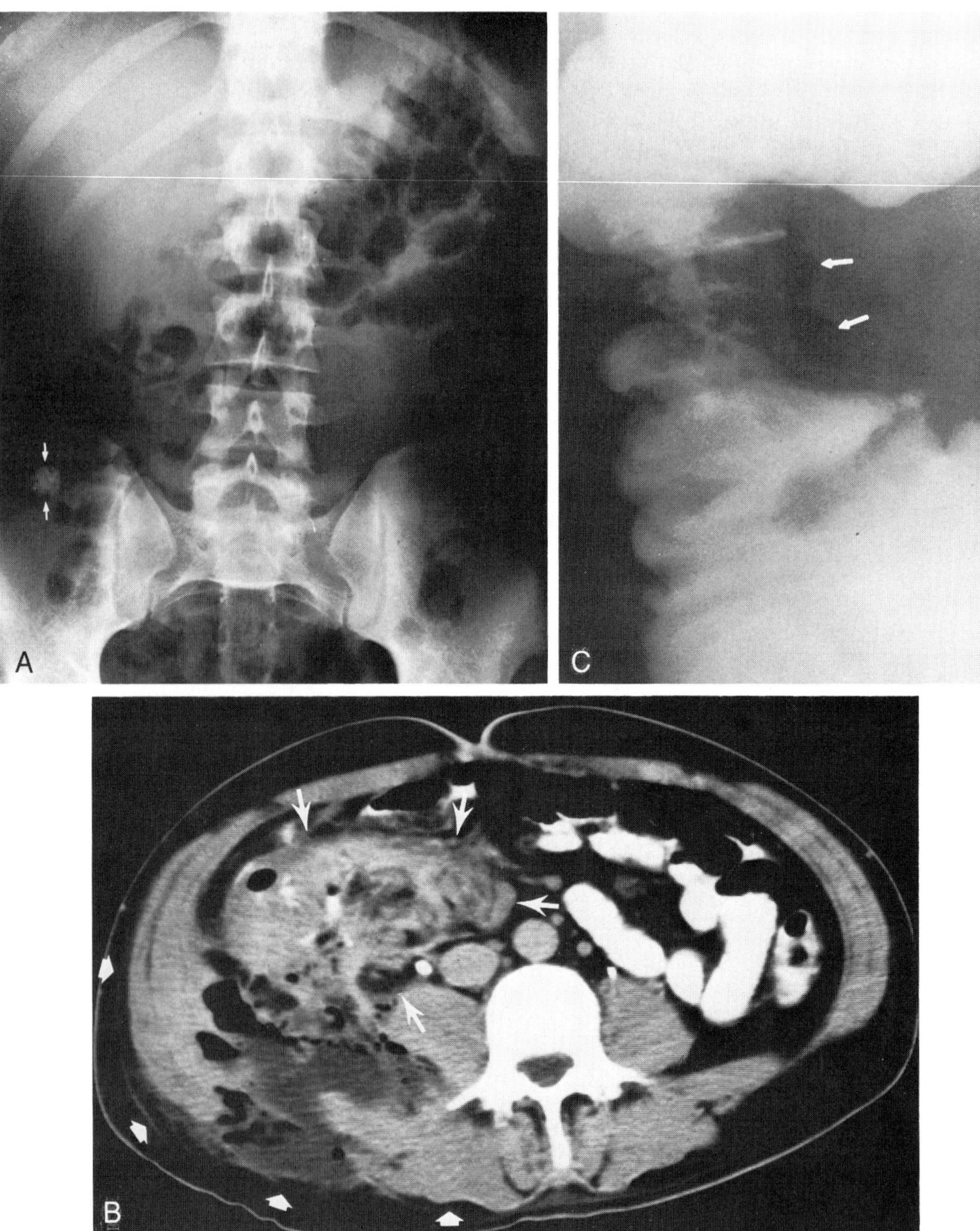

FIGURE 3–48. Appendicitis. *A.* Appendicolith. Plain film shows a solitary calcification *(arrows)* in a young man with fever and right lower quadrant pain. The radiographic and clinical findings are diagnostic of appendicitis. *B.* Periappendiceal abscess. CT of a young woman with fever and diffuse abdominal pain as a result of ruptured appendix shows an intraperitoneal inflammatory mass and gas in the anterior right lower quadrant *(arrows)*. The abscess also extends posteriorly to retroperitoneum *(arrowheads)*, where it abuts the spine and right iliac bone and displaces the right psoas muscle. *C.* Single-contrast barium enema study in a man with rupture of a retrocecal appendix shows distortion, ulceration, and spiculation. Note thickened irregular folds, luminal constriction, and extraluminal gas *(arrows)* within an abscess.

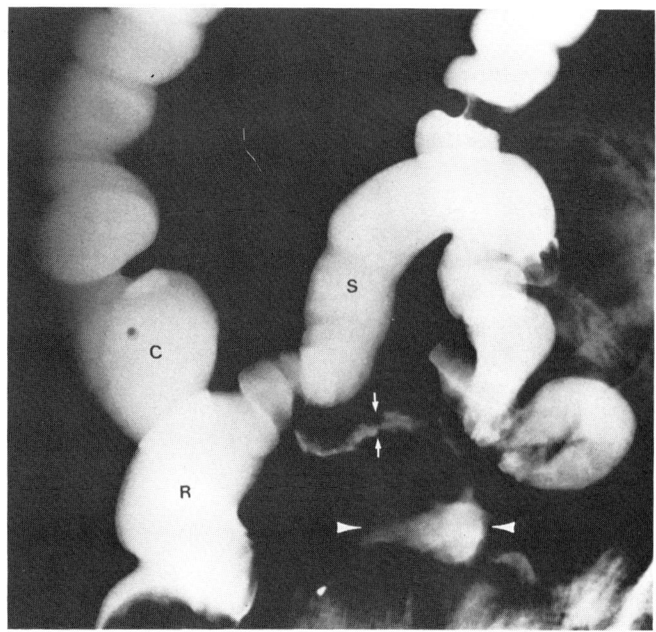

FIGURE 3–49. Tuberculosis. Small-bowel study shows marked narrowing and mucosal thickening in the terminal ileum of the bowel *(arrows)* in a man with primary tuberculosis. The amorphous collection of barium just inferior to this diseased segment of small bowel represents a fistulous cavity *(arrowheads)*. S, sigmoid; C, cecum; R, rectum.

Painless rectal bleeding is a frequent presentation. Most polyps are discovered in the rectum or the sigmoid colon. The radiographic appearance may be a sessile (flat), moundlike, or pedunculated mass projecting above the mucosal surface, which is best detected by double-contrast barium enema studies (Fig. 3–52). Pedunculated polyps (those on a stalk) are usually slow to metastasize even when they are malignant.

Adenomatous polyps must be carefully evaluated because of their malignant potential. Small ones (less than 1 cm in diameter) are unlikely to be malignant and are usually removed by colonoscopic polypectomy. Larger adenomatous polyps, and especially the villous adenoma, must be resected completely because of the much higher likelihood of malignancy. Because colonic polyps recur and have malignant potential, continuous follow-up is necessary in patients who have had a polyp. When a malignant polyp is detected, further therapy depends on whether the stalk and the colonic mucosa have been invaded.

Juvenile Polyp. The juvenile polyp is a small, pedunculated hamartoma of the colon, usually located in the rectum (75%) or the descending colon. It generally occurs in children under 10 years of age as a single lesion, manifesting with rectal bleeding in 95% of patients. Air-contrast barium enema studies usually reveal the polyp to be pedunculated. This polyp usually autoamputates and has no malignant potential.

Postinflammatory Polyps. Postinflammatory polyps (hyperplastic polyps) occur in the colon

TABLE 3–2. COLONIC POLYPS

Syndrome	Age (Years)	Malignant Potential	Location	Symptoms	Description
Adenomatous polyp	>40	Yes	Colon	Bleeding or incidental	Pedunculated, single
Villous adenoma	>35	Yes	Colon, small bowel	Bleeding or mucoid feces	Sessile, single
Juvenile retention polyp	1 to 14	No	Rectum (75%), sigmoid colon (15%)	Bleeding	Pedunculated; 85% are single
Hyperplastic (metaplastic) polyp	>20	No	Colon	None	Small, multiple
Pseudopolyp (inflammatory)	>15	No	Colon	Ulcerative colitis	Sessile, multiple, inflammatory

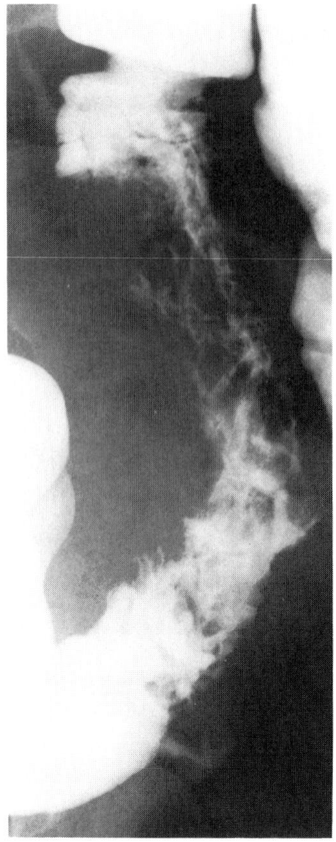

FIGURE 3–50. Amebiasis. Single-contrast barium enema study shows a markedly irregular mucosal surface in a long segment of the descending portion of the colon of a patient with bloody diarrhea.

as a result of inflammatory bowel disease, usually ulcerative colitis or regional enteritis (granulomatous colitis). The lesions are multiple and represent hyperplastic overgrowth of colonic mucosa in areas of previous inflammation. Diagnosis is made through barium enema studies, which usually reveal other evidence of inflammatory bowel disease.

Villous Adenoma. The villous adenoma is a sessile, shaggy, polypoid lesion related to the adenomatous polyp. It is usually single and occurs in patients over age 35 years. The majority of these are in the rectum or cecum. Clinical signs include rectal bleeding, diarrhea, and mucoid feces. Many patients manifest lowered serum potassium and albumin levels. Barium enema studies reveal an irregular mucosal mass (Fig. 3–53; see also Fig. 3–8). The villous adenoma has high malignant potential. Small lesions (less than 2 cm in length) have a 10% chance of malignant transformation. Larger lesions have more than a 50% chance of such degeneration. Because they are sessile, they must be treated surgically.

Lipoma. The lipoma is the second most common benign tumor of the colon. Sixty percent of all GI lipomas are in the colon, usually in the cecum or the right colon. Barium enema studies reveal a smooth submucosal or subserosal mass that changes diameter and shape when compressed. Colonic lipomas are usually found incidentally and require no therapy.

Endometriosis. Endometriosis is the spread of endometrial cells to the serosa of the colon. There, these cells continue to grow and eventually protrude into the lumen. The disease occurs in 5% of women, causing vague lower abdominal symptoms, which are usually associated with menses. Most of these lesions (85%) occur in the rectosigmoid. A barium enema study or a CT scan can reveal an extraluminal mass if it is large. Double-contrast barium enema studies best demonstrate mucosal abnormalities. Although endometriosis can cause narrowing of the bowel lumen, obstruction is rare. The lesions do not cause hemorrhage unless they penetrate the mucosa (Fig. 3–54).

Carcinoid Tumor. Most carcinoid tumors (50%) occur in the appendix, in which they are benign, do not metastasize, and do not cause the carcinoid syndrome. Carcinoid tumors of the appendix are usually incidental findings but can cause obstruction and appendicitis. Carcinoid tumors occur elsewhere in the colon, usually in the rectum (5% to 10%).

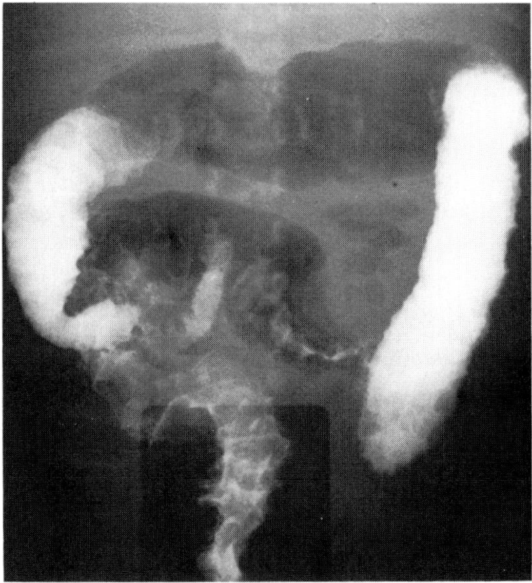

FIGURE 3–51. Pseudomembranous colitis. Barium enema study demonstrates severe mucosal ulcerations and edema throughout the colon in a child with fussiness and bloody diarrhea.

FIGURE 3–52. Colonic polyps. Double-contrast barium enema study demonstrates two pedunculated adenomatous polyps in the sigmoid colon *(arrowheads)*. The stalks are also clearly seen *(small arrows)*.

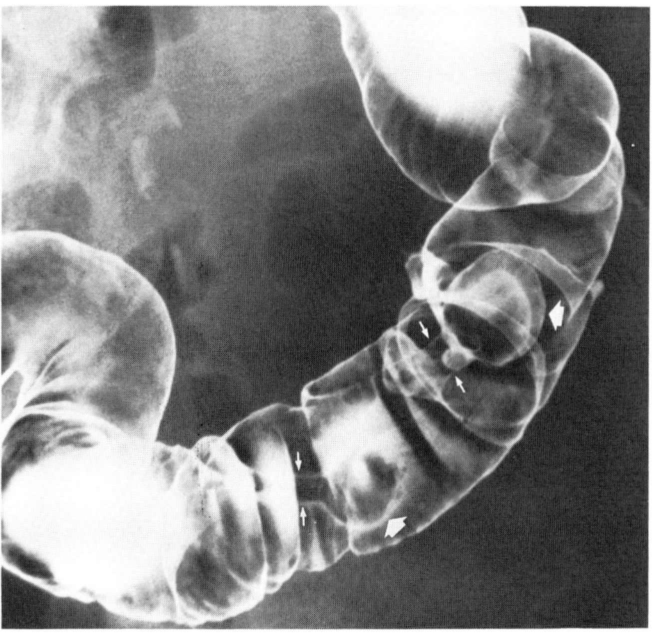

In the rectum, the lesions are usually benign. Elsewhere in the colon, they are usually invasive and malignant, penetrating the bowel wall and extending into the mesentery, in which they cause a desmoplastic reaction that restricts the motion of the bowel. Because blood from the colon passes directly to the liver, in which the serotonin is broken down, these tumors usually do not produce the carcinoid syndrome unless liver metastases are present, in which case significant amounts of serotonin reach the pulmonary and systemic circulations.

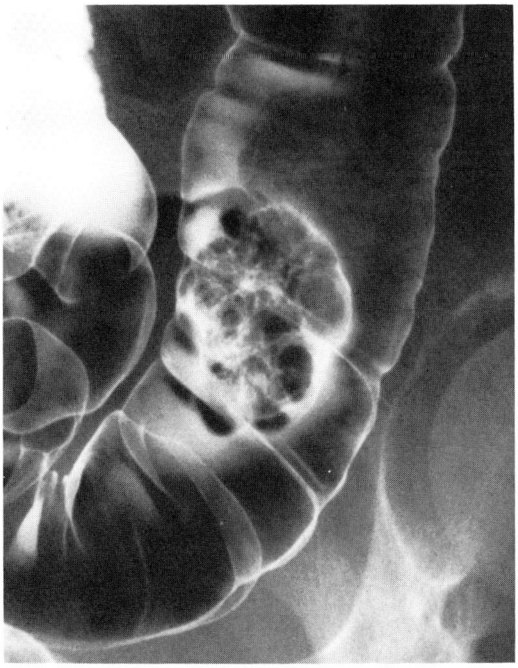

FIGURE 3–53. Villous adenoma. Spot film from a barium enema study shows a mushroom-shaped mass in the descending portion of the colon in a 55-year-old man with chronic diarrhea. Note the sessile appearance and the spiculated texture.

Adenocarcinoma. Adenocarcinoma is the most common malignant tumor of the colon and is responsible for 15% of all cancer deaths.

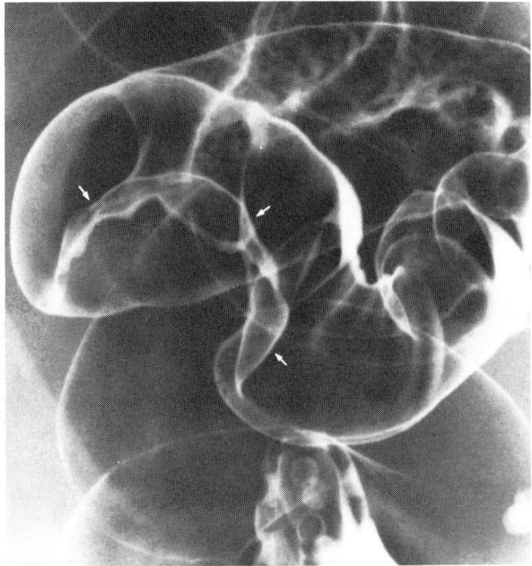

FIGURE 3–54. Endometrioma. Double-contrast colon examination with a magnified view of the sigmoid colon shows a large mass protruding into the lumen in a woman with pelvic pain related to menses. The serosa has been invaded, and the lesion has penetrated through the mucosa *(arrows)*.

The tumor occurs in equal numbers of men and women, usually occurs in people over the age of 45, and is most often located in the rectosigmoid (50% of colon carcinomas occur in the rectum and 20% in the sigmoid colon). The adenomatous polyp and the villous adenoma are the most common premalignant lesions of adenocarcinoma of the colon. Patients with some polyposis syndromes (see Table 3–1) and long-standing inflammatory bowel disease have such a high incidence of carcinoma that early colectomy is advocated.

Most patients with colon cancer notice a change in bowel habits or rectal bleeding. When the tumor is in the right colon, in which the fecal material is fluid, symptoms are usually vague and may include cramping, simulating other GI problems such as cholecystitis and appendicitis. Obstruction is uncommon unless disease is advanced. Anemia, weakness, and weight loss are common. The stool shows occult blood but not fresh blood. When the tumor is in the smaller diameter left colon, obstruction is more common, and patients experience constipation with episodes of diarrhea. Fresh blood per rectum is common with tumors of the left colon.

Adenocarcinoma of the colon is diagnosed radiographically by means of barium enema, preferably with double-contrast technique. The appearance of the tumor depends on the location and the tumor stage (Fig. 3–55). The mass may appear polypoid, infiltrative, or ulcerative. The examination can reveal a filling defect, a pedunculated mass, ulceration of the mucosa, obstruction, or, on occasion, intussus-

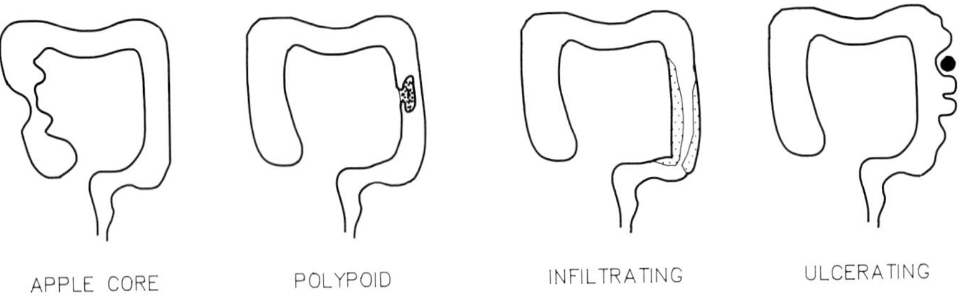

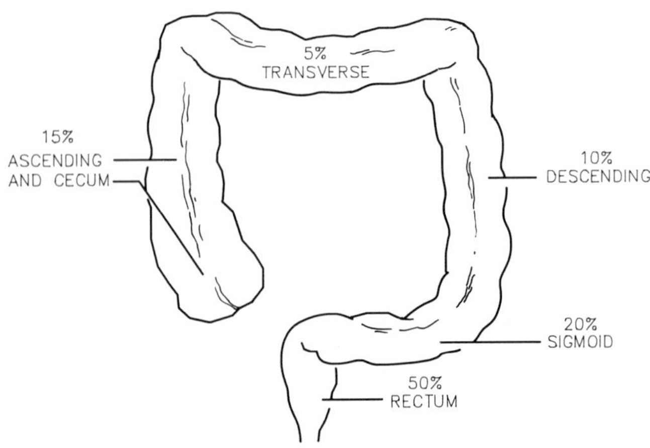

FIGURE 3–55. *A.* Appearances of colon carcinoma. *B.* Locations of colon carcinoma.

ception. Advanced lesions produce annular constriction of the bowel lumen (described as an apple-core lesion; Fig. 3–56).

CT and MRI are most valuable for determining local spread, adenopathy, liver metastases, and response to therapy. The detection and staging depends substantially on the site of tumor. Tumors in the ascending, transverse, and descending portions of the colon and in the sigmoid colon are often small when detected and grow slowly. They are usually diagnosed from clinical symptoms, results of barium enema studies, and colonoscopy findings. The primary lesion is often not detectable by CT and MRI. CT scans may show a colonic mass that does not fill with contrast and does displace the normal bowel, although focal peristaltic contraction or feces have a similar appearance.

The primary purpose of CT or MRI is to detect metastatic disease. Carcinomas from the proximal and the sigmoid colon spread rapidly to the liver. Liver metastases are often detected even when the primary tumor is very small, and they may be the first evidence of the primary tumor. Detection of liver metastases has a major impact on staging. The tumor may also extend to the mesenteric root and the omental lymph nodes. These metastatic lesions are often small and difficult to distin-

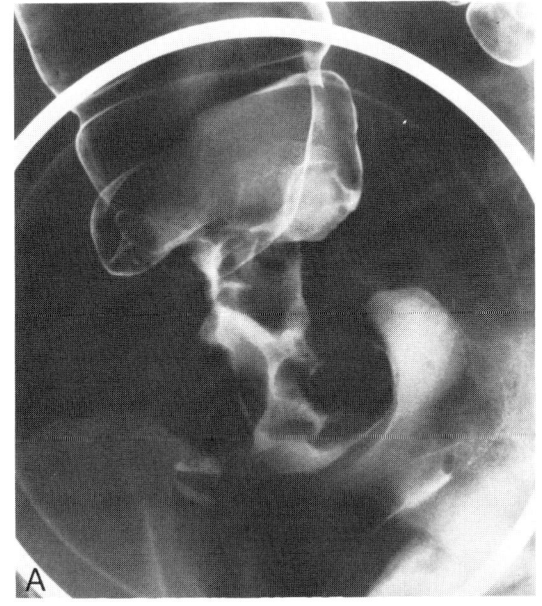

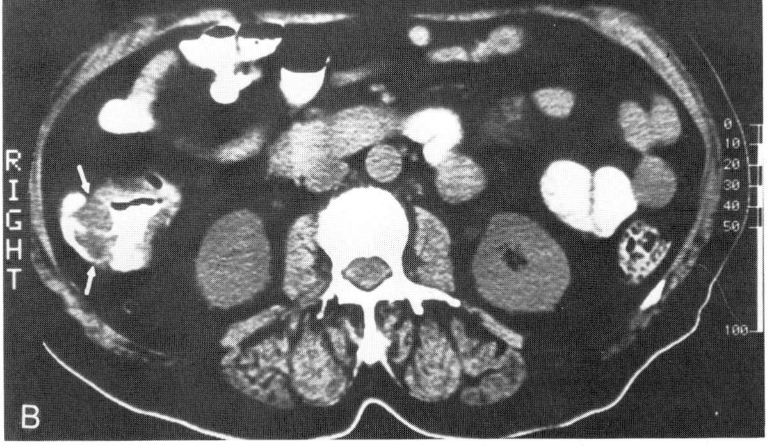

FIGURE 3–56. Colon carcinoma. *A.* Double-contrast enema study demonstrates a circumferential, constricting (apple-core) lesion in the proximal ascending colon in a 50-year-old man with anemia. *B.* CT shows adenocarcinoma infiltrating a segment of the proximal ascending colon *(arrows)*. Neither regional adenopathy nor local invasion was visible, but liver metastases were shown on higher slices.

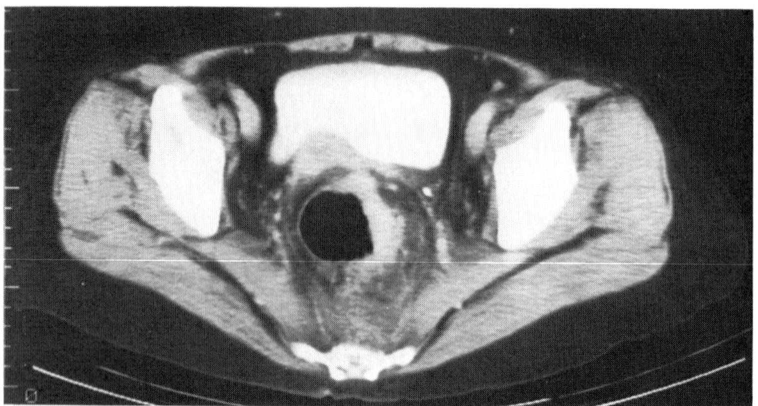

FIGURE 3–57. Colon carcinoma. Contrast CT shows thickening of the left lateral wall of the rectosigmoid with a nodular, irregular appearance in a 65-year-old man with rectal bleeding. The strand-like appearance in the posterior perirectal fat and the small but numerous nodes indicate extracolonic extension. Numerous low-density lesions were seen in the liver, which indicated hepatic metastases.

guish from normal nodes. Other staging requires chest radiography to determine the presence of pulmonary metastases, although these typically occur later than liver lesions.

When carcinoma occurs in the rectum, it is more locally invasive. The lesion causes symptoms early, especially when rectal bleeding or invasion of the rectal sphincter occurs. It is detected in CT and MRI as an invasive mass that crosses soft-tissue planes (Fig. 3–57). Adjacent pelvic lymph nodes may be invaded, including internal and external iliac nodes, obturator nodes, and, less commonly, inguinal and ischiorectal fossa nodes. Liver metastases occur much later. Staging of rectal carcinoma therefore requires evaluation for local invasion and liver metastases. Bone marrow metastases occur commonly and are readily detected in the spine and the pelvis through MRI.

Colon carcinoma is treated by wide excision, which includes lymph nodes. In advanced disease, surgical relief of obstruction is palliative. The overall 5-year survival rate is about 50%. However, local recurrence occurs in 10% of patients, and some patients develop multicentric tumor. Patients can be followed by measurement of carcinoembryonic antigen, which increases with tumor recurrence.

Other Malignancies. Squamous cell carcinoma occurs at the anus but is rare. Cloacogenic carcinoma is a rare tumor of the remnants of the cloaca and contains squamous cell, transitional cell, and mucoid cell components. Lymphoma is usually of the non-Hodgkin's type and manifests in several forms. It may be focally constricting, focally dilating (aneurysmal), fungating, or diffusely polypoid.

Vascular Diseases

Infarction. The most common vascular disease of the colon is ischemic disease, caused by atherosclerosis, vasculitis, embolism, or venous thrombosis. Patients usually develop acute abdominal pain or signs of obstruction, although the onset may be insidious and the symptoms nonspecific. Many patients have predisposing disease. The most common site of bowel infarction is the junction of the transverse colon and the splenic flexure because it receives end-arterial supply from the superior and inferior mesenteric arteries. Infarction also occurs in other parts of the small intestines and colon but is rare in the rectum because of the rich vascular supply to this area.

The radiographic diagnosis of ischemic bowel disease is made through barium enema studies, which can reveal a variety of findings, depending on the stage of the disease. Spasm and edema occur early, appearing as a narrowing of the lumen and a thickening of the bowel folds. Multiple, large indentations (thumbprints) in the bowel wall are caused by localized blood or edema and may also be detectable. By about 10 hours after ischemia, hemorrhagic infarction may occur and can be followed by necrosis and scarring. The barium enema study at these stages reveals a featureless segment of bowel, devoid of haustral markings and without peristalsis (Fig. 3–58).

Necrotizing Enterocolitis. Necrotizing enterocolitis (NEC) is an ischemic necrosis of the bowel that usually occurs in neonates (90% of cases occur during the first 10 days after birth). Most (75%) of the affected infants are premature, many have hyaline membrane disease, and the condition usually does not occur until the infant has been fed. The origin of NEC is unknown; it is probably caused by sparse blood flow to the gut. The usual signs are diarrhea, rectal bleeding, abdominal distension, and bile emesis.

The plain film findings in severe NEC are adynamic ileus, pneumatosis intestinalis (air in

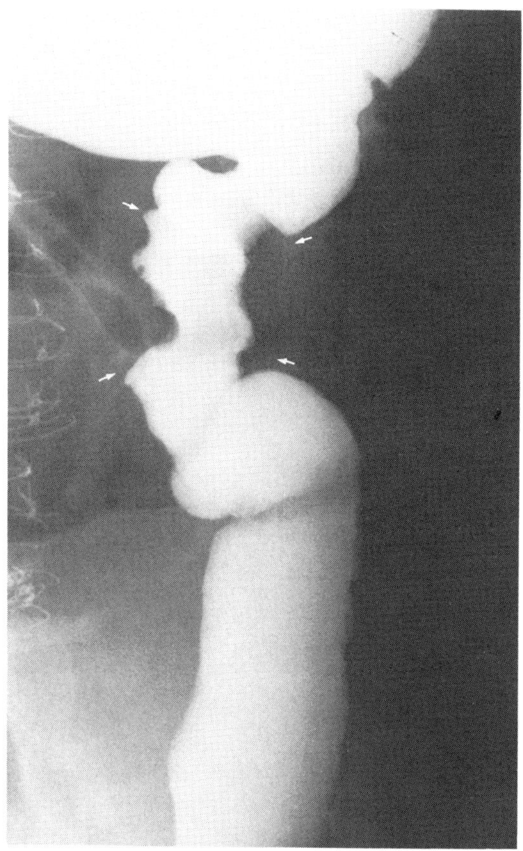

FIGURE 3–58. Bowel ischemia. Single-contrast barium enema study shows a narrowed segment of the descending colon with mucosal thickening and edema *(arrows)* in a patient with acute onset of abdominal pain.

the intestinal wall), portal venous gas, and pneumoperitoneum (Fig. 3–59). Such findings correlate with a high rate of mortality. When a newborn has signs of NEC but plain radiographs are normal, he or she should be treated presumptively; a barium enema study is not advised because of the risk of bowel perforation. The treatment of NEC includes oxygen administration, systemic antibiotics, correction of fluid and electrolyte disturbances, and elimination of bowel activity (by parenteral feeding). Surgical intervention may be necessary when there is evidence of perforation or when vital signs are unstable.

Intussusception. Idiopathic intussusception usually occurs between the ages of 6 months and 3 years. It is almost always ileocolic, the terminal ileum (the intussusceptum) passing into the cecum. Clinical symptoms are intermittent abdominal pain, bloody diarrhea, and vomiting. Plain films show a soft-tissue mass and absence of gas in the right lower or right upper quadrant. After surgical consultation, the radiologist can attempt to diagnose and also cure this condition by gently reducing the intussusception. Both air and barium given by enema can be used to push the intussuscepted ileum out of the colon. The examination must be performed under fluoroscopic control with low pressure in order not only to prevent bowel rupture but also to prevent infarction of the involved bowel.

Intussusception also occurs in adults, almost always as a result of lymphoma or polypoid

FIGURE 3–59. Necrotizing enterocolitis (NEC). Anteroposterior view of neonatal abdomen shows dilated bowel with pneumatosis intestinalis.

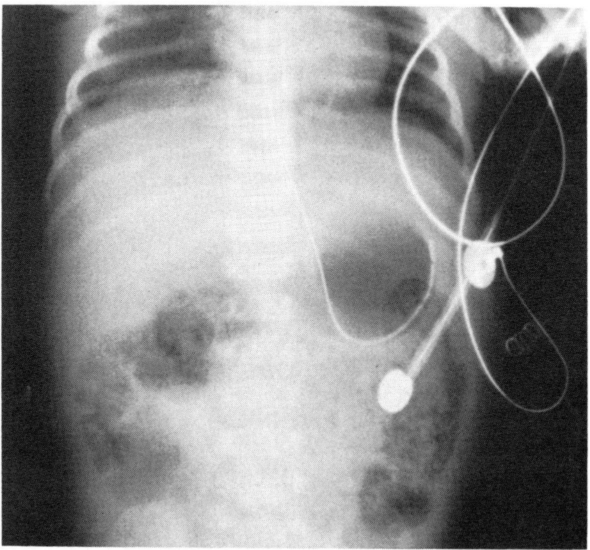

intraluminal tumor. Pathological ileocolic or colocolic intussusception in an adult is almost never reduced by barium enema, although the condition is usually diagnosed by means of this examination. CT scans can show the dilated outer bowel (the intussuscipiens) and the inner bowel (the intussusceptum) with mesenteric fat, as well as the mass that has caused the process.

Diverticular Disease

Acquired diverticula of the colon are common. They are demonstrated in half of patients over 60 years of age. Diverticula are the most common causes of a palpable colonic mass, rectal bleeding, and pain in this age group. The diverticula, which are usually multiple, are formed by herniation of the mucosa of the bowel through the muscle layer. Although they occur throughout the colon, most are in the left portion of the colon, especially the sigmoid colon. The rectum is spared. In rare instances, a single giant diverticulum (up to 20 cm in diameter) in the sigmoid or descending colon occurs.

Most diverticula are asymptomatic and are detected incidentally. Such disease without infection or symptoms is called diverticulosis. A barium enema study in a patient with diverticulosis shows multiple small sacs projecting outward from the bowel lumen and filled with barium. On air contrast examinations, they can be mistaken for polyps when they are seen end-on. Diverticula can usually be distinguished from polyps by the appearance of the barium within (see Fig. 3–17). Diverticula can also be seen on MRI scans as multiple, round, fluid-filled sacs, clearly visible against the abdominal fat (Fig. 3–60).

When a diverticulum becomes obstructed, infection can develop, resulting in abscess formation and bowel perforation. This inflammatory disease is called diverticulitis. Patients often have clinical signs and symptoms of bowel obstruction and sepsis, but the clinical manifestation can be nonspecific, particularly in older patients. Barium enema studies can reveal an inflammatory mass and multiple diverticula (Fig. 3–61). If the diverticulum has ruptured, the study may also reveal extravasation of contrast. CT is the best technique for the demonstration of a pericolic abscess. It can also show mural thickening, infiltration of mesenteric fat, and noninfected diverticula.

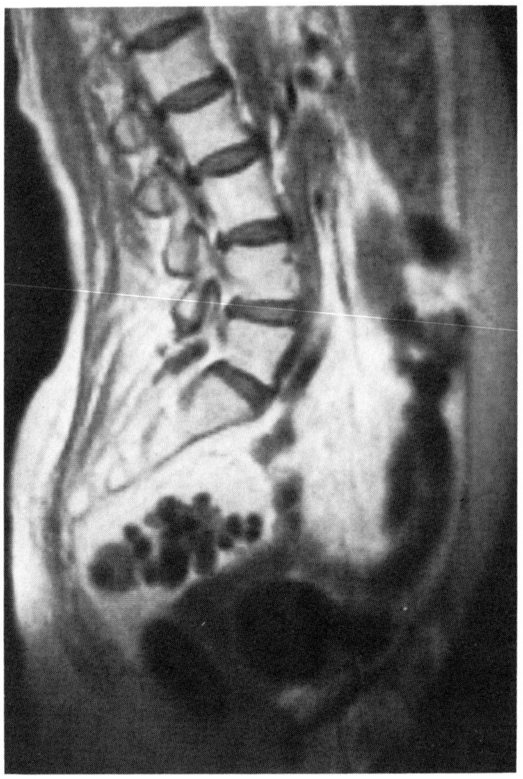

FIGURE 3–60. Diverticulosis. Sagittal T1 spin echo magnetic resonance image (MRI) of the pelvis shows multiple, air-filled (low-intensity) diverticula of the sigmoid colon, easily seen against high-intensity mesenteric fat in an 82-year-old woman evaluated for spinal cord compression. Higher slices showed multiple metastatic lesions in the spine as the cause of her symptoms. STIR images in this region showed no evidence of inflammation or infection of these diverticula.

Clinical features of sepsis and the presence of diverticula allow a presumptive diagnosis of diverticulitis even when an inflammatory mass is not seen. Making such a presumptive diagnosis is important because the therapy is nonoperative (antibiotics). Contained abscesses can be drained percutaneously under CT guidance.

Other diseases that may be confused clinically with diverticulitis are carcinoma, regional enteritis, and ulcerative colitis. Because both diverticulitis and colon carcinoma are common in the elderly population, careful diagnosis and follow-up of bowel disease is required for this age group.

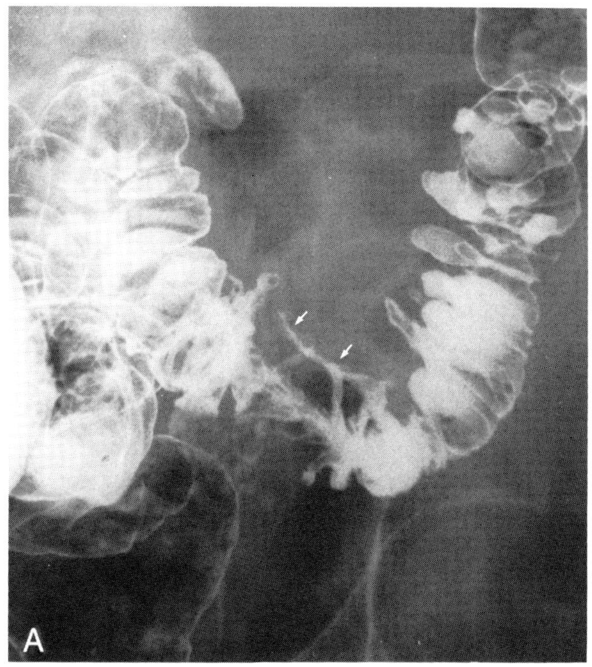

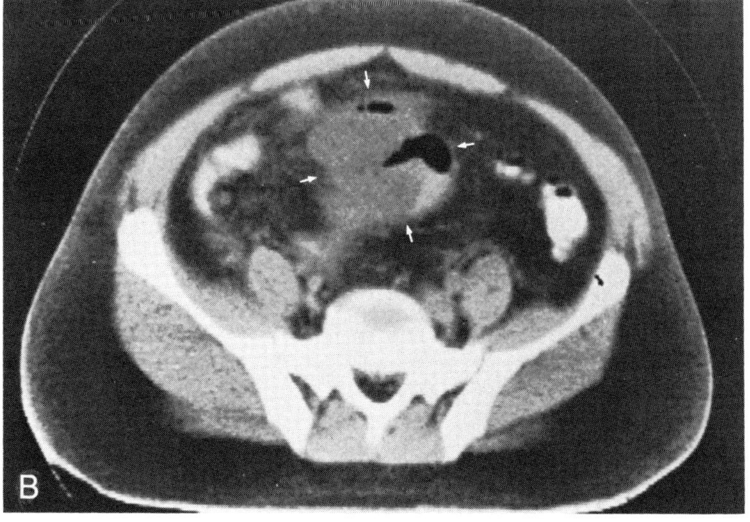

FIGURE 3–61. Diverticulitis. *A.* Double-contrast barium enema study shows a segment of the sigmoid colon that contains numerous diverticula and an intramural fistula *(arrows)* from diverticulitis. *B.* CT of the pelvis shows an abscess *(arrows).* Air is present within the bowel lumen and more peripherally in the abscess.

Part II
Solid Organs of the Abdomen

The solid organs of the abdomen—the liver and the biliary system, the pancreas, and the spleen—are discussed individually in this section. Because of their connections and proximity to the alimentary tract and vessels, diseases of these organs often involve contiguous structures or the bowel.

LIVER AND BILIARY TRACT

Trauma

The liver is second only to the spleen as the most commonly injured organ as a result of blunt trauma. Hemorrhage from such injuries is one of the most common causes of death in trauma patients. Blunt injuries generally cause compression and fracture of the liver parenchyma. Capsular disruption may then result in massive intraperitoneal hemorrhage. The most severe injuries include fractures into the major hepatic veins and the inferior vena cava. Such fractures require immediate surgery, and are therefore rarely imaged. In some cases, the mass of the liver parenchyma and its surrounding capsule tamponade the injured vessels, limiting life-threatening blood loss.

The diagnosis of liver injury is best made through CT after oral and intravenous contrast are administered (Fig. 3–62) because it shows the extent of the liver injury, the amount and the location of the blood, and injuries to other organs. CT is also important in follow-up of patients who undergo surgery and those who are managed nonoperatively. Liver fracture appears on CT as a linear or stellate-shaped, low-density area within the parenchyma. Blood has a lower density than enhanced liver and can be seen surrounding the liver and within the peritoneal cavity. In the subcapsular space, blood is best seen lateral to and flattening the liver margin. Clotted blood or contrast-filled active hemorrhage may be as dense as or denser than enhanced liver. In patients with fatty liver infiltration, a delayed scan (after 2 to 3 days) may be required to show the low-density contusions.

The mortality rate from blunt injuries to the liver is high (10% to 25%). Management depends on the extent of injury. When the amount of peritoneal blood is small, the liver lacerations are peripheral, and no other abdominal lesions are present, the patient may be managed nonoperatively. Patients who are hemodynamically unstable require immediate surgery. CT findings of deep injury involving the portal hilum, lacerations of the major hepatic veins, hemoperitoneum persisting 1 week after the injury, and progressing injury indicate a poor prognosis.

Large- (cutting-) needle liver biopsy is a common iatrogenic cause of liver hemorrhage, particularly in a patient with a clotting abnormality; this hemorrhage usually is subcapsular. A biloma, an entrapped segment of a bile duct, may occur after liver injury and appears on CT as a thin-walled cystic fluid collection.

Congenital Abnormalities

Variations in the size, the lobes, and the position of the liver are uncommon and are usually not a diagnostic problem. The liver is affected by several storage diseases that result in abnormal function (to be discussed). The majority of clinically relevant congenital abnormalities are in the biliary tract. The radiographic evaluation of such abnormalities includes ultrasonography, which can demonstrate dilatation of the biliary system and the presence of stones, and direct contrast injection of the bile ducts with the use of percutaneous or retrograde endoscopic techniques.

Biliary Hypoplasia and Atresia. Biliary hypoplasia is failure of intrahepatic ductal development that results in a small gallbladder, or the absence of one, and in poorly formed bile ducts. Several related abnormalities cause disease of connected or nearby structures. Obstruction of the common hepatic duct by the diaphragm can lead to stone formation or biliary cirrhosis. Bronchobiliary fistula can result from embryonic failure of biliary tract development, resulting in the passage of bile into the lungs. Biliary tract malformations are also associated with duodenal atresia.

Symptoms of biliary hypoplasia include clay-colored stools and jaundice in the first few months of life. Diagnosis is by nuclear medicine iminodiacetate studies (Chapter 9), which show normal liver uptake but no excretion. Treatment, which must occur before liver failure, consists of establishing drainage from the

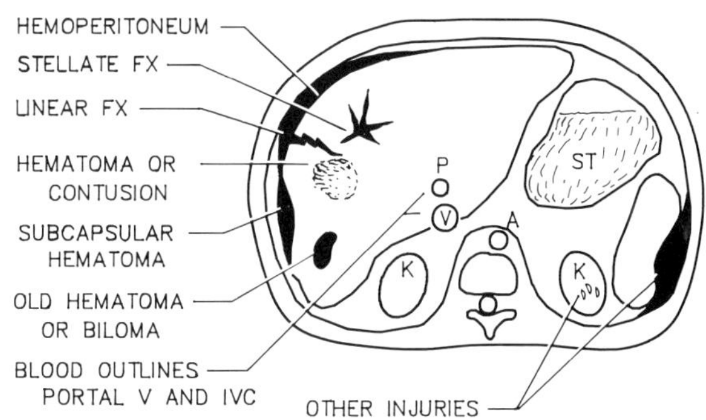

- SECOND MOST COMMONLY INJURED ORGAN
- OTHER VISCERAL INJURIES COMMON
- HEMATOMA IS LOWER DENSITY THAN ENHANCED LIVER
- HEMATOMA MAY BE SIMILAR TO FATTY LIVER
- RIGHT LOBE – ASSOCIATED LUNG, R KIDNEY INJURY
- LEFT LOBE – ASSOCIATED PANCREAS, DUODENUM INJURY
- POOR PROGNOSIS IF: DEEP LESIONS
  LARGE OR INCREASING HEMOPERITONEUM
  PERSISTENT HEMOPERITONEUM
  IVC, PORTAL HILUM, MAJOR HEPATIC VEIN INJURY

A

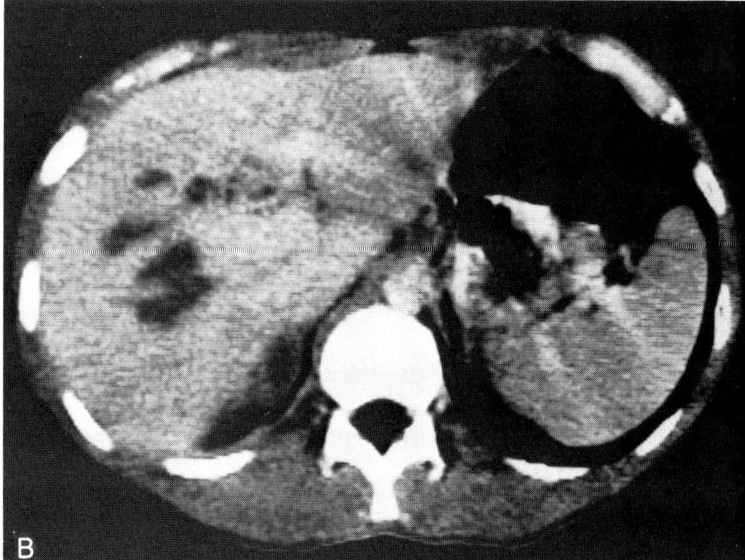

FIGURE 3–62. Liver injury. *A.* Diagram. FX, fracture; V, vena cava; portal V, portal vein; IVC, inferior vena cava; R, right. *B.* Liver fracture. Contrast CT shows several large, low-density defects in the liver from blunt trauma in a 25-year-old man injured in an automobile accident. This scan, obtained several days after the injury, shows the contusions as low density.

liver into the small bowel via a hepatoenterostomy.

Choledochal Cyst. A choledochal cyst is a congenital segmental dilatation of the extrahepatic bile duct. It usually is discovered in girls under 10 years of age when it causes biliary obstruction. Cholangitis and stone formation may result from stasis. The lesion is not a true cyst but rather an obstructed distal common bile duct or weakness of the wall of the common hepatic duct, or both. CT scans or ultrasonograms show a cystic mass. The intrahepatic ducts and, less commonly, the pancreatic ducts may be dilated in these patients as a result of obstruction.

Caroli's Disease. Caroli's disease is a familial, multifocal ectasia of the intrahepatic biliary system characterized by saccular dilatation of the ducts, stone formation, and cholangitis. Most patients are young adults when the disease is diagnosed. A cholangiogram shows the saccular dilatation of the ducts and may reveal

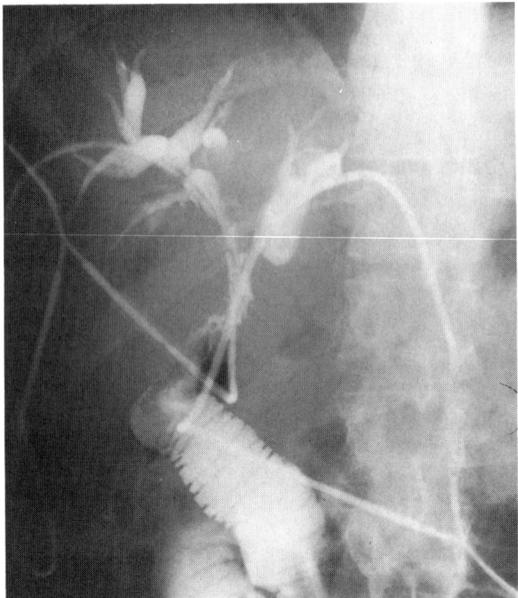

FIGURE 3–63. Caroli's disease. Percutaneous cholangiogram shows dilated intrahepatic ducts. Note drainage into the duodenum. (From King J, Orrison WW, Davis M, Kleinman R: Percutaneous choledochoscopic choledocholithotomy in Caroli's disease. Gastrointest Radiol 1990, 15:137–138.)

the stones (Fig. 3–63). Many patients develop complications such as liver abscess, biliary cirrhosis, and calculi.

Systemic Disease

Liver Disease

Because the liver is the site of detoxification, storage, and synthesis of many substances, it is commonly affected by disease related to infiltration by endogenous materials. The most important are glycogen storage disease, lipid infiltration, alpha$_1$-antitrypsin deficiency, Wilson's disease (copper deposition), and hemochromatosis (iron deposition). CT demonstrates abnormal liver density in some of these diseases and shows the complications of cirrhosis. A nuclear medicine liver-spleen scan best demonstrates reticuloendothelial liver function (see Chapter 9).

Alcoholic Liver Disease. The most common systemic liver disease is caused by excessive alcohol intake. Ingestion of alcohol in large quantities over long periods of time eventually leads to parenchymal destruction and interstitial fibrosis (cirrhosis). The clinical manifestations of alcoholic liver disease include variceal bleeding, hepatic encephalopathy, and alcoholic hepatitis.

In the early stages of alcoholic liver disease, hepatocytes become infiltrated with fat and the liver is of abnormally low density on CT scans, in comparison with portal vessels and the spleen. Ultrasonograms frequently appear normal, but the liver may be echogenic and attenuate the ultrasonic beam. At this stage, the liver is usually enlarged, but the condition is reversible if the alcohol intake is reduced or eliminated.

Later, after prolonged alcohol intake, fibrosis develops, and the liver appears scarred and shrunken and has irregular edges (Fig. 3–64). These changes cause a dense, echogenic appearance on ultrasonograms, and fewer vessels are visible. Disorganized, focal areas of regenerating liver tissue (called regenerating nodules) form. Because normal portal, biliary, and

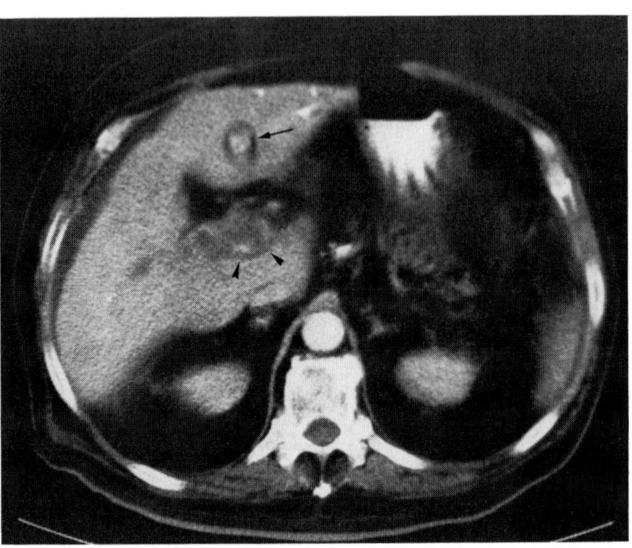

FIGURE 3–64. Alcoholic liver disease. CT with intravenous and oral contrast shows enhancement of the recanalized umbilical vein (*arrow*) and clot within the portal vein (*arrowheads*). The liver is surrounded by a thin rim of ascites and has an irregular margin as a result of cirrhosis and regeneration.

vascular architecture is not present in this disorganized tissue, liver function is poor.

In addition to liver dysfunction, stricture or obstruction of the portal vessels results in elevated portal venous pressure (portal hypertension) and shunting of unmetabolized waste products into the systemic circulation. Variceal hemorrhage may also occur. Both CT scans and ultrasonograms can show a patent or recanalized umbilical vein, which indicates portal hypertension. This vessel may enlarge, extending to the umbilicus and shunting portal blood to the superficial abdominal venous plexus (called a caput medusa). Additional findings include splenomegaly and numerous collateral vessels. Portal hypertension may be confirmed by demonstration of hepatofugal flow (flow away from the liver) on Doppler ultrasonograms. Patients who develop portal hypertension have increased risk of portal venous thrombosis. Ultrasonograms, CT scans, and MRI scans in such cases may show thrombus within the portal vein instead of flowing blood.

Patients with alcoholic liver disease are at risk for two additional life-threatening diseases. The more serious is hepatocellular carcinoma, apparently caused by the toxic effect of alcohol and the continuing regeneration and fibrotic process. Portal hypertension and resultant esophageal and gastric varices are serious, not only because of the risk of acute hemorrhage, but also because of toxicity to the brain and multiple organ injury. Portal hypertension can be partially treated by surgical procedures in which blood is shunted from the portal system to the inferior vena cava. However, when the blood is shunted past the liver, toxic materials such as ammonia enter the systemic circulation and may cause encephalopathy.

Glycogen Storage Disease. Several congenital diseases are characterized by the abnormal storage of glycogen in the liver. The glycogen by itself causes increased density on CT. However, concomitant lipid infiltration causes the density to be normal or low. Cirrhosis develops in some patients with glycogen storage diseases.

Fatty Infiltration. Fatty infiltration of the liver occurs in alcoholics, patients with adult-onset diabetes, obese patients, and jejunal-ileal bypass patients; in hyperalimentation and in many chronic illnesses; and after chemotherapy. The storage of triglycerides in the liver reflects the imbalance of protein, carbohydrates, and fat in patients with these conditions. Usually the liver is diffusely involved. In some patients, the infiltration is focal (called focal fatty infiltration); this may involve a whole segment or a lobe or may diffusely involve the entire liver. It may change in location from one examination to the next. These appearances may simulate those of other diseases, including metastatic tumor. However, in focal fatty infiltration, the vessels are in normal position (i.e., there is no displacement by a mass) and there is no enhancement. CT scans show a low-density liver (Fig. 3–65), identified by the high density of the normally enhancing vessels and in contrast to the normal-density spleen. The appearance of increased fat is not clearly shown on MRI with T1 spin echo. However, STIR images show very low intensity in areas of focal fatty infiltration, which enables easy differentiation of fat from tumor and cystic lesion.

Hemochromatosis. Hemochromatosis is an iron storage disorder that results in iron deposition in the liver and, to a lesser extent, the spleen. The disease may be primary or familial (in which case iron is deposited in the liver, the pancreas, and the heart), it may be idiopathic, or it may be secondary to the presence of excessive amounts of iron resulting from increased intake, defective erythropoiesis, multiple transfusions with red blood cell breakdown, or hemolysis. Many patients with hemochromatosis develop cirrhosis and fibrosis of the liver and, consequently, portal hypertension. Many also develop hepatocellular carcinoma.

CT and MRI yield the most informative images of hemochromatosis (Fig. 3–66). CT can show the increased density of the liver, the spleen, the pancreas, and the heart by comparison with other normal structures. It can be performed with two x-ray energies (dual-energy CT), which enable comparison and quantification of the iron content in these organs. On MRI, the involved organs have an altered appearance as a result of the paramagnetic effect of iron and other blood products. Both T1 and T2 are shortened because of this paramagnetic effect. The T2 effects dominate, and therefore the liver and other involved organs appear to have abnormally low intensity on all types of scans, whether T1- or T2-weighted.

Alpha$_1$-Antitrypsin Deficiency. Alpha$_1$-antitrypsin deficiency is a disease in which the proteolytic agent trypsin is not properly metabolized. It causes the most serious disease in

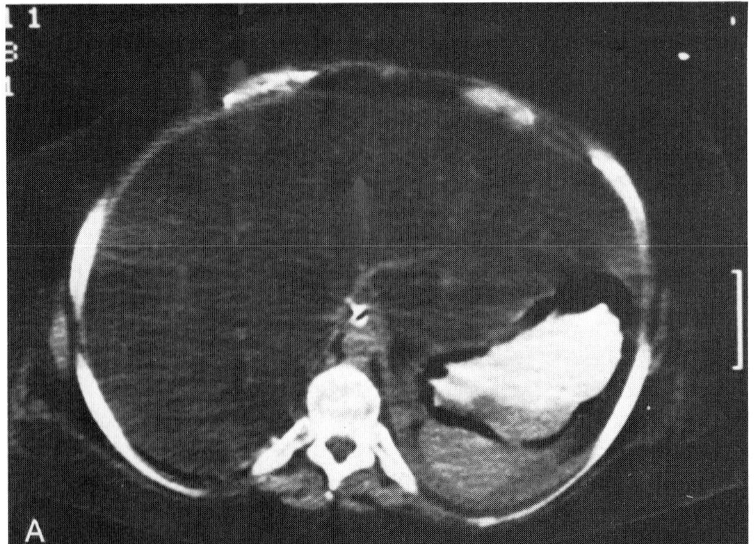

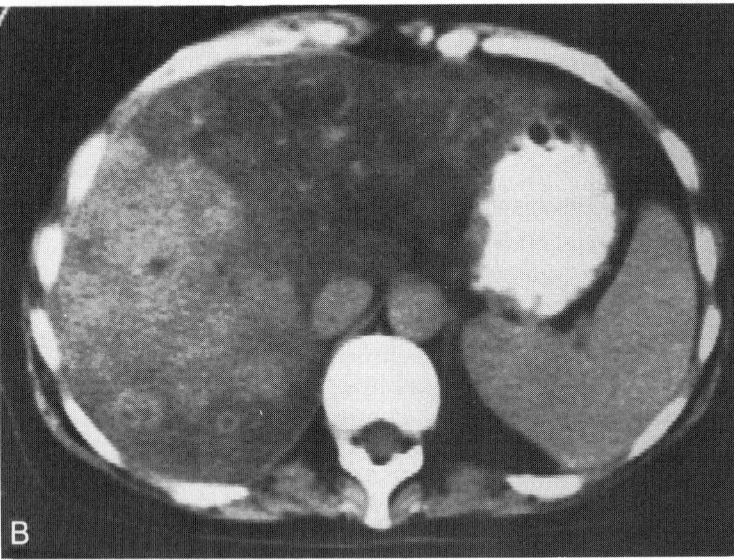

FIGURE 3–65. Fatty liver infiltration. *A.* Enhanced CT shows low density of the liver, which resulted from diffuse fatty replacement in a severely obese woman. During a surgical procedure, she suffered a hypotensive episode which led to necrosis and gastric perforation. Air can be seen within the wall of the stomach, surrounding the oral contrast. *B.* Focal-fatty liver infiltration. Enhanced CT shows low density in the left lobe and the most posterior portion of the right lobe of the liver. The normal position of blood vessels indicates that these low-density areas are focal infiltrations of fat rather than of tumor.

the lungs (see Chapter 2). However, some patients (usually children) with homozygous inheritance develop cirrhosis.

Wilson's Disease. Wilson's disease results in abnormal deposition of copper in the liver and in the basal ganglia of the brain. The liver disease may progress to cirrhosis. Abnormalities in liver density may be detectable on CT. However, in most patients the scan is normal unless cirrhosis has developed. MRI shows normal liver intensity even though copper has paramagnetic properties.

Inflammation and Infection

Generalized involvement of the liver is common in viral hepatitis but is distinctly rare in other infections, except in patients with depressed immune systems. Focal infection (abscess) can form in the liver as a result of infestation by a variety of organisms.

Bacterial Liver Abscess. Bacterial involvement of the liver is usually pyogenic and is caused by portal venous infection (40% of patients), generalized sepsis (30%), and biliary infection (20%). Such infections result in single or multiple abscesses in the liver. Patients may have fever and general malaise but may not have signs that direct attention to the liver. Many patients do not develop fever. The usual sources of liver abscesses are biliary tract disease, malignancy, and, less commonly, appendicitis. The causative organisms include the gram-negative rods (especially *Escherichia*

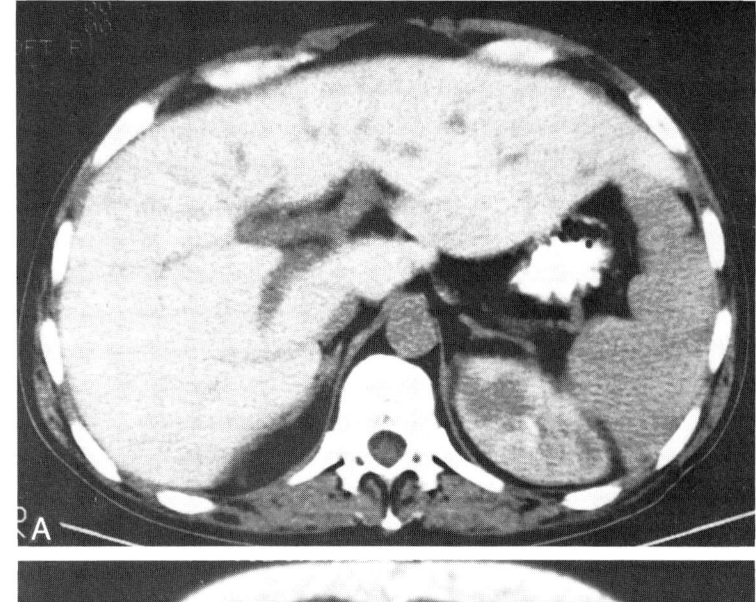

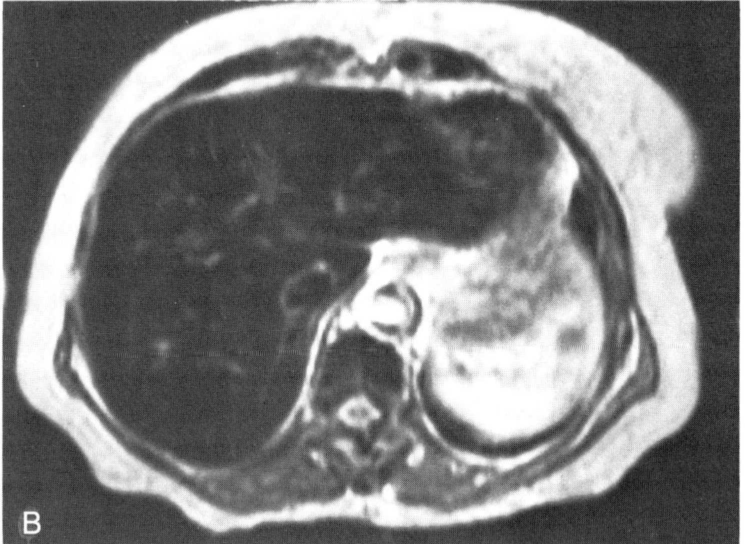

FIGURE 3–66. Hemochromatosis. *A.* Noncontrast CT shows very high density in the liver (in comparison with the normal spleen and kidney) that was caused by iron deposition in a patient with hemochromatosis. *B.* Proton density spin echo scan through the liver shows very low signal intensity as a result of infiltration of the liver by iron in a patient who had undergone multiple transfusions. The low intensity (which was shown on both T1- and T2-weighted sequences) is caused by the paramagnetic effect of iron.

coli), anaerobic bacteria, and streptococci. Fungal abscesses occur in patients with cancer and diseases that cause or are associated with immunosuppression.

The diagnosis of hepatic abscess is best made with contrast-enhanced CT, which can show the pus-filled cavity and adjacent abnormalities such as pleural effusion, subpulmonic effusion, and subdiaphragmatic or subcapsular empyema (Fig. 3–67). On CT, abscesses appear as multiple small lesions (microabscesses) or large, solitary or confluent, low-density masses (macroabscesses). Microabscesses may be uniformly scattered throughout the liver (a pattern more common in fungal than in other infections) or may be clustered (a pattern limited to enteric bacterial infection). Both micro- and macroabscesses are of lower density than enhanced liver tissue and may be septated or multilobulated, with smooth or irregular margins. Rim enhancement is uncommon (only about 5% of abscesses). Differentiation from dilated bile ducts is made by identification of a nonuniform pattern, and differentiation from metastatic liver tumor can be made when clusters of abscesses are present. Clusters of tumor are rare in metastatic disease.

Ultrasonography can also be used in detection and diagnosis of hepatic abscess but is particularly helpful in directing needle aspiration and placement of percutaneous drainage and irrigation catheters. Ultrasonograms show discrete or poorly defined hypo- or hyperechoic areas and minimal acoustic through-

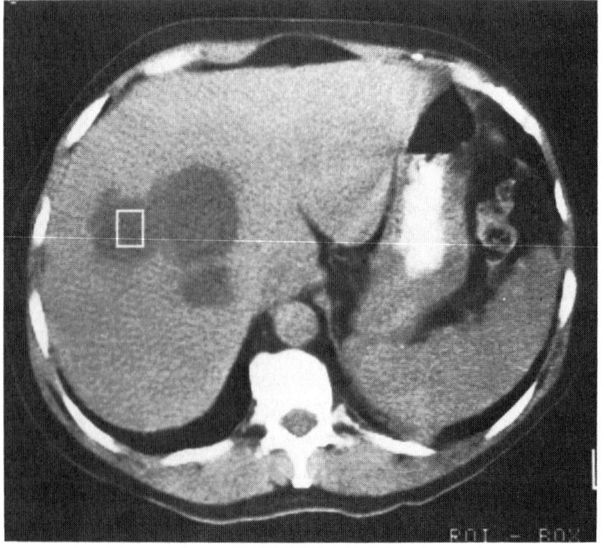

FIGURE 3–67. Pyogenic liver abscess. Contrast CT shows focal low-density areas in the liver of a man with fever and fatigue. He was unable to complete his usual regimen of three sets of tennis. These lesions were drained percutaneously under ultrasonographic guidance, which obviated the need for surgery.

transmission. Gas, complex fluid, and internal septations may be present. The cavity can usually be drained through a single catheter, apparently because the individual lesions eventually cause adjacent necrosis and then communicate. When disease is limited, percutaneous therapy allows many liver abscesses to be managed without surgery; such patients have a good prognosis. Among patients with disseminated infection, the mortality rate is high, despite surgical drainage and antibiotic therapy.

Viral Hepatitis. Viral hepatitis is usually diagnosed clinically. When CT is performed, it is usually to rule out other types of liver disease or to assess complications. The liver usually appears normal, but generalized enlargement and low density secondary to edema or fatty infiltration may be demonstrated. When hepatitis is seen in an alcoholic or a poorly nourished patient, fatty infiltration can be well demonstrated on CT. Patients with chronic hepatitis often develop hepatocellular carcinoma. MRI is less sensitive for diagnosing hepatitis.

Unusual Organisms. Mycobacteria, fungi, protozoans, and parasites also infect the liver. Hepatic tuberculosis occurs only in disseminated disease. In such cases, the need to manage the liver disease is usually less urgent than that of disease elsewhere. Candidiasis occurs in immunosuppressed patients, particularly those being treated for leukemia and lymphoma and those with AIDS (Fig. 3–68). Other fungal infections are cryptococcosis, histoplasmosis, and mucormycosis. The usual abnormality is multiple microabscess throughout the liver, best demonstrated by CT and ultrasonography. CT shows punctate, low-density areas and may show a dense rim around the lesions. MRI shows multiple punctate areas of high signal on STIR or T2-weighted images. Therapy requires an accurate diagnosis (usually by liver biopsy) and antifungal agents. The ultimate outcome often depends on the underlying disease. Splenic involvement is associated with a high mortality rate.

Hepatic schistosomiasis results when the schistosomal cercariae enter the portal circulation and lodge in the presinusoidal portal veins. Portal hypertension and, eventually, portal hepatic cirrhosis develop. CT may show calcifications of the liver and capsule. Enhancing fibrous bands radiate through the liver. *Echinococcus* infections can involve the liver, resulting in one or more round, calcified cysts that are similar to those seen elsewhere. *Ascaris lumbricoides* appears as a serpentine filling defect within the biliary system on cholangiogram, but is unlikely to be diagnosed on CT.

Amebiasis. Infection from *Entamoeba histolytica* affects 10% of the world population and is especially associated with unsanitary living conditions. The liver is involved in 8% of patients with GI tract disease. Patients have general malaise and fever, abdominal pain, and diarrhea; these symptoms are similar to those seen with other causes of liver abscess. Many of these patients have visited an endemic area just before onset of the disease. The diagnosis can be made with serological testing,

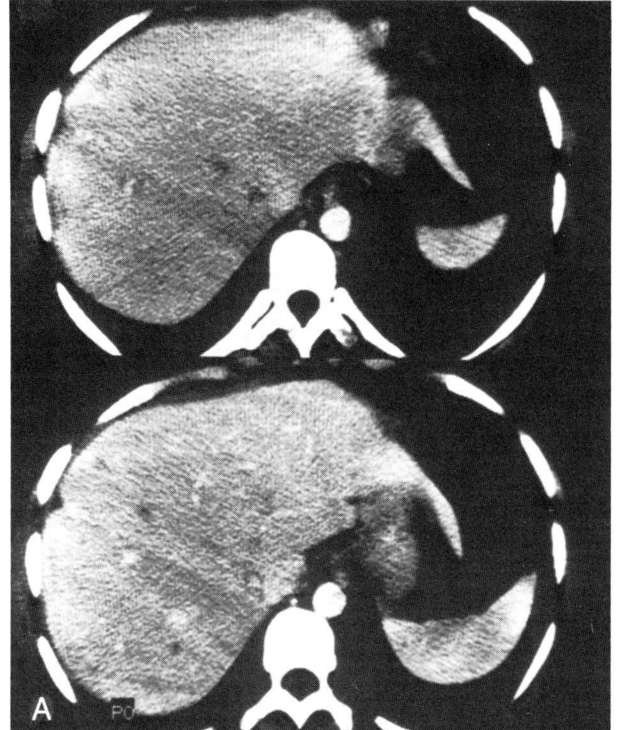

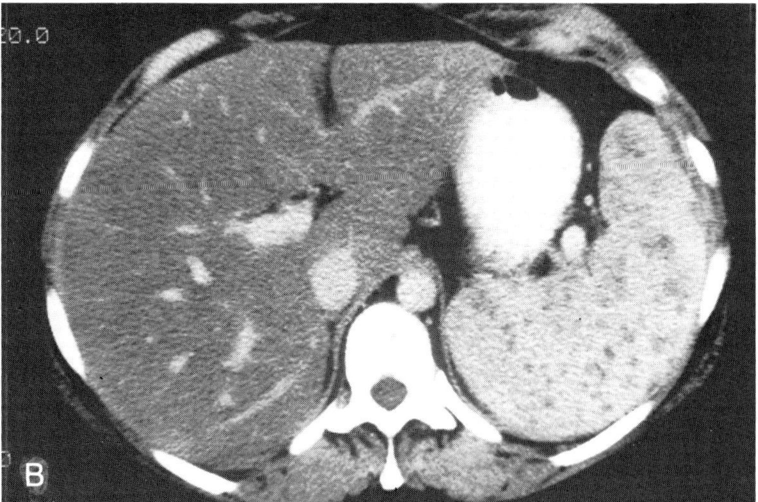

FIGURE 3–68. Microabscesses. *A.* Contrast CT viewed at narrow (liver) windows shows multiple, small, round, low-density lesions representing disseminated candidiasis in a patient with acquired immunodeficiency syndrome (AIDS). *B.* Numerous abscesses are seen in the spleen of another patient with breast carcinoma. (Courtesy of J. Smith, First Hill Diagnostic Imaging Center, Seattle.)

but because false-negative rates are high (up to 18%), aspiration is often required.

The ultrasonographic features of amebic abscess include (1) focal mass, (2) hypoechogenicity, (3) absence of wall echoes, (4) through-transmission, and (5) peripheral location near the capsule (Fig. 3–69). However, these features are not present in all cases. CT scans show a round, well-defined mass of low density in comparison with the normal-density liver. Occasionally, the abscess is of higher density than the normal liver. The abscess wall may be enhanced, and edema may be present in the marginal liver tissue. The abscess composition is variable; it may be thick and viscous but is usually a complex, watery fluid. The center contains complex fluid and may contain septations and internal debris. The abscess is seen as high intensity on MRI sequences that show high contrast between different types of tissue, such as STIR and T2 spin echo.

Patients with amebiasis respond well to antiamebic chemotherapy. They require percutaneous drainage when the lesion is not responsive and when bacterial abscess is considered. Many patients with hepatic ame-

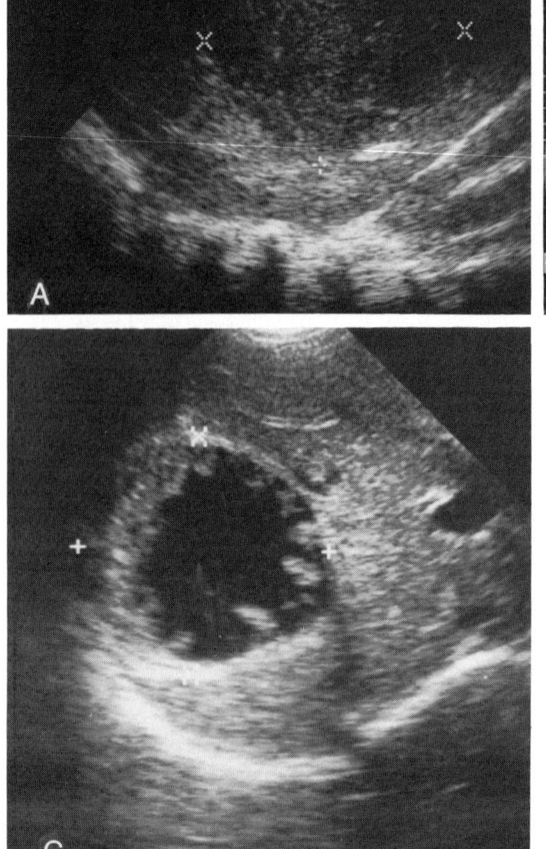

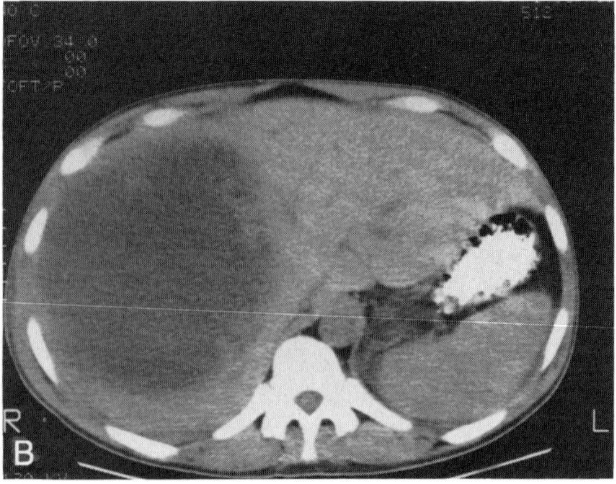

FIGURE 3–69. Amebiasis. *A.* Ultrasonogram shows an 11.6 × 10.2 cm hypoechoic lesion in the right lobe of the liver in a 26-year-old man from Vietnam. This is an amebic cyst, and it has the characteristic solid appearance of such lesions because of the proteinaceous viscous fluid within it. *B.* The same lesion on CT. *C.* Ultrasonogram of the same cyst 18 months later after treatment. It has shrunk to 7.8 cm in diameter and now has effective through-transmission and no longer resembles a solid lesion.

biasis develop infection in the chest, best diagnosed on CT; this infection also responds to therapy. Low-density liver abnormalities may persist on CT for 6 months or more after therapy.

Biliary Tract Disease

Choledocholithiasis. Biliary duct stones (choledocholithiasis) occur in 15% of patients with gallstones (cholelithiasis). They also occur in patients with bile stasis, sclerosing cholangitis, Caroli's disease, stenosis of the papilla of Vater, and recurrent pyogenic cholangitis. Stasis and obstruction caused by these stones produce jaundice (75% of patients), biliary colic (80%), and fever (30%). Patients may also develop acute pancreatitis.

CT scans show stones as being of high density (calcium bilirubinate) or water density (cholesterol), often within a dilated common bile duct. Dilated intrahepatic ducts and an enlarged gallbladder with gallstones may also be identified. Ultrasonograms easily demonstrate the common duct dilatation, whereas hepatic duct or common duct stones may be difficult to visualize (Fig. 3–70; see also Fig. 3–13).

Cholangitis

Cholangitis is a general term reflecting inflammation of the bile ducts. It may be a sclerosing process or an infection involving the walls of the bile ducts. When caused by infection, it is called recurrent pyogenic cholangitis.

Infectious (Ascending) Cholangitis. Infectious cholangitis is an ascending, often fulminant, infection of the biliary tract. It usually occurs in patients with biliary obstruction caused by stricture, tumor, or stones. The infection is the result of bile stasis and various enteric bacteria. Other causes of infectious cholangitis include Caroli's disease and chole-

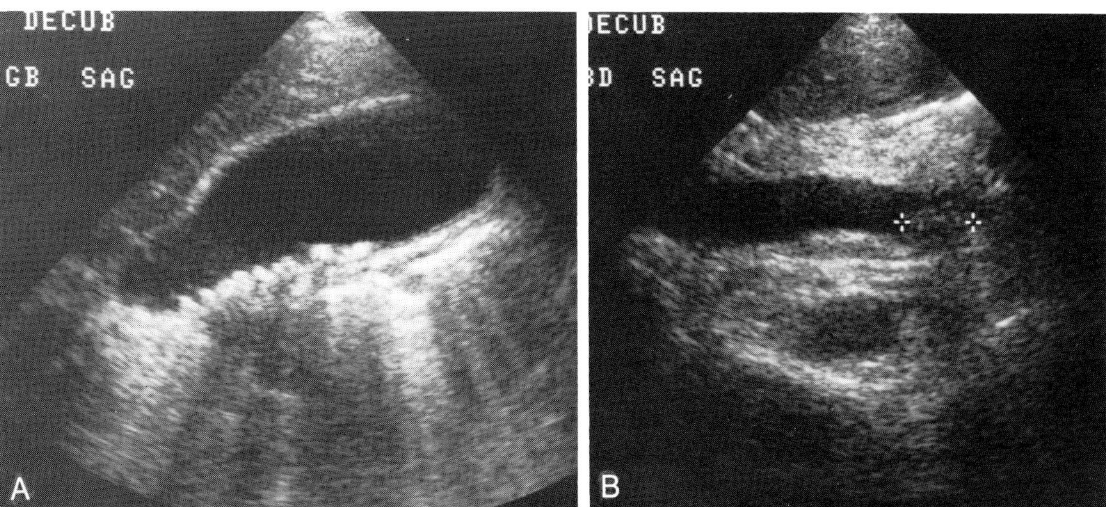

FIGURE 3–70. Dilated gallbladder and stones. *A.* A longitudinal ultrasonographic image of the gallbladder shows the characteristic appearance of multiple gallstones in a 47-year-old man. *B.* A longitudinal image of the common bile duct reveals a shadowing opacity within the duct. The duct is dilated to 17 mm. The obstruction is caused by a common bile duct stone. Although ultrasonography is not sensitive for the detection of common bile duct stones, it is quite efficient for determining whether the duct is dilated.

dochal cyst. Patients develop pain, jaundice, and fever. The white blood cell count is elevated, and blood cultures usually yield positive results. The condition can lead rapidly to generalized sepsis and shock. Diagnosis is difficult because the symptoms or findings of generalized sepsis can be confused with those of alcoholic hepatitis, renal or intestinal infection, and hepatic abscess.

Both CT and ultrasonography can help establish the diagnosis of infectious cholangitis. CT scans show the dilated ducts, the presence of biliary stones if they are dense, the presence of gallstones and a distended gallbladder, and associated hepatic abscess, dilated intrahepatic ducts, and intraductal gas. Ultrasonograms can show the same abnormalities; however, the appearance of the stones and technical artifacts associated with gas, surgical clips, and the mud-like sludge that is often in the bile ducts can cause a confusing appearance similar to that of cholangiocarcinoma. Full evaluation of the ducts and identification of isodense stones requires cholangiography, which can be performed either by retrograde endoscopic injection (see Fig. 3–9) or by percutaneous cholangiography. These techniques can simultaneously provide diagnosis and establish drainage by placement of a stent.

Sclerosing Cholangitis. Sclerosing cholangitis is an idiopathic inflammatory disease of the biliary system that usually occurs in men over 40. It may be associated with ulcerative colitis or retroperitoneal fibrosis or may be secondary to obstruction by stones or cancer. Patients develop signs of biliary obstruction and stone formation. The obstruction results in stasis of bile and, consequently, fibrosis and sclerosis. The cholangiogram shows intraductal stones; segmental, irregular narrowing of the bile ducts; and strictures. CT scans show areas of segmental biliary obstruction throughout the liver. Ultrasonograms may also show biliary obstruction and a thick-walled common bile duct. Involvement of the biliary system is patchy and results in abnormal, dilated bile ducts intermixed with normal ones.

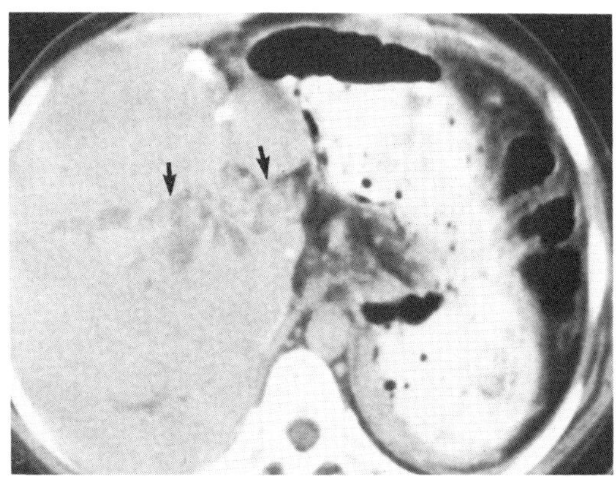

FIGURE 3–71. Pyogenic cholangitis. CT shows dilated biliary ducts with stones and debris *(arrows)*. Calcifications are present anteriorly in the left lobe. (Courtesy of R. B. Jeffrey, Stanford University, Palo Alto, California.)

Recurrent Pyogenic Cholangitis. *Clonorchis sinensis* is endemic to eastern Asia, where it is a common cause of peripheral bile duct obstruction and fibrosis. The organism is ingested when fresh-water fish are eaten, and it migrates centrally to the liver, where it causes intrahepatic biliary obstruction, cholangitis, liver abscess, and stone formation. *Escherichia coli* or *Ascaris* species may cause similar disease. Patients have multiple episodes of fever with signs of biliary obstruction. CT and ultrasonograms show dilated, pus-filled intrahepatic bile ducts and stones (Fig. 3–71). The stones of recurrent pyogenic cholangitis are of a mudlike consistency and are composed of calcium bilirubinate. The appearance may be difficult to distinguish from that of cholangiocarcinoma with obstruction.

Gallbladder Disease

Inflammation of the gallbladder (cholecystitis) may be either acute or chronic. Patients with acute cholecystitis develop fever, chills, an elevated white blood cell count, and acute onset of right upper quadrant pain and tenderness. Symptoms of chronic cholecystitis range from asymptomatic to recurrent episodes of right upper quadrant pain.

Gallstones. Real-time ultrasonography is the preferred method for the evaluation of the upper abdomen for detection of gallstones, which are present in about 8% of the general population. The presence of gallstones does not necessarily indicate cholecystitis. Stones form in the gallbladder as a result of an imbalance of the three basic components of bile: cholesterol, lecithin, and fluid. Gallstones are usually present with clinically symptomatic acute and chronic cholecystitis. On ultrasonography, gallstones move with changes in patient position and cause a shadow in the ultrasonic beam behind the stones (see Figs. 1–12 and 3–70). A shadow may not be seen if the stone is small or is not in the focal zone of the transducer or if a transducer of too low a frequency is used.

Acute Calculous Cholecystitis. When the cystic duct becomes obstructed, usually by a gallstone, the gallbladder wall becomes edematous, hyperemic, and inflamed. Patients have right upper quadrant pain, fever, and an increased white blood cell count. Such findings are often considered diagnostic of acute cholecystitis; however, many patients with right upper quadrant pain have other disease. Results of ultrasonography and nuclear medicine iminodiacetate scans (Chapter 9) are nearly 100% accurate for the diagnosis of acute cholecystitis.

In acute cholecystitis, ultrasonograms show uniform wall thickening (more than 3 mm) and a distended gallbladder (Fig. 3–72). Gallstones are present in 93% of these patients. An important diagnostic sign is extreme tenderness over the gallbladder elicited by applied pressure with the ultrasonic transducer during the examination (Murphy's sign). Fluid adjacent to the gallbladder indicates perforation and often abscess. Irregular thickening of the gallbladder wall suggests gangrene. Gas in the gallbladder wall (emphysematous cholecystitis)

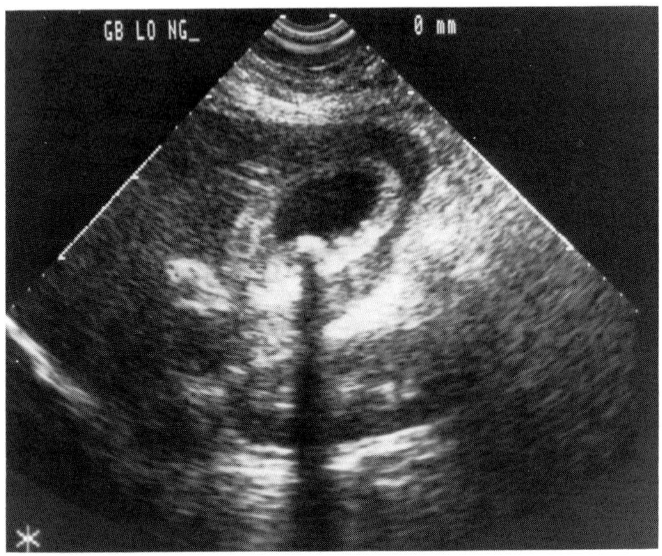

FIGURE 3–72. Acute cholecystitis. Longitudinal ultrasonogram shows a greatly thickened, highly echogenic gallbladder wall in a 36-year-old woman with acute right upper quadrant pain. The central portion of the dilated gallbladder shows the normal low echogenicity of bile. A large stone is present in the dependent portion of the gallbladder and shows posterior acoustic shadowing. The liver shows uniform echogenicity superiorly (to the viewer's left). (Courtesy of P. Lynch, Sitka, Alaska.)

indicates infection. Diagnosis includes elimination or evaluation of other diseases that can coexist with or mimic acute cholecystitis, including pancreatitis, appendicitis, ulcer disease, hepatitis, liver abscess, tumor, renal infection or stones, and even cardiac and pulmonary disease.

The inflamed gallbladder eventually ruptures if it is not removed or decompressed. Treatment of acute cholecystitis is surgical removal of the gallbladder. The surgery may be delayed until after a course of antibiotics if the patient is less ill. Patients who are too ill for surgery can be treated by percutaneous puncture and drainage of the gallbladder by a catheter or a needle.

Acute Acalculous Cholecystitis. Acalculous cholecystitis is acute cholecystitis without stones and represents about 7% of cases of acute cholecystitis. The cystic duct is not obstructed, but the gallbladder is acutely inflamed, as in acute calculous cholecystitis. Associated conditions include trauma, surgery, burns, sepsis, diabetes, debilitating disease, and hyperalimentation. Possible causes include vasculitis and bile stasis, which lead to acute inflammation. The most important ultrasonographic findings are gallbladder wall thickening, adjacent fluid, intramural gas, and sloughed mucosal membrane. Gallbladder tenderness is usually difficult to elicit because many affected patients are severely ill, debilitated, or unconscious. Nuclear medicine imaging is the most informative examination for diagnosing acalculous cholecystitis, showing absence of radioisotope in the gallbladder. However, fasting (common among ill patients) may result in a false-positive nuclear medicine scan because of physiological nonfilling of the gallbladder.

Chronic Cholecystitis. Chronic cholecystitis is the result of damage to the gallbladder mucosa from chronic irritation by stones. The chronic inflammation may cause calcification of the gallbladder wall and predisposes the patient to the development of cancer. The affected gallbladder is unable to concentrate bile. Diagnosis is made from the detection of stones, a thick gallbladder wall, and no tenderness. The patient is not acutely ill, and Murphy's sign is not present. In some cases of chronic cholecystitis, the gallbladder may be small and shrunken. Ultrasonograms then show the gallbladder wall, its echoes, and a shadow.

Neoplasms

Most benign liver masses are simple cysts filled with clear fluid. They are incidental findings on CT or ultrasonograms. Multiple cysts in the liver are commonly seen in patients with polycystic kidney disease (Fig. 3–73). Such cysts are not associated with functional impairment as occurs in the kidney. Most benign tumors of the liver are primary vascular neoplasms, highly vascular solid tumors, or nodules. The most important of these are the cavernous hemangioma, the hepatic adenoma, and focal nodular hyperplasia. Although all of these have a radiographic appearance that may

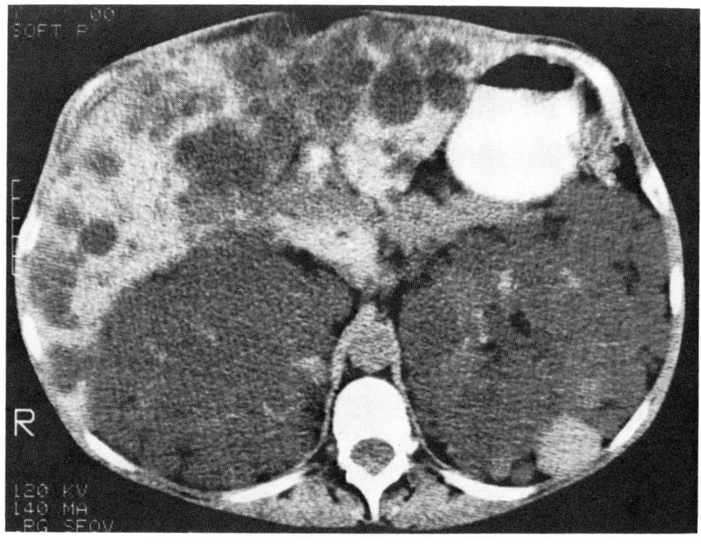

FIGURE 3–73. Multiple liver cysts. Noncontrast CT shows two large, water-density structures on each side of the spine that represent the kidneys in a young man in whom the renal parenchyma was almost totally replaced by cysts as a result of adult polycystic kidney disease. Approximately one third of patients with polycystic kidney disease also have hepatic cysts, as shown here. Cysts may also occur in the pancreas and the spleen.

be indistinguishable from that of hepatocellular carcinoma, their CT enhancement patterns, MRI appearance, and angiographic characteristics often allow differentiation among them.

Cavernous Hemangioma. The cavernous hemangioma is the most common benign tumor of the liver. It may be single or multiple. Most are detected incidentally in asymptomatic patients. Plain radiographs can show a large liver and calcification of the lesion (present in 10% of patients), but CT best identifies the mass and its location. A precontrast image shows a discrete lesion of lower density than the liver. After a bolus injection of intravenous contrast, marked, progressive characteristic enhancement occurs from the periphery to the center (see Fig. 1–6). MRI shows very high intensity on T2 spin echo and STIR sequences (Fig. 3–74). Ultrasonograms usually show an echogenic mass with increased through-transmission, but the appearance is variable, and many hemangiomas are hypoechoic or have mixed echogenicity. Arteriograms show (1) normal-sized arteries that lead to a large, rounded, vascular mass and (2) pooling of contrast in the irregular cavernous venous spaces on delayed films.

Either CT or nuclear medicine imaging with labeled red blood cells (see Chapter 9) can be used to make a specific diagnosis of hemangioma and eliminate metastatic tumor as a diagnostic possibility. A CT lesion that fills in from periphery to center after a bolus of contrast is unlikely to be metastatic tumor. On a red blood cell–labeled scan, the pooled blood in the large vascular spaces causes increasing

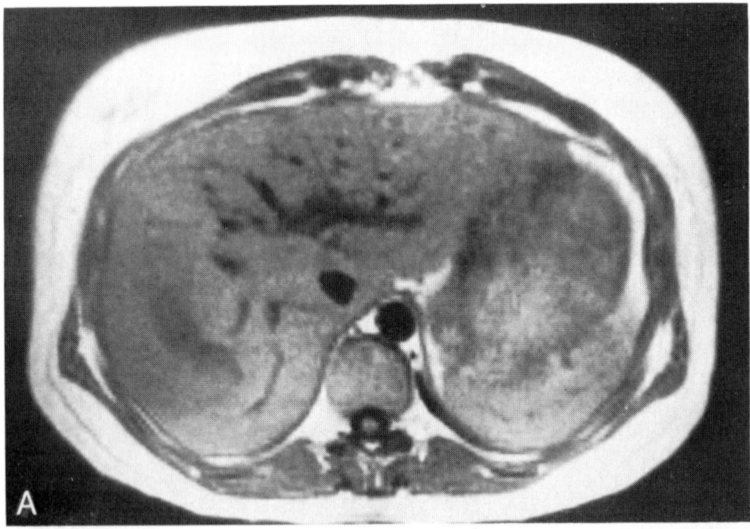

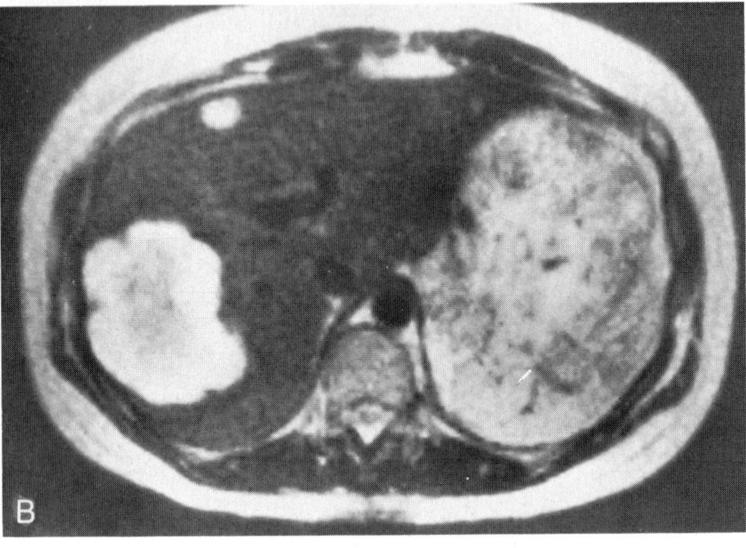

FIGURE 3–74. Cavernous hemangioma. *A.* A T1 spin echo image shows a mass in the right lobe of the liver, but the full extent of the abnormality is difficult to identify. *B.* The T2-weighted spin echo image shows low intensity of the normal liver. A large, slightly lobulated mass in the right lobe of the liver appears very bright on the T2-weighted image (it also appeared bright on STIR images). The fluid-filled stomach and the spleen are difficult to separate in the left side of the abdomen. Note also an additional hemangioma anteriorly in the medial segment of the left lobe of the liver. A CT scan of the same patient is also shown in Figure 1–6. (Courtesy of B. Porter, First Hill Diagnostic Imaging Center, Seattle.)

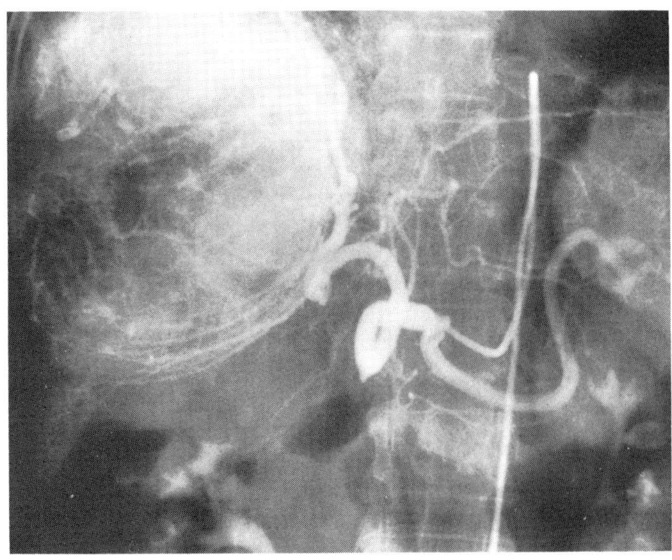

FIGURE 3–75. Hepatic adenoma. Celiac angiogram shows a round, densely vascular lesion in the liver, fed predominantly by the hepatic artery in a young, asymptomatic woman with an abdominal mass. (Courtesy of E. Ring, University of California, San Francisco.)

activity in the lesion. Metastases are generally hypovascular and do not show progressive uptake. Hemangiomas may bleed spontaneously or after abdominal trauma, but this is uncommon.

Hepatic Adenoma. Hepatic adenoma is a solitary benign tumor composed of hepatocytes but no bile ducts. It is most common in young women who have taken oral contraceptives. Men receiving androgen therapy and patients with glycogen storage disease may also develop these tumors. Histological examination shows that the mass contains hepatocytes but no bile ducts and none of the reticuloendothelial cells (notably Kupffer cells) that are normally present in liver tissue. The patient generally has no significant clinical symptoms unless hemorrhage occurs.

The hepatic adenoma is usually detected incidentally on CT or ultrasonography. CT scans show a mass, which transiently enhances after a bolus of contrast. Ultrasonograms show a mass, which is either highly echogenic or of minimal echogenicity; neither appearance is specific for hepatic adenoma. Angiograms can demonstrate (in half of patients) a highly vascular mass (Fig. 3–75). There is neovascularity without pooling of contrast. The lesion is fed by numerous arterial branches and may displace adjacent normal vessels. The appearance of the feeding artery and of numerous branching vessels around the periphery of the mass has been described as an apple on a stem. The absence of Kupffer cells results in poor or no uptake on liver-spleen scans (see Chapter 9) and can be helpful in differentiation of hepatic adenoma from other tumors, notably focal nodular hyperplasia (Fig. 3–76). Treatment is usually surgical removal because these tumors can hemorrhage spontaneously or become malignant.

HEPATIC ADENOMA

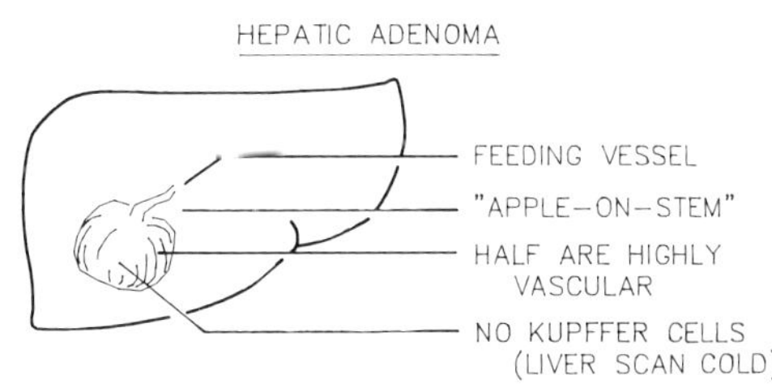

- ASSOCIATION – 99% WOMEN
  ORAL CONTRACEPTIVES
- COMPLICATIONS – HEMORRHAGE
  MALIGNANCY

FOCAL NODULAR HYPERPLASIA

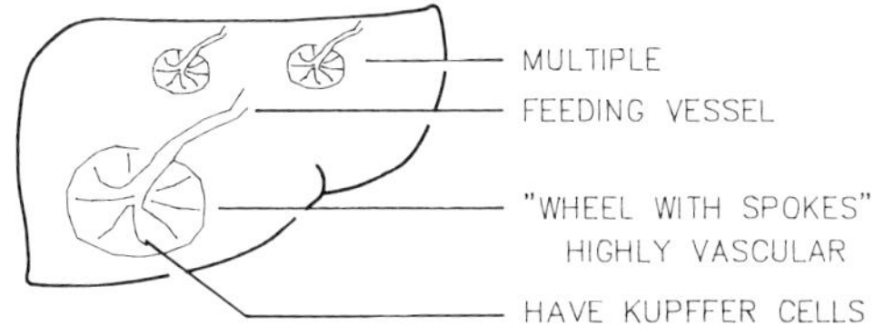

- ASSOCIATION – 80% WOMEN
  ORAL CONTRACEPTIVES ?
- COMPLICATIONS – USUALLY NONE
  SELDOM HEMORRHAGE

FIGURE 3–76. Characteristics of hepatic adenoma and focal nodular hyperplasia.

Focal Nodular Hyperplasia. The liver is capable of regenerating tissue in response to injury or other stimuli. These regenerating nodules are called focal nodular hyperplasia. Histological examination reveals that they contain all normal hepatic cell components but lack the organization of the normal liver. Like the hepatic adenoma, focal nodular hyperplasia occurs most commonly in women. Patients often have only vague right upper quadrant pain.

The masses, which are usually multiple, are shown on CT as lobular, enhancing nodules. About half have a central stellate area representing scar that does not enhance. Angiograms show highly vascular lesions with a reticular pattern but without arteriovenous shunting in nearly all cases. The feeding artery enters the center of each mass and branches into smaller vessels that radiate outward, simulating the spokes of a wheel. Because Kupffer cells are present, focal nodular hyperplasia usually takes up the radiopharmaceutical agent on a liver-spleen scan (see Chapter 9). Therefore, when uptake is demonstrated, hepatic adenoma (which seldom takes up the radiopharmaceutical agent) is largely ruled out (see Fig. 3–76). When poor or no uptake is demonstrated, the examination is less helpful. Despite the highly vascular nature of these lesions, hemorrhage seldom occurs. Ultrasonograms show a small mass or masses that are hypoechoic but may be hyper- or isoechoic with the liver, and the ultrasonograms are therefore nonspecific. Treatment is usually conservative.

Hepatocellular Carcinoma. Hepatocellular carcinoma (also called hepatoma, a poor term because it connotes a benign tumor) constitutes 75% of all primary malignant tumors of the liver. This aggressive tumor occurs in adults, is associated with hepatitis and cirrhosis of the liver, and is more common in Asia and Africa than in other parts of the world. It is also associated with malnutrition, parasitic liver disease, and recurrent pyogenic cholangitis. Cords or sheets of malignant parenchymal cells are seen in histological examination. Hepatocellular carcinoma is highly vascular and may have various forms: focal mass, multiple discrete masses, or diffuse tumor (Fig. 3–77). Focal and discrete masses often have a fibrous outer rim, which may differentiate them from metastases. Ten percent of these tumors calcify.

Patients experience pain and weight loss and have a palpable abdominal mass. If portal vein thrombosis occurs, ascites may develop. Leukocytosis is often present, and there may be a sudden elevation of alkaline phosphatase levels. Serum alpha-fetoprotein levels are measurable in about one third of patients.

Hepatocellular carcinoma is most effectively evaluated by means of CT and MRI. Multiple masses, diffuse involvement, and local invasion are important findings (Figs. 3–78 and 3–79), and there is usually transient, intense contrast enhancement. Although such findings are suggestive of the diagnosis of carcinoma of the liver, they are not specific, and so biopsy is required. Ultrasonograms may show a hypoechoic, hyperechoic, or complex mass and, if present, the fibrous capsule. On MRI scans, hepatocellular carcinoma has a low signal on T1 spin echo sequences, a high signal on T2 spin echo sequences, and very high intensity on STIR sequences. The appearance on all sequences may be complex if hemorrhage or necrosis is present. A rim of low intensity as a result of the fibrous capsule is frequently pres-

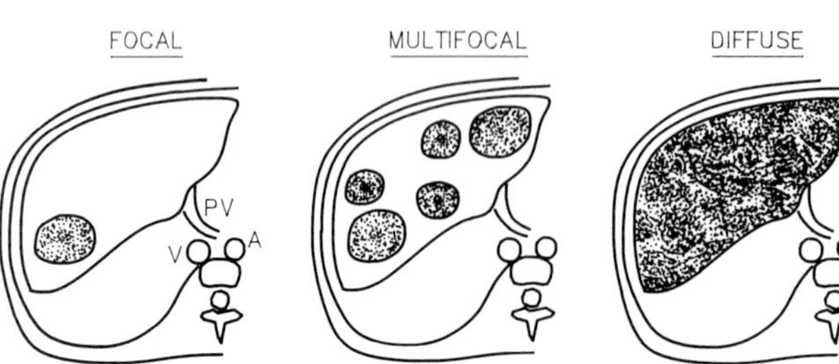

- INVADE VENA CAVA (V) AND PORTAL VEIN (PV)
- TUMOR STAIN ON ANGIOGRAPHY; HIGHLY VASCULAR
- DEFECT ON LIVER SCAN, DENSE UPTAKE ON GALLIUM SCAN
- SELDOM CALCIFY
- USUALLY HAVE A RIM OR CAPSULE

FIGURE 3–77. Forms of hepatocellular carcinoma. A, aorta.

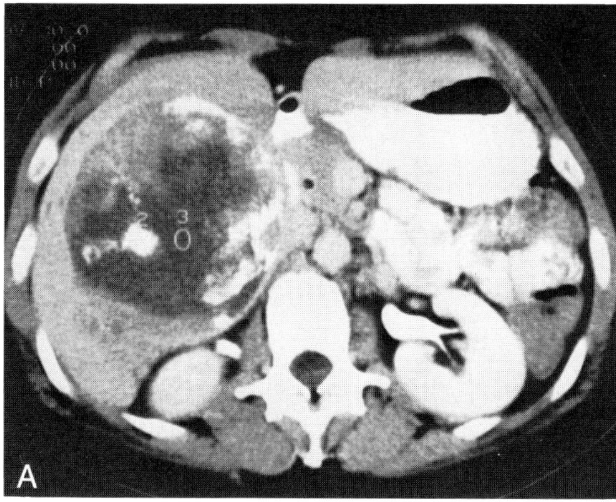
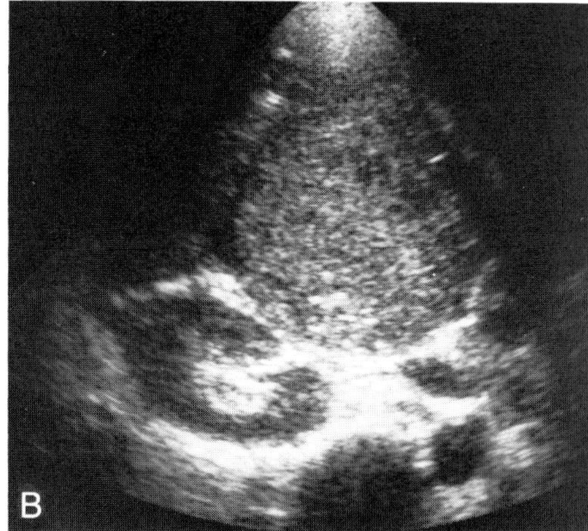

FIGURE 3–78. Hepatocellular carcinoma. *A.* Contrast CT shows patchy enhancement of a large, low-density liver lesion. *B.* The ultrasonogram is a similar transverse image through the right lobe of the liver and shows the well-circumscribed, echogenic lesion. The patient, a 31-year-old woman, developed hepatocellular carcinoma in association with parenchymal liver injury from earlier infection by *Echinococcus.*

ent. MRI can also show portal and hepatic vein invasion, an ominous prognostic sign.

Angiograms show a dense tumor stain, abnormal irregular vessels (tumor vascularity), and large draining veins. The lesion appears as a defect on liver-spleen scans because it does not take up the radiopharmaceutical agent (see Chapter 9). Gallium scanning can be helpful in selected cases for distinguishing hepatocellular carcinoma from benign lesions because the malignant tumor takes up gallium, although infection can also show gallium uptake.

Complications of hepatocellular carcinoma are liver failure, hemorrhage, and local invasion. Liver failure and biliary obstruction result in bile stasis and the accumulation of toxic materials in the blood. Hemorrhage into the richly vascularized liver occurs when the tumor invades or obstructs major vessels. Hepatocellular carcinoma commonly invades the inferior vena cava and hepatic veins, which results in pulmonary emboli or vascular occlusion. The prognosis of hepatocellular carcinoma is poor. Most patients die within 6 months after the diagnosis is made. In rare instances, single tumors are removed surgically with good results.

Hepatoblastoma. Hepatoblastoma is a malignant tumor of children that arises from em-

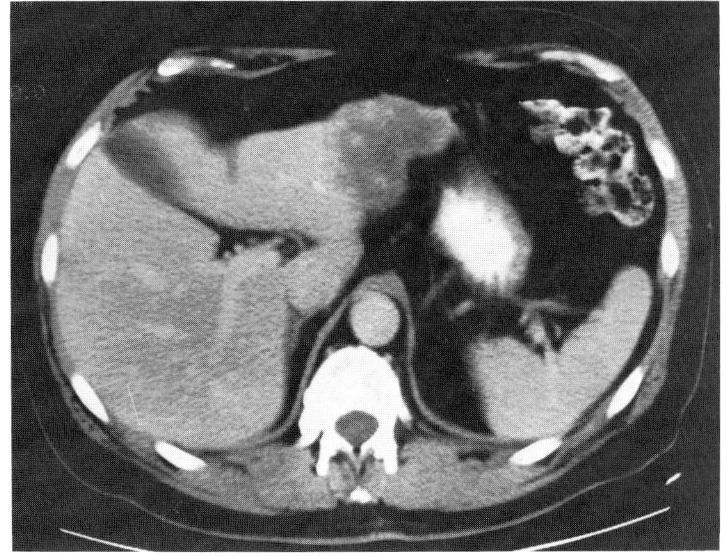

FIGURE 3–79. Hepatocellular carcinoma. Enhanced CT shows a low-density mass involving most of the lateral segment of the left lobe of the liver with patchy enhancement. There is no extension outside the liver. The only symptom of the patient, a 55-year-old man, was weight loss. (Courtesy of B. Porter, First Hill Diagnostic Imaging Center, Seattle.)

bryonal hepatic cells. The disease is usually identified between birth and the age of 3 years when a liver mass is detected. The most common signs are anorexia, anemia, thrombocytopenia, and high serum alpha-fetoprotein levels. The majority of these tumors are malignant. On CT scans, the mass has an appearance similar to that of hepatocellular carcinoma, and it is usually less dense than adjacent liver after contrast is administered. The presence of calcification (50% of patients) and the youth of the patient are helpful for differentiating hepatoblastoma from hepatocellular carcinoma (usually seen after age 5 years). MRI usually shows a well-defined liver mass that displaces normal structures. The tumor is treated by surgical resection.

Metastases. The most common liver tumors are metastases. Cells from most malignant tumors eventually enter the blood stream and are filtered by the liver. Sources of liver metastases include colon carcinoma, lung carcinoma, breast carcinoma, melanoma, carcinoid, pancreatic carcinoma, choriocarcinoma, leiomyosarcoma, and renal cell carcinoma. Most metastases are multiple, low-density masses, best diagnosed on CT and MRI. Some lesions enhance markedly, but most enhance only enough to attain a density similar to that of the normal liver (Fig. 3–80). Therefore, the use of either a rapid bolus of contrast or a combination of noncontrast/contrast is required for optimal detection of liver metastases. Adenocarcinoma metastases from the colon occasionally calcify. MRI shows metastatic tumor in the liver as high intensity on T2 spin echo or STIR sequences and as low intensity on T1 spin echo sequences. STIR imaging

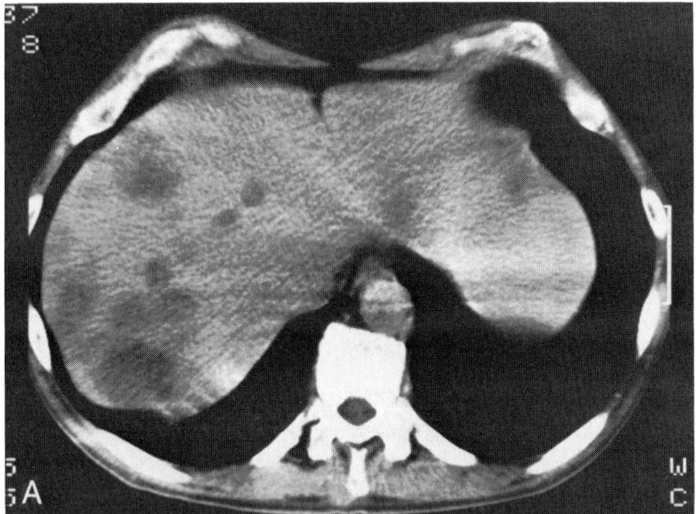

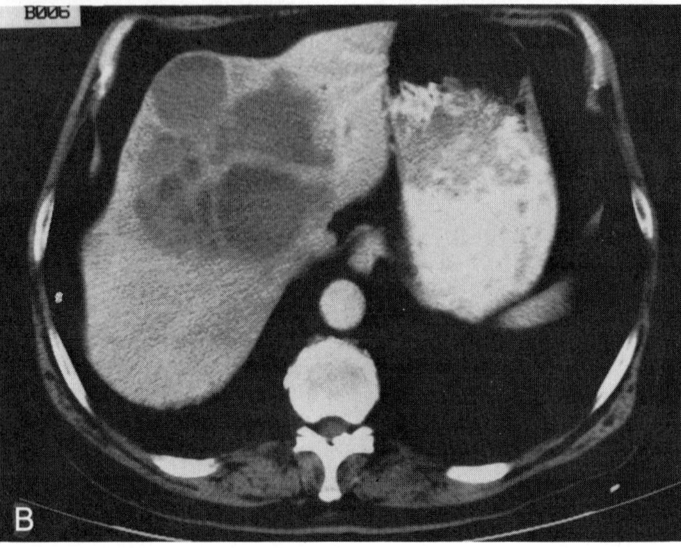

FIGURE 3–80. Liver metastases. *A.* Metastatic melanoma. Contrast-enhanced CT shows multiple, low-density areas in the liver of a 50-year-old man with melanoma. *B.* Colon carcinoma. Contrast-enhanced CT of the upper abdomen in a 61-year-old man with colon carcinoma shows multiple, cavitary lesions involving much of the right lobe of the liver and the medial segment of the left lobe. Contrast, food, and air are shown in the stomach. No adenopathy was found. The radiologist used CT to guide a percutaneous biopsy of the largest lesion.

has the added advantage of suppressing the signal from fat and showing adenopathy. A helpful finding in differentiating metastatic tumor from abscess is the clustering of small lesions that is seen in infectious liver disease.

Cholangiocarcinoma. Cholangiocarcinoma, a slow-growing, malignant tumor (usually adenocarcinoma) that arises from bile duct epithelium, is most common in the 40- to 80-year age group. It is sometimes associated with ulcerative colitis. The tumor usually arises in the large intrahepatic ducts or in the extrahepatic ducts (Fig. 3–81). Because it invades adjacent structures, it cannot be totally resected in most cases, but partial resection combined with the use of biliary drainage catheters can prolong survival without the painful and unpleasant symptoms of bile duct obstruction. These drainage catheters are usually placed percutaneously through the liver by the radiologist. Despite the efforts of surgery and interventional radiology, patients with cholangiocarcinoma survive less than 1 year after diagnosis. Portal vein invasion carries a very poor prognosis.

Gallbladder Carcinoma. When adenocarcinoma arises from the gallbladder, the tumor is highly malignant and rapidly fatal. Gallstones, obstruction, and calcification of the gallbladder predispose a patient to the development of adenocarcinoma of the gallbladder, a tumor of persons over 65. By the time of diagnosis, the tumor has usually spread to the liver and surrounding organs, and so survival is short. Ultrasonograms show the gallbladder as a large, right upper quadrant mass with associated bile duct obstruction. Early gallbladder carcinoma may appear as only a small, intraluminal gallbladder mass or even as focal wall thickening.

Vascular Disease

The liver receives blood from the portal vein and from the hepatic artery. Venous drainage is via the hepatic veins. The inferior vena cava passes through the liver in its course to the right atrium, receiving the hepatic venous drainage. The portal vein receives blood from the splenic, superior mesenteric, and inferior mesenteric veins (Fig. 3–82). The fetal circulation (see Chapter 5) directs oxygenated blood from the umbilical vein to the intrahepatic portal vein and then through the ductus venosus to the vena cava and the right atrium. It can recanalize in adults with retrograde flow when portal obstruction is present (see Fig. 3–64). The most important vascular diseases of the liver are portal venous hypertension and hepatic vein obstruction (Budd-Chiari syndrome). The liver seldom becomes ischemic because it has low oxygen requirements and dual blood supply.

Portal Venous Hypertension. Portal venous hypertension is the result of obstruction to blood flow in the portal vein, which may be either extrahepatic or intrahepatic. Extrahepatic portal hypertension occurs when the portal vein is obstructed by tumor, thrombus, or surgery. Although liver function is normal, the blood from the intestines, the stomach, and the spleen is shunted by collateral vessels past the liver. The increased portal pressure also results in bleeding esophageal and gastric varices (discussed in Part I of this chapter) and dilated hemorrhoidal and umbilical veins.

Intrahepatic portal hypertension is caused by obstruction of venous channels within the liver, usually as a result of cirrhosis from alcoholic or infectious liver disease. The blood from the portal vein and the hepatic artery normally passes through the hepatic sinusoids into the hepatic veins and then to the right atrium. Scarring or irregular regeneration of the liver from cirrhosis results in variable degrees of obstruction to portal venous flow within the liver. This obstruction leads to elevation of portal venous pressure, which then causes development of gastric and esophageal varices (Fig. 3–83). Other consequences are shunting of blood past the liver, which causes hepatic encephalopathy; the development of hemorrhoids; and umbilical artery engorgement (see also the "Alcoholic Liver Disease" section).

Portal hypertension is diagnosed clinically from the presence of hemorrhage from varices, telangiectasia, and the development of hepatic encephalopathy. Treatment is directed at eliminating the cause of the obstruction, if possible. When cirrhosis is the cause, surgical bypass of the liver or liver transplantation are the only options. Many bypass operations have been devised, but the most popular are an anastomosis of the splenic vein to the left renal vein (splenorenal shunt) and of the portal vein to the inferior vena cava (portacaval shunt). Unfortunately, these procedures may worsen the hepatic encephalopathy. Radiographic examination requires demonstration of the portal venous system and the renal veins. MRI can be used to demonstrate patency of shunt vessels.

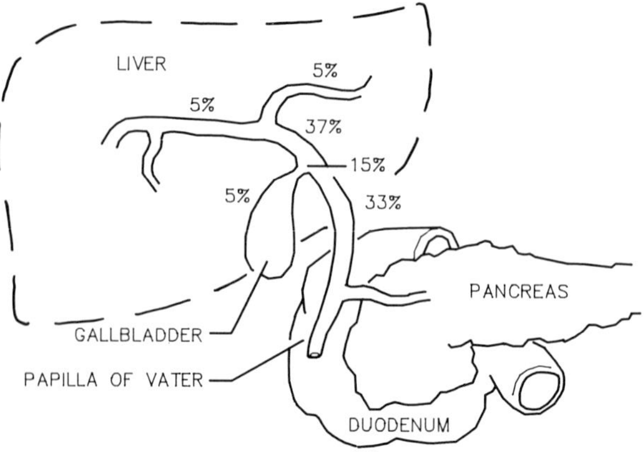

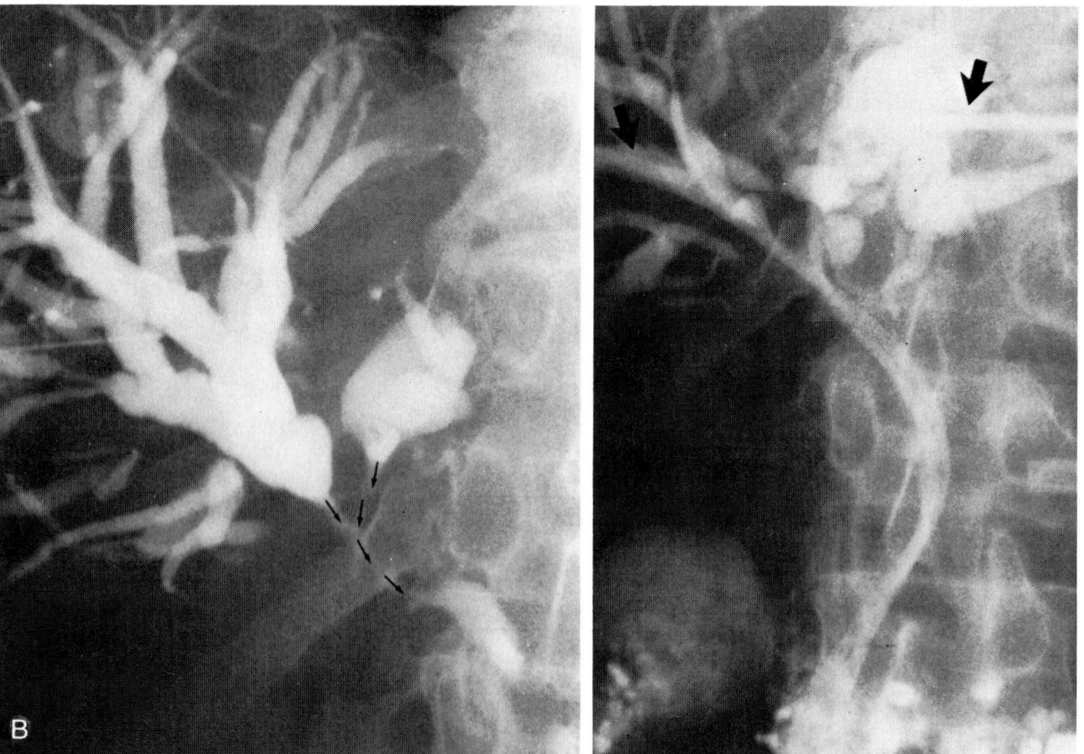

FIGURE 3–81. Cholangiocarcinoma. *A.* Diagram. *B.* Left view of the biliary system shows dilatation of the bile ducts caused by constricting cholangiocarcinoma. Arrows mark the obstructed common bile duct. Right view shows that bilateral drainage is established by percutaneous placement of catheters *(arrows)* passing into the duodenum. Note decompression of the bile ducts. (From Ring E, Kerlan R: Percutaneous transhepatic cholangiography and interventional radiology of the gallbladder and bile ducts. *In* Way LM, Pellegrini CA [eds]: Surgery of the Gallbladder and Bile Ducts, p 178. Philadelphia: WB Saunders, 1987.)

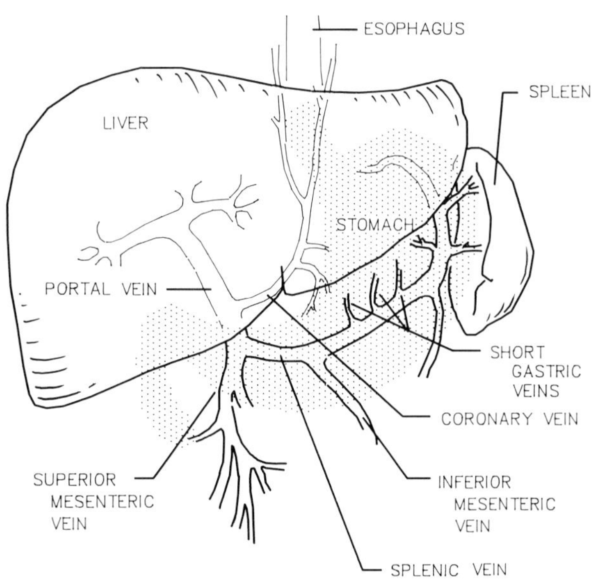

FIGURE 3–82. Portal venous blood flow.

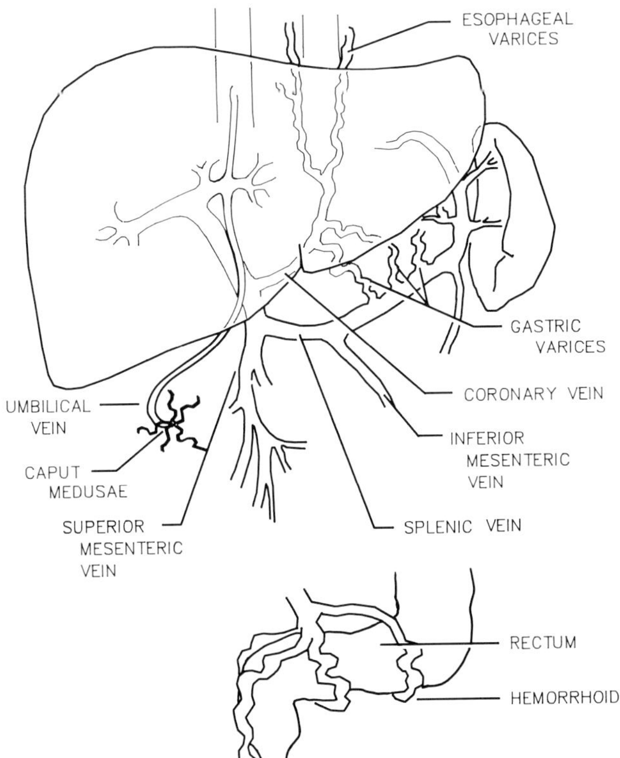

FIGURE 3–83. Complications of portal venous hypertension.

Hepatic Vein Obstruction. Obstruction of the hepatic veins or the intrahepatic vena cava (Budd-Chiari syndrome) prevents the flow of blood through the liver and can also cause portal hypertension. The veins are usually obstructed near their junction with the inferior vena cava. Causes of hepatic venous obstruction include traumatic injuries, hepatocellular carcinoma, clot or tumor in the inferior vena cava, congenital web of the vena cava, and right atrial myxoma. In many of these conditions both the hepatic veins and the inferior vena cava are obstructed. The patients have hepatomegaly and ascites and may develop jaundice and varices.

The best examination for screening patients with suspected hepatic venous thrombosis is Doppler ultrasonography, which shows the individual hepatic veins and their confluence. Hepatic venous flow and clots are readily assessed. Other important findings are thickened irregular walls of the veins, focal stenosis, and the demonstration of collateral flow.

CT with noncontrast and dynamic contrast techniques may show the hepatic enlargement and the vascular flow distribution. Because the caudate lobe (the caudal, square-shaped lobe posteriorly near the vena cava) drains directly into the vena cava, it is not enlarged and shows normal enhancement. This observation is therefore of great value for diagnosing hepatic venous thrombosis. The precontrast image shows the normal density of the caudate lobe against the low density and enlargement of the remainder of the liver and the obstructed spleen (Fig. 3–84). Infusion of contrast initially causes enhancement of the spleen and the caudate lobe and, later, redistribution to the engorged, abnormal liver.

MRI can show obliteration and lack of flow through the hepatic veins and the inferior vena cava and can demonstrate clots within the veins. The disease is diagnosed arteriographically from the demonstration of the obstruction and collateral circulation.

Portal Vein Thrombosis. Acute thrombosis of the portal vein occurs in conjunction with inflammation and obstruction. The most common causes are ascending cholangitis, hepatic vein thrombosis, pancreatitis, and splenectomy. The manifesting signs may be those of the underlying disease, but many patients have limited, nonspecific symptoms. Diagnosis on ultrasonography is made by identification of intraluminal echogenic clot and demonstration of obstruction to flow. Noncontrast CT shows the high-density clot in the portal vein. Contrast-enhanced CT shows the clot as being of lower density than the enhanced liver and outlined by the enhancing vessel wall (see Fig. 3–64).

Complications of portal vein thrombosis depend on the underlying cause and the degree of obstruction. Infectious causes can lead to fulminant sepsis. Destruction and obliteration of the portal vein lead to formation of collat-

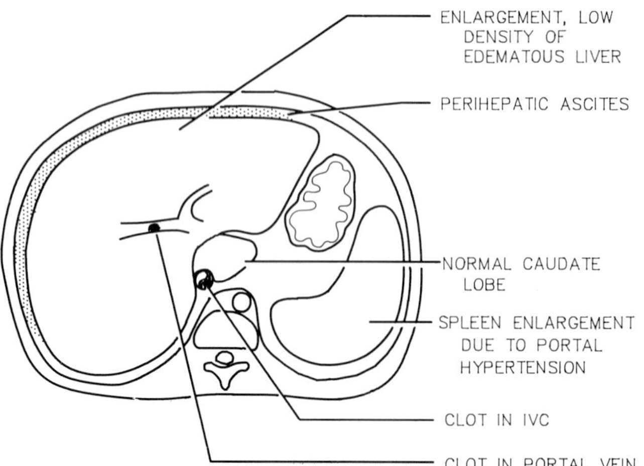

FIGURE 3–84. Hepatic venous thrombosis.

eral channels, called cavernous transformation of the portal vein. Severe portal obstruction can cause bowel infarction and sepsis.

PANCREAS

Trauma

Pancreatic injury is less common than injury to the spleen and the liver in patients with abdominal trauma. However, it is associated with a relatively high mortality rate (up to 20%). Injury to the pancreas often occurs in conjunction with other injuries; for example, because of the proximity of the pancreas to the duodenum, pancreatic injuries are commonly associated with duodenal injuries. In many patients with pancreatic injury, death is caused by injuries to other organs. Patients may have symptoms related to these other injuries or may have severe abdominal pain. The most common mechanism of injury is compression against the spine. Injuries include laceration, contusion, rupture, and transection. Complications of pancreatic injury include hemorrhage and the development of abscess and pseudocyst. Although elevation of serum amylase frequently occurs in pancreatic injuries, many patients do not show such an elevation.

The diagnosis cannot be made by means of peritoneal lavage because of the retroperitoneal location of the pancreas (and the associated portion of the duodenum). The most informative imaging test for evaluation of the gland is CT, which can show hematoma, laceration, and transection of the pancreas. In addition, it can show the other injuries associated with abdominal trauma. Because injury to the pancreatic duct results in some of the most important complications of pancreatic injury, an endoscopic retrograde pancreatic study may be required. Ultrasonography is difficult to apply in an injured patient but is valuable for follow-up and for the identification and evaluation of posttraumatic pancreatic pseudocyst or abscess.

It is difficult to identify pancreatic injury on CT because of the nonuniform texture of the pancreas and the presence of adjacent tissue swelling and hemorrhage. The most important findings are inhomogeneous density in the pancreas, cleft (indicating transection), hemorrhage, and duodenal injury (Fig. 3–85). Some patients develop posttraumatic pancreatitis, exhibiting a swollen gland with adjacent soft-tissue infiltration of the anterior pararenal space, which causes thickening of Gerota's fascia. Pancreatic pseudocysts are cystic fluid collections within, extending from, or distant from the pancreas (to be discussed). Other complications include the development of abscess; the most serious complication is autodigestion of adjacent tissue as a result of liberated digestive enzymes.

Congenital Abnormalities

Significant congenital anomalies of the pancreas are rare. The pancreas normally forms

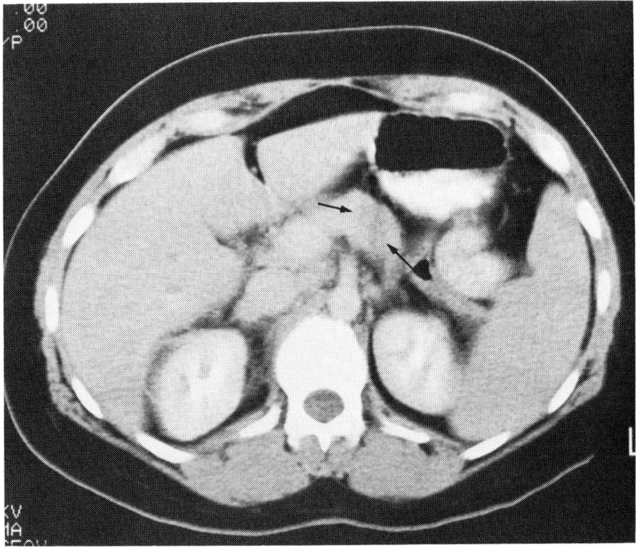

FIGURE 3–85. Pancreatic contusion. CT scan of the midabdomen shows enlargement and low density of the body of the pancreas. The contusion occurred when the patient was thrown from an inner tube sled, compressing the pancreas against the spine.

from two segments: the dorsal pancreas and the ventral pancreas (Fig. 3–86). These two segments later fuse, and the separate ducts join. When this formation is altered or interrupted, a variety of structural alterations result, the most consequential of which is annular pancreas. In most cases, simple variations of the locations and the course of the pancreatic ducts develop. These variations are usually asymptomatic but can lead to obstruction of the pancreatic or common bile ducts and pancreatitis.

Annular Pancreas. When the ventral and dorsal pancreatic buds fail to fuse, the ventral bud encircles the duodenum, resulting in annular pancreas. The lesion can cause a high-grade obstruction or may be an unimportant anatomical variation. Patients may become symptomatic at any age. An upper GI examination reveals annular, extrinsic obstruction of the descending portion of the duodenum. CT scans and ultrasonograms can show increased tissue around the duodenum, but differentiation from tumor or adenopathy may not be possible. Annular pancreas is suspected when tissue with the same density as pancreas is seen lateral to the descending portion of the duodenum.

Pancreas Divisum. The most common anatomical variant of the pancreas is pancreas divisum, which occurs when the ventral and dorsal pancreas fail to fuse, leaving two separate ducts draining into the duodenum. The inferior head of the pancreas is drained by a short pancreatic duct (the ventral duct) that joins the common bile duct before entry into the duodenum. Most of the pancreas, including the remainder of the head, the body, and the tail, is drained by the dorsal pancreatic duct, which has a separate entry into the duodenum. CT scans and ultrasonograms show increased thickness of the pancreatic head, which may be divided into dorsal and ventral portions by a plane of fat. Pancreas divisum is a frequent cause of idiopathic pancreatitis when one or both ducts become partially obstructed.

Cystic Fibrosis. Cystic fibrosis is an inherited autosomal recessive disease characterized by thick mucous secretions (therefore it is also called mucoviscidosis) by all glandular secret-

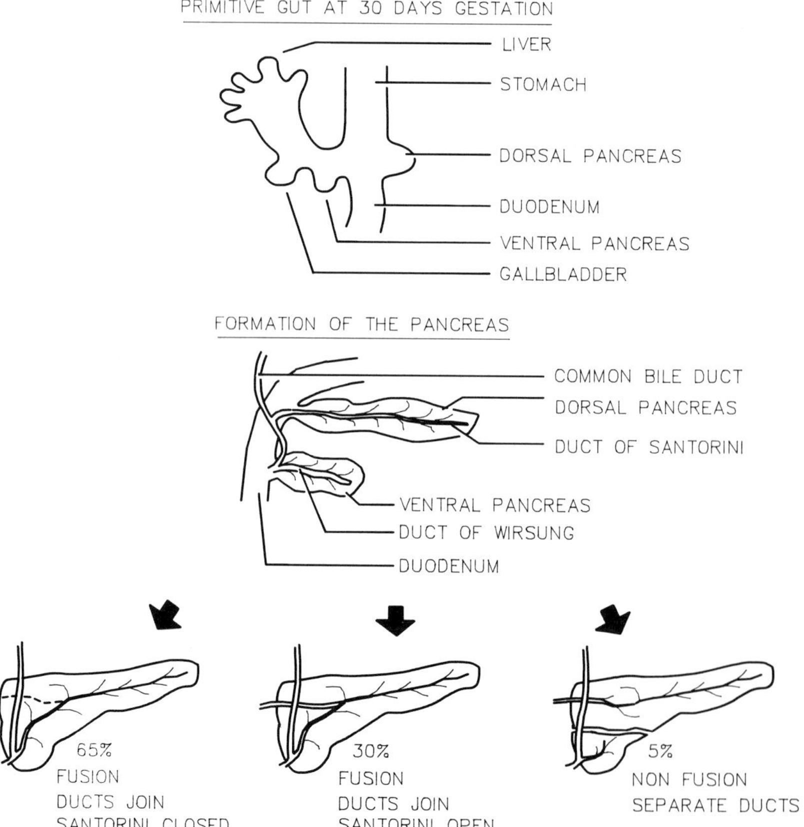

FIGURE 3–86. Development of the pancreas.

ing tissue, including the lungs (see Chapter 2), the pancreas, and the intestines. These thick secretions in the small bowel cause thickening of the duodenal folds and occasional obstruction from intussusception. Also, because the pancreas is often unable to secrete enzymes effectively, digestion and resorption are reduced. The secretions affect the function and the appearance of the colon, causing it to resemble jejunum on barium studies. CT scans show an atrophic, fatty pancreas.

Inflammation and Infection

Pancreatitis. Pancreatitis is usually a noninfectious inflammation caused by obstruction of the pancreatic ducts. The most common causes are alcoholism, obstructing gallstones, trauma, and surgery. The pathological appearance of pancreatitis may be either edematous or necrotizing. In edematous pancreatitis, the gland is enlarged and swollen and has a low-density appearance on CT scans and low echogenicity on ultrasonograms as a result of edema. Necrosis and hemorrhage are absent. The inflammation involves the parenchyma and the adjacent soft tissues. The ducts are not involved. Edematous pancreatitis has a benign but variable course, and therapy is supportive.

Necrotizing pancreatitis is more serious than edematous pancreatitis and is characterized by necrosis and hemorrhage. It involves the entire gland, including the ducts. Fat necrosis and fluid around the pancreas are also often present. In both types of pancreatitis, the pancreatic injury results from the secretion of trypsin, which then activates other digestive enzymes. These enzymes cause autodigestion of the pancreas and adjacent tissue, which results in edema, hemorrhage, and inflammation.

Patients complain of severe, upper abdominal pain radiating to the back. Most cases are diagnosed by clinical history, particularly if the patients have had previous episodes of pancreatitis. The serum amylase level is often elevated in acute pancreatitis; however, many other conditions can cause such elevation. Furthermore, elevated serum amylase is not always present in pancreatitis.

Imaging is performed to diagnose pancreatitis, to evaluate for infectious pancreatic abscess, phlegmon, or pseudocyst formation, to detect ampullary gallstones as a cause of pancreatitis, and to rule out pancreatic carcinoma. Ultrasonography is effective for identifying edema and enlargement of the pancreas and for demonstrating other factors related to the development of pancreatitis, such as the presence of gallstones and alcoholic liver disease. Ultrasonography is also effective for the identification and follow-up of pseudocyst, phlegmon, and abscess. It is best performed in patients with mild disease and preferably after the acute phase has resolved. The ultrasonographic images show decreased echogenicity of the pancreas, generalized or focal enlargement, highly echogenic punctate calcifications, and the major complication of pancreatitis, the formation of a pseudocyst (Fig. 3–87). Pseudocysts are usually close to the pancreas. However, they may extend into the abdomen anywhere and are sometimes seen in the chest or the pelvis.

CT is the primary diagnostic technique for patients with severe, acute, or complicated pancreatitis (Fig. 3–88). The CT diagnosis of pancreatitis is based on direct evidence of pancreatic inflammatory disease as well as on circumstantial evidence of predisposing factors and adjacent inflammation. CT abnormalities in pancreatitis include an enlarged gland and, sometimes, the dilatation of the pancreatic duct. Small gas bubbles, pseudocysts, and thickening of Gerota's fascia adjacent to the pancreas suggest an inflammatory process. The presence of gallstones or fatty liver infiltration (caused by alcoholism) also supports the diagnosis of pancreatitis.

In acute pancreatitis, CT shows an enlarged pancreas with diffuse or focal areas of low density. The fat around the superior mesenteric artery is preserved, although peripancreatic fat may be of higher density than usual. This finding helps to differentiate pancreatitis from pancreatic carcinoma, which can invade the fat around the superior mesenteric artery. In chronic pancreatitis, the pancreas is usually small and atrophic with scattered calcifications, but occasionally it may be enlarged. The calcifications can often be seen on plain radiographs. The most common complications of pancreatitis are the formation of pseudocysts and peripancreatic fluid collections.

Pancreatic Pseudocyst. A pancreatic pseudocyst is an encapsulated cyst, filled with fluid and pancreatic secretions. It forms when obstruction and inflammation of pancreatic ducts cause extravasation of digestive enzymes into the pancreatic parenchyma. The local autodigestion results in the formation of one or more cystic structures with fibrous walls. The pseudocyst develops weeks after the acute ep-

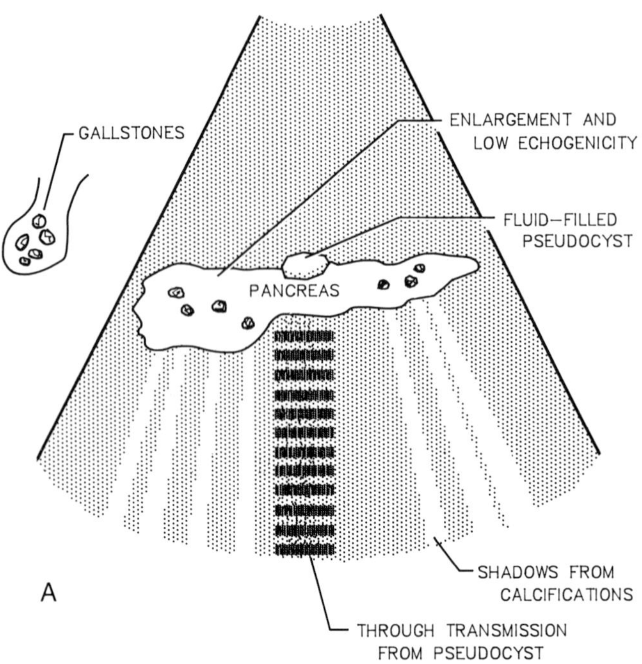

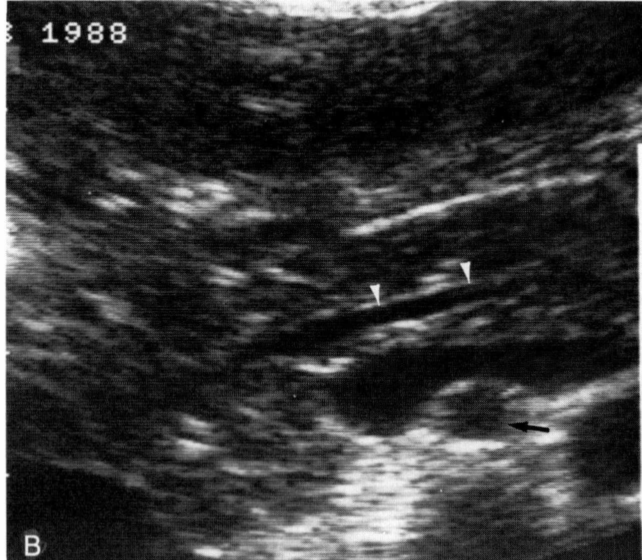

FIGURE 3–87. Pancreatitis. *A.* Diagram. *B.* Dilated pancreatic duct. Transverse ultrasonogram shows dilatation of the pancreatic duct *(arrowheads)* in a patient with acute pancreatitis. The pancreas shows low echogenicity in comparison with the liver. The linear hypoechoic structure posterior to the pancreatic duct is the splenic vein joining the superior mesenteric vein. The superior mesenteric artery *(black arrow)* is surrounded by normally echogenic fat.

isode of pancreatitis, as the capsule forms around isolated collections of fluid, hemorrhage, and pancreatic juices. It may be found outside the pancreas, especially in the area of the tail and extending into the lesser sac. When the enzymes invade tissues outside the pancreas, the pseudocyst may be adjacent to or entirely separate from the gland. The most common manifestation of a pseudocyst is persistent pain after a bout of pancreatitis.

Pseudocysts are best diagnosed with CT and ultrasonography. Both can reveal the large, dilated cystic cavities (Fig. 3–89). Ultrasonography is most practical for follow-up of a known lesion, but CT is most informative for surveying the entire pancreas and abdomen. About 30% of pseudocysts resolve spontaneously within 6 weeks, and so most are initially managed conservatively. Those that do not resolve are treated by surgical drainage into the stomach, in which the digestive enzymes do no harm. Single lesions can be aspirated or drained by catheters placed under CT or ultrasonographic guidance. Rupture of a

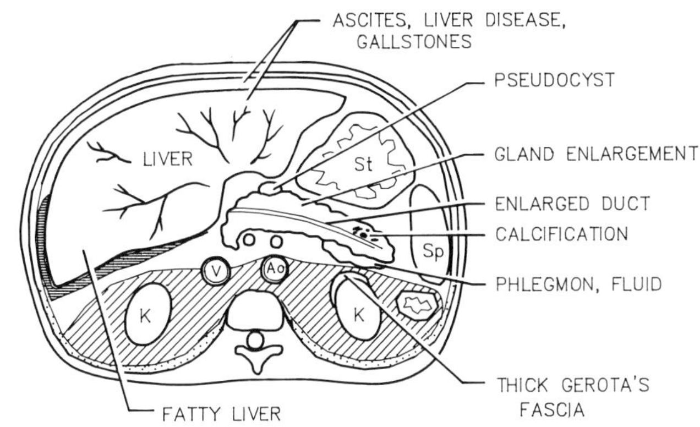

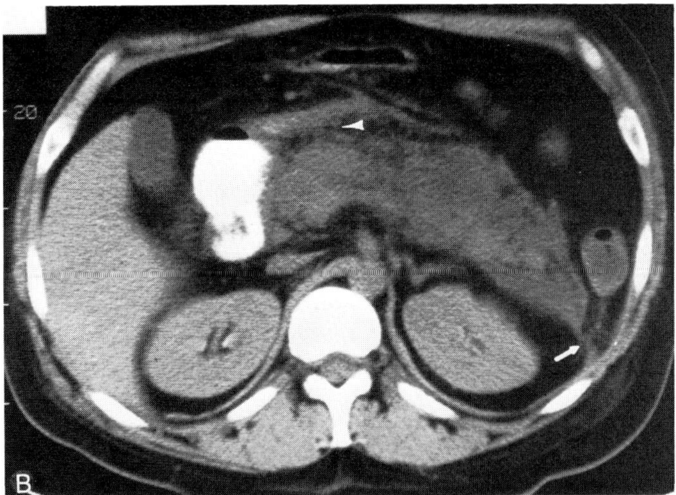

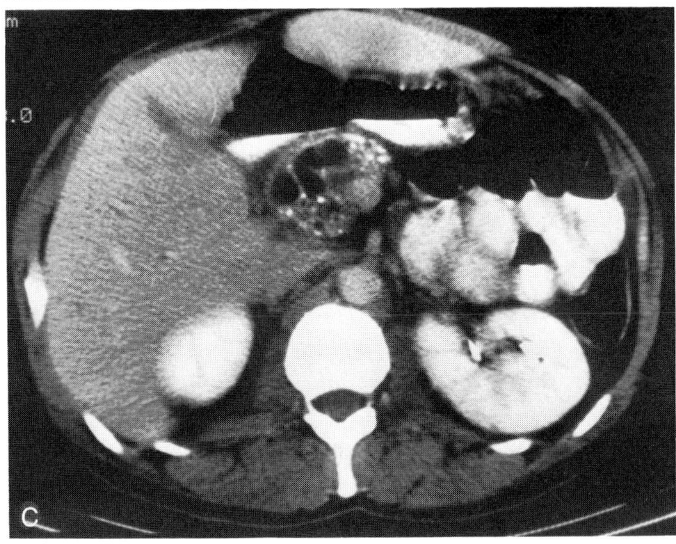

FIGURE 3–88. Pancreatitis. *A.* Diagram. *B.* Acute pancreatitis. Contrast CT shows enlargement and low density of the pancreas in a 35-year-old alcoholic who had experienced previous bouts of pancreatitis. Inflammation involving the fat anterior to the pancreas *(arrowhead)* and thickening of the lateral conal fascia *(arrow)* are corroborative findings. Note that the fat around the mesenteric vessels is preserved, which is typical of acute pancreatitis. *C.* Chronic pancreatitis. Enhanced CT shows an enlarged head and uncinate process of the pancreas with multiple punctate calcifications. The pancreatic duct is massively enlarged, showing tortuosity and segmentation (the black lumen within the gland). The fat surrounding the origin of the celiac axis is intact, which is consistent with pancreatic inflammatory disease. (Courtesy of B. Porter, First Hill Diagnostic Imaging Center, Seattle.)

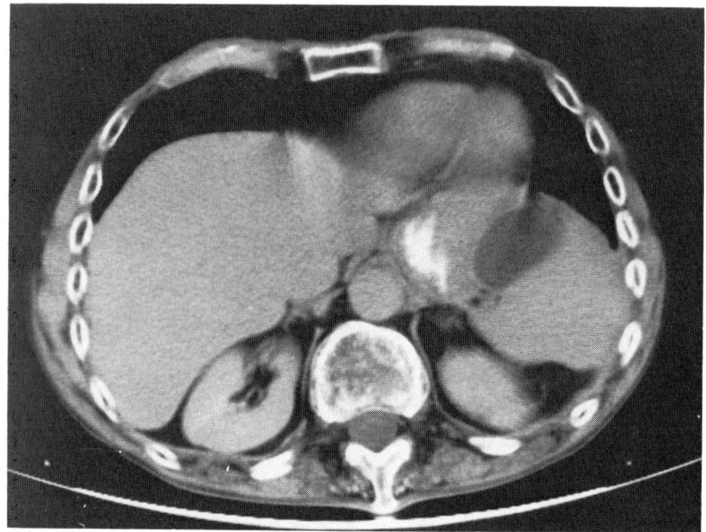

FIGURE 3–89. Pancreatic pseudocyst. CT through the upper abdomen after oral and intravenous contrast shows a water-density, rounded structure, lateral to the stomach. Although the pancreas cannot be seen on this image, lower slices showed this pseudocyst to be projecting superiorly from the tail of the pancreas. Between the pseudocyst and the contrast in the stomach is inflammatory thickening of the gastric wall.

pseudocyst into the retroperitoneum or the lesser sac causes local autodigestion of tissue, which frequently results in shock and death.

Many pancreatic pseudocysts regress spontaneously. Others stabilize over time. Pseudocysts can become infected, hemorrhage, dissect into adjacent structures, or rupture. Other fluid collections occur in the peripancreatic tissues and may extend along adjacent spaces, including the anterior pararenal space, the lesser sac, the transverse mesentery, the perirenal space, and the psoas compartment. Few of these amorphous fluid collections form discrete pseudocysts.

Pancreatic Phlegmon and Abscess. Pancreatic phlegmon is a diffuse edematous or necrotic tissue mass in or around the pancreas and is associated with inflammation or trauma. A phlegmon develops from autodigestion of the pancreas and consists of edematous tissue, inflammatory cells, and necrosed pancreas. CT scans and ultrasonograms show an amorphous soft-tissue mass within or near the pancreas. Unless the phlegmon becomes infected, no treatment is required. An infected pancreatic phlegmon or pseudocyst is often fatal.

Neoplasms

Benign tumors of the pancreas are rare. They include cystadenomas and islet cell adenomas. The most important malignant tumor of the pancreas is the adenocarcinoma. Islet cell tumors may also be malignant.

Cystadenoma. The cystadenoma of the pancreas is a rare, slow-growing cystic tumor that is usually asymptomatic. Two types occur. Microcystic adenomas occur in the older population, usually in the head of the pancreas, and have no malignant potential. They appear as poorly defined cysts without a capsule. Macrocystic adenomas (also called mucinous cystadenomas) occur in middle age, usually in women, and usually in the body or the tail of the pancreas. They are encapsulated and have abundant fibrous elements. When a macrocystic adenoma is in the head of the pancreas, it causes obstruction of the pancreatic duct or the common bile duct and is detected early. Otherwise, the tumor can grow to a large size before detection. Because a macrocystic tumor has malignant potential (a malignant macrocystic tumor is called a cystadenocarcinoma), it must be treated aggressively.

CT scans show a lobulated, septated, cystic mass in the pancreas. The septations are best evaluated on ultrasonography. A cystadenoma can be difficult to distinguish from pancreatic pseudocyst, cystadenocarcinoma (Fig. 3–90), and adenocarcinoma of the pancreas. The latter two commonly metastasize to the liver.

Islet Cell Adenoma. Tumors of the pancreatic islet cells are rare but are important because they can cause endocrine imbalances. These tumors include insulinoma (in 60% to 75% of islet cell tumors), gastrinoma (20%), vipoma (vasoactive intestinal peptide), glucagonoma, and somatostatinoma. Approximately 15% of islet cell tumors do not secrete hormones and are therefore detected as large masses or metastases. The hormonally active,

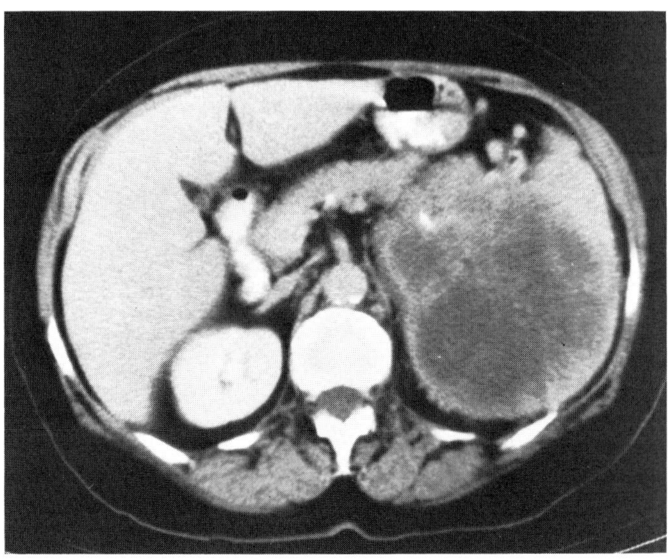

FIGURE 3–90. Cystadenocarcinoma of the pancreas. Contrast CT shows a multilobulated, complex, predominantly cystic mass involving the majority of the left upper quadrant. This and lower scans showed the lesion arising from the tail of the pancreas and secondarily invading the spleen. The body and head of the pancreas are normal. Other slices suggested adjacent invasion of the posterior wall of the stomach and involvement of the left adrenal gland.

symptomatic tumors are usually less than 2 cm in diameter when detected but can often be shown by CT (Fig. 3–91). Insulinomas are usually very small, hypervascular masses and are less easily detected.

Islet cell adenomas are hyperdense after contrast in comparison with the adjacent pancreas and may be calcified. Gastrinomas have the highest rate of malignancy (50% to 80%). Their associated high level of serum gastrin results in ulceration anywhere in the stomach, the duodenum, or the small bowel. CT-based diagnosis of islet cell tumors is improved by a scan with thin (3- to 5-mm) slices, performed immediately after rapid intravenous injection of contrast.

A thorough work-up of patients with endocrine abnormalities referable to the pancreas is indicated for several reasons. Islet cell tumors may be associated with the multiple endocrine neoplasm type I syndrome. These patients therefore require clinical investigation and, if indicated, imaging tests to identify pituitary, parathyroid, and adrenal abnormalities. In addition, about 15% of insulinomas, 60% of gastrinomas, and 60% of glucagonomas are malignant. If the tumor cannot be located on CT scans or ultrasonograms, angiograms may show a hypervascular area in the pancreas.

Adenocarcinoma. The most common malignant tumor of the pancreas is the adenocarcinoma. It occurs twice as often in men as in women, usually after the age of 40. Symptoms depend on the location of the mass. In the head of the pancreas, it obstructs the pancreatic duct and common bile duct, which results in jaundice and symptoms of obstruction. In the body and the tail of the pancreas, it may be asymptomatic until it becomes large enough to compress adjacent structures. Many patients experience weight loss, abdominal pain, and a change in bowel habits. Some patients develop deep venous thrombosis.

Early clinical suspicion and imaging evaluation of pancreatic adenocarcinoma are essential if small tumors are to be detected and treated. Advanced disease is frequently untreatable at the time of diagnosis. Pancreatic carcinoma can be confused with pancreatitis if the latter is localized. However, the inflammation of pancreatitis often extends anteriorly. Posteriorly, pancreatitis thickens Gerota's fascia and the lateral conal fascia but does not usually encase the mesenteric arteries (see Fig. 3–88).

Pancreatic adenocarcinoma is evaluated by means of CT and ultrasonography. Both can demonstrate a mass in the head, the body, or the tail of the pancreas and can also demonstrate erosion of fat around the superior mesenteric artery, adjacent spread, liver metastases, adenopathy, and peritoneal implants of tumor (Fig. 3–92). Both CT and ultrasonography can be used for guiding needle biopsy of a pancreatic mass and enabling the diagnosis of pancreatic carcinoma to be made without surgery. Ultrasonograms show a sonolucent lesion that causes pancreatic enlargement (Fig. 3–93). Dilatation of the common bile ducts and the pancreatic ducts can be demonstrated on ultrasonograms in most cases. CT scans

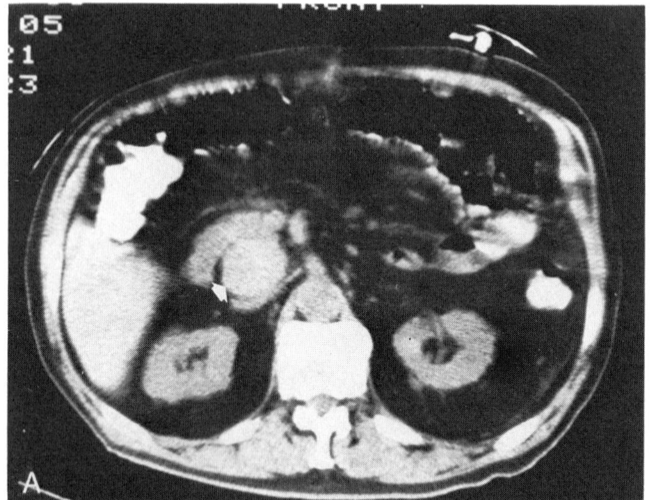

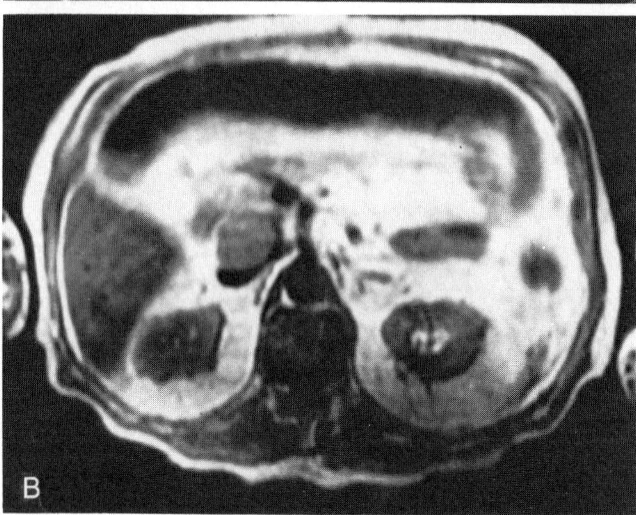

FIGURE 3–91. Gastrinoma in the head of the pancreas. *A.* CT shows a soft-tissue mass in the head of the pancreas *(arrow)*. The compressed inferior vena cava, which is directly posterior, and the duodenum, which is lateral, show that the mass is in the head of the pancreas. *B.* Proton density MRI shows the mass and its relation to the inferior vena cava and the superior mesenteric artery. This tumor manifested with perforation of a jejunal ulcer as a result of excess gastrin secretion.

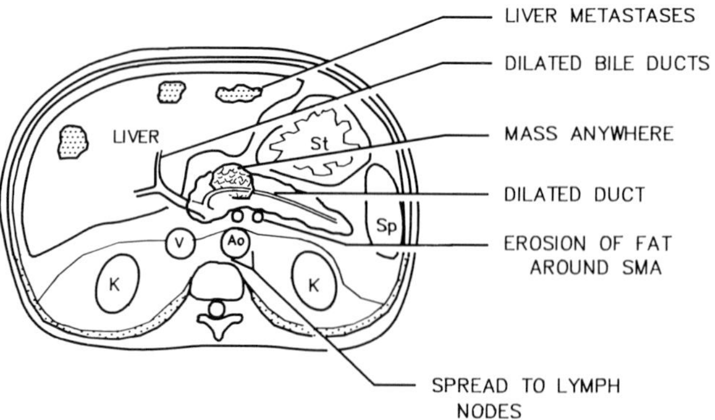

FIGURE 3–92. Pancreatic carcinoma. *A.* Diagram. SMA, superior mesenteric artery; St, stomach; Sp, spleen; V, vena cava; Ao, aorta; K, kidney.

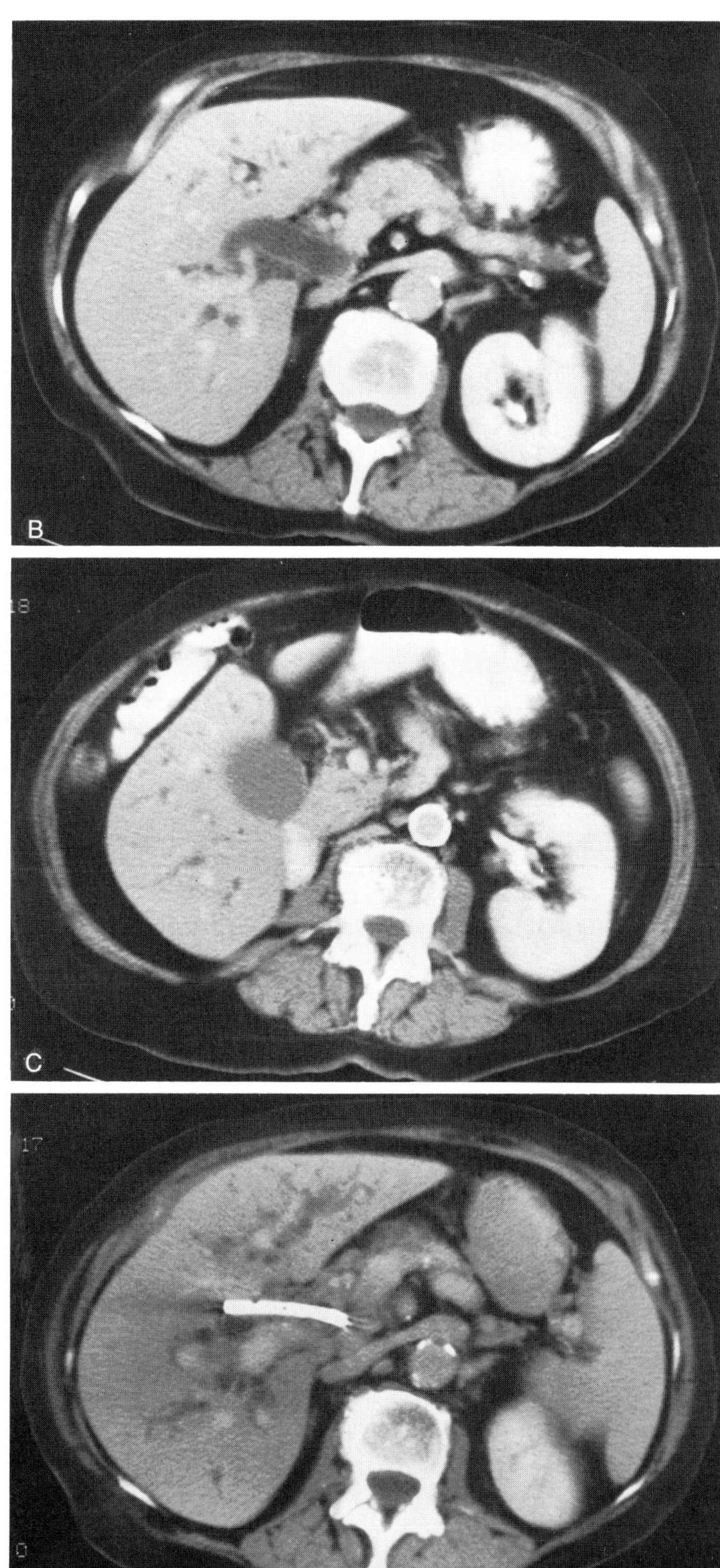

FIGURE 3–92 *Continued B.* Contrast CT of the upper abdomen shows dilated intrahepatic ducts (low density). Dilatation of the common bile duct (1.5 cm) is also present in an 82-year-old woman with painless jaundice. *C.* The common duct ends abruptly in the head of the pancreas as shown on a lower slice. Note also compression of the duodenum, enlargement of the gallbladder, and congenital absence of the right kidney. *D.* The common bile duct and the pancreatic duct were drained by an indwelling stent placed during surgery for an ampullary carcinoma of the pancreas.

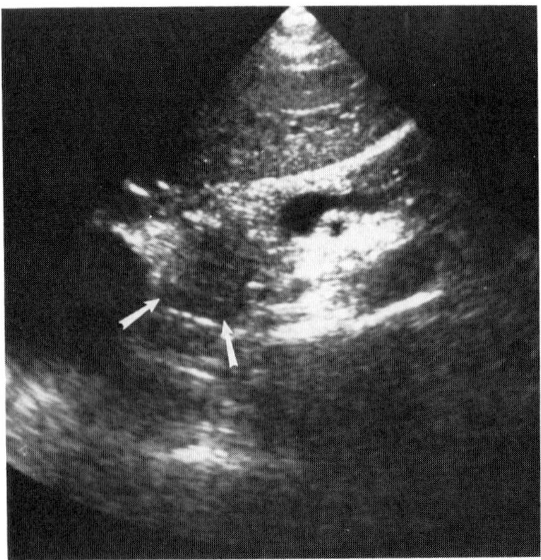

FIGURE 3–93. Pancreatic carcinoma. Transverse ultrasonogram shows a hypoechoic mass in the head of the pancreas *(arrows)*. The location of the mass is defined by the relationships of the splenic vein and the superior mesenteric artery and vein (see Fig. 1–11).

with thin slices and a bolus of contrast show the different densities of tumor and normal pancreas. Adenocarcinoma is usually of lower density than the normal pancreas after administration of contrast. MRI can show the mass but its usefulness is limited by spatial resolution and motion artifact.

Treatment and survival depend on the size and extent of tumor at the time of diagnosis. The tumor is aggressive and usually has spread to adjacent organs at the time of diagnosis. Survival is limited; most patients die within 6 months after the diagnosis is made.

SPLEEN

Trauma

The spleen is the abdominal organ most frequently injured by blunt trauma. Rupture of the spleen is particularly serious because of its high amount of blood flow and large vessels. Injuries include contusion, laceration, transection, and pedicle rupture. Patients may have signs of blood loss and peritoneal irritation in the left upper quadrant, but many have no localizing signs.

Plain films can show hemoperitoneum and left lower rib fractures. CT is most effective in the diagnosis of splenic injury (95% sensitivity). If splenic rupture or laceration has occurred, blood can usually be seen (although the presence of peritoneal lavage fluid may be confusing). CT scans generally show the blood as having decreased density in comparison with the enhanced spleen. Active bleeding often has very high density because of extravasation of contrast. Hemorrhage from the spleen is usually of highest density in or near the spleen, in comparison with more distant and diluted blood. This sign, the sentinel clot sign, occurs because the fresh blood near the spleen is most dense; it is helpful for diagnosing splenic hemorrhage as the cause of hemoperitoneum. A subcapsular splenic hematoma is confined and causes flattening of the adjacent splenic tissue. In some cases, blood dissects to the retroperitoneal space, thickening the lateral conal fascia and the left anterior pararenal fascia. Splenic laceration appears as a low-density cleft or an amorphous heterogeneous area of the spleen (Fig. 3–94), usually on the lateral aspect of the spleen. Congenital clefts are usually on the medial side of the spleen. A contusion has mixed high and low density.

Treatment of splenic injury depends on the hemodynamic status of the patient. Many patients can be managed conservatively when CT and clinical findings are limited. The risk of delayed rupture was formerly used to justify immediate splenectomy in victims of abdominal trauma. However, CT experience suggests that delayed hemorrhage is rare and that splenic injuries can be managed on the basis of initial CT findings and clinical features. Consequently, most splenic injuries are managed conservatively, especially in children. In severe hemorrhage, emergency surgery is performed. In some patients, angiographic embolization is effective treatment. Complications of these therapies include delayed rupture, transfusion hepatitis, and compromised immune competence.

Congenital Abnormalities

Congenital diseases of the spleen are caused by morphological and functional abnormalities. Accessory splenic tissue is found in up to 30% of autopsy specimens and is generally of no significance, although it may simulate adenopathy. Patients with additional splenic tissue who have undergone splenectomy for trauma or other problems are fortunate to have such tissue. The most common sites of this tissue are medially along the splenic artery, the greater omentum, and the splenorenal liga-

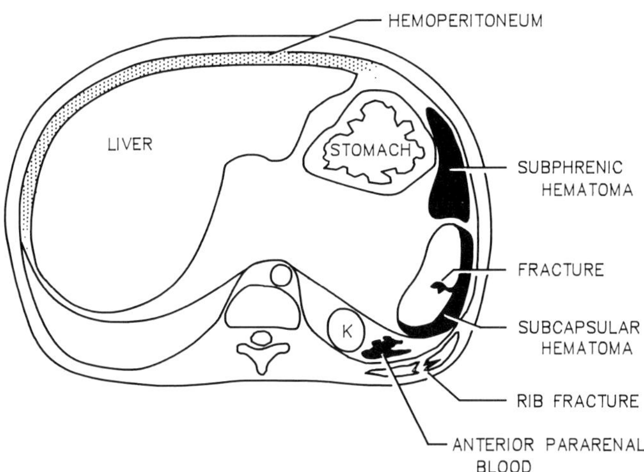

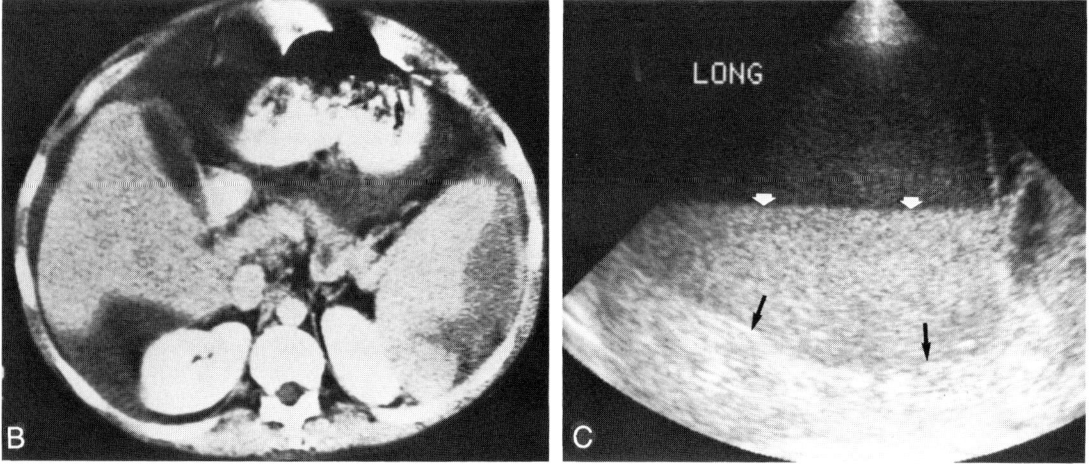

FIGURE 3–94. Splenic trauma. *A.* Diagram. K, kidney. *B.* Contrast CT shows a cleft in the posterolateral spleen, which indicates laceration. Intraperitoneal hemorrhage is present laterally. This blood is of lower density than the enhanced spleen and is of higher density than hemoperitoneum around the liver; this appearance identifies the spleen as the site of hemorrhage (the sentinel clot sign). *C.* Ultrasonogram shows a layer *(white arrows)* between plasma and red blood cells. Deep to the hematoma is the spleen *(black arrows).*

ment. It is best demonstrated by a nuclear medicine liver-spleen scan (see Chapter 9). Asplenia and polysplenia syndromes are associated with cardiac abnormalities (see Chapter 5).

Abnormalities of function of the spleen include idiopathic thrombocytopenic purpura, polycythemia vera, and hereditary spherocytosis. Most hematological disorders of the spleen result in sequestration of abnormal blood cells. Therefore, the primary radiographic finding is splenic enlargement. Such diseases are best diagnosed on CT, which demonstrates the enlargement and overall density of the spleen (Fig. 3–95). The spleen is normally posterior to the midline and extends no more than 15 cm vertically. Its enhanced CT density is equal to or slightly higher than that of the liver. Assessment of the spleen can be difficult if the liver is abnormal. Size and function of the spleen can be assessed on a nuclear medicine liver-spleen scan. The spleen is more difficult to assess on ultrasonography and MRI because of its location and cellular

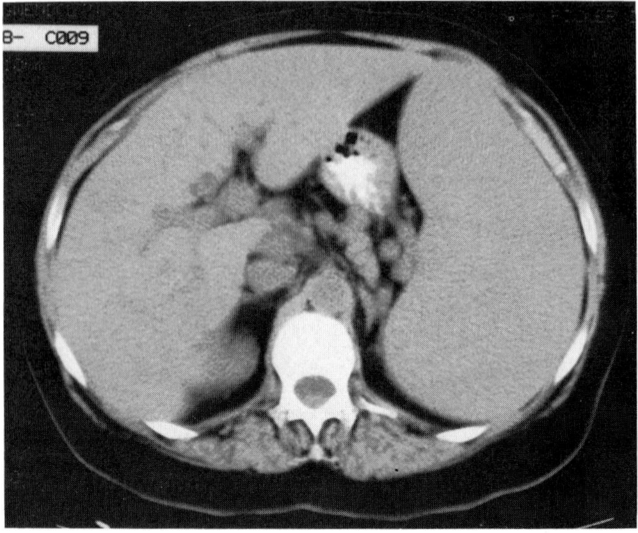

FIGURE 3–95. Hypersplenism. Massive enlargement of the spleen is evident on noncontrast CT in a patient in whom consumption of platelets and red blood cells by the spleen resulted from idiopathic hypersplenism.

contents. In T2 spin echo and STIR images, the normal spleen has high intensity, like tumors and other pathological tissues, and this makes it difficult to identify pathological processes. Many patients with hematological splenic disorders are treated by splenectomy or partial splenic embolization.

Inflammation and Infection

Inflammatory disease of the spleen is unusual. When it does occur, it is usually with generalized sepsis in immunocompromised patients, particularly those with AIDS. Splenic enlargement may be the only abnormality identified. Microabscesses appear as multiple, low-density abnormalities (see Fig. 3–68*B*). Involvement of the spleen in conjunction with liver abscesses carries a very high mortality rate. Echinococcosis can involve the spleen and cause a large, circumscribed cyst similar to that seen elsewhere in the body. The wall of the cyst, if calcified, can be seen on plain films. Histoplasmosis, when disseminated, can involve the spleen and leave multiple, residual scattered calcifications, a common finding on CT. Tuberculosis can have a similar appearance.

Neoplasms

Benign neoplasms of the spleen include cysts, cystic lymphangiomas, and dermoid tumors. They are usually discovered incidentally and are of no consequence.

The most important malignant neoplasm involving the spleen is lymphoma. Splenic involvement is frequent and is important in the staging of the disease, in which CT, or in some cases MRI, is used. Both can demonstrate splenic enlargement, but neither can provide a reliable assessment of actual involvement by the lymphoma. In non-Hodgkin's lymphoma, splenomegaly usually indicates tumor involvement, but this is not true in Hodgkin's disease. Coronal STIR images provide excellent means of diagnosis, staging, and follow-up of lymphoma by demonstrating adenopathy as high intensity against the low-intensity or black appearance of other tissues (see Figs. 4–9 and 4–74). However, diffuse lymphomatous involvement of the spleen may not be detected because of the similar signal characteristics of splenic and lymphomatous tissue.

Metastases to the spleen are uncommon. Primary tumors that spread to the spleen include melanoma, lung carcinoma, breast carcinoma, colon carcinoma, and renal cell carcinoma. Such lesions are usually of low density on CT in comparison with the enhanced normal spleen.

Vascular Disease

Splenic Infarction. Splenic infarction occurs when branches of the splenic artery are occluded. The most common cause is emboli from the heart. Pancreatitis and splenic torsion are also associated with splenic infarction. In young patients, splenic infarction is caused by sickle cell anemia, thalassemia, and polycythemia. Patients may also develop splenic infarction as a complication of bacterial endocarditis. Most have left upper quadrant pain, but many have no immediate symptoms. CT scans show a wedge-shaped peripheral area of low density in most patients. The abnormalities may also be nodular. Outer margin enhancement and, in chronic infarction, calcification and retraction may also be seen. In sickle cell anemia and other hemoglobinopathies, the abnormal cells cause multiple vascular occlusions and, subsequently, infarctions. Over time, the spleen becomes small and scarred with multiple calcifications.

Portal Hypertension. Splenic enlargement occurs as a direct effect of portal venous obstruction (discussed earlier with diseases of the liver). The obstruction to venous drainage causes massive enlargement of the spleen and vascular engorgement. Diagnosis is most easily made on CT, which can show other effects and complications of liver disease. MRI can show the large spleen and flow characteristics in the splenic and portal systems (Fig. 3–96).

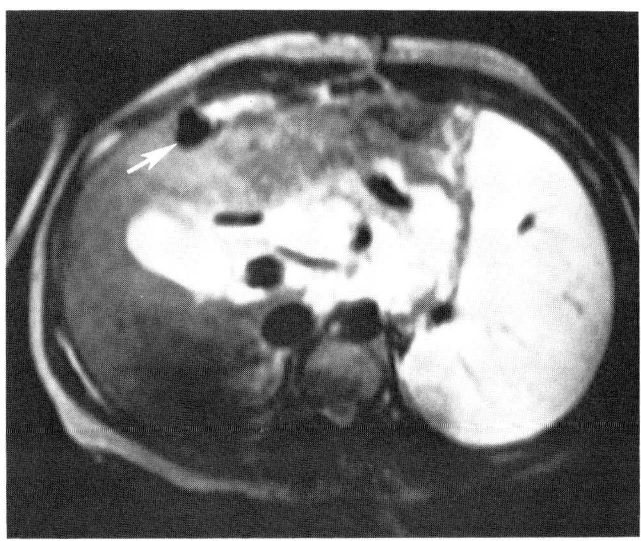

FIGURE 3–96. Alcoholic liver disease with portal hypertension. T2-weighted spin echo scan shows an enlarged, hyperintense spleen and a recanalized umbilical vein *(arrow)*, which appears black because of high flow, in this 40-year-old chronic alcoholic. The enlarged spleen is a result of hepatofugal blood flow caused by increased vascular resistance within the liver.

Part III
General Abdominal Imaging

Most diseases of the abdomen, especially those of the solid organs, cause specific symptoms and can be evaluated with the techniques described in Parts I and II of this chapter. In many instances, however, disease affects more than one organ, involves the abdominal spaces, or spreads to adjacent organs. Evaluation of such processes requires a general approach to cross-sectional imaging. The most important disease categories that require this more general approach are trauma, infection, and tumor, including metastatic disease and lymphoma.

ABDOMINAL TRAUMA

Trauma to the abdomen can result in hemorrhage, direct injury to solid organs, and injury to the bowel. In both penetration and blunt trauma, the injury frequently occurs in more than one area. CT is ideal for evaluation of blood collections and injuries to the solid organs because it shows the entire abdomen. CT has replaced peritoneal lavage at most trauma centers as the most rapid and effective method of evaluating intraperitoneal hemorrhage because it allows direct measurement of the amount of blood and shows the injured organs. Many patients who would formerly have undergone exploratory surgery are treated conservatively as a result of CT findings.

For a patient with abdominal trauma, CT should be performed with contiguous 1-cm slices after the administration of oral and intravenous contrast. The oral contrast prevents confusion between hemorrhage and bowel, and the intravenous contrast produces enhancement of the liver, the spleen, the kidneys, the collecting system, and the large vessels, allowing better determination of the location of hemorrhage and contusion. Even a small amount of dilute oral contrast (250 to 400 ml of dilute, water-soluble contrast) is effective because the most significant injuries are in the duodenum and proximal jejunum. It can be given by nasogastric tube to an ill or comatose patient.

Fluid and blood in the abdomen are easily detected by their appearance and location. Fluid, as might be seen in intraperitoneal bladder rupture, is of low (water) density. Blood is higher in density but appears dark on CT in comparison with enhanced organs when displayed at the window settings used for abdominal imaging (see Fig. 3–94*B*). This appearance is distinguished from the dense appearance of blood in the brain when viewed at narrow brain windows. When active bleeding occurs during scanning, the concurrent extravasation of contrast gives the blood a very high density. Dilution or breakdown of blood can cause a variable appearance. Blood of the highest density is nearest the site of bleeding.

Blood or fluid may be intraperitoneal, retroperitoneal, or intrapleural. The location of these collections can be determined from knowledge of the anatomical spaces in the abdomen (see Fig. 3–11), physical relationships of structures (see Fig. 3–10), and the characteristics of fluid within these spaces (Fig. 3–97). Intraperitoneal fluid shows clear margins with the liver and spleen and no medial extension posteriorly. Pleural fluid shows indistinct margins with the liver and spleen and extends medially to the spine.

Evaluation of abdominal injury requires attention to the individual organs and to the real and potential spaces of the abdomen and peritoneum. Injuries caused by motor vehicle accidents are often multiple. Contusion and fracture should be sought in the liver, the pancreas, the spleen, the duodenum, and the kidneys (Fig. 3–98). Small amounts of blood are detectable on CT scans and should be sought in the paracolic gutters, the lesser sac, and the subhepatic space (Morison's pouch). Such blood collections are not visible on plain films and may not be detected on peritoneal lavage. Thickening of the bowel wall or of the mesentery indicates hematoma. Retroperitoneal or intraperitoneal air indicates bowel rupture.

Only rarely are other examinations necessary for evaluation of abdominal trauma. Barium studies are, in general, required for assessing injury to the alimentary tract. Cystogram is the most informative examination for the evaluation of bladder injury. MRI can show hemorrhage and solid organ injury but is not accessible to most traumatically injured patients.

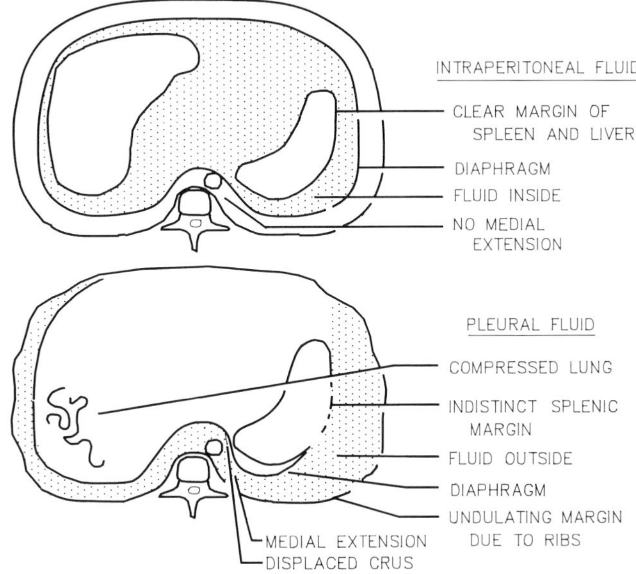

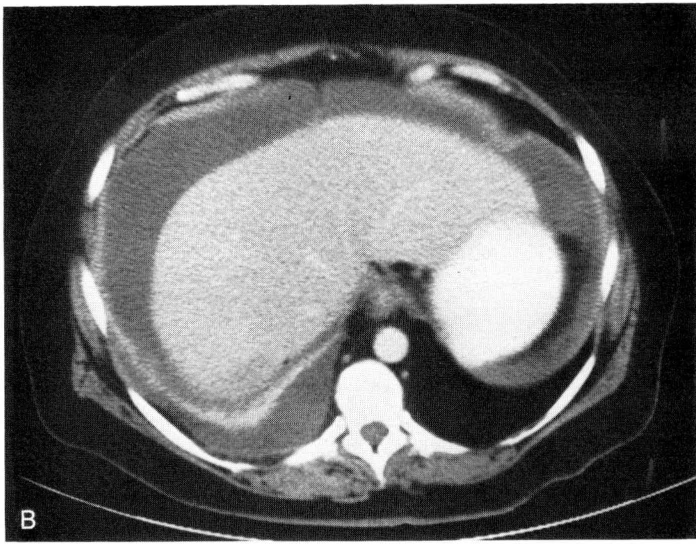

FIGURE 3–97. Pleural and intraperitoneal fluid. *A.* Diagram. *B.* Contrast CT shows both pleural effusion and intraperitoneal ascites in a middle-aged woman with ovarian cancer. On the right, the enhanced diaphragm separates the peritoneal fluid from the pleural fluid. The posterior medial extension of fluid indicates fluid in the pleural space because fluid cannot pass behind the liver.

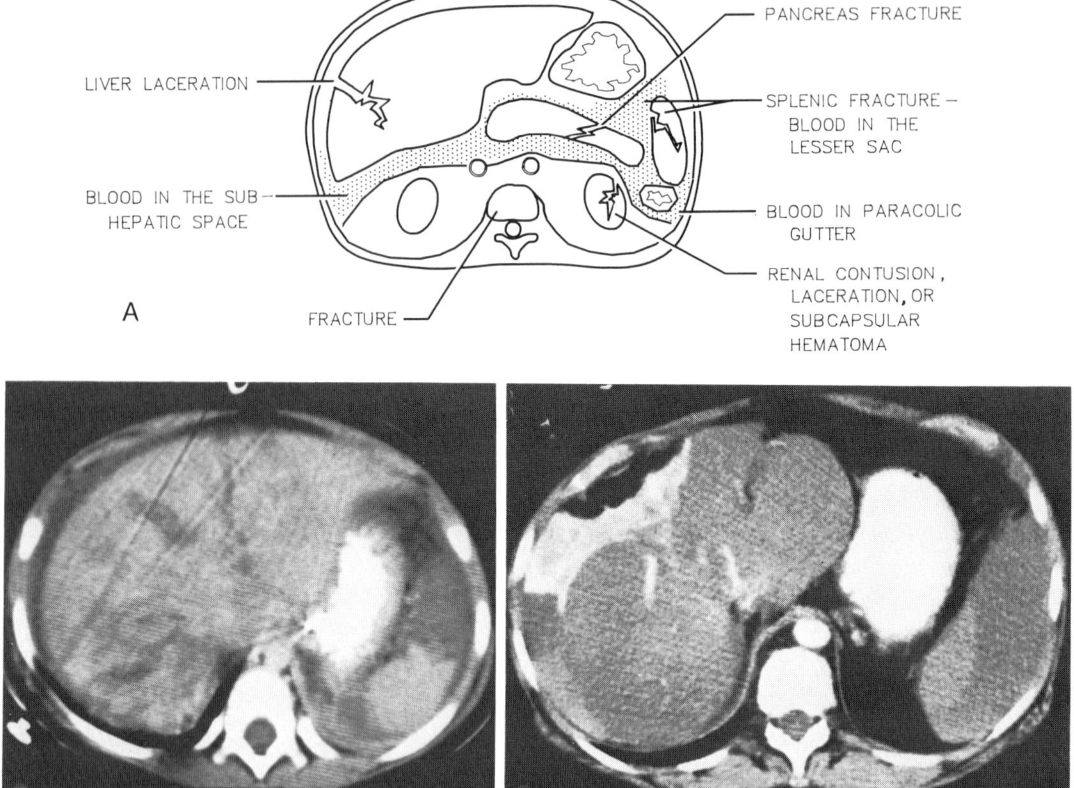

FIGURE 3–98. Abdominal trauma. *A.* Diagram. *B.* CT with intravenous and oral contrast shows low-density blood in the anterior splenic space, which indicates splenic rupture, in a 16-year-old girl injured in an automobile accident. The higher-density, smoothly marginated tissue posteriorly is normally perfused splenic tissue. There are also multiple fractures throughout the liver, and blood surrounds the outer margins of it. On abdominal CT scans, blood is of lower density than the normally enhanced spleen and liver. *C.* Contrast CT through the upper abdomen shows a wide rim of low-density blood surrounding the spleen. Accumulated, extravasated contrast is evident around the periphery of the liver and also along a line separating the right lobe from the left lobe. The deeper portions of the liver do not enhance normally as a result of injury of large deep vessels. Diagnosis at surgery included liver fracture, necrosis, and splenic rupture. The patient died of massive blood loss.

ABDOMINAL INFECTION

Many infections begin in single organs or anatomical spaces within the abdomen and are discussed in detail in the previous sections. The necrosis and destruction that ensues leads to local spread and involvement of adjacent structures if early, effective treatment is not given. Infection can pass throughout the peritoneal cavity and reach remote sites such as the subhepatic space (Morison's pouch) and the lesser sac. Both paracolic gutters and the retrovesical space may be involved. Retroperitoneal infection from renal abscess or pancreatic pseudocyst can extend superiorly or inferiorly.

Contrast GI examinations are necessary when bowel infection is present or when involvement of the bowel must be ruled out. They may also assist when fistulous tracts are present, such as with regional enteritis and stab wounds. In addition, direct injection of external drainage sites during plain film examination can show areas of communicating infection.

The evaluation of abdominal infection, like that of trauma, is performed most effectively by means of CT with both oral and intravenous contrast. Rectal contrast may also be necessary if the infection is near the rectum or the sigmoid colon. The considerations are similar to those for abdominal trauma but also include the possible paths of spread through the peritoneal cavity and the tissue planes of the

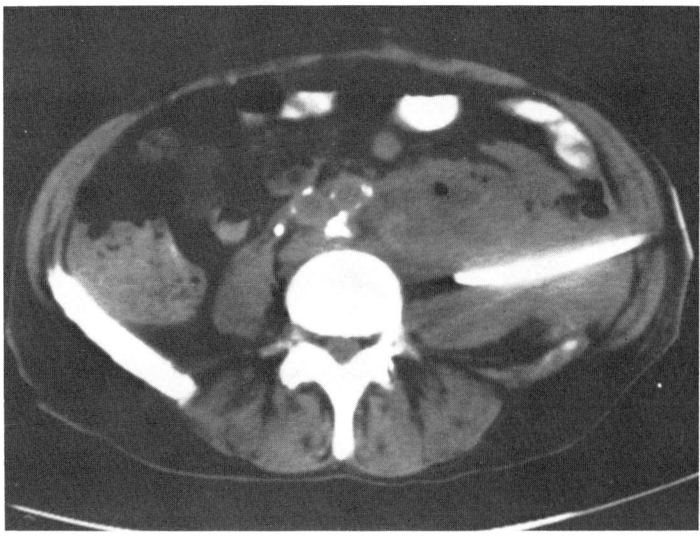

FIGURE 3–99. Abscess drainage. CT shows a catheter in the left paracolic gutter placed under CT guidance to drain a left lower quadrant abscess in a patient who developed signs of infection after prosthetic aortic graft surgery. The calcified iliac limbs of the graft can be seen just anterior to the spine.

retroperitoneal spaces. Important diseases that require such extensive evaluation include diverticulitis with abscess, bowel rupture with subsequent infection, pancreatic pseudocyst, liver abscess, appendicitis, renal abscess, and psoas muscle abscess. These are discussed in previous sections or in Chapter 4 as specific infections.

Evaluation of generalized infection requires attention to the normal appearance of solid organs, clear opacification of the bowel, and abnormal fluid collections and abnormal areas of enhancement. Because an abscess may contain gas or loculated fluid, repeat scans with the patient in a decubitus position or after additional oral or rectal contrast may clarify a possible area of abnormality. Abscesses appear as fluid collections with gas. The identification of gas assists in distinguishing infection from serous fluid and blood.

Ultrasonography can be used to further evaluate areas that are incompletely seen on CT scans. An abscess can be drained under CT or ultrasonographic guidance (Fig. 3–99). In these cases, portable, real-time ultrasonography has several advantages: it is generally faster and more convenient, it allows easy access to patients, and it is less expensive.

MRI is not as practical as CT for diagnosing acute infections of the abdomen, but it is effective for assessing chronic infection. Areas of infection or edema such as osteomyelitis, muscle abscess, loculated collections, and smoldering infection in soft-tissue planes can be easily shown with high-contrast sequences (STIR and T2 spin echo). Coronal or sagittal planes can be chosen for the best presentation of the anatomical compartment that contains the abnormality (see Fig. 4–10). Knowledge of the anatomical structures, aided by a T1 spin echo sequence, allows precise identification of the lesion, which can then be aspirated percutaneously or investigated surgically.

ABDOMINAL TUMOR

Many malignancies of the abdomen have advanced beyond the boundaries of the tissue of origin when symptoms become severe enough to warrant radiographic evaluation. Such tumors may have crossed tissue planes, invaded adjacent organs, and spread to lymph nodes. Lymphoma can arise primarily within an organ or a segment of bowel, or it may arise from lymph nodes along the central axis. Metastatic disease from abdominal viscera outside the abdomen may involve solid organs, lymph nodes, and the bones. In addition to defining anatomical structural relationships, evaluation requires knowledge of characteristic patterns of tumor spread, including typical patterns of progression through the lymphatic vessels.

The lymphatic vessels of the abdomen ultimately drain to the retroperitoneum and then to lymph node groups adjacent to the inferior mesenteric, superior mesenteric, and celiac arteries. These groups then drain through the diaphragm to the chest via chains of small lymphatic vessels or to the thoracic duct. The lymphatic vessels of the descending colon lead to the inferior mesenteric nodes, whereas those of the ascending and transverse portions of the colon drain to the superior mesenteric nodes. The jejunum and the ileum drain to superior mesenteric nodes, whereas the duodenum lymphatics drain to celiac and superior mesenteric nodes. The lymph nodes of the stomach, the pancreas, and the spleen connect predominately to celiac and gastrohepatic recess nodes. The liver drains to nodes in the porta hepatis and then to celiac nodes. Some lymphatic flow occurs across the diaphragm to the mediastinum, especially from the bare area (dome of the right lobe) of the liver. Abnormal abdominal lymph nodes are those larger than 1.0 to 1.5 cm in diameter.

Several abdominal and retroperitoneal tumors invade the venous system and cause thrombosis of the vena cava and the large veins. Renal carcinoma most notably causes renal vein invasion; tumor thrombus can continue into the inferior vena cava. Hepatocellular carcinoma invades hepatic veins, portal veins, and the inferior vena cava. Ascites may occur with any type of hepatic dysfunction but also indicates intraperitoneal tumor. Often, the cause is peritoneal or serosal metastases, commonly from ovarian carcinoma.

Many abdominal malignancies spread to characteristic locations (Table 3–3); therefore, knowledge of the primary tumor type can allow the examination of the abdomen to be tailored to the areas of most interest. For example, the adrenal glands and the spine must be examined for metastatic involvement in a patient with lung carcinoma. The spleen is of interest in a patient with lymphoma or melanoma. Gastric carcinoma metastasizes to nodes of the porta hepatis and the celiac plexus. Pancreatic carcinoma metastasizes to regional lymph nodes and then to the liver. Carcinomas of the bowel spread to the liver and to retroperitoneal and mesenteric lymph nodes.

TABLE 3–3. ABDOMINAL METASTATIC DISEASE

Metastatic Site	Primary Site
Liver	Gastrointestinal tract, ovary, lung, breast
Spleen	Lymphoma, melanoma
Pancreas	Uncommon
Adrenal glands	Lung
Kidneys	Other kidney, lung
Bowel	Melanoma, carcinoid, lymphoma
Peritoneum and omentum	Ovary
Spine	Prostate, breast, lung, colon, lymphoma, thyroid

Abdominal Lymphoma. The typical manifestation of Hodgkin's lymphoma is neck adenopathy with or without fever and other constitutional symptoms. The tumor is usually in the form of clusters of enlarged, lymphomatous nodes. In many cases, there is continuous caudal extension into the mediastinum and the retroperitoneum (see Fig. 4–9). When the abdomen is involved, the upper retroperitoneal (celiac) nodes are most affected. The spleen is involved in about one third of patients with Hodgkin's disease. However, splenomegaly in Hodgkin's disease does not necessarily indicate tumor involvement. The lymphomatous spleen may also be normal in size. Focal tumor nodules within the marrow and epidural, paraspinous tissues also occur with Hodgkin's lymphoma. Such findings indicate extensive disease.

In non-Hodgkin's lymphoma, nodes may also be demonstrated on CT scans. The nodes tend to be bulkier, and celiac, portal, superior mesenteric, and periaortic nodes are more often involved, than in Hodgkin's lymphoma (see Fig. 4–74). Patients with non-Hodgkin's lymphoma who have splenomegaly have a high probability of tumor in the spleen.

CT evaluation for suspected malignancy requires contiguous sections after intravenous and oral contrast. Each organ is carefully assessed for enlargement, abnormal contour, and inhomogeneity. The esophagus, the splenic vein, and the pancreas must be carefully evaluated in order to determine whether excess tissue is present. The periaortic and pericaval areas are next reviewed for the presence of adenopathy. The bowel may be easily differentiated from adenopathy if it is fully opacified with contrast. Additional scans with the patient in different positions and with additional contrast may be necessary to verify an abnormality near the bowel.

MRI evaluation has greatly changed the rate of detection and the characterization of tumors in the abdomen. The high spatial resolution of T1 spin echo sequences and the availability of coronal scanning provides excellent detail of the abdomen, particularly when motion artifact can be reduced. The key to abdominal evaluation is an image with high tissue contrast to detect the possible abnormalities. The highest contrast is obtained on STIR sequences. This technique also provides an intense tumor signal and suppression (cancellation) of the signal from surrounding fat. T2 spin echo sequences can alternatively be used to provide high contrast, but in the abdomen these scans are time consuming, have lower contrast than T1 spin echo or STIR images, and are easily degraded by abdominal motion.

The coronal STIR images provide extremely sensitive detection of abdominal tumors because the fat signal is suppressed and because muscle also has low signal intensity. The only high-intensity objects in these images are tumors (including malignant adenopathy), the spleen and the kidneys, and fluid in the bowel or the bladder. This high-yield survey scan can be made more productive with a matched T1 spin echo sequence in the same plane. Recurrent tumor can be assessed and differentiated from radiation or surgical changes by the relative intensity on STIR or heavily T2-weighted images. Adenopathy and bone marrow metastases are easily shown (see Chapter 7).

Effectively treated tumors, such as lymphoma, are detectable as masses on CT scans or T1 spin echo MRI. They are dark on STIR or T2 spin echo images. Recurrence is detectable by either enlargement or return of high signal intensity.

Paramagnetic contrast is less helpful in the abdomen than in the spine and the brain because the interstitial spaces also enhance, obscuring the tumor to some extent. Adenopathy can be similarly obscured when its enhanced intensity becomes similar to that of surrounding fat.

Part IV

Special Topics in Pediatric Radiology

The majority of pediatric gastrointestinal diseases are discussed within the main chapter in the sections on congenital, neoplastic, and inflammatory disorders. The following gastrointestinal diseases require special pediatric expertise for performing and interpreting the examinations.

ACUTE PEDIATRIC GASTROINTESTINAL DISEASE

Most acute GI diseases in infants and children manifest with abnormal feeding, bowel dysfunction, or rectal bleeding. The age of the child and the nature of symptoms, along with the appropriate radiographic examinations, can usually provide a specific diagnosis (Table 3–4). NEC (discussed in Part I) is usually associated with prematurity, particularly in infants with severe hyaline membrane disease. If seen in a full-term infant, underlying conditions such as Hirschsprung's disease, congenital heart disease, or midgut volvulus should be considered.

NEC is caused at least in part by decreased perfusion of the bowel. Other acute bowel diseases that manifest at birth are meconium ileus, meconium plug syndrome, neonatal small left colon, and atresias of the alimentary tract. Thirty percent of patients with meconium plug syndrome have Hirschsprung's disease and therefore require biopsy.

Other GI diseases that occur in the first month of life are midgut volvulus (one third of these manifest in the first week of life), pyloric stenosis, and incarcerated hernia. All are characterized by symptoms of bowel obstruction. Midgut volvulus causes bilious vomiting. Projectile, nonbilious vomiting indicates pyloric stenosis.

The most common causes of a small-bowel obstruction in infants are intussusception, appendicitis, and incarcerated inguinal hernia. Intussusception is usually ileocolic; no lead point is found if the patient is between 3 months and 4 years of age. Appendicitis can cause an adynamic ileus that has the appear-

TABLE 3–4. CHILDHOOD GASTROINTESTINAL DISEASE

Age	Disease	Symptoms
Premature infant	Necrotizing enterocolitis	Feeding intolerance, bloody stools
Neonate	Esophageal atresia	No feeding
	Duodenal atresia	Vomiting
	Aganglionosis/meconium plug syndrome	Failure to pass meconium within first 24 hr after birth
	Imperforate anus	No passage of meconium
	Meconium ileus	Vomiting, constipation
Birth to 2 weeks	Incarcerated hernia	Vomiting
	Midgut volvulus	Bilious vomiting
2 to 6 weeks	Pyloric stenosis	Projectile vomiting
	Malrotation	Asymptomatic unless volvulus is present
	Volvulus	Bilious vomiting
3 to 30 weeks	Intussusception	Rectal bleeding, sometimes vomiting, episodic abdominal pain
Older infants	Appendicitis	Pain, sepsis

ance of a small bowel obstruction. Inguinal hernia is much more common in boys than in girls.

Gastrointestinal Bleeding. Gastrointestinal bleeding in children can have a variety of causes (Table 3–5). In neonates, rectal bleeding is most frequently caused by anal fissures and formula allergies. In children under 2 years of age, intussusception and Meckel's diverticula usually account for rectal bleeding. The peak age for the occurrence of juvenile polyps is 5 years; they are very rare before the age of 1 year and after the age of 14 years. Intussusception can be diagnosed through ultrasonography but is most frequently identified and treated in barium enema examination. Symptomatic Meckel's diverticulum can be seen on nuclear medicine scans. Suspected polyps should be evaluated by double contrast enema.

Meconium Disease. Meconium is the normal viscous material present in the bowel of the fetus and is passed in the first few hours after birth. The most important diseases associated with meconium are aspiration during birth, meconium ileus, and meconium plug syndrome. Additional uses of the word refer to less severe problems and can be confusing. The common uses of terms relating to meconium are described as follows.

TABLE 3–5. CAUSES OF GASTROINTESTINAL BLEEDING IN CHILDREN

Below Age 2 Years
Anal fissures (50%)
Intussusception (40%)
Necrotizing enterocolitis
Meckel's diverticulum
Older Children
Polyps (50%)
Ulcer disease
Colitis
Portal hypertension

Meconium ileus is an impaction of the small bowel in the neonate by meconium and thick secretions associated with cystic fibrosis. Meconium ileus equivalent is a bowel obstruction in older patients with cystic fibrosis, when meconium is no longer present.

Meconium peritonitis is the result of an in utero vascular insult and is often caused by intussusception or volvulus. Extravasation of meconium into the peritoneal cavity causes a chemical peritonitis. Calcification of the peritoneum is evident at birth but disappears shortly thereafter. The chemical peritonitis usually causes no long-term effects. However, 15% to 40% of patients have cystic fibrosis.

Meconium plug syndrome is the failure of an infant to pass the meconium by about 24 to 48 hours after birth. An enema consisting of a high-osmolality fluid successfully clears the rectum. However, meconium plug syndrome is frequently associated with Hirschsprung's syndrome and can be associated with cystic fibrosis.

Meconium aspiration occurs when the meconium is expelled before or during birth. It may be aspirated into the lungs, where it causes a severe, often fatal, chemical pneumonitis (see Chapter 2).

RADIOGRAPHIC DIFFERENTIAL DIAGNOSIS

Frequently a single radiographic finding or pattern can suggest a limited list of diagnoses. Additional findings and clinical history can then assist in further limiting the list or in making a firm diagnosis. The following approaches to evaluation of radiographic findings can provide assistance in differential diagnosis. Diseases are listed in order of importance.

NARROWING OF THE DISTAL ESOPHAGUS

Narrowing of the distal esophagus can be caused by dysfunction, congenital anomaly, or mass lesion. The appearance on barium esophagram and CT can often provide the correct diagnosis. Fluoroscopic evaluation during the passage of the barium through the abnormal area can be especially helpful for functional assessment.

Reflux esophagitis with stricture
Caustic ingestion
Achalasia
Alcohol-induced esophagitis
Stricture from chronic nasogastric tube
Carcinoma, lymphoma
Crohn's disease
Zollinger-Ellison syndrome

LARGE GASTRIC FOLDS

Large rugal folds in the stomach may be normal, particularly if the stomach is not fully distended. They often indicate inflammatory disease or infiltration by tumor.

Normal variation
Hypertrophic gastritis
Ménétrier's disease
Peptic ulcer disease
Zollinger-Ellison syndrome
Gastric varices
Eosinophilic gastritis
Caustic ingestion
Radiation injury
Regional enteritis (Crohn's disease)
Multiple polyps
Carcinoma
Lymphoma
Amyloidosis
Tuberculosis
Pancreatitis

DILATION OF THE SMALL BOWEL

Dilation of the small bowel (wider than 3 cm) can result from obstruction or conditions that diminish the tone of the bowel.

Obstruction
Celiac disease
Nontropical sprue
Scleroderma
Diabetes
Anticholinergic therapy
Vagotomy
Ileus
Gastroenterostomy
Hypothyroidism

ABNORMALITIES OF THE TERMINAL ILEUM

Abnormalities in the region of the terminal ileum are usually caused by infection, inflammation, or tumor.

1. Infection
    Yersinia
    Tuberculosis
    Actinomycosis
    Salmonella and *Shigella*
2. Inflammatory
    Regional enteritis
    Back-wash ileitis
    Behçet's syndrome
    Eosinophilic gastroenteritis
3. Neoplasm
    Lymphoma, leukemia
    Carcinoma
    Carcinoid tumor
    Metastases

SMALL-BOWEL MASSES

Masses in the small bowel are manifestations of tumor, abscess, and blood. Findings in the bowel or elsewhere in the abdomen can help distinguish these diseases.

Lymphoma
Pancreatic abscess
Intramural hematoma
Abdominal abscess
Regional enteritis
Primary tumor
Metastatic tumor

SMALL-BOWEL TUMORS

Tumors in the small bowel are usually benign. In most cases they are difficult to distinguish from one another.

Benign tumors
Polyposis syndromes
Carcinoid tumor
Metastasis
Lymphoma
Adenocarcinoma
Leiomyosarcoma

CAUSES OF INFECTIOUS COLITIS

Infectious colitis is increasingly common, particularly in immunosuppressed patients. Sexually transmitted organisms are now among the most common causes of infectious colitis. The location of disease can be helpful in suggesting the diagnosis.

Shigella (rectum and sigmoid)
Salmonella (usually proximal colon)
Campylobacter (anywhere)
Tuberculosis (cecum, and occasionally skip areas in the colon)
Amebiasis (cecum, and occasionally skip areas in the colon)
Gonococci (rectum and anus)
Lymphogranuloma venereum (rectum and anus)
Cytomegalovirus, herpes
Yersinia
Clostridia

GAS IN THE BOWEL WALL

Gas in the bowel wall may result from a vascular insult, or it may indicate bowel infection. Both types of conditions are serious and require early diagnosis and therapy.

Ischemic colitis
Volvulus
Intussusception
Intestinal obstruction
Disseminated intravascular coagulation
Necrotizing enterocolitis
Bowel infection
Inflammatory bowel disease
Peptic ulcer disease

LARGE LUMINAL GAS COLLECTIONS

A large air-filled mass in the abdomen is usually an obstructed loop or segment of bowel. The location of the air within the bowel lumen helps rule out pneumoperitoneum.

Transverse colon volvulus
Sigmoid volvulus
Cecal volvulus
Giant sigmoid diverticulum
Large necrotic tumor
Toxic megacolon
Adynamic ileus

STRUCTURES BETWEEN THE AORTA AND THE SUPERIOR MESENTERIC ARTERY

The space between the aorta and the superior mesenteric artery normally contains only three structures. Awareness of the anatomical structures in this location can be helpful in the evaluation of CT scans and ultrasonograms.

Third portion of the duodenum
Uncinate process of the pancreas
Left renal vein

OBSTRUCTION AT THE AMPULLA OF VATER

Obstruction at the ampulla of Vater can be caused by a stone, an inflammatory process, or a tumor. The appearance of the narrowing on cholangiography can be helpful for making the diagnosis. CT, ultrasonography, and biopsy are often necessary for full evaluation.

Stone (smooth, rounded border)
Pancreatitis (smooth narrowing)
Ampullary carcinoma (irregular stricture)
Cholangiocarcinoma (irregular stricture)
Pancreatic carcinoma (smooth or irregular narrowing)

Suggested Readings

Bragg DG, Rubin P, Youker JE (eds): Oncologic Imaging. New York: Pergamon, 1985.
Jeffrey RB Jr: CT and Sonography of the Acute Abdomen. New York: Raven Press, 1989.
Lee JKT, Sagel SS, Stanley RJ (eds): Computed Body Tomography With MRI Correlation (2nd ed). New York: Raven Press, 1989.
Margulis AR, Burhenne J (eds): Alimentary Tract Radiology (3rd ed). St Louis: CV Mosby, 1983.
Meyers MA: Dynamic Radiology of the Abdomen. New York: Springer-Verlag, 1988.
Sanders RC, Campbell J, Guidi SM (eds): Clinical Sonography (1st ed). Boston: Little, Brown, 1984.
Taveras JM, Ferrucci JT, Buonocore E (eds): Radiology Diagnosis-Imaging-Intervention. Philadelphia: JB Lippincott, 1991.

4

Genitourinary Radiology

Gary K. Stimac
Fred A. Mettler, Jr.

Genitourinary imaging is a complex area of radiology encompassing several organ systems and therefore requires several imaging methods. The urinary tract is examined with contrast studies, ultrasonography, nuclear medicine, and the cross-sectional methods of computed tomography (CT) and magnetic resonance imaging (MRI). The adrenal gland is evaluated with CT and MRI. The genital system is most effectively studied through ultrasonography, CT, and MRI. General imaging of the pelvis and inferior retroperitoneum, also described in this chapter, involves primarily cross-sectional imaging methods and requires a familiarity with the relationships of structures in these areas.

This chapter is organized in three parts. The first part covers the urinary tract and the adrenal glands, and each component is discussed separately. The second part covers the genital system, and again each group of organs is discussed separately. The third part covers general imaging of the pelvis in cases of trauma, infection, and tumor, all of which often involve several organs in addition to the structural tissues of the pelvis. The Basic Evaluation and Radiographic Differential Diagnosis sections are in their usual places within the chapter. Cross-sectional imaging of the abdomen and the upper retroperitoneum are discussed in Chapter 3.

BASIC EVALUATION

Plain Film Interpretation

Obtaining supine and upright abdominal views is often the first step in evaluating genitourinary trauma or other disease; a supine projection is the first view obtained in intravenous urography. Assessment of these plain radiographs is performed as described in Chapter 3 (see Figs. 3–2 and 3–3). Of particular interest when genitourinary disease is suspected is the presence of calcifications in the kidneys and along the paths of the ureters, which suggests the presence of calculi.

Contrast Examinations

Excretory urography is often the initial radiographic examination for urinary pain, hematuria, urinary tract infection, acute obstruction, some renal masses, urolithiasis, nephrocalcinosis, and congenital abnormalities. This examination provides essential anatomical information and demonstrates function of the entire urinary tract. Excretory urography is complemented by CT, MRI, and ultrasonography, which provide additional anatomical information and can depict characteristics of a mass lesion. In general, the tubular urinary tract is best evaluated in contrast examinations because they reveal the appearance of the lumen and the flow characteristics of fluid.

There are many methods of performing excretory urography. A typical examination includes a scout film, a film that immediately follows administration of contrast material (immediate or zero-minute film), a film 5 minutes after administration of contrast material, and filled and postvoid films of the bladder. Oblique or tomographic views of the kidneys are often obtained, depending on the clinical circumstances. Fewer films are obtained for children than for adults. The scout film demonstrates the locations of calcifications and abdominal abnormalities and indicates the optimal radiographic technique. The immediate postinjection film shows the enhancement of vascular and renal cortical structures and demonstrates the outlines of the kidneys. The 5-minute film shows filling of the collecting system and the ureters. The bladder views show the bladder contour and postvoid residual urine.

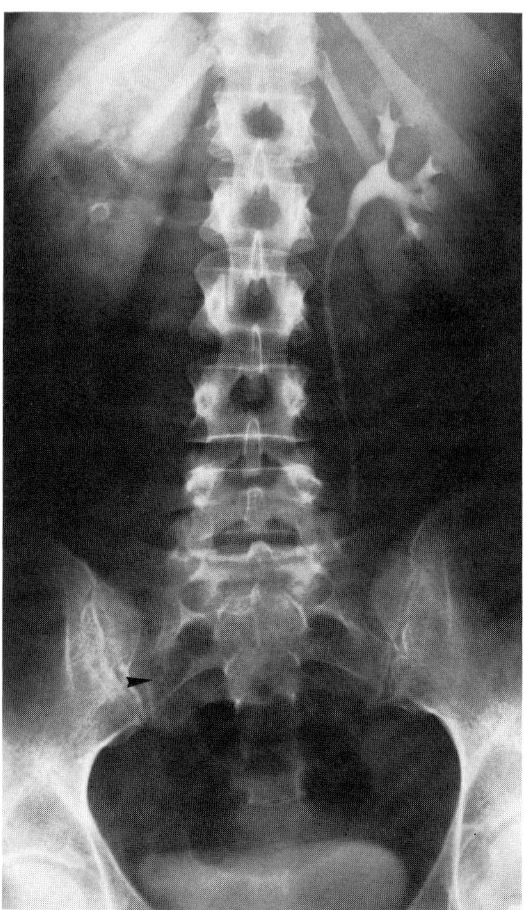

FIGURE 4–1. Renal evaluation. Excretory urography film obtained 10 minutes after contrast injection shows delayed function of the left kidney caused by ureteral obstruction in a 35-year-old woman with previous episodes of kidney stones. In the normal right kidney, note the enhancement of the parenchyma showing the renal outlines. Note also the path of the ureter and the filling of the bladder. A stone is shown on the left side overlying the inferior sacrum *(arrowhead)*.

Excretory urography allows the assessment of renal size, axis, outline, and symmetry of function (Fig. 4–1). The length of the kidney depends on the age, sex, and physique of the patient but is usually equal to the height of three or four vertebral bodies. Partially duplicated or single kidneys (shown later in Fig. 4–16) are larger. The renal axis, an imaginary line through the upper and lower poles of the kidney, is usually angled about 15 degrees laterally in the caudal direction. A different orientation of the renal axis can result from a congenital or an acquired abnormality. The renal outlines should be entirely visible and smooth. Lobulations are usually normal variations. The kidneys should function promptly and simultaneously; relative delay in function can suggest poor perfusion or obstruction. The intrarenal collecting systems should show symmetrical filling of the papillae without distention or filling defects.

The ureters often are not visible in their entirety despite intensive efforts to show them with the patient in various positions. On an anteroposterior film, they usually appear along the transverse processes, turn laterally at the sacroiliac joints, and enter the bladder posteriorly and laterally.

The bladder is evaluated for size and contour (it should be round and smooth), volume after voiding (normally less than 100 mL), prostatic or uterine impression, and irregularities of the inner wall (best seen on the postvoid film). The urethra can be demonstrated on a voiding film of the excretory urogram, but the contrast material is normally diluted by urine and so the image is poor.

Retrograde urography is performed (usually by the urologist) by cystoscopic, retrograde placement of ureteral catheters and injection of contrast material. This procedure is indicated in patients with obstruction or renal nonfunction in whom the renal pelvic collecting system and the ureters must be examined. It provides the best visualization of small filling defects (areas of nonfilling by the contrast material) of the renal pelvis and the ureters.

Cystography is performed by injecting dilute contrast material into the bladder through a urethral or suprapubic catheter. Images are obtained during filling, when the bladder is filled, and during voiding. The voiding films must be full sized, showing the bladder, the ureter, and the kidneys in order to demonstrate vesicoureteral reflux, which often occurs so rapidly that the refluxed contrast material is visible only in the renal pelvis. Fluoroscopy of the bladder and ureters is usually performed during voiding to demonstrate reflux. The Valsalva maneuver is not helpful in causing reflux because it increases both bladder pressure and intra-abdominal pressure equally and does not cause contraction of the detrusor muscle.

Voiding urethrography can be performed with cystography and is the only method of demonstrating the prostatic urethra (Fig. 4–2). The distal urethra is also well shown by this technique, but it can also be evaluated by means of retrograde urethrography.

Arteriography and Venous Digital-Subtraction Angiography

Renal arteriography is important for diagnosing suspected renal pedicle trauma, for evaluating the donor for renal transplantation, and for evaluating renovascular hypertension caused by fibromuscular hyperplasia, atherosclerotic disease, or masses affecting the renal vessels. When renal vessels need to be clearly defined, a selective arterial injection is recommended with the use of either conventional or digital-subtraction filming (Fig. 4–3). Venous injection of contrast material and digital-subtraction filming of the kidneys can be used in patients in whom an arterial examination might produce an unacceptably high risk of complications (such as those with advanced atherosclerotic disease), but the superior quality of the arterial injection examination is preferred. Although angiography rarely contributes more to the diagnosis of renal tumors than does CT, angiographic embolization of highly vascular renal tumors with particles, metal coils, or alcohol can be performed preoperatively to reduce the risk of hemorrhage and facilitate the resection.

Ultrasonography

In the urinary system, ultrasonography is the most informative examination for evaluating subacute and chronic obstruction, azotemia, nephrocalcinosis, and medical renal disease. It is used in conjunction with excretory urography and CT in assessing renal masses and cystic renal disease. The kidneys have a uniform peripheral echo appearance that corresponds to the cortex. The pyramids are less echogenic than the cortex, particularly in children. The renal pelvis is highly echogenic

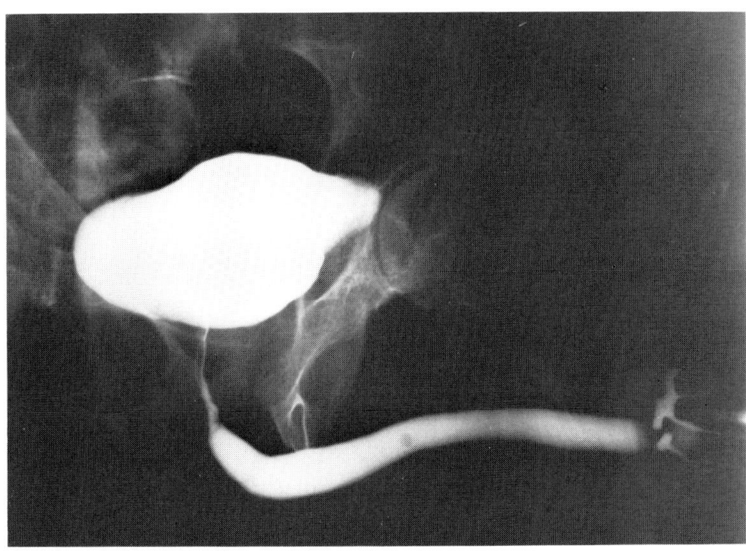

FIGURE 4–2. Urethrogram. Retrograde injection demonstrates the entire urethra and shows filling of the bladder of a 21-year-old man. The narrow prostatic urethra is normal, as are the filled membranous and the penile portions. Note also the clamp used to hold the penis during the injection.

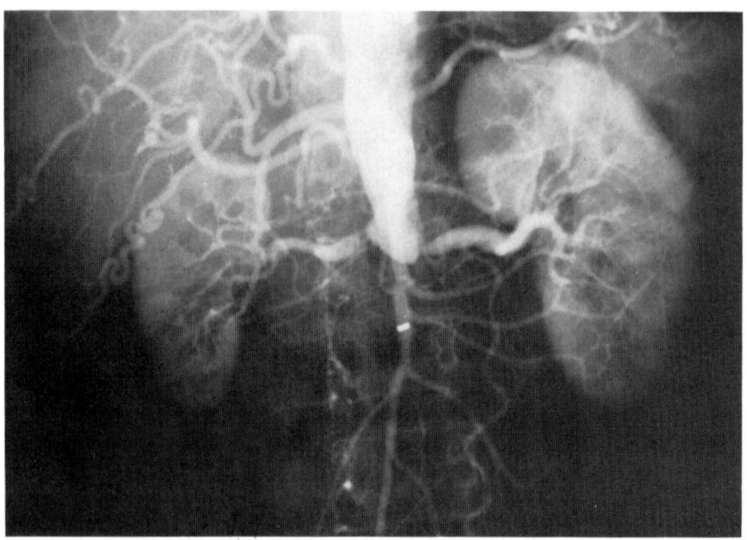

FIGURE 4–3. Renal artery stenosis. Conventional arteriogram performed through the left axillary artery shows atherosclerotic occlusion of the inferior abdominal aorta in a 55-year-old man with severe atherosclerotic disease and hypertension. Marked narrowing of the right renal artery at its origin has resulted in a small kidney. The left renal artery origin is slightly narrowed. Both kidneys show a normal vascular blush. Numerous arterial collaterals have formed to supply the lower abdomen, the pelvis, and the lower extremities.

because of the presence of pericalyceal peripelvic fat (see Fig. 1–11*A*).

On ultrasonograms, the right kidney is more easily seen than the left because the liver allows optimal sound transmission. The left kidney is seen best when an enlarged spleen provides a good transmission medium, but it is also seen well in general. Nondilated ureters are not shown well on ultrasonography. The bladder is easily evaluated when filled with fluid. Ultrasonograms can reveal residual urine volume, bladder-wall thickening, and prostatic enlargement. In general, ultrasonographic evaluation of bladder tumors is poor; they are best evaluated by cystoscopy, CT, and MRI.

Ultrasonography is one of the most important methods for imaging the female pelvic organs, and it is the primary method for imaging obstetrical conditions and diseases. Cystic lesions of the ovaries and masses in the uterus can be evaluated in conjunction with CT and MRI in order to determine the composition and, in many cases, the tissue of origin.

The uterus is easily identified on ultrasonograms. It displays moderate echogenicity and, occasionally, a central echo caused by mucus or blood. Uterine fibroids appear as masses with reduced echogenicity and poor acoustical transmission. Adnexal masses and free fluid also can be easily evaluated with ultrasonography. Although the sensitivity is high, the accuracy is poor, and it may be difficult to determine whether a complex adnexal mass represents a tumor, inflammation, or an extrauterine (ectopic) pregnancy.

In the first trimester, ultrasonography is used to assess fetal presence, number of fetuses, viability or demise, age, and whether the fetus is intrauterine or extrauterine (ectopic). Blighted ovum and missed abortion can also be diagnosed. Gestational age can be determined to within 4 to 7 days from the crown-to-rump length (Fig. 4–4). Major anomalies

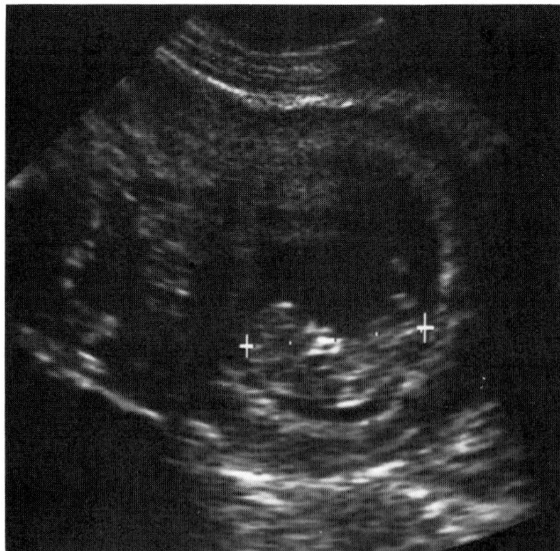

FIGURE 4–4. Crown-to-rump measurement. Longitudinal ultrasonogram shows the developing fetus deep in the amniotic fluid, which is of low echogenicity. The cursors mark the fetal head (at the left of the view) and the fetal rump. The bright echoes centrally reflect the fetal mandible. Parts of the lower extremities can be seen superior to the rump. The measurement of 41 mm indicates a gestational age of 11.1 weeks.

such as anencephaly and conjoined twins can be identified during this period. Other abnormalities in the mother rather than the fetus, such as pelvic masses, uterine fibroids, corpus luteum cysts, and trophoblastic disease also can be assessed.

During the second trimester, ultrasonography is used to identify other fetal anomalies, the location of the placenta, and the amount of amniotic fluid. Normal structures of the fetus, including the stomach, the bladder, the heart, and the brain, are visible. Fetal dating according to the biparietal diameter of the brain is accurate to approximately 10 to 14 days (Fig. 4–5). During the third trimester, ultrasonography is used to assess fetal age (accurate to within 2 to 3 weeks), relative proportions of the fetal head and body, possible intrauterine growth retardation, and factors that could affect delivery, such as the location and maturation of the placenta, the amount of amniotic fluid, and fetal weight.

Interpretation of genitourinary and obstetrical ultrasonograms requires a full understanding of the relative positions of organs, the echo "textures" of the structures, and the appearances of common disease processes. It also requires an awareness of the many congenital anomalies that can be diagnosed in utero.

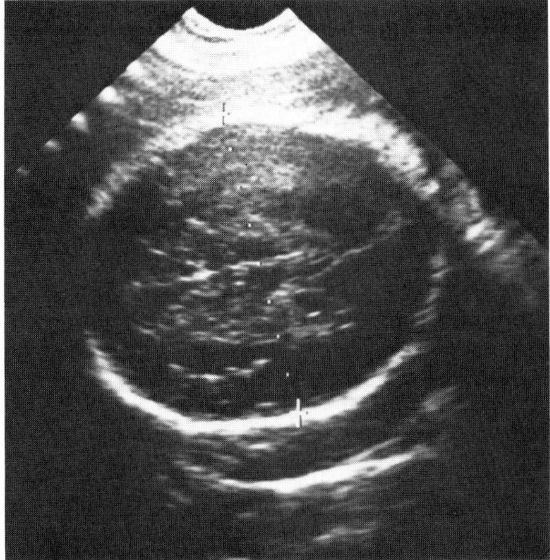

FIGURE 4–5. Biparietal diameter (BPD) measurement. Transaxial ultrasonogram through the fetal head shows the midline falx. The cerebral peduncles are areas of low echogenicity in the center of the scan. The BPD of 79 mm indicates a gestational age of approximately 32 weeks.

Computed Tomography

CT of the pelvis allows imaging of the solid organs, the tissue planes, the lymph nodes, and the vessels. Because it shows the anatomical relationships of the structures, it is valuable for assessing trauma, infection, and spread of tumor. CT is also used with ultrasonography and MRI in the evaluation of solid masses of individual organs.

The examination is performed with scans of contiguous slices of 1-cm thickness after the administration of intravenous contrast material. When venous obstruction is considered (as in the evaluation of renal cell carcinoma), the contrast can be injected into the lower leg or the foot in order to maximally opacify the vena cava. When the bladder is the primary area of evaluation, the lowest slices are obtained either without contrast or during the initial stage of contrast injection so that the bladder is not opacified by dense contrast. Rectal contrast can be used for assistance in the evaluation of disease near the rectum, the prostate, and the female reproductive organs. Oral contrast material is essential for imaging the upper pelvis, in which the bowel in the lower peritoneal cavity could cause confusion. A tampon is placed in the vagina so that the vagina and the location of the cervix are clearly shown.

Interpretation of pelvic CT requires attention to the individual organs, the soft tissue planes and retroperitoneal compartments, and the lymph nodes. Tumor masses and adenopathy are the most important findings in most cases. Detection of these abnormalities requires knowledge of structural relationships and identification of normal structures such as loops of bowel and vessels. After these normal structures are noted, questionable areas can be further evaluated by means of repeat scanning with additional oral contrast or a change of the patient's position to establish that an abnormality is not merely an unopacified loop of bowel.

Evaluation of the lymph nodes in the pelvis is important for detection of primary lymphoma and metastatic disease. The lymph node chains include the periaortic, aortocaval, internal iliac, presacral, and obturator chains (Fig. 4–6). Any lymph node larger than 1 cm in diameter or the presence of numerous small nodes must be considered as representing tumor. Adenopathy that is bilateral or above the aortic bifurcation indicates a more advanced

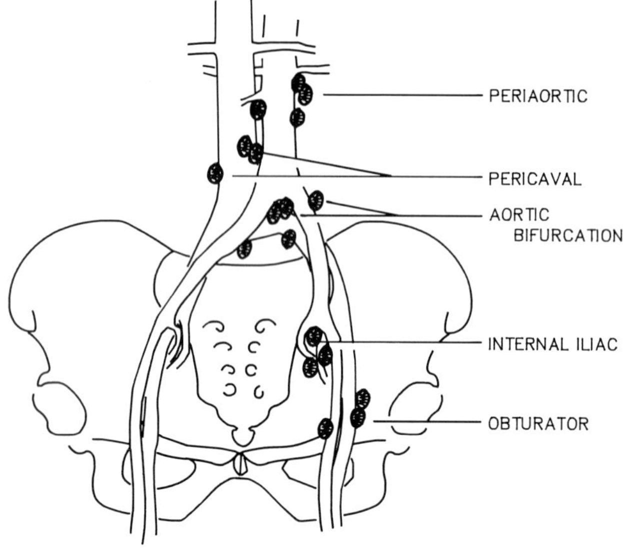

FIGURE 4–6. Characteristics of pelvic lymph nodes.

stage of disease. Inguinal nodes are often numerous and usually indicate previous infection rather than tumor involvement.

CT slices of the upper pelvis (Fig. 4–7, slices 10, 12, and 14) show the inferior part of the kidneys with enhanced collecting systems, loops of bowel with air and contrast, and the lower edge of the liver. The superior mesenteric artery and vein are anterior (slice 10) and the inferior vena cava and aorta are posterior to the duodenum, directly anterior to the spine (see also Figure 3–12). The psoas muscles are on either side of the spine. The kidneys are evaluated for smooth contour, uniform parenchymal enhancement, absence of renal or extrarenal masses, and nondilated, undeviated ureters. Cysts are easily identified on CT. The borders of small cysts are not well demarcated because of volume averaging of the curved wall of the cyst and the adjacent renal tissue. The adrenal glands are trefoil- or tadpole-shaped. The right adrenal gland is superior to the right kidney and posterior to the inferior vena cava between the liver and the crus of the diaphragm. The left adrenal gland is anterior, medial, and superior to the left kidney. Important areas to evaluate for adenopathy are the periaortic, paracaval, and mesenteric regions.

More inferiorly (Fig. 4–7, slices 16, 19, and 22), the fat of the mesentery occupies the center of the lower abdomen, and the vena cava and the aorta bifurcate into iliac vessels. The psoas muscle merges with the iliacus to form the iliopsoas. Enlarged iliac and mesenteric nodes would be identified after each vessel is identified. The next lower slices (24 and 27) show the inferior loops of opacified bowel. Posterior and lateral to these loops of bowel are the iliopsoas muscles. The iliac vessels pass anteriorly along the medial border of the muscles toward the superior pubic ramus.

The lowest slices (Fig. 4–7, slices 30, 32, 34, and 36) show the anterior midline bladder (with a urine/contrast level) and, posteriorly, the rectosigmoid. Bladder tumors generally cause thickening of the bladder wall; extravesical spread appears as an extrinsic mass. In the male, the seminal vesicles (slice 32) and prostate gland (slices 34 and 36) are between the inferior bladder and the rectum. The obturator muscles pass laterally from the inner acetabula toward the obturator foramen. Pelvic fat can assist in CT depictions of obturator nodes and in definition of the prostate and seminal vesicles.

In the female pelvis, the lower slices show the uterus inferior and posterior to the blad-

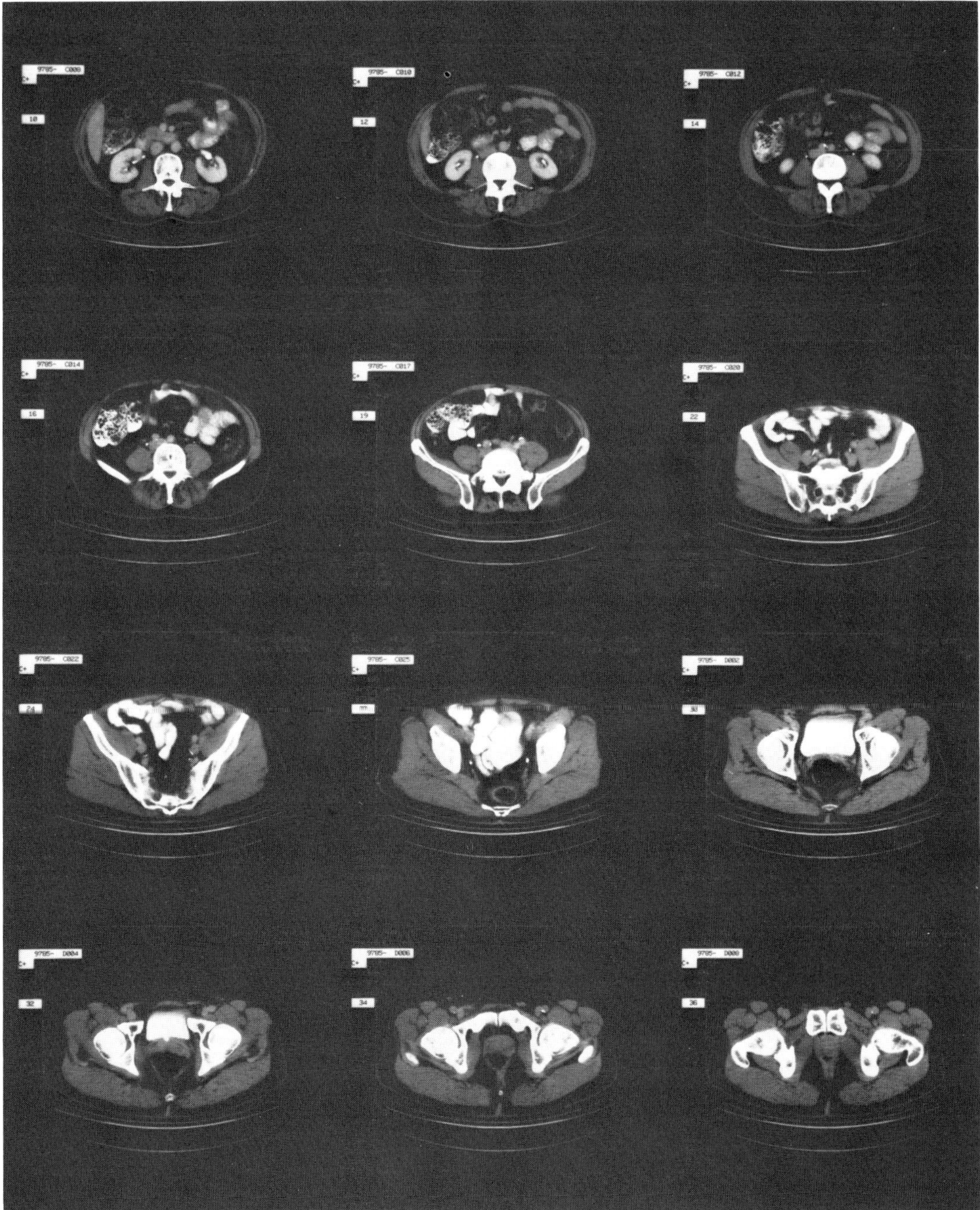

FIGURE 4–7. Pelvic computed tomographic (CT) interpretation. Selected slices (approximately every 2 cm) from a 53-year-old man with localized, stage 1 prostatic carcinoma show normal structures and demonstrate the approach to pelvic CT interpretation (see text). In this patient, microscopic disease was found on transrectal ultrasonographic biopsy. Minimal fluid is present near the prostate as a result of the biopsy. Slice numbers are to the left of each image. (Courtesy of B. Porter, First Hill Diagnostic Imaging Center, Seattle.)

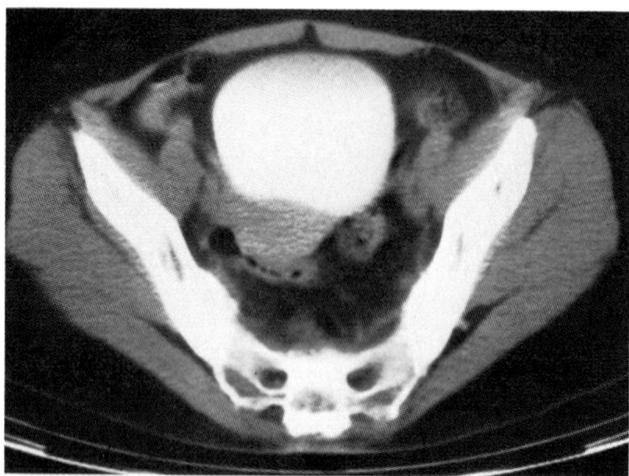

FIGURE 4–8. CT of normal female pelvis. The density of the uterus is similar to that of other soft tissue structures. The uterus is posterior to the bladder and, in this woman, slightly to the right of midline. The right adnexa is shown as a lateral extension from the uterus.

der, usually asymmetrically positioned (Fig. 4–8). The size of the uterus changes with the stages of the menstrual cycle, and the uterus shrinks after menopause. Because the density of uterine tumors is similar to that of the normal uterus, enlargement is often the first indication of carcinoma on CT. The density of the adnexa and the ovaries is similar to that of the uterus; these structures can usually be identified laterally. Cystic areas in the ovaries may be physiological corpus luteum cysts, benign cysts, or carcinoma. Normal follicles may be as large as 2.5 cm in diameter. The vagina and the cervix can be seen when air is present in the external os or when they are defined by a tampon. A small amount of fluid may be present in the cul-de-sac.

Magnetic Resonance Imaging

MRI provides excellent images of the kidney, the retroperitoneum, the bladder, the prostate, the seminal vesicles, and the female reproductive organs. MRI is better than CT in that it more clearly identifies the tissue of origin of many pelvic masses and provides coronal and sagittal imaging to demonstrate tumors, adenopathy, and infection. In the evaluation of specific organs, successful imaging depends on the location and the tissue composition. The kidneys, like the spleen, have a high water content and show similar intensity for both normal tissue and pathological lesions. Adrenal neoplasms are well demonstrated on MRI, appearing as high-intensity masses on high-contrast scans such as T2 spin echo and short TI inversion recovery (STIR) sequences. As with CT, MRI is not usually capable of differentiating benign adrenal neoplasms from malignant ones.

In the pelvis, the identification of soft tissues planes, the high contrast of tumor and adenopathy in comparison with that of pelvic fat and muscle, and the ability to image in sagittal and coronal planes enables identification of abnormalities and determination of their tissue of origin. The latter capability is especially important for the staging of pelvic neoplasms. MRI enables the evaluation of tumors of the male and female genital organs and the identification of local invasion. The bladder wall is clearly shown by MRI, which facilitates detection of bladder-wall neoplasms.

One of the most important applications of MRI in the pelvis is the detection of adenopathy from tumor invasion or primary lymphoma. The STIR sequence shows diseased lymph nodes as high intensity against a dark background of fat and muscle (Fig. 4–9; see also Fig. 4–74*B*). In addition, soft tissue tumors and metastatic disease in the bone marrow are best detected and evaluated on MRI.

Interpretation of pelvic MRI requires the same knowledge of cross-sectional anatomical relationships needed in CT evaluation. In ad-

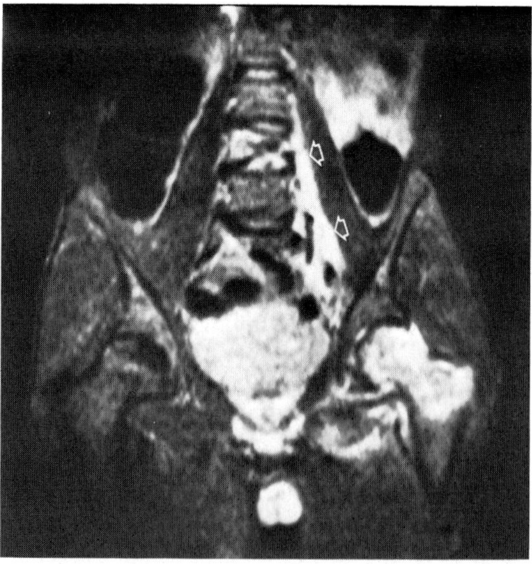

FIGURE 4–9. Pelvic adenopathy. Coronal short TI inversion recovery (STIR) image shows a chain of abnormal lymph nodes in the left paraspinous region *(arrows)* in a patient with Hodgkin's disease. In addition, this patient has bone marrow involvement of the left femoral head and a midlumbar vertebral body. Note normal high intensity in the left abdominal fluid-filled bowel, the bladder, and the testicles. Muscle and fat are of low intensity. Gas in the bowel is black.

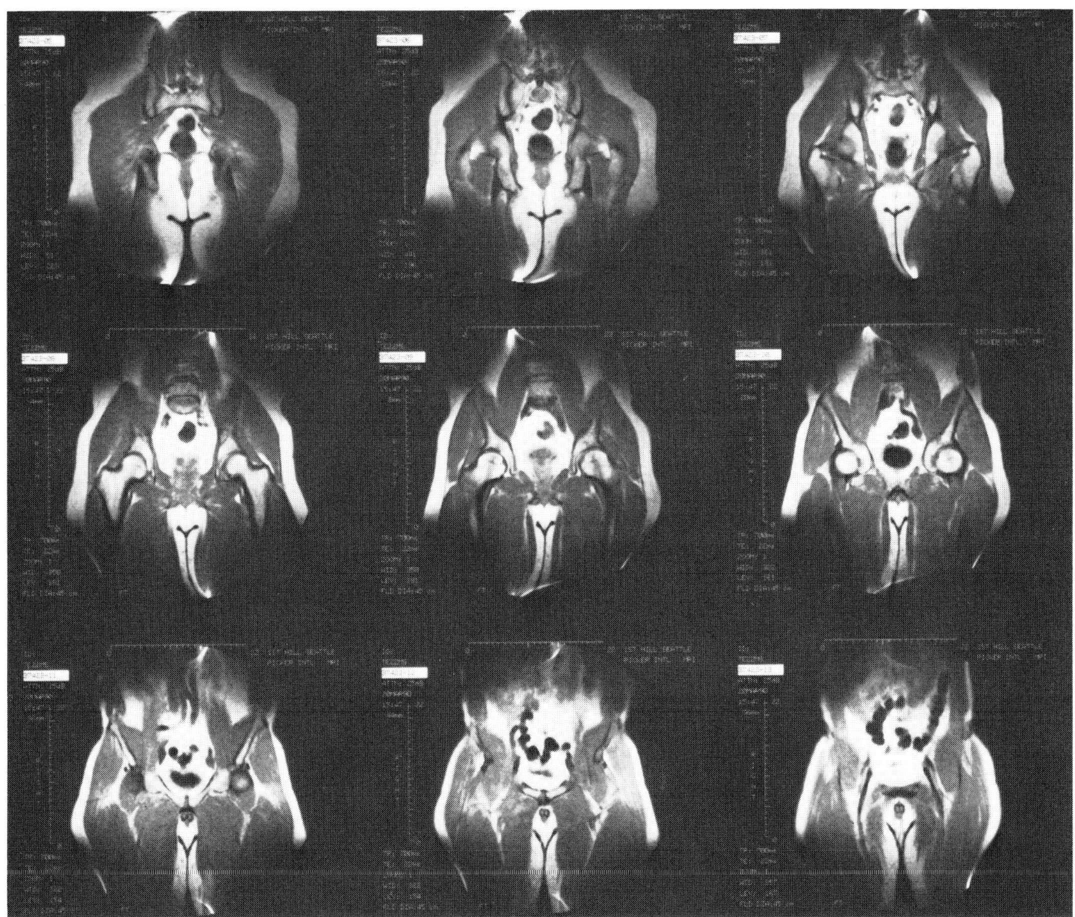

FIGURE 4–10. Coronal magnetic resonance image (MRI) of the pelvis. A series of T1 spin echo images shows the locations and intensities of normal structures. Fat appears bright, marrow is light gray, muscle is dark gray, and air and fluid are dark. Posterior slices *(top row)* show the muscles of the buttocks and back, the marrow of the sacrum, and the rectum. More anteriorly *(middle row)*, the pelvic organs and the mesenteric fat are seen in the midline. The bone marrow of the ilium, the acetabula, and the femurs are well shown for analysis of metastatic disease and avascular necrosis of the hip joint. The anterior slices *(bottom row)* show the bowel and bladder. This scan is used to define the anatomical position of abnormalities seen on STIR images.

dition, familiarity with the coronal and sagittal planes is important (Fig. 4–10). Coronal views are ideal for imaging of the prostate, the uterus, the adnexa, and the bladder and for the identification of lymphadenopathy and of bone marrow invasion. Sagittal views are used in evaluation of the spine and other midline structures.

Part I
Urinary Tract and Adrenal Glands

URINARY TRACT

Overview

Disease of the urinary tract is caused by parenchymal lesions in the kidneys (and the adrenal glands) and abnormalities of the walls and the lumen of the lower tubular system. In the kidneys and the adrenal glands, tumor and infection can result in local effects of the mass and in dysfunction. There may be distal effects of hormone abnormalities related to the tumors. In the ureters, the bladder, and the urethra, the manifesting symptoms and signs are usually caused by obstruction of the tubular tract. Common causes of obstruction include tumor, infection, clot, and stone formation.

Trauma

Trauma to the upper urinary system can be caused by penetration, blunt, or toxic injuries. The considerations in evaluating trauma from penetration injuries, such as knife and bullet wounds, are the same as those discussed for other parts of the body (see the section on traumatic diseases of the chest, Chapter 2). Entrance and exit sites must be clearly marked on the radiograph, and injury to the organs in this path must be suspected. Closed renal biopsy often produces a hematoma.

Blunt injury may affect the kidneys and the full bladder and is most often caused by a motor vehicle accident. Plain film findings can suggest possible areas of injury. Fractures of the lower ribs should arouse suspicion of renal, hepatic, and splenic injury. Fractures of the transverse processes suggest renal or ureteral injury. Pelvic fractures make bladder evaluation mandatory. Blunt trauma to a full bladder can result in rupture without other abnormalities. Free intraperitoneal air or fluid indicates abdominal injury. The psoas margin can assist in the identification of a retroperitoneal injury but is of diagnostic value only when clearly defined in its cephalad and caudal portions and when indistinct in the midportion.

Decisions for further evaluation of the urinary system after injury are based on urinalysis, plain film findings, CT examination, and clinical suspicion of injury. The presence of gross hematuria that is not found to be of urethral origin is well correlated with significant injury to the kidneys, the ureters, or the bladder. Although excretory urograms in major renal injuries usually show abnormalities, CT scans better characterize those abnormalities and often show additional unsuspected injuries in the kidneys and other organs. Therefore, all patients with suspected intra-abdominal injury should undergo CT. Rupture of the bladder is best depicted on cystograms.

The presence of microscopic hematuria is poorly correlated with abnormality on excretory urograms or cystograms. On occasion, a severe injury (such as renal pedicle transection) causes only minimal or no hematuria, and so any clinical suspicion of such an injury should prompt imaging examinations. Injury to the urethra is evaluated by means of retrograde urethrography, particularly if gross hematuria is present.

Congenital Abnormalities

Congenital anomalies occur more commonly in the genitourinary system than in any other organ system because of the complex formation of these organs. A description of the embryological development of this system elucidates the origins and nature of these anomalies.

Early stages of the primitive kidneys include the pronephros and the mesonephros forms. Later, the permanent kidney (the metanephros) begins to form from the ureteric bud and from the metanephrogenic cap (Fig. 4–11). At 2 months of gestation, the ureteric bud arises from the caudal mesonephric (wolffian) duct. This bud forms the ureter, the calyces, and the collecting tubules. The metanephrogenic cap arises from the intermediate cell mass in the pelvis and forms the glomeruli and the tubules. By 5 months of gestation, the kidney is fully formed and ascends cranially and rotates because of the different growth rates of the lower abdomen and pelvis. Blood to the kidneys is supplied first by the continuation of the aorta (the middle sacral artery), then by successively higher branches of the aorta (lateral splanchnic arteries), and finally by the renal arteries.

The cloaca is divided by the urorectal septum into the anterior portion, which becomes the bladder, and the posterior portion, which

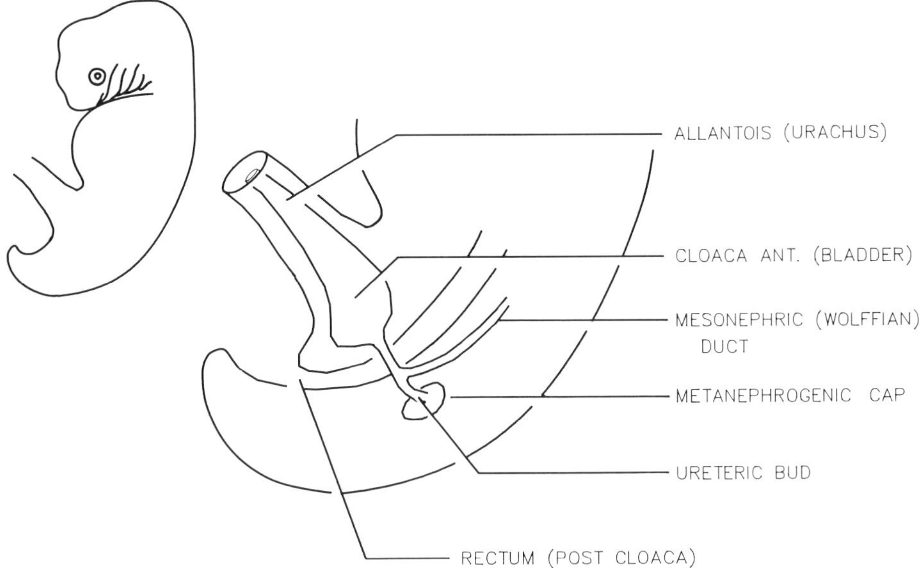

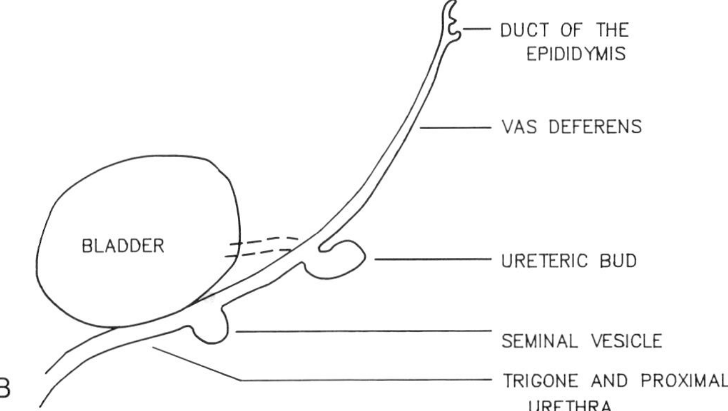

FIGURE 4–11. *A.* Origin of the urinary system (lateral view of developing pelvis). Ant., anterior. *B.* Derivation of the mesonephric (wolffian) ducts.

becomes the rectum. The apex of the bladder (which is continuous with the allantois) is obliterated, leaving a fibrous cord, the urachus, which extends from the bladder to the umbilicus. When the urachus becomes completely closed, it becomes the medial umbilical ligament. The ureter extends caudally to enter the bladder, and, in the male, the mesonephric (wolffian) ducts extend to form the ejaculatory ducts, the vas deferens, and the ducts of the epididymis to the developing testes. The most caudal portions of the mesonephric ducts fuse to form the trigone of the bladder and the proximal urethra.

In the male, the distal urethra and the prostate are formed largely from the urogenital sinus (the most caudal portion of the bladder), and the müllerian ducts disappear by the 6th week of gestation after forming the prostatic utricle (a cavity in the center of the prostate, the analog of the uterus). In the female, the mesonephric ducts disappear after forming the ureteric bud, the trigone, and the proximal urethra. The paired müllerian ducts form the uterine tubes, the uterus, and the upper portion of the vagina.

Congenital anomalies that cause severe impairment are usually identified at birth. Minor anomalies or normal variants often do not cause dysfunction. Diagnosis is most often made in contrast examinations, which reveal the location of the aberrant tubular tract. Congenital abnormalities can cause confusing images on CT or MRI because masses may appear in unusual locations.

Inflammation, Infection, and Neoplasms

Inflammation, infection, and tumor have similar appearances and manifestations in the urinary tract. In the kidneys and the adrenal glands, these diseases appear as mass lesions. In the lower portion of the tract, irregularity with narrowing and obstruction are the usual findings in contrast examinations. Cross-sectional images are required for evaluation of abscess or tumor mass and for demonstrating contiguous spread.

Obstruction, Stones, and Motility Disorders

Stone formation in the kidneys can cause direct renal injury or obstruction in the renal pelvis, in the ureter, in the bladder, or in the urethra. Most (about 80%) renal calculi are radiopaque. Stones are best identified on plain films, and the obstruction is most clearly demonstrated in contrast examinations.

KIDNEYS

Trauma

Blunt Injury. The kidney is the third (after the liver and the spleen) abdominal organ most commonly traumatized after blunt injuries. These injuries are graded according to severity, which can range from mild contusion to stellate fracture (Fig. 4–12). Patients may have pain and hematuria. Excretory urograms usually appear normal except when extraparenchymal damage occurs. However, these examinations can show conditions that predispose the patient to injury, such as horseshoe kidney, adult polycystic kidney disease, hydronephrosis, renal ectopia, or tumor. A nonfunctioning kidney can simulate absence of a kidney on excretory urograms, and so an additional examination (usually CT) is necessary for full evaluation.

Excretory urographic findings suggestive of renal injury include indistinct or enlarged renal outlines, delayed enhancement of vascular and renal cortical structures, filling defect or nonopacification in a portion of the collecting system, nonfunction, and extravasation of contrast (Fig. 4–13). Subtle, local changes in perfusion and excretion are difficult to interpret, even from film tomography, because of overlying bowel gas and normal renal variations. CT enables accurate, noninvasive assessment

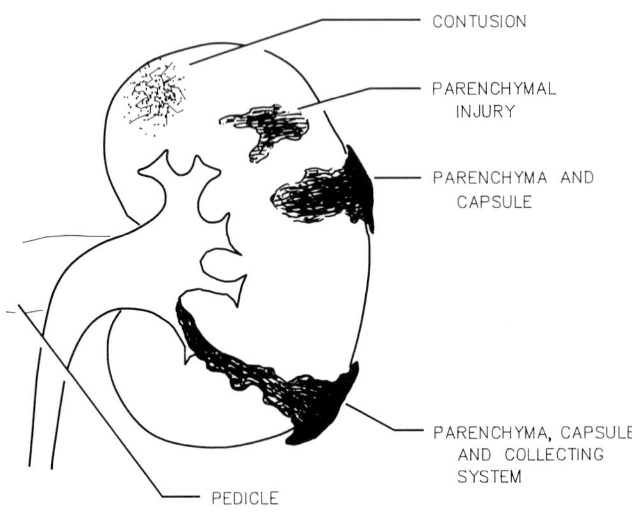

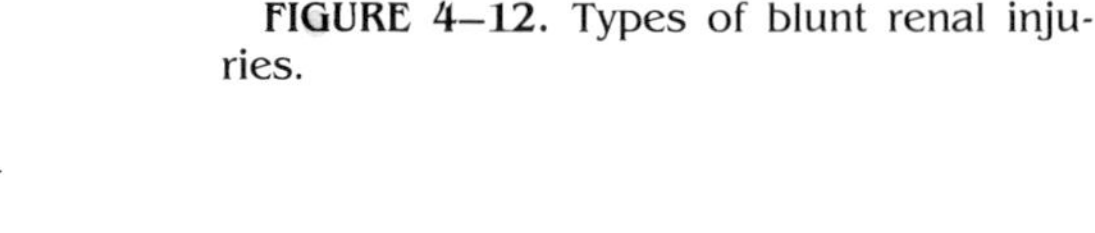
FIGURE 4–12. Types of blunt renal injuries.

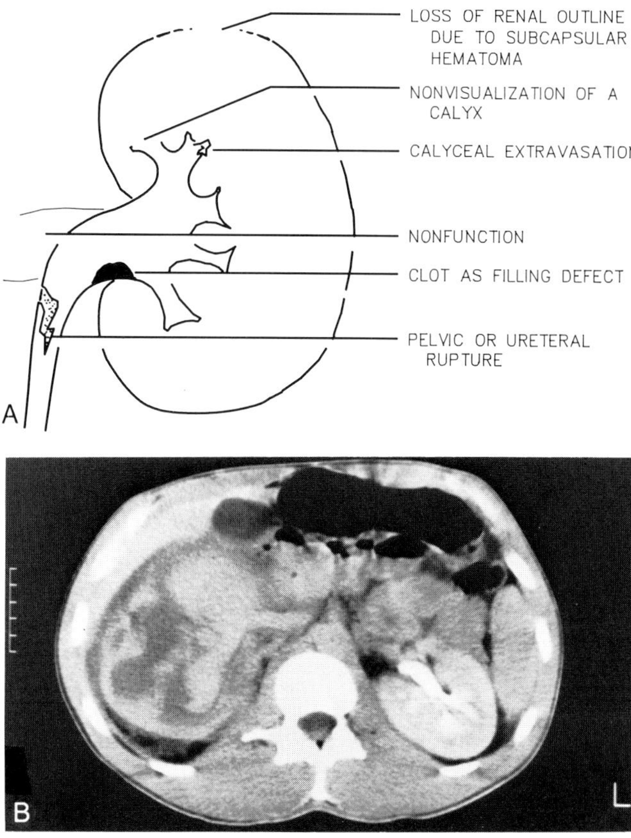

FIGURE 4–13. Renal trauma. *A.* Renal lesions seen on excretory urogram (diagram). *B.* CT demonstrating right renal fracture with marked increase in renal size. There is both intraparenchymal hemorrhage as well as hemorrhage and clot in the collecting system.

of renal injuries and provides the urologist with a reliable means of monitoring them. Retrograde pyelography is seldom used when there is renal trauma except to evaluate a nonfunctioning kidney. Arteriography is used only to evaluate the sequelae of renal injury, notably infarction, arteriocalyceal fistula, pseudoaneurysm, and expanding hematoma. Late results of renal injury are hydronephrosis, cyst formation, calcification, and fibrosis.

Retrograde Renal Injuries. The kidney can be injured from within by pressure on the collecting system, which causes retrograde flow of urine from the renal pelvis to, first, the renal tubules and then, by extravasation, into the parenchyma. This type of pressure can be caused by blunt injury to a hydronephrotic or obstructed kidney, bladder compression when the ureterovesical valves are incompetent, overdistention from retrograde urography, bladder distention with reflux, or ureteral obstruction. The radiographic appearance of this injury ranges from a brush-like filling of the collecting tubules to parenchymal or subcapsular collection. Recurrent pyelotubular reflux may be the cause of chronic pyelonephritis.

Toxic Renal Injury. Toxic injury to the kidneys can be caused by chemical agents (notably lead, chloroform, or heavy metals), aminoglycoside antibiotics, abuse of analgesic agents, and radiographic contrast material. These substances can cause acute tubular necrosis, a cessation of function of the renal tubular cells in which acute peritubular edema and parenchymal cell death cause obstruction of renal blood flow (Fig. 4–14). When the edema subsides (after about 3 days), renal function may return. In some patients, the impairment is permanent.

Aminoglycoside antibiotics cause renal failure less commonly because they are used infrequently (and dosage is reduced) in patients with renal impairment. Radiographic contrast can cause renal failure, especially in patients with poor renal function (see Appendix 1–1 in Chapter 1). Hydration of patients has virtually eliminated intravenous contrast as a cause of renal failure in patients with normal and nearly normal renal function. However, in patients with moderate to severe renal failure, radiographic studies with intravenous contrast material are contraindicated because they may cause irreversible damage to the kidney. Ul-

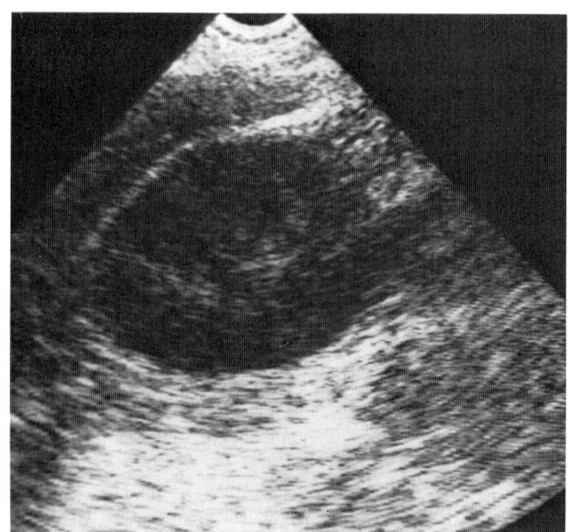

FIGURE 4–14. Acute renal failure. Longitudinal ultrasonogram of the right kidney shows generalized enlargement and loss of visualization of the corticomedullary junction in a middle-aged woman with acute renal failure caused by antibiotic therapy. Compare with Figure 1–11*A*.

trasonograms in patients with chronic renal failure show increased echogenicity of the cortex and usually a small kidney. Nuclear medicine scanning of the kidneys is used to evaluate function in such patients (see Chapter 9).

Papillary Necrosis. Papillary necrosis, the death of cells lining the renal papillae, generally results from toxic injury. The appearance of the papillae on the excretory urogram is highly variable, depending on the extent of disease, and ranges from mild blunting to extensive destruction of the calyces (Fig. 4–15). Papillary necrosis is often associated with pyelonephritis, obstruction, diabetes, sickle cell anemia, and phenacetin abuse.

Congenital Abnormalities

Renal Agenesis. Renal agenesis can result from absence of the mesonephric duct, the ureteric bud, or the metanephrogenic cap or

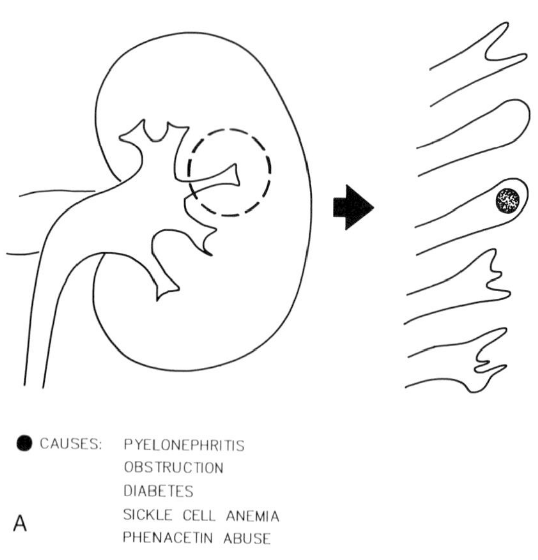

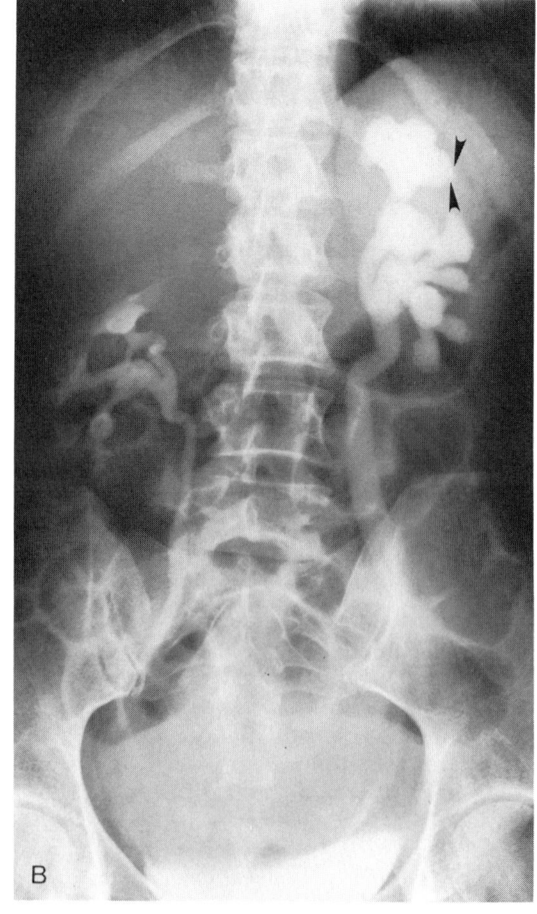

FIGURE 4–15. Papillary necrosis. *A.* Appearance of calyceal injury. *B.* Excretory urogram shows papillary necrosis as small central contrast collections at the end of the dilated calyces *(arrows)*, a result of left ureteral obstruction in a 40-year-old female.

from failure of these developing structures to unify. Approximately 1 of every 1000 people has a single kidney. Other anomalies are often present. The diagnosis can usually be made from excretory urograms that show unilateral absence of vascular, renal, cortical, and collecting structure enhancement and a normal, hypertrophied kidney on the opposite side (Fig. 4–16). The adrenal gland is usually (90% of the time) in the normal location. Renal agenesis is of no clinical significance unless other anomalies of the genitourinary system are present or unless illness or trauma compromises the normal kidney.

In some patients, a kidney fails to ascend to the normal location and remains in the pelvis.

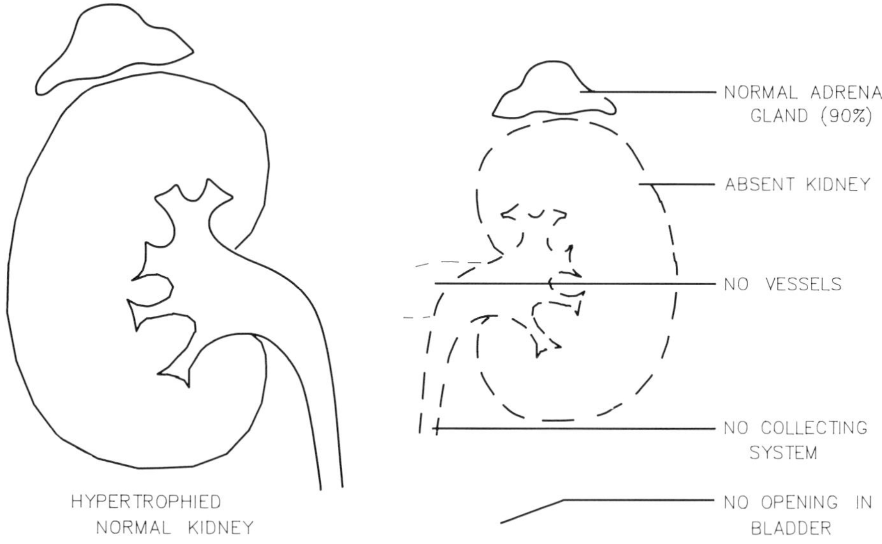

- INCIDENCE 1:1000 (BILATERAL 1:5000)
- CAUSE: EMBRYOLOGICAL FAILURE
- OTHER ANOMALIES COMMON
  FEMALES (70%) – APLASTIC VAGINA, UTERINE MALFORMATION, ABSENT OVARIES AND TUBES
  MALES (20%) – ABSENT TESTIS AND SEMINAL TRACT, HYPOSPADIAS, CLEFT SCROTUM
- CONSIDER: PELVIC KIDNEY, TRANSPLANT

A

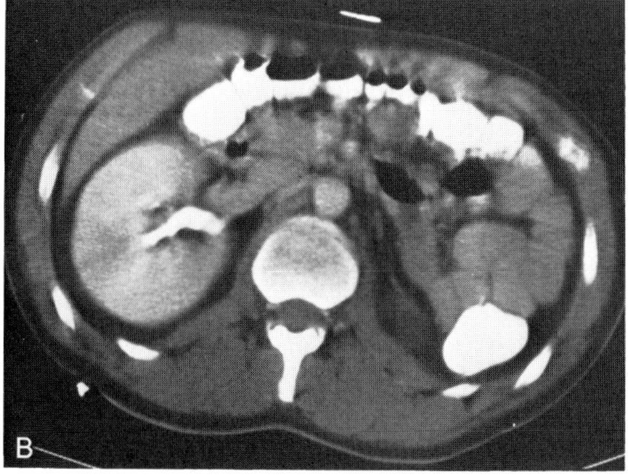

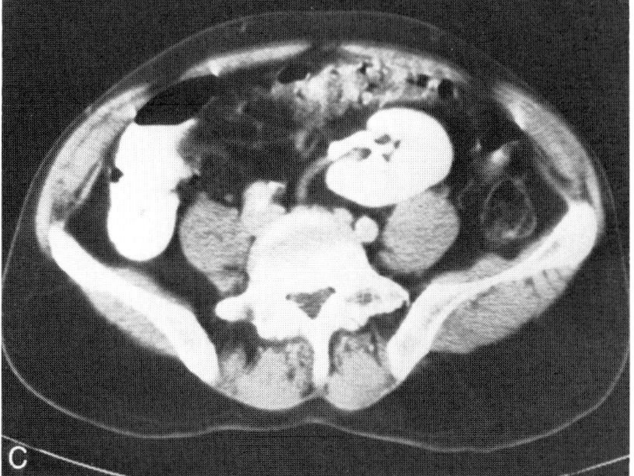

FIGURE 4–16. Absent kidney. *A.* Diagram. *B.* CT shows a large, normally functioning kidney on the right and no kidney on the left side of a young man evaluated for pelvic trauma. *C.* A different patient evaluated for pelvic mass showed "nonfunctioning" left kidney and enhancing pelvic mass on intravenous urogram. CT shows a pelvic kidney.

This can cause a confusing appearance on intravenous urograms that suggests both a nonfunctioning kidney and a pelvic mass (Fig. 4–16*C*). Associated problems of a pelvic kidney are stasis, infection, and calculi resulting from abnormal urinary drainage. One cause of a pelvic kidney is renal transplantation.

Renal Duplication. Duplication of the ureteric bud or early branching of the developing ureter can result in the development of additional renal tissue. Although the formation of multiple, separate kidneys is rare, duplications and partial duplications of a collecting system are common. In the case of complete ureteral duplication, a single, compound kidney arises from two (or more) ureters formed from separate ureteric buds. Because parts of the bladder grow at different rates, the ureter from the upper pole of the kidney inserts at a location lower than normal, often ectopically, in the bladder or elsewhere (Fig. 4–17). The upper-pole ureter often becomes obstructed, which results in a nonfunctioning upper pole. Therefore, a superior renal mass must be suspected of being the obstructed upper pole of a duplicated or partially duplicated kidney. Partial duplication, called attempted duplication, can appear as a hump on the upper, outer renal border and should not be confused with a tumor mass.

Ectopic and Fused Kidneys. The kidneys can fail to rotate or ascend, fuse, or cross the midline, or they can overascend to the diaphragm or chest. Ectopic kidneys are often malrotated, have ectopic blood supplies, and are usually located in the pelvis where they are difficult to interpret on plain radiographs (see Fig. 4–16*C*). Fusion of the kidneys can occur at any time during their ascent.

Horseshoe Kidney. Horseshoe kidney, the most common type of fusion, is characterized by connection of the lower poles of the kidneys by a fibrous band or an isthmus of renal tissue. This connection halts the ascent of the kidneys when it becomes trapped between the aorta and the inferior mesenteric artery. Horseshoe kidney is easily identified on excretory urograms by the medial position of the lower poles of the kidneys and, when present, the functioning renal tissue connecting them (Fig. 4–18). This anomaly is usually of no clinical significance, but the ureters can become obstructed either by compression as they pass over the isthmus or by compression from persistent lateral splanchnic arteries (which cross anterior to the ureters to supply the kidneys). The location of the kidneys near the midline renders them vulnerable to injury. The diagnosis of horseshoe kidney may limit employment or insurance coverage.

Congenital Enlarged Calyces. Many people have enlarged calyces that could be confused with hydronephrosis or renal parenchymal disease. This congenital variation can usually be differentiated from hydronephrosis by the normal cupping of the calyces and the normal appearance of the renal cortex.

Congenital Syndromes Involving the Kidneys

Most congenital diseases that involve the kidneys cause cystic abnormalities. Cystic renal diseases, including those that are congenital, are discussed at the end of this section. Two additional congenital syndromes that involve the kidney are retinocerebellar hemangiomatosis and abdominal muscle deficiency syndrome.

Retinocerebellar Hemangiomatosis. This disorder (also called von Hippel-Lindau disease) is an inherited autosomal dominant neurocutaneous syndrome involving predominantly mesodermal elements. The disease is characterized by multiple hemangioblastomas of the central nervous system and the retina and by tumors and cysts of the genitourinary system. The early symptoms of the disease are usually caused by the retinal and cerebellar hemangioblastomas and manifest in the second or third decade (see Chapter 8).

Because the retinal and cerebellar tumors grow slowly and do not metastasize, the clinical course of the disease depends on the presence of malignant tumors of the genitourinary system. The most common genitourinary tumors are cysts, angiomyolipomas, adenomas, and carcinomas of the kidneys; pheochromocytomas of the adrenal glands; and cysts and adenomas of the epididymis (Fig. 4–19). Renal cell carcinoma and pheochromocytoma are the most important of these tumors. The diagnosis is made by the identification of the hemangioblastomas, particularly in patients with family histories of the disease. Such patients must be evaluated for the presence of genitourinary tumors.

Abdominal Muscle Deficiency Syndrome. The syndrome of absent abdominal muscles, undescended testes, and various urinary anomalies is a rare, inherited disease of males, probably with x-linked recessive transmission. Because the abdomen appears wrinkled (like a prune), this disease is called prune-belly

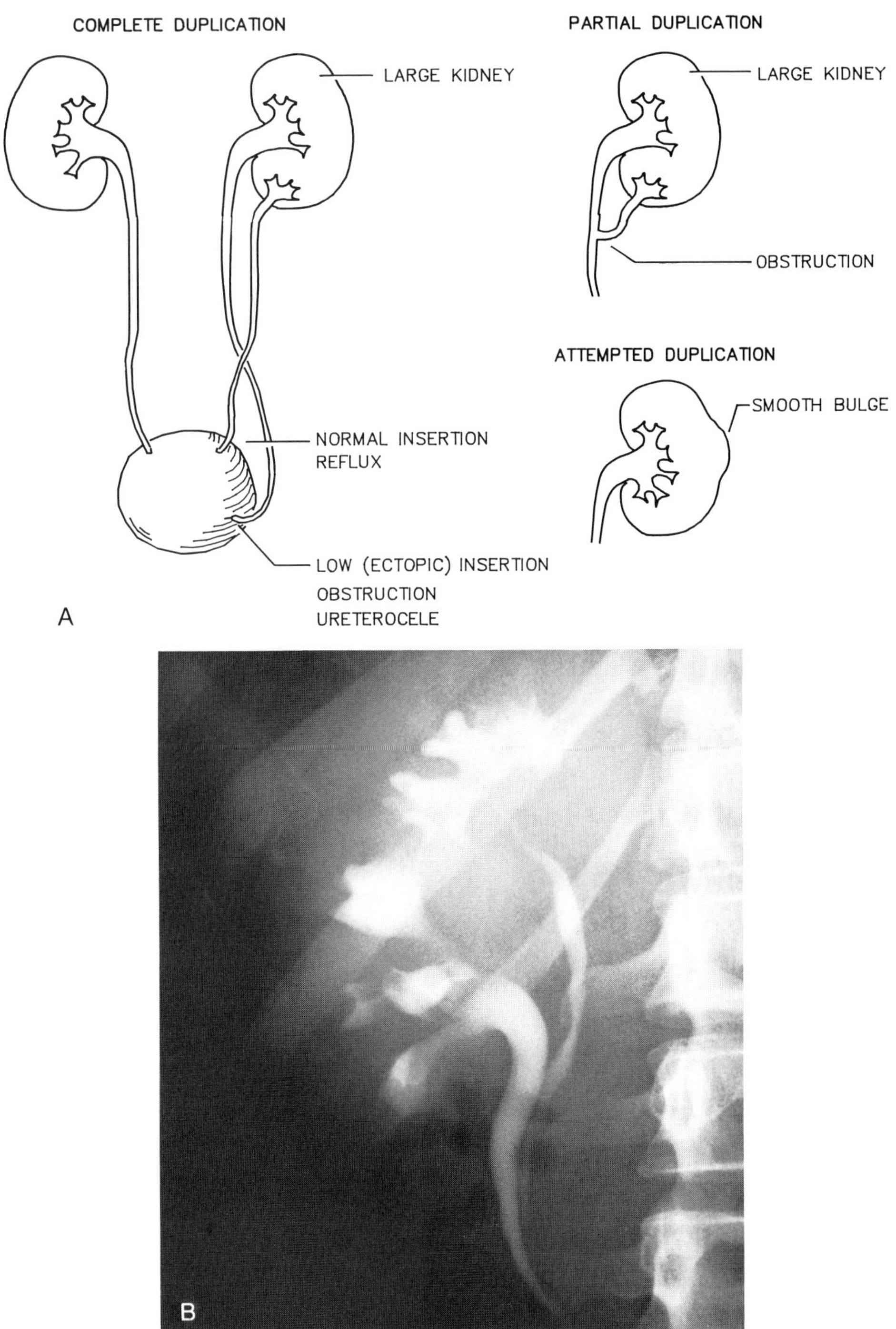

FIGURE 4–17. Renal duplication. *A.* Diagram. *B.* Excretory urogram 15 minutes after administration of contrast material shows two ureters and two separate collecting systems in this 40-year-old man with renal colic. The upper-pole calyces are blunted as a result of partial obstruction of the upper-pole ureter.

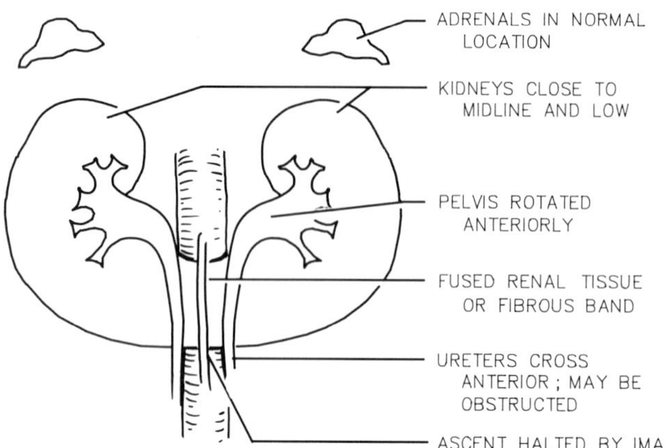

FIGURE 4–18. Characteristics of horseshoe kidney. IMA, inferior mesenteric artery; GU, genitourinary.

syndrome. Genitourinary anomalies include hydronephrosis, dilated ureters, ureterovesical reflux, dilated prostatic urethra, urachal abnormalities, and cryptorchidism.

Systemic Diseases

Medical renal disease encompasses the many systemic diseases that cause diffuse renal parenchymal injury and resultant deterioration of renal function. These diseases are grouped together because they have similar clinical and radiographic manifestations. Even renal biopsy is inconclusive in most cases.

Causes of medical renal disease are collagen vascular diseases, metabolic abnormalities, and toxic injuries. The radiographic appearance of the kidney usually does not enable differentiation among these causes. Early in the course of the disease, the excretory urogram merely shows enlarged, poorly functioning kidneys. Later in the course, the kidneys become small and shrunken. Excretory urography may be contraindicated at this stage. Ultrasonography is a more informative, safer

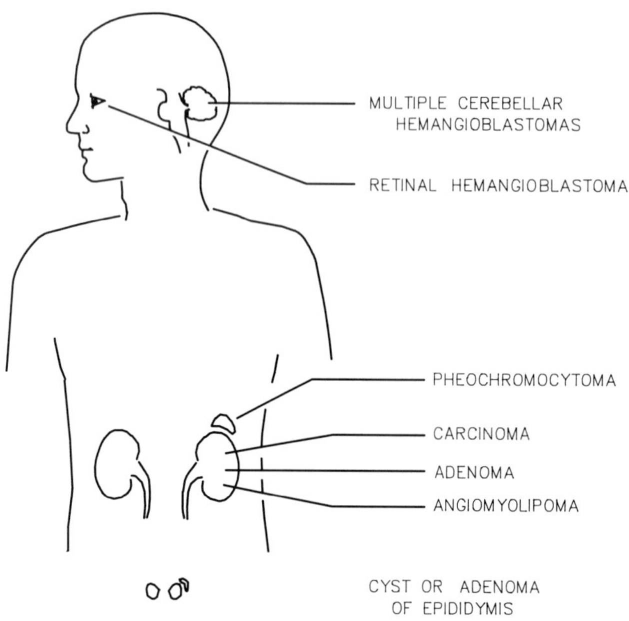

FIGURE 4–19. Characteristics of retinocerebellar hemangiomatosis (von Hippel-Lindau disease).

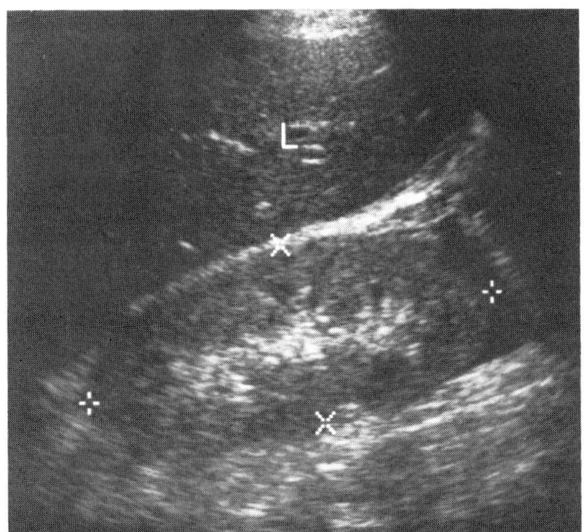

FIGURE 4–20. Medical renal disease. Longitudinal ultrasonogram shows the cortex and the medulla of the kidney as more echogenic than the adjacent liver, which is consistent with medical renal disease. The cursors indicate the kidney; L, liver.

technique for such evaluation. In advanced disease, ultrasonograms show small, highly echogenic kidneys (Fig. 4–20).

Diseases of the immune system, such as Wegener's granulomatosis, Goodpasture's syndrome, systemic lupus erythematosus, and other diseases characterized by vasculitis often affect the kidneys. The general manifestations of these diseases are discussed in Chapter 2. Excretory urograms, CT scans, and ultrasonograms show the nonspecific findings of medical renal disease when the kidneys are involved.

Nephrocalcinosis, the deposition of calcium in the medullary portion of the kidney, often results from abnormalities of calcium metabolism caused by cancer, hyperparathyroidism, sarcoidosis, hypervitaminosis D, and renal dysfunction. Injuries to the medullary portion of the kidneys can also cause nephrocalcinosis.

Infection

Infectious diseases involving the urinary tract are usually diagnosed by means of clinical examination and urinalysis. Plain film radiographs, excretory urograms, and arteriograms are seldom of help except for following the course of chronic infection. CT scans can show single or multiple abscesses within the kidneys and in the perirenal space.

Acute Pyelonephritis. Acute pyelonephritis is usually caused by gram-negative organisms and is believed to result from ascending infection from the lower urinary tract. Such infections are common in girls; urinary tract infection in a boy should raise suspicion of a genitourinary anomaly. Severe parenchymal infection with abscess probably occurs hematogenously and is usually caused by *Staphylococcus aureus* or other cocci. Diagnosis is usually straightforward, but in some cases radiographic studies are indicated in order to differentiate infection from acute obstruction, vascular thrombosis, and infiltrative tumor. In approximately 50% of patients, excretory urogram, if performed early in the course of the disease, can demonstrate large kidneys with poor opacification and a spider-like collecting system. Otherwise, the examination reveals no abnormalities. Inflammatory abnormalities within the renal parenchyma are usually less echogenic than the renal cortex on ultrasonograms and less dense than the normal kidney on CT scans. A perirenal or renal abscess, if large enough, may cause displacement of the kidney. Intravenous urograms may suggest pressure on or deviation of the calyces.

Chronic Pyelonephritis. Chronic pyelonephritis is the diagnosis derived from the clinical and radiographic findings of recurrent urinary tract infection. Like acute pyelonephritis, this infection has been assumed to be of the ascending type. However, an equally consequential causative factor may be recurrent extravasation of urine into the interstitium of the kidney as a result of reflux, obstruction, or a congenital anomaly. Early in the course of the disease, the poles of the kidney, rather than the midportion, are affected. Late in the disease, the excretory urogram shows a small, scarred kidney with caliectasis and loss of cortex (Fig. 4–21).

A focal infection sometimes causes a localized irregularity of the renal outline. A focal area of pyelonephritis or tuberculosis can cause such an appearance, but infarct, calyceal obstruction, and fetal lobulation (a normal variation of formation) should also be considered. The appearance of the calyces and the renal cortex usually help establish the diagnosis (Fig. 4–22). A defect in the cortex over a calyx is usually caused by pyelonephritis, whereas a defect between calyces is often an infarct.

Xanthogranulomatous Pyelonephritis. Xanthogranulomatous pyelonephritis represents an uncommon response to renal parenchymal infection in which the kidney becomes filled with lipid-laden macrophages (xanthoma cells). It occurs most commonly in diabetics. There is usually a predisposition to infection (stones or obstruction), which results in abscess forma-

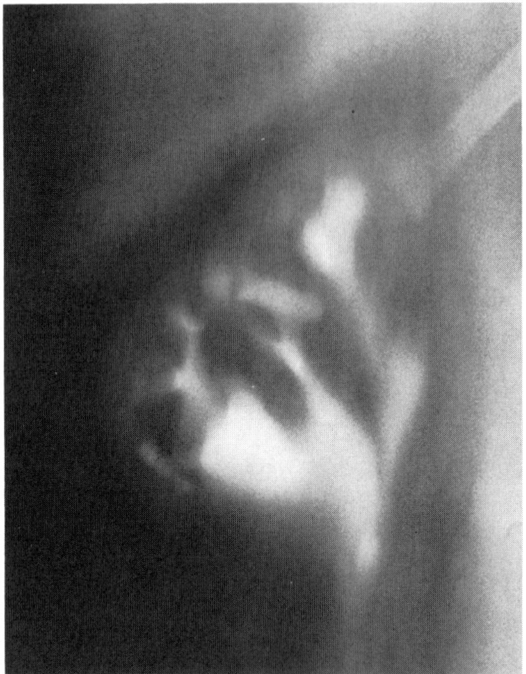

FIGURE 4–21. Chronic pyelonephritis. Tomogram of the right kidney at 15 minutes of intravenous urography shows a small kidney with irregular outline, loss of cortex, and blunted calyces. The patient, a 79-year-old immigrant from the Middle East, had a long history of kidney infections.

tion as the primary disease process. Gram-negative organisms are found in the kidney and the urine, but the true causative agent or agents are not known. The xanthomatous process is secondary.

Intravenous urograms, CT scans, and MRI scans show a large, nonfunctioning kidney and an appearance similar to that of renal cell carcinoma (Fig. 4–23). The presence of stones, microabscesses, and other evidence of infection can help establish the diagnosis of xanthogranulomatous pyelonephritis. Arteriography is not usually performed, but it can reveal an inflammatory vasculitis rather than the neovascularity of renal cell carcinoma. Patients are usually treated by nephrectomy in order to remove the source of infection.

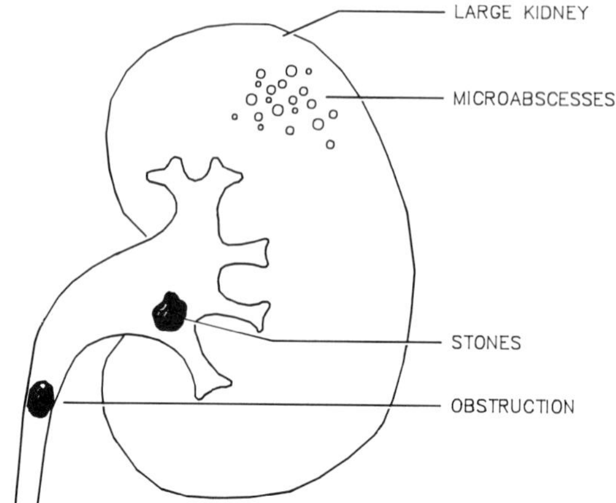

- CAUSE – GRAM-NEGATIVE BACTERIA
- CHRONIC INFECTION CAUSES XANTHOGRANULOMATOUS RESPONSE
- LOOKS LIKE CARCINOMA
- NO FUNCTION

FIGURE 4–23. Characteristics of xanthogranulomatous pyelonephritis.

Brucellosis. Infection with *Brucella* species uncommonly involves the kidney. If the infection is severe, it produces a distinctive radiographic pattern of diffuse calcification, cicatrization, and calyceal dilatation. Such infections are rare because of the widespread use of antibiotics and the eradication of the disease in cattle, the most common carrier.

Tuberculosis. Tuberculosis of the genitourinary system has become rare in the United States since antimycobacterial therapy became available. It is common in many other parts of the world, especially Southeast Asia, and many immigrants bring this disease to the United States. Tuberculous involvement of the kidney is by hematogenous spread, usually from lung lesions. The chest radiograph shows no abnormality in 50% of patients with extrapulmonary tuberculosis. The glomeruli and cortex are affected first, but the infection spreads down the tubules into the collecting system to involve the calyces, the renal pelvis, and the ureters. Genitourinary tuberculosis is characterized

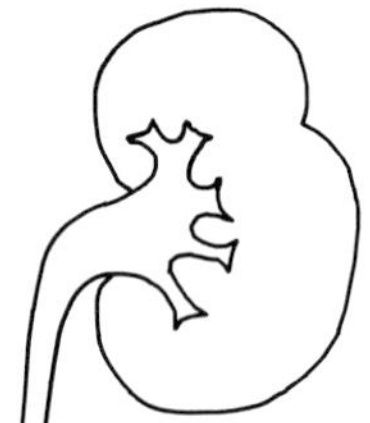

CONDITION	CALYCES	CORTEX
FETAL LOBULATION	NORMAL	NORMAL
INFARCT	NORMAL	DESTROYED
CALYCEAL OBSTRUCTION	DILATED	NORMAL
INFECTION	ENLARGED	DESTROYED

FIGURE 4–22. Characteristics of focal cleft in the kidney simulating chronic pyelonephritis.

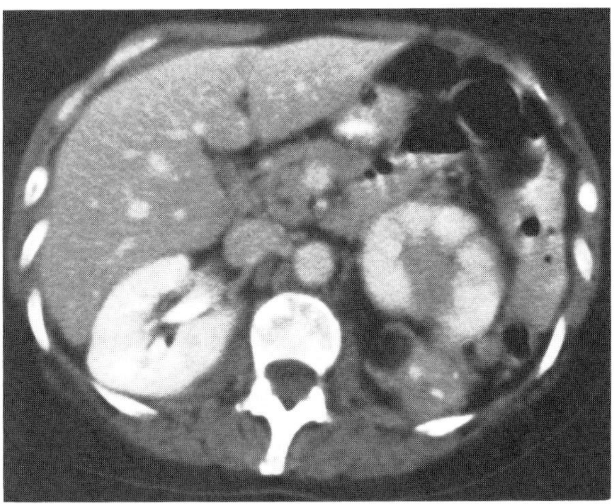

FIGURE 4–24. Renal tuberculosis. Contrast CT shows a normal right kidney. The left kidney, behind a loop of opacified bowel, is scarred and shrunken and shows internal calcification. The patient, an Asian immigrant, had pulmonary tuberculosis and renal involvement.

radiographically by parenchymal destruction and calcification (Fig. 4–24). The destruction of renal parenchyma results in a scarred, shrunken kidney. Calcification is common in the kidneys, the ureters, and the bladder and can help establish the diagnosis.

Candidiasis. Renal infection by *Candida albicans* occurs with immunosuppression, prolonged antibiotic therapy, malignancy, and diabetes. The infection spreads hematogenously. A frequent sequela is papillary necrosis. In general, the kidneys are swollen, and CT reveals many small abscesses.

Echinococcosis. The kidney is involved in 2% of cases of *Echinococcus granulosis* infestation. This infestation is primarily hematogenous. Large echinococcal cysts form in the kidneys, displacing parenchyma and collecting structures. The cysts are similar to those seen elsewhere in the body (see Chapter 2): they are characterized by a thick wall (which often calcifies), a low-density center, and the presence of internal daughter cysts.

Neoplasms

Benign tumors of the kidney are rare and usually of no clinical significance. The most important of these are renal adenomas and angiomyolipomas. Malignant renal tumors are much more common than benign tumors; most are metastases. Most malignant primary tumors of the kidney are renal cell carcinomas.

Renal Adenoma. Renal adenomas are small, nodular masses, sometimes cystic, that occur in the renal cortex. They arise from the proximal tubule. The pathological appearance of the renal adenoma may resemble that of a carcinoma. Renal adenomas may be early forms of renal cell carcinoma. Most are asymptomatic and are discovered incidentally at autopsy. On CT scans or ultrasonograms, they can appear as small nodules, indistinguishable from complex cysts or small malignant tumors (Fig. 4–25).

Angiomyolipoma. Angiomyolipomas are hamartomas composed of vascular, muscular, and fatty tissue. They are rare in the general population, but they occur in most patients with tuberous sclerosis, who often have bilateral tumors. They occur slightly more often among females than among males in the general population. The radiographic appearance depends on the amount of each kind of tissue present. Most angiomyolipomas are hypervas-

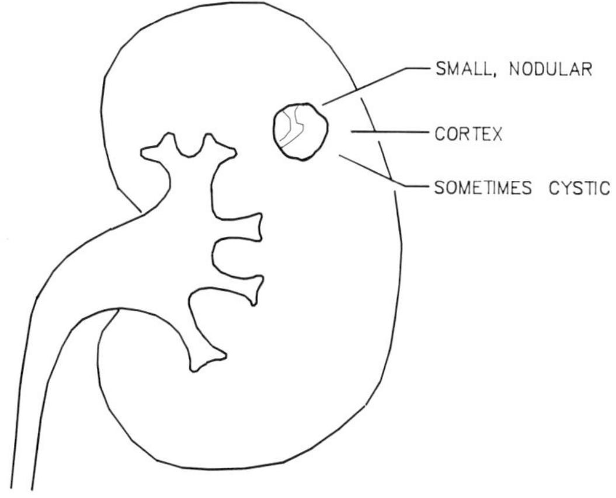

FIGURE 4–25. Characteristics of renal adenoma.

cular, noncalcified masses (Fig. 4–26). Because of the similarity of their appearance to that of renal cell carcinoma, biopsy is often required for correct diagnosis. Both CT and MRI scans can show the typical appearances of fat, a finding that greatly helps establish the diagnosis of benign angiomyolipoma. These tumors do not metastasize.

Mesoblastic Nephroma. Mesoblastic nephromas are hamartomas of the kidney that appear as renal masses, often at birth and always before 6 months of age. The lesions are usually avascular, unilateral masses that may contain calcification. They are indistinguishable radiographically from Wilms' tumor (to be discussed). The diagnosis is usually made on the basis of the findings of a renal mass in an infant less than 6 months old. Nephrectomy or local excision is curative. The tumor does not metastasize.

Renal Cell Carcinoma. Renal cell carcinomas (also called hypernephromas and clear cell carcinomas) constitute 85% of primary renal tumors. They are twice as common in males as in females and usually occur between the ages of 40 and 70 years. The tumors arise in the proximal tubule cells and bear many similarities to renal adenomas. Histological examination reveals that the tumors are composed of clear, granular, spindle-shaped cells

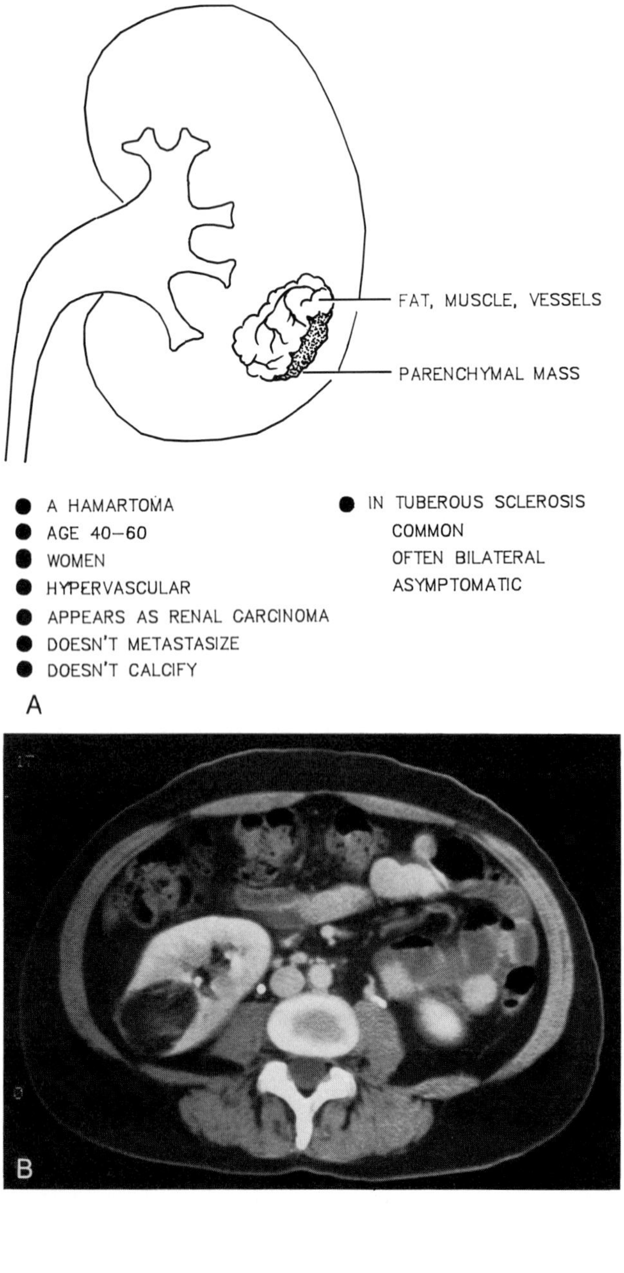

FIGURE 4–26. Angiomyolipoma. *A.* Diagram. *B.* Enhanced CT shows a fat-density, well-demarcated oval lesion in the right kidney in a 40-year-old woman. The fat, the stranding, and the vascular enhancement are pathognomonic of angiomyolipoma. (Courtesy of B. Porter, First Hill Diagnostic Imaging Center, Seattle.)

arranged in various patterns: solid, cystic, tubular, or papillary. Patients usually have hematuria (the most common sign), flank pain, or a mass. These are not always present. Other signs include fever, anemia, weight loss, erythrocytosis, hypercalcemia, and hypertension. A scrotal varicocele can indicate renal vein obstruction by tumor. Among patients with retinocerebellar angiomatosis (von Hippel-Lindau disease), the incidence of renal cell carcinoma is high (and many of them die of this disease).

Most renal cell carcinomas are highly cellular, vascular masses that distort the renal outline and displace the collecting structures. Some lesions are cystic, some are hypovascular, and some show central necrosis. Although they grow slowly, most metastasize early to the lungs, the lymph nodes, the liver, the bones, the adrenal glands, and the other kidney. Early local invasion of the renal vein and the inferior vena cava is common (10% of patients). When the tumors spread to the brain, they cause dense contrast enhancement, edema, and frequently hemorrhagic lesions (see Fig. 8–11).

Renal carcinomas that arise in the renal pelvis have different histological characteristics (transitional and squamous cell types) and are usually hypovascular. These carcinomas constitute approximately 15% of renal carcinomas and are usually of the transitional cell type. Patients with transitional cell tumors have a better prognosis than do patients with squamous cell tumors because transitional cell tumors are less invasive. Because they can spread locally down the ureters and are often multifocal, resection of the ureter is important.

Endocrine secretion by renal tumors is common. Forty percent of renal cell carcinomas produce renin, which causes hypertension; 10% produce parathyroid hormone, which causes abnormalities of calcium metabolism; and 2.5% produce erythropoietin, which results in polycythemia.

On intravenous urograms and CT scans, renal cell carcinoma appears as a nonfunctioning mass that distorts the renal outline and compresses the adjacent collecting structures. Calcification, especially if it is amorphous or central, suggests a malignant tumor. Even peripheral calcification suggests malignancy. These findings are well shown on intravenous urograms. However, the diagnosis is best confirmed by CT, which reveals the mass and local abnormalities, including invasion of the renal vein and the inferior vena cava (Fig. 4–27). The most important findings are a soft tissue mass, enhancement, hemorrhage and necrosis, and calcification. MRI can show the local invasion and demonstrate involvement of the renal vein and the vena cava (Fig. 4–28). In most patients, MRI findings are similar to those of CT. MRI has advantages in that it enables detection of tumor in the poles of the kidneys (through the use of coronal scans), detection of vascular obstruction, identification of the organ of origin, and detection of contiguous spread.

Most renal cell carcinomas are hypervascular, and abnormal vessels can be identified on angiograms. Correct diagnosis of renal cell carcinoma requires attention to radiographic and clinical factors (Table 4–1). Angiomyolipoma (described earlier) can have a similar appearance of a mass with abnormal vascularity. Xanthogranulomatous pyelonephritis (also discussed earlier) can also show a kidney mass and nonfunction.

Renal cell carcinoma is treated by radical nephrectomy, including the regional (renal hilar) lymph nodes. The 5-year survival rate depends on the stage of disease. It is as high as 80% for patients with localized disease, varies from 30% to 50% for patients with regional lymph node or vascular invasion, and is dismal for patients with distant metastases.

Wilms' Tumor. Wilms' tumor is the second most common solid childhood tumor (the most common is neuroblastoma). It occurs in children aged 3 months to 6 years. A renal mass in an infant under 6 months of age is usually a mesoblastic nephroma (described earlier), a benign tumor whose radiographic and histological appearances are similar to those of Wilms' tumor. Wilms' tumor differs histologically from renal cell carcinoma in that it is of mesodermal origin and shows sarcomatous features. Hypertension, hematuria, and a flank mass are the most common manifesting signs.

Plain film radiographs, excretory urograms, and CT scans show a renal mass and distortion of the collecting system (Fig. 4–29). Some (15%) of the tumors have calcification. Ten percent are bilateral, and metastases to the lungs and liver are common. Patients treated with surgery, chemotherapy, and radiation have a good chance of survival: the rate of 2-year survival, which appears to represent cure, is 90%. The approximate 5-year survival rate is above 80%.

Mesenchymal Tumors. Malignant forms of renal mesenchymal tumors arise from the various vascular and connective tissues of the kidneys. These tumors are uncommon, and

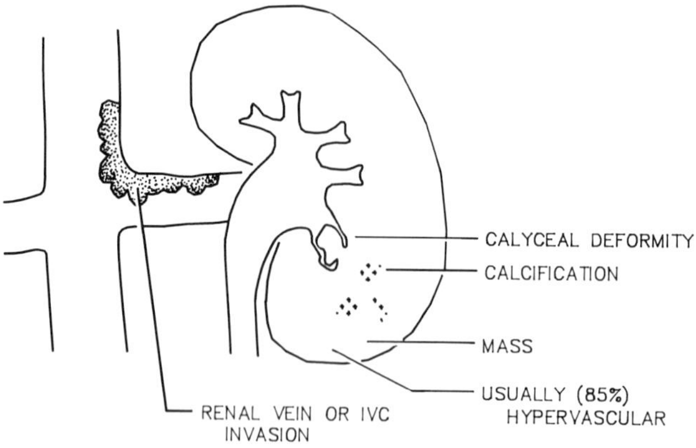

- 85% OF PRIMARY RENAL TUMORS
- AGE 40–60, M:F 2:1
- HEMATURIA, PAIN, MASS
- HORMONE STIMULATION
- METASTASIZE EARLY

A

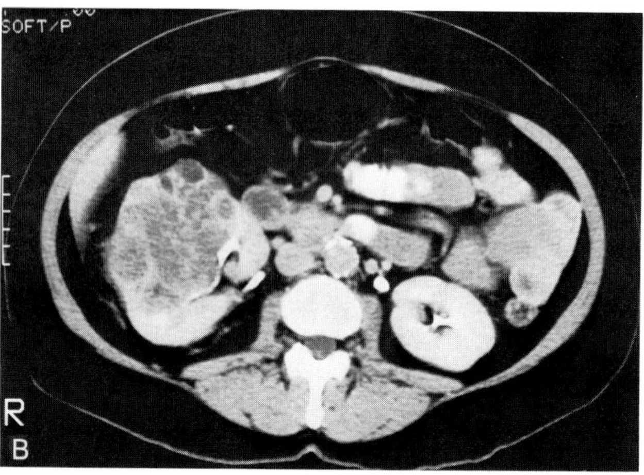

FIGURE 4–27. Renal cell carcinoma. *A.* Diagram. IVC, inferior vena cava; M:F, male:female ratio. *B.* Contrast CT shows a large mass occupying the middle and lower portions of the kidney and displacing the collecting structures. Adenopathy is present medially. In the patient, a 44-year-old woman, brain metastases were the first manifestation of disease.

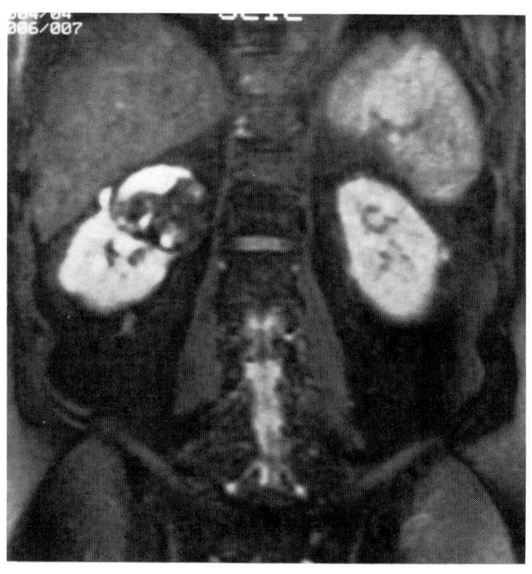

FIGURE 4–28. Renal cell carcinoma. Coronal STIR image shows a complex, superior pole mass in the right kidney of a 71-year-old man with hematuria and flank pain. Hemorrhage, necrosis, and tumor caused the complex appearance of the mass. Note the high intensity of the normal kidney, the spleen, the normal intervertebral discs, and the cerebrospinal fluid on this high-field (1.5 T) STIR image. All other tissues are of low intensity, which renders abnormalities easy to identify.

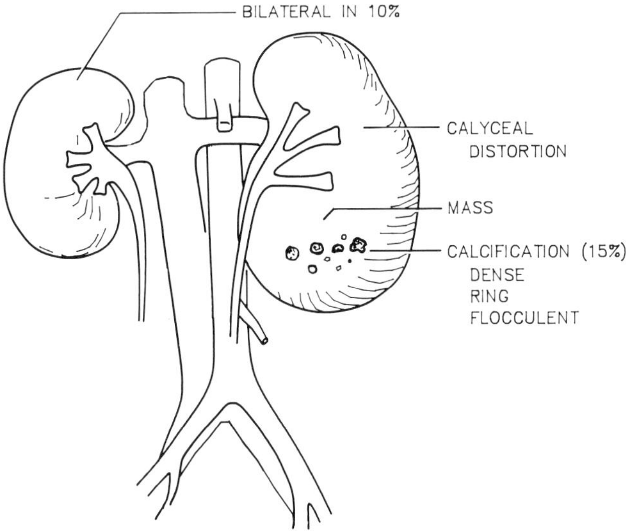

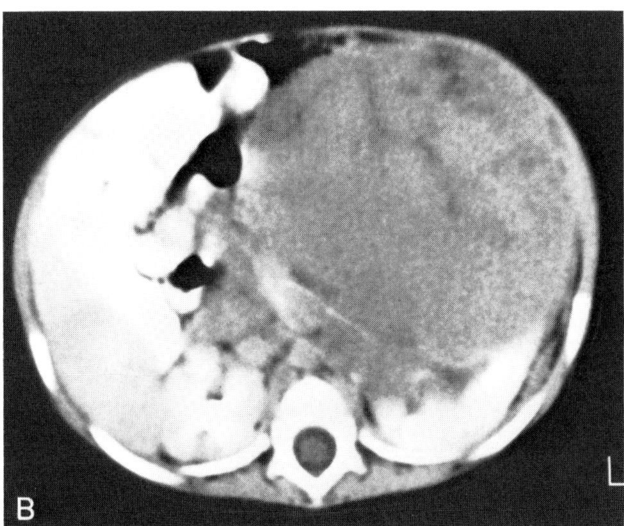

FIGURE 4–29. Wilms' tumor. *A.* Diagram. MO., months; YR., years; GU, genitourinary. *B.* CT. An extremely large mass occupies the left side of the abdomen. It splays the contrast-enhanced collecting system of the left kidney, and displaces it posteriorly.

TABLE 4–1. RADIOGRAPHIC AND CLINICAL FINDINGS IN RENAL CELL CARCINOMA

Clinical Signs
Hematuria
Mass
Flank pain
Endocrine Abnormalities
Hypercalcemia (parathyroid hormone secretion)
Hypertension (renin secretion)
Polycythemia (erythropoietin secretion)
Radiographic Findings
Nonfunctioning mass
Distorted collecting system
Central or peripheral calcification
Tumor vascularity
Hemorrhage or necrosis
Metastasis
Lungs
Lymph nodes
Liver
Bones
Adrenal glands
Opposite kidney
Differential Diagnosis
Angiomyolipoma
Xanthogranulomatous pyelonephritis

because they can also arise from the retroperitoneum, the tissue of origin is often indeterminate. The appearance on radiographs and CT scans is a mass in the region of the kidneys that is often continuous with adjacent structures. MRI, because it has superior resolution, can often delineate the boundaries of these tumors and assist in therapy.

Leukemia and Lymphoma. Involvement of the kidneys by leukemia is common and results in diffuse renal enlargement. Lymphoma involves the kidney in approximately 50% of patients, and its radiographic appearance varies from diffuse enlargement to a discrete, focal mass or multiple, nodular lesions (Fig. 4–30). These abnormalities can be shown on intravenous urograms, CT scans, and MRI scans.

Metastasis. Two thirds of renal tumors are metastases. Lymphoma and lung carcinomas are the most common tumors of origin, followed by breast and gastric carcinomas. The clinical course of the disease is determined by the type of primary tumor, and so the metastases are usually incidental. Renal function is usually normal. Radiographic evaluation shows that these lesions are hypovascular and usually bilateral.

Vascular Diseases

Most renovascular diseases manifest as hypertension. However, because hypertension is rarely of renal origin, the evaluation of hypertension should focus initially on extrarenal causes. After these causes are ruled out, a vascular lesion of the renal pedicle or large renal vessels should be suspected. Digital and conventional angiography provide the best evaluation of renovascular disease by demonstrating vascular irregularity or stenosis. Measurement of renal vein renin can be done at the time of arteriography and is also helpful for establishing the diagnosis of renovascular hypertension. The most prevalent causes of renovascular hypertension are atherosclerosis and fibromuscular dysplasia.

Atherosclerotic Disease. The most common cause of renovascular hypertension is atherosclerotic disease, which generally occurs in elderly patients. Atherosclerotic disease affects

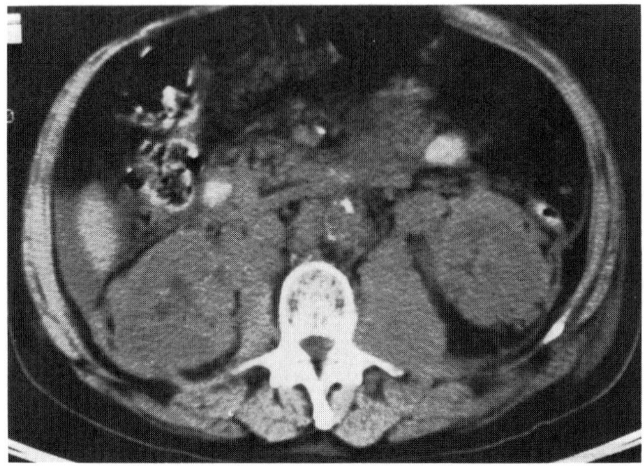

FIGURE 4–30. CT of diffuse lymphoma involving retroperitoneal spaces and both kidneys. There is extensive adenopathy in the root of the mesentery anterior to the aorta in the periaortic region, and, in addition, both kidneys have a lobular appearance.

predominantly the abdominal aortic bifurcation, the carotid bifurcations, the vessels of the lower extremities, and the coronary arteries. The renal and intracranial arteries are less often involved. The disease is more severe in diabetic patients. In the kidneys, the usual abnormality is an irregular narrowing of the renal artery at its origin from the aorta. Atherosclerotic disease is usually evident elsewhere in the abdominal aorta and the iliac arteries.

Angiography with digital or direct film techniques best demonstrates the narrowing of the arteries (see Fig. 4–3). Renal vein sampling for renin secretion can be performed as part of the angiographic examination. The narrowed segment can be treated surgically, or it can be dilated by the radiologist by means of a balloon catheter (Fig. 4–31).

Fibromuscular Dysplasia. Fibromuscular dysplasia is a disease of young women characterized by dysplastic changes in the walls of various arteries, most commonly the renal, extracranial carotid, and iliac arteries. This dysplasia produces a pattern of regularly alternating narrowing and dilatation of the arteries. Renal artery involvement usually is in the middle and distal thirds. Arteriograms show the alternating narrowed and widened arteries, which give the vessels the appearance of a string of beads (Fig. 4–32). The disease is progressive, despite the temporary efficacy of surgical or angiographic angioplasty.

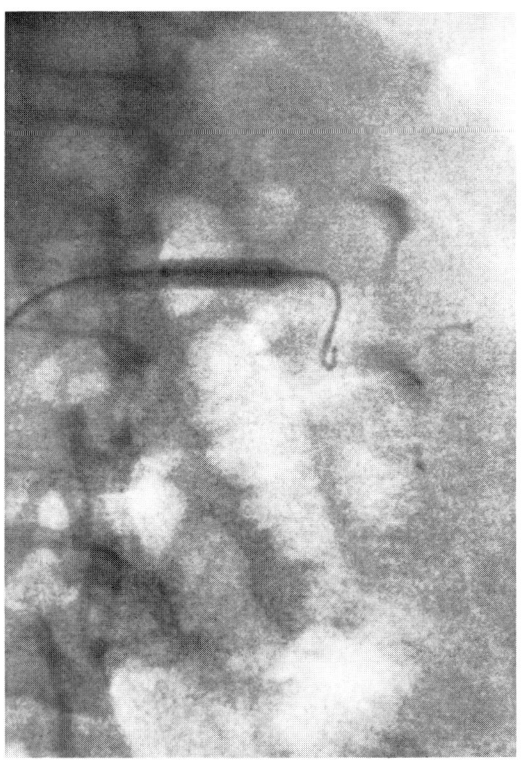

FIGURE 4–31. Balloon catheter dilatation of renal artery atherosclerotic disease. Video monitor view of the left kidney shows an inflated balloon catheter dilating a stenotic renal artery. Contrast (which appears black on the video image) can be seen in the calyces of the kidney. (Courtesy of J. King, University of New Mexico, Albuquerque.)

Neurofibromatosis. Neurofibromatosis occasionally produces intimal fibrosis at the origin of the renal arteries. This fibrosis is caused by an abnormality of the arterial intima, not by neurofibroma. The radiographic appearance is a nonspecific narrowing at the origin of the renal artery.

Other Causes of Hypertension. Several other conditions less commonly cause hypertension. Retroperitoneal fibrosis (to be discussed) can encase the renal arteries. Trauma can cause narrowing of the renal vessels and, in turn, hypertension. Intrarenal fibromuscular dysplasia, atherosclerosis, and localized infarction can also lead to increased renin production and hypertension.

Renal Vein Thrombosis. Renal vein thrombosis most commonly occurs when tumor, usually from renal cell carcinoma, invades the vein (see Fig. 4–27*A*). Blood flow is obstructed, and venous drainage of the kidneys is impaired. The kidneys become swollen, and function deteriorates. The clinical signs may suggest renal infection, acute tubular necrosis, acute glomerular nephritis, or obstructing stone. Excretory urogram shows a nonfunctioning or poorly functioning kidney. Angiograms can show the obstruction in the renal vein and the inferior vena cava.

Less common causes of renal vein thrombosis are chronic glomerulonephritis, hypercoagulability of the blood, and severe dehydration. The right renal vein drains directly into the inferior vena cava without collateral veins, and so obstruction cannot be alleviated by reverse collateral flow. The left renal vein receives the paravertebral, phrenic, and gonadal veins and can therefore drain by reverse collateral flow. Thus the right kidney is more likely than the left kidney to be injured by renal vein thrombosis.

Cystic Renal Disease

Cystic disease of the kidneys is common. The assessment can be difficult because of the many descriptions and classifications of cystic

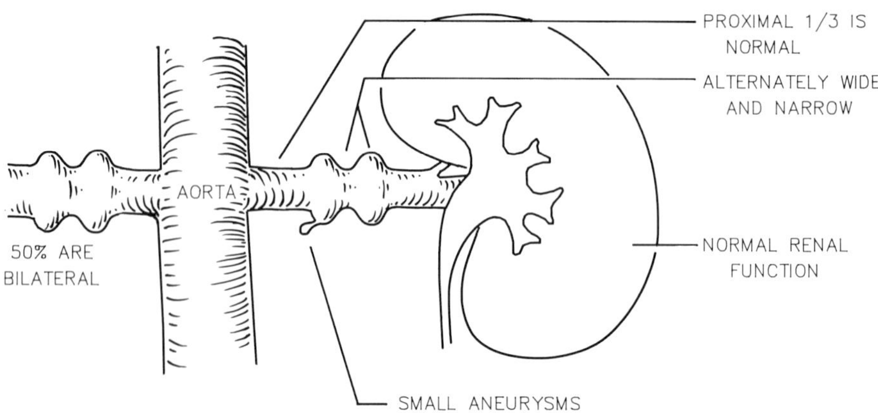

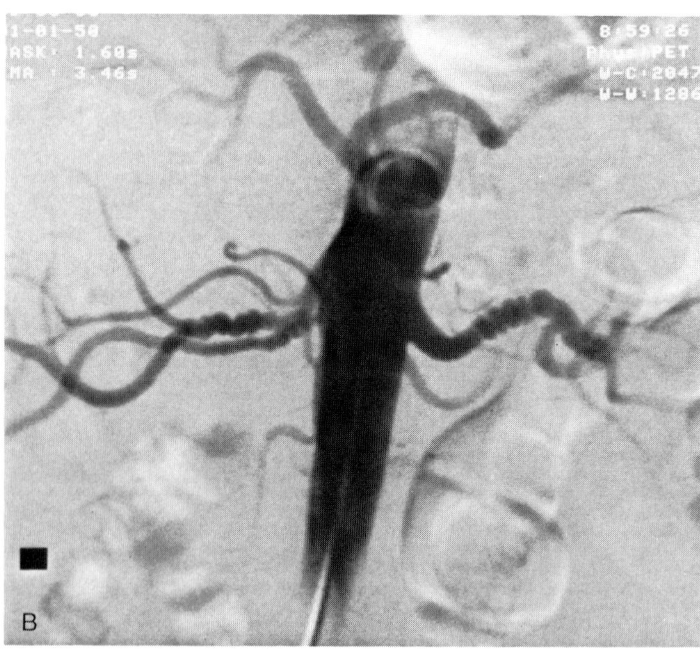

FIGURE 4–32. Fibromuscular dysplasia (FMD) of the renal artery. *A.* Diagram. SMA, superior mesenteric artery. *B.* Digital aortogram shows a string-of-beads appearance of the renal arteries in a middle-aged woman with renovascular hypertension. (Courtesy of J. King, University of New Mexico, Albuquerque.)

disease, but it is important to differentiate cystic disease from carcinoma. Cystic lesions are considered (and easily recalled as) either tubular or parenchymal.

Tubular Cystic Disease

Benign Tubular Ectasia and Medullary Sponge Kidney. The least severe tubular abnormality is benign tubular ectasia, a slight dilatation of the collecting tubules in an asymptomatic patient (Fig. 4–33*A*). This condition should be considered a variation of normal. In patients with such findings, the disease does not usually progress.

In some patients, however, the dilatations become cystic, and the papillae acquire a sponge-like appearance and can form calcified

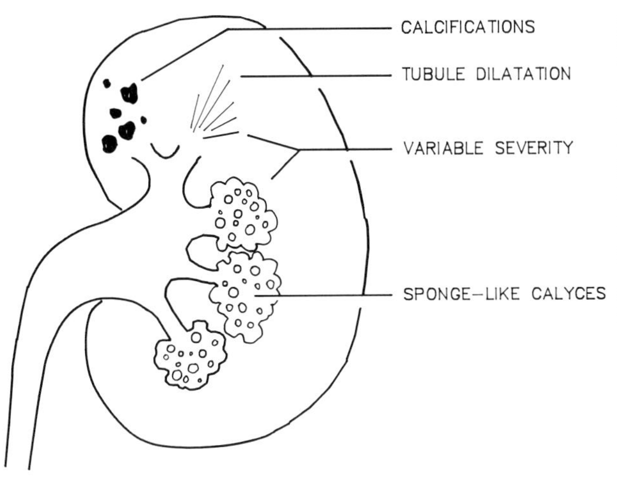

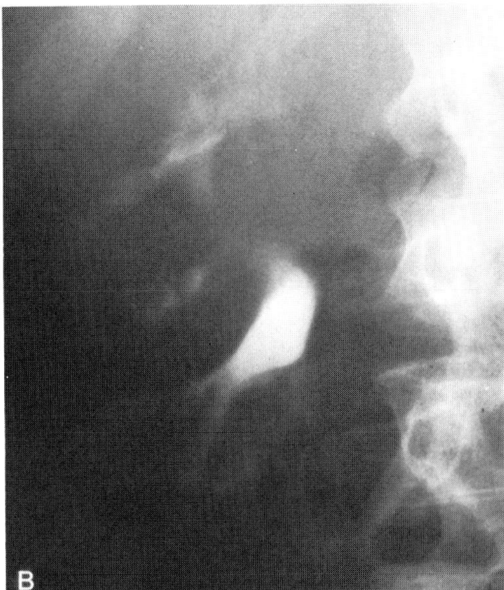

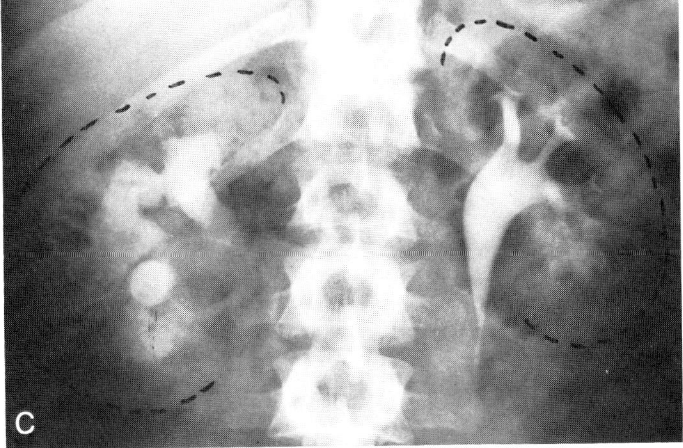

FIGURE 4–33. Spectrum of tubular ectasia. *A.* Diagram. *B.* Benign, tubular ectasia. The collecting system of the right kidney is clearly demonstrated; however, peripheral to the calyx, there is in each case a diffuse, fan-like collection of contrast in the tubule. *C.* Medullary sponge kidney. Large, sponge-like concretions are present in both kidneys, more severely on the right side.

concretions (Figs. 4–33*B* and 4–33*C*). This more advanced disease is termed medullary sponge kidney. Benign tubular ectasia seems to be the benign end of the spectrum of medullary sponge kidney. Because a diagnosis of the latter can significantly affect a patient's employment and insurability, the term "medullary sponge kidney" should be used only when definite findings of advanced disease are present. Among patients with medullary sponge kidney, the incidence of renal infections and stones is high.

Medullary Cystic Disease. Uremic medullary cystic disease is a rare, rapidly fatal uremic syndrome of adolescents. It is characterized by uremia and rapid loss of salt in the urine. Proteinuria is minimal or absent. Multiple cysts are present in the medullary portion of the kidneys (Fig. 4–34) and can be well demonstrated by CT or ultrasonography. Often, the cysts are microscopic and are not detectable. The kidneys are contracted rather than enlarged.

Infantile Polycystic Kidney Disease and Congenital Hepatic Fibrosis. Infantile polycystic kidney disease and congenital hepatic fibrosis also represent a spectrum of tubular disease. The polycystic kidney disease is manifested in infancy, and the hepatic fibrosis appears in teenagers who have had minimal (nonfatal) polycystic kidney disease.

Infantile polycystic kidney disease manifests

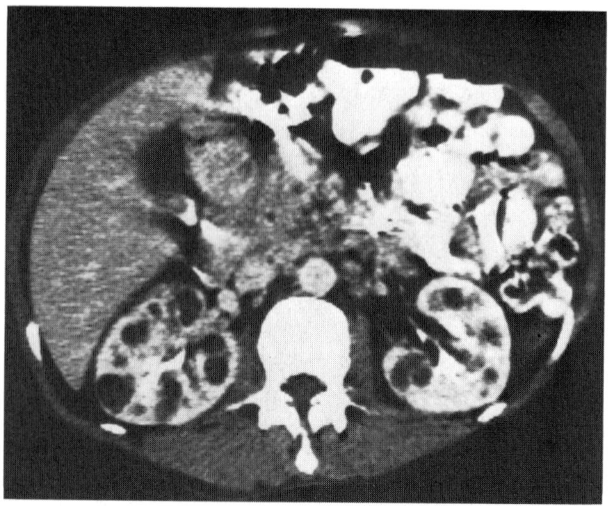

FIGURE 4–34. Medullary cystic renal disease. Contrast CT shows multiple, small cysts in a young man with uremia. The cysts do not affect the outer cortex, which indicates their medullary location. Also, the kidneys are not enlarged.

as massive, poorly functioning kidneys in newborn infants. These kidneys are characterized pathologically as having saccular and tubular cysts of the collecting tubules. Nephrons and glomeruli are normal. On intravenous urograms, the kidneys appear enlarged with poorly defined borders (Fig. 4–35). Rays of contrast enhancement are seen in the dilated collecting tubules.

Congenital hepatic fibrosis manifests during the teen years as periportal fibrosis, which leads to gastric and esophageal varices. Hemorrhage is the usual cause of complications or death. Renal and bile duct cysts are present to a lesser degree than in infantile polycystic kidney disease. Liver function is normal, and jaundice and ascites are absent. Patients can live a normal life span.

Parenchymal Cystic Disease

Simple Cyst. The most common parenchymal cystic disease is the simple cyst. Contrast examinations and CT can often reveal a large cyst clearly (Fig. 4–36), but ultrasonograms confirm the diagnosis when they show a well-circumscribed, anechoic mass (see Fig. 1–10). If the cyst contains inhomogeneous fluid or septations, it can simulate a solid mass. One percent of renal cysts have calcification in the wall and, although most of them are benign, 20% represent carcinoma. When calcification

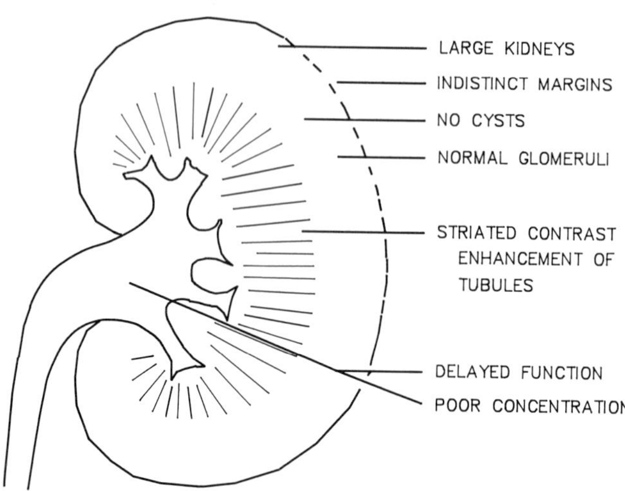

FIGURE 4–35. Characteristics of infantile polycystic kidney disease.

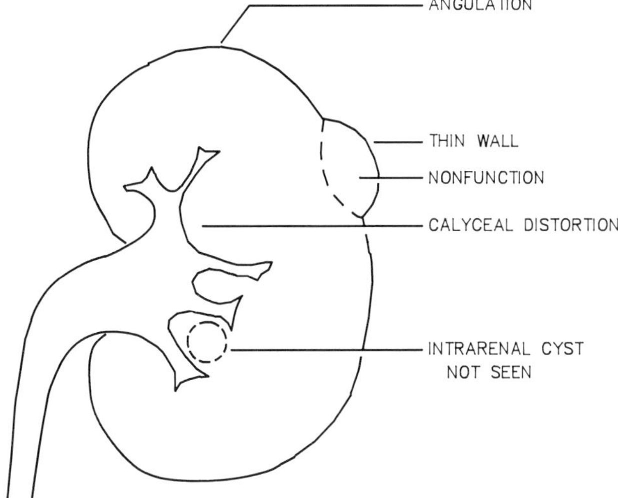

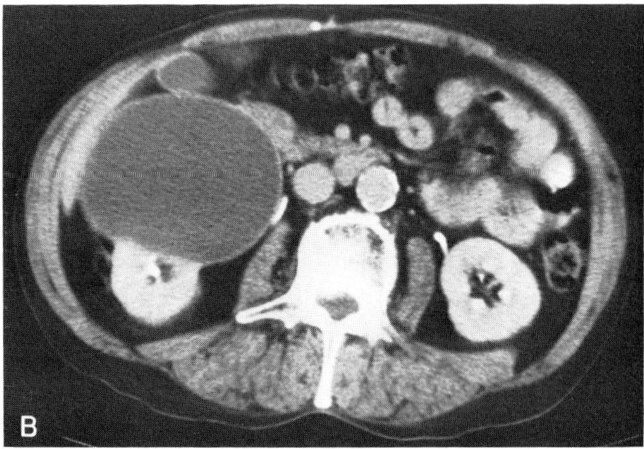

FIGURE 4–36. Simple renal cyst. *A.* Diagram. *B.* Contrast CT shows an 8-cm–diameter cyst of the right kidney in a 60-year-old man with rectal carcinoma. The cyst is an incidental finding. Note the smooth margin, the extension from the kidney, and the simple fluid contents. Note also calcification of the aorta.

in the cyst is diffuse, the lesion is overwhelmingly likely to be carcinoma (90%). CT and MRI do not reveal well-defined borders between the cyst and the parenchyma unless the cyst is large.

Multiple Renal Cysts. Multiple renal cysts are common and are usually of no clinical significance. When the cysts are associated with adult polycystic kidney disease (to be discussed), they compress the renal parenchyma and ultimately result in renal failure.

Multiloculated Renal Cysts. Multiloculated renal cysts are rare, multiple, septated cysts in one portion of a kidney. They are composed of mesenchyme, and therefore a better term for them is "benign multilocular cystic nephromas" (Fig. 4–37). They often occur in children and are not hereditary. Multiloculated renal cysts have no malignant potential, although the lesions bear some histological resemblance to Wilms' tumor and mesoblastic nephroma.

Adult Polycystic Kidney Disease. Adult polycystic kidney disease is an inherited autosomal dominant failure of nephron and tubule formation, which results in expansile cysts that eventually compress the normal renal parenchyma to cause renal failure (Fig. 4–38). Patients often also have cysts in the liver (see Fig. 3–73) and other organs, and many die as a result of rupture of an associated intracranial aneurysm. Trauma or increasing cyst size can cause bleeding into the cyst or the renal col-

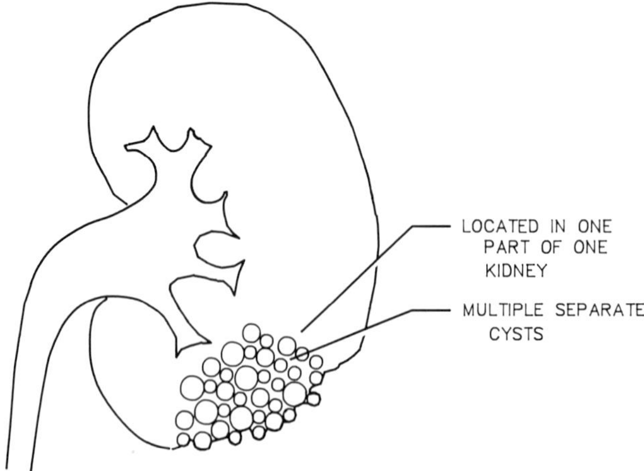

FIGURE 4–37. Characteristics of multiloculated renal cyst.

lecting system. The disease usually becomes clinically significant at about age 45 years when the patient develops renal failure, but it can manifest in infants.

Multicystic Dysplastic Kidney. Multicystic dysplastic kidney is the most common cause of a renal mass in a newborn. It is a failure of renal development that results in multiple parenchymal cysts and absence or incompleteness of the renal collecting system. It is usually unilateral and manifests in infancy but is not hereditary. Intravenous urograms and CT scans show a nonfunctioning renal mass with an amorphous appearance that resembles a bunch of grapes (Fig. 4–39). The mass has no malignant potential.

Other Cystic Lesions. Other conditions can have an appearance similar to that of a renal cyst. The most important distinction is between a benign cyst and a cystic tumor. Tumor cysts often have thick walls, internal hemorrhage, necrosis, and calcification. Complex cysts therefore often mandate biopsy. On ultrasonograms, hydronephrosis is commonly confused with renal cysts. On intravenous urograms, a calyceal diverticulum can be confused with cystic renal disease and also prompts consideration of renal tuberculosis and papillary necrosis. In children, Wilms' tumor, lymphoma, and hydronephrosis must be considered in the evaluation of any renal mass. Inherited diseases that cause cystic renal lesions are tuberous sclerosis (multiple renal cysts and angiomyolipoma), retinocerebellar angiomatosis (multiple renal cysts and renal cell carcinoma), and Meckel's syndrome (encephalocele and renal cysts).

URETERS AND RENAL PELVIS

Trauma

The ureter is seldom injured because it is deep within the retroperitoneum. Except for gunshot and knife wounds, the injuries are usually iatrogenic, including ligation or transection at surgery and perforation during retrograde pyelography. Chronic obstruction, reflux, and infection caused by stasis of urine can functionally impair the ureters.

Congenital Abnormalities

Ureteral anomalies include ureteral duplication (discussed earlier with renal duplication), ureteral diverticulum, retrocaval ureter, ectopic distal insertion, ureterocele, and adynamic distal ureter.

Ureteral Diverticulum. A ureteral diverticulum occurs as a blind pouch during formation of the ureter. When it fills on excretory urogram, it is easily identified. The appearance, however, is not specific. Tumor and infection can also cause such a radiographic appearance.

Retrocaval Ureter. Normally, the inferior vena cava forms from vascular segments pos-

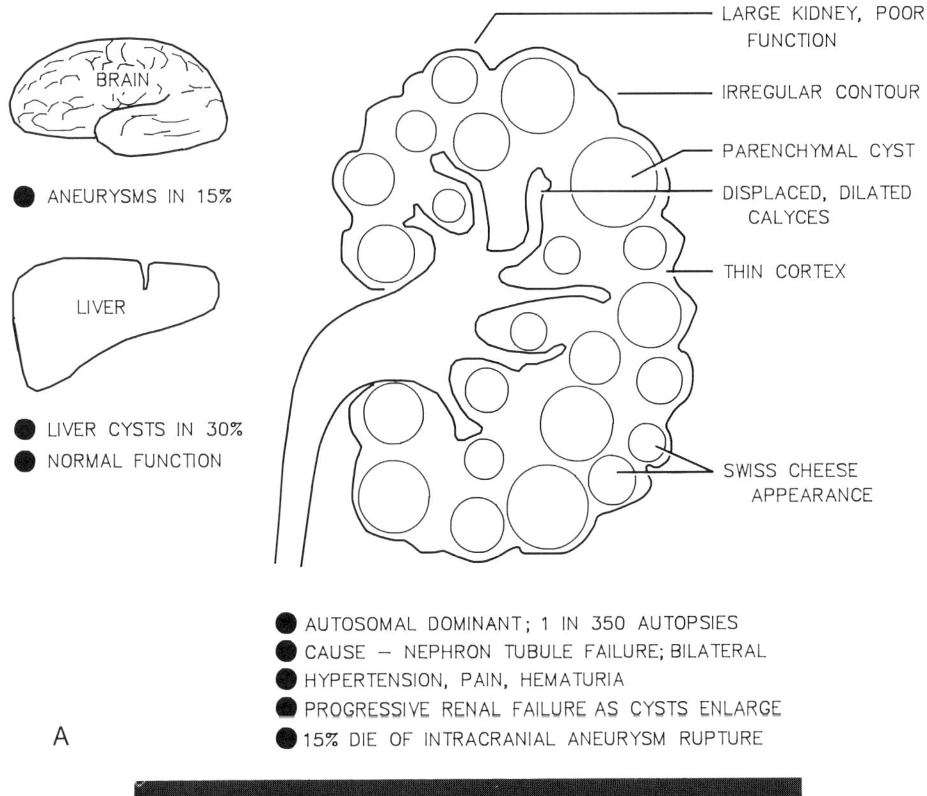

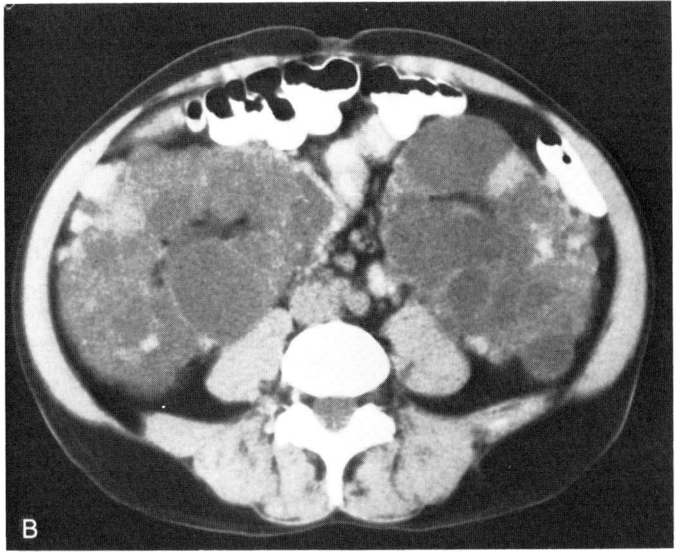

FIGURE 4–38. Adult polycystic kidney disease. *A.* Diagram. *B.* Noncontrast CT in a 49-year-old man with renal failure shows compression of the renal parenchyma by the numerous large cysts.

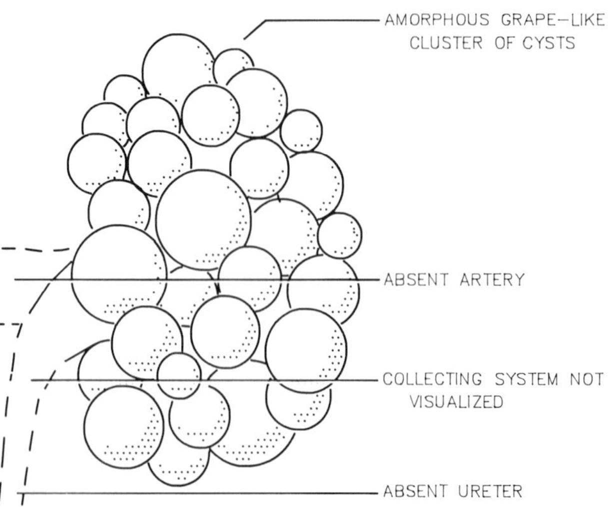

FIGURE 4–39. Characteristics of multicystic dysplastic kidney.

terior to the ureter. When a portion of this vessel forms from ventral segments, the ureter passes behind it and crosses anteriorly to enter the bladder. Retrocaval ureter can be seen on radiographs as an abrupt medial deviation of the midportion of the ureter as it passes behind the inferior vena cava (Fig. 4–40). The appearance on CT scans can be confusing and requires careful study of successive slices to delineate the path of the ureter. Such a ureter occasionally becomes mechanically obstructed.

Ectopic Distal Insertion. Ectopic insertion of the distal ureter is a rare failure of migration of the caudal portion of the ureter. In women, the ureter can insert into any pelvic structure, most commonly the vestibule (the lowest vaginal segment), the urethra, and the vagina. In men, it can insert into the urethra and seminal vesicles (Table 4–2). In women, the ectopic ureter is almost always associated with ureteral duplication.

Ureterocele. A ureterocele is a diverticulum of the ureter at its insertion into the bladder. It can compress the ureteral lumen to cause obstruction, but it is usually asymptomatic. It does not cause reflux. On excretory urograms, cystograms, and CT scans, it often appears as a filling defect in the bladder if it does not initially fill with contrast material. Late films, especially after the patient has voided, show the contrast-filled diverticulum. The appearance of the contrast-filled ureter, with its widened insertion, resembles that of a cobra. The so-called ectopic ureterocele is a refluxing, dilated ureteral orifice; it occurs primarily in infants and young children and is usually associated with ureteral duplication.

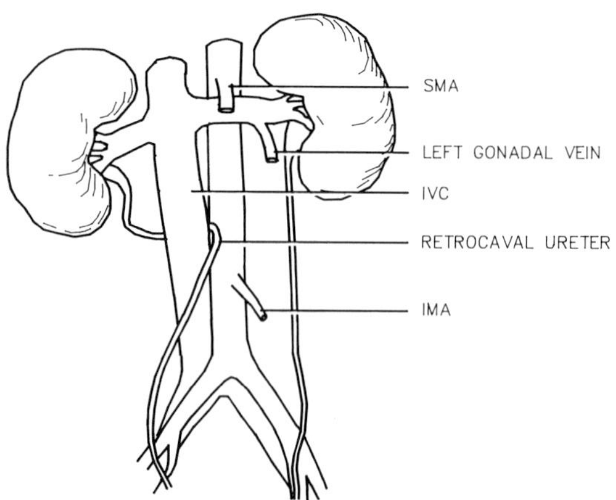

FIGURE 4–40. Characteristics of retrocaval ureter. SMA, superior mesenteric artery; IVC, inferior vena cava; IMA, inferior mesenteric artery.

TABLE 4–2. SITES OF ECTOPIC URETER INSERTION

Site	Comments
Female (90%)	
Vestibule (38%) Urethra (32%) Vagina (27%) Uterus (3%) Ovaries, fallopian tubes (0.1%)	In women, ectopic ureteral insertion is associated with ureteral duplication, and usual symptom is incontinence; insertion into ovaries or fallopian tubes occurs only with severe congenital anomalies
Male (10%)	
Posterior urethra (54%) Seminal vesicle (28%) Vas deferens (10%) Ejaculatory ducts (8%)	Present with infection, infertility, obstruction; usually occurs without ureteral duplication
Either Sex (0.1%)	
Rectum	Occurs only with severe congenital anomalies

Adynamic Distal Ureter. Adynamic distal ureter (also called megaureter) occurs when congenital absence of peristalsis in the distal ureter causes functional obstruction. The result is urinary stasis and proximal ureteral enlargement. On excretory urograms, the ureter appears enlarged and obstructed. The abnormality may be unilateral or bilateral. Stasis of urine can lead to infection.

Infection

Most infections of the ureters and the renal pelvis are ascending infections. Many of them are the result of chronic infection and also involve the bladder. These chronic infections are discussed later with infectious disease of the bladder.

Neoplasms

Benign tumors of the ureter and renal pelvis are rare. The most notable is ureteral polyp, which may cause obstruction. Malignant tumors of the renal pelvis and the ureters are transitional and squamous cell carcinomas. The terms "papillary" and "invasive" applied to these tumors relate to pathological diagnosis, not to radiographic appearance.

In the renal pelvis, malignant tumors are usually of the transitional cell type (85%) and appear as small filling defects in an otherwise normal renal pelvis (Fig. 4–41). The less common squamous cell tumor shows more aggressive characteristics, including invasion beyond the renal pelvis. Stones or infection often accompany squamous cell carcinoma. Either type of lesion can be multiple or single, can be bilateral or unilateral, and can show various grades of aggressiveness. Angiograms show that the tumors are avascular.

Tumors of the ureters are usually of the transitional cell type and cause an irregular filling defect. The ureter below the tumor is often dilated, in contrast to the narrowing seen in ureteral stricture. An extraluminal mass can be demonstrated by CT or MRI. Metastatic involvement of the ureters and the renal pelvis occurs by direct spread from retroperitoneal tumors such as lymphoma, carcinoma of the pancreas, carcinoma of the cervix, and colon cancer.

Dilatation and Obstruction

Dilatation of the ureters and the renal pelvis can be nonobstructive or obstructive and is a common diagnostic problem. No treatment is necessary for this condition if there is no obstruction; therefore, nonobstructive causes

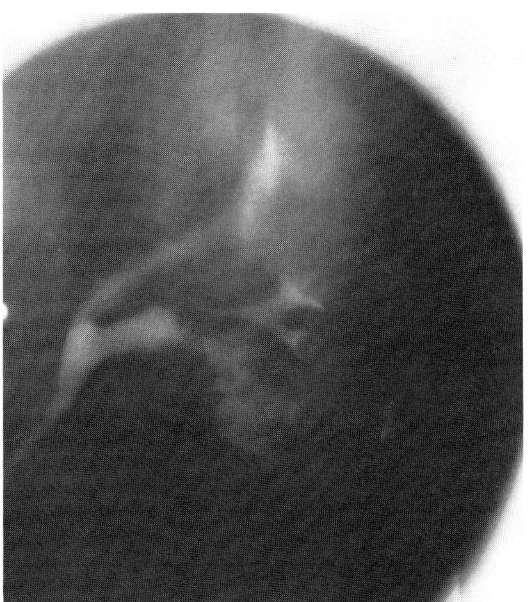

FIGURE 4–41. Transitional cell carcinoma of the renal pelvis. Tomogram from intravenous urogram shows distortion of the renal pelvis and filling defect within the lower-pole collecting system.

should be ruled out first. These include high urine flow, pregnancy, postobstructive atrophy, infection, megaureter (described earlier), and congenital megacalyx (increase in size and number of calyces without associated abnormality). Obstructive causes of dilatation of the ureters and the renal pelvis are tumor (discussed earlier), stone, and stricture. Reflux caused by an incompetent ureterovesical sphincter also can result in dilatation of the ureter and renal pelvis.

Ureteral Stones. Eighty-five percent of ureteral stones are radiodense because they contain calcium compounds, including calcium phosphate and calcium oxalate. A careful search of the plain radiograph of a patient with renal colic often reveals a stone in the expected path of the ureter. Other stones, predominantly cystine, urate, and struvite, are not sufficiently dense to be seen on plain radiographs (see Figs. 3–2 and 4–1). In a patient with suspected renal stones who has not undergone previous radiographic evaluation, an excretory urogram is required for establishing the diagnosis. Usually the point of obstruction can be demonstrated. Treatment is initially conservative. Many patients pass the stone spontaneously with hydration. Surgery or lithotripsy is used when the stone is not passed.

Stricture. Stricture can result from radiation, surgery, trauma, retroperitoneal fibrosis, inflammatory disease, or endometriosis. It usually appears as an irregular narrowing of the ureter on excretory urogram.

BLADDER

Trauma

Bladder injury often occurs with pelvic fracture, usually when the bladder is full. Occasionally, the bladder is ruptured during cystoscopy or transurethral resection of the prostate. Rupture can be extraperitoneal (80%) or intraperitoneal (20%; more common in children). Extraperitoneal extravasation is of no immediate consequence but can eventually lead to infection. Intraperitoneal rupture is an emergency because urinary products accumulate in the systemic circulation. The plain radiograph or cystogram can show the pelvic fracture, free intraperitoneal fluid, and compression of the bladder by hematoma (Fig. 4–42). CT is less reliable for diagnosing bladder rupture.

Chronic injury to the bladder occurs when it becomes obstructed as a result of prostatic hypertrophy or urethral stricture. The bladder enlarges, and the muscle consequently thins. Outpouchings of the bladder can then occur in areas where the muscle is weakest (Fig. 4–43). These outpouchings are called cellules or bladder diverticula.

Congenital Abnormalities

Anomalies of the bladder include patent urachus, urachal cyst, exstrophy, and bladder duplication. Although the urachus becomes a

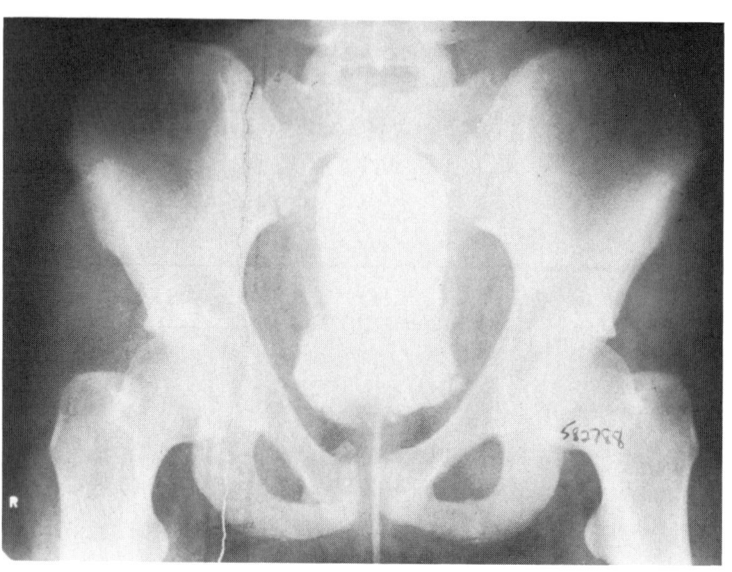

FIGURE 4–42. Bladder rupture. Cystogram shows extravasation of contrast from the filled bladder. Fluid and blood compress the bladder bilaterally. A right pubic ramus fracture is also shown.

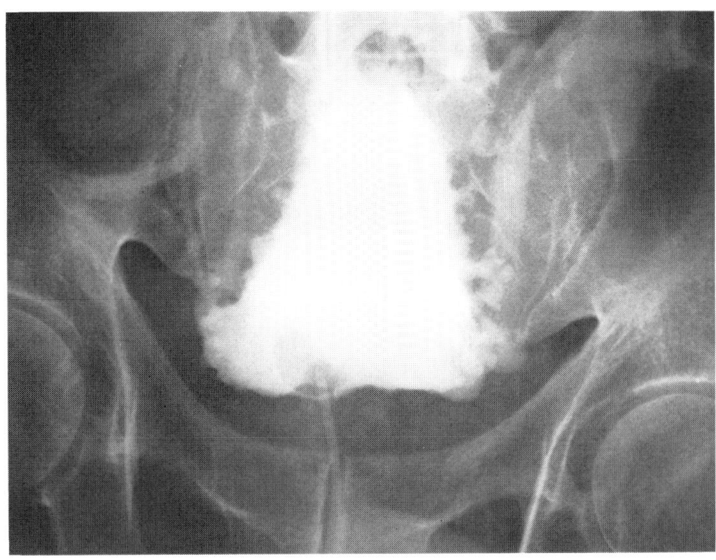

FIGURE 4–43. Bladder diverticula. The bladder is contracted and shaped somewhat like a Christmas tree. Along the lateral margins of the bladder, contrast is seen extending into cellules.

fibrous band in most adults, a persistent lumen lined with transitional epithelium remains in some people. Urachal abnormalities range from free communication between the bladder and the umbilicus to discrete urachal cyst.

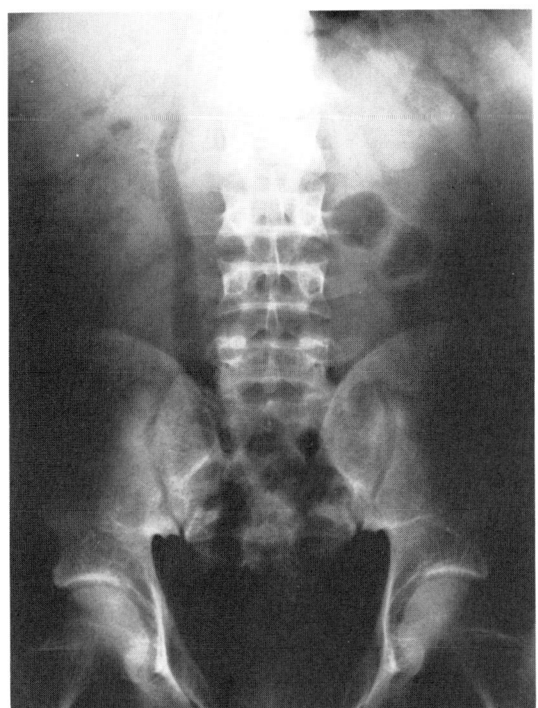

FIGURE 4–44. Exstrophy of the bladder. Abdominal plain film shows separation of the pubic bones as a result of the open midline and the exposed bladder. The mass at the pubic symphysis is the splayed penis (epispadias). The vertical air column to the right of the spine is the ureter, connected to the sigmoid colon by a ureterosigmoidostomy to divert the urine away from the bladder.

Bladder duplication is rare; it varies from formation of two separate bladders to a septated single cavity.

Exstrophy of the Bladder. Exstrophy is a rare anomaly of midline fusion affecting the bladder, the pelvic bones, the abdominal musculature, the penis, and, occasionally, the lower gastrointestinal tract (Fig. 4–44). These structures fail to fuse anteriorly in the midline, leaving an exposed, open bladder. The abdom inal radiograph shows outward rotation of the iliac bones, separation of the pubic bones, an open bladder, and epispadias. Excretory urograms can show evidence of recurrent renal infection. Patients require urinary diversion because attempts to close the bladder are unsuccessful. Most patients die of renal infection.

Infection

Acute infections of the bladder are usually diagnosed clinically. Radiographic examinations are used to rule out a structural or congenital abnormality or to evaluate possible ascending infection of the kidney. They also are often used to evaluate chronic infections.

Bacterial Cystitis. Bacterial cystitis is usually caused by *Escherichia coli.* It is most common in young girls and can continue into adulthood. The diagnosis is made clinically. An excretory urogram is performed only to rule out a structural lesion.

Chronic Infections of the Renal Pelvis, the Ureters, and the Bladder. Chronic irritation caused by recurrent urinary tract infections can lead to inflammatory disease of the walls of the collecting structures in the renal pelvis, the ureters, and the bladder. The inflammatory response may be cystic, may be associated with histiocytic infiltration, and may be characterized by narrowing and irregularity. Emphysematous cystitis results from infection of the bladder wall by gas-forming organisms, usually *E. coli;* it occurs primarily in diabetic patients. Infection by mycobacteria and fungi generally affect the kidneys in addition to the ureters and the bladder (discussed earlier).

Schistosomiasis. Schistosomiasis is the most common urinary parasitic infection worldwide; it is particularly prevalent in Africa, western Asia, and southern Europe. It is unusual in the United States. The disease is caused by infestation of pelvic veins by *Schistosoma haematobium.* The organisms enter the pelvic veins and infest the ureters and the bladder. Eggs laid along the bladder wall cause calcification and hyperplasia. The bladder is involved in 85% of cases of urinary tract schistosomiasis. Radiographs show thin calcifications and, in advanced cases, full-thickness fibrosis of the bladder wall.

The ureter is involved in 45% of patients, in whom similar changes of fibrosis and calcification occur. Strictures and obstruction of the ureterovesical junction are common. The results are ureteral obstruction, bladder outlet obstruction, and a shrunken, noncontractile, fibrotic bladder. The infection predisposes the patient to the development of bladder carcinoma, which can be of either squamous cell (75%) or transitional cell (25%) type.

Neoplasms

Benign tumors of the bladder are rare. They include pheochromocytoma, chemodectoma, neurofibroma (in neurofibromatosis), nephrogenic adenoma (metaplastic renal tissue in the bladder), hemangioma, and lymphangioma. Malignant tumors of the bladder are primarily transitional cell type (95%) but also include squamous cell carcinoma (5%).

Bladder Carcinoma. Carcinoma of the bladder is second only to prostate carcinoma as the most common genitourinary tumor. Men are afflicted three times as often as women, and most patients are over 50 years of age. It occurs more often in patients exposed to carcinogens, namely tobacco and aniline dyes. Among patients with chronic bladder infections such as schistosomiasis, there is also a high incidence of bladder cancer. The most common clinical finding is gross hematuria. Tumors near the trigone can cause obstruction.

TABLE 4–3. STAGING OF BLADDER CARCINOMA

Stage	Tumor Location
0	Superficial tumor confined to the mucosa
A	Superficial tumor confined to the submucosa
B	Muscle invasion; superficial (B1) or deep (B2)
C	Extension through serosa or perivesical fat
D	Metastases to local lymph nodes (D1) and to distant nodes or other tissues (D2)

Most bladder carcinomas are of the transitional cell type and commonly occur at the base of the bladder. Involvement may be limited to a papillary intravesicular mass that can be resected cystoscopically, or it may be a full-thickness infiltrating mass of the bladder wall. Both the grade of the tumor (the degree of differentiation) and the stage (extent) of involvement (Table 4–3) influence the course of therapy and the prognosis. The most important therapeutic distinction is between stages B (confined to the bladder wall) and C (local invasion). The radiographic evaluation can quickly determine whether the patient is beyond stage B by showing adenopathy or distant metastases (stage D).

Several imaging techniques are often used in addition to clinical findings and cystoscopy in the evaluation of patients with bladder cancer. The usual radiographic findings are thickening of the bladder wall, a filling defect, and a mass (Fig. 4–45). Radiographic diagnosis of a small, curable lesion or even a full-thickness lesion is difficult because of the normal trabeculation of the bladder wall. Advanced lesions are easily identified. Intravenous urograms can show obstruction and a filling defect, which is best seen on the postvoid film. Ultrasonograms can show an intraluminal mass and abnormal echogenicity of the bladder wall. CT scans can show a mass, bladder wall abnormalities, and extension of the mass to adjacent tissues (Fig. 4–46). MRI, because it can demonstrate soft tissue planes to best advantage, is the best technique for detecting bladder wall invasion (see Fig. 1–24) and is as effective as CT for identifying lymph node involvement, usually involving the obturator and lower periaortic nodes. MRI is also best for detecting distant bone metastases. These latter findings can de-

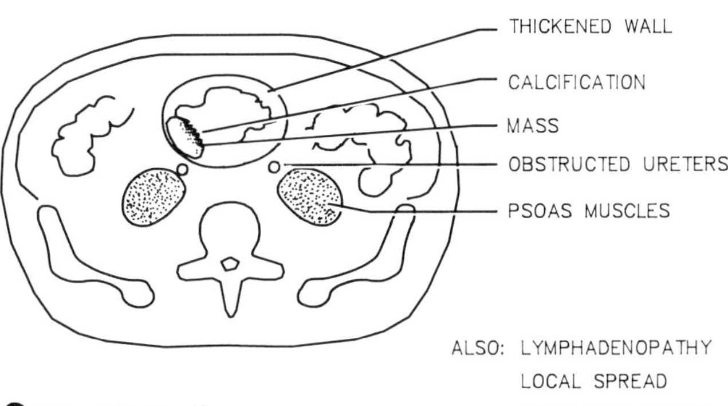

FIGURE 4–45. Characteristics of carcinoma of the bladder.

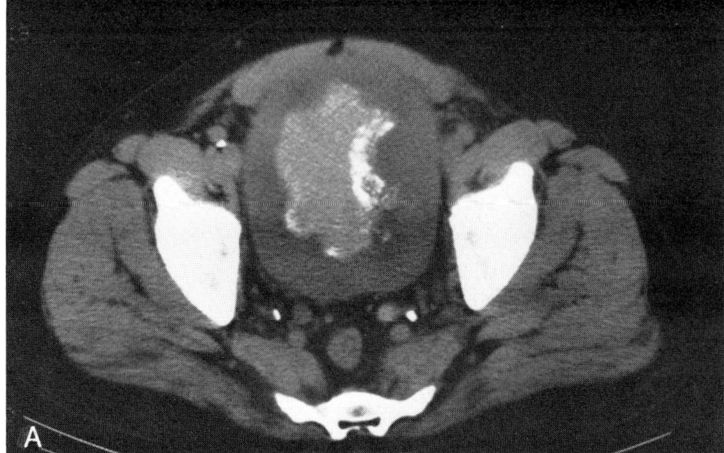

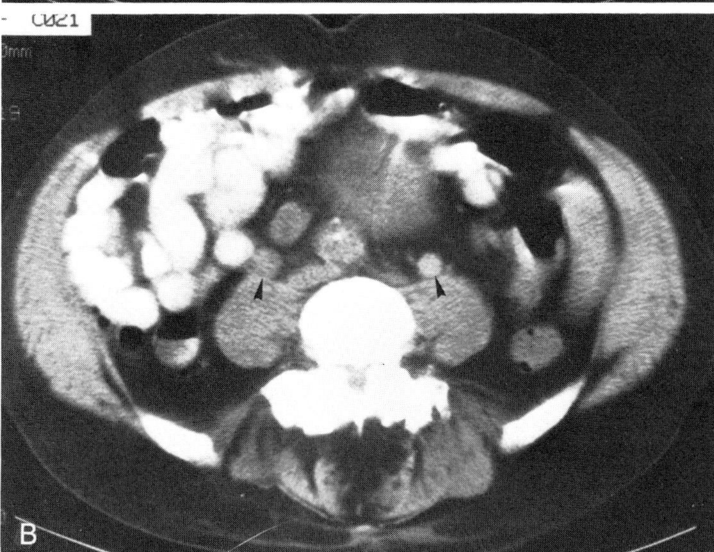

FIGURE 4–46. Transitional cell carcinoma of the bladder. *A.* CT 4 hours after intravenous urography shows thickening of the bladder wall to up to 5 cm and extensive left-sided calcification in this 48-year-old man with hematuria, renal dysfunction, and a pelvic mass. The irregular central cavity of the bladder is shown by the contrast material from the intravenous urogram. Numerous obturator nodes are shown lateral to the internal iliac vessels. *B.* Higher slices show the dilated, obstructed ureters (*arrowheads*), just anterior to the psoas muscles. (Courtesy of B. Porter, First Hill Diagnostic Imaging Center, Seattle.)

tect stage D disease and eliminate uncertainty regarding local perivesical extension of the tumor.

Prognosis depends on the grade of the tumor and the stage of involvement. Intravesical lesions often can be totally removed cystoscopically. More invasive lesions are difficult to resect. The radiographic examination is therefore critical for therapy planning.

Other, less common tumors of the bladder are squamous cell carcinoma (about 5% of bladder tumors) and metastatic tumors to the bladder, including melanoma (most common) and stomach, breast, kidney, and lung carcinomas. Squamous cell carcinoma is indistinguishable radiographically from transitional cell carcinoma and carries a very poor prognosis.

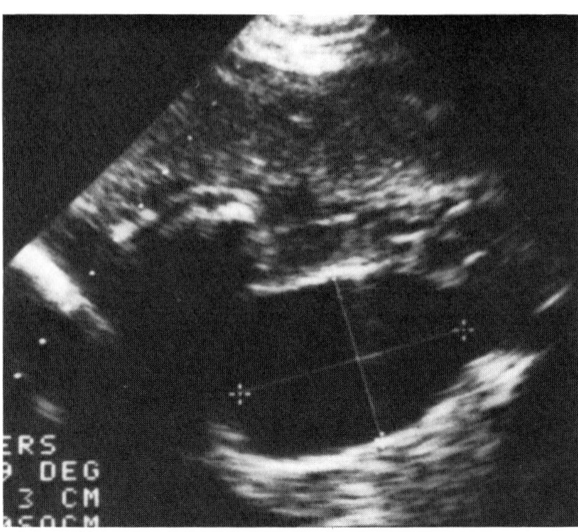

FIGURE 4–48. Urethral valves. Longitudinal in utero ultrasonogram shows the distended bladder, caused by urethral valves.

URETHRA

Trauma

Urethral injury can involve the prostatic, membranous, or penile portions (Fig. 4–47; see also Fig. 4–2) and can result from pelvic fracture, blunt injury, or catheterization. Any patient suspected of having a urethral injury (inability to void, blood at the meatus) should first be evaluated by means of retrograde urethrography. The injury can range from a partial tear, demonstrated by minor extravasation, to complete transection. The treatment of urethral injuries is controversial; some surgeons advocate early, and some late, repair.

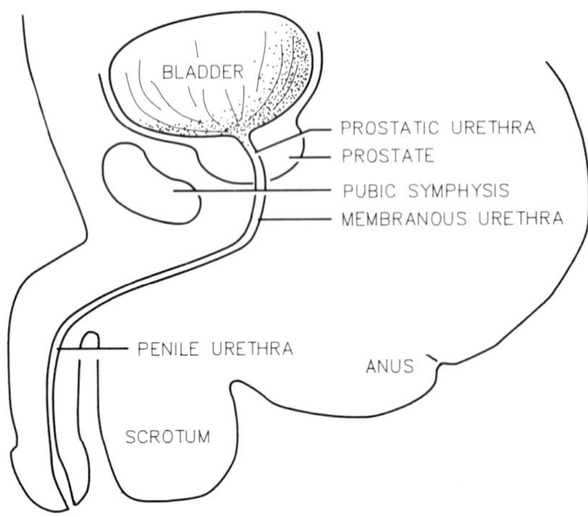

FIGURE 4–47. Anatomical structure of the urethra with sites of extravasation.

Congenital Abnormalities

Valves and Diverticula. Valves and diverticula of the urethra can cause urinary obstruction in the developing fetus and, consequently, renal destruction, abdominal distention, and diminished development of the thorax. Such obstruction can be diagnosed in utero by ultrasonographic demonstration of the paucity of amniotic fluid (oligohydramnios) and the presence of a large, fluid-filled, thick-walled fetal bladder and hydronephrosis (Fig. 4–48). Therapeutic shunting can relieve the obstruction in utero. Diverticula of the urethra can also compress and obstruct the normal urinary channel.

Müllerian Duct Remnants. Müllerian duct remnants in males are rare. The most common are pelvic cysts and an enlarged prostatic utricle. The müllerian duct cyst occurs in the midline at the base of the bladder adjacent to the trigone. It lies above the prostate and is connected to it by fibrous material. It may communicate with the urethra. Patients may have dysuria or obstruction. This cyst can be detected on cystograms or ultrasonograms. CT scans may show the midline cyst attached to the base of the bladder. An abnormally large prostatic utricle (the analog of the uterine cavity) is always associated with undescended testis and hypospadias.

Neoplasms

Tumors of the urethra are rare but can occur anywhere along its course. They include squamous cell carcinoma (70%), transitional cell carcinoma (30%), and adenocarcinoma (rare). Urethral tumors are more common in women than in men (5:1). They are difficult to diagnose in women because of the difficulty in evaluating the urethra. Bleeding and obstruction are the most common signs. Retrograde urethrography and voiding cystography can show irregularity, narrowing, and extravasation, but these findings are not specific for the tumor. The diagnosis is usually made by means of biopsy.

ADRENAL GLANDS

Overview

The adrenal glands are located within Gerota's fascia. They form separately from the kidney and are usually in normal position despite genitourinary anomalies. The adrenal cortex produces steroids (glucocorticoids and mineralocorticoids). The adrenal medulla, derived from chromaffin cells, produces sympathomimetics. The adrenal cortex is controlled by the pituitary gland, and so pituitary abnormalities must be considered when abnormalities of adrenocorticotropic hormones (ACTH) are encountered. The normal adrenal glands are best demonstrated with CT, which shows a tadpole- or trefoil-shaped gland anterior, superior, and medial to the kidneys (Fig. 4–49; see also Fig. 3–10). Large adrenal masses can be seen on excretory urogram or ultrasonogram, but CT is the best method for detecting and characterizing them. In general, the contour rather than the size of the adrenal gland is used to evaluate disease. Most adrenal abnormalities do not enhance, in comparison with enhancement of the normal kidneys and the inferior vena cava. Calcification can be seen as a result of previous infection, hemorrhage, or tumor.

Small adrenal masses, less than 3 cm in diameter, most likely represent adenomas, whereas lesions larger than 5 cm in diameter likely represent malignant tumors. Because the adrenal glands are frequently the site of metastasis, they are routinely examined in patients with pulmonary malignancies. Overall, CT is somewhat more informative than MRI for adrenal evaluation; both methods are relatively nonspecific.

Trauma

The adrenal glands are protected deep in the abdomen. They are surrounded by fat and are deep to the kidneys. They are therefore seldom injured in blunt trauma. Other injuries to the kidneys, the vessels, or the upper abdominal organs are always more severe.

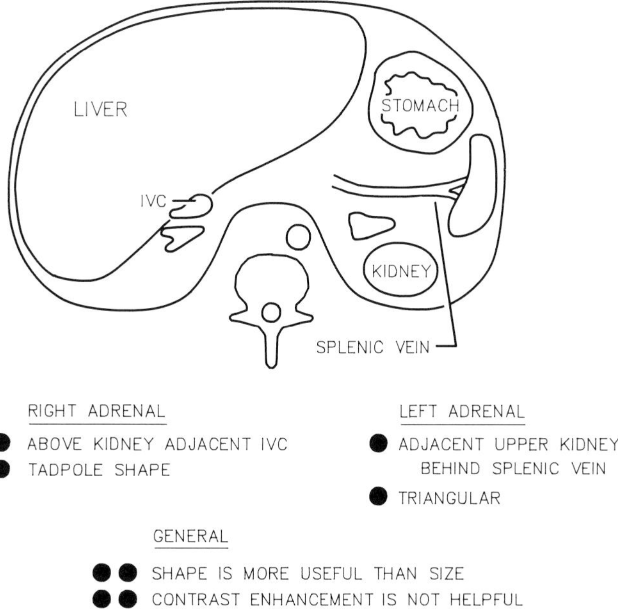

FIGURE 4–49. Adrenal gland anatomy. IVC, inferior vena cava.

Congenital Abnormalities

Congenital lesions of the adrenal glands are rare. Even in the case of genitourinary anomalies, such as renal agenesis, the adrenal glands are usually in the normal location (see Fig. 4–16*A*).

Systemic (Endocrine) Disease

The most important hormones secreted by the adrenal gland are cortisol, aldosterone, and epinephrine. Endocrine diseases affecting the adrenal glands include pituitary hypersecretion or hyposecretion of ACTH and hypersecretory states of the adrenal medulla.

Cushing's Syndrome. Cushing's syndrome is the overproduction of cortisol by the adrenal glands, which results in changes in body habitus, fat distribution, hair growth, muscle strength, glucose tolerance, bone mineralization, and mood. In most cases (85%) the cause is adrenal hyperplasia, the result of excessive secretion of ACTH by the pituitary gland. This excess is usually caused by a pituitary adenoma. Primary adrenal adenoma and primary adrenal carcinoma are much less common causes of Cushing's syndrome in adults but are the main causes of the syndrome in children. Ectopic ACTH production by tumors of the lung (especially oat-cell carcinoma), the kidneys, and the pancreas cause a small number of cases of Cushing's syndrome.

When Cushing's syndrome is caused by adrenal hyperplasia, the diagnosis is strongly supported by biochemical abnormalities and response to administration of ACTH and steroids. CT scans show diffusely enlarged adrenal glands bilaterally without focal bulges (Fig. 4–50). No contrast enhancement is demonstrated. In an elderly patient, a chest radiograph should be obtained in order to rule out a lung tumor. Also, CT evaluation of the kidneys and pancreas can rule out an ACTH-secreting tumor.

Adrenal Hyposecretion. Adrenal hyposecretion (Addison's disease) usually causes no detectable adrenal abnormality because smallness of the adrenal glands is considered a variation of normal.

Infection

Infection of the adrenal gland is uncommon. Usually, other organs are affected more severely. However, septicemia caused by pyogenic organisms, particularly meningococci (meningococcemia), can result in life-threatening infection of the adrenal gland. The richly vascularized adrenal medulla can rupture and cause fatal hemorrhage (Waterhouse-Friderichsen syndrome). After such an event, calcification in the adrenal gland may be visible on plain films. Histoplasmosis and tuberculosis affect the adrenal gland but not without affecting other parts of the body. Radiographs are seldom obtained for evaluating adrenal infection.

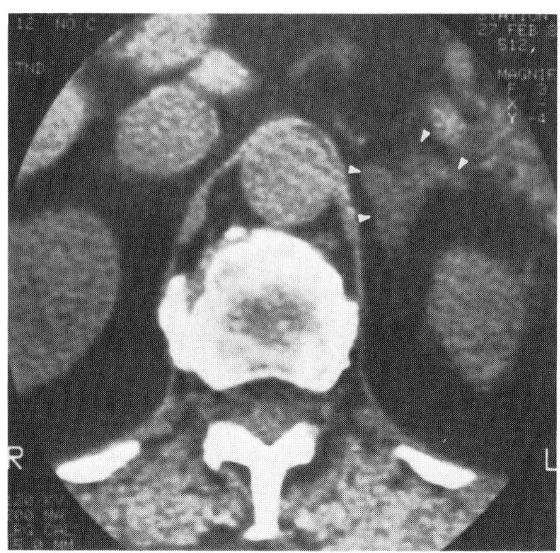

FIGURE 4–50. Adrenal hyperplasia. Noncontrast CT shows diffuse enlargement of the left adrenal gland, which maintains its triangular shape (*arrowheads*). The right adrenal gland was similarly enlarged as a result of an ACTH secreting pituitary adenoma.

Neoplasms

Tumors of the adrenal gland manifest as palpable masses or as a clinical syndrome related to endocrine disturbance. CT best identifies these tumors by demonstrating a focal mass, but this finding does not usually help establish a specific diagnosis. Most adrenal masses are isodense or of low density on CT scans and are not enhanced with intravenous contrast material. Knowledge of whether the lesions are unilateral or bilateral (Table 4–4) can assist in narrowing the differential list of possibilities.

In general, adrenal cortical tumors produce symptoms early and are therefore small at the time of detection. Medullary tumors and primary carcinomas are often large at the time of

TABLE 4–4. UNILATERAL AND BILATERAL ADRENAL MASSES

Unilateral
- Adenoma (most common; low density; early symptoms)
- Pheochromocytoma (90%; can have calcification, size 3 to 6 cm)
- Adrenal carcinoma (large mass)
- Metastasis (usually unilateral)
- Neuroblastoma

Bilateral
- Hyperplasia
- Pheochromocytoma
- Histoplasmosis (usually with calcification)
- Tuberculosis
- Metastases (from lung and breast carcinomas and from melanoma)
- Lymphoma
- Hemorrhage

detection. When the mass is large, it can be difficult or impossible to determine whether the tumor arises from the liver, the kidney, the spleen, or other adjacent organs. Ultrasonography or MRI may help establish such a distinction. The most important primary adrenal tumors are pheochromocytoma, neuroblastoma, adrenal cortical adenoma, and adrenal carcinoma. Tumor metastases from lung carcinoma are common.

Pheochromocytoma. Pheochromocytoma is a tumor of the adrenal medulla that secretes norepinephrine, epinephrine, and other catecholamines. Hypertension, headache, weight loss, and decreased gastrointestinal motility are the most common signs and symptoms. Pheochromocytoma accounts for 1% of cases of hypertension.

Diagnosis is often suggested by clinical signs and biochemical tests, but CT can demonstrate the adrenal mass (Fig. 4–51). Most pheochromocytomas are large (3 to 6 cm) when detected as inhomogeneously enhancing tumors, 90% of which are unilateral. Calcification and central necrosis may be evident. Large tumors may be difficult to distinguish from the kidney or the liver. MRI can show the tissue of origin by demonstrating the capsule, fat, and tissue planes separating these organs. Arteriography is not usually helpful in the evaluation of pheochromocytoma and could precipitate a hypertensive crisis when the injection of contrast causes secretion of catecholamines. However, intravenous contrast is often used with CT in the evaluation of such lesions without adverse effect. Ninety percent of pheochromocytomas are benign and can be completely resected.

Neuroblastoma. Neuroblastomas are primitive tumors of neural crest cells. Seventy percent arise in the abdomen near the midline; half of these arise in the adrenal medulla. Other sites include the cervicothoracic area (20%), the perispinal area (5%), and the pelvis (5%). Most are detected in children under the age of 6 years from the presence of a flank mass, cutaneous flushing, diarrhea, and, if metastasis has occurred, bone pain.

CT or MRI scans can show a retroperitoneal mass that usually enhances because of hypervascularity (Fig. 4–52). This hypervascularity can be detected on angiograms. Microscopic

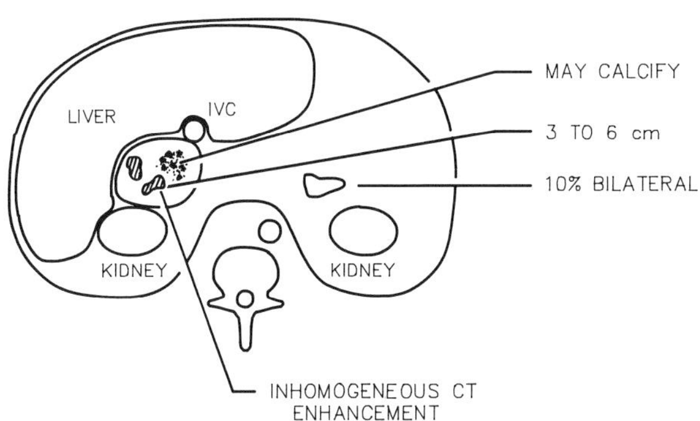

FIGURE 4–51. Characteristics of pheochromocytoma. IVC, inferior vena cava; GI, gastrointestinal.

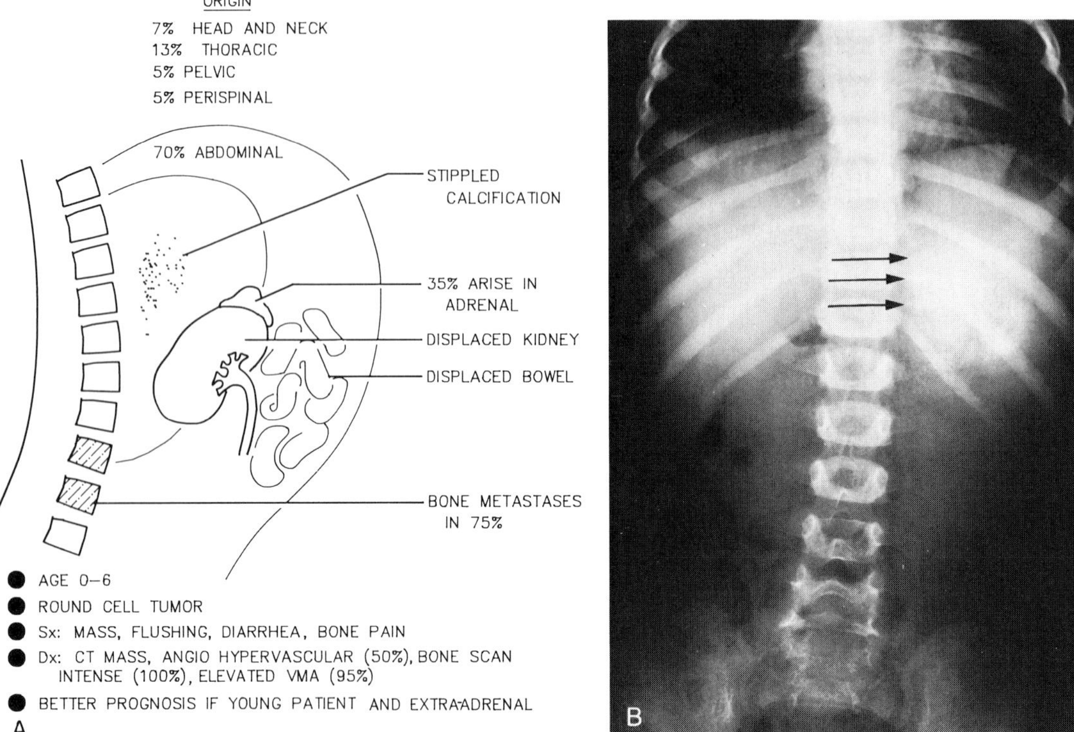

FIGURE 4–52. Neuroblastoma. *A.* Diagram. Sx, symptoms; Dx, diagnosis; VMA, vanillylmandelic acid level. *B.* Plain film shows a vague left upper quadrant mass (*arrows*) in a young child.

calcification is common in neuroblastomas, and thus many such lesions are shown on technetium 99m phosphate nuclear medicine images. These images also show bone metastases. Both neuroblastomas and pheochromocytomas can be detected on nuclear medicine scans through the use of iodine 131 metaiodobenzylguanidine. This radiopharmaceutical agent has an affinity for tumors of neuroectodermal origin. Prognosis of neuroblastoma is best if the patient is young (birth to 2 years of age) and the tumor is extra-adrenal.

Adrenal Carcinoma and Cortical Adenoma. Adrenal carcinoma is rare and can affect any

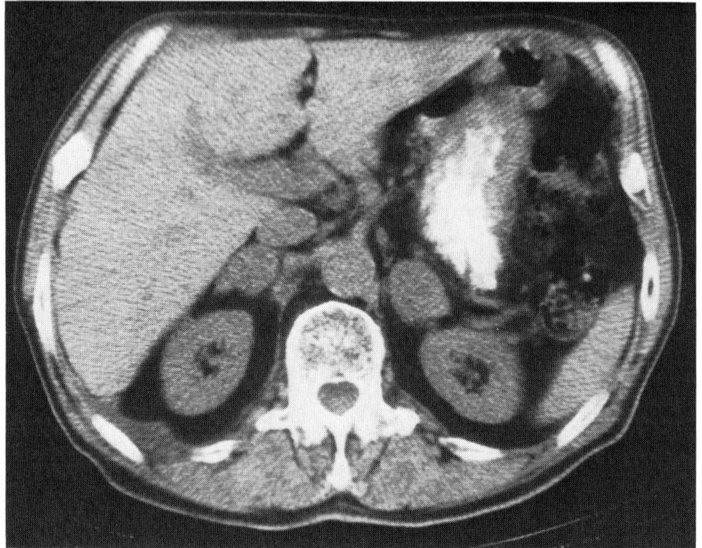

FIGURE 4–53. Bilateral adrenal metastases. Noncontrast CT of an 82-year-old man with lung carcinoma (shown on chest CT in Fig. 2–67) shows bilateral adrenal masses. The masses are inhomogeneous, and their outline is slightly irregular.

type of cell in the gland. Primary adrenal carcinomas are always unilateral, and most are large (more than 6 cm in diameter) when detected.

The adrenocortical adenoma is a rare, benign tumor, usually discovered incidentally. A functioning adenoma can cause an increase in levels of corticosteroids.

Metastatic Tumor. The most common tumors of the adrenal glands are metastases from lung carcinoma. These metastases are often bilateral and do not enhance with intravenous contrast (Fig. 4–53). When the tumor mass is unilateral or shows irregular outlines, malignancy can be distinguished from adrenal hyperplasia (see Fig. 4–50). CT evaluation for lung carcinoma should include scans of the adrenal gland. Metastases also arise from breast carcinoma and melanoma.

Part II
The Genital System

MALE GENITAL SYSTEM

CT and MRI scans enable the organs of the male genital system to be identified easily and usually enable disease to be located within one of these organs. The more important and most common diseases involve the prostate. Infectious prostatitis is a chronic process that is difficult to treat. In elderly patients, the prostate is affected by benign hyperplasia and malignant carcinoma, both of which cause obstruction of the bladder outlet. Symptoms and signs of such obstruction include frequency of, urgency of, and difficulty in urination. Such chronic obstruction can result in injury to the bladder and the kidneys (Table 4–5). In the testicles, a variety of mass lesions can develop; they are most easily evaluated clinically but can be imaged effectively by ultrasonography and MRI.

Prostate

The prevalence of prostatic carcinoma requires accurate screening and staging techniques. Transrectal ultrasonography, CT, and MRI are all applied, along with clinical tests. The radiographic diagnosis is based in part on the location of a mass. The prostate is divided into three zones: central, transitional, and peripheral. The central zone is cone-shaped, being widest at the bladder base and narrower inferiorly. This zone occupies 20% of the prostate in young men and decreases in size with age. The transitional zone occupies about 5% of the prostate in young men but enlarges in

TABLE 4–5. GENITOURINARY ABNORMALITIES CAUSED BY BLADDER OUTLET OBSTRUCTION

Early
Hypertrophy of detrusor muscle
Trabeculation of bladder wall
Formation of diverticula
Ureteral obstruction
Late
Muscular dysfunction
Urinary stasis
Hydronephrosis
Renal infection

older men, resulting in benign prostatic hyperplasia. Carcinoma usually arises in the peripheral zone. On ultrasonograms, carcinoma is usually hypoechoic but may be hyperechoic or isoechoic with the normal prostate.

On MRI, the zonal anatomical structure of the prostate is shown on T2 spin echo and STIR images as a bright signal in the peripheral zone and a lower signal intensity in transitional and central zones. Anterior and lateral to the prostate is the periprostatic plexus that also shows intense signal. On T1 spin echo images, the prostate is relatively homogeneous. Benign prostatic hypertrophy usually shows a mixed, intermediate to high signal in an enlarged transitional zone. However, this condition may be difficult to distinguish from malignancy, which has similar MRI intensity.

Infection

Prostatitis. Inflammatory disease of the prostate is common and can be caused by bacterial, tuberculous, and fungal organisms. In chronic prostatitis, calcification within the prostate can be seen on plain films and CT scans. Tuberculosis can affect the prostate, the epididymis, and the seminal vesicles. Retrograde urethrography and voiding cystoureterography are helpful in evaluation of these types of involvement.

Neoplasms

Benign Prostatic Hyperplasia. The most common cause of obstruction of the bladder outlet in men is prostatic hyperplasia, an apparently normal aging process in which the transitional zone of the prostate enlarges, causing compression of the prostatic urethra. The condition develops in most men over the age of 50. Outlet obstruction results in progressive bladder dysfunction and, eventually, renal damage, unless the obstruction is alleviated.

The effects of the obstruction and the enlarged prostate can be demonstrated well on excretory urography and cystography. Findings associated with benign prostatic hyperplasia are a mass at the base of the bladder (the hyperplastic prostate), bladder trabeculation, the formation of bladder diverticula, and a large postvoid residual (Fig. 4–54). CT and ultrasonography can be helpful in the evaluation of prostatic hyperplasia or tumors that spread from adjacent organs to invade the prostate. MRI may facilitate the determination of the site of the mass, whether other organs are infiltrated, and possibly the tissue of origin, enabling the distinction between hyperplasia and tumor to be made. Benign prostatic hyperplasia is effectively treated by transurethral resection of a portion of the gland. It has no malignant potential.

Prostate Carcinoma. Carcinoma of the prostate is one of the most common tumors of elderly men (aged 60 to 80) and affects a large proportion (25%) of men over the age of 70. It is commonly found incidentally in scrapings from transurethral resection of the prostate. Occasionally, it is found in younger men (aged 40 to 50) in whom the tumor appears to be more aggressive and invasive. The cause of the tumor is not known, but its growth is strongly

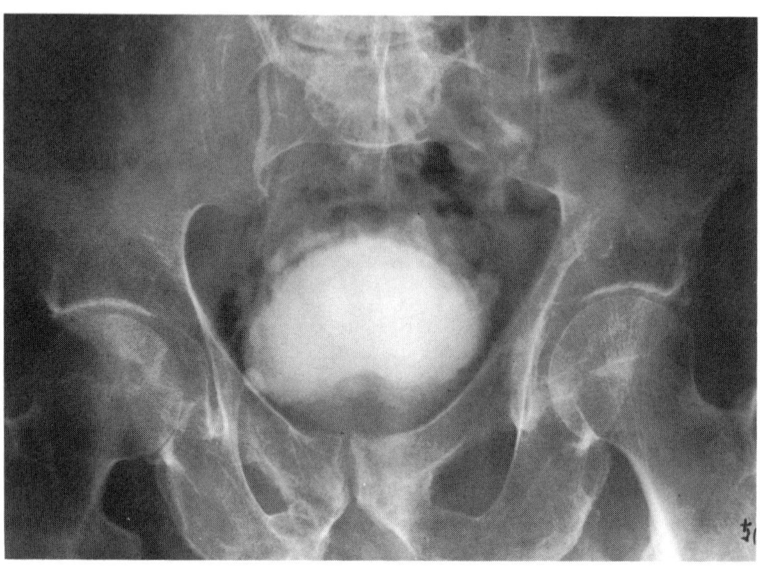

FIGURE 4–54. Prostatic hyperplasia. Excretory urogram shows indentation of the inferior bladder as a result of prostatic enlargement in an older man.

influenced by androgens. The tumor is an adenocarcinoma. In staging, a classification similar to that of bladder carcinoma is used. The most important distinction is whether the tumor is confined to the gland. Patients with microscopic disease are asymptomatic. Patients with advanced disease develop urinary obstruction or infection. The prostate-specific antigen can indicate the presence of prostatic carcinoma in patients with microscopic or advanced disease. Serum acid phosphatase levels are usually elevated when tumor has spread beyond the prostatic capsule.

Radiographic evaluation depends on the extent of the tumor. Local disease, suggested by a prostatic nodule and an elevated level of prostate-specific antigen, is initially evaluated with transrectal ultrasonography, which provides comprehensive evaluation of the prostate. This method enables small lesions to be identified and allows guided needle biopsy for tissue diagnosis. In advanced disease, diagnostic tests focus on the findings of bladder outlet obstruction and on the identification of the prostatic mass, local invasion, adenopathy, and distant metastases. CT and MRI scans can show the mass and invasion of the bladder and the pelvic lymph nodes (Fig. 4–55). Large masses can be demonstrated by cystography, CT, and MRI.

Local invasion can be suspected when the margin between the levator ani (which passes from the pubic bone past the prostate and forms a sling around the rectum) and the prostate is indistinct. Further lateral extension is shown when the tumor is continuous with the internal obturator muscle. Enlargement, change of tissue density or intensity, and effacement of margins of the seminal vesicles also suggest local invasion. Local invasion is well shown by CT scans, but MRI is more effective because it shows soft tissue planes more clearly.

Staging of prostate carcinoma is greatly facilitated by CT and MRI. Adenopathy from prostate carcinoma initially develops near the gland in the obturator and iliac nodes. Spread above the aortic bifurcation indicates advanced disease. Both MRI (especially STIR sequences) and CT show adenopathy well. The identification of metastasis is important because it eliminates uncertainty over local pen-

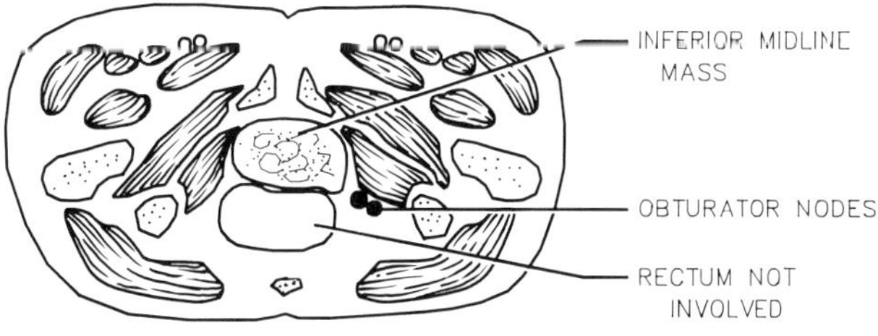

- ASSOCIATED WITH HORMONES
- SYMPTOMS OF URINARY OBSTRUCTION
- ADENOCARCINOMA
- ELEVATED SERUM ACID PHOSPHATASE IN ADVANCED DISEASE

A

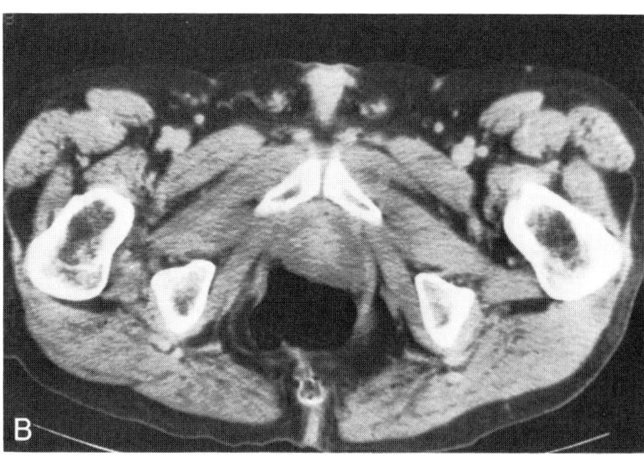

FIGURE 4–55. Prostate carcinoma. *A.* Diagram. *B.* Contrast CT shows a large mass anterior to the air-filled rectum and inferior to the bladder in a 75-year-old man. The margins between the prostate and the levator ani are indistinct, which indicates extension to the seminal vesicles. (Courtesy of B. Porter, First Hill Diagnostic Imaging Center, Seattle.)

etration of the prostatic capsule. Plain films, MRI scans, and bone scans can show the sclerotic bone metastases.

Treatment methods include surgery, radiation therapy, and hormonal chemotherapy. Because prostate carcinoma occurs deep in the pelvis, it is difficult to treat without affecting urinary and sexual function. The prognosis depends on the extent of disease at the time of diagnosis and on the grade of the tumor. Patients with localized disease have a good prognosis. Unfortunately, many men have incurable lesions at the time of diagnosis; many are not candidates for radical therapy because of their age. Patients with metastatic disease die of extensive bone marrow disease, despite local control of the tumor.

Testis

Mass lesions in the testis range from benign cystic collections to the most highly malignant of all carcinomas. Therefore, several conditions must be suspected when an abnormal mass is found in the scrotum. Most of these conditions can be differentiated from each other and, in particular, from carcinoma by clinical and ultrasonographic examinations (Fig. 4–56). MRI can show the location of the lesion and indicate whether it is cystic, solid, or vascular. The most common lesions are carcinoma, traumatic contusion, torsion, varicocele, and hydrocele.

Trauma

Injury to the testis includes contusion from blunt force, compression from hematoma, torsion of the spermatic cord, and laceration. Contusion of the testis is associated with severe pain but does not require imaging tests or surgical treatment unless laceration results in hemorrhage. Torsion of the spermatic cord can cause a testis to become strangulated and nonfunctional if not corrected within 2 hours. Diagnosis of traumatic injury is usually made from clinical history, physical examination, and nuclear medicine perfusion studies. Routine and Doppler ultrasonography can demonstrate parenchymal injuries, fluid collections, and poor blood flow.

Inflammation

Epididymitis. Inflammation of the epididymis is caused by prostatitis (the most common cause), transurethral surgery, and reflux of urine down the vas deferens. The epididymis becomes swollen and indurated. Although the testis does not become involved, passive congestion and the swelling of the epididymis result in general scrotal enlargement. Patients experience onset of acute, severe pain and a swollen, inflamed testicle. The diagnosis is generally made clinically on the basis of the history of prostatitis or recent transurethral surgery. However, ultrasonography can assist by demonstrating the enlarged, inflamed epididymis. Infiltration of the spermatic cord by a local anesthetic controls the initial phase, after which the prostatitis is treated.

Neoplasms

Benign tumors of the testis are extremely rare. Malignant tumors develop from all of the structural and germ-cell components of the testis. These tumors represent approximately

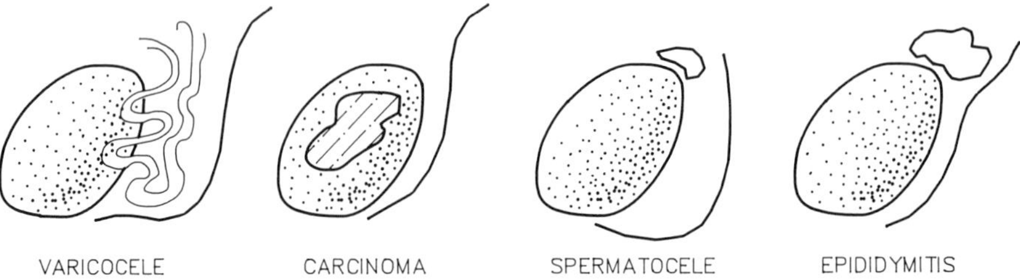

FIGURE 4–56. Types of testicular masses.

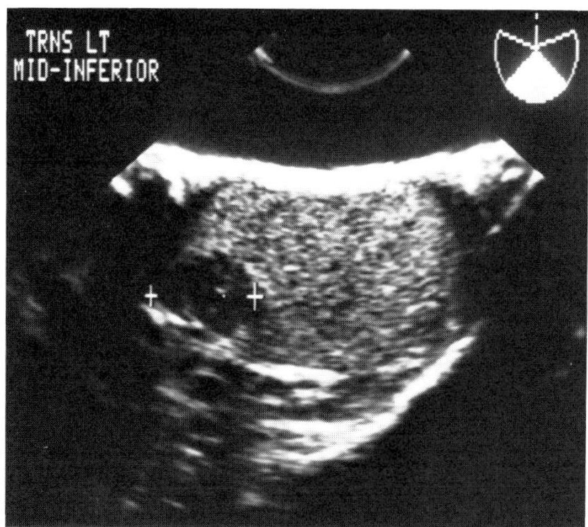

FIGURE 4–57. Testicular carcinoma. Transverse ultrasonogram of the midinferior testis shows a hypoechoic mass lesion in the medial portion of the left testis. This lesion represented metastatic testicular carcinoma from the opposite testis.

1% of all tumors in males and are of several tissue types, ranging from the relatively benign seminoma to the highly malignant embryonal cell carcinomas. Lymphoma may also involve the testis (see Fig. 4–58).

Testicular Carcinoma. Testicular carcinoma is the most common cancer of young men. It is especially common in undescended testes. Cell types include seminoma (40%), which carries a favorable prognosis if detected and treated early, and germ-cell tumors (embryonal carcinoma, teratoma, teratocarcinoma, and choriocarcinoma), which carry a much poorer prognosis. Diagnosis is usually made from findings of clinical examination and surgical excision, but ultrasonography of the testis can be helpful in evaluation of a testicular mass (Fig. 4–57). MRI clearly shows tumor as distinctly different (Fig. 4–58). CT or MRI examination of the abdomen is crucial because the lymphatic drainage from the testis is directly to the level of the kidneys.

Vascular

Varicocele. A varicocele is a dilatation of the pampiniform venous plexus above the testis, usually on the left side, that is caused by incompetent valves. Gravitational force and the more complex drainage into the left renal vein via the left gonadal vein result in dilatation of the veins posterior and superior to the testis. The mass of veins is often painful and becomes distended with the Valsalva maneuver. Clinical examination and ultrasonography reveal a worm-like collection of vessels. If pain, infertility, or testicular atrophy is of concern, a varicocele can be successfully treated by spermatic vein ligation. A new varicocele (especially on the right side) in an adult should raise the suspicion that a tumor is obstructing the renal vein or the vena cava, as in renal cell carcinoma.

Fluid Collections

Hydrocele. A hydrocele is a simple fluid collection within the tunica or the processus vaginalis. Causes include communication with the peritoneal cavity and testicular infection. The symptoms of a hydrocele depend on its cause; a congenital hydrocele is painless. It is detected clinically and ultrasonographically as a fluid collection around the testis (Fig. 4–59). MRI can also clearly show the fluid separately from the testis. If the hydrocele causes com-

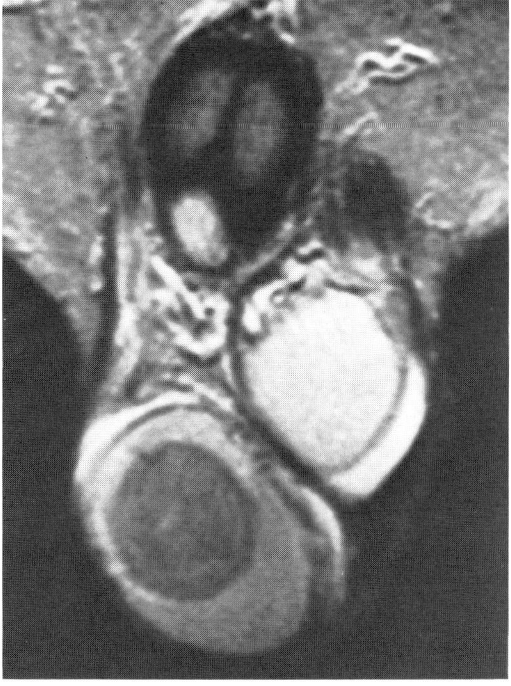

FIGURE 4–58. Testicular lymphoma. T2 spin echo coronal MRI of the testicles shows the corpora cavernosa and the spongiosa in cross-section superiorly. The left testicle has a normal smooth appearance with a small amount of fluid. The right testicle shows a large, well-circumscribed focal central abnormality of low intensity. Surgical removal in the patient, a 64-year-old man, showed large cell lymphoma. (Courtesy of E. Dienes, Venice MRI Center, Venice, Florida.)

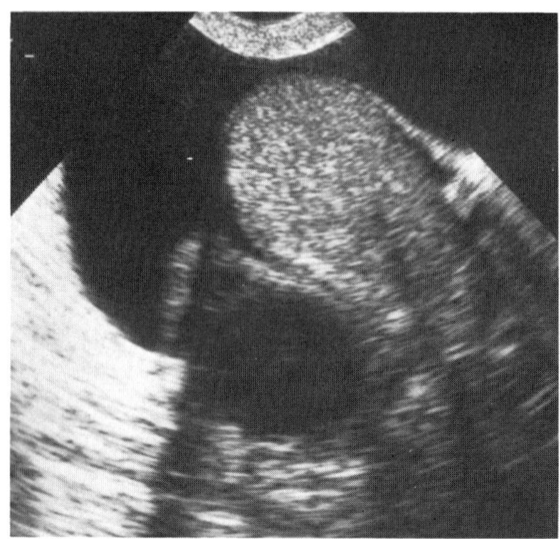

FIGURE 4–59. Hydrocele. Transverse ultrasonogram of the scrotum shows uniform dense echoes of the testis. Posteriorly (on the viewer's left) is a large anechoic hydrocele; note the dense through-transmission, which indicates that this is simple fluid. The hydrocele and dilatation of the epididymis (low echogenicity deep to the testis) were caused by obstruction as a result of prostate surgery.

pression of the testis, it can be aspirated, or the tunica vaginalis can be resected.

FEMALE GENITAL SYSTEM

The female genital organs are best imaged by CT, MRI, and ultrasonography. Disease is usually easily identified by its tissue of origin, although this can be difficult to determine in large lesions. Important diseases involve the uterus, the cervix, and the ovaries. Infectious disease, called pelvic inflammatory disease, is common but difficult to detect unless a well-defined abscess is present. Pregnancy and its complications are important considerations in premenopausal women. Tumors occur in all age groups: they are usually ovarian and cervical neoplasms in younger women and endometrial tumors in older women. The symptoms of pelvic malignancy include pain, uterine bleeding, and effects from compression or invasion of the urinary or alimentary tract.

The most important clinical factors in evaluation are age, the menstrual history, presence or absence of fever, and the result of a sensitive pregnancy test. In young women, masses in the pelvis are usually abscesses, cysts, or pregnancy-related conditions, but ovarian and cervical carcinomas also occur. These conditions cannot always be differentiated by imaging studies, but the radiographic findings together with the clinical findings are usually diagnostic. In a postmenopausal woman, uterine bleeding or a pelvic mass is usually the result of a neoplasm, most commonly uterine leiomyoma (fibroid), endometrial carcinoma, ovarian carcinoma, or cervical carcinoma.

MRI, CT, and ultrasonography are the best radiographic methods for assessing the female reproductive system. In obstetrical evaluation, ultrasonography is used almost exclusively. Transvaginal ultrasonography is more effective than transabdominal ultrasonography for evaluating adnexal masses and early pregnancy because there is less tissue to attenuate the sound beam. Also, because the area of interest is closer to the transducer, the resolution is better.

Interpretation requires an understanding of the anatomical structure of the pelvis in the axial, sagittal, and coronal planes (discussed earlier in the Basic Evaluation section). The most informative view of the uterus is the sagittal projection (Fig. 4–60). The coronal plane provides the best overview of the adnexal region and the lateral pelvis. The objectives of CT and MRI include identifying the organ of origin and showing local invasion;

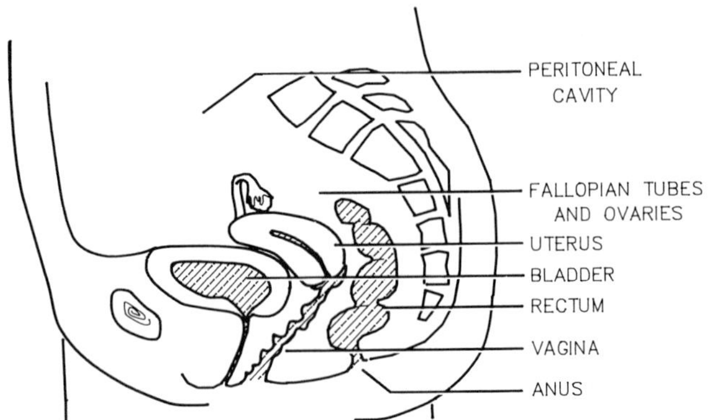

FIGURE 4–60. Female pelvic anatomical structure in the sagittal plane.

adenopathy; involvement of the rectum, the bladder, and the ureters; and distant metastatic spread. In general, solid pelvic lesions are of uterine origin and cystic lesions are of ovarian origin. Advanced tumor and infection are difficult to differentiate because either may cross tissue boundaries. Fluid or blood, adenopathy, bowel contents, and involvement of the omentum cause similar appearances for a tumor or an abscess and limit detailed evaluation by CT and MRI. Evaluation can be particularly difficult in patients whose tumors have been treated surgically or by radiation therapy.

Trauma

The female reproductive organs are rarely injured because they are protected deep within the pelvis. Usually, injuries to these organs accompany more life-threatening injuries to the adjacent pelvic and abdominal organs.

Infection

Tubo-Ovarian Abscess. Tubo-ovarian abscess typically appears in patients who have an intrauterine device, those who have had infection (particularly gonorrhea), or who have had previous bouts of pelvic inflammatory disease. A patient's signs may include only leukocytosis, a slightly elevated erythrocyte sedimentation rate, and a mild fever. The ultrasonographic findings of a variably echogenic pelvic mass and associated fluid in a young woman who is not pregnant are highly suggestive of pelvic abscess (Fig. 4–61). The clinical findings of fever and pain usually differentiate abscess from cystic tumor. Rupture of a tubo-ovarian abscess results in spread of purulent material into the peritoneal cavity, which can lead to fatal peritonitis.

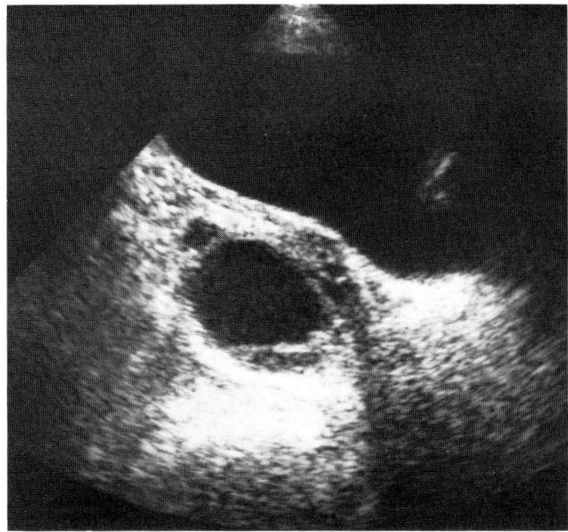

FIGURE 4–61. Tubo-ovarian abscess. Ultrasonogram demonstrates a complex adnexal mass with fluid debris level in pelvic inflammatory disease.

Neoplasms

Endometriosis. Endometriosis, the presence of endometrial tissue outside the uterus, commonly causes symptoms in women 20 to 30 years old. The usual locations of this ectopic tissue are the ovary, the uterosacral ligament and the cul-de-sac, the colon and the rectum, the bladder, and the abdominal cavity; less common sites are the cervix, the vagina, and the pleura. Usually, multiple areas are involved. Patients have pelvic pain, but this is helpful neither for diagnosing nor for locating the abnormality. Symptoms correlate well with the monthly onset of menses. The radiographic appearance of endometriosis depends on which organ is affected. In most cases, the lesions are small, multiple, and not easily distinguished from normal tissue on scans. Lesions near the ovaries are usually bilateral and cystic, and scarring from previous hemorrhage is present. Implants in the uterosacral ligaments are numerous small shot-like masses. Larger lesions near the rectum and the bladder appear as smooth submucosal masses that are indistinguishable from tumor (see Fig. 3–54). In some patients, endometriosis appears as a complex adnexal mass or, in other rare instances, as a constricting lesion of the ureter or as filling defects in the colonic or bladder wall.

Uterine Leiomyoma. Uterine leiomyomas (fibroids) are benign, smooth-muscle tumors of the uterine wall and are the most common pelvic tumors. These tumors, which are usually multiple, develop as focal, intramural, spherical masses (Fig. 4–62). They increase in size in response to estrogen and thus enlarge during pregnancy and involute after menopause. The tumors become fibrotic as a result of atrophic and degenerative changes, and they frequently calcify. Uterine leiomyomas that extend to the broad ligament can compress vessels and ureters, and they are difficult to distinguish from ovarian tumors. Five percent of them involve the cervix. When they enlarge and develop vascular engorgement, they can cause uterine hemorrhage, a complex diagnostic problem in either a pregnant or a nonpregnant woman.

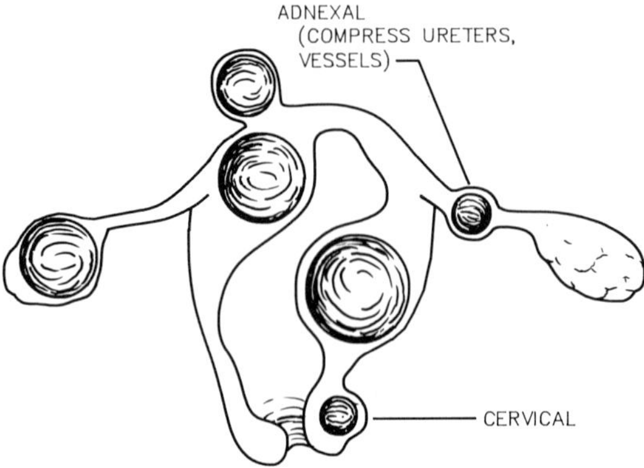

- SMOOTH MUSCLE TUMOR
- LAYERS OF FIBROSIS AND CALCIFICATION
- ALWAYS MULTIPLE
- INCREASE IN SIZE DUE TO ESTROGEN (PREGNANCY)
- RARE TRANSFORMATION TO LEIOMYOSARCOMA

A

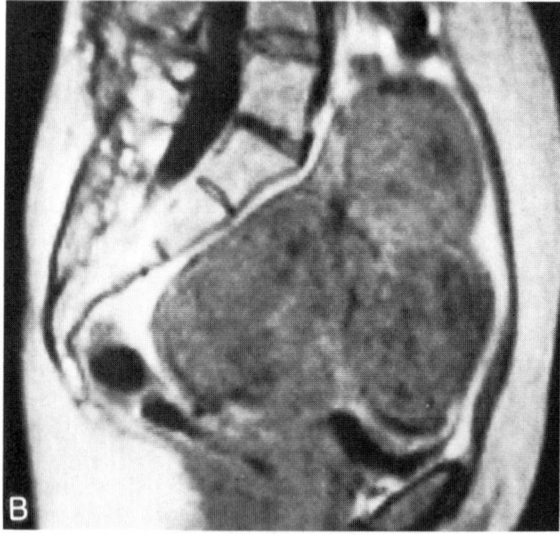

FIGURE 4–62. Uterine leiomyoma. *A.* Diagram. *B.* Sagittal T1 spin echo MRI shows several large round lesions in the pelvis superior and posterior to the bladder (which appears as a black crescent, just above the pubic bone). The patient, a 49-year-old woman, was found on physical examination to have a fixed pelvic mass, shown to be multiple, large uterine leiomyomas. (Courtesy of B. Porter, First Hill Diagnostic Imaging Center, Seattle.)

Most leiomyomas are small and asymptomatic. Pain during menses and pressure on the bladder, the colon, and the small bowel are most common but are not of much assistance in diagnosis.

A uterine leiomyoma appears as a soft tissue or calcified mass on plain films or CT scans and as an area of low echogenicity with poor sound transmission on ultrasonograms. Plain films show a characteristic calcified mass. MRI shows low intensity on T1 and T2 spin echo and STIR sequences because of the fibrosis or the composition of the calcification (Fig. 4–62*B*). The appearance is more complex when hemorrhage or cellular change is present.

Leiomyomas of the uterus are easily separated from surrounding tissue at surgery. Some demonstrate a highly cellular appearance that results in a diagnosis of leiomyosarcoma (Fig. 4–63). These tumors may be degenerating benign tumors or primary malignant sarcomas. They are not as aggressive as sarcomas that arise from other tissues, such as the endometrium.

Dermoid Tumor. The dermoid tumor of the ovary is a common pelvic neoplasm. It can have a variety of appearances, depending on its composition. The major constituent is a semisolid sebaceous material, but matted hair, teeth, and skin are also often present. The solid components usually arise from one portion of the cyst wall. Patients develop pelvic pain as a result of pressure, torsion, or leakage of the liquid contents into the peritoneal cavity. Ultrasonography may demonstrate a characteristic hair-fluid level within the tumor. Ultrasonograms, CT scans, and MRI scans can show the mass and help determine its origin from the ovary. CT scans and radiographs can show teeth or other calcified material. MRI scans show signal characteristics that are distinct from other neoplasms (Fig. 4–64). The tumor is benign, except for rare development of squamous cell carcinoma in one of the elements of the cyst.

Endometrial Carcinoma. The endometrium is the fourth leading site of cancer (after the lungs, the breasts, and the cervix). The tumor is usually an adenocarcinoma, and there is an increased incidence of such tumors among postmenopausal women who have received prolonged estrogen stimulation. It usually arises as a discrete lesion but later penetrates the uterine wall and spreads to the peripelvic tissues. The mass appears similar to muscle on CT scans and appears solid on ultrasonograms. MRI scans show widening of the endometrial cavity or uterine masses that have high-intensity signals on T2 spin echo and STIR images.

The prognosis for endometrial carcinoma is generally good because bleeding occurs early and most lesions are detected in early stages. Lesions arising in the lower third of the uterus are more likely to be squamous cell carcinoma or aggressive adenocarcinoma and carry a poorer prognosis, like that of cervical carcinoma. Metastases from endometrial carcinoma

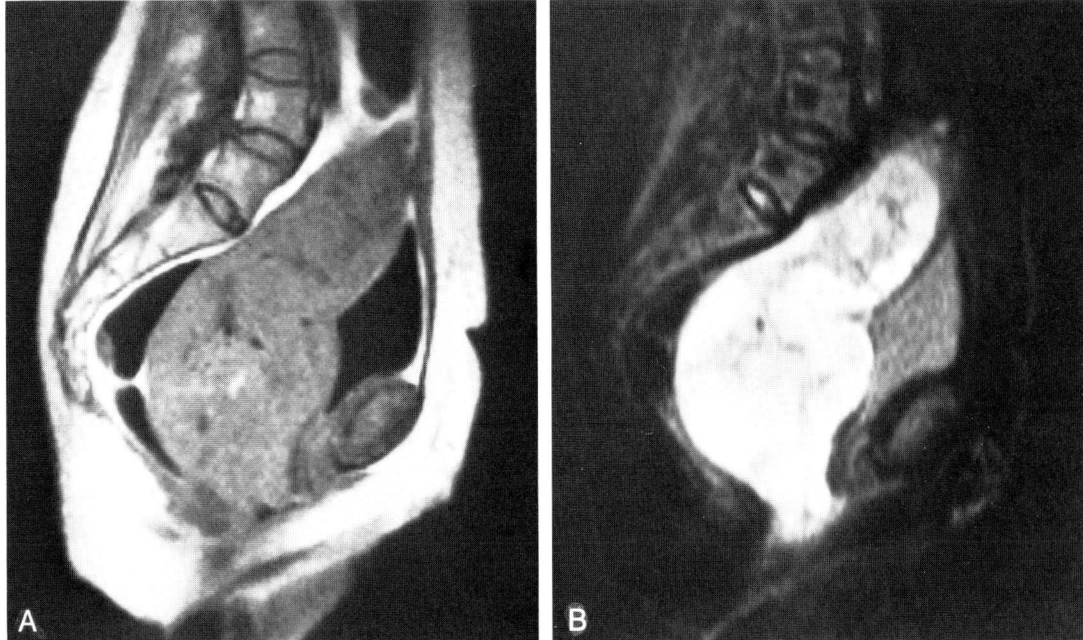

FIGURE 4–63. Leiomyosarcoma. *A.* Sagittal T1 spin echo sequence shows a large uterine mass that includes the cervix and extends superiorly above the bladder in a 74-year-old woman being staged for therapy of a malignant pelvic mass. This image allows clear identification of the rectum posteriorly and the diamond-shaped bladder anteriorly. *B.* Matching STIR image shows extremely high tissue contrast of the tumor, a leiomyosarcoma. (Courtesy of B. Porter, First Hill Diagnostic Imaging Center, Seattle.)

are most often found in the lungs, the liver, the brain, and the bones.

Benign Ovarian Tumors. Benign cystic lesions of the ovary are common. When they contain simple fluid, they are similar to cysts seen elsewhere in the body. Cyst types include follicular cysts and corpus luteum cysts. These appear as well-circumscribed, water-density cysts in the ovaries (Fig. 4–65*A*). There is no contrast enhancement on CT or MRI. Multiple cysts bilaterally can have a complex appearance, designated polycystic ovarian disease

FIGURE 4–64. Ovarian dermoid tumor. Coronal STIR image posterior to the uterus shows a high intensity mass in the right ovary in a 21-year-old woman with an ovarian mass. More anterior slices showed areas of fat and calcification and clearly separated the mass from the cervix and the uterus. (Courtesy of B. Porter, First Hill Diagnostic Imaging Center, Seattle.)

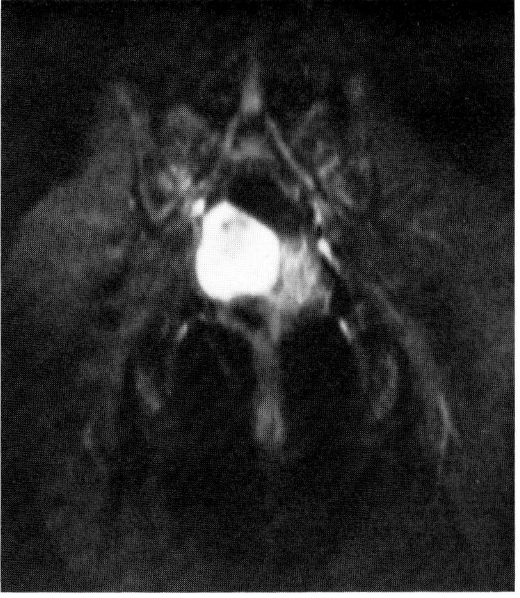

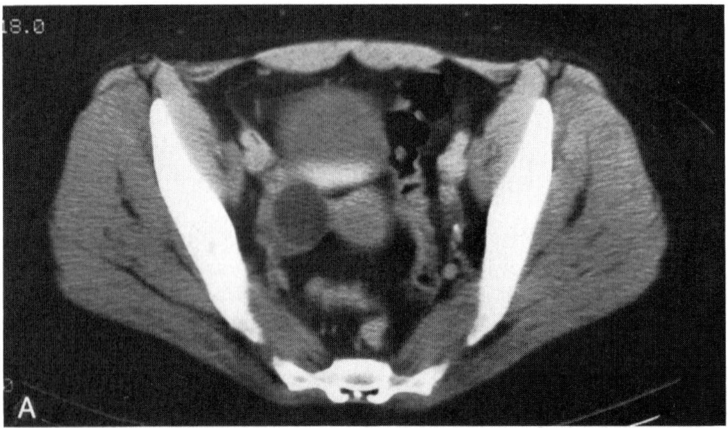

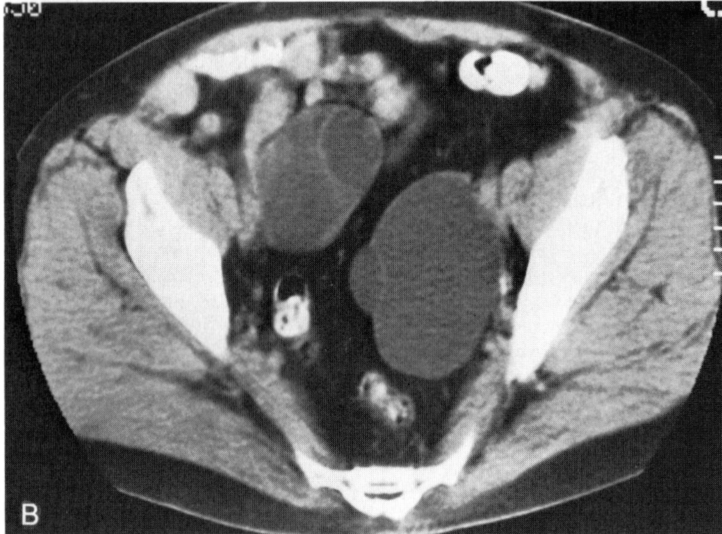

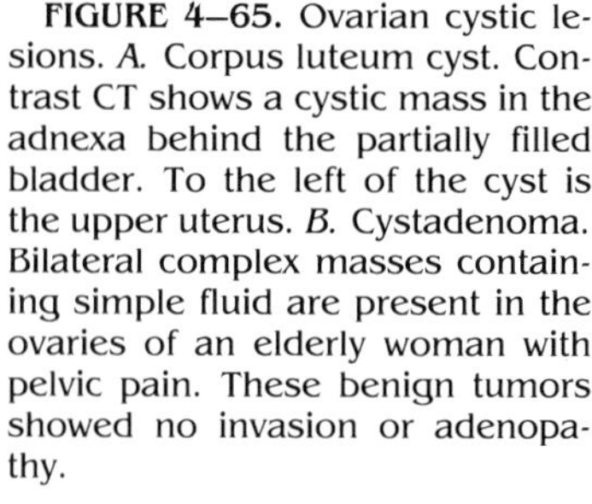

FIGURE 4–65. Ovarian cystic lesions. *A.* Corpus luteum cyst. Contrast CT shows a cystic mass in the adnexa behind the partially filled bladder. To the left of the cyst is the upper uterus. *B.* Cystadenoma. Bilateral complex masses containing simple fluid are present in the ovaries of an elderly woman with pelvic pain. These benign tumors showed no invasion or adenopathy.

(Stein-Leventhal syndrome). Because of the complexity of the cysts, this appearance can be similar to that of malignant ovarian tumors.

A cystadenoma of the ovary is a septated, usually large cystic lesion in one or both ovaries. The serous cystadenoma has water density (Fig. 4–65*B*). These lesions often have multiple septations and may have thick walls. Calcification or a soft tissue component may also be present. The mucinous cystadenoma has a higher density. Because of the complex appearance of these lesions, they are usually indistinguishable from malignant ovarian neoplasms. The absence of adjacent invasion or hemorrhage, of adenopathy, of omental implants, and of distant spread can suggest a benign process. However, an ovarian malignancy could have a similar appearance.

Ovarian Carcinoma. Ovarian carcinomas are among the 10 most common solid malignant tumors and consist of a variety of cell types, the most common being adenocarcinoma. These tumors usually occur in young women and are of various grades of malignancy. Clinical symptoms include weight gain and increasing abdominal girth. In general, these tumors are cystic and usually are extensive at the time of detection (Fig. 4–66). It is not uncommon for bilateral tumors to be present. Important diagnostic findings of advanced disease are mesenteric edema, mesenteric nodularity, omental implants, and abdominal ascites. Treatment is limited; most patients are treated with surgery and chemotherapy.

Cervical Carcinoma. Cervical carcinoma, which constitutes 15% of all cancers in women, is associated with herpes simplex type 2 infection early in life. The virus appears to affect the developing cervix in a way that leads to cancer approximately 30 years later. The mor-

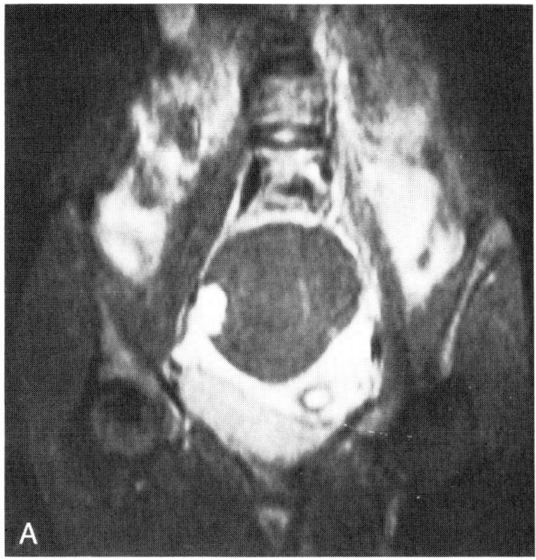

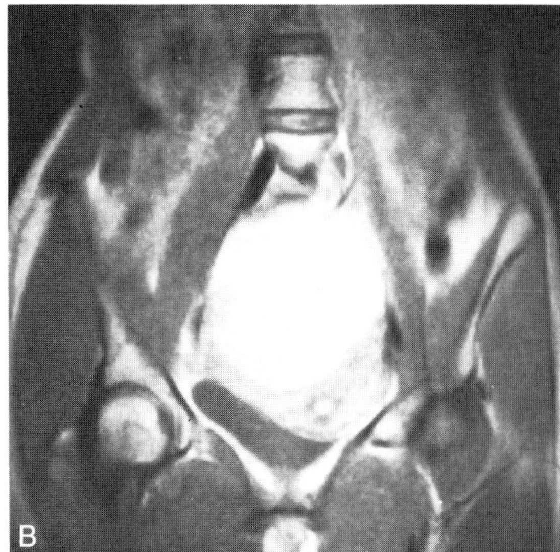

FIGURE 4–66. Ovarian carcinoma. *A.* Coronal STIR image shows a large, round, low-intensity ovarian cyst (intermediate gray) posterior and superior to the bladder in a 33-year-old woman with a pelvic mass. The right-sided focus of high intensity proved to be clear-cell carcinoma of the ovary. *B.* The cyst is of high intensity on T1 spin echo sequences (much higher than that of fat), which indicates the presence of complex fluid containing, in this case, hemorrhage. (Courtesy of B. Porter, First Hill Diagnostic Imaging Center, Seattle.)

bidity and mortality rates of cervical cancer have markedly decreased because of early detection by the pap smear; radiographs are not usually obtained. Most early tumors can be cured. Advanced disease spreads to contiguous structures and invades internal iliac lymph nodes. Distant metastasis is to the lungs, the liver, the brain, and the bones. MRI and CT can be helpful in the assessment of local and distant spread. As with other malignancies in the pelvis associated with pain, compression by tumor mass, and bleeding, symptoms can be alleviated by angiographic embolization of the hypogastric artery.

Obstetrical Conditions and Diseases

Pregnancy. Intrauterine pregnancy is best and most safely assessed through ultrasonography. The earliest ultrasonographic signs of intrauterine pregnancy are generalized uterine enlargement and the presence of a gestational sac. This sac appears as a small, echo-free fluid collection within the uterine cavity and is first seen at 3 weeks of fetal age (5 weeks after the last menstrual period). A yolk sac and a fetal pole, the first identifiable longitudinal views of the fetus, are seen in transvaginal ultrasonograms at 5½ weeks of fetal age. The beating heart, the first evidence that the fetus is alive, can be imaged at about 4 to 5 weeks of fetal age. Pregnancy can be followed to term, and renal, cardiac, gastrointestinal, and central nervous system abnormalities can be diagnosed by means of ultrasonography (Fig. 4–67). The crown-to-rump length and the biparietal and

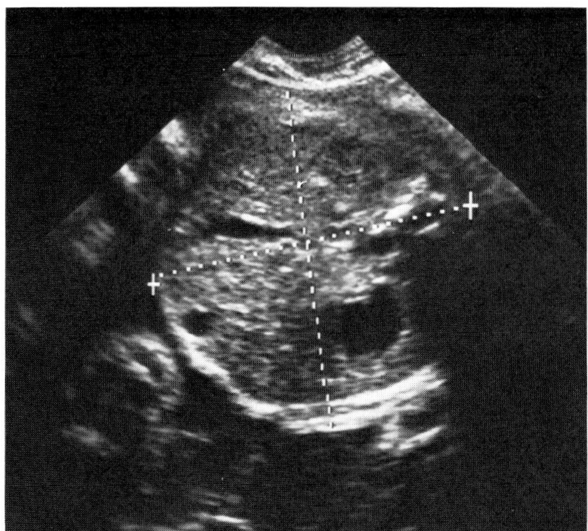

FIGURE 4–67. Fetal abdomen. Transverse ultrasonogram through the fetal abdomen shows low echogenicity in the stomach (lower right), the umbilical vein (lower left), and the linear gallbladder (upper right). High echogenicity is present in the fetal spine (to the viewer's right on the axis). Other views showed a normal heart, kidneys, spine, and placenta. The measurement of the size of the abdomen was concordant with the biparietal diameter.

TABLE 4–6. FETAL AGE ASSESSMENT

Definitions

Biparietal diameter (BPD) = head diameter across the thalami (cm)
CR = crown-to-rump distance (cm)
Gestational age (GA) = no. weeks since last menstrual period
Fetal age (FA) = no. weeks since fertilization
GA = FA + 2 weeks

Calculation of Gestational Age (in Weeks)

= CR (cm) + 6
= BPD (cm) × 4 + 2, if less than 15 weeks
= BPD (cm) × 4 + 1, if between 15 and 20 weeks
= BPD (cm) × 4, if older than 20 weeks

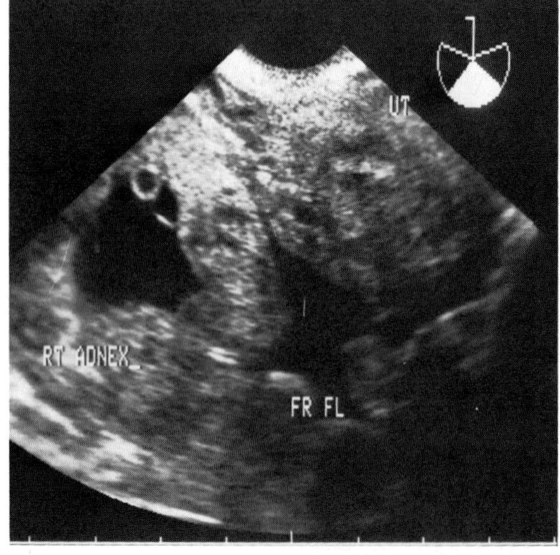

FIGURE 4–68. Ectopic pregnancy. Transverse ultrasonogram shows no evidence of intrauterine (UT) gestational sac in a 33-year-old woman with a positive pregnancy test result. Deep to the uterus, there is fluid or blood in the cul-de-sac (FR FL). The right adnexa (to the viewer's left) shows a ring-shaped area of decidual reaction surrounding the amniotic cavity. A yolk sac is seen superiorly. Other scans showed the 8-week extrauterine fetus.

abdominal diameters of the fetus are the standard measurements, and reliable charts correlate these measurements with fetal age (Table 4–6; see also Figs. 4–4 and 4–5). Assessments of the fetal and placental positions and maturation, as well as the amount of amniotic fluid, are also made by means of ultrasonography. The standard examination also includes assessment for intrauterine growth retardation and fetal anomalies.

Ectopic Pregnancy. Ectopic pregnancy requires early diagnosis because of the risk of fatal hemorrhage. It is most reliably diagnosed through the use of ultrasonography in conjunction with a sensitive pregnancy test and clinical history. Typical ultrasonographic findings are an adnexal mass and absence of an intrauterine pregnancy (Fig. 4–68). Additional findings may include fluid in the cul-de-sac, the identification of the extrauterine gestational sac, the decidual reaction, and endometrial changes.

Hydatidiform Mole. A hydatidiform mole is an abnormal proliferation of chorionic tissue. It occurs at a rate of 1 in 2000 pregnancies in the United States. The usual manifestations are a product of conception too large for the date and hyperemesis gravidarum. The diagnosis in the first trimester is difficult because the mole may have the same ultrasonographic appearance as a degenerating intrauterine pregnancy. By the second trimester, the ultrasonogram shows hydropic villae (Fig. 4–69). Theca-lutein cysts of the ovaries are seen in 20% to 50% of cases. Surgical evacuation of the mass is usually curative, but 3% of these masses become choriocarcinoma. Choriocarcinoma in women responds well to methotrexate. Metastases are to the lungs and the brain.

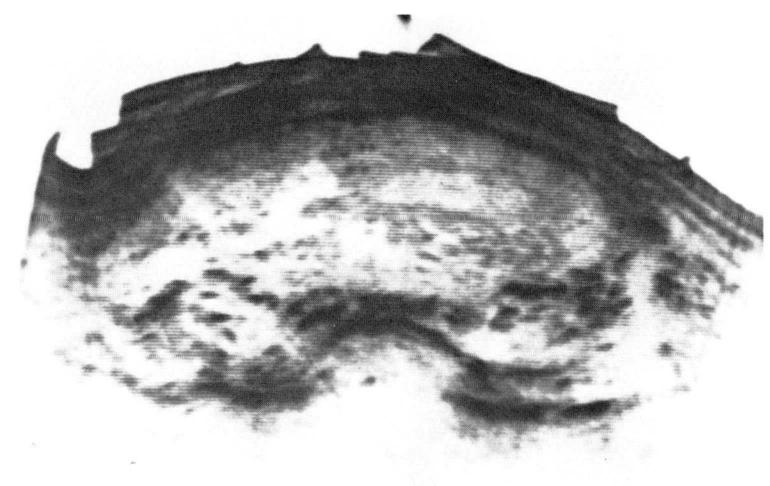

FIGURE 4–69. Ultrasonographic appearance of a second-trimester hydatidiform mole. This compound scan taken transversely through the uterus shows the uterus disrupted by multiple, irregular echolucencies from hydropic villae in a 27-year-old female. This appearance is typical of a hydatidiform mole.

Part III

General Imaging of the Pelvis and the Retroperitoneum

Disease of the pelvis can manifest in a variety of ways because of effects of compression or invasion of the rectum, the bladder, and the reproductive organs. Internal bleeding often helps determine the affected organ; pelvic pain is not usually noteworthy unless it correlates with menses. Lesions involving single organs are described in Parts I and II of this chapter. Intraperitoneal disease is discussed in Chapter 3. When disease spreads throughout the pelvis, a general approach to pelvic and retroperitoneal imaging is required. This approach is most often required for the evaluation of infection, advanced or recurrent tumor (including lymphoma), and retroperitoneal disease.

PELVIC INFECTION

Retroperitoneal Abscess. Abscess can develop in any part of the peritoneal or retroperitoneal space (see Fig. 3–11). The location is the best indicator of the origin of the infection. CT provides the most informative evaluation. Regional enteritis and diverticulitis cause infection in the posterior pararenal space; pancreatic infection involves the anterior pararenal space; and renal infection spreads to the perirenal space. Initially, an abscess remains confined to the space of origin, but eventually it crosses to adjacent spaces. CT provides the most informative evaluation of psoas abscess and hematoma. Coronal MRI scans provide high tissue contrast and a view in the psoas muscle plane (Fig. 4–70).

Retroperitoneal Fibrosis. Retroperitoneal fibrosis is a disease with several causes in which extensive fibrous tissue encases the aorta, the vena cava, and the iliac vessels in the regions of their bifurcations. The disease can extend laterally to involve other structures, especially the ureters, which then become obstructed. Urine extravasation, infection, drugs (such as methysergide), and chronic bleeding are all associated with retroperitoneal fibrosis.

Radiographs show encasement of the aorta, the vena cava, and the iliac vessels by abnormal tissue (Fig. 4–71). The ureters are displaced medially and may be obstructed. The bladder has a pine-tree appearance if it also is encased. Treatment includes discontinuation of drugs, administration of steroids, surgical

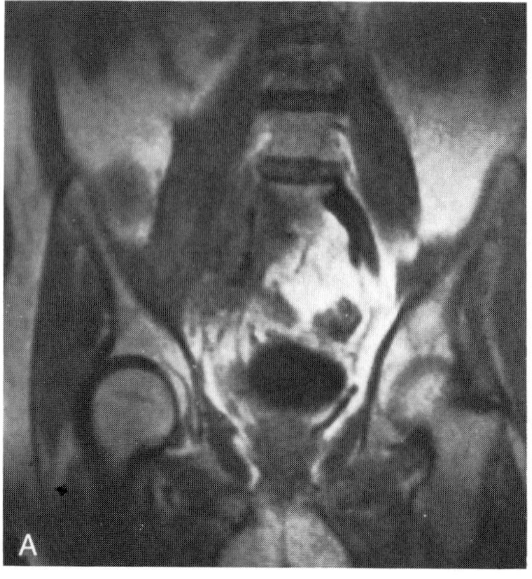

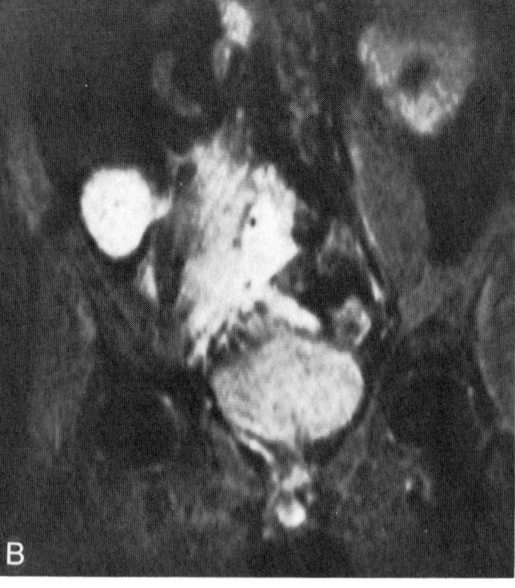

FIGURE 4–70. Retroperitoneal abscess. *A.* Coronal T1 spin echo sequence shows abnormal appearance of the psoas margin, the lower spinal marrow, and the pelvic fat on the right side. *B.* Matching coronal STIR image shows edema surrounding the psoas muscle. A high-intensity abscess mass is present, involving the lower lumbar vertebrae and the deep pelvic structures and displacing the psoas muscle laterally. The patient developed *Klebsiella* abscess after renal transplant. (Courtesy of B. Porter, First Hill Diagnostic Imaging Center, Seattle.)

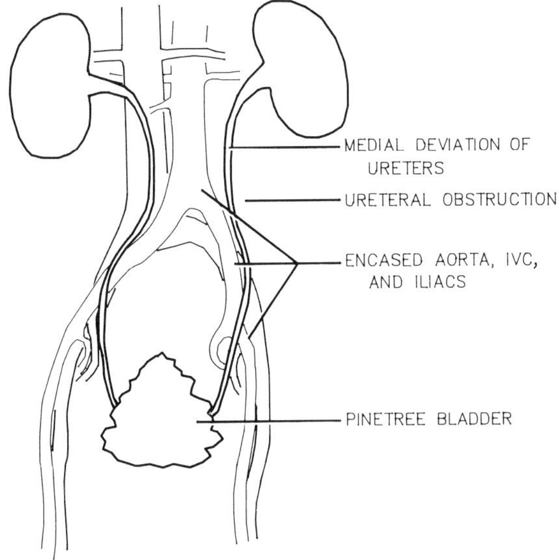

FIGURE 4–71. Characteristics of retroperitoneal fibrosis. IVC, inferior vena cava.

lysis, and, if necessary, ureteral diversion. The disease is usually self-limiting, and the fibrous tissue can be completely resorbed.

NEOPLASMS

Diagnosis of tumor extension or recurrent tumor in the pelvis is one of the most difficult radiologic evaluations. Cross-sectional imaging techniques are primarily used for assessing invasive tumor, adenopathy, scarring, and changes associated with therapy. Such techniques are essential for diagnosing recurrence, metastasis, and adenopathy from primary tumors and from lymphoma.

The most easily detected pelvic abnormality in tumor extension is ascites. The fluid is confined to the peritoneal cavity, clearly outlines abdominal and pelvic organs, and displaces the bowel (Fig. 4–72). The most common tumor to cause ascites is ovarian carcinoma. Other findings of importance are tumor implants to the omentum, extension through the serosa of the organ of origin, regional adenopathy, and extension into the retroperitoneum. Such findings indicate extension outside the primary organ and, in most cases, a much worse prognosis. MRI and CT are both used to assess tumor extension. MRI can show tissue planes and lymphadenopathy. When surgery has been performed or when scarring or radiation changes are present, diagnosis of small areas of recurrence is difficult.

Retroperitoneal Tumors. Retroperitoneal tumors are distinctly rare. They may arise from any of the various retroperitoneal structures, including those that are mesodermal, neurogenic, and embryonic. The most common benign and malignant retroperitoneal tumors are listed in Table 4–7. Thorough knowledge of the cross-sectional anatomical structure of the retroperitoneum is essential for the identification and evaluation of tumors in this area (see Chapter 3). Both CT and MRI are used in the evaluation of retroperitoneal tumors. CT provides excellent spatial resolution but does not always demonstrate soft tissue planes. In addition, tumor and normal tissue have similar densities on CT scans. MRI is limited by motion and spatial resolution but can show soft tissue planes, can demonstrate the tumor in the coronal and sagittal planes, and can show high contrast between tumor and muscle or fat (Fig. 4–73).

Lymphoma. Diagnosis of lymphoma in the pelvis requires an approach similar to that used in the upper abdomen (see Chapter 3). The

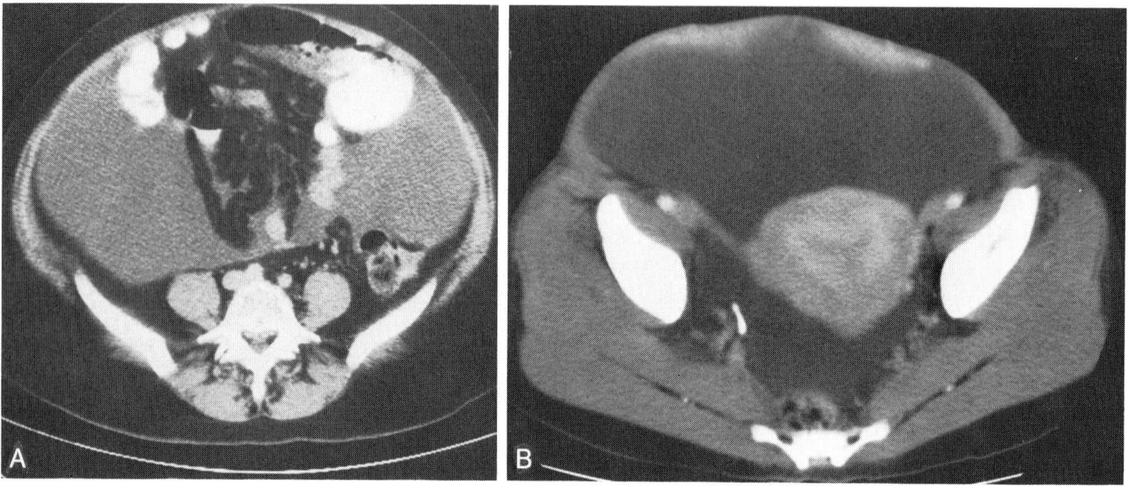

FIGURE 4–72. Pelvic peritoneal ascites. *A.* Malignant ascites. Contrast CT of the pelvis shows marked ascites with bowel and mesentery floating centrally. The patient, a 51-year-old woman, had malignant ascites caused by recurrent ovarian carcinoma. At that time, CT demonstrated omental implants, which are characteristic of ovarian carcinoma and were resected at surgery. *B.* Ascites caused by liver failure. CT shows marked pelvic extension of ascites outlining the uterus and the broad ligaments. The enhancing structures laterally are the iliac arteries. Note fluid in the pouch of Douglas, the space between the uterus and the rectosigmoid.

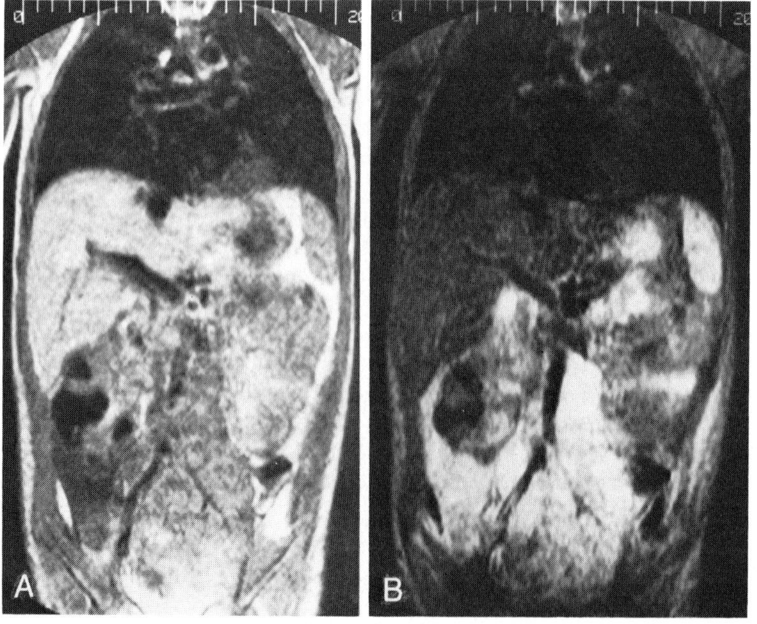

FIGURE 4–73. Retroperitoneal rhabdomyosarcoma. *A.* T1 spin echo image shows a flow void in the aortic bifurcation and the iliac vessels. Air is shown in the right colon. The remainder of the pelvis is filled with a nondescript soft tissue intensity that is similar to bowel (in the left middle and upper quadrants) and liver (on the right). *B.* STIR images show marked increased intensity in the soft tissue abnormality in the pelvis, which was shown to be disseminated pelvic rhabdomyosarcoma, in a 10-year-old girl. The iliac vessels, the aorta, and the bowel are all surrounded by tumor.

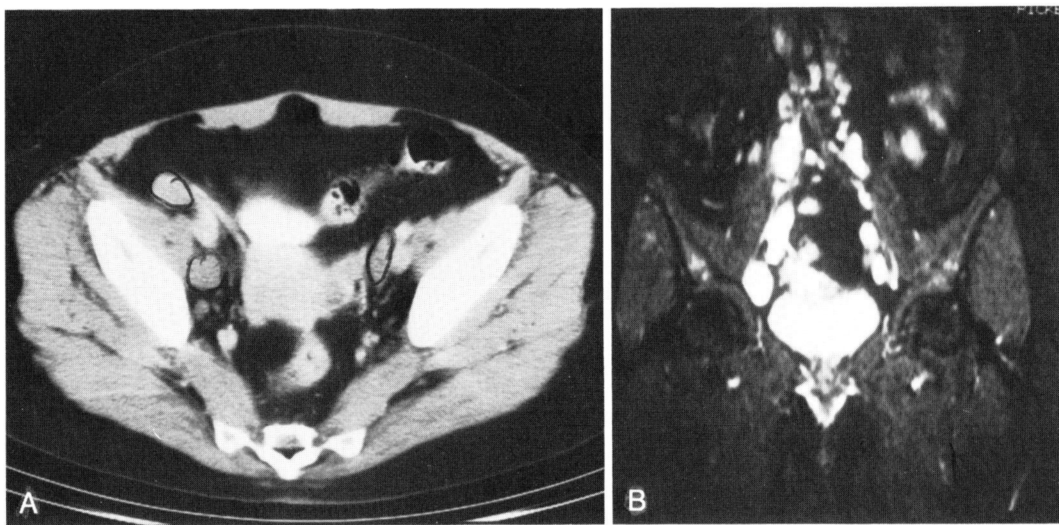

FIGURE 4–74. Non-Hodgkin's lymphoma. *A.* Contrast-enhanced CT of the pelvis shows obturator lymph nodes that are enlarged as a result of lymphomatous involvement in a 41-year-old woman with non-Hodgkin's lymphoma involving the neck, the chest, the abdomen, and the pelvis. The abnormal nodes are graphically enhanced in order to distinguish them from muscle tissue and vessels, which have a similar appearance on CT. *B.* Coronal STIR image shows multiple lymph nodes of the iliac chains bilaterally. (Courtesy of B. Porter, First Hill Diagnostic Imaging Center, Seattle.)

primary areas of interest are the aortocaval and iliac chains, which are most clearly seen on coronal images (see Fig. 4–6). Deep in the pelvis, the obturator and the iliac nodes are best seen on axial views. Both CT and MRI can be used to diagnose pelvic lymphoma. On CT, the nodes have a density and a size similar to those of vessels, and so the iliac branches must first be delineated. The para-aortic and paracaval areas are easily evaluated because of the normal presence of fat in these areas. Coronal MRI with STIR sequences is ideal for evaluation of pelvic adenopathy because the nodes are of very high intensity against low-density fat, muscle, and bone marrow (Fig. 4–74). The bladder and the bowel, which also appear bright on STIR images, are easily differentiated from other areas of tumor involvement, including the bone marrow (see Fig. 4–9).

TABLE 4–7. INCIDENCE OF BENIGN AND MALIGNANT RETROPERITONEAL TUMORS

Type of Tumor	Incidence
Benign	
Cyst of caudal gut	21%
Pheochromocytoma	18%
Granular cell myoblastoma	16%
Neurofibroma	8%
Leiomyoma	8%
Xanthogranuloma	7%
Ganglioneuroma	6%
Lipoma	6%
Other	10%
Malignant	
Lymphosarcoma	18%
Leiomyosarcoma	18%
Liposarcoma	12%
Hodgkin's disease	10%
Embryonal cell carcinoma	7%
Sympathicoblastoma	5%
Hemangiopericytoma	5%
Metastatic disease	5%
Other	20%

Pelvic Lipomatosis. Pelvic lipomatosis is a rare disorder of unknown cause in which proliferation of normal fatty tissue in the pelvis elevates and compresses the bladder and the rectum. The disease is most common in middle-aged adults. The most important radiographic findings are an increase in perivesical fat, a pear-shaped bladder, and asymptomatic elevation of the rectum. These findings can be demonstrated in excretory urography, barium enema studies, and CT. The disease is usually self-limiting; only rarely do patients require urinary diversion for obstruction.

RADIOGRAPHIC DIFFERENTIAL DIAGNOSIS

Frequently, a single radiographic finding or pattern can suggest a limited list of diagnoses. Additional findings and clinical history can assist in narrowing the list or in making a firm diagnosis. The following approaches to evaluation of radiographic findings can provide assistance in differential diagnosis. Diseases are listed in order of importance.

CAUSES OF BILATERALLY ENLARGED KIDNEYS

When both kidneys are enlarged, a generalized process is involved. The causes are obstruction, infiltration, edema, and proliferation.

1. Obstruction
   - Hydronephrosis
   - Venous thrombosis
   - Adult polycystic kidney disease
2. Infiltration
   - Lymphoma
   - Leukemia
   - Amyloidosis
3. Edema
   - Nephrotic syndrome
   - Acute glomerulonephritis
   - Acute tubular necrosis
4. Proliferation
   - Collagen vascular disease (early stages)

CAUSES OF A UNILATERALLY AND DIFFUSELY ENLARGED KIDNEY

When only one kidney is diffusely enlarged, a local process is the cause. When a patient has only a solitary kidney, it shows compensatory hypertrophy. A partially duplicated kidney is the most common cause of renal enlargement.

Renal duplication
Single kidney
Hydronephrosis
Lymphoma
Renal vein thrombosis
Xanthogranulomatous pyelonephritis
Acute glomerulonephritis

CAUSES OF BILATERALLY SMALL KIDNEYS

Small kidneys are the result of a loss of renal parenchyma from infection or vascular disease. The kidneys appear shrunken and scarred, and the cortex is thinned, as manifested by the relative proximity of the calyces to the outer renal border.

Chronic pyelonephritis
Chronic glomerulonephritis
Collagen vascular disease (late stages)
Atherosclerosis
Infarction

NONFUNCTIONING RENAL MASS

Renal cell carcinoma must first be considered when a nonfunctioning renal mass is identified. Two other important lesions, angiomyolipoma and xanthogranulomatous pyelonephritis, have nearly identical appearances and, being benign, must be ruled out before aggressive tumor therapy is begun. Metastasis is the most common renal tumor.

Metastasis
Renal cell carcinoma
Angiomyolipoma
Xanthogranulomatous pyelonephritis
Abscess

CAUSES OF A FLANK MASS IN AN INFANT

Sixty percent of abdominal masses in children are in the kidneys. Hydronephrosis and Wilms' tumor are the most common. All except mesoblastic nephroma can be bilateral.

Hydronephrosis (25%)
Wilms' tumor (20%)
Cystic renal disease (15%)
Neuroblastoma (15%)
Retroperitoneal tumors,
  mesoblastic nephroma,
  mesenchymal tumors

CAUSES OF BLUNTED CALYCES

Blunting or rounding of the calyces must be diagnosed from a radiograph for which compression (to distend the ureters) was not used. Blunting of the calyces can be caused by parenchymal, papillary, or ureteral abnormalities.

Obstruction
Papillary necrosis
Endstage pyelonephritis
Tuberculosis

CAUSES OF NEPHROCALCINOSIS

The deposition of calcium in the medullary portion of the kidneys is called nephrocalcinosis. It is found in only a limited number of diseases. Abnormalities of calcium metabolism include cancer, hyperparathyroidism, sarcoidosis, hypervitaminosis D, and renal disease.

Medullary sponge kidney
Renal tubular acidosis
Papillary necrosis
Metabolic abnormalities of calcium

CAUSES OF RENAL CORTICAL CALCIFICATION

Calcification in the renal cortex is usually caused by infection or tumor.

Chronic pyelonephritis
Tuberculosis
Chronic glomerulonephritis
Xanthogranulomatous pyelonephritis
Tumor
Simple cyst

CAUSES OF MIDURETERAL STRICTURE

Narrowing of the ureter is normal near the renal pelvis, near the pelvic brim, and at the entrance to the bladder. Narrowing of other portions of the ureter can be caused by intrinsic or extrinsic lesions.

Trauma
Tumor
Endometriosis
Retroperitoneal fibrosis
Radiation injury
Retrocaval ureter
Tuberculosis
Schistosomiasis

CONDITIONS ASSOCIATED WITH RETROPERITONEAL FIBROSIS

The cause of retroperitoneal fibrosis is currently unknown. Immunity-related, infectious, toxic, and neoplastic causes have been suggested.

Ergot therapy
Chronic infection
Leakage from abdominal aortic aneurysm
Malignancy
Vasculitis

CAUSES OF A TESTICULAR MASS

Testicular masses have a variety of forms ranging from highly malignant tumors to benign fluid collections. The clinical examination can usually distinguish these. Ultrasonograms and MRI clearly show the location and the composition of the mass. Nearly all solid painless masses are malignant tumors.

Carcinoma
Spermatocele, hydrocele
Epididymitis
Varicocele
Orchitis
Infarction
Trauma

5 Cardiovascular Radiology

Robert J. Telepak
Michael F. Hartshorne
Gary K. Stimac

Cardiovascular radiology involves not only the heart but also vascular structures throughout the body. In the chest, heart disease has a major impact on the pulmonary system. Many forms or manifestations of heart disease are therefore considered in Chapter 2 (Chest Radiology). Other cardiovascular diseases are discussed with diseases of specific organs in other chapters under the major heading "Vascular Diseases." This chapter addresses primarily the heart and the great vessels.

The major emphasis in this chapter is on congenital heart disease (CHD), including the embryological and later development of the heart. The cardiac diseases of adulthood that require imaging are discussed in a section on acquired heart disease. Trauma to the heart, being a relatively minor consideration, is discussed in that section also.

BASIC EVALUATION

The radiologist has three main responsibilities in the imaging of cardiovascular disease. First, the radiologist is sometimes the first person to identify cardiovascular disease. Plain film findings are usually not definitive but may suggest the presence of cardiac disease and the need for additional evaluation by other imaging tests. The most common finding is an enlarged cardiac silhouette that can be further evaluated by cardiac series or ultrasonography to identify specific chamber enlargement. For example, calcifications within the coronary arteries correlate well with extensive atherosclerotic plaque and luminal stenosis (Fig. 5–1).

Second, the radiologist is often asked to provide additional information about a patient with known heart disease. Finally, the radiologist has a role in therapy of extracardiac vascular disease. Examples include balloon angioplasty of an atherosclerotic peripheral arterial lesion or treatment of gastrointestinal bleeding by infusion of vasopressin.

Complementary imaging examinations are especially informative in cardiovascular radiology. Whereas one imaging study may suggest a diagnosis, others help to more fully characterize the problem. The radiologist is often in the best position to identify abnormalities and suggest additional imaging examinations. For example, a chest radiograph showing a widened mediastinum might be followed by computed tomography (CT) to document dissection of the aorta. An aortogram would then be necessary in order to assess aortic valvular

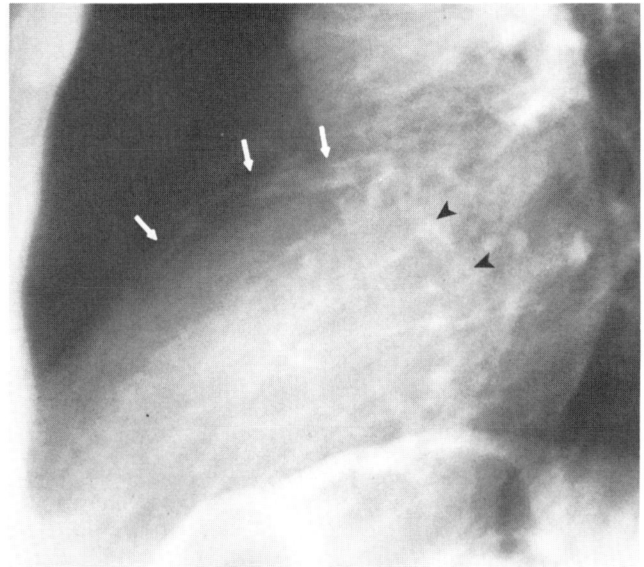

FIGURE 5–1. Coronary artery calcification. Close-up view from a lateral chest radiograph shows extensive calcification along the left anterior descending artery (*arrows*) and the left circumflex coronary artery (*arrowheads*) in a middle-aged male with severe atherosclerotic disease. Calcifications this extensive are an ominous sign of atherosclerosis that also involves smaller coronary branches. The likelihood that a cardiac event will occur is high.

regurgitation or involvement of the coronary arteries by the dissection. Multimodality evaluation is also necessary when multiple problems are present or when there are complications of an initial problem. For example, a newborn for whom a chest radiograph shows congestive heart failure (CHF) may require an echocardiogram or an angiogram to determine the type of CHD responsible for the secondary CHF. The standard abbreviations for normal structures and most forms of heart disease are used throughout this chapter and are listed in Table 5–1.

Plain Film and Fluoroscopic Evaluation

Plain film evaluation of the chest (discussed in Chapter 2) includes consideration of overall heart size and individual chamber enlargement and assessment of pulmonary vascularity. Other important findings are calcifications of the pericardium, the myocardium, the valves, the aorta, and the coronary vessels. The situs (the locations of the heart and abdominal organs) is also assessed. The cardiac series consists of posteroanterior, lateral, and oblique radiographs combined with a barium swallow. This technique permits better characterization of specific chamber enlargement than does the standard radiograph. Fluoroscopy is used to observe motion of cardiovascular structures (especially if they contain calcifications) and may help determine their location.

Plain film findings in the lungs often assist in the assessment of heart disease. The most important is CHF, the failure of the left chambers of the heart to pump blood into the systemic circulation (Fig. 5–2). The pulmonary findings include increased size of pulmonary vessels, upward redistribution of blood flow, Kerley's B lines, and pleural effusion (see Fig. 2–77).

Angiography

The definitive examination to detect anatomical defects, vascular insufficiency, and most functional abnormalities of the heart is cardiac angiography. Femoral (or brachial) artery or vein catheters are placed in a chamber or outflow tract of the heart. The coronary arteries can be injected directly in order to evaluate perfusion or occlusion. Knowledge of the arterial supply is essential for interpreting the results of these examinations (Fig. 5–3). When orientation poses a problem, the three primary arteries—the right coronary artery (RCA), the left anterior descending (LAD), and the left circumflex artery (LCX)—can be modeled with the use of the thumb, index, and middle fingers of the left hand, respectively.

Cardiac angiography is often accompanied by functional tests such as the use of exercise or drugs to induce changes in cardiac function. Consequently, because of the risk of cardiac arrhythmia or infarction, the examiner is usually an angiography-trained cardiologist.

Angiography also helps evaluate chamber

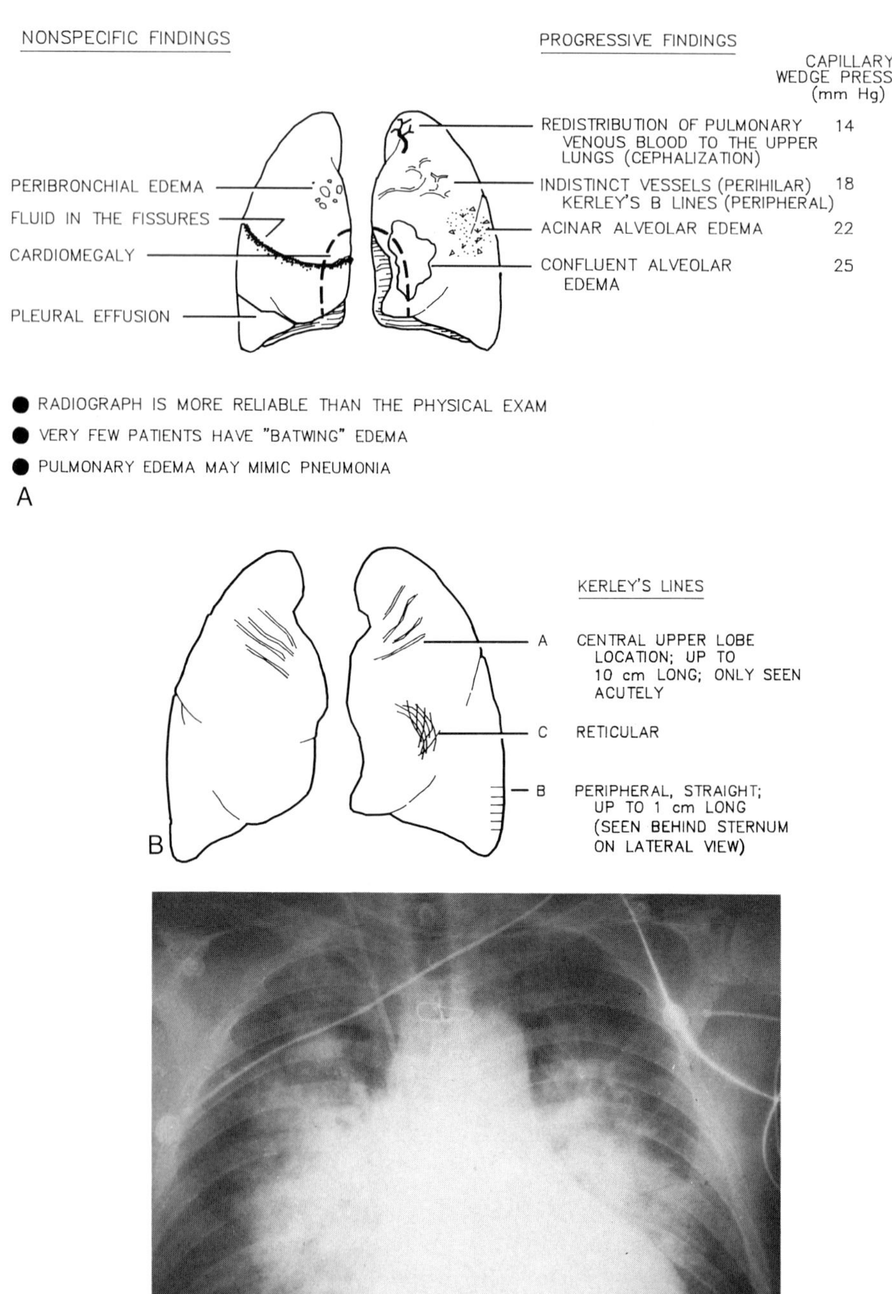

FIGURE 5–2. Congestive heart failure. *A.* Radiographic findings. *B.* Kerley's lines, types A, B, and C. *C.* The heart is enlarged even after magnification of anteroposterior projection is accounted for. The left ventricular muscle has failed, causing both chamber dilatation and pulmonary edema.

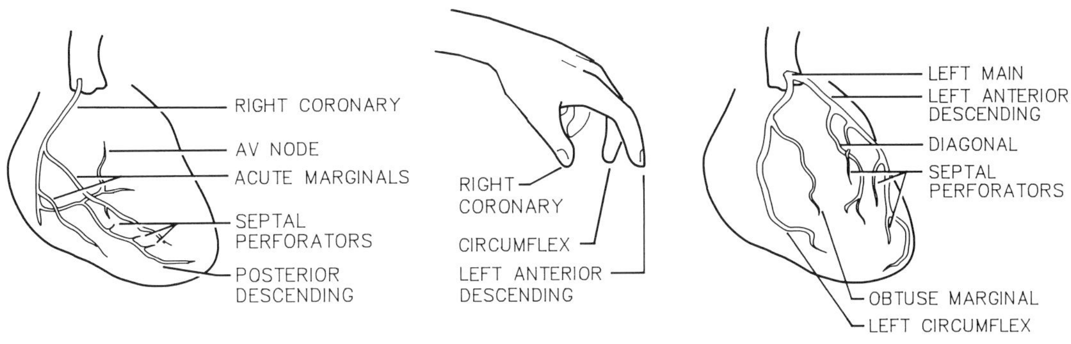

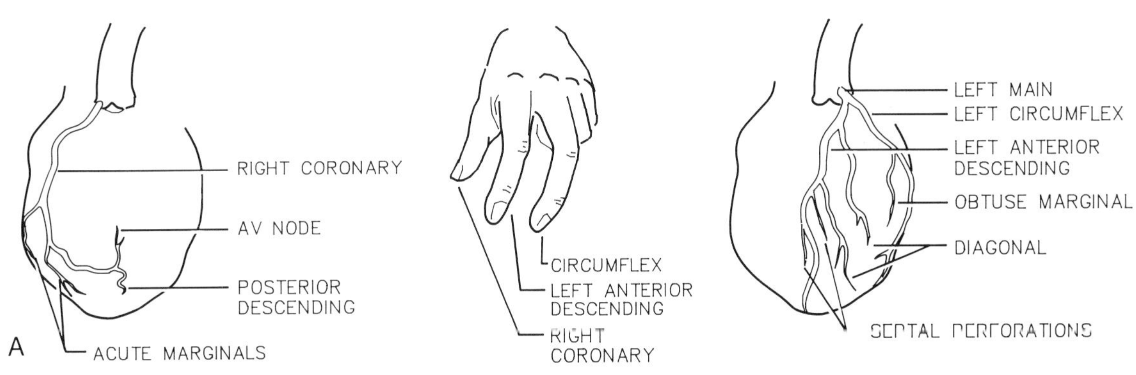

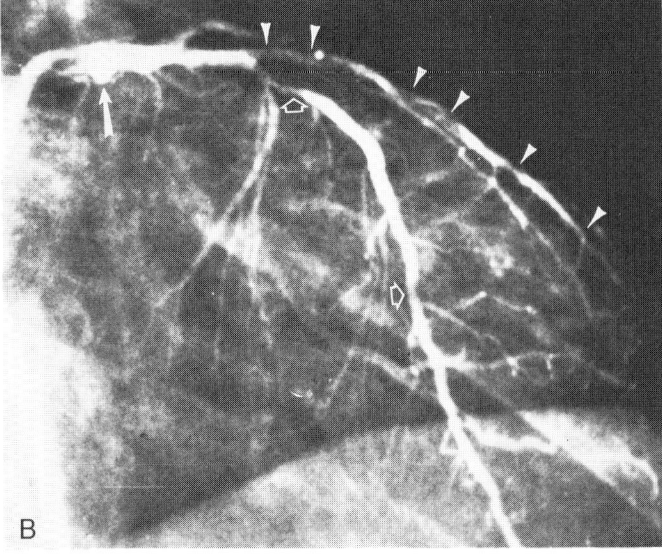

FIGURE 5–3. Coronary angiography. *A.* Diagram. AV, atrioventricular. *B.* Arteriogram in the right anterior oblique projection with contrast injected into the left main coronary artery shows atherosclerotic disease. The circumflex branch is 100% obstructed at its origin (*arrow*). There are sequential high-grade stenoses in the left anterior descending artery (*arrowheads*). Two stenotic lesions mark the large diagonal branch (*open arrowheads*). Smaller branch arteries elsewhere show irregular lumens. (Courtesy of L. Pupa, MD, Brooke Army Medical Center, Fort Sam Houston, Texas.)

size and position, wall motion, and abnormal interconnections between the chambers. Stenosis, aneurysms, dissections, and disruptions in the extracardiac vascular system can be identified through angiography.

TABLE 5–1. COMMON ABBREVIATIONS IN CARDIOVASCULAR RADIOLOGY

AI	Aortic (valvular) insufficiency
APVR	Anomalous pulmonary venous return
AR	Aortic (valvular) regurgitation, or aortic insufficiency
AS	Aortic (valvular) stenosis
ASD	Atrial septal defect
CAD	Coronary artery disease
CHD	Congenital heart disease
CHF	Congestive heart failure
COARCT	Coarctation of the aorta
CTGV	Corrected transposition of the great vessels
CUSHION	Endocardial cushion defect
DORV	Double-outlet right ventricle
IVC	Inferior vena cava
LA	Left atrium
LAD	Left anterior descending (coronary artery)
LAE	Left atrial enlargement
LCA	Left (main) coronary artery
LCC	Left common carotid (artery)
LCX	Left circumflex (coronary artery)
LPA	Left pulmonary artery
LSCA	Left subclavian artery
LV	Left ventricle
LVE	Left ventricular enlargement
LVH	Left ventricular hypertrophy
MI	Myocardial infarction or mitral insufficiency
MR	Mitral (valvular) regurgitation
MS	Mitral (valvular) stenosis
PDA	Patent ductus arteriosus
PS	Pulmonic (valvular) stenosis
RA	Right atrium
RAE	Right atrial enlargement
RCA	Right coronary artery
RCC	Right common carotid (artery)
RHD	Rheumatic heart disease
RPA	Right pulmonary artery
RSCA	Right subclavian artery
RV	Right ventricle
RVE	Right ventricular enlargement
RVH	Right ventricular hypertrophy
SBE	Subacute bacterial endocarditis
SV	Single ventricle; also stroke volume
SVC	Superior vena cava
TA	Tricuspid (valvular) atresia
TAPVR	Total anomalous pulmonary venous return
TGV, TGA	Transportation of the great vessels (arteries)
TOF	Tetralogy of Fallot
TRILOGY	Trilogy of Fallot
TRUNCUS	Persistent truncus arteriosus
TS	Tricuspid (valvular) stenosis
VSD	Ventricular septal defect

Ultrasonography

Ultrasonography of the heart can be performed in patients of any age. At most medical centers, in utero ultrasonography (including cardiac evaluation) is performed by a radiologist. Cardiac ultrasonography (called echocardiography) of infants, children, and adults is usually performed by a cardiologist in conjunction with patients' clinical history and examination, electrocardiogram, and nuclear medicine examinations as part of a general assessment of the heart. A sonographer is occasionally asked to evaluate the hepatic venous drainage into the right atrium or to diagnose pericardial effusion.

In utero screening for cardiac and other congenital defects has improved diagnosis and treatment of such abnormalities. In the fetus there is usually no difficulty in determining the location of the heart, the stomach, and the aorta, which are normally all on the left side (Fig. 5–4). Occasionally, septal defects and vascular abnormalities can be identified. Echocardiography enables the cardiologist to image the pericardium, chambers, valves, and outflow tracts and allows real-time scanning of the valves. Through Doppler techniques, the direction and magnitude of flow, the presence of stenosis, and the presence of valvular regurgitation can be determined.

Computed Tomography

CT is applied to intra- and extracardiac evaluation. Conventional CT is used to assess chamber size and position, wall thickness, and pericardial effusions. It also can demonstrate the presence, the position, and the extent of calcifications in the aorta, the cardiac valves, and the pericardium. Ultra-fast cineangiographic CT scanners show wall motion and provide measurement of functional parameters such as stroke volume, ejection fraction, and coronary blood flow (Fig. 5–5*A*). Tumors and thrombus in the chambers, valvular regurgitation, and areas of myocardial infarction can also be detected and measured. CT density measurements can be used to assess cardiac involvement in hemochromatosis.

Nuclear Medicine

Nuclear cardiological examinations are effective for evaluating cardiac function, ische-

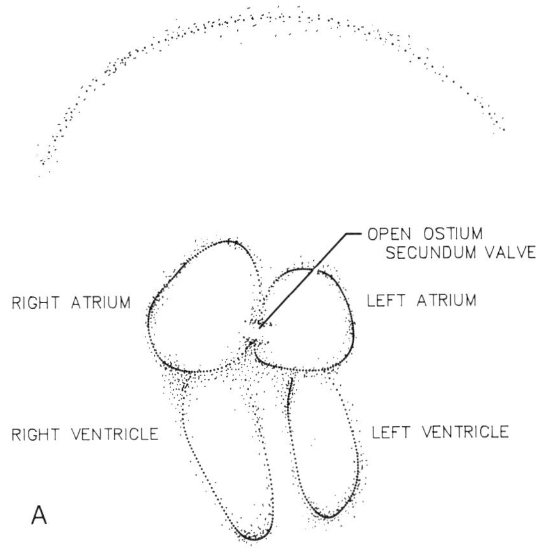

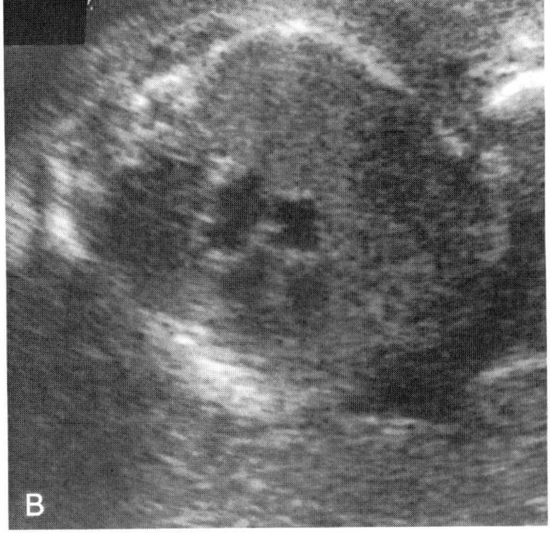

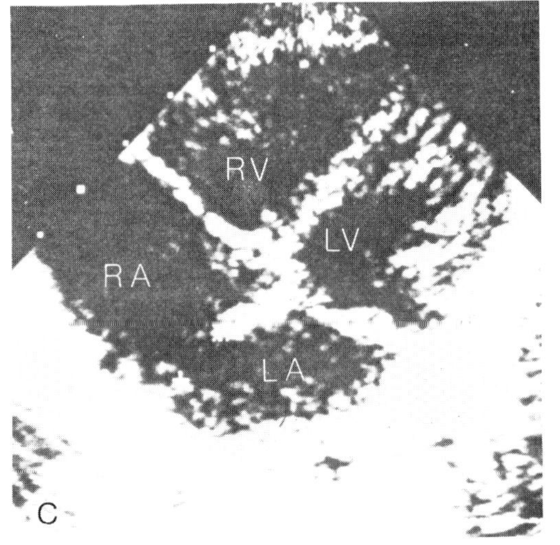

FIGURE 5–4. Ultrasonographic cardiac examination. *A.* Diagram. *B.* Real-time ultrasonographic examination during the second trimester of pregnancy shows a slice across the thorax in a four-chamber projection. The labeled diagram (*A*) corresponds to the image (*B*). Note the open ostium secundum valve between the atria. Real-time image quality is superior to a freeze-frame image such as this. *C.* Image taken from a real-time echocardiogram shows the four chambers of the heart. Viewing the right ventricle (RV), left ventricle (LV), right atrium (RA), and left atrium (LA) in motion on video display makes assessment of wall motion and of valve motion possible. Doppler flow techniques can color-code direction of blood flow and superimpose that on the display.

mia, and the presence of infarction. Such examinations (see Chapter 9) are usually a cooperative effort by a cardiologist and a nuclear medicine specialist. The scans provide functional assessment of myocardial perfusion through the use of thallium or isonitril agents. Wall motion and functional parameters of the heart, such as ejection fraction, can be quantitatively measured with the use of gated blood pool studies. Acutely infarcted tissue can be detected by means of pyrophosphate. The presence and magnitude of intracardiac shunts also can be measured by means of nuclear medicine techniques.

Magnetic Resonance Imaging

MRI is potentially the most comprehensive of all imaging examinations used in the evaluation of the heart. Its ability to image in any plane (including off-axis) enables the examiner to see normal and abnormal cardiac structure, contributing to a diagnosis of CHD. Flow-void phenomenon on spin echo T1 images and flow enhancement on gradient-refocused cineangiographic MRI images are used to evaluate and characterize blood flow (including coronary artery flow) and obstructions to it. Ventricular functional parameters and volumes can be determined by volumetric methods similar to those used in ultra-fast cineangiographic CT.

The cardiac chambers and the great vessels appear either black or white, depending on the sequence used, in marked contrast to myocardium and vessel walls. When the imaging sequence is gated to the cardiac cycle, this marked contrast difference provides sharp images demonstrating the intracavitary blood and

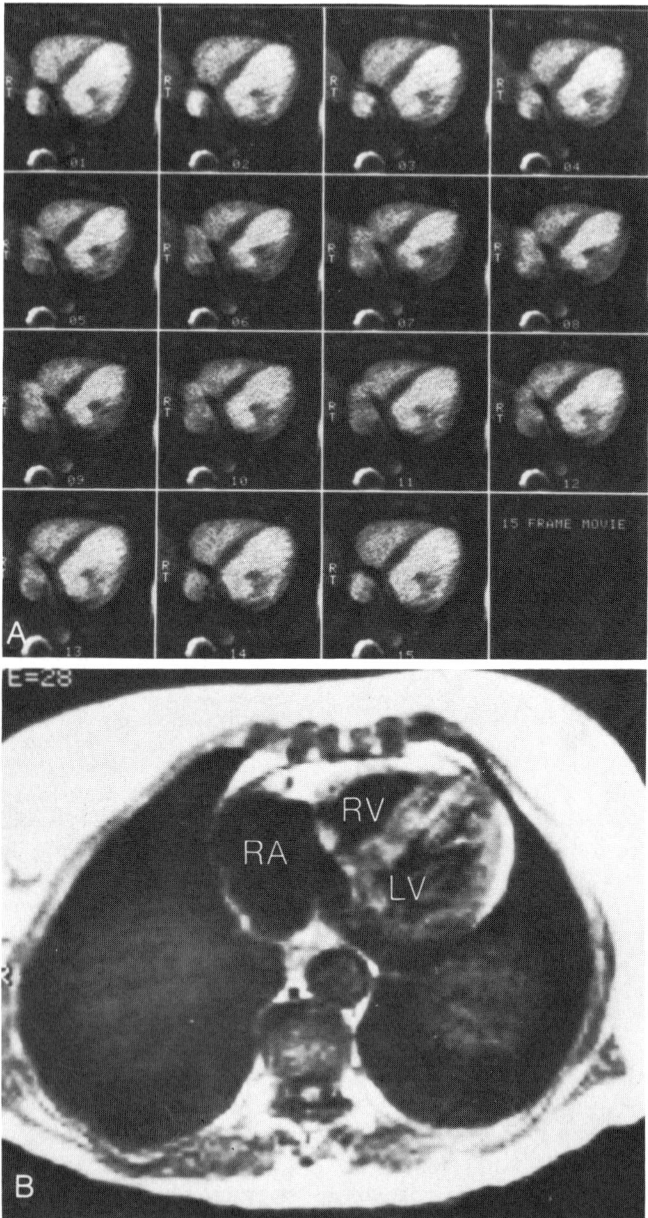

FIGURE 5–5. Sequential cardiac computed tomographic (CT) images and magnetic resonance imaging (MRI) scans. *A.* A sequence of 15 images from an ultra-fast CT scanner shows the right and left ventricles contracting during systole (frames 1 to 6) and then dilating during diastole (frames 7 to 15). The left ventricle contains a greater concentration of contrast and appears whiter than the right ventricle. The dark area within the left ventricle is a papillary muscle. *B.* A slice from a gated MRI examination of another patient's mediastinum shows the left ventricle (LV) to have a thicker wall than the more anterior right ventricle (RV). High-signal pericardial fat surrounds both ventricles. The thin-walled chamber to the patient's right is the right atrium (RA).

the cardiac walls. Therefore, MRI demonstrates the thickness and homogeneity of the myocardium, the size of the chambers, and the internal cardiac structure (Fig. 5–5*B*). Images of the heart at systole and diastole are compared in order to assess myocardial contraction. Patency and flow in coronary arteries also can be assessed. The pericardium, which is of low signal intensity, is easily demonstrated because it is bordered by mediastinal and epicardial fat.

CONGENITAL CARDIOVASCULAR DISEASE

Embryology

An embryological description of the step-by-step development of the fetal cardiovascular system elucidates the many aspects of CHD.

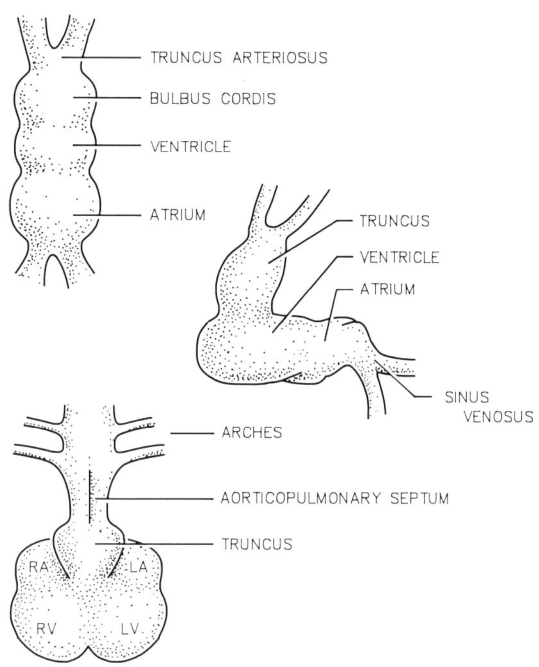

FIGURE 5–6. Development of the heart.

Development of the Heart

Angiogenic tissue capable of developing into blood vessels and tubular structures first begins to form in the third week of gestation and develops into a cluster of vessels with a tubular structure anteriorly. This tube moves forward, rotates, and flexes to form two lateral heart tubes. This tissue, destined to become the heart, is suspended within the developing pericardial cavity. Interruption or failure of any of these developments results in cardiac anomaly.

Chambers begin to develop and share a common center (Fig. 5–6). This common area, the endocardial cushion, later develops into the mitral and tricuspid valves and adjacent septal structures. The sinus venosus develops and directs oxygenated blood to the embryonic heart. Additional vessels that later become the inferior (IVC) and superior (SVC) venae cavae develop. At the same time, the conus cordis is developing to become the outflow tracts of both ventricles. The interatrial and interventricular septae further develop to make a four-chambered heart. The foramen ovale, a one-way flap valve, forms within the interatrial septum. The aortic and pulmonic valves form within the ventricular outflow tracts. The pulmonary outflow tract, the aorta, and the great vessels develop as a series of arches (to be discussed).

Lack of proper development of one or more structures within the heart leads to a congenital anomaly. The most extreme abnormalities are incompatible even with fetal life and result in miscarriages. Improper formation of the internal structures such as the septae leads to atrial septal defect (ASD) or ventricular septal defect (VSD). Lack of normal regression of an interim structure can likewise cause problems. Patent ductus arteriosus (PDA) is the most common example.

The fetal circulation transfers oxygenated blood preferentially to the brain. Four anatomical structures unique to the fetal circulation system are present: the placenta, the ductus venosus, the foramen ovale, and the ductus arteriosus. They control the circulation in the fetal system and regress after birth. The most important features of this circulation are oxygenation of blood by the placenta, bypass of the liver via the ductus venosus, bypass of the lungs via the ductus arteriosus, and shunting of oxygenated blood through the foramen ovale to the left chambers of the heart and then to the brachiocephalic vessels (Fig. 5–7). This fetal system may persist after birth, or it may recanalize under various conditions. The single umbilical vein carries oxygenated blood, and the paired arteries carry deoxygenated blood. The systemic and pulmonary circulations are essentially in parallel. Although the fetal lungs receive limited blood flow to help their development, they are nonfunctional. Vascular resistance is opposite to normal, the pulmonary circuit being relatively high and the systemic circuit being low.

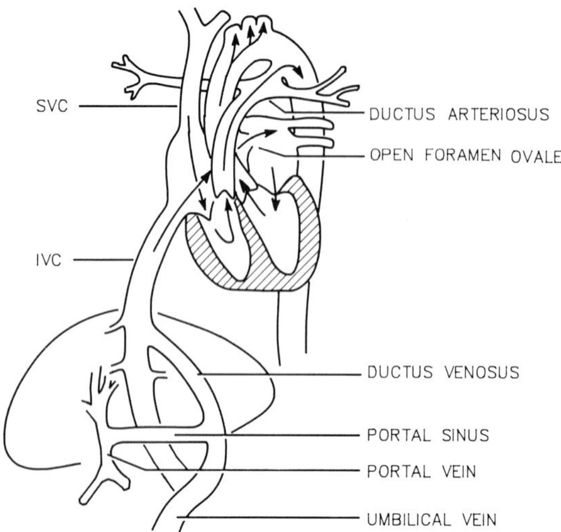

FIGURE 5–7. Fetal circulation. IVC, inferior vena cava; LA, left atrium; SVC, superior vena cava; RV, right ventricle.

Marked changes occur at birth. Elimination of the placenta causes the systemic vascular resistance to increase. As the lungs expand, increased oxygen levels decrease vasoconstriction and pulmonary vascular resistance. Increased blood return to the left atrium from the lungs causes the foramen ovale to functionally close within minutes after birth and to be sealed in 75% of children within the first year of life. Blood flow changes direction in the ductus arteriosus, which then usually functionally closes within 1 day after birth and anatomically closes within 10 days. The ductus venosus closes within 3 to 7 days. Problems arise when functional or anatomical closure does not occur properly. The best-known examples of such problems are PDA and ostium secundum type ASD.

Aorta and Great Vessels

While the heart is developing, the truncus arteriosus forms over the outlets of the right and left ventricles. An internal septum develops, dividing the truncus into the main pulmonary and aortic trunks. Lack of proper development of the septum and associated aortic and pulmonic valves leads to the varieties of truncus anomalies. The septum is not straight but spirals as it ascends. If it fails to form properly, various forms of transposition of the great vessels (TGV) can occur.

From the upper part of the truncus arteriosus, there arise dorsal and ventral aortas that are interconnected by six pairs of vascular arches, which form at different times during the developmental cycle (Fig. 5–8). Some of these arches persist and enlarge, whereas others regress entirely. Of the arches that remain, the paired third arches become the internal carotid arteries, the left fourth becomes the (normal) left aortic arch, and the right fourth becomes the proximal right subclavian artery. The proximal part of the sixth pair becomes the pulmonary arteries, and the distal part becomes the ductus arteriosus. Errors in this process can lead to three varieties of right aortic arch, a double arch, or varieties of aberrant or isolated subclavian arteries. The aorta usually descends on the same side as the arch. The ductus arteriosus is on the same side as the arch. If an aberrant subclavian artery is present, it is always on the side opposite that of the arch.

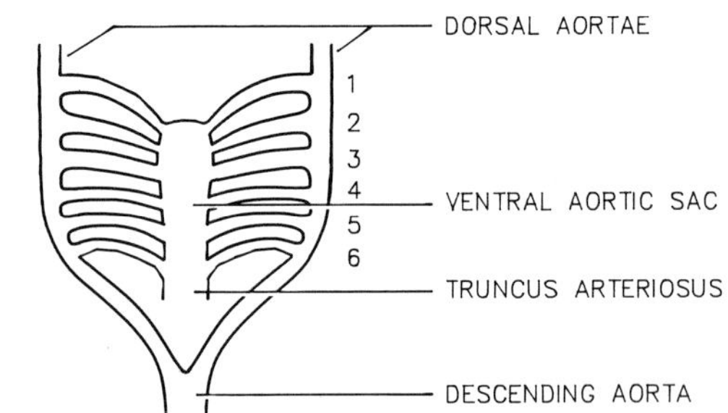

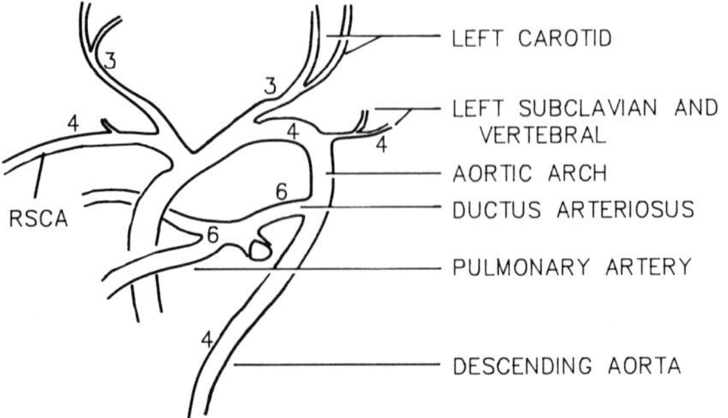

FIGURE 5–8. Origin of vessels. RSCA, right subclavian artery; PA, pulmonary artery.

The origins of the great vessels can also be understood as the development of a vascular ring connecting the ascending and descending aortas. The great vessels develop from branches of the ventral (ascending) aorta. Anomalies of the brachiocephalic vessels are the result of abnormal interruptions of this ring. The location of interruption of this ring determines the positions of the brachiocephalic vessels and explains the anomalous courses of vessels, such as aberrant subclavian artery and pulmonary sling.

Congenital Heart Disease

The incidence and relative frequency of CHD depends on the population investigated. The *relative* frequencies of the many types of CHD in the general population have been estimated from the data from a large number of sources and are shown in Table 5–2.

Evaluation of CHD requires attention to both clinical and radiographic factors. The age of the patient is important in that most diseases manifest during specific age ranges. Cyanosis is not always obvious and may not be identified by the radiologist, but it greatly assists in diagnosis. Whereas cyanosis may be obvious clinically in some patients, it may not be evident in others because of compensating effects of coexisting lesions. Cyanosis develops when the oxygen saturation of the blood falls below 92%. The lower the saturation is, the worse the cyanosis is. Cyanosis develops as a result of right-to-left shunting or admixture lesions.

In a right-to-left shunt, the lungs become oligemic, and the patient becomes cyanotic because most of the blood bypasses the lungs.

TABLE 5–2. THE RELATIVE FREQUENCY OF CONGENITAL HEART DISEASE (CHD)

CHD	%
VSD	27
VSD and PS	15
PDA	12
ASD	9
PS	8
AS	7
COARCT	6
CUSHION	6
TOF	5
TGV	4
All others combined	1
Total	100%

For explanation of abbreviations, see Table 5–1.

TABLE 5–3. CAUSES OF CYANOTIC CHD

% of Cases	Cause
40	TOF
15	TGV
10	TRUNCUS
10	TA
5	TRILOGY
20	All other types of CHD

For explanation of abbreviations, see Table 5–1.

The most common lesions in this category are tetralogy of Fallot (TOF), tricuspid atresia (TA), pulmonary atresia (PA), Ebstein's anomaly, and any type of CHD with pulmonic stenosis (PS). The last group of lesions is called TOF physiology because they are similar to TOF.

In admixture lesions, deoxygenated venous blood is mixed with oxygenated arterial blood and pumped into the systemic circulation. The degree of cyanosis in admixture lesions is generally less than that with right-to-left shunts. The amount of pulmonary blood flow seen is increased with admixture lesions, in some cases because of return of oxygenated blood to the lungs and in other cases because of left-to-right shunts from associated or compensatory lesions such as ASD, VSD, or PDA. The most common causes of admixture lesions are TGV, persistent truncus (TRUNCUS), single ventricle, total anomalous pulmonary venous return (TAPVR) type III, and double-outlet right ventricle (DORV). The most common causes of cyanotic CHD (Table 5–3) are easily remembered because all the terms begin with the letter T.

On radiographs the position of the aortic arch, the cardiac apex, and the abdominal organs (situs) should be noted in any child. The size of the cardiac silhouette, identification of specific chamber enlargement, and the assessment of pulmonary vascularity are the foundations of the radiographic interpretation.

Radiographic evaluation of CHD requires a systematic approach that is based on assessing the aorta; the position, size, and shape of the heart; the location of abdominal viscera; and the appearance of the pulmonary vessels. Although congenital heart anomalies are definitively diagnosed by means of angiography and echocardiography, the radiologist has an important role: differentiating lung disease from heart disease, suggesting a congenital heart defect in a patient with nonspecific symptoms, and suggesting an alternative diagnosis for a patient with equivocal findings or an erroneous diagnosis. The last task is particularly important because the surgical expectations or approach can be altered by the suggestions of the radiologist.

The Aorta

The position of the aortic arch is one of the most important factors in assessment of CHD. A right-sided aortic arch results when the right dorsal aorta persists; it directly affects the origins of the brachiocephalic vessels and is often associated with other cardiac anomalies. On chest radiographs, a normal left aortic arch is seen to displace the trachea to the right; in an infant, it moves farther to the right with expiration. On a barium swallow study, the normal left arch is seen to displace the esophagus to the right. With a right aortic arch, the trachea is displaced to the left, and in an infant, it is splinted on the right by the aorta; it therefore does not move normally to the right with expiration. A right aortic arch extends more superiorly than a normal left arch. The descending aorta is usually (but not always) on the same side as the arch. Because of the normal thymic shadow in infants, it may be impossible to determine the side of the aortic arch and the descending aorta from the chest film.

Many types of CHD affect the aorta, causing either enlargement or shrinkage (Table 5–4).

TABLE 5–4. CAUSES OF ABNORMAL SIZE OF THE AORTIC ARCH IN A CHILD

Size of Aortic Arch/CHD	Cause
Enlarged Arch	
AS	Poststenotic dilation
AI	Increased volume
PDA	Increased volume
COARCT	Obstruction
TOF	Right-to-left shunt
Systemic hypertension	Renal disease, other causes
TRUNCUS	Mimics an enlarged aorta
Diminished Arch	
Septal defects	Left-to-right shunt
Supravalvular AS	Obstruction
Hypoplastic left heart syndrome	Obstruction
TAPVR	Obstruction, low flow

For explanation of abbreviations, see Table 5–1.

TABLE 5–5. TYPES OF CONGENITAL HEART DISEASE ASSOCIATED WITH RIGHT AORTIC ARCH

Congenital Disease	% of Patients With Disease Who Have Right Arch
Asplenia	40
Persistent truncus arteriosus	32 to 35
Tetralogy of Fallot (TOF)	25 to 28
Transposition of the great vessels (TGV) with pulmonic stenosis	5 to 10
Tricuspid atresia (TA)	5
Ventricular septal defect (VSD)	2

Note: When a right aortic arch is detected, VSD, and TOF, being more common, are the most likely causes (see text).

Enlargement of the aorta usually is the result of increased flow or poststenotic dilatation. A small aorta is usually caused by shunting of blood away from the aorta. The normal aortic arch is difficult to see on chest films in children up to about age 3 years. When a definite aortic arch is seen in a child less than 3 years old, enlargement must be suspected.

Right Aortic Arch

The incidence of a right aortic arch is 1 per 2500 births. Complicated classifications of right aortic arches exist, but for practical purposes, there are two major varieties. In the first case, the aorta descends on the right side, and there is no retroesophageal segment. Usually this is the result of mirror-image aorta, and the brachiocephalic arteries originate in reverse order. The second type, in which the descending aorta is on the left side, results in a retroesophageal course of the aorta.

Many forms of CHD are associated with a right aortic arch (Table 5–5). The relative incidence of the disorder is expressed as a percentage of patients with the disease. On an absolute basis, VSD is so common that most of the cases of right aortic arch seen are in VSD patients. Conversely, 80% to 90% of cases of right arch and CHD are TOF. Because VSD is a part of TOF, these numbers are intertwined. It is clear that when a patient with CHD is seen to have a right aortic arch, the chances that VSD or TOF is present are extremely high. The other types of CHD are certainly possible but much less likely. For example, asplenia and TRUNCUS are commonly associated with a right aortic arch, but these conditions are rare in comparison with VSD and TOF.

Right Aortic Arch With Aberrent Arteries. Various aberrant arteries and veins occur in association with a right-sided aortic arch. The right aortic arch with aberrant left subclavian artery is the most common type of right aortic arch. The left subclavian artery in such cases arises as the first rather than the last of the great vessels and passes in front of the esophagus to the left side of the body (Fig. 5–9). This type of aorta usually descends on the left, and the incidence of associated CHD is very low (less than 5%). In a rare subtype of right aortic arch with aberrant left subclavian artery, the left subclavian is isolated; that is, it does

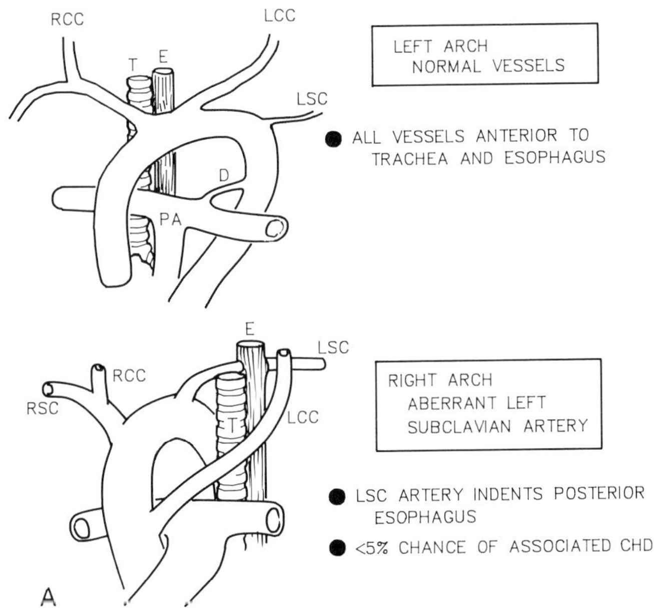

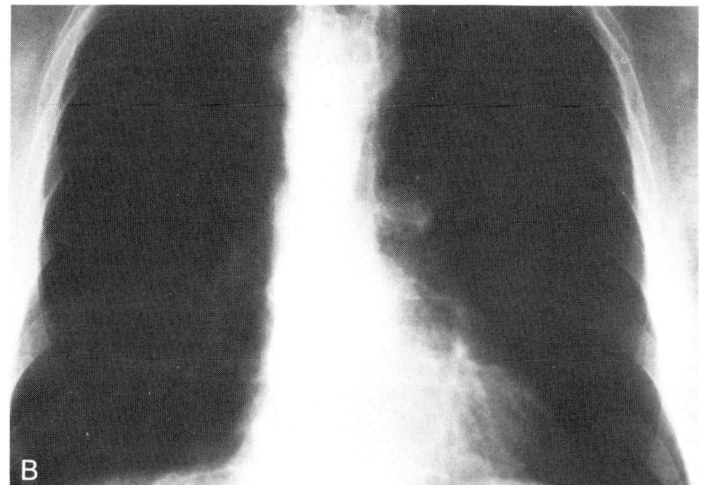

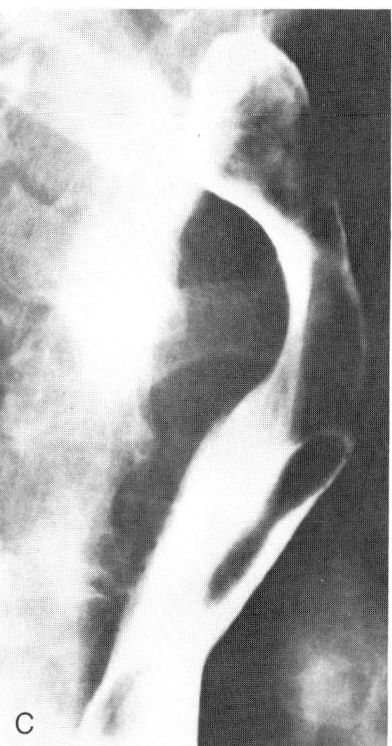

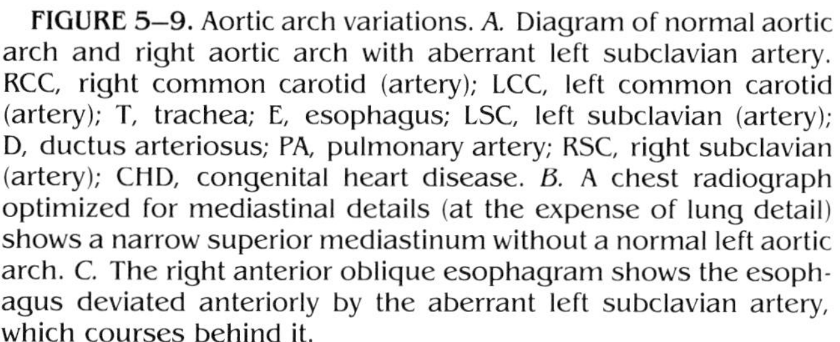

FIGURE 5–9. Aortic arch variations. *A.* Diagram of normal aortic arch and right aortic arch with aberrant left subclavian artery. RCC, right common carotid (artery); LCC, left common carotid (artery); T, trachea; E, esophagus; LSC, left subclavian (artery); D, ductus arteriosus; PA, pulmonary artery; RSC, right subclavian (artery); CHD, congenital heart disease. *B.* A chest radiograph optimized for mediastinal details (at the expense of lung detail) shows a narrow superior mediastinum without a normal left aortic arch. *C.* The right anterior oblique esophagram shows the esophagus deviated anteriorly by the aberrant left subclavian artery, which courses behind it.

not branch off the aorta but, rather, arises from the left vertebral artery. Most patients with this variety of right aortic arch also have a ductus arteriosus that completes the ring around the esophagus and the trachea. However, it is a loose ring, and patients rarely have constrictive symptoms. In general, aberrant arteries pass behind the esophagus, aberrant veins pass anterior to the trachea, and the pulmonary sling (anomalous origin of the left pulmonary artery from the right pulmonary artery) passes between the esophagus and trachea.

Mirror-Image Right Aortic Arch. The mirror-image right aortic arch is much less common. The aorta forms in such a fashion that the arch is on the right and the great vessels arise in reverse order. The aorta usually descends on the right. The incidence of CHD with mirror-image right aortic arch is very high (more than 95%). Ninety percent of CHD patients with a right aortic arch have the mirror-image type.

Double Aortic Arch. The double aortic arch is the most common and most serious form of complete vascular ring because it causes symptomatic constriction. A double arch occurs when the fourth arch and the dorsal aortic roots on both sides persist. The trachea and the esophagus are completely encircled by the aortic arches and their vascular derivatives. In contrast to other types of vascular rings, which are completed by the ductus arteriosus, this ring is completed by the second arch. CHD is rarely associated with double arch.

In severe cases, symptoms begin almost at birth. With less constrictive double arches, they may be delayed. Symptoms may be caused by tracheal compression (coughing, wheezing, tachypnea) or esophageal compression (dysphagia, choking, or aspiration). On a posteroanterior chest film, the trachea is midline and indented on both sides (Fig. 5–10). On the lateral film, the trachea may be anteriorly displaced and narrowed. The barium swallow examination shows the esophagus to be indented bilaterally. On the lateral view, the barium-filled esophagus shows deep indentation posteriorly where the two arches unite.

On angiogram, the right arch is usually lower and larger (75% of cases), whereas the left arch is smaller (often being atretic), posterior, and higher. Coronal MRI may show both arches and where they join inferiorly. The constriction around the trachea and the esophagus is relieved by surgically dividing the smaller of the two arches.

Heart Size

Assessment of heart size (also discussed in Chapter 2) is essential in the evaluation of cardiac disease, especially CHD. The closer the heart is to the film, the less it is magnified. Posteroanterior and left lateral plain chest films yield the least distorted measure of heart size. Anteroposterior and right lateral views cause the heart to appear falsely larger by 5% to 10% or more.

The most commonly used measurement of heart size is the cardiothoracic ratio, in which the width of the heart is compared with the width of the thorax on the posteroanterior film (Fig. 5–11). These measurements are not made along a single horizontal line through the heart and lungs, and this ratio is only a relative indication of heart size. The maximal heart width should be less than half of the maximal thoracic width. Falsely high ratios may be obtained if the orientation of the film is anteroposterior, if the patient takes an insufficiently deep breath, or if the film is taken during expiration. The cardiothoracic ratio is most useful in the follow-up of a patient, with the earlier examinations serving as a control. It is essential to realize that the cardiac silhouette includes the heart and the pericardium (Fig. 5–12).

When cardiac enlargement is detected, it is also important to attempt to determine which specific chamber or chambers are enlarged. This information in turn leads to determination of the cause of the chamber enlargement and ultimately to the diagnosis. Advanced imaging methods such as CT, ultrasonography, and MRI effectively identify enlarged cardiac chambers. The traditional cardiac series is seldom used but is still valuable as a basic step in chamber evaluation.

In the assessment of chamber size, it is important to differentiate enlargement and hypertrophy. Although they sometimes occur together, they are significantly different. Enlargement is most easily identified and is almost always caused by passage of excess blood volume through a chamber. All four heart chambers can enlarge. Isolated chamber enlargement is less common than simultaneous multichamber enlargement. Ventricular enlargement also occurs as a compensatory mechanism for failure. By dilating, the left ventricle stretches the myocardial wall and provides greater contractility by the Starling effect.

Left atrial enlargement may be caused by either volume overload (as occurs with mitral

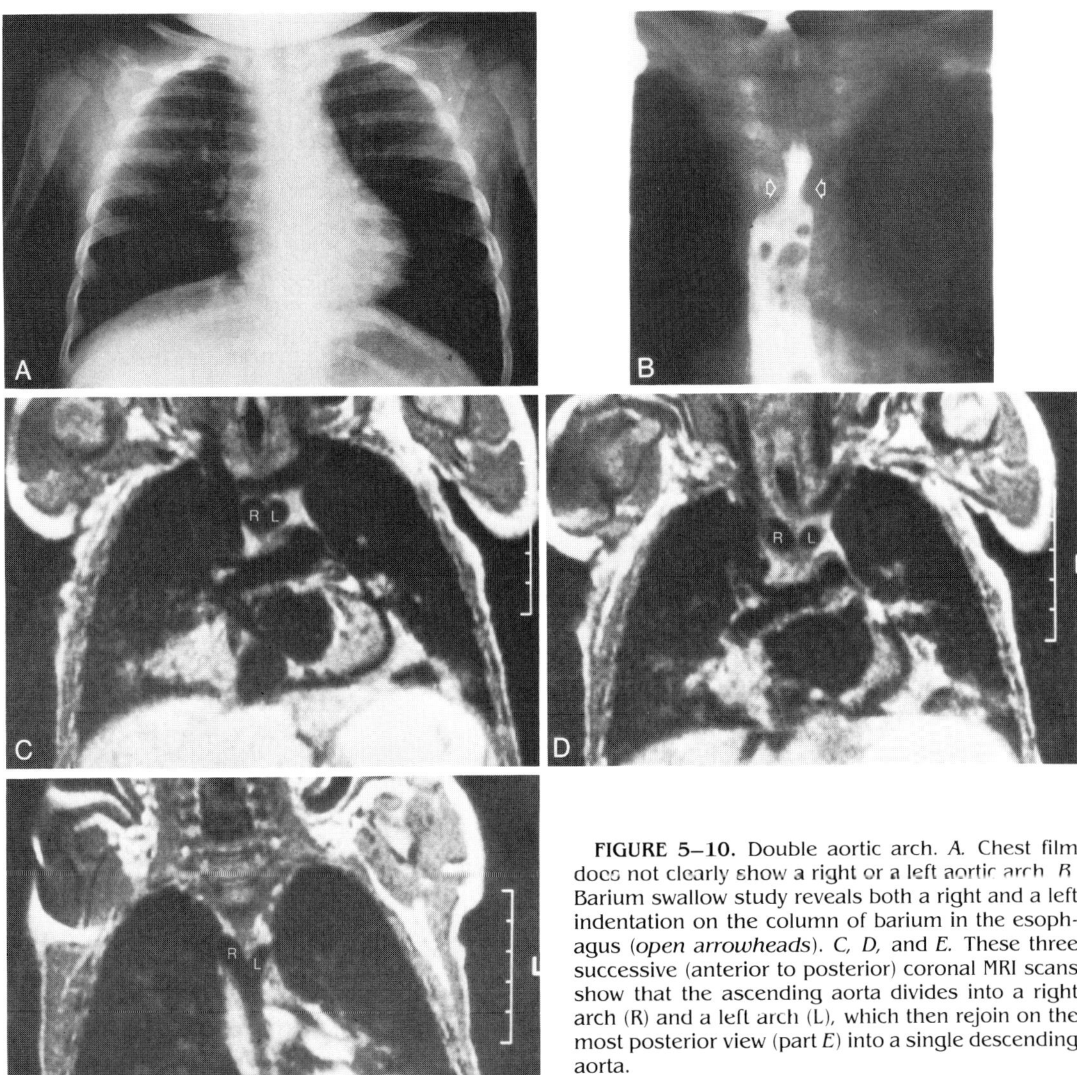

FIGURE 5–10. Double aortic arch. *A.* Chest film does not clearly show a right or a left aortic arch. *B.* Barium swallow study reveals both a right and a left indentation on the column of barium in the esophagus (*open arrowheads*). *C, D,* and *E.* These three successive (anterior to posterior) coronal MRI scans show that the ascending aorta divides into a right arch (R) and a left arch (L), which then rejoin on the most posterior view (part *E*) into a single descending aorta.

insufficiency) or increased pressure (as occurs with mitral stenosis). The effect of mitral insufficiency is greater than that of mitral stenosis. The combination of the two produces the greatest dilation. Plain film findings include elevation of the left main bronchus on the posteroanterior view and posterior extension of the left atrium on the lateral and right anterior oblique views. A double density of the enlarged left atrium is often seen on the posteroanterior view, but this can also be seen in normal patients.

Right ventricular enlargement is best seen on the left anterior oblique view in the form of a rounded right lateral margin. This view and the lateral view can show a narrowed space between the anterior heart margin and the sternum and posterior displacement of the inferior vena cava. Right ventricular enlargement also causes a more prominent and rounded right lower heart border, best seen on the posteroanterior view.

Left ventricular enlargement results in a downward displacement of the apex. It can be caused by aortic stenosis (AS), as a result of pressure, or by aortic insufficiency (AI), as a result of volume. AI causes the greatest degree of enlargement.

Hypertrophy results from increased pressure load over time. Only chambers with thick muscular walls are capable of hypertrophy. Thus only the right and left ventricles can

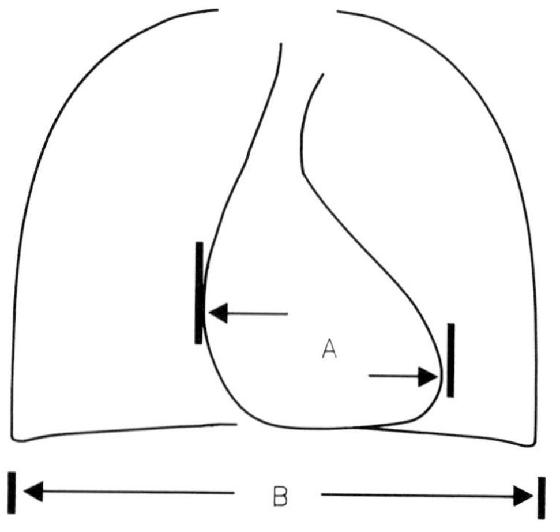

FIGURE 5–11. Measurement of the cardiothoracic ratio.

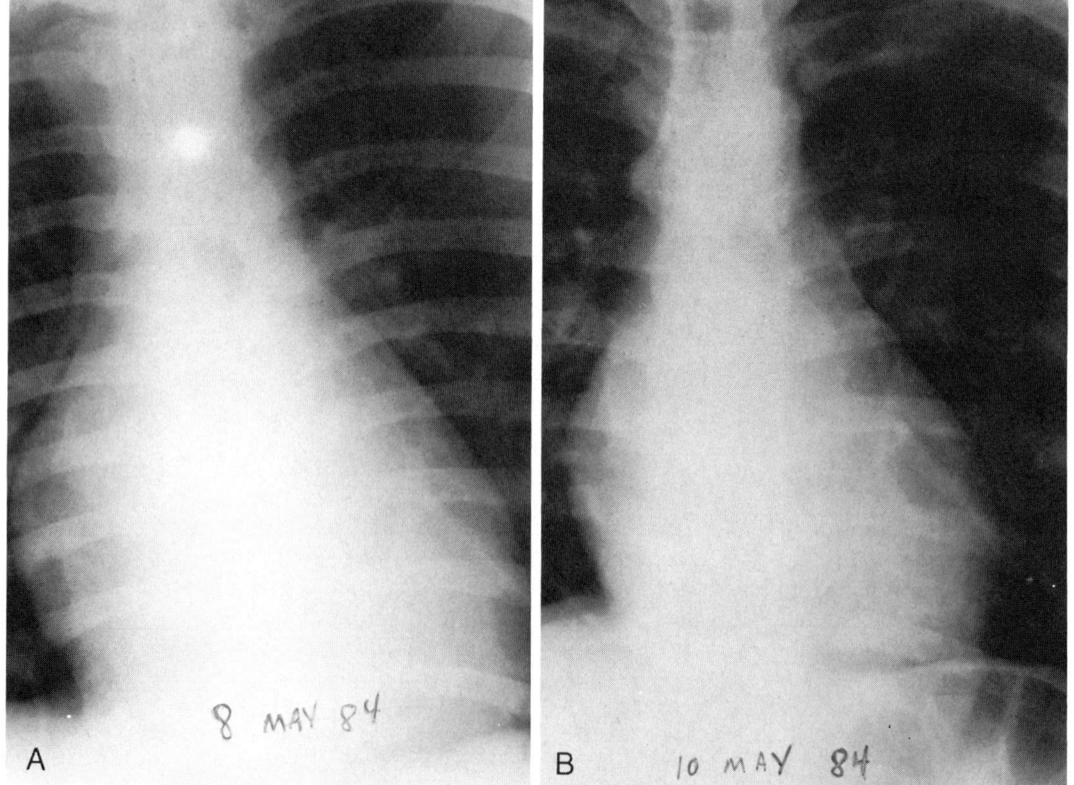

FIGURE 5–12. Cardiac silhouette enlargement from pericardial effusion. *A.* A posteroanterior film shows an appearance suggestive of an enlarged heart. However, the enlargement was the result of a pericardial effusion in a patient with systemic lupus erythematosus (SLE). *B.* After pericardiocentesis, the silhouette is normal.

hypertrophy. They do not necessarily enlarge in volume at the same time that they hypertrophy. For example, a patient with severe AS can have severe left ventricular hypertrophy and yet have a normal overall heart size. However, in a patient with severe AI, the left ventricle is significantly enlarged as a result of the high volume overload. Left ventricular hypertrophy is characterized initially by rounding of the apex and by normal heart size. In AS, hypertrophy occurs initially and left ventricular enlargement develops later, when the heart begins to fail. Right ventricular hypertrophy is difficult to diagnose and is usually suggested by associated findings of pulmonary hypertension or PS. Elevation of the apex and straightening of the upper left heart border are imprecise findings in right ventricular hypertrophy.

Situs

Situs refers to the positions of the atria and the abdominal viscera. It is important because certain kinds of situs arrangements are associated with a high incidence of CHD. The atria are not seen on chest radiographs, but they are almost always on the same side as the aortic arch. The side of the stomach bubble indicates the side of the visceral organs. An understanding of the sometimes confusing terms used to describe congenital cardiac anomalies is essential for communication between the radiologist and the primary care clinician (Table 5–6).

Determination of the situs allows prediction of the likelihood of CHD. Situs solitus is the normal situation with the arch (atria) and the stomach bubble on the left. Among such persons, the incidence of CHD is low (less than 1%). Whenever the chest or abdominal film demonstrates that the gastric air bubble and the cardiac apex are on opposite sides of the midline, the patient is presumed to have CHD until proved otherwise. Whenever films demonstrate a confusing situs (i.e., the gastric air bubble and the cardiac apex are on opposite sides of the midline, or a midline liver is present), the differential diagnosis must include the polysplenia and asplenia syndromes (to be discussed), and associated CHD must be considered likely. Several other specific kinds of situs must be considered.

In situs inversus, both the aortic arch and the stomach bubble are on the right, and the incidence of CHD among such patients is high. It should be appreciated that the most common reason for the diagnosis of situs inversus (dextroconfusion) is a mislabeled film. There are several kinds of situs inversus, each of which carries a different risk of associated CHD. (1) In situs inversus with mirror-image dextrocardia (also called mirror-image), the heart is on the right side of the chest, and the positions of the ventricles and atria are reversed. Among patients with mirror-image type situs, the incidence of CHD is very low (3%), but it is still greater than that of the general population (1%). (2) In situs solitus with dextrocardia, the arch (atria) and the stomach bubble are normal (on the left). However, the ventricles (cardiac apex) are on the right. Among such patients, the incidence of CHD is high (more than 95%). (3) In situs inversus with levocardia, the arch (atria) and the stomach bubble are on the right, and the ventricles (apex) are on the left. Among patients with this type of situs, the incidence of CHD is essentially 100%.

Situs ambiguous (indeterminatus) occurs when the arch (atria) and the stomach bubble are on opposite sides (this is not the same

TABLE 5–6. TERMS USED TO DESCRIBE ORGAN POSITIONS IN CONGENITAL HEART DISEASE

Situs	Positions of heart chambers, vessels, and abdominal organs in relation to one another
Situs solitus	Normal positions of atria, cardiac apex, aortic arch, stomach, and spleen on left side and of liver on right side
Situs inversus	Lateral transposition of these organs
Situs ambiguous	Indeterminate situs; atria and stomach on opposite sides
Dextroposition	Displacement of normal heart (and mediastinum) to right
Dextroversion	Location of heart in right hemithorax with cardiac apex on left and with left ventricle remaining on left but lying anterior to right ventricle
Dextrocardia	Location of heart in right hemithorax with cardiac apex on right, often with abnormal positioning of other viscera
Dextroconfusion	Apparent situs inversus (attributable to mislabeling of radiograph)
Mirror image	
Heart	Same as dextrocardia
Vessels	Left-to-right reversal of course of aortic arch and order of origins of brachiocephalic vessels

TABLE 5–7. FEATURES OF THE ASPLENIA AND POLYSPLENIA SYNDROMES

Feature	Asplenia	Polysplenia
Symmetry	Bilateral right-sidedness	Bilateral left-sidedness
Lung: minor fissure	Bilateral (3-lobed lungs bilaterally)	None (2-lobed lungs bilaterally)
Bronchi	Bilateral eparterial (both bronchi pass over pulmonary arteries)	Bilateral hyparterial (both bronchi pass under pulmonary arteries)
Spleen	None	More than one, on one or both sides
Red blood cell scan	No splenic tissue seen	Multiple spleens on one or both sides
Age at onset of symptoms	Newborn	Adult
Sex	Males slightly more	Females predominantly
Cyanosis	Severe	Absent
Pulmonary blood flow	Usually decreased	Normal, occasionally increased
CHD	Severe (PS or PA, common atrium, SV, TGV, or TAPVR)	Usually none, moderate degree if present (ASD, common atrium, or APVR)
Abdominal aorta	Frequently on same side as IVC	Normal
IVC	Normal	May be normal or interrupted below liver with azygos continuation
Azygous vein	Unapparent	May be quite large if IVC is interrupted
SVC	Usually present bilaterally	Usually present bilaterally

For explanation of abbreviations, see Table 5–1.

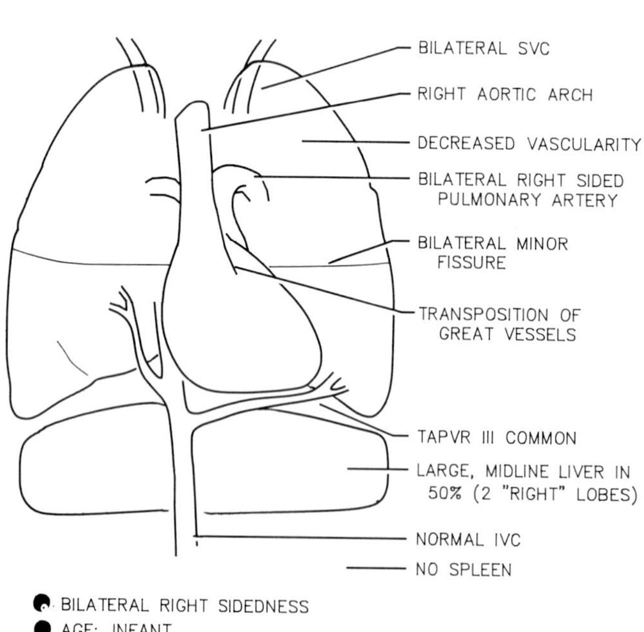

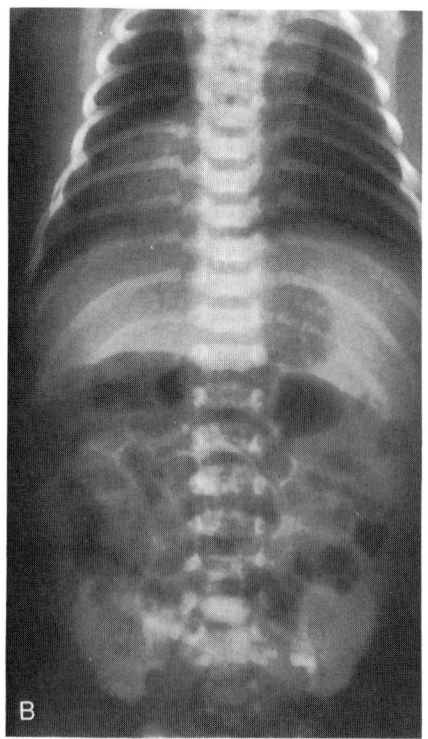

FIGURE 5–13. Asplenia. *A.* Diagram. SVC, superior vena cava; TAPVR, total anomalous pulmonary venous return; IVC, inferior vena cava; CHD, congenital heart disease. *B.* A full-body x-ray shows a large midline liver in a cyanotic premature infant. The stomach bubble is indeterminate as to which side it is on. The heart is, in this case, in the right side of the chest, and the aorta appears to be on the right side. The shadow in the left mediastinum represents the thymus. The pulmonary vessels are small. (Courtesy of R. Brasch, Department of Radiology, University of California, San Francisco.)

configuration as the apex and stomach bubble's being on opposite sides). There are two variations, the asplenia and polysplenia syndromes, whose presence depends on the location of splenic tissue (Table 5–7). CT or a nuclear medicine (technetium 99m–labeled) heat-damaged red blood cell scan can confirm the presence or absence of splenic tissue.

Asplenia. The asplenia syndrome can be characterized as bilateral development of structures that are normally right-sided. The liver is on both sides of the midline, and the spleen is absent. A middle lobe is present in each lung. Among asplenia patients, the incidence of CHD is very high. TGV is almost always present (Fig. 5–13), and TAPVR type III is often present. Infants with asplenia are cyanotic, and treatment is directed toward correction of the transposition.

Polysplenia. The polysplenia syndrome can be characterized as bilateral development of structures that are normally left-sided. Splenic tissue is present bilaterally, and, as in asplenia, the liver is on both sides of the midline. The lungs have a lingular segment bilaterally, and the inferior vena cava is often interrupted, venous return being carried by the (left-sided) azygos vein. Among polysplenia patients, the incidence of CHD is slightly higher than that among normal persons, but not as high as that among asplenia patients. Cardiac disease is less severe than in asplenia, and so the condition is not diagnosed until later in life. The most common congenital disease is ASD. Patients who have the polysplenia syndrome are usually not cyanotic. Chest radiographs show a midline liver, absence of minor fissures in the lungs, and normal or increased pulmonary vascularity (Fig. 5–14).

Dextroposition. Dextroposition, the displacement of the heart into the right side of the chest, can also be caused by skeletal, diaphragmatic, or pulmonary abnormalities. Skeletal abnormalities such as severe scoliosis, pectus deformity, or asymmetry of the thoracic cage can cause dextroposition. Skeletal abnormalities may suggest the presence of a genetic disease, many of which are accompanied by congenital heart defects. Diaphragmatic herniation and hypogenetic right lung syndrome are two other common causes of dextroposition.

Diaphragmatic Herniation. Diaphragmatic herniation, usually left-sided, is one of the more common causes of dextroposition (see Fig. 2–17). The abdominal contents enter the left side of the chest and displace all structures to the right.

Hypogenetic Right Lung Syndrome. Hypogenetic right lung syndrome occurs when hypoplasia of the right pulmonary artery results in hypoplasia of the right lung and the diaphragm. The heart and the mediastinum shift to the right. Usually there is partial anomalous pulmonary venous return (APVR), which proceeds from the right lung to the inferior vena cava via a curved (scimitar-shaped) pulmonary vein along the right border of the heart. The heart and the mediastinum consequently are shifted to the right (Fig. 5–15). The disease is therefore also called scimitar syndrome and partial APVR. The arterial supply to the hypoplastic lung, which is often from the aorta, can be demonstrated angiographically.

Pulmonary Blood Flow

The next major factor to consider in the evaluation of CHD is pulmonary blood flow. The two objectives are to quantify the flow (i.e., to determine whether flow is normal, increased, or decreased) and to determine the type of flow abnormality. The flow abnormality may be active congestion, resulting from arterial flow, or passive congestion, resulting from pulmonary venous obstruction. Distinguishing arteries from veins can be difficult but is facilitated by their course, origins, branching, and distinctness (Table 5–8).

Increased pulmonary blood flow can be assessed in several ways (Fig. 5–16). In the absence of a large shunt, the descending right pulmonary artery along the bronchus inter-

TABLE 5–8. DISTINGUISHING PULMONARY ARTERIES FROM VEINS

Pulmonary Veins
Run more vertically in upper portion of lung, horizontally in lower portion
Less sharply defined than arteries
Branch less than arteries
Lower confluence in mediastinum of pulmonary veins at right atrium
Passive congestion causes veins to be large, indistinct
Pulmonary Arteries
Run more horizontally in upper portion of lung, vertically in lower portion
More sharply defined than veins
Branch more than veins
Originate from higher point in mediastinum
Increased flow causes arteries to be large, distinct

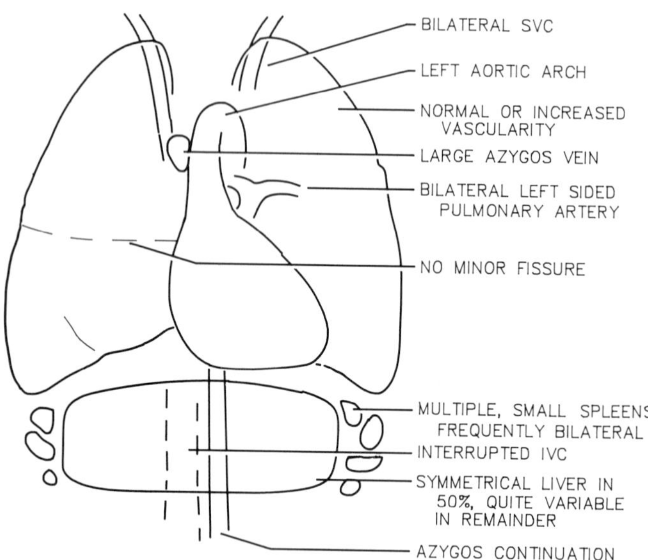

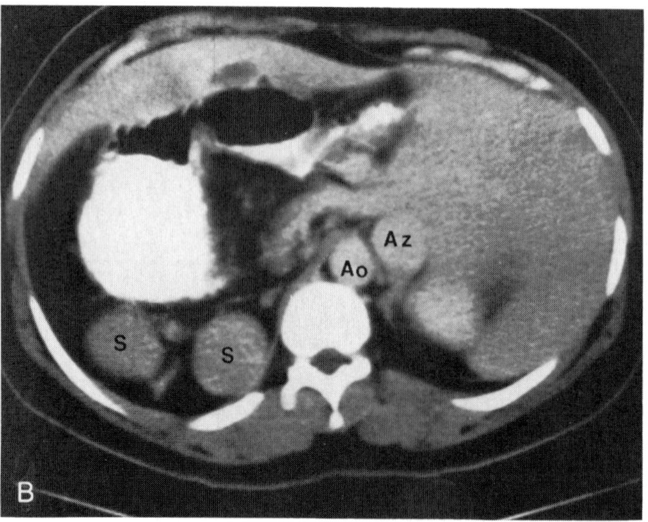

FIGURE 5–14. Polysplenia. *A.* Diagram. SVC, superior vena cava; IVC, inferior vena cava; CHD, congenital heart disease. *B.* A CT slice of the upper abdomen shows the liver predominantly on the left side. Multiple, round lumps of splenic tissue (S) are seen posterior to the white, contrast-filled stomach on the right side. Between the normal aorta (Ao) and the liver is the enlarged azygos vein (Az). No inferior vena cava is seen.

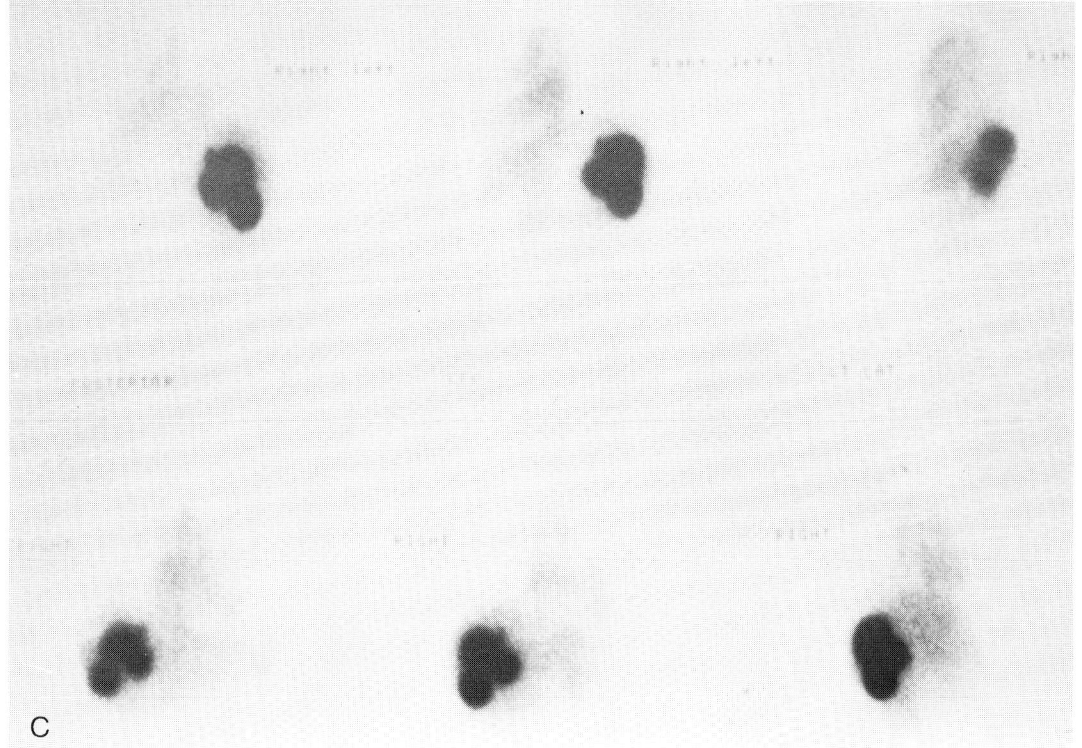

FIGURE 5–14 *Continued C.* Technetium 99m–tagged red blood cell scan shows intense sequestration of the damaged red cells in multiple, right-sided lumps of spleen.

medius is never larger in diameter than the trachea. In other words, if the right pulmonary artery is smaller than the trachea, there is no detectable shunt. A second method is to compare vessels seen end-on with their companion bronchi. If the vessels are larger than the bronchi, the ratio of pulmonary artery to systemic blood flow is at least 2:1, which is the smallest ratio at which a shunt is identifiable on plain radiographs. A third method is to compare the vessels with those of other patients of similar age, height, and physique. The criteria for normal pulmonary vascularity change with age. For example, in newborns the absolute size of the vessels is very small. An appearance of pulmonary markings that is normal by adult standards probably means that their size is at least mildly increased in a newborn. Accurate assessment of pulmonary vascularity on chest films requires considerable experience.

Normal Pulmonary Vessels. CHDs that do not result in shunting of blood or mitral valve obstruction do not usually affect the pulmonary vessels. The most important of these diseases are coarctation of the aorta, PS, congenital AS, endocardial fibroelastosis, and congenitally corrected transposition of the great arteries. TOF patients who have a mild degree of PS have only mild cyanosis (therefore the condition is called pink TOF) and normal pulmonary vascularity.

Small Pulmonary Vessels. When blood flow is decreased, the lungs are relatively oligemic. The two major causes of this decrease are right-to-left shunts and pulmonary hypertension.

PS is the most common cause of right-to-left shunt, either isolated or in conjunction with other (usually congenital) heart problems. The venous blood is restricted from leaving the right side of the heart to enter the lungs. The pulmonary vessels are much smaller in size and apparently fewer in number. Other diseases that cause obstruction to flow to the lungs are TOF, TA, and Ebstein's anomaly. Single ventricle with PS and TRUNCUS type IV (to be described) are less common congenital defects that can cause decreased caliber of the pulmonary vessels.

There are two varieties of pulmonary hypertension. Primary pulmonary hypertension is caused by an idiopathic narrowing of the medium-sized and small pulmonary arterial

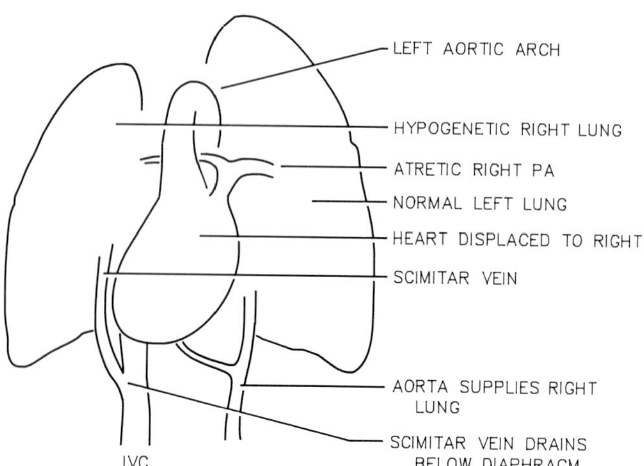

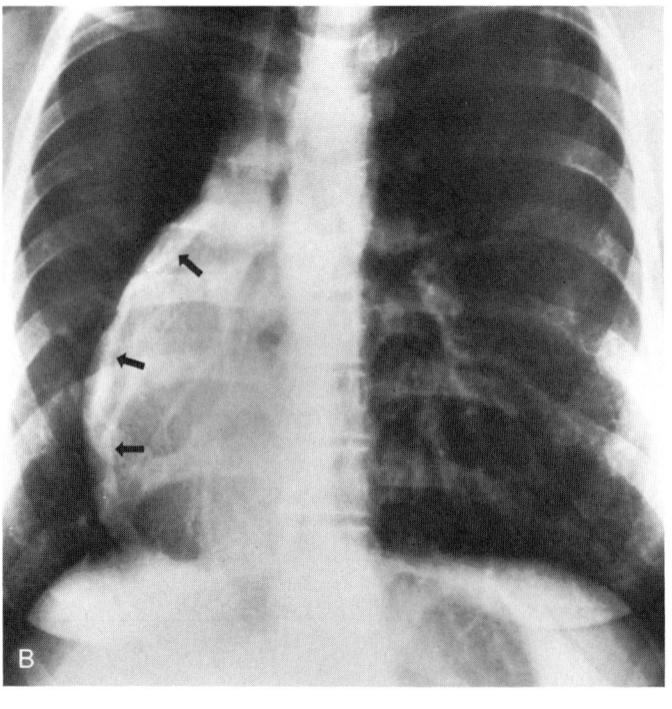

FIGURE 5–15. Hypogenetic right lung (scimitar) syndrome. *A.* Diagram. PA, pulmonary artery; IVC, inferior vena cava; CHD, congenital heart disease; ASD, atrial septal defect; VSD, ventricular septal defect. *B.* Posteroanterior chest film shows marked vascular attenuation in the right lung. The heart is displaced to the right side of the chest (dextroposition, not dextrocardia). Along the right border of the heart (*arrows*), a curvilinear pulmonary vein passes from the right lung through the diaphragm. This form of partial anomalous venous return is sometimes called scimitar or venolobar syndrome.

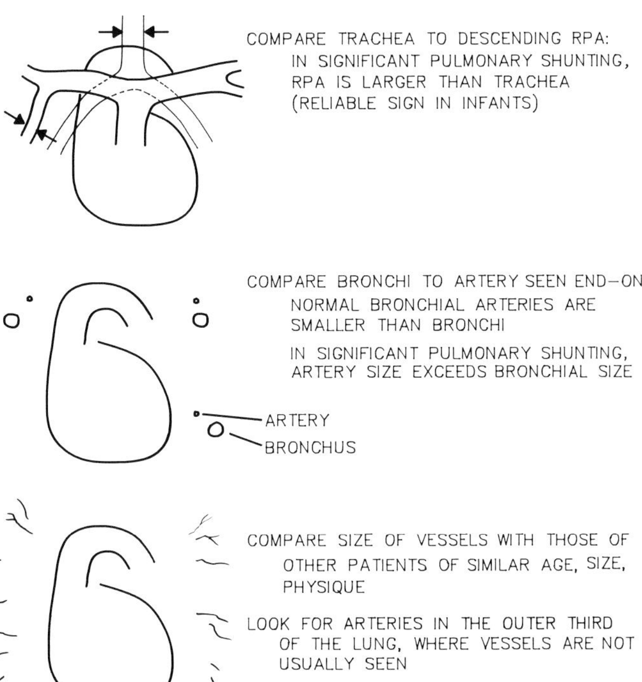

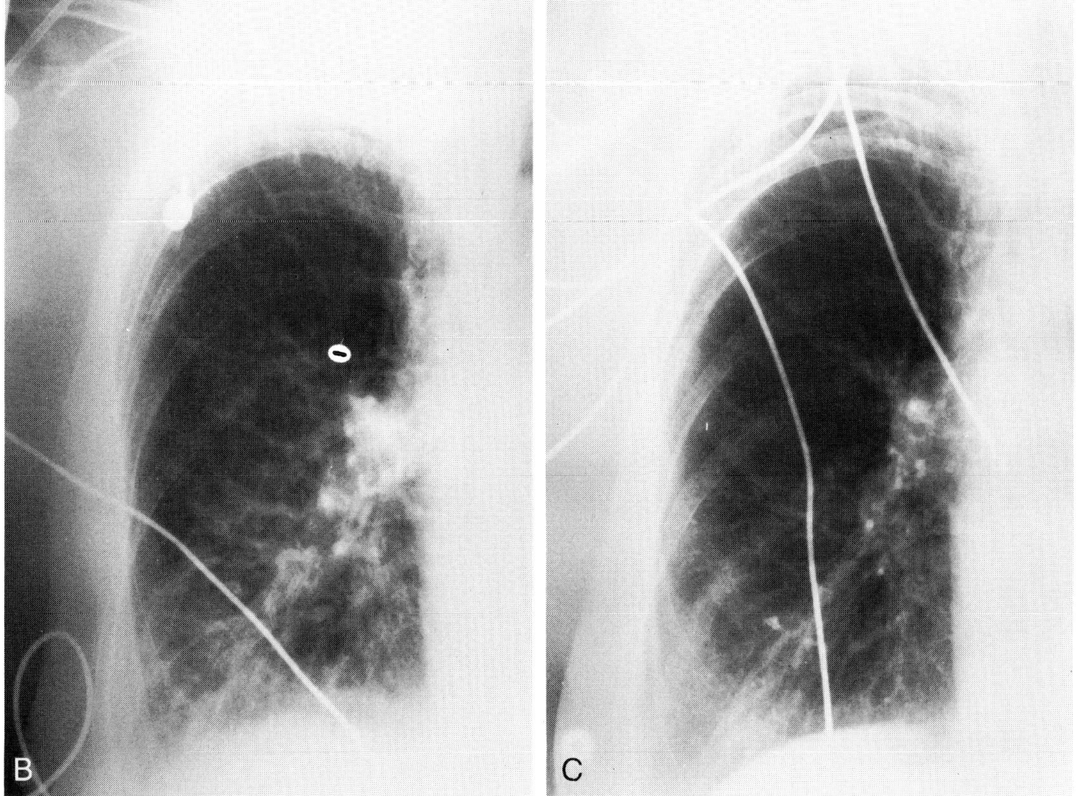

FIGURE 5–16. Increased pulmonary blood volume. *A.* Diagram. RPA, right pulmonary artery. *B* and *C.* Venous distention in a patient with congestive heart failure (*B*) is relieved after diuresis (*C*). The caliber of the blood vessels has decreased, and the edges of these vessels are more distinct in the normal state.

TABLE 5–9. CAUSES OF PULMONARY VENOUS CONGESTION

Normal Heart Size
Mitral stenosis
Mitral atresia
Cor triatriatum
Left atrial myxoma
Pulmonary veno-occlusive disease
TAPVR type III
Hypoplastic left heart syndrome
Cardiac Enlargement
Mitral regurgitation
Left ventricular failure from any cause

TAPVR, total anomalous pulmonary venous return.

branches. The central pulmonary arteries are moderately larger than normal and taper gradually so that the peripheral lung zones are oligemic.

Secondary pulmonary hypertension is most often caused by Eisenmenger's syndrome, in which a previous, large left-to-right shunt overperfuses the lungs for a long time. The increased pressure and volume of blood causes secondary pulmonary hypertension. The central pulmonary arteries are dilated and taper rapidly, causing the peripheral portions of the lungs to become markedly oligemic.

Actively Enlarged Pulmonary Vessels. CHDs in which the pulmonary vessels appear enlarged and distinct on radiographs are caused by overcirculation of blood through the lungs, usually the result of a left-to-right shunt. These CHDs are divided into acyanotic and cyanotic groups, although the diagnosis can often be made in the absence of knowledge of the arterial blood gas values. Sometimes the blood gas values are equivocal or inconsistent with the presumptive diagnosis. In such instances, the radiologist may suggest an alternative diagnosis or indicate that the lesion is more complicated than suspected on clinical findings. The most common acyanotic diseases are ASD, VSD, and PDA.

Passive Congestion. There are numerous causes of increased pulmonary vascularity attributable to passive venous congestion (Table 5–9; see also Table 2–7). They are all results of either physical or functional obstruction that causes blood to back up into the pulmonary veins. Causes of passive congestion include CHF and lesions that prevent return of pulmonary venous blood to the left ventricle, such as mitral stenosis, left atrial myxoma, or cor triatriatum. Radiographs show enlarged, indistinct vessels (veins), redistribution of blood flow to the upper lungs, pleural effusion, and Kerley's lines (Fig. 5–17; see also Fig. 5–2). CHF is discussed later and in Chapter 2.

TYPES OF CHD

A method of organizing the many CHD conditions is essential for diagnosis. The method used in this chapter is to categorize the diseases first by cyanosis, then by the appearance of the pulmonary vascularity, and finally by heart size (Fig. 5–18).

Individual congenital diseases are presented according to this format, which also assists in organization and application of this information. The three major considerations of this approach are, therefore, the presence or absence of cyanosis, the type of pulmonary blood flow (i.e.,

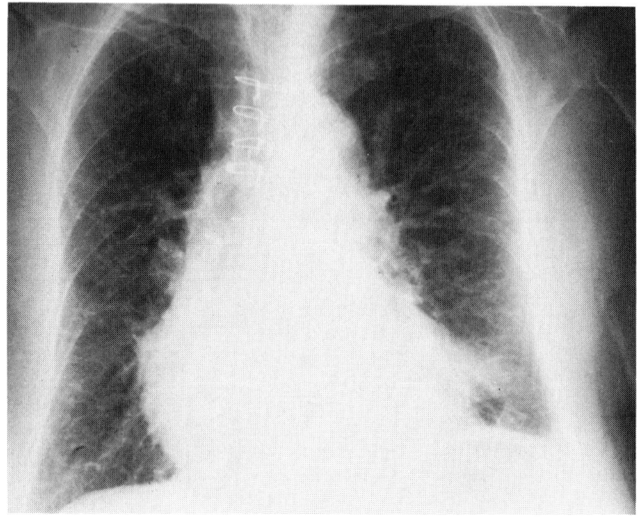

FIGURE 5–17. Congestive heart failure in an adult. The heart is enlarged, the perihilar vessels are indistinct, the lungs are marked with a reticular pattern that includes Kerley's B lines, and there is a small, left pleural effusion that blunts the left lateral costophrenic angle. The patient's left ventricle is failing, even after coronary artery bypass grafting.

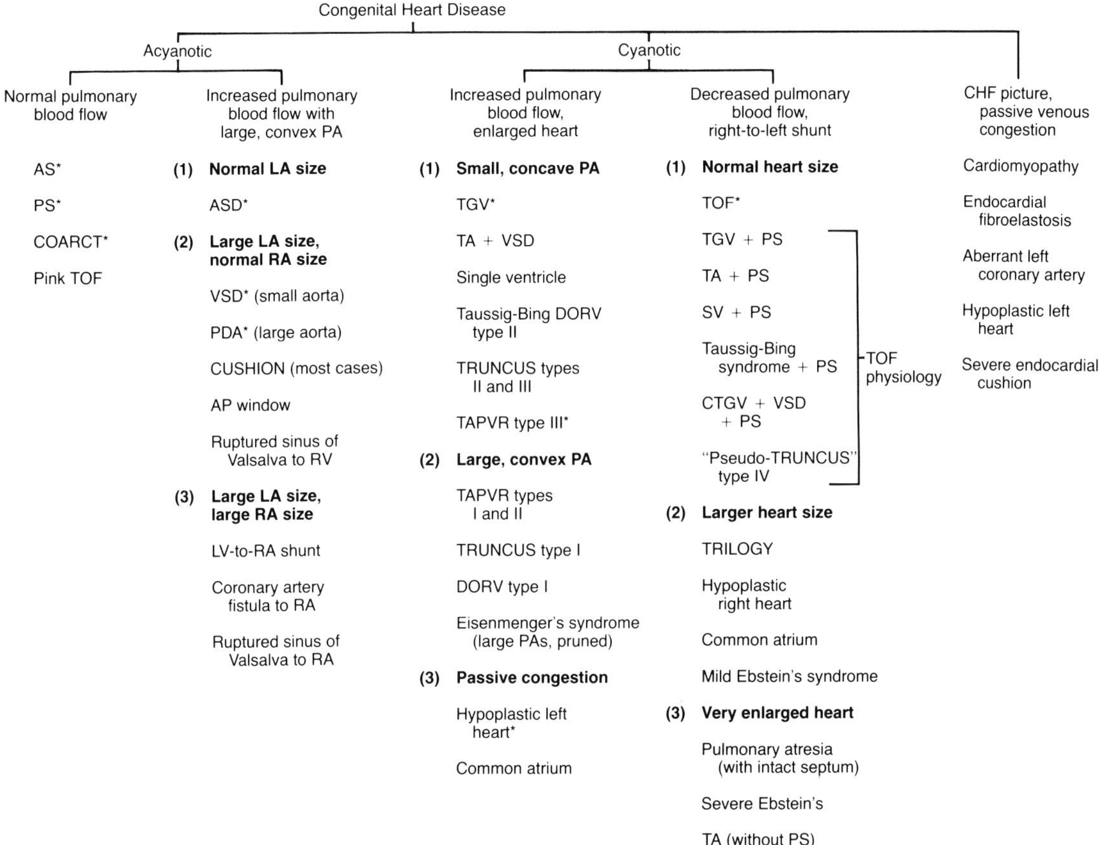

FIGURE 5–18. Schema for the evaluation of congenital heart disease. Asterisks indicate common causes. PA, pulmonary artery; AP, aortopulmonary. For explanation of other abbreviations, see Table 5–1.

normal, decreased, or increased), and heart size (normal or enlarged). Knowledge of even one of these factors helps limit the differential diagnosis. Use of this method reduces an extremely complex diagnostic problem to a much shorter and workable differential diagnostic list.

Presentation: Acyanotic, Normal Heart Size, Normal Pulmonary Vascularity (Column 1 of Fig. 5–18)

Acyanotic CHD with normal pulmonary vascularity is the result of some type of outflow obstruction. The obstruction may cause hypertrophy but not enlargement. The most important diseases in this group are coarctation, PS, and AS (Fig. 5–19). Mild TOF, in which PS is present but not severe and which is called pink TOF, has a radiographic appearance similar to that of PS. Cyanosis is minimal, and the patient appears pink, as opposed to cyanotic (blue).

Aortic Stenosis. Aortic stenosis (AS) is the most common type of CHD with this clinical presentation. It can be congenital or acquired. The discussion of AS is presented later in the section "Acquired Diseases."

Pulmonic Stenosis. Isolated PS is rare. More commonly, it is associated with other anomalies. The most common, and important, of these is TOF. PS can be associated with any of the cyanotic heart diseases. In such cases, however, the pulmonary vasculature is decreased because of the low blood flow to the lungs. In the most severe cases of PS, an ASD and a PDA are needed to augment the severely limited blood flow to the lungs. A VSD may also be present but is not essential for survival. In mild to moderate PS, patients are asymptomatic. Patients with severe, isolated PS are

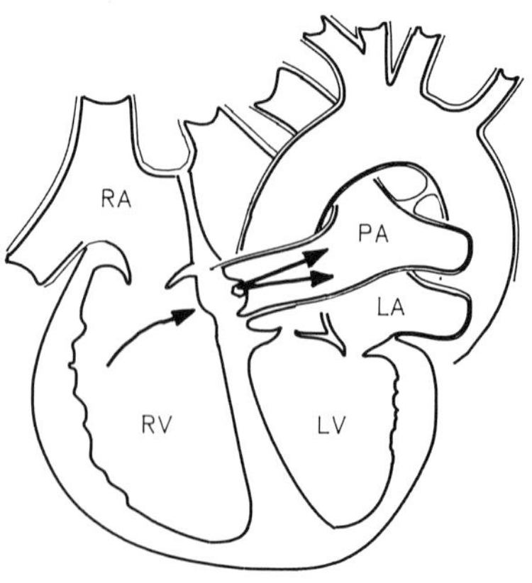

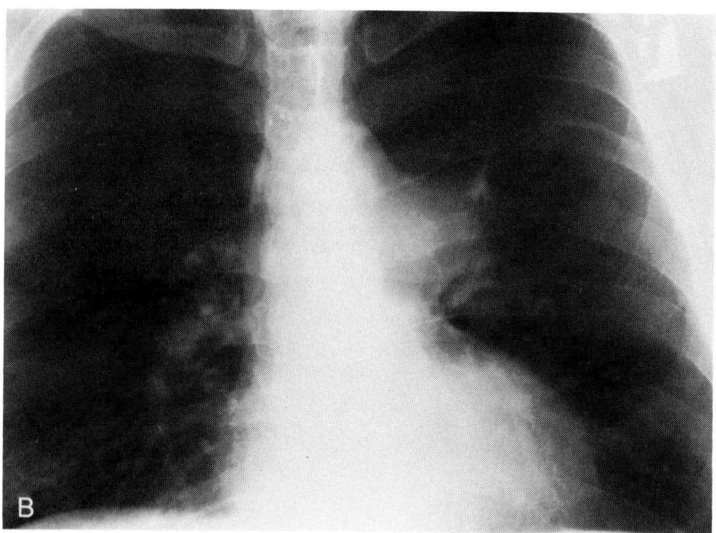

FIGURE 5–19. Pulmonic stenosis. *A.* Diagram. *B.* Marked poststenotic dilation of the central pulmonary artery in an adult male makes a prominent bulge over the left hilar region.

not cyanotic. They have symptoms of fatigue, dyspnea on exertion, and eventually right heart failure that produces cor pulmonale, an enlarged liver, and pedal edema.

Radiographs usually show normal pulmonary vascularity, a small pulmonary artery, and usually a normal heart size (Fig. 5–19). The jet effect caused by the stenotic valve can produce marked enlargement of the left pulmonary artery. Absence of the pulmonary valve results in massive enlargement of the main pulmonary artery.

Coarctation of the Aorta. The two major types of coarctation of the aorta, infantile and adult, represent opposite ends of a spectrum (Table 5–10). The site of the coarctation is usually described in relation to where the ductus arteriosus enters the aorta (preductal or postductal). The infantile, or neonatal, type of coarctation is much less common but by far the more severe type. This lesion is preductal in position and is much longer than the adult type. It can appear alone as a long segment lesion of the ascending aorta, as a generalized hypoplastic aorta, or as complete interruption of the aortic arch. It is frequently associated with the hypoplastic left heart syndrome and could therefore be considered part of the spectrum of that disease. The adult type of coarctation is more common. The lesion is postductal with thickening of the aortic wall and narrowing of aortic diameter over a short segment just beyond the ligamentum arteriosum. Pseudocoarctation is a kink at the site of the ligamentum arteriosum. It is usually seen in older adults and has no pressure gradient.

TABLE 5–10. FEATURES OF COARCTATION OF THE AORTA

Characteristics	Type of Coarctation: *Infantile/Neonatal*	*Adult*	*Pseudo-Coarctation*
Age at diagnosis	Neonate	Several weeks to late adulthood	Usually older, but can be seen in younger people
Site	Preductal	Postductal	Kink at ligamentum arteriosum
Severity	Very severe	Mild to moderate	None
Chest film	Small ascending aorta and arch, large PA, CHF	Rib notching, "3" sign on aorta, "Ɛ" sign on barium swallow, prominent ascending aorta	High aortic arch
Lesion	Long segment or hypoplastic ascending aorta	Short segment Thickened wall, narrow diameter at coarct site	No lesion Aortic arch positioned higher than usual; kinked aorta; no obstruction
Pressure gradient	High grade or total obstruction	Moderate to severe pressure gradient	No gradient
Associated diseases	Hypoplastic left heart syndrome PDA (compensatory lesion)	Bicuspid aortic valve (80%) PDA (35%) VSD (15%) Turner's syndrome Secondary LV hypertrophy	Adult: none Child: increased incidence of PDA and VSD

For explanation of abbreviations, see Table 5–1.

CHF is the most common manifesting symptom of infantile coarctation. It usually occurs in the neonate after the first week of life, when the PDA closes. In the adult type, symptoms, if any, do not appear until the child is several years old and often not until quite late in adult life. The most recognizable symptoms of adult coarctation are headache and claudication of the lower extremities. The blood pressure is decreased in the lower extremities and increased in the upper extremities.

Chest films in infantile coarctation show CHF and a small aorta. When hypoplastic left heart syndrome is also present, the PDA remains open, producing a large pulmonary outflow tract, which can be mistaken for the aortic arch. The blood flow in the PDA is from right to left (i.e., from the pulmonary to the systemic circulation), opposite to the flow in typical PDA.

In adult type coarctation, chest films show a high aortic arch with an indentation (the coarctation), which gives it a "3" configuration (Fig. 5–20). On barium swallow examination, the indentation makes an "Ɛ" configuration. Also shown are enlargement of the ascending aorta and rib notching (which occurs only in the postductal type of coarctation). This notching is usually seen after age 8 years and involves the inferior surface of the posterior third to ninth ribs. It is caused by increased retrograde flow through the intercostal arteries back to the descending aorta. Cardiac catheterization measurements reveal a mild to severe pressure gradient across the coarctation. Secondary left ventricular hypertrophy is seen in severe cases. MRI with the use of off-axis planes makes it possible to visualize the exact site of the coarctation.

The overall prognosis for infantile coarctation is extremely poor; 75% of affected infants die within 1 month. Adult coarctation is treated by surgical resection of the coarcted segment and substitution of a graft.

Presentation: Acyanotic, Increased Pulmonary Vascularity with Large Convex Pulmonary Artery, Cardiac Enlargement (Column 2 of Fig. 5–18)

Acyanotic CHD with actively increased pulmonary vascularity results from overcirculation of blood through the lungs. The overcirculation is caused by a left-to-right shunt that mixes oxygenated blood and venous blood in the right side of the heart or in the pulmonary artery. The blood that enters the systemic circulation is fully oxygenated, and so there is no cyanosis. The most important diseases in this group are ASD, VSD, and PDA. In all three of these diseases, there is cardiac enlargement, but the type of enlargement depends on the location of the shunt.

Atrial Septal Defect. ASD is the sixth most common CHD, accounting for about 7% of CHD cases. Because of the complex formation

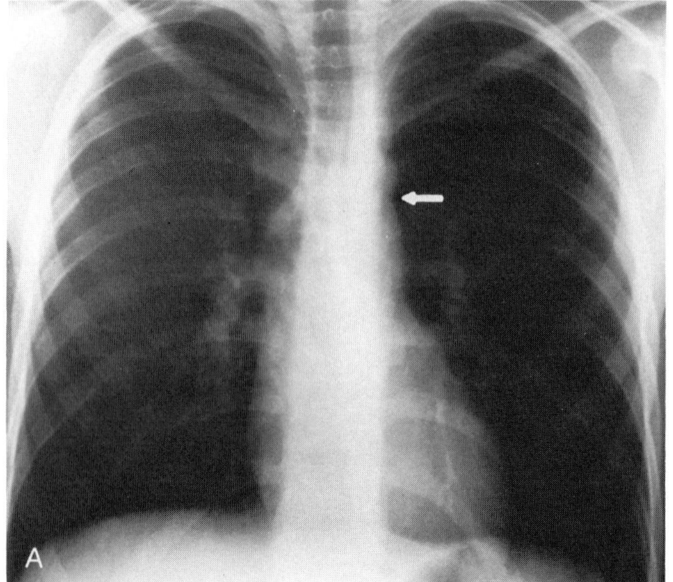

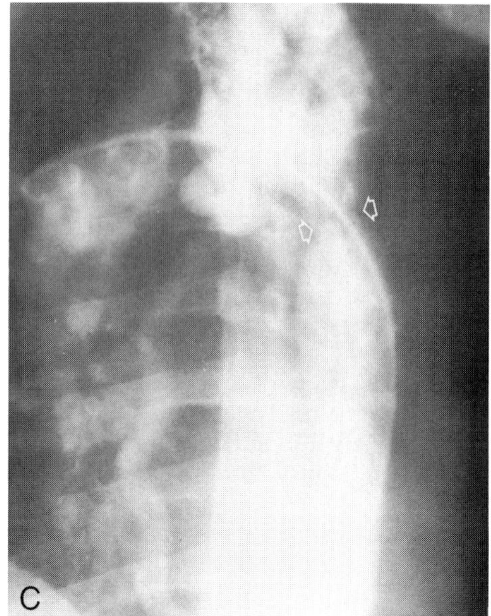

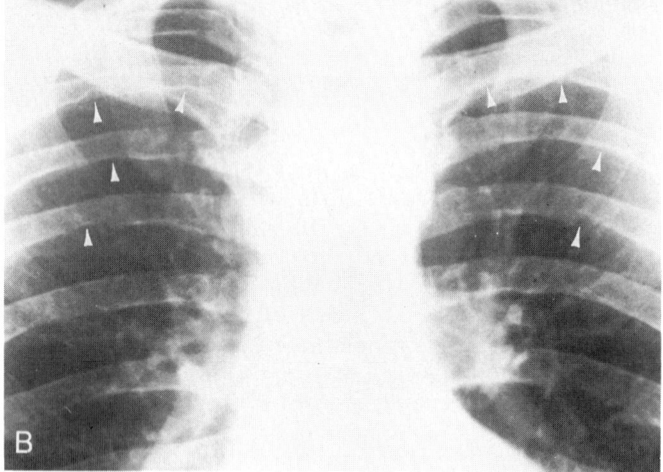

FIGURE 5–20. Coarctation of the aorta. *A.* Posteroanterior chest film shows a notch in the descending aorta (*arrow*) caused by coarctation in a 10-year-old boy. (Courtesy of R. Brasch, Department of Radiology, University of California, San Francisco.) *B.* Another patient with a long-standing coarctation developed notches (*arrowheads*) in the inferior margins of the upper ribs, where engorged costal arteries serving as collateral vessels have become tortuous and pulse against the ribs. *C.* An arteriogram of the aortic arch opacifies its major vessels and shows the coarct (*open arrowheads*) as an abrupt constriction of the lumen of the aorta.

of the atrial septum, the partition between the right and left atria has potential for abnormal communication in three separate places (Fig. 5–21).

The sinus venosus type of ASD is located superior and posterior in the interatrial septum, where the pulmonary veins enter. It is frequently seen in association with partial anomalous venous return of right upper lobe pulmonary veins into the superior vena cava. This type of ASD is uncommon and is seen usually in neonates.

The ostium secundum type of ASD is in the midportion of the atrial septum anteriorly, at the fossa ovalis. This is the site of the foramen ovale, which in fetal life functions as a one-way flap valve that opens preferentially from the right atrium into the left atrium. This valve functionally closes shortly after birth, and the result is a thin septal membrane. The ostium secundum ASD occurs when this thin membrane is defective and the valve remains patent. It is the most common type of ASD, accounting for two thirds of all cases. As infants, patients tolerate the left-to-right shunt because the shunt is of low pressure. The shunt is often detected at a much older age (late teens) when a murmur is heard on physical examination. The prognosis is favorable because the problem is usually isolated and is not associated with valvular abnormalities.

The ostium primum type of ASD is most inferior in the atrial septum and is almost always associated with abnormalities of the adjacent mitral and tricuspid valves. It is frequently part of the endocardial cushion defect

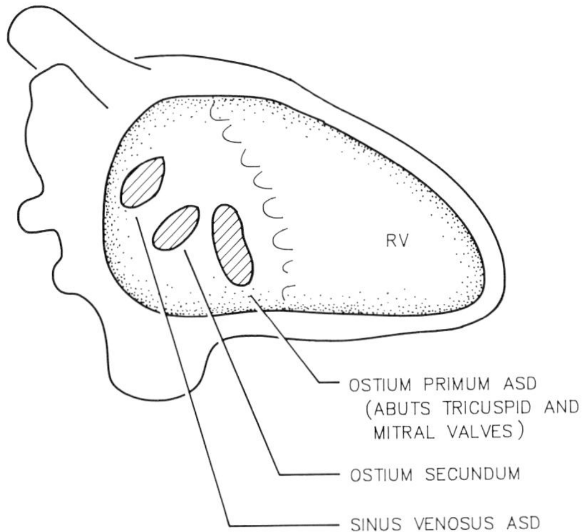

FIGURE 5–21. Types of atrial septal defects (ASD). RV, right ventricle.

(to be described). Ostium primum manifests in early childhood, especially if it is part of the endocardial cushion defect.

ASD patients are not usually cyanotic, except for those with severe ostium primum ASD or with the endocardial cushion defect, in which cyanosis develops as a result of shunting from the left ventricle to the right atrium. Late in the course of severe ASD, the excess blood flow to the lungs from the left-to-right shunt results in intimal proliferation of the pulmonary arteries and secondary pulmonary hypertension. The end stage is Eisenmenger's syndrome, in which pulmonary artery pressures exceed systemic pressures and the shunt reverses to become right-to-left. When Eisenmenger's syndrome develops, the patient may become cyanotic, a condition called tardive cyanosis.

Chest radiographs in mild cases of ASD are often entirely normal. Increased pulmonary blood flow is visible if the shunt magnitude is greater than 2:1. The proximal pulmonary arteries may be enlarged. There may be enlargement of both the right atrium and the right ventricle (i.e., right-sided enlargement) (Fig. 5–22), but not of the left atrium; this finding differentiates ASD from VSD and PDA. When Eisenmenger's syndrome occurs, the central pulmonary arteries become very large and the peripheral portions of the lungs become oligemic. On angiography, the catheter passes across the ASD from the right side of the heart to the left. The ASD itself is frequently not well seen with contrast injection into the left atrium. The diagnosis is usually proved by a demonstration that the oxygen saturation of blood taken from the right atrium exceeds a similar sample from the superior vena cava. Ultrasonography provides direct visualization of ASD lesions. However, in normal patients, loss of echo reception (echo dropout) can cause a normal septum to be misinterpreted as ASD. Therefore, multiple views and Doppler techniques are necessary for confirming the diagnosis.

Treatment is surgical closure of the ASD. This must be done before Eisenmenger's syndrome develops because closure of the ASD in the face of severe pulmonary hypertension causes right-sided heart failure and death.

Ventricular Septal Defect. VSD is overall the most common single type of CHD, accounting for 27% of all CHD cases. VSD can occur alone or can accompany other cardiac lesions (Table 5–11), most commonly PS, endocardial cushion defect, and TOF. The greater contractile force of the left ventricle ensures that shunting is from left to right unless other conditions, such as PS or pulmonary hypertension, are present. As a result, mixed right- and left-sided cardiac enlargement and pulmonary overcirculation occur.

The interventricular septum consists of a large muscular portion centrally and anteriorly and a thin membranous portion posteriorly near the tricuspid valve. There are three major forms of VSD: membranous, muscular, and supracristal (Fig. 5–23). The membranous type is the most common, accounting for 80% of all cases. It is the type of VSD involved in the endocardial cushion complex. Because of its proximity to the tricuspid valve, the membranous type of VSD can allow left-to-right shunting of blood directly from the left ventricle into the right atrium. The muscular type of VSD is much less common and usually small. There may be a single defect or multiple de-

TABLE 5–11. CHD THAT MAY BE ASSOCIATED WITH VSD

Pulmonic valve stenosis	15%
Endocardial cushion defect	6%
Tetralogy of Fallot	5%
Subaortic stenosis	<5%
Corrected TGV	<5%
Coarctation of the aorta	<5%
Interruption of the aortic arch	<5%
DORV	<5%
TRUNCUS	<5%
AP window	<5%
ASD	<5%
PDA	<5%
Hypoplastic RV	<5%

For explanation of abbreviations, see Table 5–1.

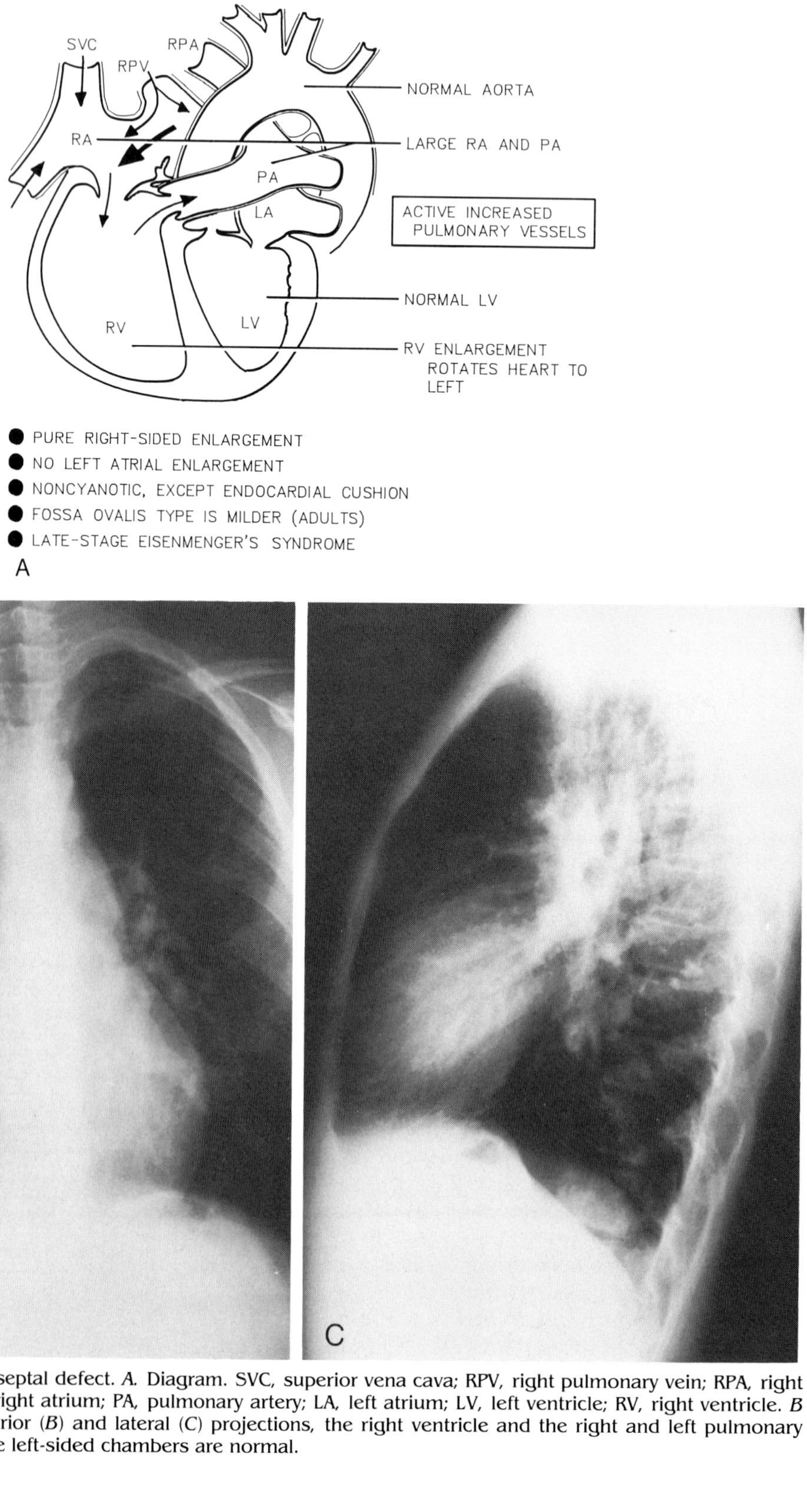

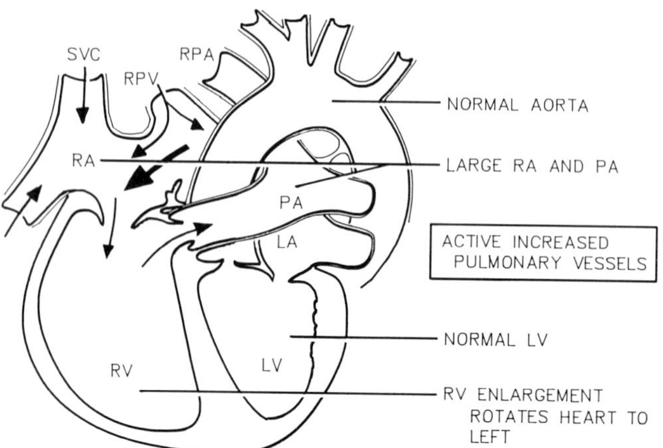

- PURE RIGHT-SIDED ENLARGEMENT
- NO LEFT ATRIAL ENLARGEMENT
- NONCYANOTIC, EXCEPT ENDOCARDIAL CUSHION
- FOSSA OVALIS TYPE IS MILDER (ADULTS)
- LATE-STAGE EISENMENGER'S SYNDROME

A

B

C

FIGURE 5–22. Atrial septal defect. *A*. Diagram. SVC, superior vena cava; RPV, right pulmonary vein; RPA, right pulmonary artery; RA, right atrium; PA, pulmonary artery; LA, left atrium; LV, left ventricle; RV, right ventricle. *B* and *C*. On posteroanterior (*B*) and lateral (*C*) projections, the right ventricle and the right and left pulmonary arteries are dilated. The left-sided chambers are normal.

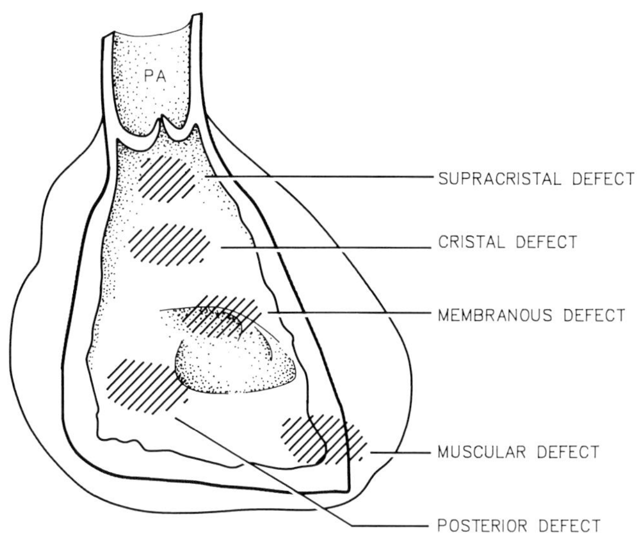

FIGURE 5–23. Appearance of ventricular septal defect. PA, pulmonary artery.

fects in the muscular septum, which tend to close partially as the septum contracts. This type of VSD is usually seen in children, and at least 30% of the defects spontaneously close by age 2 years. The supracristal type (also called the bulbar type) of VSD is least common and is located high in the membranous portion of the septal wall. It results from a defect in the conus portion of the truncus arteriosus in the aortic outflow tract. It is therefore associated with TOF, TGV, and TRUNCUS.

As with ASD, there is a left-to-right shunt, the magnitude of which is proportional to the size of the defect. A systolic murmur can be heard. Shortness of breath and dyspnea develop at a much earlier age (although not in the immediate neonatal period) than do symptoms caused by ASD because of the much higher pressure of the ventricular system. There is usually no cyanosis unless the VSD is associated with an endocardial cushion defect. Cyanosis caused by Eisenmenger's syndrome occurs as a later complication in a fashion similar to that described for ASD. However, it develops at a much earlier age because the process is driven by the higher ventricular pressures.

Chest radiographs show increased pulmonary flow if the magnitude of the shunt is greater than 2:1 (Fig. 5–24). The right ventricle is enlarged because of the excess blood volume shunted to it from the left ventricle. The right atrium is not enlarged because the shunt occurs at the ventricle level. Unlike ASD, in which the left atrium can decompress by shunting its excessive volume into the right atrium, the left atrium must pump the entire blood volume into the left ventricle, and consequently it enlarges. Therefore, the cardiac appearance is mixed right- and left-sided enlargement (especially left atrial enlargement), a finding that is essential for differentiating VSD from ASD. The left atrium may become smaller later because its volume load decreases. Decreased size of the left atrium is a bad prognostic sign because it indicates reversal of blood flow in the shunt.

In angiography, the catheter passes across the VSD from the right ventricle to the left ventricle; contrast injected into the left ventricle usually reveals the lesion in the interventricular septum. Angiograms may show more than one VSD. Cardiac ultrasonography shows the septal defect; scans can be falsely positive, because of echo dropout effect, as described in ASD detection. Doppler flow studies can show the shunting of blood. Chamber sizes can be easily measured by ultrasonography.

Nearly a third of VSDs (especially the muscular type) close spontaneously and need no treatment. Definitive therapy for significant VSD lesions is surgical closure of the abnormal opening in the septum. In an infant with significant VSD, the Dannan procedure (banding one of the pulmonary arteries) protects one of the lungs from the high systemic pressures and minimizes or delays the development of pulmonary hypertension. This temporizing procedure allows closure of the VSD when the child is older.

Endocardial Cushion Defect. The endocardial cushion is the tissue responsible for forming adjacent structures in the central portions of the heart chambers. These structures include the more inferior parts of the interatrial septum, the septal leaflet portions of the mitral

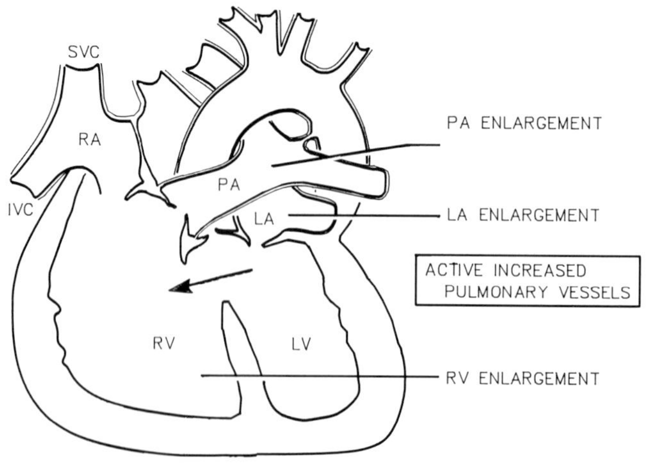

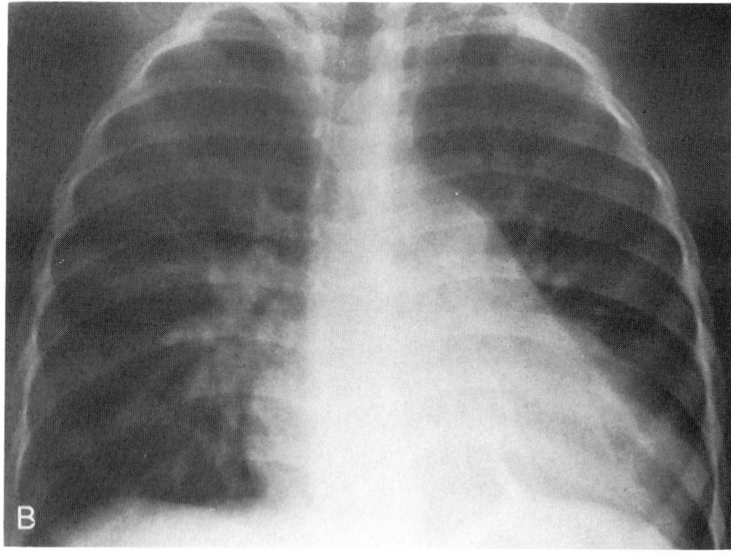

FIGURE 5–24. Ventricular septal defect (VSD). *A.* Diagram. SVC, superior vena cava; RA, right atrium; PA, pulmonary artery; IVC, inferior vena cava; LA, left atrium; RV, right ventricle; LV, left ventricle. *B.* Posteroanterior chest film shows mixed left- and right-sided enlargement. The vessels are large and distinct.

and tricuspid valves, and the superior portions of the interventricular septum (Fig. 5–25). Depending on the severity of the malformation, all or part of the defect may be present. Overall, endocardial cushion defect is less common than ASD or VSD, except among patients with Down's syndrome.

Mild and intermediate defects are functionally similar to ASD (i.e., left-to-right shunt), with additional mitral regurgitation caused by the cleft mitral valve leaflet. Patients have heart murmurs and increased pulmonary blood flow because of the shunt, but they are acyanotic. Symptoms are mild during childhood.

Intermediate and severe defects are functionally similar to VSD. Patients develop symptoms at an earlier age because the VSD component of the syndrome becomes dominant. The usual symptoms are poor weight gain during infancy, recurrent respiratory infections, systolic cardiac murmur, and CHF.

Severe cushion defects include a direct shunt from the left ventricle to the right atrium, a condition that is much more serious because the shunting is from a high-pressure chamber into a low-pressure chamber. Affected patients may be cyanotic as a result of the mixing of venous and arterial blood. Electrocardiograms

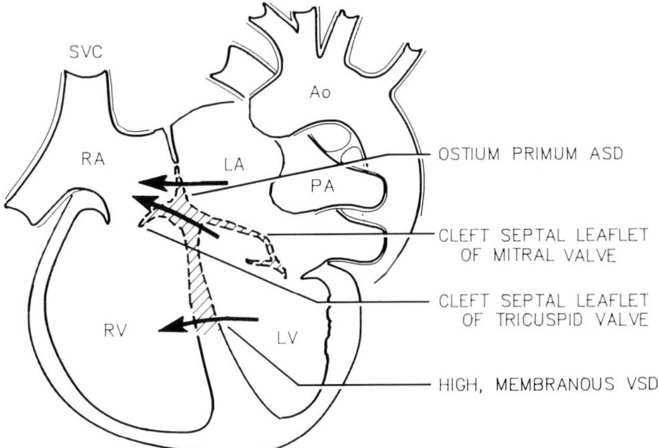

- MILD DEFECT RESEMBLES ASD
- SEVERE DEFECT RESEMBLES VSD
- USUALLY ACYANOTIC
- SEVERE DEFECT SHUNTS LV TO RA AND CAUSES CYANOSIS
- HIGH ASSOCIATION WITH DOWN'S SYNDROME
  50% OF CUSHION DEFECT PATIENTS HAVE DOWN'S
  15% OF DOWN'S HAVE CUSHION DEFECT
- OSTIUM PRIMUM ASD (LEAST SEVERE) PRESENT IN ALL CASES
- CLEFT SEPTAL LEAFLET OF MITRAL VALVE (PRESENT IN MODERATELY SEVERE CASES) CAUSES MITRAL REGURGITATION
- HIGH, MEMBRANOUS VSD PRESENT IN SEVERE CASES

A

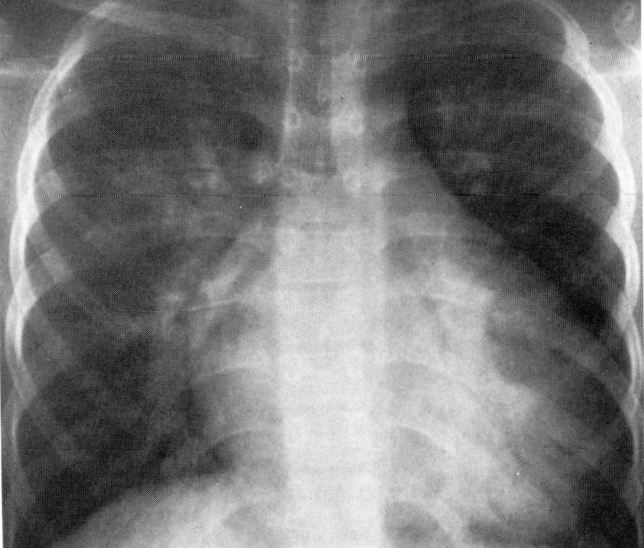

FIGURE 5–25. Endocardial cushion defect. *A.* Diagram. SVC, superior vena cava; Ao, aorta; RA, right atrium; LA, left atrium; PA, pulmonary artery; ASD, atrial septal defect; RV, right ventricle; LV, left ventricle; VSD, ventricular septal defect. *B.* Posteroanterior chest film shows a massively enlarged heart with a prominent proximal pulmonary artery segment. Pulmonary vessels are markedly enlarged and distinct. The patient, a 12-year-old girl, was not cyanotic. (Courtesy of R. Brasch, Department of Radiology, University of California, San Francisco.)

often reveal left-axis deviation, not because of the large size of the left ventricle, but because the ventricular conducting system is directed along the malformed cushion.

The chest film appearance is similar to that of ASD. In addition, some degree of left atrial enlargement is frequently present, as a result of mitral regurgitation. Angiograms show a narrowing of the left ventricle outflow tract (the goose-neck deformity, seen only on the anterior view) caused by the malformed mitral valve. Cardiac ultrasonography shows a much larger defect in the central portion of the heart than in either ASD or VSD alone.

Surgical treatment is limited by the absence of important structures in the central part of the heart. Furthermore, involvement of the mitral and tricuspid valves causes additional difficulty in repair. The prognosis depends on the severity of disease.

Patent Ductus Arteriosus. PDA, persistent patency of the ductus arteriosus, is the third most common cause of CHD, accounting for approximately 12% of cases. In fetal life the ductus arteriosus carries blood from the right ventricle to the aorta for oxygenation via the placenta. After birth the ductus arteriosus normally constricts within several days and then fibroses to become the ligamentum arteriosum. Persistent patency of the ductus arteriosus after birth results in a reversal of blood flow (i.e., from aorta to pulmonary artery) because of high systemic pressure and low pulmonary pressure. The result is redundant blood flow through the lungs, the left side of the heart, and the aorta.

The failure of the ductus arteriosus to close is often the result of another abnormal congenital condition, such as coarctation of the aorta, VSD, AS, PS, or pulmonary hypertension. Another rare CHD that causes similar abnormal circulation is the aortopulmonary window.

The clinical presentation depends on which, if any, other conditions are present. The condition often goes undiagnosed until patients reach adulthood, when pulmonary hypertension develops. In severe cases, patients become symptomatic by about 1 or 2 years of age, but in mild cases, patients may not become symptomatic until later life, even into the fifth decade. Patients with isolated PDA are acyanotic. Because the shunt functions during both systole and diastole, the murmur is pansystolic and has a machinery-like to-and-fro character.

In diseases that cause increased pulmonary pressure, such as infantile respiratory distress syndrome in the neonate or pulmonary hypertension in the adult, the shunting remains right-to-left, resulting in cyanosis. A similar situation occurs with hypoplastic left heart and infantile type coarctation syndromes, in which a PDA is necessary for survival.

On chest radiographs, PDA is characterized by increased pulmonary blood flow and enlargement of both the left atrium and the left ventricle (Fig. 5–26). There may be an additional finding of prominence of the ascending aorta, caused by the increased blood volume of the shunt. The process is therefore entirely left-sided. Right-sided heart chambers are not enlarged because they are excluded from the shunt. On angiograms, injection of contrast into the aortic arch shows the pulmonary arteries and the lungs immediately. The PDA most often enters the aorta distal to the takeoff of the left subclavian artery, and so a contrast injection into the upper portion of the descending aorta also shows the pulmonary arteries. The PDA itself may be directly visible on angiograms and occasionally on cardiac ultrasonograms.

As in ASD, VSD, and endocardial cushion defect, the dreaded complication in PDA is Eisenmenger's syndrome. Treatment is surgical closure of the PDA and must be conducted before Eisenmenger's syndrome develops. This is most commonly accomplished within the first year of life by placement of a surgical clip across the PDA.

Presentation: Cyanosis, Increased Pulmonary Vascularity, Cardiac Enlargement (Column 3 of Fig. 5–18)

Cyanotic CHDs associated with actively enlarged pulmonary vessels often have a characteristic radiographic appearance that allows diagnosis when clinical data are inconclusive or unavailable. This cyanotic group consists of TGV, single ventricle variants, TRUNCUS, TA with VSD, and TAPVR.

Transposition of the Great Vessels. In the development of the normal fetus, the truncus arteriosus spirals. If this spiraling does not occur, the aorta and the main pulmonary artery do not attach properly to the left and right ventricles. This results in TGV (also called transposition of the great arteries [TGA]). The lesion causes no problem in utero because oxygenated blood from the placenta enters first the right ventricle and then the systemic circulation. At birth, however, the patient becomes severely cyanotic because the venous and arterial circuits separate and function in parallel. A left-to-right shunt must be present in order to maintain life. Therefore, ASD, VSD, PDA, or combinations of these conditions are usually present. A large ASD and a large PDA best enable the patient to survive. Overall, about 90% of patients have an ostium secundum type of ASD, and 50% have a high supracristal type of VSD. Blood can also reach the lungs via large collateral bronchial arteries.

TGV is the most common cause of cyanosis in the first week of life. Severity of symptoms (shortness of breath and dyspnea) depends on

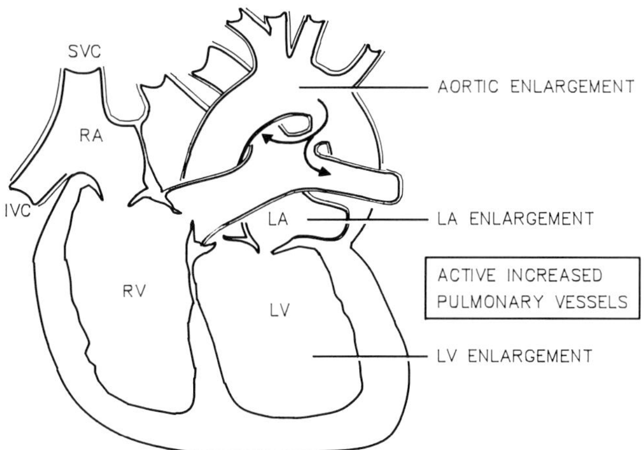

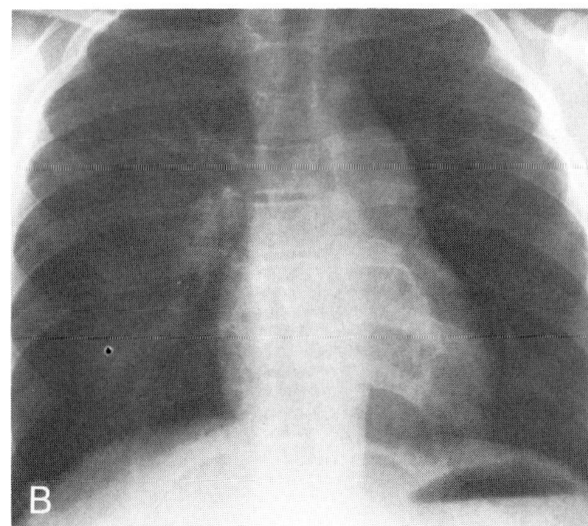

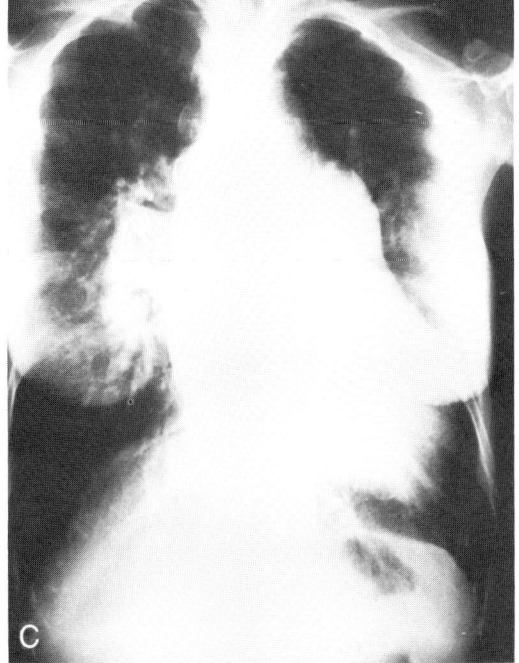

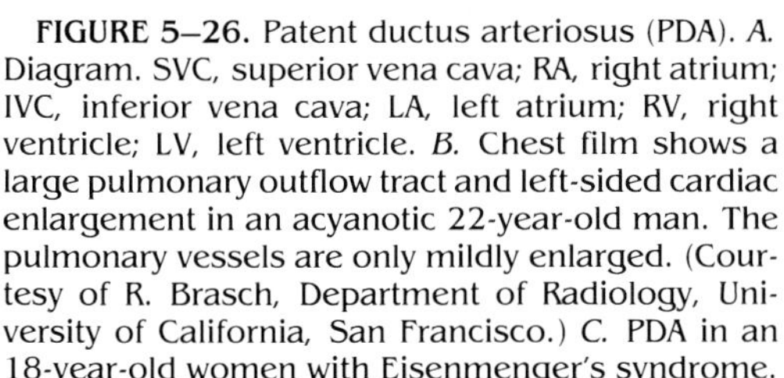

FIGURE 5–26. Patent ductus arteriosus (PDA). *A.* Diagram. SVC, superior vena cava; RA, right atrium; IVC, inferior vena cava; LA, left atrium; RV, right ventricle; LV, left ventricle. *B.* Chest film shows a large pulmonary outflow tract and left-sided cardiac enlargement in an acyanotic 22-year-old man. The pulmonary vessels are only mildly enlarged. (Courtesy of R. Brasch, Department of Radiology, University of California, San Francisco.) C. PDA in an 18-year-old women with Eisenmenger's syndrome. The pulmonary artery forms a large bulge over the left hilum. The right pulmonary artery is dilated centrally, and both right and left pulmonary branches are pruned peripherally. This is characteristic of a PDA that has led to pulmonary arterial hypertension and reversal of the left-to-right shunt. The patient is now cyanotic.

how well the associated lesions compensate for the TGV. Patients with less left-to-right shunting become severely cyanotic earlier.

On chest radiographs, 80% of patients show increased pulmonary blood flow. The proximal pulmonary arteries, especially on the right side, may be very prominent and elevated, suggesting the appearance of a waterfall. The area of the great vessels appears narrowed because the transposed aorta and pulmonary artery overlap in the anteroposterior view. The narrowness is even more pronounced when thymic tissue is small as a result of the stress of the CHD. Cardiomegaly may be present within a few days of birth but more often develops over a few months. The cardiomegaly, along with the overlap of the pulmonary artery and the aorta, give the heart the appearance of an egg on its side (Fig. 5–27). The other 20% of patients with complete TGV have pulmonic stenosis or atresia in addition to the TGV and therefore have decreased pulmonary blood flow and a normal heart size. On chest radiographs, the condition resembles TOF.

On lateral-view angiograms, an injection of contrast into the more anterior ventricle (the more heavily trabeculated right ventricle) causes visualization of the brachiocephalic arteries, which confirms that the right ventricle is misconnected to the aorta. In the normal lateral view, the more anterior great vessel emanating from the heart is the pulmonary artery.

The recommended immediate treatment of TGV is augmentation of the shunt. The Rashkin balloon septostomy, performed by passing a catheter across the foramen ovale, inflating the balloon, and pulling it back through, creates or enlarges the ASD. More definitive operative procedures may also be performed.

Double-Outlet Right Ventricle. An incomplete form of TGV consists of a completely transposed aorta but an incompletely transposed pulmonary artery. The result is that both great vessels come off the right ventricle, hence the name "double-outlet right ventricle" (DORV) syndrome. The mediastinal silhouette is wider than in complete TGV because the incompletely rotated aorta and the pulmonary artery are more side-by-side (Fig. 5–28). Associated PS is more common, present in approximately 50% of cases. In the Taussig-Bing form of DORV, the VSD is subpulmonic, which results in direct shunting from the left ventricle to the pulmonary trunk.

Corrected TGV. Corrected transposition of the great vessels (CTGV) is a natural correction that is, in effect, a double transposition. In addition to the aorta and the pulmonary artery being transposed, the right and left ventricles are inverted, causing the anatomical right ventricle to be on the patient's left side and the anatomical left ventricle to be on the right. The atria remain in their normal positions. The mitral and tricuspid valves and the coronary arteries follow the ventricles. The path of blood flow (Fig. 5–29) allows normal oxygenation. Venous blood returning to the right atrium goes to the anatomical left ventricle, which functions as a right ventricle and pumps it into the pulmonary artery. Oxygenated blood from the lungs returns to the left atrium and then goes to the anatomical right ventricle, which functions as a left ventricle and pumps it into the aorta. The right ventricle effectively adapts in order to pump blood at high pressure into the systemic circulation.

Theoretically, patients with CTGV can function normally, and a few do. Symptoms develop in these patients as a result of the presence of one or more associated lesions. These include PS, VSD, malformations of the mitral valve, and complete heart block. As in other conditions, PS is the most common lesion and has greatest effect on clinical symptoms. The appearance of the pulmonary vascularity depends on which of the associated lesions are present.

Persistent Truncus Arteriosus. TRUNCUS accounts for 2% of all congenital heart diseases and occurs when the aorticopulmonary septum, which normally divides the primitive aorta into the aorta and the pulmonary artery, fails to form. The aortic, pulmonic, and coronary circulations have a common origin. A common aorticopulmonic valve is present with two to seven valve cusps (usually, there are three). One third of patients with TRUNCUS have a right-sided aortic arch. A high membranous type of VSD is always present, causing a left-to-right shunt and showing increased pulmonary blood flow on chest radiograph. The failure to pump oxygenated blood into the systemic circulation, in addition to the admixing of arterial and venous blood, causes clinical symptoms of cyanosis. The blood flow to the pulmonary arteries is from various parts of the aorta and is classified into four types according to the origin of the vessels (Fig. 5–30).

In TRUNCUS type I (50% of cases), the principal feature is a common origin of the

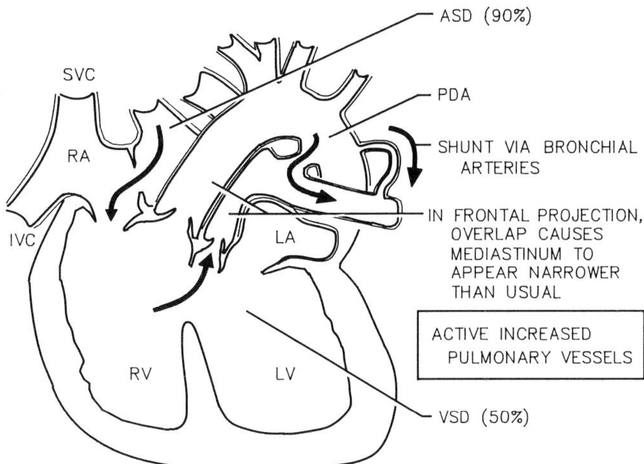

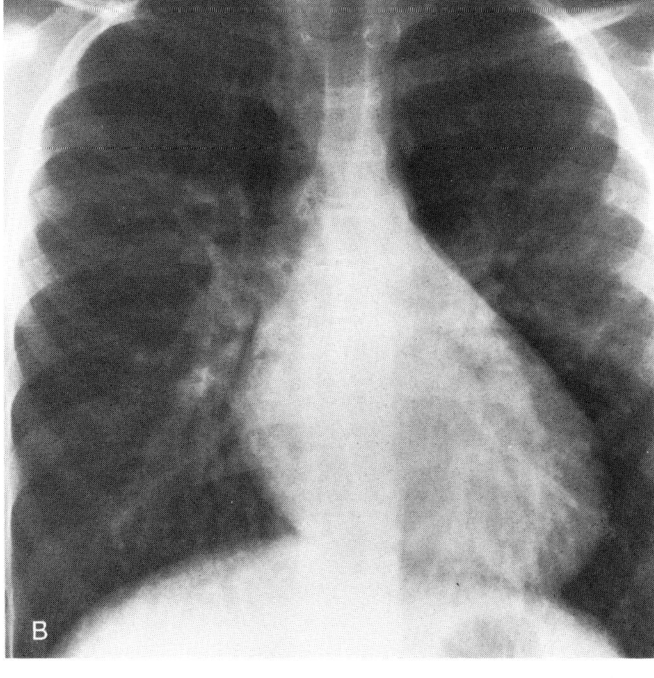

FIGURE 5–27. Transposition of the great vessels. *A.* Diagram. ASD, atrial septal defect; PDA, patent ductus arteriosus; SVC, superior vena cava; RA, right atrium; IVC, inferior vena cava; LA, left atrium; RV, right ventricle; LV, left ventricle; VSD, ventricular septal defect. *B.* PA chest film of a 6-year-old with cyanosis shows an egg-shaped heart and a narrow mediastinum. The mediastinum is narrowed because the pulmonary artery is in front of the aorta. The pulmonary vascularity is distinct and increased. (Courtesy of R. Brasch, Department of Radiology, University of California, San Francisco.)

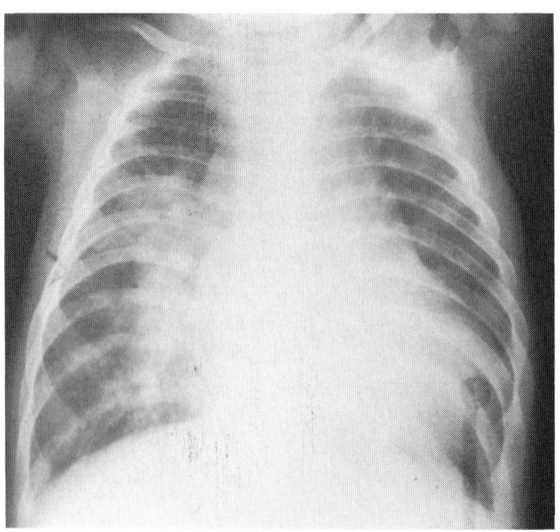

FIGURE 5–28. Double-outlet right ventricle (DORV) with ventricular septal defect. Chest film shows increased pulmonary vascularity. The mediastinal silhouette is widened because the incompletely rotated aorta and pulmonary artery lie side by side. (Courtesy of B. Cunningham, Brooke Army Medical Center, Fort Sam Houston, Texas.)

aorta and the main pulmonary artery. The left and right pulmonary arteries originate normally from the main pulmonary artery. In TRUNCUS type II (25% of cases), there is no main pulmonary artery segment, and separate left and right pulmonary arteries originate from the posterior wall of the truncus. In TRUNCUS type III (10% of cases), the pulmonary arteries originate from the lateral ascending aorta. In TRUNCUS type IV (15% of cases), there are no pulmonary arteries coming off the truncus or the ascending aorta. Arteries to the lungs are from the descending aorta. As such, they really are enlarged bronchial arteries rather than pulmonary arteries. Because of the pulmonary atresia in TRUNCUS type IV, there is markedly decreased pulmonary blood flow, a right-to-left shunt, and marked cyanosis. TRUNCUS type IV is also called pseudo-TRUNCUS because it is not a true persistent truncus but rather a severe form of TOF with pulmonary atresia either at or just beyond the pulmonic valve.

Cyanosis is less severe in type I than in the other types and usually occurs when the child is crying or distressed. In severe cases, CHF develops by 2 to 3 weeks of age. The clinical manifestations of pseudo-TRUNCUS are similar to those of TOF.

The radiographic appearance depends to some extent on the type of defect. Usually the heart is oval because of right ventricular enlargement, and the mediastinum is narrow because of the absence of the main pulmonary artery segment. The aortic arch is superior and, in 30% of cases, right-sided. In TRUNCUS type I, the main pulmonary artery segment causes a left hilar convex bulge; in the other types of TRUNCUS, the mediastinum is narrow as a result of the absence of a main pulmonary artery. On angiograms of TRUN-

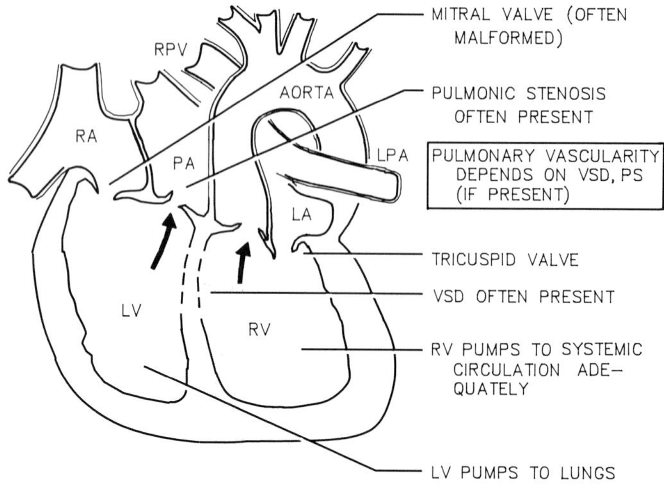

FIGURE 5–29. Corrected transposition of the great vessels. RPV, right pulmonary vein; RA, right atrium; PA, pulmonary artery; VSD, ventricular septal defect; ASD, atrial septal defect; LPA, left pulmonary artery; LA, left atrium; LV, left ventricle; RV, right ventricle; PS, pulmonary stenosis.

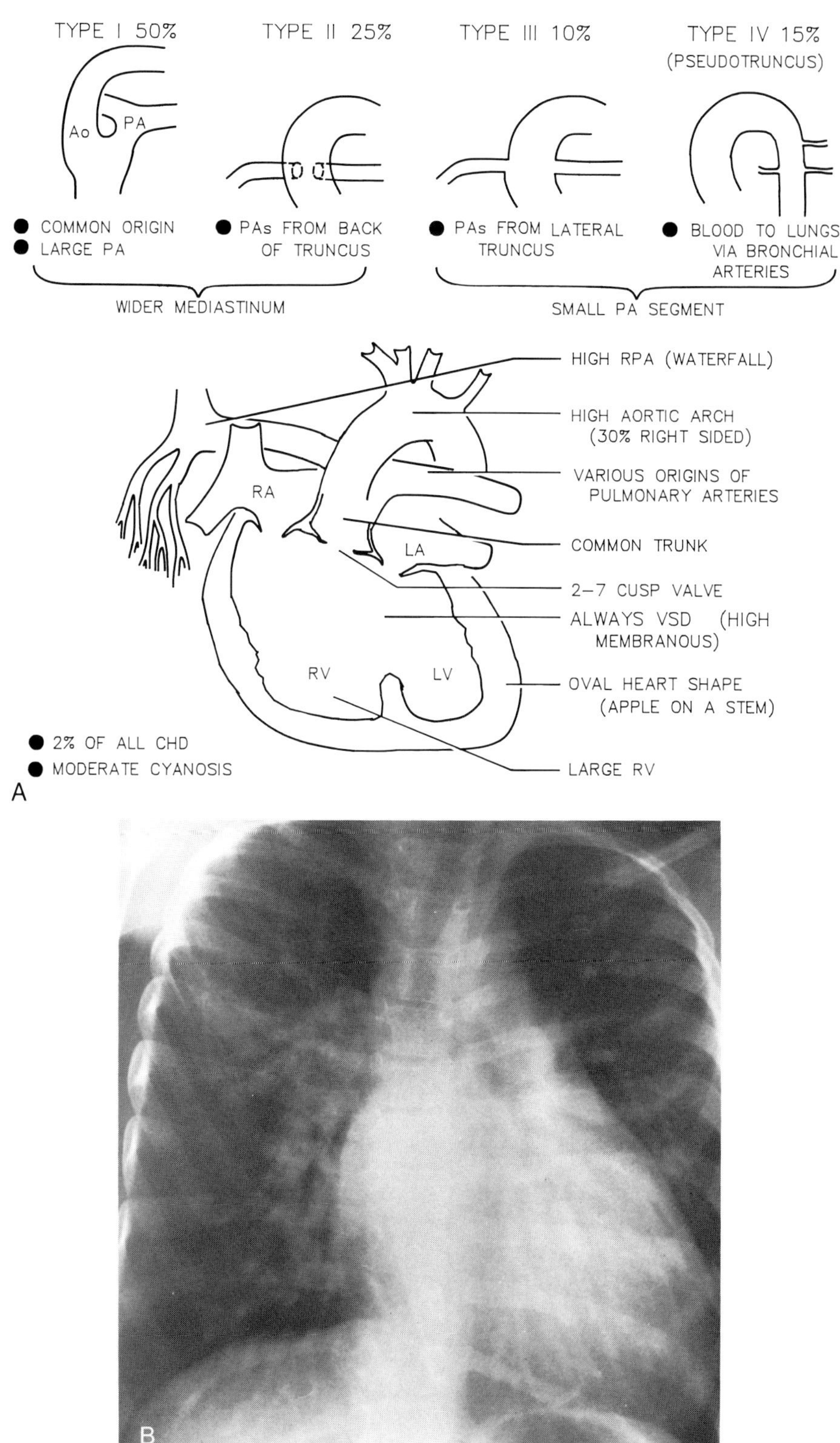

FIGURE 5–30. Persistent truncus arteriosus type I. *A.* Diagram. Ao, aorta; PA, pulmonary artery; RPA, right pulmonary artery; RA, right atrium; LA, left atrium; RV, right ventricle; LV, left ventricle; VSD, ventricular septal defect; CHD, congenital heart disease. *B.* Posteroanterior chest film shows marked cardiac enlargement in a young cyanotic girl. The common trunk shows as a wide mediastinum. Pulmonary vascularity is markedly increased and distinct. It is also asymmetrical, being more prominent in the right upper lobe. (Courtesy of R. Brasch, Department of Radiology, University of California, San Francisco.)

CUS type I, an injection of contrast into the left ventricle causes simultaneous visualization of the pulmonic and systemic circulations. Unfortunately, this is by no means a unique characteristic because a large, high VSD or an aorticopulmonary window can cause the same angiographic appearance. On angiograms, types II and III appear very similar. The chest film appearance of pseudo-TRUNCUS is similar to that of TOF. Filling of the lungs is via bronchial arteries.

Rastelli's procedure is the surgical correction most often used for TRUNCUS. In this procedure, a prosthetic pulmonary valve is placed in the right ventricle outflow tract, and a Dacron graft is continued to the pulmonary arteries. The VSD is then closed. On chest radiographs, the metal ring of the valve is clear evidence that this procedure has been performed.

Tricuspid Atresia. Tricuspid atresia (TA) prevents blood from flowing in its normal path from the right atrium to the right ventricle. Pure tricuspid atresia is incompatible with life because no venous blood can return to the lungs. Oxygenation is therefore achieved by the presence of compensating lesions. The radiographic and clinical appearances of TA are variable, depending on which of the associated abnormalities are present and how severe they are.

A minority of cases of TA (TA with VSD) cause cyanosis and increased pulmonary vascularity (Column 3 of Fig. 5–18). In TA with VSD, there is shunting of venous blood across an ASD, which is also always present. The VSD causes recirculation of venous and arterial blood through the lungs. The radiographic appearance is enlargement of the pulmonary artery, the peripheral pulmonary vessels, and the right ventricle (Fig. 5–31). The arteriovenous mixing in the left atrium produces cyanosis.

TA with PS mimics tetralogy of Fallot, to be described later with diseases that cause cyanosis and decreased pulmonary blood flow. TA with neither PS nor VSD is also possible, but rare.

Total Anomalous Pulmonary Venous Return. TAPVR results from an abnormal connection between the pulmonary circulation and the right side of the heart. As a result, oxygenated venous blood returning from the lungs is returned either partially or totally to the venous system rather than to the left atrium. In all types of TAPVR, the patient must have either an ASD or a VSD to survive. The direction of the blood flow through the ASD or the VSD is opposite that for isolated septal defects (i.e., is right-to-left). In patients with TAPVR, ASD is the most common associated CHD. Conversely, 25% of patients with ASD of any type have a partial APVR; 90% of patients with the sinus venosus type of ASD have partial APVR.

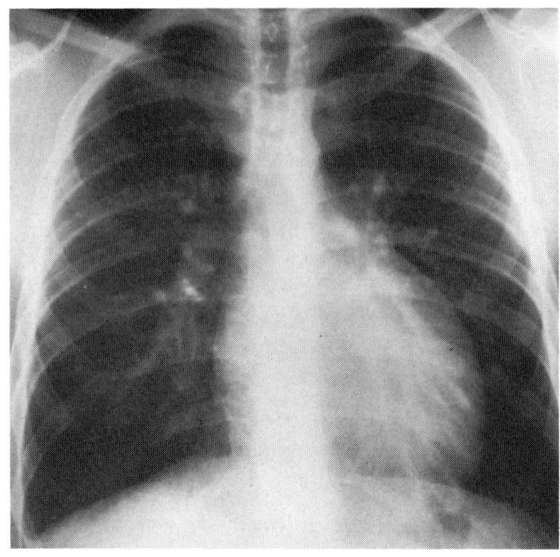

FIGURE 5–31. Tricuspid atresia with ventricular septal defect. Posteroanterior chest film in an 18-year-old male with cyanosis shows enlargement of the heart with enlargement of the pulmonary outflow tract. The pulmonary vessels are enlarged and distinct. (Courtesy of R. Brasch, Department of Radiology, University of California, San Francisco.)

There are three major subtypes of TAPVR (Fig. 5–32*A*). Type I accounts for 50% of all cases and is an anomaly of the cardinal veins. The abnormal connection is at the supraclavicular level, where the pulmonary veins connect to a left-sided vertical vein instead of to the left atrium (Fig. 5–32*B*, *C*). Blood travels upward through this vertical vein first to the left subclavian vein and then to the superior vena cava. In TAPVR type II (30% of cases), the abnormal connection is at the cardiac level, usually to the coronary sinus but, in some cases, directly to the right atrium.

In TAPVR type III (20% of cases), the blood returning from the lungs enters the venous system below the diaphragm, usually into the portal vein, but almost any vein such as the gastric vein or even the inferior vena cava can be involved. There is frequently obstruction to flow as the anomalous vessel passes through the diaphragm. Type III is clinically the most severe. A subcategory of type III is the venolobar syndrome, a partial APVR type

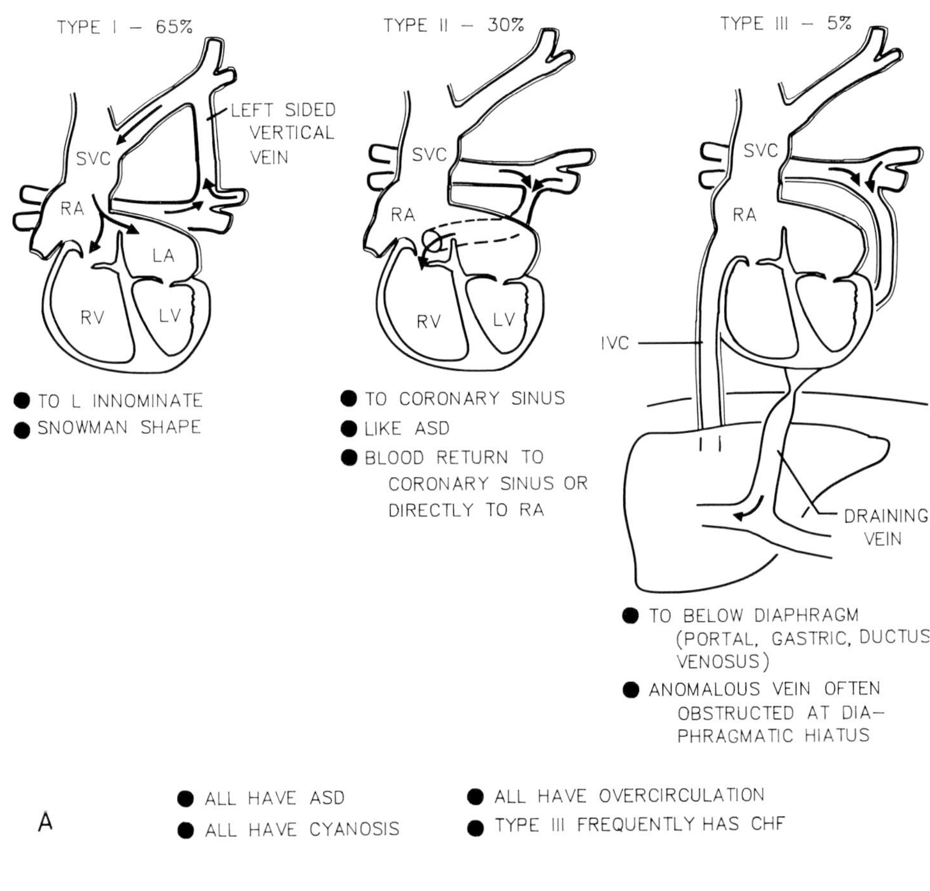

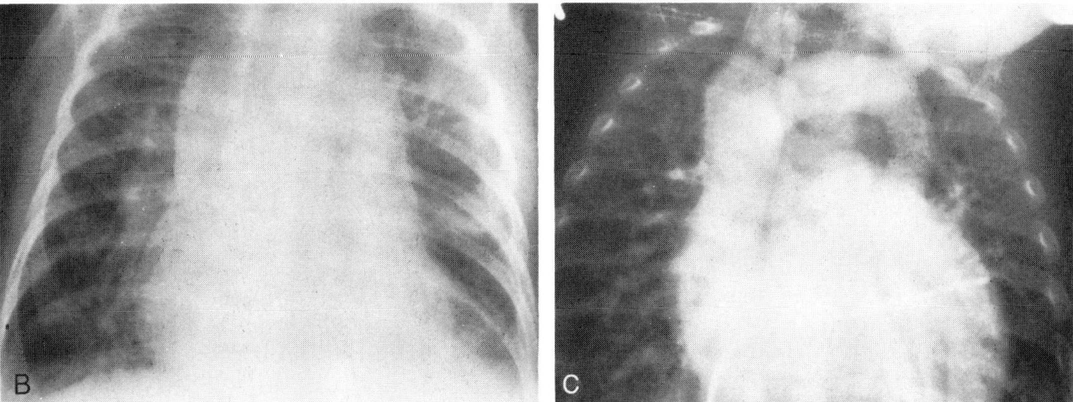

FIGURE 5–32. Total anomalous pulmonary venous return (TAPVR). *A.* Diagram of types I, II, and III. SVC, superior vena cava; RA, right atrium; LA, left atrium; RV, right ventricle; LV, left ventricle; L, left; ASD, atrial septal defect. *B.* Chest film of a mildly cyanotic newborn with TAPVR type I shows the snowman-like appearance of the heart. The upper portion, appearing as a wide mediastinum, includes a large vertical vein on the left side that carries the anomalous pulmonary venous return to the left innominate vein. The enlarged right superior vena cava makes up the right side of the mediastinal silhouette. The pulmonary vessels are actively enlarged. (Courtesy of R. Brasch, Department of Radiology, University of California, San Francisco.) *C.* A second case of type I TAPVR is studied as a dextrophase arteriogram. The image is performed after contrast injected into the right ventricle has passed through the pulmonary arterial circulation and is progressing through the left-sided vertical vein back into the engorged superior vena cava (refer to part *A*).

III in which the venous drainage of the right lower lung enters the venous system below the diaphragm (see Fig. 5–15).

TAPVR causes cyanosis primarily because of a lack of sufficient oxygenated blood entering the systemic circulation. The right-to-left shunt further contributes to cyanosis as a result of admixture of venous blood. Type I patients are usually not very cyanotic at birth because of the protective effect of the ASD; cyanosis often does not develop for many months. In some mild cases, the diagnosis is not made until adulthood. Like type I, type II entails no obstruction of flow, and because an ASD is usually present, cyanosis may not develop until many months to years after birth. Newborns with type III develop the most severe symptoms and do so early. Pulmonary venous congestion and CHF are manifested as cyanosis and are frequently brought on by feedings.

The radiographic appearance depends on the type of TAPVR and the severity of disease. On plain films, Type I characteristically has a snowman, or figure 8, appearance of the mediastinum. The left side of the snowman's head is the vertical vein, and the right side is the enlarged superior vena cava. The body is the enlarged right atrium and right ventricle. The vertical vein is usually obscured by the normal thymic shadow, and so this diagnosis is not commonly made in neonates. Pulmonary blood flow is actively increased as a result of recirculation of blood through the lungs.

In type III, passive pulmonary venous congestion may be superimposed on the active overcirculation as a result of the obstruction of blood flow as it crosses the diaphragm. For this reason, TAPVR type III is the second most common cause of CHF (after hypoplastic left heart syndrome) in the neonatal period. On chest radiographs, the heart is enlarged, and the CHF is seen as reticular infiltrate that develops within the first few days after birth. It may be confused with hyaline membrane disease. The only definitive treatment is surgical redirection of blood as necessary.

Hypoplastic Left Heart Syndrome. Hypoplastic left heart syndrome is the most common cause of CHF in the first day of life and the most common cause of death due to CHD in the first week of life. It represents a group of left-sided lesions that includes mitral atresia, hypoplastic left atrium and left ventricle, and aortic atresia. All these result in a hypoplastic left ventricle. The entire cardiac output is pumped by the hypertrophied and dilated right ventricle, and the entire systemic flow passes through a PDA. Patients have cyanosis and an ashen-gray pallor. Radiographic findings are a large heart and severe pulmonary edema (Fig. 5–33). No corrective surgical techniques are available. Many of these infants die within a few days after birth.

Presentation: Cyanosis, Decreased Pulmonary Vascularity, and Normal-Sized or Enlarged Heart, Right-to-Left Shunt (Column 4 of Fig. 5–18)

Tetralogy of Fallot. Decreased pulmonary vascularity most commonly results from CHD that includes PS (see Fig. 5–18). The most common syndrome is TOF. In most of these syndromes, the heart is normal-sized or slightly enlarged. If PS is present to a significant degree together with other abnormalities, the PS tends to dominate both the clinical and radiographic pictures; this process is called TOF physiology. These diseases therefore have a chest film appearance similar to that of TOF. Two other diseases in this category, Ebstein's anomaly and hypoplastic right heart syndrome, simulate PS by restricting flow through the right ventricle.

TOF accounts for 40% of cases of cyanotic CHD detected after the neonatal period. The age range of most patients is from less than 1 year to adolescence. In variants of TOF, called the trilogy and pentalogy of Fallot, the primary lesion is PS, but the associated defects vary (Fig. 5–34).

The most important of the components in all of these syndromes is PS. The worse the degree of PS is, the worse is the cyanosis and the earlier in life the patient becomes symptomatic. In a minor subgroup called pink TOF, the PS is mild; consequently, cyanosis is absent except during exercise.

Several types of PS can be present. In typical TOF, it is infundibular: that is, within the right ventricle outflow tract below the pulmonic valve. In trilogy of Fallot, it is more often valvular. A related anomaly, supravalvular stenosis, may be present in the main pulmonary artery or a branch of it. This may be frank atresia of a pulmonary artery segment. Unequal pulmonary blood flow can result. The previously described syndrome of pseudo-TRUNCUS could be considered the most severe variant of this type of abnormality. A portion of a pulmonary artery that is very stenotic (or atretic) causes the lung on that side to have markedly decreased pulmonary vascularity in comparison with the other side.

The other findings in TOF contribute to the physiological and radiographic presentation.

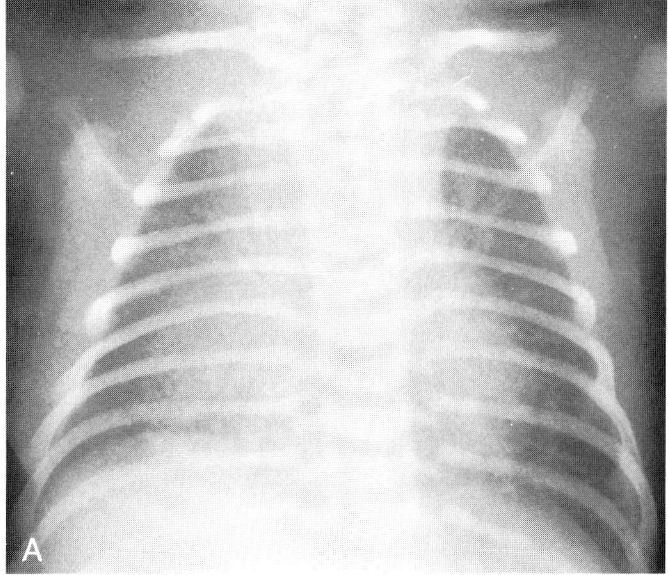

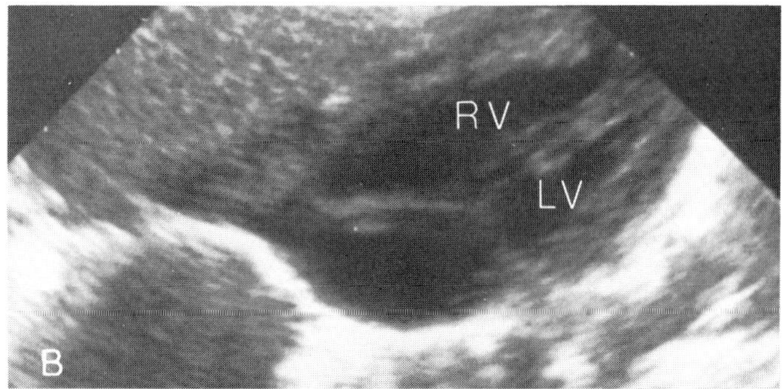

FIGURE 5–33. Hypoplastic left heart syndrome. *A.* Rapidly worsening congestive heart failure in a newborn has produced pulmonary edema, which is seen as a diffuse opacification of the lungs. *B.* An echocardiogram shows the lumen of the right ventricle (RV) and the left ventricle (LV) surrounded by walls of equal thickness. The normal left ventricular wall is thicker than the right. The left ventricular chamber size is significantly smaller than normal.

Right ventricular hypertrophy develops in response to the high pressures against which it must pump. This situation exists because of both the PS and the systemic pressures across the VSD. The VSD is of the high supracristal type. The overriding position of the aorta is more of a secondary finding that is attributable to the high VSD. The relative lack of importance of this finding is evident in TOF, in which the VSD is absent and obviously not essential.

The degree of cyanosis is directly proportional to the severity of PS and the consequent amount of right-to-left shunting. The PDA is initially beneficial, allowing blood to pass from the aorta to the pulmonary arteries. However, when it closes within a few weeks after birth, cyanosis develops. Clubbing of the fingers may be present in severe cases of cyanosis. Patients also have fatigue, dyspnea on exertion, and failure to thrive as infants. They symptomatically learn to assume a squatting position, which increases the systemic pressure and decreases the shunt.

Chest radiographs show oligemia of the lungs that is caused by the PS and the right-to-left shunting through the VSD (or the ASD). The heart is enlarged in a boot-shaped configuration (Fig. 5–34). Right ventricular hypertrophy may make the right heart border prominent. Left ventricular enlargement may result from the excess blood volume shunted to the left and may make the left heart border prominent. The right suprahilar area may be convex because of a right aortic arch, which is present in 25% to 35% of TOF cases. The left suprahilar area is usually concave because the main pulmonary artery is small. In trilogy of Fallot, the left suprahilar area may appear prominent because of poststenotic dilation, which is caused by the jet effect of the valvular PS.

An angiographic injection of contrast into the right ventricle may reveal the infundibular

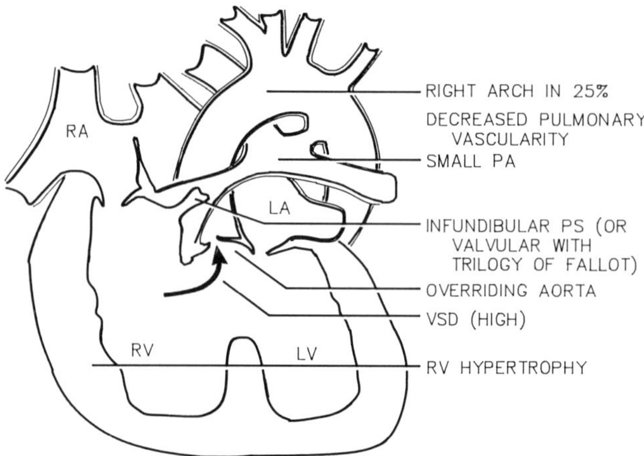

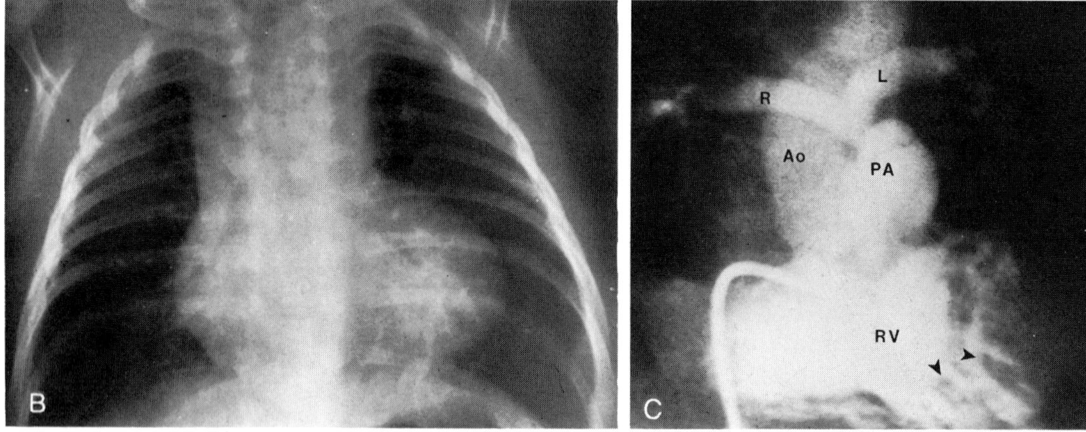

FIGURE 5–34. Tetralogy of Fallot (TOF). *A.* Diagram. PA, pulmonary artery; RA, right atrium; LA, left atrium; PS, pulmonary stenosis; VSD, ventricular septal defect; RV, right ventricle; LV, left ventricle; ASD, atrial septal defect. *B.* Posteroanterior chest film in a 1-month-old infant shows the typical boot-shaped heart. The pulmonary vessels are small and attenuated. The aortic arch in this patient is left-sided. (Courtesy of R. Brasch, Department of Radiology, University of California, San Francisco.) *C.* In a second patient, an arteriogram performed after contrast is injected in the right ventricle (RV) shows thick trabeculations of the right ventricle (*arrowheads*) indicating right ventricular hypertrophy. The pulmonary artery (PA) is small and malformed with small right (R) and left (L) pulmonary artery branches. The normal caliber aorta (Ao) is seen because contrast is shunted right to left by the VSD.

stenosis. Both the pulmonary artery and the aorta are visualized simultaneously as a result of the VSD and the overriding aorta, but the pulmonary artery is usually small. Right ventricular pressures measured at catheterization are very high because of the PS. Oxygen saturation of the aortic arterial blood is low (about 75% instead of the usual 97%).

There are at least five types of major operative therapies for TOF. The principal goal of these operations is to restore blood flow to the lungs. Without surgery, only 50% of severe TOF patients survive to age 7 years and only 10% to age 20.

TOF Physiology. If PS is present to a significant degree together with other abnormalities, the PS tends to dominate both the clinical and radiographic pictures. This is the cause of the six CHD varieties shown in column 4 of Figure 5–18 and labeled TOF physiology. They all mimic TOF on chest radiographs because, like TOF, they include PS as the most important abnormality.

Ebstein's Anomaly. Ebstein's anomaly, or, a more proper term, Ebstein's malformation of the tricuspid valve, is a developmental abnormality of the tricuspid valve in which both the septal and posterior leaflets are inserted well below the tricuspid annulus (Fig. 5–35). A dysplasia of the chordae tendineae and the papillary muscles may also be present. In effect, part of the right ventricle becomes part of the right atrium, a so-called atrialization of the right ventricle. Tricuspid regurgitation occurs with resultant marked right atrial enlargement. Although PS is not present, the dysfunctional right ventricle and the tricuspid regurgitation cause an equivalent obstruction

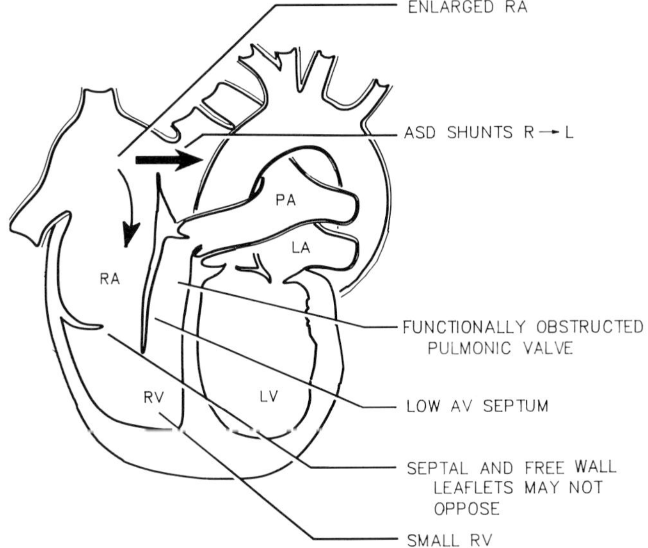

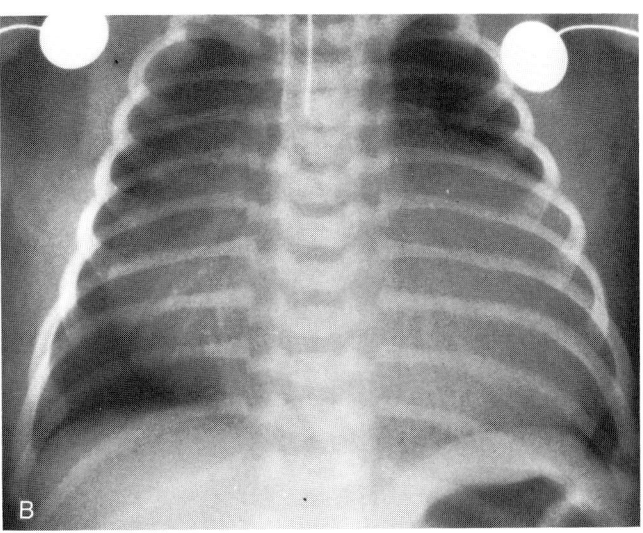

FIGURE 5–35. Ebstein's anomaly. *A.* Diagram. RA, right atrium; ASD, atrial septal defect; R, right; L, left; PA, pulmonary artery; LA, left atrium; AV, atrioventricular; RV, right ventricle; LV, left ventricle; PS, pulmonary stenosis. *B.* Posteroanterior chest film of a 1-day-old premature infant shows massive enlargement of the heart. The right side of the heart extends well into the right chest because of the enlarged right atrium. The thymic shadow obscures the upper chest. The pulmonary vascularity is normal or mildly decreased. (Courtesy of R. Brasch, Department of Radiology, University of California, San Francisco.)

of blood flow. In Ebstein's anomaly, poor contraction of the right ventricle and obstruction of blood flow caused by the abnormal tricuspid valve position restrict emptying of the right ventricle. An ASD is almost always present.

Symptoms are similar to those produced by pulmonic stenosis. Severely affected patients are usually cyanotic as newborns. They may have cardiac arrhythmias, especially Wolff-Parkinson-White syndrome. Occasionally, mild cases of Ebstein's anomaly go undetected until adulthood.

Chest films show marked enlargement of the cardiac silhouette (primarily because of a huge right atrium) and decreased pulmonary blood flow. The differential diagnosis of such an appearance includes PS with intact septum and a large pericardial effusion. On angiogram, a right atrial injection shows the huge right atrium as well as the ASD, shunting in the right-to-left direction. The right ventricle is small.

Hypoplastic Right Heart Syndrome. Failure of proper development of right-sided heart structures can lead to a complex set of CHDs, including TA, tricuspid stenosis (TS), pulmonic atresia, and hypoplasia of the right ventricle. The most common (and most complicated) type is TA, in which the tricuspid valve fails to form from the endocardial cushion. An ASD with blood flow from right to left must be present in order for blood to bypass the obstructed tricuspid valve to reach the left side of the heart. A PDA or a VSD is necessary in order for at least some blood to get back to the lungs. The most common subtype of TA is characterized by normal great vessels and PS. In a less common subtype, TGV is present, but PS is usually minimal. Almost all patients with hypoplastic right heart that includes TA are cyanotic and exhibit decreased pulmonary blood flow on chest films. Overall heart size and individual chamber enlargement depends on the size and the types of shunts present.

Presentation: CHF Picture, Passive Venous Congestion (Column 5 of Fig. 5–18) As noted earlier, the most common cause of CHF in the first day of life is hypoplastic left heart syndrome. In children a few months old, it is severe COARCT.

CHD presenting with signs and symptoms of CHF in older children can be due to a variety of diseases. These include cardiomyopathy, endocardial fibroelastosis, aberrant left coronary artery syndrome, hypoplastic left heart syndrome, and severe cases of endocardial cushion.

SYSTEMIC DISEASES

Endocrine Diseases

Endocrine diseases do not affect the heart directly. Thyrotoxicosis can cause heart failure when the increased metabolic rate requires increased cardiac work for prolonged periods of time. Cushing's disease can increase the demands of the heart when electrolyte disturbances alter blood pressure. Abnormalities of calcium metabolism can affect contractility. Radiographic findings in patients with these conditions are nonspecific.

Metabolic Diseases

Metabolic diseases affect the heart when abnormal materials are deposited in the myocardium. Such conditions, called storage diseases, include hemochromatosis and glycogen storage diseases.

Hemochromatosis, whether primary or secondary to multiple blood transfusions, can result in uptake of hemosiderin by the myocardial cells and cause myocardiopathy. Arrhythmia caused by conduction abnormalities and CHF, which is refractory to medical management, also occurs. CT obtained at two x-ray energies can demonstrate and quantify the increased iron content of the heart and the liver (the liver being the organ most commonly affected in hemochromatosis; see Fig. 3–66). MRI of the heart and the liver in hemochromatosis shows low intensity as a result of the paramagnetic effects of the iron.

Glycogen storage diseases produce cardiomegaly because of deposition of glycogen in the myocardial cells. CHF usually occurs during the first year of life, and survival is only for a few years. Sudden death caused by arrhythmia is not uncommon.

Alcohol affects the heart. Toxicity may lead to a cardiomyopathy in which the four chambers of the heart become dilated and cardiac wall motion is symmetrically reduced. There are no specific radiographic signs of this cardiomyopathy.

Diseases of the Immune System

Of the autoimmune diseases, the most common one that affects the heart is systemic lupus erythematosus, which does so by deforming and destroying the mitral and tricuspid valves, a process called Libman-Sacks endocarditis. The radiographic findings are dependent on valve function and are not specific.

In patients with rheumatoid arthritis, the heart valves are rarely involved. Scleroderma affects all layers of the heart with fibrosis, resulting in a restrictive cardiomyopathy. The conducting tracts of the heart are often involved, which results in arrhythmias and conduction defects. The radiographic findings of scleroderma relate to lung disease and pulmonary hypertension. In rare instances, Reiter's syndrome causes aortic insufficiency and medial necrosis of the aortic root. Periarteritis nodosa can affect the coronary arteries and cause myocardial infarction.

INFECTION

Infection can occur in the heart, the pericardium, and the vessels. Infection can destroy the heart valves, resulting in severe cardiac dysfunction. The most important infectious cardiac diseases are rheumatic fever and bacterial endocarditis.

Rheumatic Fever. Rheumatic fever is an uncommon sequel to respiratory infection by group A beta-hemolytic streptococci. About 3% of patients with rheumatic fever subsequently develop heart disease. There is little evidence that the organism itself infects the heart. Some evidence supports the possibility that toxins from the streptococci damage the heart. The most likely explanation is that the immune system creates antibodies against the bacteria that cross-react with tissues such as the valves of the heart and mediate the damage.

Rheumatic fever usually involves and destroys the mitral valve and, less commonly, the aortic valve, causing serious dysfunction that ultimately requires surgical intervention. This destruction can lead to mitral valve stenosis (the most common valvular lesion of rheumatic mitral valve disease), mitral valve insufficiency (the most common cause of cardiac decompensation in patients with rheumatic mitral valve disease), or both. These complications are discussed later in the section on acquired heart disease. Less commonly, rheumatic fever manifests as carditis, a nonspecific self-limiting inflammation of the myocardium and the pericardium.

Bacterial Endocarditis. Bacterial endocarditis is an infection of the endocardium that results from septicemia. It most seriously affects abnormal valve leaflets (usually in the tricuspid valve) and prosthetic valves (especially the aortic valve). Turbulence caused by the valve abnormalities facilitates infestation by bacteria. Acute bacterial endocarditis, usually caused by *Staphylococcus aureus,* is a severe infection that causes rapidly progressive valve destruction and septic emboli. Subacute bacterial endocarditis is usually caused by *Streptococcus viridans* and has a more insidious course, characterized by fever and heart murmur. Both forms of endocarditis are common in drug abusers who inject drugs intravenously. Infectious aneurysms (mycotic aneurysms) can form in arteries of the brain (see Chapter 8) and in the splenic artery when the infected material seeds the vasa vasorum of these vessels. When mycotic aneurysms rupture in the brain, they usually cause fatal hemorrhage.

Pericarditis. Inflammation of the pericardium, called pericarditis, has a variety of causes. The most common are infectious agents (especially viruses, but also tuberculosis), uremia (often predisposing the patient to fatal cardiac tamponade), autoimmune reaction to infarcted myocardial tissue (Dressler's syndrome), other autoimmune diseases such as systemic lupus erythematosus (see Fig. 5–12), and cardiac surgery (postpericardiotomy syndrome). Patients experience chest pain, which often changes with posture. If the pericarditis is constrictive, patients have dyspnea and CHF. Echocardiography is the best method for diagnosis of a pericardial effusion associated with pericarditis. On radiographs, the heart size may be small or normal. Fifty percent of patients with pericarditis have some calcification of the pericardium. If pericardial effusion is present, the cardiac silhouette is enlarged and globular.

Echinococcosis. Echinococcosis, infestation by *Echinococcus granulosus,* in rare instances affects the heart, in which it produces a large cyst, usually in the left ventricle. The cyst can rupture into the ventricle or the pericardium. The echinococcal cyst appears similar to those seen elsewhere in the body.

Chagas's Disease. Chagas's disease is a parasitic infestation of the heart, the esophagus (see Chapter 3), and other organs by *Trypanosoma cruzi.* The disease is most common in South America. In the heart, the organism proliferates, destroys muscle tissue, and forms connective tissue. This connective tissue, in conjunction with an inflammatory response, increases heart size. The disease also destroys autonomic nerve fibers in the heart, which leads to conduction abnormalities, most notable of which are atrioventricular block, bundle-branch block, and premature ventricular contractions. The usual clinical symptom is palpitations caused by the conduction abnormalities. The most common radiographic finding is cardiomegaly, which is nonspecific.

NEOPLASMS

Primary tumors of the heart are extremely rare. They are seen in about 1 in 5000 autopsies. They can obstruct flow through the heart. Most are benign and can be safely removed surgically. The most common tumor involving the heart is metastatic disease from a primary tumor, most frequently lung or breast carcinoma. Metastases to the heart are 10 to 20 times more common than primary tumors of the heart. Metastatic disease to the myocardium almost always also involves the pericardium, frequently causing pericardial effusion. Metastatic tumors to the heart are usually of little consequence in comparison with the effects of the primary tumor or of metastases to other organs.

Myxoma. The myxoma is the most common primary tumor of the heart, making up more than half of all primary cardiac tumors. It is usually benign, with an extremely small malignant potential. The tumor is three times more common in women than in men, and the peak age is between 40 and 60 years. Myxomas frequently are pedunculated masses that usually originate from a site on either the interatrial or the interventricular septum. About 90% originate in the atria and are four times as common in the left atrium as in the right. The left atrial myxoma usually originates near the fossa ovalis.

Ninety percent of patients have some constitutional symptoms such as recurrent fevers (without leukocytosis), malaise, sweats, and anemia. Because the tumor frequently is pedunculated, it can move within the chamber during the cardiac cycle. If the stalk is long enough, it can partially or totally obstruct the flow of blood through the mitral or tricuspid valve and even protrude through it. This may cause variable heart murmurs. In addition, parts of the tumor can break off and become systemic emboli. One third of patients with atrial myxoma have symptoms of emboli, half of which are to the central nervous system. A left atrial myxoma embolizes mainly to the brain and the kidneys, the organs with the highest blood flow. Right atrial myxomas embolize to the lungs as tumoral pulmonary emboli.

On chest radiographs, left atrial myxoma may resemble mitral stenosis. Half of patients have an appearance of CHF that is caused by left atrial obstruction, not left ventricular failure. Although myxomas can sometimes be visualized on both CT and MRI, ultrasonography is the diagnostic method of choice (Fig. 5–36). The tumor and its motion can be imaged, and Doppler measurements can show obstruction to flow. Surgical removal of the myxoma is curative.

Other Cardiac Tumors. Rhabdomyoma rarely occurs in the heart except in patients with tuberous sclerosis. Fibroma and angioma, other benign tumors of the heart, are distinctly rare. Malignant primary tumors of the heart consist of poorly differentiated spindle-cell sarcoma, histiocytic lymphoma, and rhabdomyosarcoma.

ACQUIRED HEART DISEASE

Cardiac Dysfunction

Congestive Heart Failure. CHF is the failure of the left side of the heart to pump effectively, which results in pulmonary venous congestion (see also Chapter 2). The inability of the left ventricle to pass on the blood that it receives from the lungs is a functional obstruction and has the same effect as the physical obstruction by mitral stenosis, a left atrial myxoma, or cor triatriatum. The causes of left-sided heart failure are many (Table 5–12). They may or may not be identifiable on plain films. Chest films show progressive vascular congestion that worsens as pulmonary venous (wedge) pressure increases (see Fig. 5–2).

TABLE 5–12. CAUSES OF LEFT-SIDED HEART FAILURE

Ischemia	Atherosclerotic coronary artery disease
Hypertension	High pressure afterload
Aortic valvular disease	Aortic stenosis, aortic insufficiency, or both
Myocardiopathy	Viral, diabetic, alcoholic
Other	Endocardial fibroelastosis, glycogen storage disease

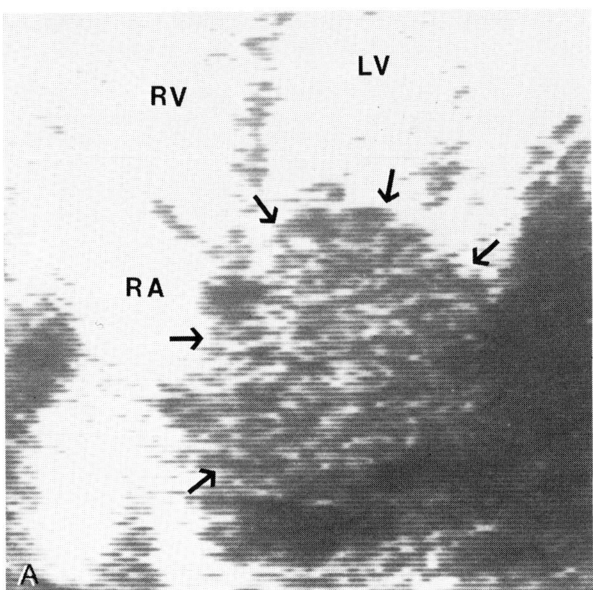

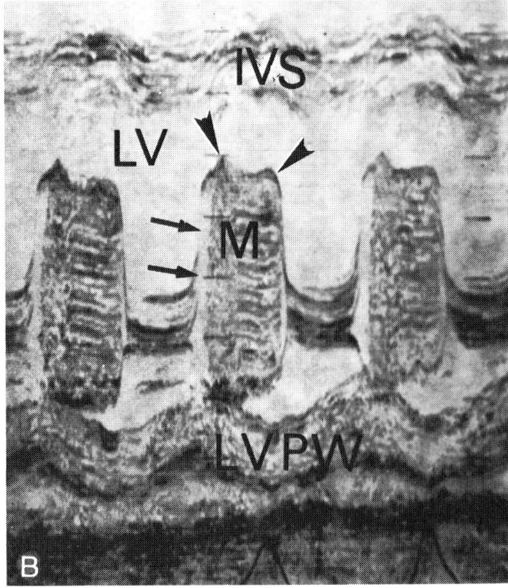

FIGURE 5–36. Left atrial myxoma. *A.* A freeze-frame from an apical four-chamber echocardiogram shows a normal right ventricle (RV), left ventricle (LV), and right atrium (RA). The myxoma mass (*arrows*) fills the entire left atrium and obstructs blood flow to the left ventricle. *B.* Atrial myxoma. An M-mode echocardiogram displays the mitral valve. The interventricular septum (IVS), the left ventricular chamber (LV), the left ventricular posterior wall (LVPW), and the anterior mitral valve leaflets (*arrowheads*) as well as the massive echoes from the atrial myxoma (M) are seen. There is a thin gap (*arrows*) between the mass and the leaflet where a thin stream of blood still flows around the tumor, which is jammed behind the valve leaflet.

The upper limit of normal pulmonary venous pressure is approximately 12 to 13 mm Hg. As the pressure rises above this level, various abnormalities develop on chest film. CHF generally proceeds in a fairly orderly fashion. Because of the effect of gravity on the body in the upright position, the upper-lobe pulmonary veins are normally smaller in caliber than those in the lower lungs. Pleural effusion frequently implies that right-sided failure is also present. The chest film may show less severe effects in patients with long-standing CHF, even when the pulmonary wedge pressure is over 30 mm Hg. In acute myocardial infarction, the chest film abnormalities occur at a pressure about 5 mm lower than usual. Heart size usually remains normal on chest radiographs in acute myocardial infarction.

Myocardial Infarction. Myocardial infarction, death of a portion of the myocardium, is the result of interruption of the oxygen supply to the heart, which is usually caused by atherosclerotic narrowing, embolic obstruction, or spasm of the coronary arteries. Although chest radiographs usually show no abnormality, these studies are always obtained in patients suspected of having myocardial infarction because findings of coronary artery atherosclerosis or CHF are associated with poor prognosis and require prompt therapy. Rupture of a papillary muscle, a myocardial wall, or the interventricular septum in patients with myocardial infarction is rare and often fatal.

Calcification of the coronary arteries can often be identified on plain chest radiographs (see Fig. 5–1) and is strongly correlated with ischemic disease. Because coronary artery atherosclerosis causing cardiac arrhythmia is the most common cause of sudden death from cardiac disorder, patients who exhibit such findings and in whom myocardial infarction is suspected are monitored closely.

On occasion, the heart fails to pump effectively in the acute stages of myocardial infarction, and the patient develops prompt CHF. Vigorous treatment is indicated in order to prevent extension of the infarction. The only radiographic abnormality in such patients is central pulmonary edema. In contrast to other causes of heart failure, the heart in this case remains normal in size, and pleural effusion is uncommon.

Rupture of the left ventricle occurs in fewer than 5% of patients with myocardial infarction. It usually occurs within the first 5 days of infarction. As hemorrhage into the myocar-

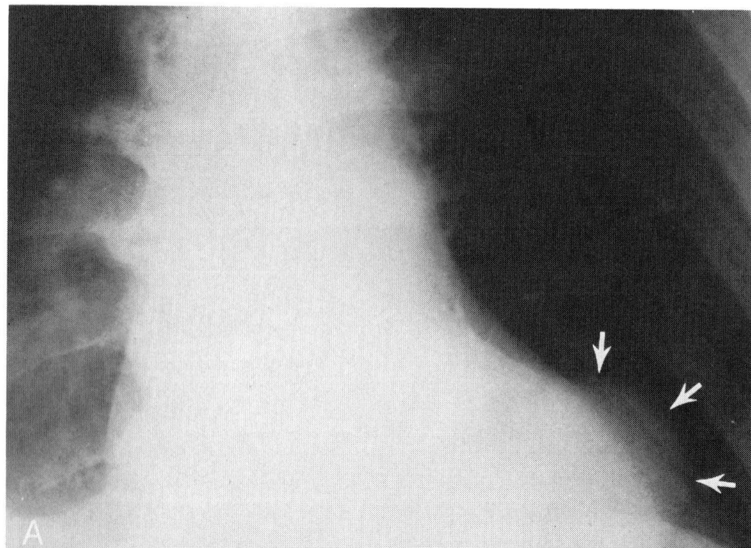

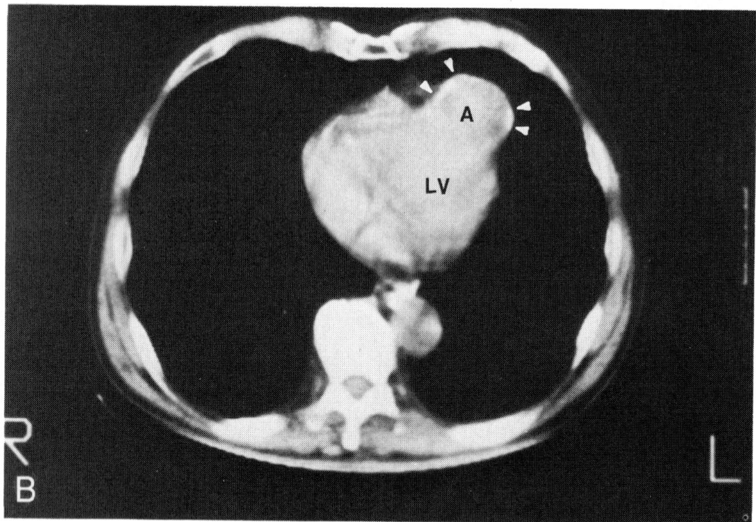

FIGURE 5–37. Left ventricular aneurysm. *A.* A bulge at the apex of the left ventricle (*arrows*) is an aneurysm that developed after a myocardial infarction. *B.* A CT image through the left ventricle (LV) shows the aneurysm (A) with a rim of calcification (*arrowhead*).

dium progresses, the wall softens over a 2- to 3-day period. Dissection eventually reaches the pericardium. The rupture is uniformly fatal.

The mitral papillary muscle can become infarcted and rupture in 1% of patients, resulting in severe mitral valve insufficiency and death. Rupture of the intraventricular septum in myocardial infarction is distinctly rare (0.5%) but fatal.

The most important delayed sequela of myocardial infarction is the formation of a cardiac aneurysm. The infarcted muscle becomes replaced by scar tissue and becomes an akinetic portion of the myocardium. It is most common in the left ventricle and develops weeks to months after myocardial infarction (Fig. 5–37). The diagnosis of cardiac aneurysm is best made by means of cardiac ultrasonography, angiography, or nuclear medicine scanning (see Chapter 9). Chest radiographs usually show a focal bulge in the left ventricular wall and may show a calcified rim.

Aortic Valvular Disease

The normal aortic valve has three independent semilunar cusps: the right cusp, the left cusp, and the posterior (or noncoronary) cusp. There are three commissures, which are the sites of attachment of the cusps to the aortic wall. Because the free edges of the cusps are longer than the straight-line distances between the commissures, there is good apposition of the cusp edges when the valve is closed and yet a wide area for unimpeded blood flow when it is open. The two major abnormalities of the aortic valve are stenosis and insufficiency (also called regurgitation).

Aortic Stenosis. AS comprises several types of lesions obstructing aortic outflow. AS may be congenital, rheumatic, or senescent in origin. The site of AS is most commonly valvular (more than 75% of cases) but can also be subvalvular (fewer than 20% of cases) or supravalvular (fewer than 5% of cases). Congenital valvular AS is rare. It can occur as a valvular dome in which the cusps are fused with only a small aperture for blood flow. Alternatively, a unicuspid valve in which the orifice is eccentrically placed may be present. This type of abnormality is seen in infants with critical AS. The dome and unicuspid varieties account for fewer than 5% of all cases of congenital valvular AS, whereas 95% of cases are associated with a bicuspid aortic valve.

A bicuspid aortic valve is the most common cardiac anomaly of any kind and is present in 1% to 1.5% of all live-born infants. Males are affected three times as often as females. It is caused by commissural maldevelopment. Most patients lead completely normal lives because the bicuspid valve is not originally stenotic. However, with advancing age (usually over 45 years), the bicuspid valve cusps can develop fibrosis and thickening with secondary calcification and stenosis. The fibrosis and thickening occur in part because the two valve cusps are of unequal size, which results in a relative jet effect that is worse over the short cusp. Further fibrosis then develops with worsening of the stenosis and an even greater jet effect. Bicuspid valves are also prone to the development of bacterial endocarditis and are associated with coarctation of the aorta.

Until the development of antibiotics, the most common cause of AS was rheumatic fever. In more recent decades and in countries where medical care and antibiotics are available, nonrheumatic causes are more common. The most common presentation is involvement by rheumatic disease of the mitral valve alone; the next most common is involvement of the combination of mitral and aortic valves, and least common is involvement of the aortic valve alone. Rheumatic fever indirectly causes AS. The patient initially has an infection, usually in the pharynx from group A beta-hemolytic streptococci, that incites an immunological antigen-antibody reaction, which secondarily affects the valves. The result is thickening and fibrosis of the valve cusps, verrucous vegetations, calcific deposits, and eventual fusion of the commissures, causing AS (and usually concomitant AI). Even if the acute infection occurs in childhood, patients usually do not develop symptoms until after age 30 years.

Valvular AS can also be caused by aging (usually seen in patients older than 65) and is called degenerative or senile calcific AS or aortic sclerosis. Equal numbers of males and females are affected. The valve leaflets become less compliant with advancing age, and dystrophic calcifications may develop within the cusps. However, there is no fusion of the cusps (Fig. 5–38).

Subvalvular AS is of two major varieties. The common form is caused by a form of hypertrophic cardiomyopathy in which fibromuscular thickening of the myocardial wall obstructs the outflow of blood from the left ventricle. This process frequently extends downward to involve the anterior leaflet of the mitral valve, resulting in mitral regurgitation. The subvalvular stenosis is worse during systole when the left ventricular chamber walls thicken. This syndrome, previously called idiopathic hypertrophic subaortic stenosis, is now termed asymmetrical septal hypertrophy. A rare cause of subvalvular AS is formation of a discrete congenital subvalvular membranous diaphragm or a fibrous ridge beneath the valve.

Supravalvular AS is rare. It is caused by a congenital narrowing of the aorta or a diaphragm in the aortic segment just above the valve. Williams' syndrome (infantile hypercalcemia and characteristic facies) is frequently present in these cases.

In all cases of AS, forward flow of blood is restricted by a decrease in real or effective cross-sectional area. To maintain cardiac output, the flow velocity increases, causing both a high-pitched systolic murmur and a jet effect that results in poststenotic dilation of the ascending aorta. The normal cross-sectional area of the open aortic valve is 2.5 to 3.0 cm^2. Stenosis is considered mild when the cross-sectional area is between 1.5 and 0.75 cm^2, moderate when the area is between 0.75 and 0.5 cm^2, and severe (critical) when the area is smaller than 0.5 cm^2. As the stenosis worsens, the pressure on the left ventricular side of the stenosis increases, causing a large pressure gradient across the stenotic area. This gradient can be measured directly through cardiac catheterization or indirectly by means of Doppler cardiac ultrasonography as a shift of the peak systolic frequency.

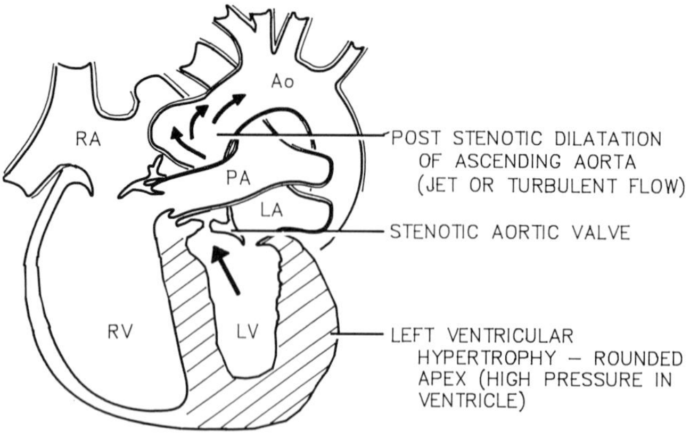

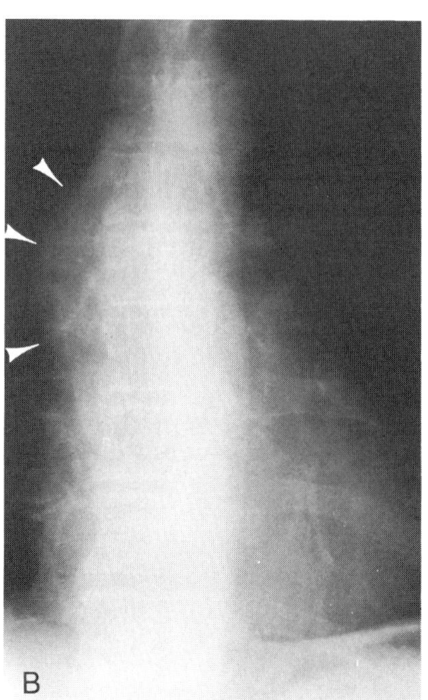

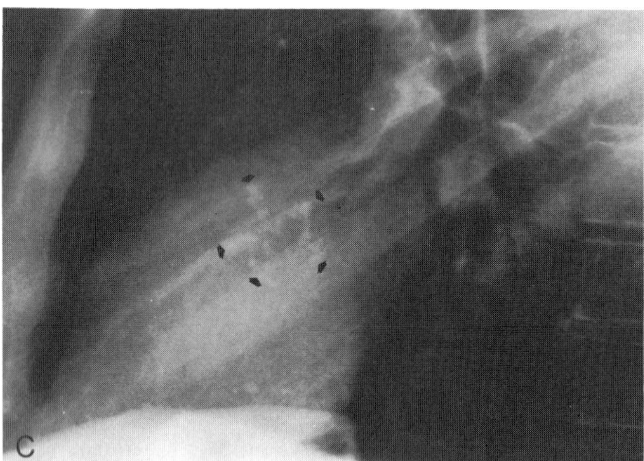

FIGURE 5–38. Aortic stenosis. *A.* Diagram. Ao, aorta; RA, right atrium; PA, pulmonary artery; LA, left atrium; RV, right ventricle; LV, left ventricle. *B* and *C.* The posteroanterior view (*B*) shows the poststenotic dilatation of the ascending aorta (*arrowheads*). The lateral view (C) shows calcifications in the area of the aortic valve (*arrowheads*). Hypertrophy of the left ventricle produces little or no observable change in the cardiac silhouette.

Patients may live for many years without symptoms because the heart tolerates a systolic pressure burden much better than a diastolic volume burden (as is seen in AI). When AS patients become symptomatic, they frequently do so rapidly. The appearance of the symptomatic triad of angina, CHF, and syncope is ominous, and the incidence of death within 2 years is high among such patients left untreated. Sudden death is not uncommon. Physical examination often reveals a crescendo-decrescendo systolic murmur and decreased pulse intensity.

Three important findings are seen on chest films in patients with AS: (1) calcifications in the region of the aortic valve, (2) poststenotic dilation of the ascending aorta, and (3) rounding of the left ventricular apex caused by left ventricular hypertrophy. Valvular calcifications are seldom visible on the frontal view, in which the valve overlies the spine; they are better seen on the lateral view (Figs. 5–38, 5–39). Valvular calcifications may be well shown by CT. The calcium is deposited in degenerated tissue, a process that takes many years to develop and is therefore normally seen in older patients. Definite valvular calcifications on chest films in a patient less than 55 years of age indicates clinically significant AS. In general, the more calcifications that are present, the worse the stenosis is. Patients with AS caused by congenital bicuspid valve de-

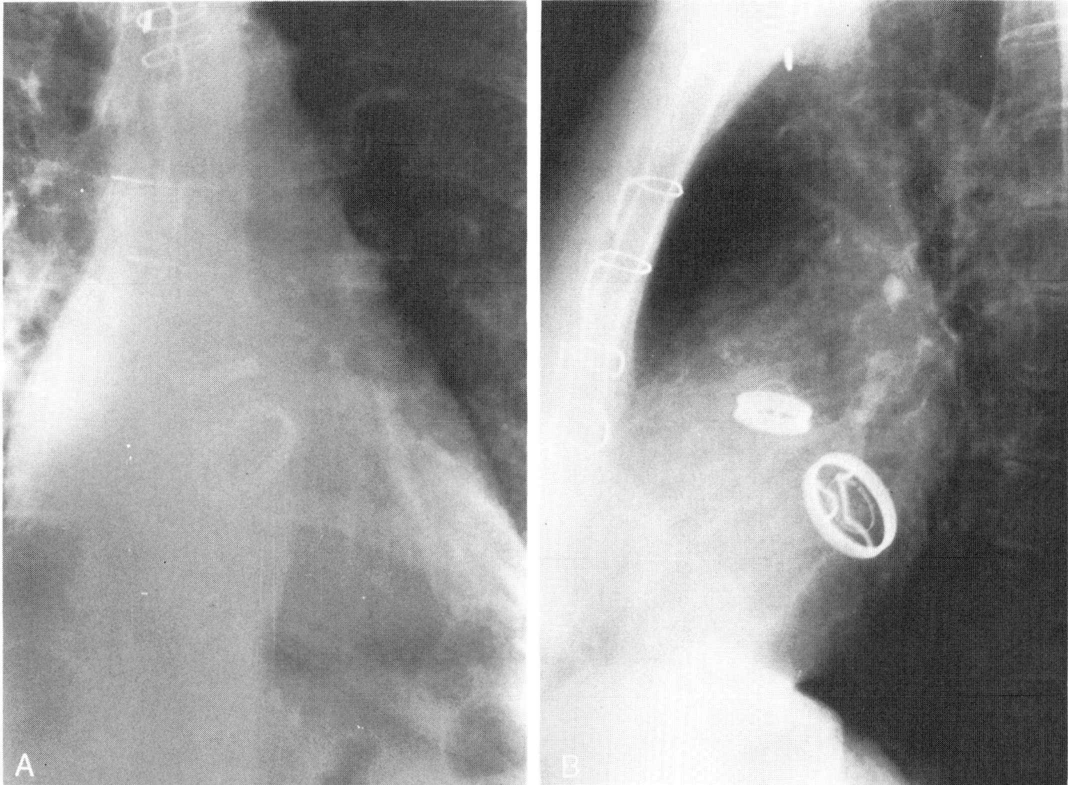

FIGURE 5–39. Aortic and mitral valve positions. The posteroanterior (*A*) and lateral (*B*) chest radiographs of a patient with a prosthetic aorta and mitral valves show the characteristic valve positions and orientation. The smaller valve is the aortic valve. Valvular calcification is difficult to photograph and so is not seen here. These areas should be searched for valvular calcification.

velop more valvular calcifications and do so at an earlier age than do patients with rheumatic AS.

Valvular AS causes a jet effect that tends to dilate the ascending aorta, a finding that is informative if present but does not exclude the diagnosis if absent. It is said to be present in up to 90% of patients with rheumatic AS but in only 70% of patients with bicuspid aortic valve AS. Subvalvular and supravalvular AS usually do not have ascending aorta dilation.

In the early and moderate stages of AS, the heart size is normal. The increasing pressure gradient across the stenotic valve causes left ventricular hypertrophy to develop as an initial response. It may, as mentioned earlier, be seen as rounding of the apex of the left ventricle. The overall left ventricular size, however, remains relatively normal, showing little or no indication on chest films that the left ventricular wall is thickened. Rapid left ventricular enlargement in a patient with AS usually denotes a failing left ventricle. This enlargement may also be caused by associated AI, which develops because a stenotic valve that cannot completely open cannot completely close, either.

Cardiac ultrasonography can measure the left ventricular wall thickness and the ascending aortic diameter and can show thickened aortic valve leaflets and decreased leaflet motion. Doppler ultrasonography can detect and quantify both the stenotic turbulent flow of AS and the presence of AI. It can also be used to indirectly measure the valve cross-sectional area through peak systolic flow measurements. Through cardiac catheterization, the decreased movement of the thickened valve leaflets can be demonstrated. Also left ventricular chamber size and wall thickness and the left ventricular ejection fraction can be assessed, and associated AI and coronary artery disease can be shown. Overall, ultrasonography is believed to be more informative than catheterization for assessing the severity of AS.

Medical treatment of AS is only symptomatic and temporizing. Although aortic valvulotomy and balloon-dilation valvuloplasty have been used, the definitive treatment is valve replacement. Aortic valves made of synthetic materials have a longer life span but require anticoagulation therapy. Natural biosynthetic valves such as cadaver, porcine, fascial, or pericardial valves do not last as long but also do not require anticoagulation. The patient's prognosis is much better if surgery is performed early than later after the onset of symptoms. The chances of morbidity and mortality increase significantly as the patient becomes more symptomatic.

Aortic Valvular Insufficiency. AI occurs when the valve leaflets are incompetent, allowing retrograde flow of blood from the aorta to the left ventricle during diastole. Whereas AS is a pressure-related problem for the left ventricle, AI is a volume-related problem. As the end-diastolic volume of the left ventricle increases, so does the end-diastolic pressure. This causes the left ventricle to fail and to respond to the increasing volume by dilating. This dilation is achieved by a stretching of the myocardial fibers, which causes a more effective contraction. The degree of left ventricular chamber dilation can become very high.

Much later in the course of the disease, as left ventricular failure becomes even worse, the enlargement of the left ventricle dilates the mitral valve annulus, causing mitral valvular regurgitation. The excess volume is then passed to the left atrium, which also responds to volume overload by enlarging. Finally, the volume is passed back to the lungs, resulting in pulmonary venous congestion. Unlike AS, which is almost always a chronic problem, AI can be either acute or chronic. There are many causes of AI (Table 5–13); overall, rheumatic endocarditis is the most common.

The heart does not tolerate volume overload as well as pressure overload, and so symptoms develop more quickly in AI than in AS. The incompetent valve cannot support a diastolic pressure, and so there are both a bounding pulse with a large pulse pressure and a diastolic murmur. The patient develops shortness of breath as CHF progressively develops.

The most notable chest film finding is an enlarged cardiac silhouette caused at first by left ventricular enlargement and later made worse by left atrial enlargement (Fig. 5–40). CHF develops progressively. The ascending aorta is often dilated when the disease affects primarily the ascending aorta, rather than the valve.

TABLE 5–13. CAUSES OF AORTIC (VALVULAR) INSUFFICIENCY (AI)

Acute AI

Damage to Aortic Valve
- Bacterial endocarditis
- Defective prosthetic valve

Damage to Aortic Valve Root
- Aortic dissection
- Marfan's syndrome
- Blunt trauma

Chronic AI

AS Causing Secondary AI
- Rheumatic fever
- Bicuspid aortic valve

Congenital
- Bicuspid aortic valve

Connective Tissue Disease
- Marfan's syndrome
- Ehlers-Danlos syndrome
- Osteogenesis imperfecta

Aortitis Damaging the Valve and Annulus
- Syphilis
- Rheumatoid arthritis
- Rheumatoid variants (ankylosing spondylitis, Reiter's syndrome)

Other
- Hypertension
- Atherosclerosis
- Myxomatous degeneration
- Aneurysm at sinus of Valsalva

Cardiac ultrasonography can show left ventricular, left atrial, and aortic root enlargement. The presence of regurgitation can be clearly shown by Doppler ultrasonography or by angiography with injection of contrast into the aortic root. The amount of regurgitation cannot be measured exactly by any means; rather, it is graded in severity in a semiquantitative fashion.

Similar to the situation with AS, medical therapy is useful for temporizing until definitive surgical replacement of the valve can be accomplished. The sooner that the surgery is done, the better the outcome is for the patient.

Mitral Valvular Disease

The mitral valve has two leaflets. The anterior (or septal) leaflet is smaller and immediately next to the aortic valve. The posterior leaflet is larger. As with the aortic valve, the commissures are the areas where the leaflets

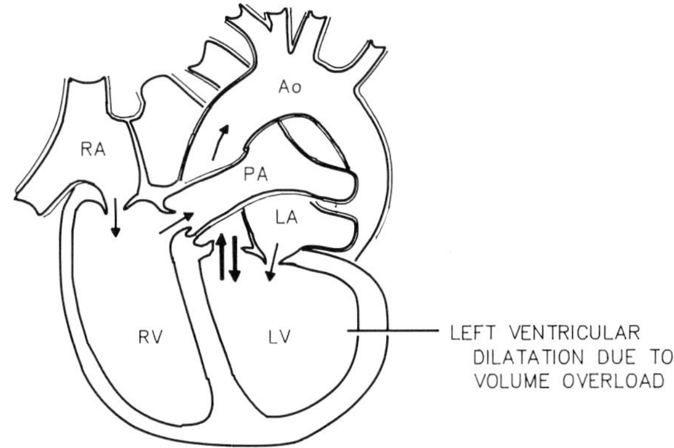

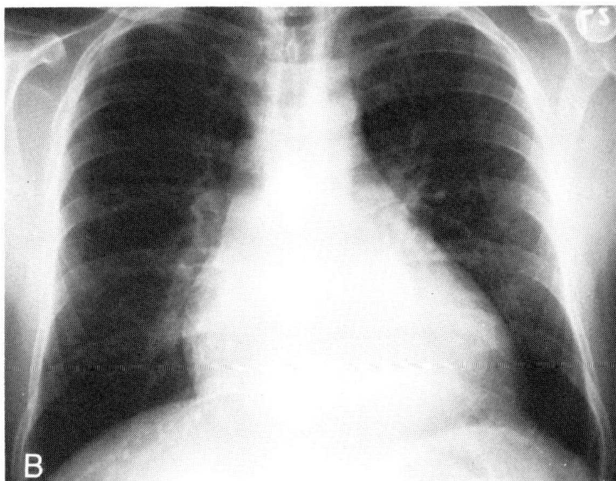

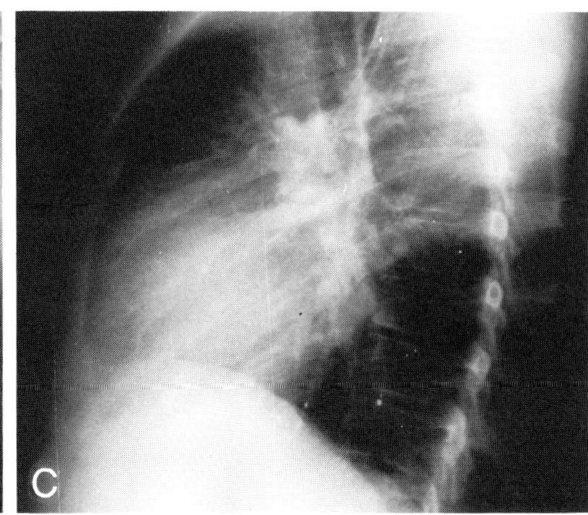

FIGURE 5–40. Aortic insufficiency. *A.* Diagram. Ao, aorta; RA, right atrium; PA, pulmonary artery; LA, left atrium; RV, right ventricle; LV, left ventricle. *B* and C. Posteroanterior *(B)* and left lateral *(C)* films show an enlarged cardiac silhouette in a patient with bacterial endocarditis that destroyed the aortic valve. This abrupt onset of volume overload caused dilatation of the left ventricle.

contact when the valve is closed. The papillary muscles and the chordae tendineae provide a restraint type of support system for the leaflets when they are in the closed position. The normal mitral valve cross-sectional area is 4 to 6 cm^2. The two major abnormalities of the mitral valve are mitral stenosis and mitral regurgitation (also called mitral insufficiency).

Mitral Stenosis. Nearly all cases of mitral stenosis (MS) are of rheumatic origin, although only half of the patients provide a history of rheumatic fever. Females are affected twice as often as males. Just as with rheumatic AS, the immunological antigen-antibody reaction set off by the preceding streptococcal infection causes calcifications within the leaflets as well as fibrous thickening of the leaflets and commissures that makes them much less compliant. Eventually the commissures progressively fuse, and the valve cross-sectional area decreases. The chordae may become fibrosed and, consequently, shortened. As with AS, a stenotic mitral valve usually cannot close well, and so mitral regurgitation (MR) develops to some degree in most cases of MS.

Congenital stenosis of the mitral valve can result from short parachute-like chordae that restrict leaflet opening, but this is very rare. Atherosclerotic calcifications of the mitral valve occur in the mitral annulus. They can be quite extensive, at times in the shape of a C or a J (Fig. 5–41). However, this does not affect the leaflets and so does not cause stenosis, although there may be a slight increase in the risk of subacute bacterial endocarditis.

The obstruction of blood flow causes left atrial enlargement, the primary chest radiograph finding in mitral stenosis. Blood then backs up into the lungs, producing pulmonary venous congestion. This leads first to pulmonary capillary hypertension and then to arterial hypertension, which eventually result in cor

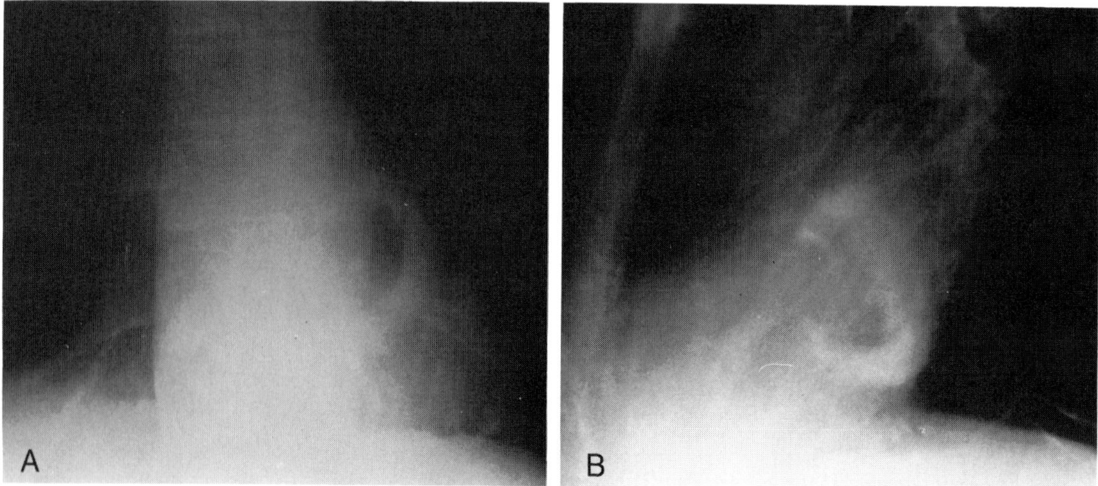

FIGURE 5–41. Mitral annulus calcification. The posteroanterior (*A*) and lateral (*B*) chest radiographs show a C-shaped ring of calcification around the mitral annulus. It is impressive but inconsequential in this case.

pulmonale (right-sided heart failure from pulmonary arterial hypertension).

The latent period between the episode of acute rheumatic fever and the onset of clinical symptoms is usually 15 to 20 years. Intermittent symptoms brought on by exercise develop when the valve area decreases to 1.5 to 2.0 cm^2. Symptoms of critical mitral stenosis develop when the area decreases to 0.5 to 1.0 cm^2. The symptoms are those of CHF: shortness of breath, dyspnea on exertion, cough (sometimes with hemoptysis), cyanosis, and pedal edema. Atrial arrhythmias (paroxysmal atrial tachycardia and atrial fibrillation) are also common, probably resulting from stretching of the conducting system in the walls of the dilated left atrium. A low-pitched, rumbling diastolic murmur is heard. The appearance and severity of symptoms are directly related to left atrial pressure (clinically measured as pulmonary wedge pressure).

A variety of calcifications occur in mitral stenosis. Calcifications in the walls of the left atrium may develop. Coarse calcifications of the mitral annulus are common. Speckled or nodular calcifications of the mitral valve leaflets may be seen in rheumatic cases. The pulmonary venous hypertension can cause small sites of microhemorrhage within the lungs that results in hemosiderin deposits and miliary nodular microcalcifications.

The principal findings on chest radiographs are chamber enlargement (especially of the left atrium and the right ventricle), valvular calcifications (leaflets and annulus), signs of CHF, pulmonary microcalcifications caused by mitral hemosiderosis, and sometimes calcifications within the left atrial wall itself (Fig. 5–42).

Mitral stenosis causes enlargement not only of the left atrium but also of the left atrial appendage. The highest degree of left atrial appendage enlargement occurs with rheumatic mitral stenosis. Right ventricular hypertrophy may be present as a result of pulmonary artery hypertension and appears as rounding and uplifting of the cardiac apex. Right ventricular enlargement is more common and is caused by right-sided heart failure. Left ventricular enlargement is not seen in pure mitral stenosis because the left ventricle is protected by the stenotic mitral valve.

Cardiac ultrasonography can show thickened and nodular mitral valve leaflets. Poor leaflet motion can be demonstrated on M-mode scans and directly visualized on real-time ultrasonography. Doppler ultrasonography can indirectly measure the pressure gradient across the valve by the shift in maximal frequency. Cardiac catheterization is not very useful in mitral stenosis except to detect coronary artery disease, which may affect the risk of surgery.

Mitral commissurotomy is still sometimes performed. However, with the availability of prosthetic and biosynthetic mitral valves, valve replacement is the treatment of choice. As with all other cardiac valve surgery in adults, the sooner it is performed before severe symptoms develop, the better the outcome is for the patient.

Mitral Regurgitation. Mitral regurgitation occurs when the mitral valve leaflets are unable

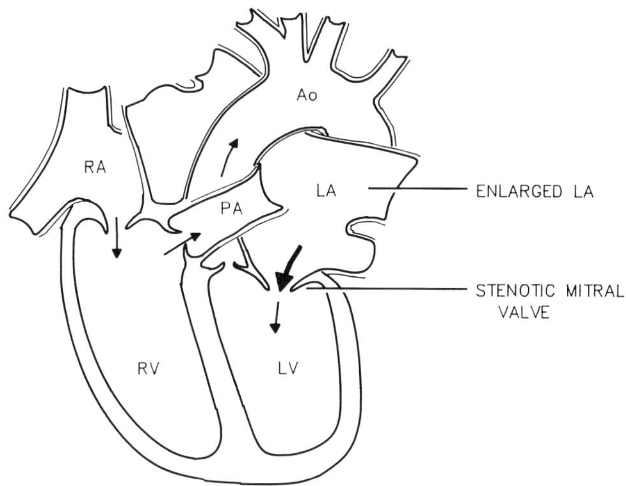

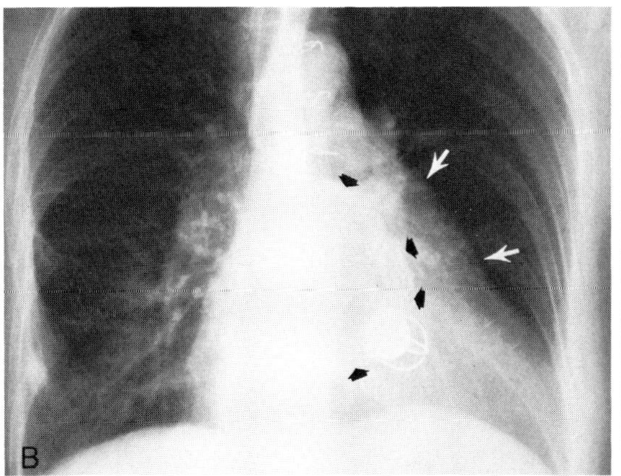

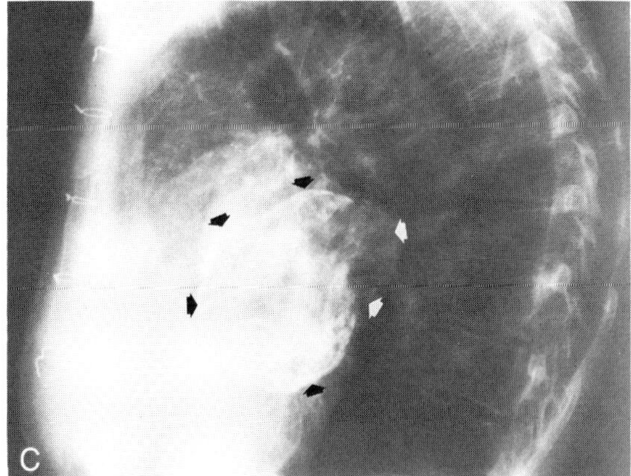

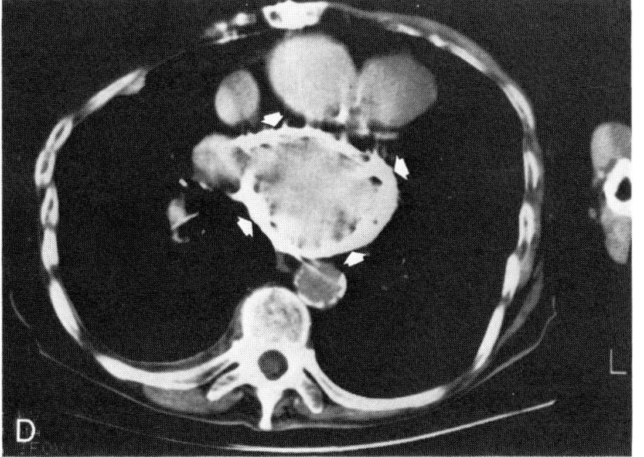

FIGURE 5–42. Mitral stenosis. *A.* Diagram. Ao, aorta; RA, right atrium; PA, pulmonary artery; LA, left atrium; RV, right ventricle; LV, left ventricle. *B, C,* and *D.* A prominently calcified, dilated left atrium is seen on the posteroanterior (*B*) and lateral (*C*) views as well as on the CT (*D*) (*arrowheads*). The left atrial appendage is also prominent on the posteroanterior view (*arrows*). The stenotic mitral valve has been replaced by a Star-Edwards ball valve prosthesis.

TABLE 5–14. CAUSES OF MITRAL VALVE REGURGITATION

Causes	Effect
Congenital	
Congenitally short chordae tendineae	Hold leaflets open
Marfan's syndrome	Myxomatous degeneration of the valve and dilation of ring
Endocardial cushion defect	Cleft mitral (and tricuspid) valve
Mitral prolapse syndrome	Congenital flaccidity of the mitral leaflets
CTGV with Ebstein's anomaly	Ebstein's anomaly usually affects the tricuspid valve, but in CTGV the ventricles and valves are turned around, and so mitral valve is affected
Acquired	
Rheumatic fever	Causes acute regurgitation, later mitral stenosis
Infective endocarditis	Gram-positive bacterial organisms destroy the mitral valve
Papillary muscle/chordae tendineae dysfunction	Acute MI causes ischemia or necrosis of the papillary muscles
Cardiomyopathy	Dilates the LA and LV chambers, enlarges the annulus
LV dilation	Any cause of LV chamber dilation such as CHF, AI
Idiopathic hypertrophic subaortic stenosis/asymmetrical septal hypertrophy	Irregular increase of the LV muscle mass of the septum can interfere with mitral valve closure
Calcified mitral annulus	In rare cases, the calcified mass of the annulus immobilizes the posterior leaflet

For explanation of abbreviations, see Table 5–1.

to properly close the mitral orifice during systole. Mitral regurgitation results in flow of a large fraction of the left ventricular blood backwards into the left atrium. As a result, the left ventricle must pump a large volume in order to ensure that a sufficient amount of blood enters the aorta. The left atrium must accommodate the large volume required to fill the left ventricle and the force of the regurgitant flow.

Mitral regurgitation has a large number of causes (Table 5–14); the most common is rheumatic heart disease, and the next most common is bacterial endocarditis. When rheumatic heart disease is the cause, mitral regurgitation is always associated with mitral stenosis. Any process that causes severe dilation of the left ventricle can also dilate the mitral valve annulus to the point of causing valve incompetence.

If caused by acute bacterial endocarditis or an acute myocardial infarction, mitral regurgitation symptoms can appear rapidly, even within days. The symptoms are those of CHF and sometimes atrial fibrillation. In cases of rheumatic fever origin, symptoms may not appear until several years later, when a low-pitched diastolic murmur may be heard.

Chest films show dilation of the left atrium and the left atrial appendage. The overall heart size is enlarged, usually because of left ventricular enlargement, which causes the apex to be pointed somewhat downward. Mild to moderate pulmonary venous congestion is often present (Fig. 5–43). On angiography, a regurgitant jet of contrast can be seen entering the left atrium from an injection into the left ventricle. Doppler cardiac ultrasonography can show this regurgitant jet and also measure the size of the dilated chambers.

The definitive treatment is prosthetic replacement of the mitral valve. Posteromedial annuloplasty can be attempted for a dilated annulus. Ruptured chordae tendineae or papillary muscles can be surgically repaired.

Traumatic Heart Disease

Blunt Trauma. Traumatic effects on the heart range from pericardial hemorrhage to rupture of the ventricle. Contusion simulates myocardial infarction clinically. There is hemorrhage into the myocardium, which can heal with little scar formation if the injury is mild. Extensive injury can result in rupture of the myocardium, which is usually fatal. Valve injury can result in tearing of the leaflets or rupture of the chordae tendineae. In rare instances, coronary arterial injury may result in thrombosis, especially if there is underlying atherosclerotic disease. Abnormal cardiac wall motion is characteristic of contusion and can be detected by gated radionuclide ventriculography (see Chapter 9) or echocardiography.

Penetrating Trauma. Penetrating wounds to

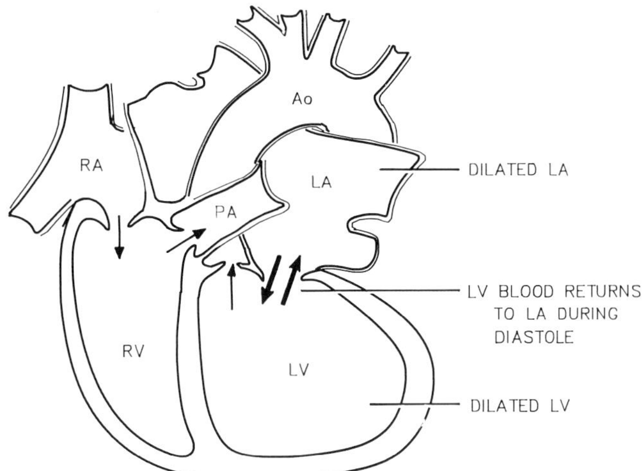

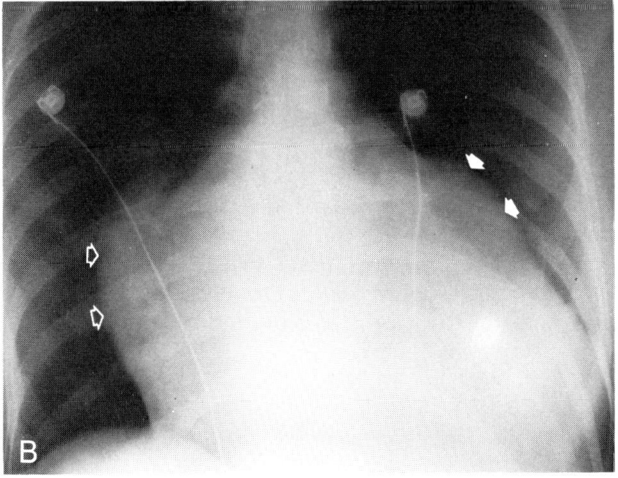

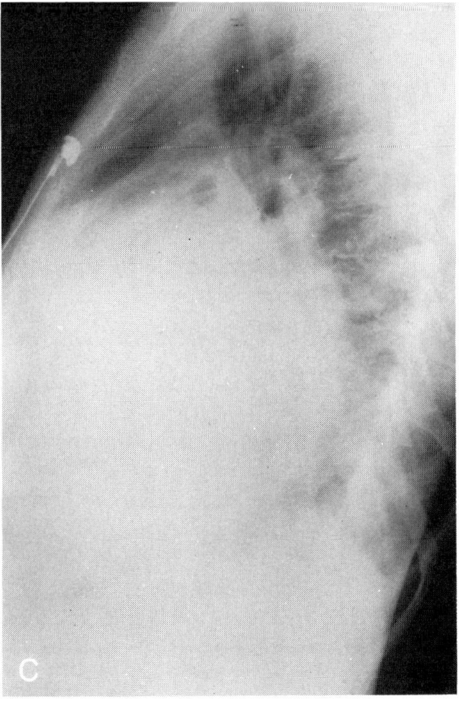

FIGURE 5–43. Mitral regurgitation. *A.* Diagram. Ao, aorta; RA, right atrium; PA, pulmonary artery; LA, left atrium; RV, right ventricle; LV, left ventricle. *B* and *C.* The posteroanterior (*B*) and lateral (*C*) views show extreme dilatation of the left ventricle. The left atrium is so dilated that it forms the right heart border on the posteroanterior view (*open arrowheads*). Note how the left atrial appendage is also prominent on the same view (*closed arrowheads*).

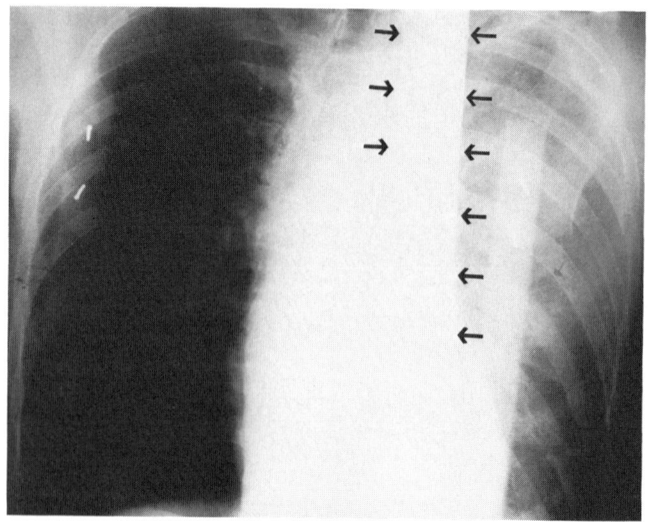

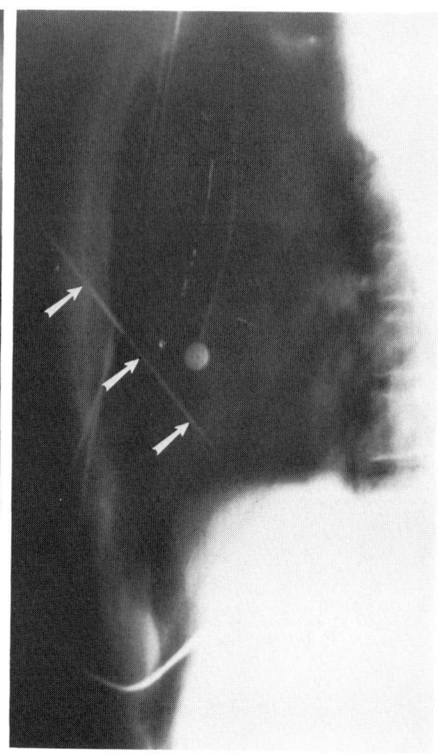

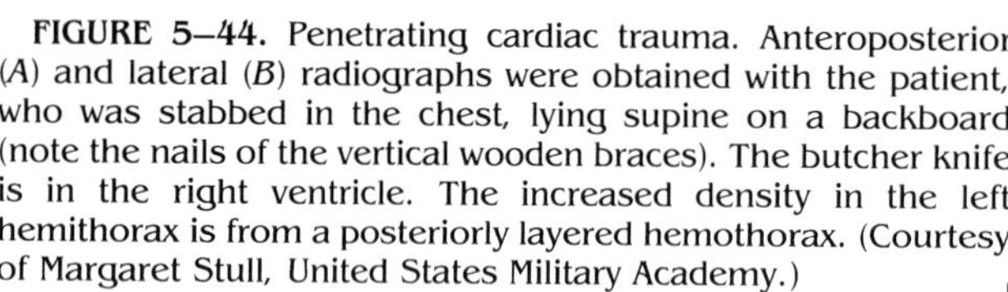

FIGURE 5–44. Penetrating cardiac trauma. Anteroposterior (*A*) and lateral (*B*) radiographs were obtained with the patient, who was stabbed in the chest, lying supine on a backboard (note the nails of the vertical wooden braces). The butcher knife is in the right ventricle. The increased density in the left hemithorax is from a posteriorly layered hemothorax. (Courtesy of Margaret Stull, United States Military Academy.)

the heart are an obvious cause of trauma, frequently fatal. Some patients survive long enough to be radiographed (Fig. 5–44).

EXTRACARDIAC VASCULAR DISEASE

Aortic Dissection. The aorta has three layers (intima, media, and adventitia). An aortic dissection occurs when the innermost of the three layers, the intima, is disrupted. Arterial blood under pulsatile systemic pressure can then dissect under the intima, causing a false lumen parallel to the true lumen. The dissection may re-enter the true lumen at one or more points or not at all.

The dissection can occur at any point in the aorta and can proceed proximally, distally, or both ways. As it proceeds down the descending aorta, it does so in a spiral fashion, following the fibers of the aortic wall. The dissection may stop at any point or proceed down to and sometimes involve the origins of the renal and more proximal arteries coming off the abdominal aorta (Fig. 5–45). The left renal artery is more often involved than the right. Proximal spread from the arch can involve the origins of the coronary arteries. Such involvement can pinch off the origins of these vessels, causing markedly decreased flow or cutting off flow completely. Distal tissues such as the kidney or the myocardial muscle can become ischemic or even infarcted. The dissection can also dilate the aortic valve annulus, causing aortic valvular regurgitation.

The dissections are classified according to location and extent (Table 5–15). There are two classifications of aortic dissection: the DeBakey and the Stanford classifications. Any aortic dissection involving the ascending aorta is a Stanford type A dissection. The Stanford

TABLE 5–15. CLASSIFICATION SYSTEMS FOR AORTIC DISSECTION

Portions of Aorta Involved	% of Patients	DeBakey	Stanford
Ascending, arch, and descending	45	I	A
Ascending only	30	II	A
Descending only	25	III	B

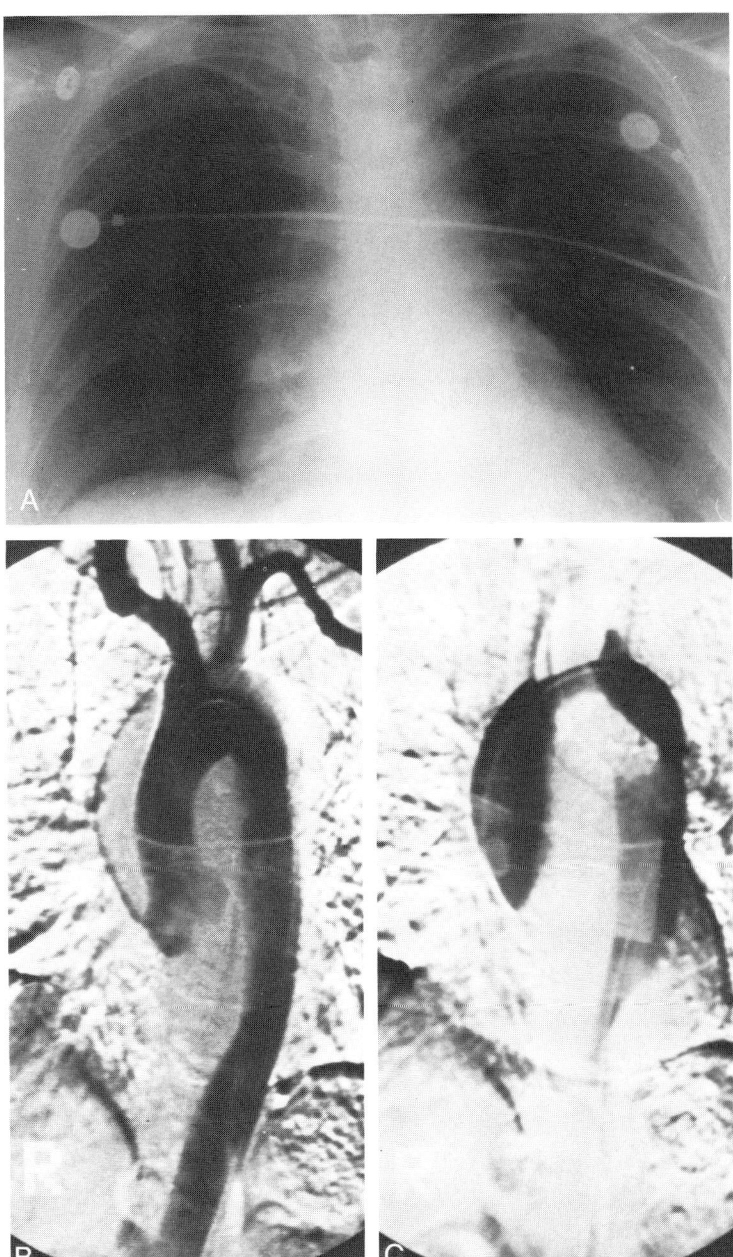

FIGURE 5–45. Aortic dissection type I. Appearance on a supine chest radiograph (*A*) is within normal limits, but the aortic arch arteriogram is grossly abnormal. For the first injection (*B*), the catheter is in the true lumen, and contrast flows through the brachiocephalic, left carotid, and left subclavian arteries. In a second study (*C*), the catheter injects contrast into the false lumen. The dissection extends from the aortic valve across the entire arch.

classification is more useful therapeutically than the DeBakey classification because type A lesions usually have to be surgically treated, whereas type B lesions are usually treated medically.

Standard posteroanterior and lateral chest films are usually the first imaging tests for aortic dissection. The two major imaging methods that should be considered are CT and angiography. The most important consideration in choosing between these two studies is whether the patient is a candidate for surgery. The study of choice for suspected surgical candidates (Stanford A) is angiography. Its advantages are that it can best define the extent of the dissection, show involvement of branch arteries such as the renal and coronary arteries, and show aortic regurgitation. Disadvantages are that it is invasive and requires large amounts of contrast.

CT is noninvasive, involves less contrast, and can show thrombus or contrast in the true or false lumens. Its disadvantages are that it cannot define the extent of disease as well as angiograms, cannot show valvular regurgitation, and cannot show branch artery involvement as well as angiograms.

Traumatic Aortic Disruption. Traumatic injury to the aorta is a serious clinical concern in any patient who has sustained blunt chest trauma. The most common mechanisms of injury are collision of the chest with a steering wheel or dashboard or any collision characterized by rapid deceleration. Patients may have numerous associated injuries, such as rib fracture, lung contusion, and pneumothorax, that account for the patient's pain, respiratory difficulty, or hemodynamic instability. The injury most often occurs at locations of aortic attachment (Fig. 5–46*A*). The most common location of traumatic aortic rupture is at the attachment of the ligamentum arteriosum.

The radiographic diagnosis of traumatic aortic rupture can be confusing on initial evaluation because of associated injuries, inability of the patient to take a deep inspiration, and the necessity of obtaining the radiographs with the patient in the supine position. Patients without aortic rupture frequently have a wide-appearing mediastinum because of these factors. When this appearance is coupled with a history of blunt chest trauma, further evaluation with upright chest films or angiography is mandatory.

Several findings on the chest radiograph are of assistance in diagnosing traumatic aortic disruption. The most conclusive are (1) a mediastinal width of more than 8 cm at or above the level of the aortic arch, (2) apical pleural density (capping) representing blood above the apical portion of the lung, (3) deviation of a nasogastric tube to the right of the T4 vertebral body, and (4) widening of the right paratracheal stripe (greater than 5 mm) (Fig. 5–46*B*). Less reliable signs are poor definition of the aortic arch, a mediastinal/thoracic ratio of more than 0.25, deviation of the trachea to the right, left pleural effusion (presumably hemothorax) without rib fracture, and aorticopulmonary window opacification. When the aortic wall is calcified and such calcifications are seen

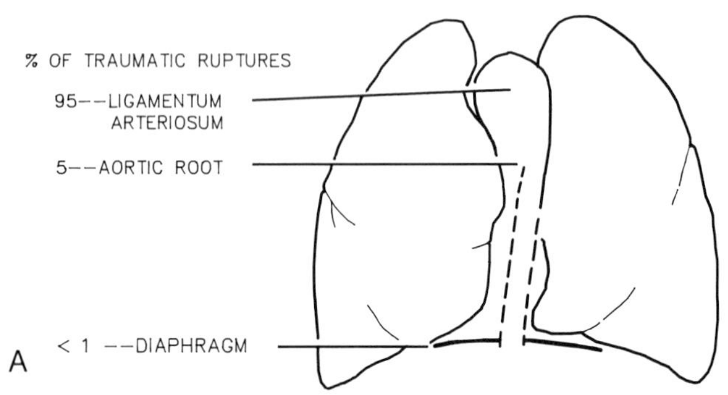

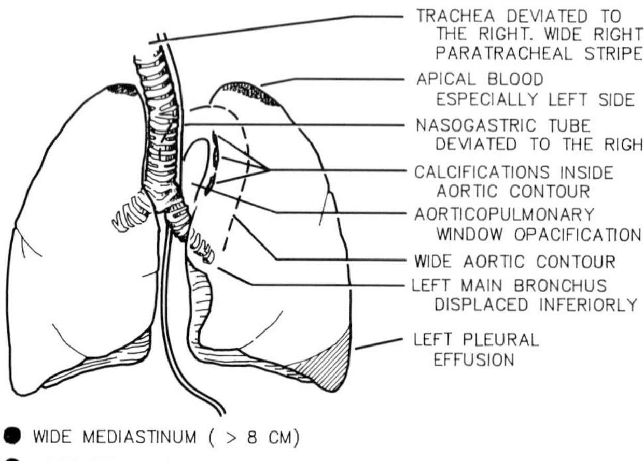

FIGURE 5–46. Traumatic aortic disruption. *A.* Sites of aortic rupture. *B.* Plain film findings.

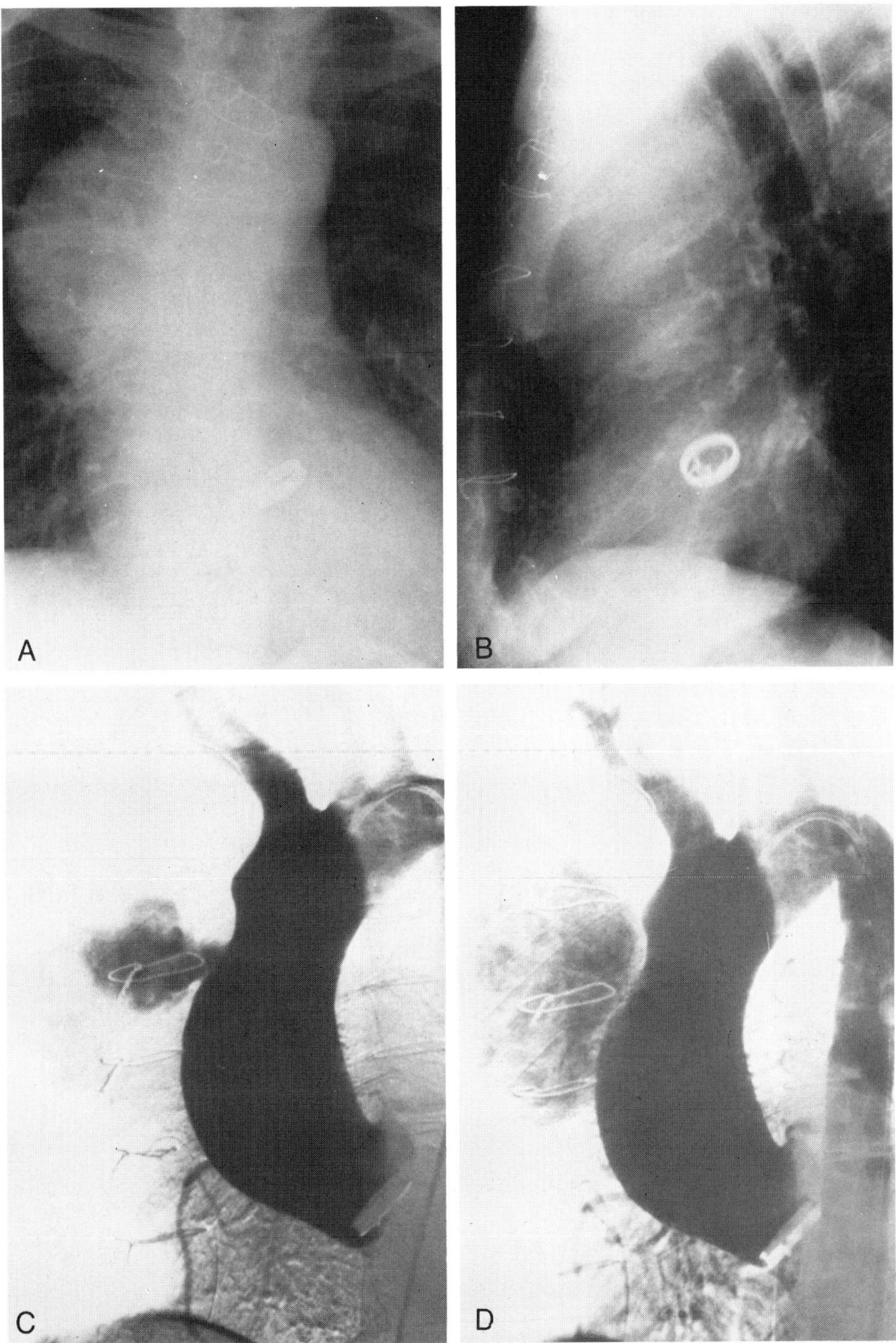

FIGURE 5–47. Pseudoaneurysm of the ascending aorta. Posteroanterior (*A*) and lateral (*B*) chest radiographs of a patient in whom the aortic valve was replaced by a prosthetic valve and in whom a prominent anterior mediastinal mass bulges to the right. Early (*C*) and late (*D*) films from an aortogram show contrail jetting into a large, round pseudoaneurysm that formed at the site where a cannula from the bypass pump had been placed into the aorta during surgery.

within the aortic contour, aortic rupture with a false lumen can be suspected.

Diagnosis in suspected cases is established by angiography. Because 5% of traumatic ruptures occur at the aortic root, it is important to inject near the aortic valve and demonstrate filling of the coronary arteries. Normal flow and opacification of these and the brachiocephalic vessels is important in identifying a false lumen or tear. CT scanning is not as effective as aortography in diagnosing traumatic rupture, particularly in that it does not assist with surgical planning. Patients frequently develop false aneurysms as a result of traumatic aortic injury. Because these aneurysms can hemorrhage at a later time, patients with suspected aortic injury require early evaluation and therapy.

Aortic Aneurysm. Aortic aneurysms are usually caused by atherosclerotic disease but are also seen in cystic medial necrosis, Marfan's syndrome, syphilis, hypertension and as sequelae to traumatic aortic injury. The aneurysms are usually elongated and can involve the origins of the brachiocephalic or visceral arteries. Involvement of the coronary arteries is rare. Aneurysms can dissect, creating a false lumen, or they can rupture into the mediastinum or the pericardium. Profuse hemorrhage into the pericardium or left pleural space is the most common cause of death in rupture of an ascending aortic aneurysm, for which the mortality rate is 70%. The diagnosis requires angiography.

A true aneurysm involves all three wall layers of the aorta. Aneurysmal dilation is usually fusiform or saccular. Pseudoaneurysms (also called false aneurysms) can occur. They involve a relatively narrow-necked penetration of at least two, and frequently all three, aortic wall layers. When only two layers are penetrated, the blood is contained by the adventitial layer. When all three layers are involved, only the surrounding tissues hold the blood. This is a life-threatening situation that requires immediate surgery (Fig. 5–47).

Infectious (Mycotic) Aortic Aneurysm. Infectious aneurysm is an uncommon infection of the aorta and most often affects the descending portion of the vessel. It usually occurs in drug addicts and is often associated with subacute bacterial endocarditis or septicemia. *Sal-*

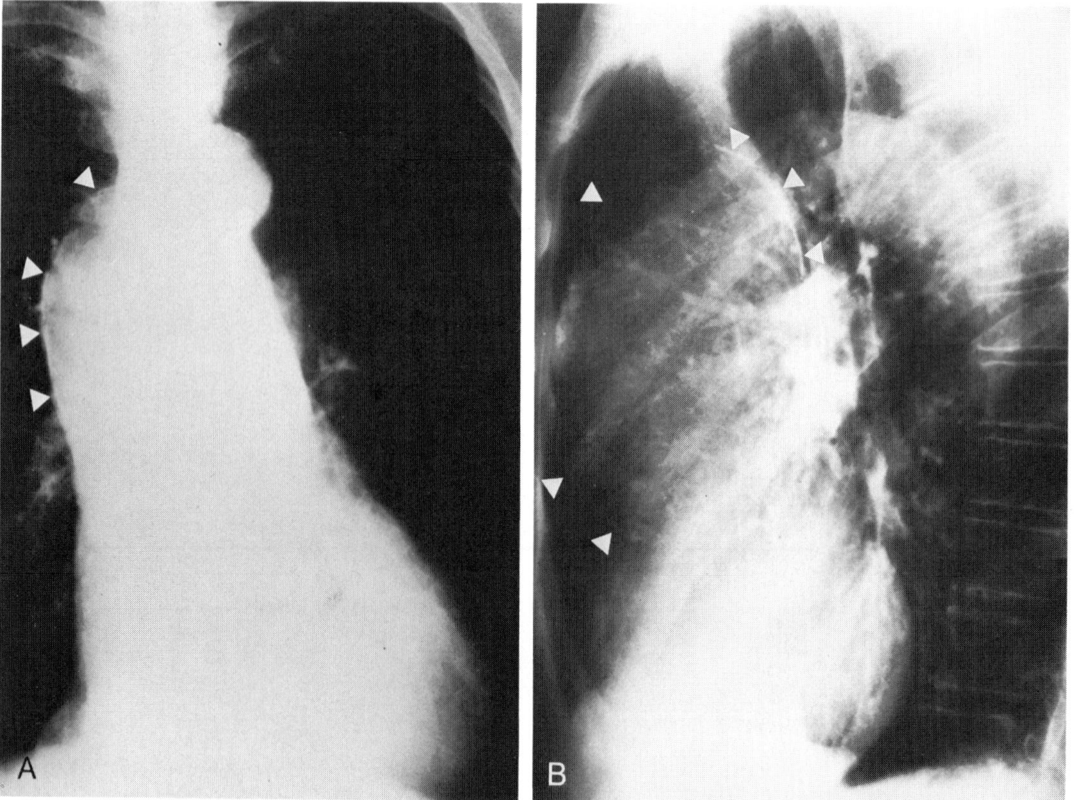

FIGURE 5–48. Syphilitic aortic aneurysm. Posteroanterior (*A*) and lateral (*B*) chest radiographs show a dilated ascending aorta with calcification along its walls (*arrowheads*).

monella, *Streptococcus*, and *Mycobacteria* are the usual infecting organisms.

Syphilis and Aortic Aneurysm. About 10% of patients with syphilis develop an aortitis 5 to 25 years after infection with *Treponema palladium*. As with other infections, the pathway of spread to the wall of the aorta is through the vasa vasorum. The intact endothelium effectively resists infection during bacteremia. The condition starts as an endarteritis of those vessels in which the wall of the aorta is attacked from within. Aneurysm, aortic regurgitation, and coronary ostial disease are common sequelae (Fig. 5–48).

Marfan's Syndrome: Effects on the Aorta. Severe degeneration of the media of the aorta, typically worst in the root of the aorta, is seen in Marfan's syndrome. Loss of some elastic and smooth muscle fibers in the media of the aortic wall is normal with aging. This loss can become tortuosity and ectasia of the aorta in the elderly. Myxomatous transformation of the aortic and mitral valves can also occur in Marfan's syndrome with subsequent aortic insufficiency and mitral regurgitation. Radiographs show aneurysmal dilatation of the ascending aorta. The term "cystic medial necrosis" is applied to this condition, but it is misleading because no necrosis is involved.

RADIOGRAPHIC DIFFERENTIAL DIAGNOSIS

Single radiographic findings or patterns frequently suggest a limited list of diagnoses. Additional findings and the clinical history can then assist in further limiting the list or in making a firm diagnosis. The following approaches to evaluation of radiographic findings can provide assistance in differential diagnosis. Diseases are listed in order of importance.

ASYMMETRICAL PULMONARY VASCULARITY

When pulmonary vascularity is unequal, a wide variety of causes must be considered. CHD is important, but many mechanical or structural abnormalities indicate lung or mediastinal disease as the cause of the asymmetrical pulmonary vascularity.

Swyer-James syndrome	The lucent lung is smaller
Tension pneumothorax	Involved side is lucent
Bronchial obstruction	The lucent, obstructed lung is larger
Absent pectoralis muscle	Apparent lucency
Pulmonary sling	Right-sided lucent lung in 50%
Pulmonary embolus	Oligemia of the lung due to PA obstruction (Westermark's sign)
Asymmetrical pulmonary edema	Frequent in COPD patients or in dependent lung
Hilar mass	PA compression by tumor
Congenital heart disease:	
TOF with pulmonary artery atresia	Atresia is on the side opposite the aortic arch
Isolated pulmonary artery stenosis	Occurs without other CHD
Truncus arteriosus	Increased pulmonary blood flow usually on the right (waterfall sign)
Pseudo-TRUNCUS (TRUNCUS type IV)	TOF physiology due to severe PS
After shunt procedure for TOF	Shunt sends more blood to one side
Pulmonary valvular stenosis	Dilatation of the left PA with increased flow to the left lung
Scimitar/venolobar syndrome	Right lung is hypoplastic
PDA	Very large left PA bulge results in hypoperfusion of the left upper lobe

CONGESTIVE HEART FAILURE IN THE NEWBORN

CHF at birth is usually caused by a severe obstructive lesion. In storage diseases, CHF is the consequence of cardiomyopathy caused by muscle infiltration. The mechanism of how neonatal CHF is caused by maternal diabetes is complex and not thoroughly understood.

Hypoplastic left heart syndrome
Coarctation
TAPVR type III
Cor triatriatum
Storage diseases
Maternal diabetes

CONGENITAL HEART DISEASE IN THE ADULT

The presence of CHD in the adult indicates either that the lesion is not severe enough to cause major problems in hemodynamics and oxygenation or that a coexisting, protective lesion is present. The list of possible causes is short.

PS
ASD
VSD
PDA
Congenital aortic valve disease
Coarctation of the aorta
Corrected transposition (without other significant abnormalities)

CONGENITAL SYNDROMES ASSOCIATED WITH CARDIOVASCULAR DISEASE

Syndrome	*Associated Cardiovascular Disease*
Cornelia de Lange's	VSD in 15% of cases
Down's (trisomy 21)	CHD in 40% of cases (large number of cases with endocardial cushion defect; other cases with ASD, VSD, PDA, or TOF)
Ellis–van Creveld	ASD in 50% of cases
Holt-Oram	ASD or VSD in 60% of cases
Hurler's	Heart disease in 70% of cases, usually biventricular hypertrophy, thickened heart valves, intimal proliferation of pulmonary artery and coronary arteries
Ivemark's	Situs indeterminatus, asplenia, visceral symmetry, CHD (pulmonary atresia or PS, common atrium, single ventricle, TGV, or TAPVR)
Kartagener's	Mirror-image heart in all cases (situs inversus and dextrocardia)
Kawasaki's	Some heart involvement in 20% of cases (myocarditis, pericarditis, coronary arteritis or vasculitis, coronary artery aneurysm with thrombus)
Lutembacher's	Mitral or aortic valvular stenosis seen in 5% to 10% of patients with ASD
Marfan's	Secondary ascending aortic aneurysm, dissection, or pericardial tamponade or a combination of these
Noonan's	PS and septal defects
Pompe's	Infiltrative glycogen storage disease of heart muscle
Turner's	CHD in 20% of cases (coarctation of aorta in 70%, ASD or VSD in 30%)
Uhl's	Partial or complete absence of right ventricle; huge right atrium
von Gierke's	Same as those of Pompe's disease
Williams'	Supravalvular AS and peripheral PS

6

Mammography

Robert D. Rosenberg
Juleann Cottini Gandara
Gary K. Stimac

BASIC EVALUATION

Breast cancer accounts for 130,000 new cases of cancer and 40,000 deaths yearly. Only as recently as the 1980s was it exceeded by lung cancer as a cause of cancer death in women. Currently, one in nine women eventually develops breast cancer. The primary risk factors for breast cancer are sex, age (Table 6–1), personal history of breast cancer, family history of breast cancer (especially in premenopausal first-degree relatives), and biopsy showing atypical cell growth. Other risk factors of lesser importance include age at first pregnancy, lactational history, and menstrual history (ages at menarche and menopause). The early detection of breast cancer is best made by clinical physical examination, breast self-examination, and mammography. *Definitive* diagnosis of breast cancer is made through biopsy of breast tissue.

There are two distinct types of mammographic examinations: screening and diagnostic examinations. The purpose of screening mammography is the early detection of breast cancer. This examination has a limited role in evaluation of benign breast diseases and is only moderately useful in the evaluation of patients with breast symptoms. Thus, screening mammograms are used to identify nonpalpable early breast tumors in asymptomatic patients. Diagnostic mammograms are used for patients with specific signs or symptoms (such as a mass or a discharge) to determine whether the clinical abnormality is mammographically suspected for malignancy, to identify suspicious-looking lesions elsewhere, or to follow up a previously noted abnormality. A normal mammogram in this setting does not exclude the possibility of breast cancer and should not preclude biopsy of a palpable abnormality. Biopsy may be avoided when mammography or ultrasonography clearly proves a

TABLE 6–1. BREAST CANCER INCIDENCE BY AGE

Age Range	Risk*
30 to 39	27
40 to 49	127
50 to 59	212
60 to 69	322
70 to 79	404
80 to 89	435

*Number of new cases per year per 100,000 women in 1988.

palpable abnormality to be a benign lesion, such as a simple cyst.

Mammography is, at best, 90% sensitive for detecting breast cancer. A normal mammogram therefore does not exclude the possibility of cancer, especially when a suspicious palpable mass has been identified by experienced clinicians. From a practical viewpoint, the purpose of mammography is not the diagnosis of cancer but the selection of patients for breast biopsy. Thus patients are sent for biopsy when they have a breast lesion suitable for needle localization and when the probability of breast cancer is above a certain threshold. Because about 25% of breast biopsies in the United States yield positive results for cancer, patients with lesions who have a perceived risk above 10% to 15% are sent for biopsy. In Europe, the rate of positive biopsy results is higher (around 50%). In large screening populations, the risk of cancer is about 0.5% (0.3% to 0.7%, depending on the population of patients and whether they have had a previous recent screening examination), and so the approximate rate of biopsy recommendations in the United States should be about 2% in a pure screening population. In practice in the United States, the screening population is a self-selected group that probably has higher-than-average risk factors or has signs and symptoms that raise suspicions of cancer.

Screening mammography has decreased the rate of mortality from breast cancer by approximately 30% as a result of diagnosis at an earlier stage. On average, mammography identifies cancer 2 years earlier than does physical examination (or other clinical presentation) in patients under the age of 50 and approximately 3½ to 4 years earlier in patients over the age of 50. This earlier detection results in improved long-term survival.

Screening Mammography Recommendations

Current American Cancer Society recommendations for screening mammography are a baseline mammogram between ages 35 and 40, mammograms yearly or every other year from ages 40 to 50, and mammograms yearly after age 50.

No upper limit of age is recommended in the United States, whereas in Sweden, screening ends at age 75. Patients with a family history of early breast cancer may benefit from screening before age 40. Given the more aggressive nature of many breast cancers found in younger patients, yearly screening mammograms may be advisable in patients in the 40-to-49 age group, especially in those women with a strong family history of breast cancer, with dense breast tissue, or with inconclusive results of a clinical breast examination.

Imaging Technique

Mammographic detail and accuracy are highly sensitive to technique. Adequate technique requires proper angulation of the x-ray tube for each view, optimal positioning of the patient, and adequate compression of the breast and proper exposure. Lack of adequate compression results in poor visibility of small masses, more frequent appearances of pseudotumors, and increased irradiation of the patient. Proper technique also requires imaging as much of the breast tissue as possible in each view. Consistency of technique facilitates comparison of new and old examination findings. Obtaining proper exposure is more difficult than in routine radiography because mammography film has high contrast and, therefore, a more narrow exposure latitude.

Mammography requires a dedicated mammography unit to provide proper geometry of the x-ray source, a small focal spot, a good compression device, and the low constant kilovolt peak capability necessary for producing adequate contrast and sharpness. Most mammography machines have phototimers to produce consistent exposures. Mammographic x-ray grids are generally used for all patients and are required for those with dense breast tissue.

Mammography is performed either by film-screen technique or with the use of specialized xeromammography units. Film-screen technique is more commonly used, although either can provide an adequate examination. Standard film-screen views for a screening examination are a medial-lateral oblique view and a cranial-caudal (CC) image for each breast (Fig. 6–1). If abnormalities are suspected on the screening images, other views may be obtained, such as a straight medial-lateral view, an exaggerated CC view (emphasizing medial or lateral portions of the breast), other oblique views, and spot compressions. Magnification techniques with or without focal compression are used to evaluate mass lesions and to better characterize microcalcifications. Special views (such as pinch views) are used in some patients

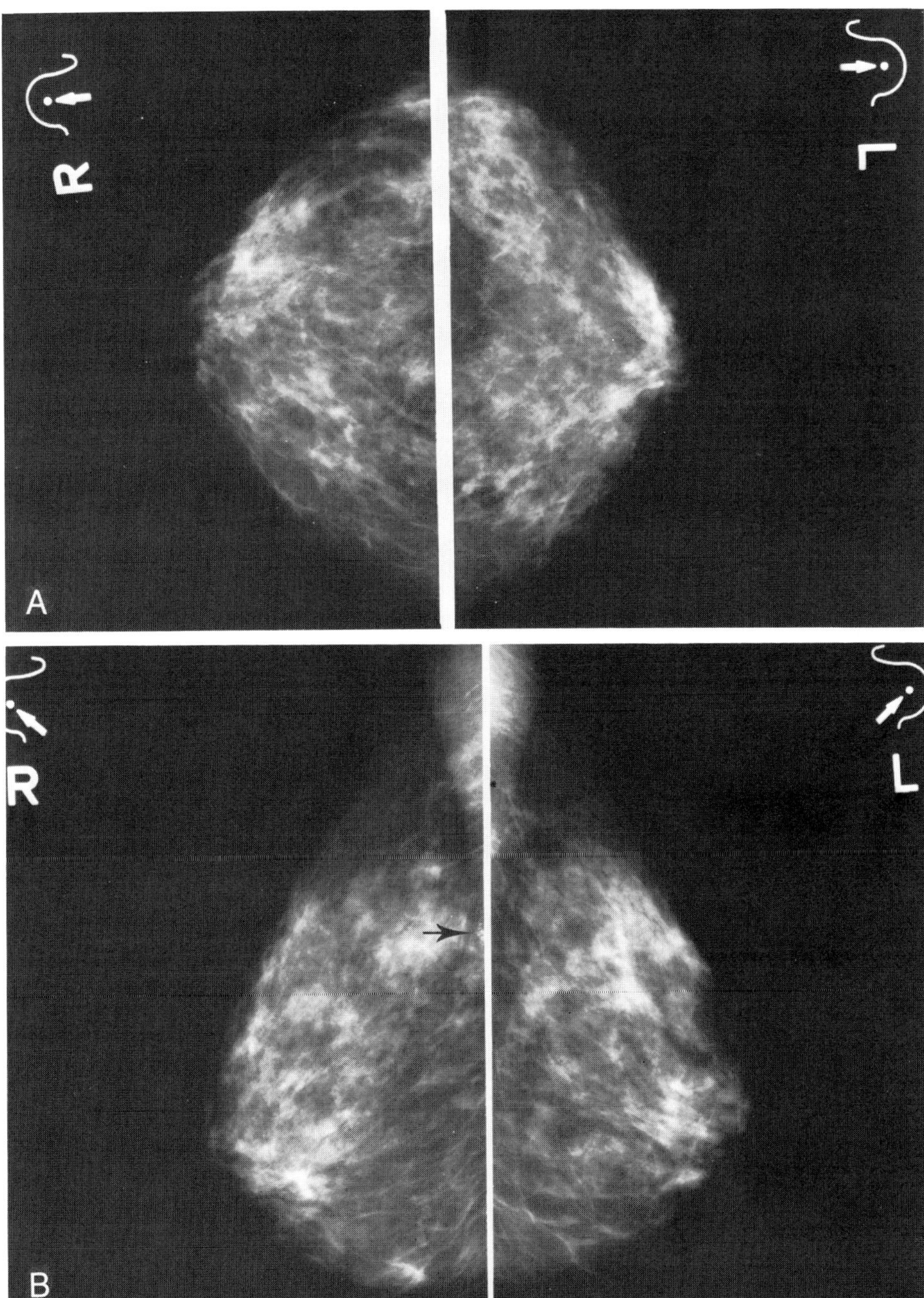

FIGURE 6–1. Routine bilateral mammogram. *A.* In the cranial-caudal (CC) view, markers are used on the lateral side of each breast. *B.* In the medial-lateral oblique view, markers are used on the superior side of the breast. The normal glandular structure appears as linear and dense parenchyma converging at the nipple in a 55 year-old-woman. Grouped microcalcifications are seen deep on the right axillary view only (*arrow*). These are on the very edge of the mammogram, which emphasizes the importance of including as much breast tissue as possible.

who have breast prostheses, in order to separate the glandular breast tissue from the radiodense prosthesis.

The effective focal spot size for mammography depends on the design of the equipment (see Chapter 1); the spot should be approximately 0.2 to 0.5 mm in diameter for routine mammographic images, and less than 0.2 mm diameter for magnification images (the small focal spot setting). The usual kilovolt peak for film-screen mammography is 25 to 28 (higher for xeromammography), with a source–to–

image-receptor distance of at least 50 cm to enable high resolution.

Specialized mammography screens and film are also necessary for providing contrast and detail. Dedicated film processors provide improved consistency and may allow improved film speed and contrast. Technical factors that influence mammographic interpretation include proper exposure, proper positioning, and optimal compression. The exposure should produce good contrast and penetration in the image without overexposure. The skin line is usually not seen without a bright light in most film-screen images. Motion blurring (usually from breathing) and grid lines should be eliminated. On the oblique image, the pectoralis muscle line should end near the level of the nipple. On the CC view, the pectoralis muscle may be seen on the deep margin of the film and should not be confused with a lesion.

The radiation dose to the breast varies according to whether film-screen mammography or xeromammography is used and, in film-screen mammography, the specific film speed and screens used. In general, the dose from film-screen technique is lower than that from xeromammography. The dose to each breast in a two-view examination is best expressed as the mean glandular dose in rad. It must be less than 1.0 rad per breast per examination, and is generally much less than 0.5 rad per breast. The theoretical increase in breast cancer caused by these doses is very small in view of the clinical utility of mammography. Also, the time between radiation exposure and the observed increase of breast cancer for high doses is more than 15 years. The risk of breast cancer caused by mammography is further minimized by the low radiation sensitivity of breast tissue in the population undergoing the examination (i.e., women over 35 years of age).

Interpretation

The normal breast shows great variation on mammograms, depending on the age, the parity, the genetic background, and the hormonal status of the patient. In the young, premenopausal woman, dense fibroglandular tissue occupies most of the mammographically visible breast volume. The amount of fibroglandular tissue is gradually replaced by fat in most patients. The dense parenchyma decreases with age and parity, starting medially and inferiorly; the breast becomes predominately adipose after menopause.

Because the breasts are usually similar in parenchymal distribution, comparison of both breasts greatly assists in evaluation. Previous films are of even more value for comparison, however, because total symmetry is rare and interval change is easier to detect. The primary sign of breast cancer is a discrete mass. Other (secondary) signs include malignant calcifications, increased density, architectural distortion, focal asymmetries, skin thickening, and nipple retraction. Masses, asymmetries, and microcalcifications must be carefully examined in order to determine whether they have benign or malignant characteristics. Benign calcifications and apparent masses are common. Calcification analysis requires a magnifying glass and magnification spot views. Abnormalities shown on screening images must be evaluated with additional views or ultrasonography. This further evaluation (work-up examination) consists of (1) spot compression or magnification views or both in order to better see or exclude masses and to evaluate characteristics of calcifications; (2) views at varying angles; and (3) ultrasonograms in order to differentiate solid from cystic lesions (Figs. 6–2, 6–3, 6–4). True masses should be seen on two views. The second view may need to be tailored in order to demonstrate the mass when it is in a location not shown on the initial image (lateral CC, exaggerated views, and so forth).

Skin lesions are frequently seen on mammograms and are a potential source of confusion. They may be seen on one or both views. Warts may contain malignant-appearing calcifications. Placement of radiopaque markers over a skin lesion and filming with the marker tangent to the lesion reveal the relationship of the skin lesion to the mammographic abnormality. Therefore, the physical examination conducted at the time of mammography should include evaluation of the skin for lesions (moles, warts, and so forth), retraction, and scars.

Xeromammography

In xeromammography, an electrical plating technique is used to produce an image. As a result, it is most sensitive to the detection of edges ("edge enhancement") and is therefore advantageous for identifying calcifications. On the other hand, large masses with relatively uniform density are less easily detected than on film mammography. Clear superiority of

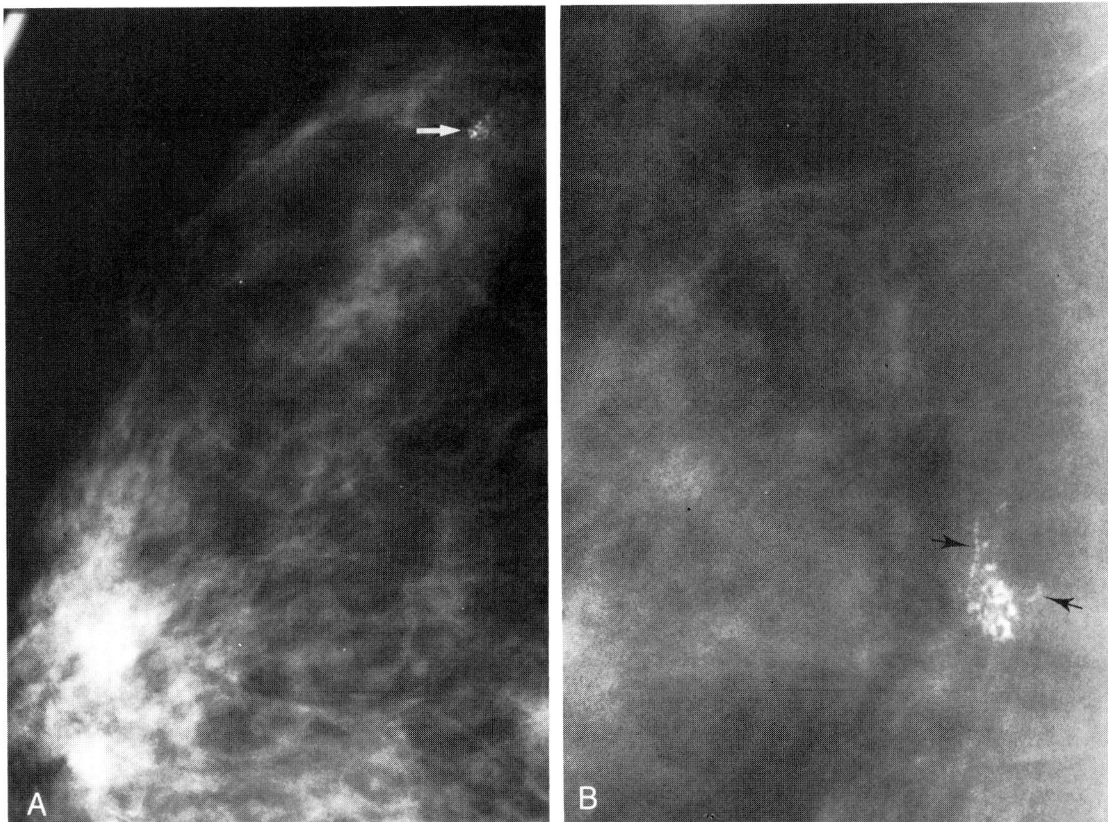

FIGURE 6–2. Work-up evaluation of patient in Figure 6–1. *A*. Exaggerated lateral CC view. More of the lateral breast is included on this image than on a routine CC view; lateral location of the calcifications is shown (*arrow*). *B*. Magnification of axillary view shows characteristics suspicious for malignancy, including branching (*arrows*) and irregularity of the density, size, and borders of the calcifications.

either xeromammography or film mammography for identification of breast cancer has not been established.

Ultrasonography

Ultrasonography has an important but limited role in breast imaging. It can show whether a mammographic mass is a simple benign cyst (Fig. 6–4); however, the benign-versus-malignant nature of solid masses is not easily assessed by ultrasonography. As in film mammography, solid masses with poor margins are more likely to represent malignancy than are well-marginated ones. Ultrasonography is also used in imaging palpable masses not seen on mammography and for patients with clinical infection or abscess. It is less sensitive to early breast cancer than is mammography and is therefore not used in routine screening for cancer (see also Figs. 6–10, 6–12).

Needle Localization Procedure

The radiologist must be able to localize nonpalpable lesions for biopsy. There is a variety of prebiopsy needle localization techniques and devices. One commonly used method involves needle placement through a fenestrated compression device (Fig. 6–5). Most radiologists prefer this method because the needle can be placed parallel to the chest wall (either horizontally or vertically), which significantly decreases the risk of chest wall penetration in comparison with perpendicular needle placement. The technique is also quickly learned and quickly performed with minimal needle repositioning. The imaging plane is chosen for minimizing the distance from skin to lesion. In the initial needle placement, the needle traverses the lesion. After confirmation of good needle position in the first plane, images are made in a second plane (usually at right angles), and then needle depth

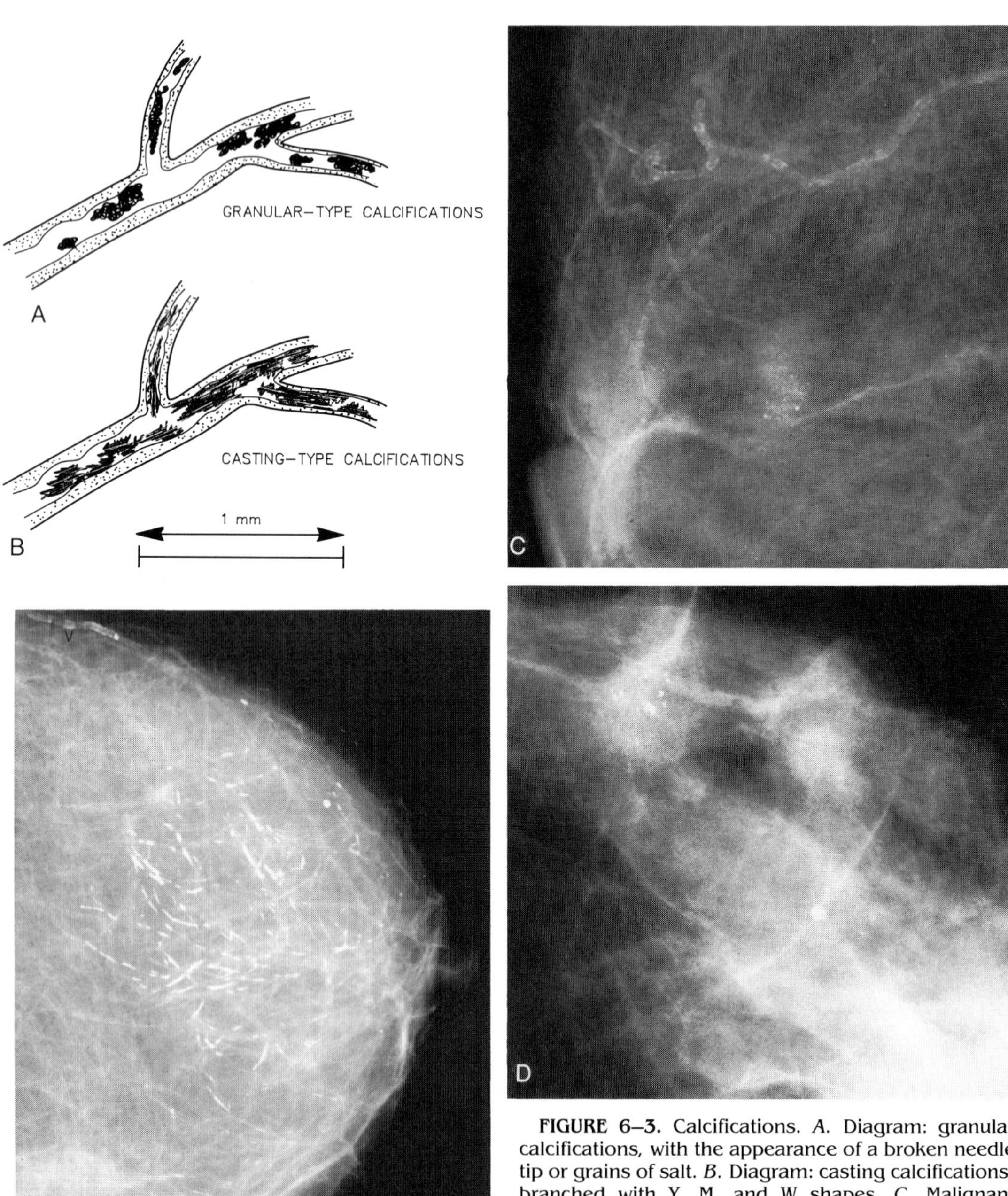

FIGURE 6–3. Calcifications. *A.* Diagram: granular calcifications, with the appearance of a broken needle tip or grains of salt. *B.* Diagram: casting calcifications, branched with Y, M, and W shapes. *C.* Malignant calcifications. These are usually grouped microcalcifications with marked variations in size, shape, and density and some of which may be branched. *D.* Malignant calcification. Very fine, clustered, punctate shapes are highly variable in density. *E.* Benign secretory calcifications. These are dense and well-marginated.

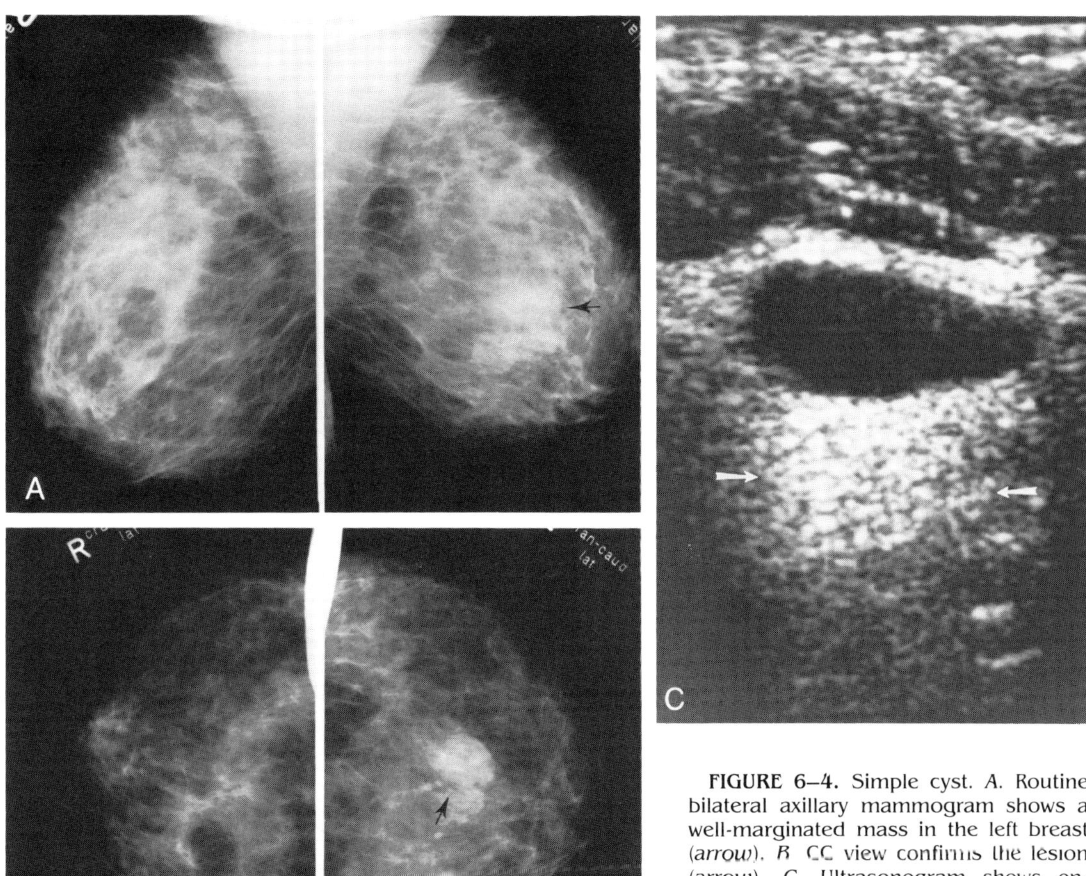

FIGURE 6–4. Simple cyst. *A.* Routine bilateral axillary mammogram shows a well-marginated mass in the left breast (*arrow*). *B.* CC view confirms the lesion (*arrow*). *C.* Ultrasonogram shows enhanced through-transmission (*arrows*), well-defined walls, and no internal echoes.

is adjusted. It is better for the needle to be slightly through the lesion than short of it.

A hooked wire is inserted through the needle, and the needle is withdrawn, leaving the hook within 5 to 10 mm of the lesion. A radiograph of the excised biopsy specimen confirms that the radiographic lesion was excised (Fig. 6–6). If there is doubt as to whether the lesion was removed, follow-up mammograms may be necessary several months after resolution of the surgical changes to confirm that excision was successful. Needle localization procedures require coordination and agreement between the radiologist and the surgeon. The surgeon is greatly assisted by marked copies of the final localization films indicating the area to be excised and clarifying the relationship of the wire to the lesion.

Galactography

Galactograms are occasionally performed for patients with a clinical history of nipple discharge. To be clinically significant, nipple discharge should be spontaneous, persistent, and nonlactational.

Discharges of surgical significance (suspicious for malignancy) are serous, serosanguineous, sanguineous, and watery. Purulent, milky, or multicolored discharges are usually related to benign conditions and generally can be treated medically. The draining duct is cannulated by means of a small-bore, blunt needle, and water-soluble contrast is injected (Fig. 6–7). Mammography images are obtained with slight compression and are examined for intraluminal filling defects or duct obstruction

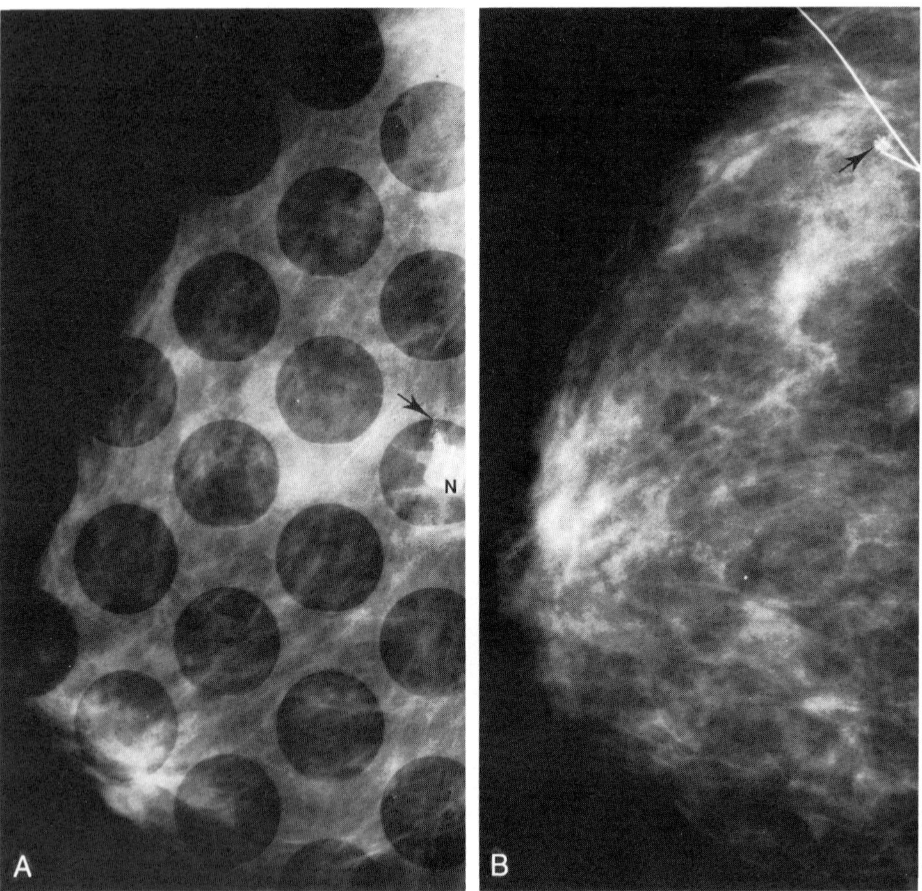

FIGURE 6–5. Needle localization procedure. *A.* Compression mammogram with the use of a fenestrated localization paddle shows the needle (N) passing through the paddle into the calcifications (*arrow*). The needle was inserted from the lateral aspect of the breast, the closest approach. The needle and its hub are seen end-on. *B.* The needle has been withdrawn after insertion of a hooked wire. The tip of the wire is at the calcifications (*arrow*).

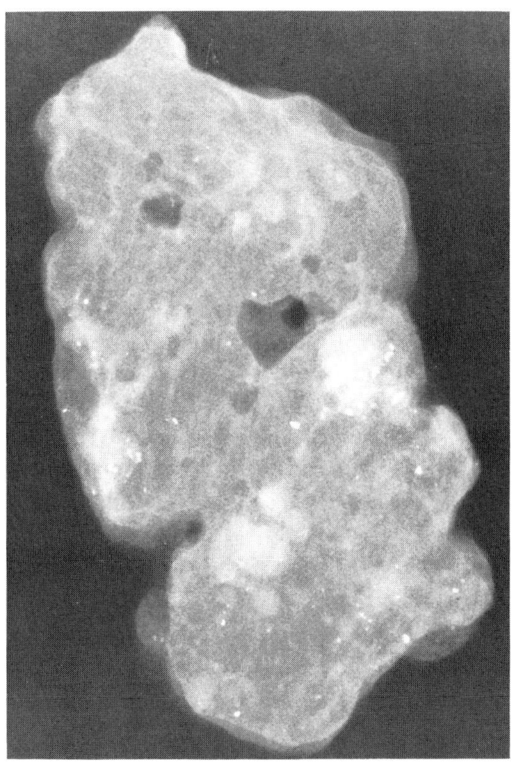

FIGURE 6–6. Specimen radiograph of excised tissue with multiple calcifications. This tissue contained carcinoma.

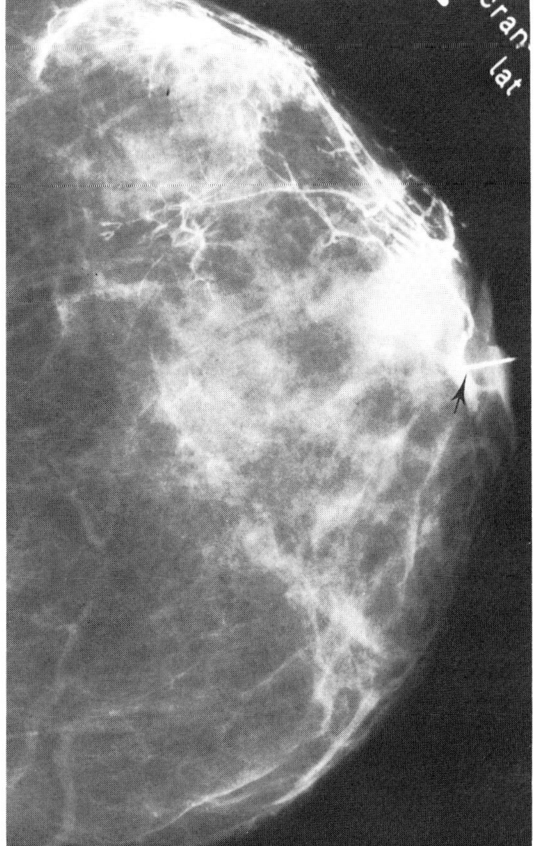

FIGURE 6–7. Galactogram: CC view of the left breast of a 45-year-old woman with a clear, watery discharge. A blunt needle enters a duct (*arrow*) that fills part of the lateral ductal system. No areas of obstruction or narrowing are identified.

by extrinsic masses or diffuse tumor. Care must be taken not to introduce air into the system because air bubbles may simulate intraluminal filling defects. Most intraluminal defects are intraductal papillomas.

TRAUMA

Breast trauma can have several appearances. Acute breast trauma, especially from surgery, frequently produces a mass attributable to hematoma. Blunt trauma and surgery cause necrosis, which can appear indistinguishable from malignancy. Fat necrosis may produce a spiculated mass and may cause microcalcifications. These microcalcifications are often linear and amorphous, appearing in the surgical bed (postoperatively) or the area of trauma and are occasionally bizarre in shape. A history of surgery or trauma, correlated with, for example, a surgical scar or ecchymosis, aids in determining the nature of the calcifications. Malignant calcifications tend to be small, variable in size (0.5 mm or smaller in diameter), and tightly clustered (five or more in a 1-cm^2 area) and may be granular or exhibit a needletip appearance and branching. Irregularity in size, density, and configuration is more suggestive of malignant calcifications than of benign calcifications. A common manifestation of trauma is oil cysts, which are small, low-density, circumscribed masses that represent a form of fat necrosis. They may develop rim calcification (Fig. 6–8).

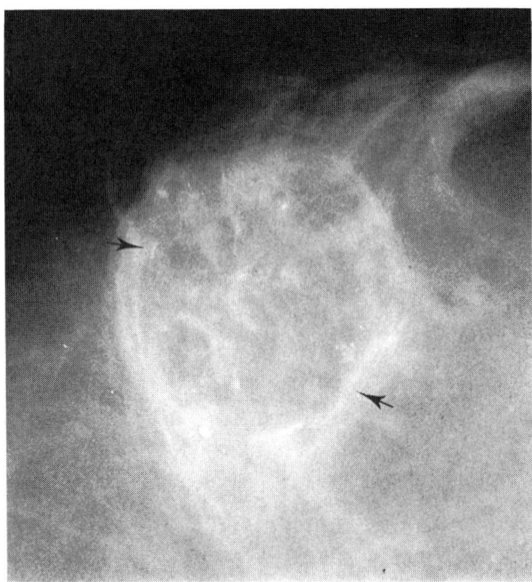

FIGURE 6–8. Fat necrosis (oil cyst). Magnification mammogram shows a focal mass in a woman who had recently undergone reduction mammoplasty. The low-density center of the mass is necrosed fat. Small calcifications are present at the margins (*arrows*).

Postoperative changes may be confusing, regardless of whether surgery was performed for benign or malignant disease. In general, these benign areas (masses, focal densities, focal architectural distortions) remain unchanged or decrease in size with time. However, the number and the size of calcifications caused by fat necrosis usually increase, and coalescence often occurs. Multifocal or incompletely excised lesions may develop shortly after surgery, whereas recurrent carcinoma usually takes several months or years to become visible. A unilateral mammogram is necessary six months after surgery for estabishing a new baseline. If there is doubt about the completeness of excision, serial, semiannual examinations beginning 6 months after surgery may be necessary.

CONGENITAL DISEASE

Few congenital diseases involve the breast. Breast sizes are often asymmetrical (the left breast is usually larger), and occasionally there is even absence of a breast. Mild parenchymal asymmetry is common. When the parenchyma are markedly asymmetrical (particularly focal), mammographic evaluation can be difficult. Most large areas of asymmetry caused by malignancy are palpable. Asymmetry of normal breast parenchyma generally does not result in a palpable mass, and its appearance usually changes depending on the view. Accessory nipples may occasionally be seen (along the "milk line") and may be associated with accessory breast tissue that is hormonally responsive.

SYSTEMIC DISEASE

The breasts are subject to hormonal influence, and any alteration of hormonal status or lactation may cause a temporal variation in breast tissue density. Such changes are generally bilateral because of the systemic nature of such a process. Exogenous hormones (such as those given to relieve symptoms of menopause) can cause breast tissue proliferation and may stimulate cyst production or possibly fibroadenomatous growth. Breast edema can develop from any cause of systemic edema, such as congestive heart failure. This edema can cause increased breast tissue density and an extended reticular pattern of breast parenchyma and skin thickening. Radiation therapy may cause skin thickening and diffuse breast tissue density.

Cellular tissue changes occur during the menstrual cycle. The mammographic significance of these changes, however, has not been established, although premenstrual tenderness in some patients may prevent adequate compression, which results in a suboptimal mammogram. During pregnancy and lactation, the ducts enlarge and the breast tissue becomes denser; therefore, mammography may be of somewhat limited usefulness during those times.

INFLAMMATION AND INFECTION

Infection involving the breast is a frequent occurrence and may include abscess. It can cause mammographic abnormalities that mimic cancer; however, the clinical circumstances usually enable correct interpretation (Fig. 6–9). Ultrasonography may assist in the identification and drainage of an abscess.

NEOPLASMS

The most important distinction in mammography is differentiation of benign or normal breast parenchyma from carcinoma. Although no findings in malignant and benign diseases are pathognomonic, general guidelines allow adequate specificity that enable decisions regarding biopsy to be made. General characteristics of benign masses in approximate order of importance are (1) smooth, well-marginated borders, (2) relatively low density, and (3) homogeneity (Table 6–2). Malignant lesions usually have irregular (especially spiculated) borders and are more dense than benign lesions or normal breast parenchyma. Malignant lesions often cause distortion of the surrounding breast architecture (called desmoplastic reaction) and may distort the adjacent skin line or parenchymal borders.

A true mass is one seen on more than one projection of a mammogram. Summation of normal fibroglandular breast tissue may appear mass-like, particularly on a single view. With additional projections (with slightly different angles), these pseudotumors or composite shadows can usually be differentiated from true masses. Pseudotumors generally have

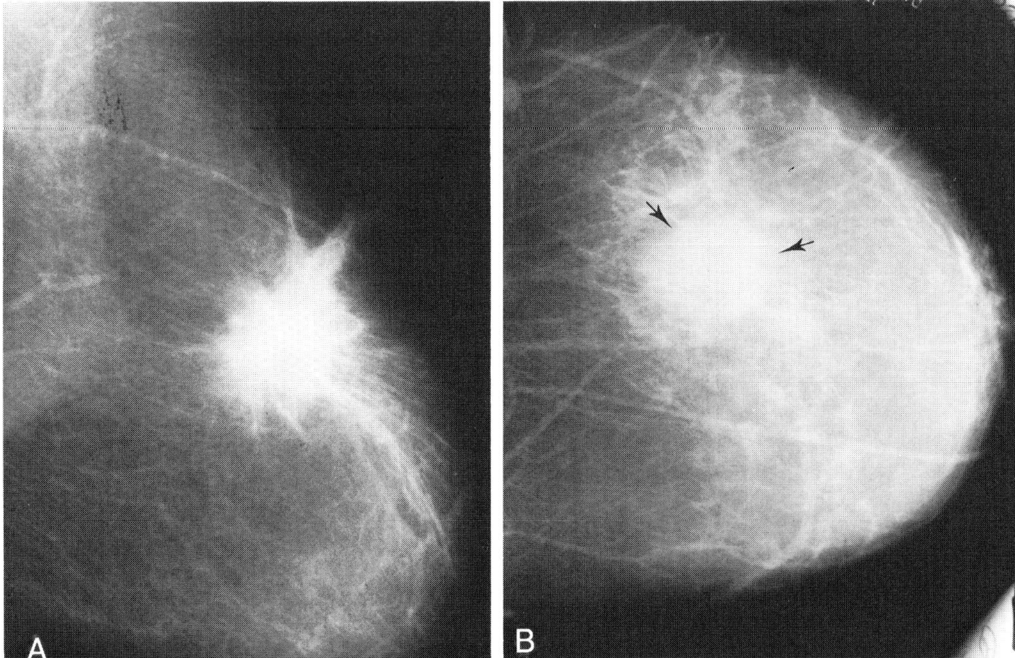

FIGURE 6–9. Inflammatory disease. *A*. Axillary mammogram shows a spiculated breast mass in a young woman who had focal redness and pain. This radiograph is indistinguishable from one of cancer. A biopsy of the mass was therefore performed, and infection was diagnosed. *B*. CC view shows a mass with irregular borders (*arrows*) in another woman with quadrant edema and tenderness. It also required biopsy, which revealed an abscess.

TABLE 6–2. CHARACTERISTICS OF BREAST MASSES

Malignant Characteristics
Radiographically dense for size
Spiculated margins
Enlargement over time
Local architectural distortion
Microlobulated
Benign Characteristics
Well-defined margins
Halo (low-density rim surrounds mass)
Low density for size
Umbilicated (lymph node)
Stable over time
Diminishes over time
Round or lobulated

scalloped, concave (inward) contours, are more amorphous in shape than are true tumors, and have fatty elements interspersed. In contrast, true masses tend to have convex (outward), spiculated, and multilobulated or microlobulated borders and do not show associated (interspersed) linear fat lines. In addition, pseudotumors lack other features suggestive of malignancy, such as spiculation, lobulation, and microcalcification. Alternately angled view and spot-compression views are extremely useful for differentiating pseudotumors from true masses.

Calcifications are commonly seen in the breast. The analysis of these calcifications is one of the most important aspects of mammographic interpretation (Table 6–3). Benign calcifications generally are round or large and linear with distinct borders, are of similar size, and are denser and larger than malignant calcifications. Benign calcifications also may be scattered through the breast whereas malignant calcifications are usually clustered or grouped. Malignant calcifications tend to be very small and irregular in shape, are infrequently round or oval, and tend to vary in size. They usually have a variety of shapes and sizes within a group. Typical malignant calcifications have an appearance of a broken needle or grains of salt, or they are branched, or both. Numerous small calicifications in the shape of ducts are also suggestive of malignancy.

Some groups of calcifications have indeterminate shapes fitting into neither clearly malignant nor clearly benign categories. In general, groups of calcifications are characterized by the appearance of the most malignant-looking calcifications, not by the average or the most benign looking ones. There is no lower limit for the number of calcifications that generates concern, although it has been suggested that fewer than three or five calcifications in a 1-cm^2 area have low malignant potential, unless they demonstrate clear malignant characteristics such as branching. Milk of calcium in microcysts has characteristic features. It is the result of layering calcifications that have different shapes on different views: round with slowly fading borders on CC views and linear or crescentic shape in axillary views.

Another sign of malignancy is focal architectural distortion of the breast tissue. This distortion may produce retraction of the nipple or the skin. It may also involve other overlying and adjacent parenchyma, distorting the margin of the otherwise smooth parenchyma of the breast. Skin thickening may be seen in some malignancies that infiltrate the lymphatic system and indicates advanced disease.

Nipple discharge is also an important diagnostic feature of breast disease. The most common cause of discharge is an intraductal papilloma, which is a benign tumor. Nipple discharge that is turbid or milky has a low association with malignancy. Bloody discharges (and sometimes clear discharges) are more highly correlated with malignancy in patients at risk. Pain is generally a sign of benign breast disease such as cysts or infection, although malignant disease may cause pain or other focal sensations such as a burning sensation or itching.

Benign Masses

Breast Cysts. Simple cysts of the breast are common and occur from time to time in many women. They are the most common breast

TABLE 6–3. MAMMOGRAPHIC APPEARANCE OF CALCIFICATIONS

Benign Characteristics
Distinct
Round
Scattered
Dense
Large
Malignant Characteristics
Irregular density, size, and shape
Clustered
Ductal casts
Branched (Y-, M-, N-, W-shapes)
Broken needle
Crushed stone
Sand-like

masses and probably arise from fluid accumulation behind an obstructed duct. Simple cysts may become large and palpable and may appear on physical examination as hard masses. They may come and go with menses. On ultrasonography, a simple cyst has enhanced through-transmission, no internal echoes, and smooth walls (see Fig. 6–4). Small, true cysts (less than 1 cm in diameter), complex cysts (bloody, septated), or deep small cysts may not be conclusively diagnosed by ultrasonography.

Fibrocystic Change. The development of fibrous and cystic changes in the breast, called fibrocystic changes—previously misnamed "fibrocystic disease"—is a common breast parenchymal response to hormonal stimulation. It varies greatly in degree and effect. Its manifestation on breast physical examination and on mammograms varies greatly as well. Density changes, nodularity, adenosis, fibroadenomas, papillary growths, and cystic responses are found in varying degrees.

Various theories of etiology and exacerbation, such as that of caffeine intake, have been postulated without demonstration of a conclusive cause-and-effect relationship. Fibrocystic changes also may vary greatly in clinical manifestations, and patients may be asymptomatic.

Fibroadenoma. The fibroadenoma is a benign tumor of the breast. It generally has smooth margins, may be slightly lobulated, and usually has a density similar to that of normal breast tissue. It is usually a well-marginated mass and may develop coarse, benign-appearing calcifications. Involuting shrinking fibroadenomas may develop irregular margins and may form small, malignant-appearing microcalcifications, particularly at their periphery. These calcifications often coalesce to form the dense characteristic popcorn calcifications. Fibroadenomas are a frequent false-positive indication for biopsy.

Other Benign Masses. Low- and mixed-density masses that are benign lesions include lipomas and hamartomas. Medium- and higher-density benign tumors include cystosarcoma phylloides (which may occasionally be malignant) and giant fibroadenomas (Fig. 6–10).

Malignant Masses

Adenocarcinoma. Adenocarcinoma is, for all practical purposes, the only primary malignancy of the breast. Metastatic disease to the breast rarely occurs, and equally rare are other types of malignant primary breast tumors. Most carcinomas arise from the ductal epithelium and are referred to as ductal carcinomas (Fig. 6–11). A subtype of the ductal carcinoma is the medullary carcinoma (Fig. 6–12). A small minority of tumors arise in the lobules and are referred to as lobular carcinoma (Fig. 6–13). Some carcinomas have features of both ductal and lobular tumors. The ductal carcinomas are believed to arise in the extralobular portion of the terminal ducts and spread within the ducts before becoming invasive. This initial spread is often associated with microcalcifications in the necrotic intraductal tumor debris. Such calcifications are often branched as well as small and irregular in shape (see Figs. 6–1, 6–2). Invasive tumors may lose these initial calcifications as they destroy the ducts and grow, or they may be accompanied by an increase in the number of malignant calcifications.

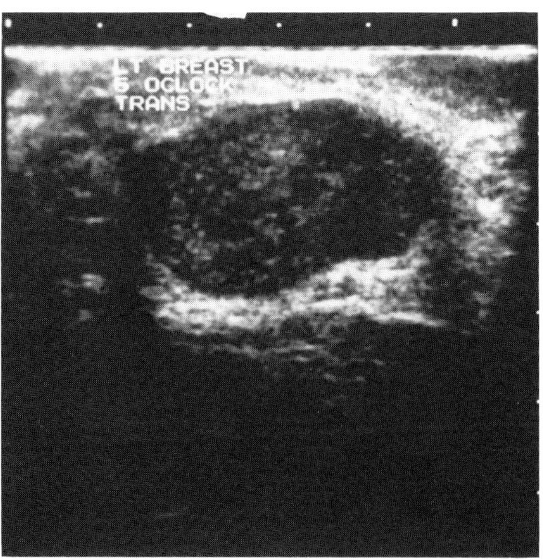

FIGURE 6–10. Fibroadenoma. Ultrasonogram of a mammographic mass in the breast of a 30-year-old woman shows a homogeneous mass with internal echoes and well-defined margins. The mass was palpable, but there were no associated abnormalities.

Ductal carcinoma in situ is commonly diagnosed in screening mammography and represents the earliest detectable tumor. It was seldom diagnosed before the advent of mammography. The diagnosis of in situ and early invasive ductal carcinoma has led to the improvement in morbidity and mortality rates for breast cancer patients. Lobular carcinoma in situ is occasionally diagnosed on biopsy of a larger, suspicious-looking abnormality. However, lobular carcinoma in situ is not a mammographic diagnosis. Invasive lobular carci-

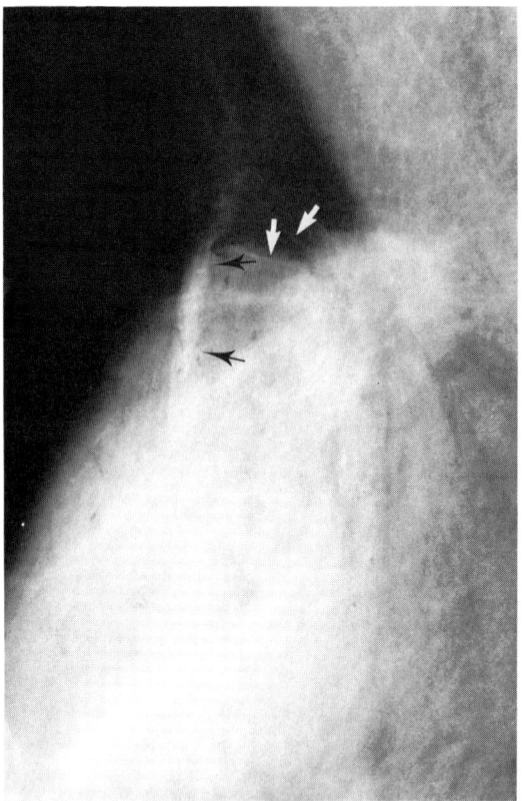

FIGURE 6–11. Invasive ductal cancer. Axillary mammogram shows spiculations on a mass (*white arrows*) and skin retraction and thickening (*black arrows*), findings of advanced carcinoma. This mass was palpable and painless.

noma may have the same mammographic appearance as invasive ductal carcinoma, but it is more difficult to diagnose mammographically and is a relatively common cause of mammographically missed breast cancer.

Metastatic Breast Cancer. Many breast carcinomas metastasize. The most common initial site of metastatic spread is the axillary lymph nodes. Lymph nodes seen on mammography are very common, and unless they are striking in size and asymmetry or density, they are not considered suspicious-looking. Other common sites of spread of breast cancer are the chest, particularly the lungs and the pleura; the bones; the liver; and the brain. Metastatic disease to the contralateral breast is occasionally noted, although a second primary tumor in either the same breast or the other breast is more common. Less metastatic disease is found at the time of diagnosis when breast cancer is diagnosed early (by mammography) than when diagnosed late. Malignant pleural effusion, metastatic disease to the bones, or brain metastases are occasional initial manifestations of breast cancer. Multicentric breast cancer or breast cancers with nearby satellite lesions are not uncommon.

Metastatic disease to the breast rarely occurs. The most common primary lesions to metastasize to the breast are malignant melanoma and lung cancer. The mammographic appearance of a metastatic breast mass is not

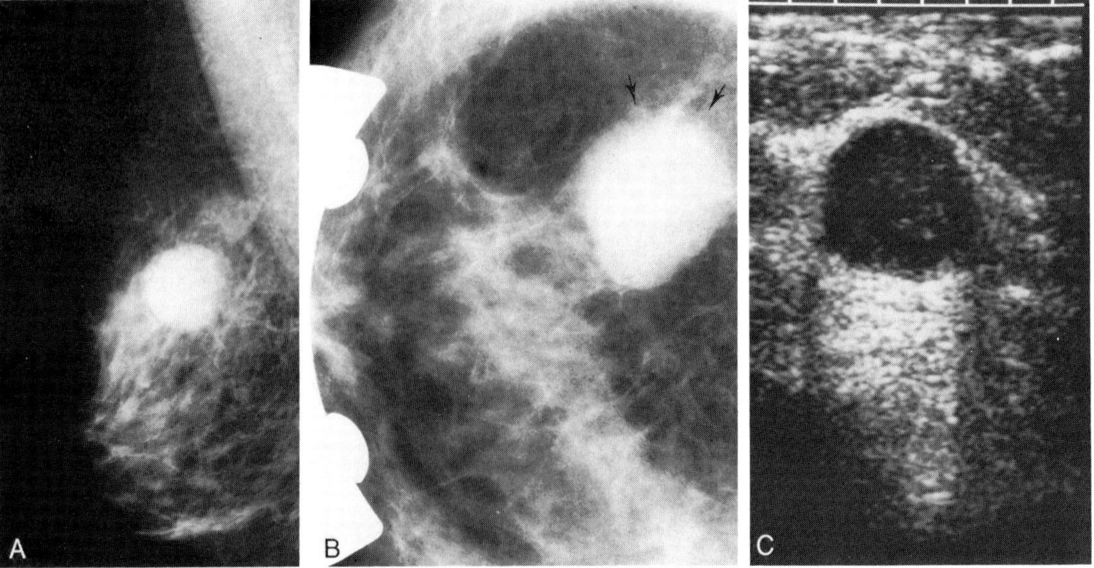

FIGURE 6–12. Medullary carcinoma. *A*. Routine mammogram of a breast with fatty replacement shows a large mass on the right. *B*. Magnification/compression view of mass shows an irregular deep margin (*arrows*) and lobulation of the mass. *C*. Ultrasonogram shows the mass to be hypoechoic with enhancement and through-transmission; however, definite internal echoes are present.

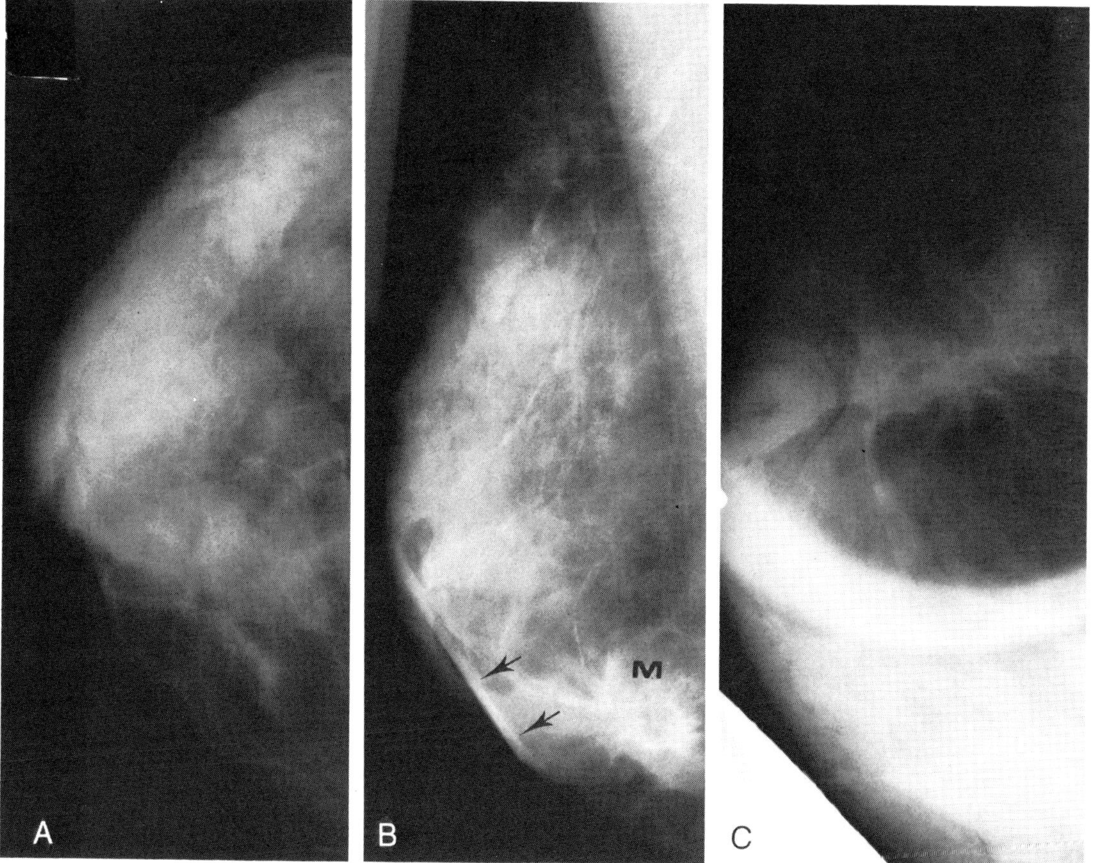

FIGURE 6–13. Invasive lobular cancer. *A*. CC view shows a possible medial mass. *B*. Axillary view shows skin retraction. *C*. On lateral compression view, the mass is less rigid than a ductal cancer, but it demonstrates spiculated margins, which indicate malignancy.

distinguishable from primary breast cancer, although metastatic lesions generally are multiple, bilateral, and small.

VASCULAR DISEASE

Calcification of the arteries in the breast is very common and is rarely a source of confusion. These calcifications often have a railroad-track appearance and are of no clinical significance (see Fig. 6–3). Confusion may arise when arterial calcifications are viewed end on, sometimes creating the impression of clustered microcalcifications. Additional views with varying angles are usually sufficient to clear up the confusion.

RADIOGRAPHIC DIFFERENTIAL DIAGNOSIS

A single radiographic finding or pattern can frequently suggest a limited list of diagnoses. Additional findings and clinical history can then assist in further limiting the list or in making a firm diagnosis. The following approaches to evaluation of radiographic findings can provide assistance in differential diagnosis. Diseases are listed in order of importance.

LOW-DENSITY BREAST LESIONS*

Low-density lesions are almost always benign.

Lipoma
Fat necrosis (some have calcified rim)
Galactocele
Hamartoma (fibrolipoma)

*Same density as fat.

MEDIUM-DENSITY BREAST LESIONS

Medium-density lesions have a variety of causes. The appearances of the margins are often helpful in diagnosis. The density is similar to that of breast parenchyma.

Well-Marginated

Lymph nodes (mostly upper outer quadrant, frequently have some fatty area within, and often umbilicated; sharp margins)
Fibroadenoma (may calcify, sometimes densely; usually sharp margins)
Cysts (sharp margins; occasionally are septated and therefore appear as lobulated masses)

Irregular Margins

Cancer (usually high density)
Radial scar
Degenerating fibroadenoma
Hematoma
Inflammation
Surgery or trauma

HIGH-DENSITY BREAST LESIONS

A mass with a density greater than similar-sized areas of breast parenchyma is always considered suspicious for cancer.

Cancer
Abscess
Hematoma
Cystosarcoma phylloides
Radial scar

CHARACTERISTICS OF CALCIFICATIONS

The appearance of calcification often allows a diagnosis. The most important distinction to be made is between benign and malignant disease.

Lesions With Characteristic Patterns

Type of Calcification	*Cause*
Single, large, dense, popcorn	Fibroadenoma
Railroad-tracking	Vascular calcification
Dense, linear	Benign ductal-secretory calcification
Small, round, dense, scattered	Plasma cell mastitis
Changing calcifications	Milk of calcium
Lobular calcifications	Fibrocystic change
Ring-shaped calcifications	Fat necrosis
Group, irregular microcalcifications	Malignancy
Irregular or branching calcifications	Malignancy
Irregular, crushed-stone shapes	Malignancy

BENIGN CAUSES OF MALIGNANT-APPEARING CALCIFICATIONS

Several benign diseases cause small, irregular calcifications that appear malignant. Additional findings can assist in ruling out malignancy, but any suspicious-looking lesion should be examined in biopsy.

Skin lesions (moles or warts)
Breast atypia
Involuting fibroadenoma
Fat necrosis
Fibrocystic change

Suggested Readings

Kopans D: Breast Imaging. Philadelphia: JB Lippincott, 1990.
Tabar L, Dean PB: Teaching Atlas of Mammography, 2nd ed. New York: Thieme Medical Publishers, 1985.

7

Musculoskeletal Radiology

Gary K. Stimac

BASIC EVALUATION

Plain Film Interpretation

Plain radiographs of the bones provide excellent spatial resolution and density discrimination. They provide both the convenient rapid evaluation necessary for diagnosis of traumatic fractures and the fine detail required for the diagnosis of subtle changes of arthritis, infection, and tumor. Because plain films are obtained as the first radiographic evaluation in traumatized patients, general guidelines are helpful for making such assessments for each part of the body. These guidelines are summarized in the Appendix 7–1.

Plain films of the skull can show fractures of the cranium, the facial bones, and the jaw; metabolic abnormality; metastatic tumor; congenital anomaly; and sinus disease. Such examinations are most often used for evaluating acute head injury, but computed tomography (CT) and magnetic resonance imaging (MRI) are preferred when intracranial injury is suspected. Even acutely, most facial fractures are better demonstrated by CT, which also shows associated injury to soft tissues and to the brain.

Evaluation of skull films requires attention to the continuous lines of the normal structures and identification of opacification of sinuses, air in the orbits, and abnormal density of the bones. Interpretation requires experience in viewing the complex and overlapping lines. The most important findings on skull films are (1) fracture as evidenced by displacement, discontinuity, or overlap of bone margins; (2) sinus opacification; (3) orbital emphysema; and (4) bone defect from metabolic, neoplastic, or infectious disease (Fig. 7–1).

Plain films of the spine are also used predominantly for evaluation of acute trauma because they can show most fractures and can be obtained quickly without moving the patient. Suspected or confirmed fractures can be further evaluated with CT. Evaluation of metastatic tumors and degenerative diseases can be made with plain films, but CT, myelography, and MRI better show the bone and soft tissue abnormalities.

Plain film evaluation is particularly important in the evaluation of the cervical spine. Interpretation requires searching for fractures, alignment abnormalities, soft-tissue injuries or masses, degenerative osteophytes, and congenital or cortical defects. Trauma evaluation re-

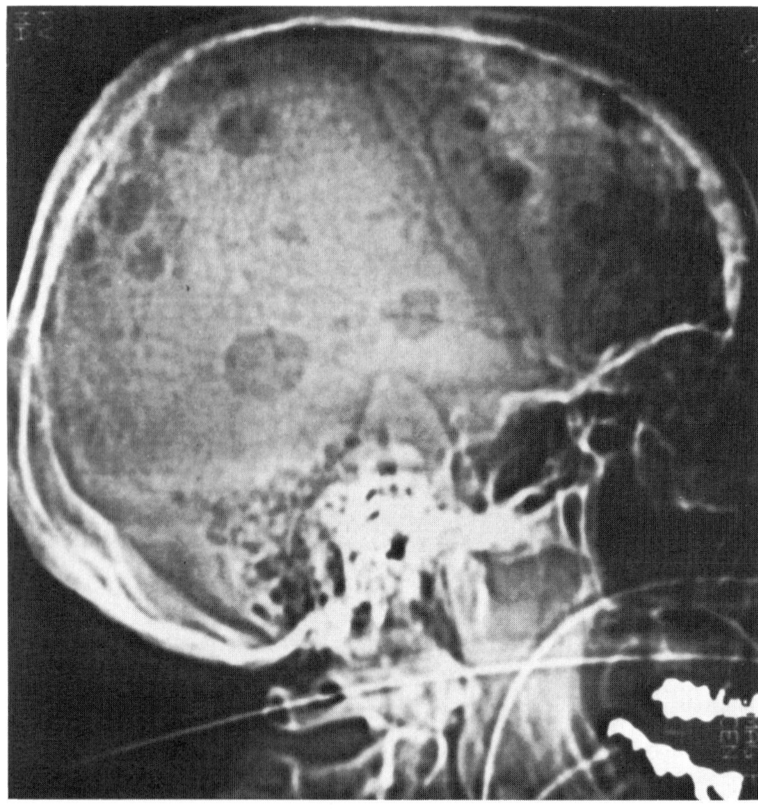

FIGURE 7–1. Skull metastases. Lateral computed tomographic (CT) scout film is, in effect, a digitized lateral plain film of the skull. It shows multiple well-circumscribed (punched-out) lesions throughout the skull in a 60-year-old man with unexplained obtundation. The lesions, typical of myeloma, which was subsequently diagnosed, were obvious on bone windows but not shown on standard brain windows.

quires identification of fractures in the vertebral bodies, spinous processes, and facets. The most useful view in cervical evaluation is the lateral view. Fractures at the upper levels not shown on the lateral view may be visible on the odontoid view. Abnormal alignment is determined from alteration of the anterior and posterior margins of the vertebral bodies, the back of the spinal canal, and the positions of the spinous processes (Fig. 7–2). When subtle or nondisplaced fractures are suspected, stress views (i.e., flexion and extension) and plain film polytomography may be helpful. Oblique views show the neural foramina and are often the first examinations obtained for evaluating osteophytic disease. Any suspected fracture or unexplained neurological deficit should be further evaluated with high-resolution CT scanning.

Plain film evaluation of the bones in the chest, the abdomen, and the pelvis is discussed in Chapter 2 (Chest Radiology) and Chapter 3 (Gastrointestinal Radiology).

Evaluation of the bones of the extremities requires two or three views. Optimal projections of each bone or joint ensure that subtle fractures and dislocations are not missed. When radiographs of the extremities are taken, it is important to limit the view to the bone in question and to indicate the precise location of pain or deformity (see Appendix 7–1). Important findings are soft-tissue swelling, fracture, altered bone density, cortical and periosteal erosion, and joint space abnormality (Fig. 7–3). Careful inspection of each portion of the film under a bright light (an intense light used to transilluminate dark areas of a film) ensures that each part of the bone is viewed and can reveal subtle abnormalities. In addition to standard views, oblique views, stress views, or magnified radiographs can be obtained as indicated.

The evaluation of extremity films requires a systematic review of (1) the soft tissues, in order to identify swelling or the presence of a foreign body; (2) the cortical margins, in order to see fracture; (3) the trabecular pattern, in order to identify tumor or metabolic disease; and (4) the joint space, in order to assess alignment abnormality or arthritis. An understanding of the normal appearance (and the normal variation) is essential and can be gained from texts on normal anatomy and anatomical variants or from comparison with the patient's

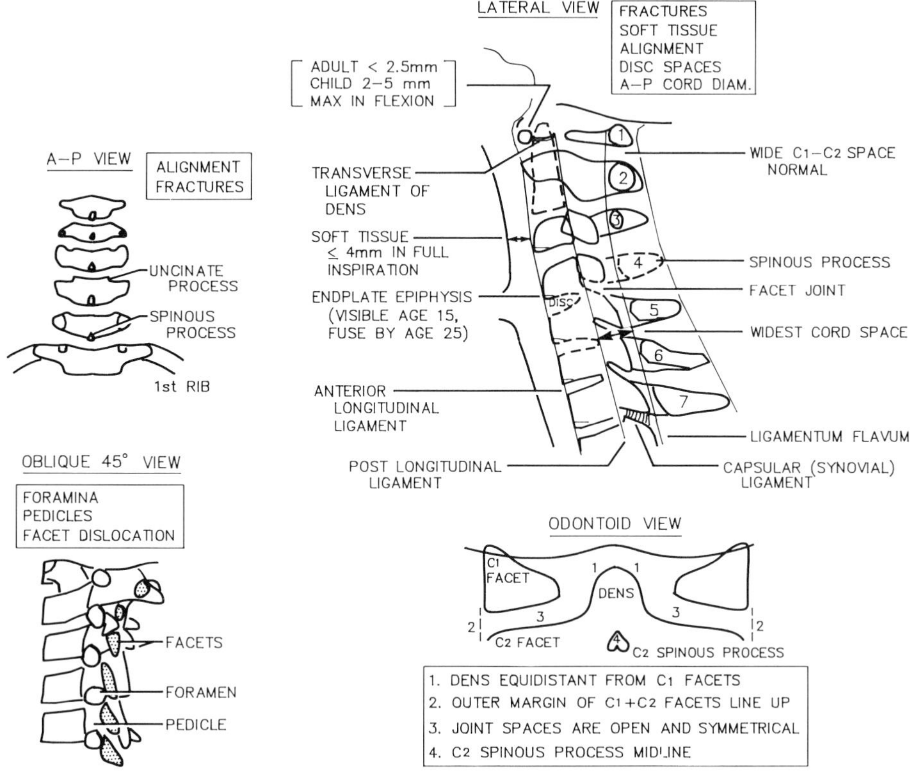

FIGURE 7–2. Cervical spine evaluation.

normal side and normal films of other patients. A skeleton should always be available to assist in interpretation.

Arthrography

Arthrography, the evaluation of the joint spaces with the use of injected contrast material, can be employed for all the large joints and many of the small joints of the body. Radiopaque material and air (often both) can be injected and followed by plain film or CT evaluation. This technique has the advantages of providing contrast enhancement and allowing sampling of the joint-space fluid. However, these tests are invasive and show only the inside of the joint space. The ability of MRI

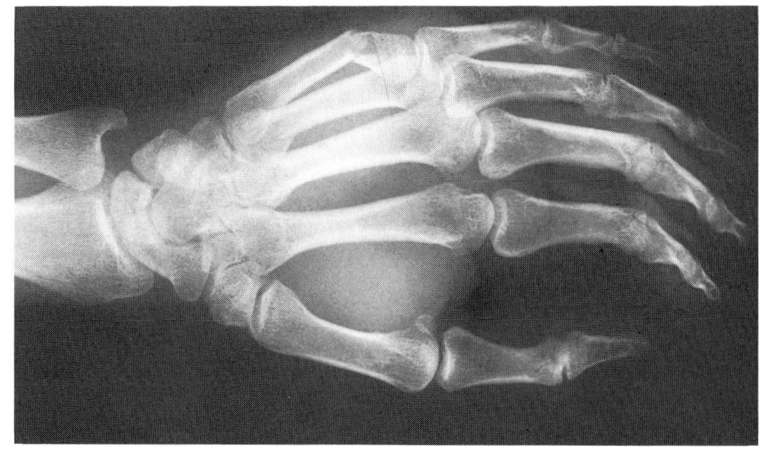

FIGURE 7–3. Evaluation of extremity films. Oblique view of the hand shows a fracture of the distal fifth metacarpal and associated soft-tissue swelling in a young man after a fist fight. The fracture (called a boxer's fracture) does not extend into the joint. Note the regular soft-tissue margin around the remaining bones and the uniform joint space margins.

to fully image the bone marrow, the soft tissues, the articular cartilage, the meniscus, and the joint space has resulted in replacement of arthrography of the knee, the shoulder, the hip, and the temporomandibular joint for most applications. Plain film arthrography is also often replaced by MRI in the imaging of smaller joints.

Arthrography is still used for diagnosing complex injuries and in the identification of loose bodies within the joint and of articular cartilage injury. Assessment requires knowledge of the normal joint anatomical structure and attention to interruptions of the margins, filling defects, and imbibition of contrast by abnormal cartilage. In the shoulder and the wrist, extravasation of contrast into separate joint cavities enables diagnosis of joint disruption (Fig. 7–4).

Computed Tomography

CT is useful for evaluation of fractures and contiguous spread of bone abnormalities into the soft tissues or into the medullary cavity. It can be helpful in the assessment of the intramedullary location of bone lesions, but plain films and MRI are generally more effective. CT is also used to evaluate bone density

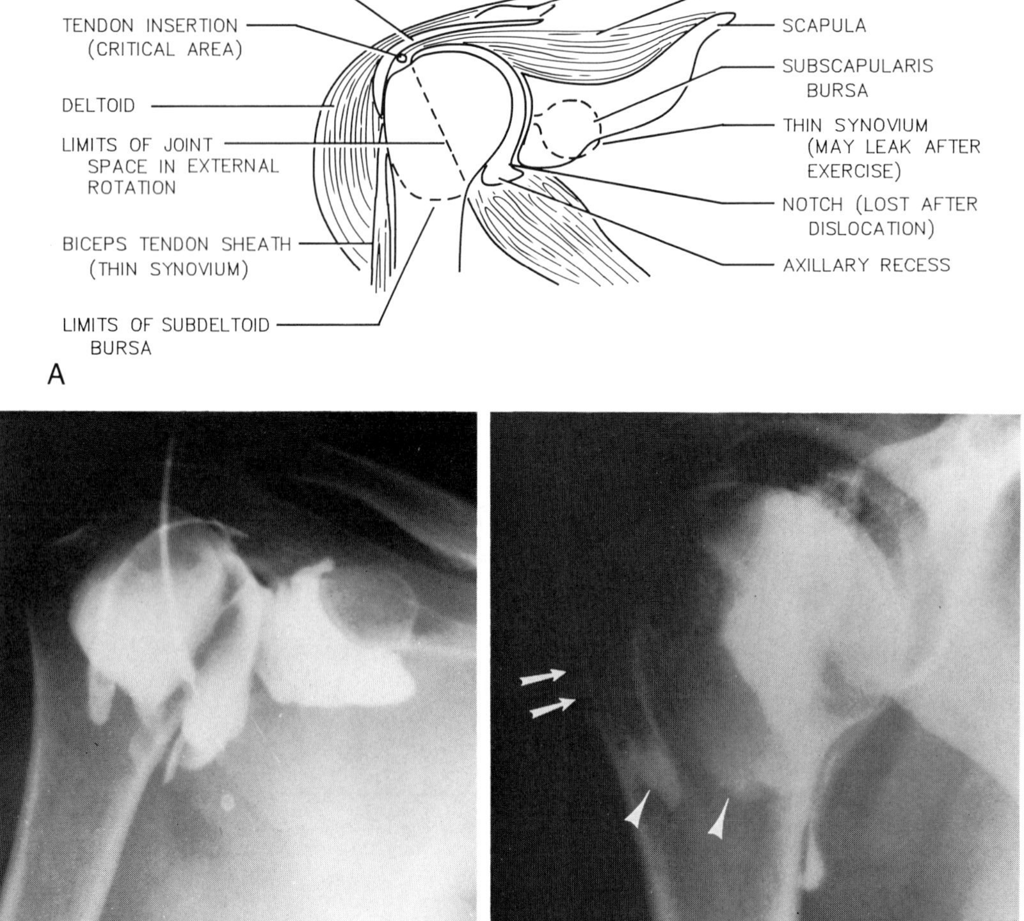

FIGURE 7–4. Shoulder arthrography. *A.* Diagram of normal shoulder joint. *B.* Internal rotation shoulder arthrogram shows a normal joint space. Note the limits of the joint space laterally and inferiorly. *C.* Rotator cuff tear. Internal rotation view of a shoulder arthrogram shows contrast within the joint and separately in the subacromial-subdeltoid bursa *(arrows)*. The contrast inferolaterally *(arrowheads)* is not in the joint space but in the bursa.

changes associated with aging and medical therapy.

CT of the skull is especially advantageous in evaluation of the face, the orbits, the temporal bone, and the skullbase. In the cranial skull, plain films are more effective in showing fractures, metabolic abnormalities, and metastatic tumors, but CT better shows the associated intracranial abnormality. In the face, the orbits, the temporal bone, and the skullbase, CT best demonstrates fractures, tumors, infections, sinus disease, and orbital disease and can provide views in the axial and coronal planes. The use of thin slices (1 to 2 mm) and bone algorithms allows unambiguous identification of abnormalities.

Transnasal endoscopic sinus surgery requires direct coronal, high-resolution imaging to show the architecture of the sinuses, specifically the ostiomeatal complex (the structures surrounding the ostium of the maxillary sinus). Sinus or nasal disease near this complex can obstruct the maxillary, anterior ethmoid, or frontal sinuses. Such high-resolution CT images enable the surgeon to remove only a small segment of bone, polyp, or mucus and relieve the obstruction, obviating the need for radical surgery (Fig. 7–5).

Interpretation of sinus CT images requires attention to bone margins for fracture or erosion, opacification within the sinuses or the nasal cavity, pterygopalatine masses, and extension of possible abnormalities to the alveolar ridge, the orbits, or the pituitary fossa. Far lateral extension of the sphenoid sinuses, a septated (hidden) antrum of the maxillary sinuses, and the intrasphenoid position of the carotid arteries are important findings both for diagnosis of occult sinus disease and for surgical planning.

In the temporal bone, high-resolution CT provides detail of the middle ear, the mastoid air cells, and the petrous apex. Axial and coronal thin-slice (1 to 2 mm) bone technique is capable of showing infections and tumors and allows precise delineation of middle ear structures. Associated soft tissue abnormalities such as tumor extension, cerebellopontine angle mass, or contiguous neck abnormality can be shown in soft tissue CT views or MRI.

Interpretation of CT images of the temporal bone is complex because of the small but numerous structures of the middle ear. It is important to have an understanding of the temporal bone in the axial plane (best for showing acoustic neuroma) and in the coronal plane (best for showing cholesteatoma) (Fig. 7–6). Basic anatomical guidelines for the temporal bone are as follows: (1) the cochlea and the carotid artery are anterior structures; (2) the jugular vein and the vestibular apparatus are posterior; (3) the facial (seventh) nerve is above the cochlear (eighth) nerve, and both are anterior (7-Up, Coke down); (4) the vestibular nerve (superior and inferior divisions) is posterior (and enters the posteriorly located vestibule); and (5) the scutum (the sharp upper bone for attachment of the tympanic membrane) is best seen on coronal views and is destroyed early by cholesteatoma.

CT of the alveolar ridge and the mandible can be used to evaluate facial trauma. It is also used for evaluation of jaw implants and to identify landmarks for the placement of metallic prostheses.

In the cervical spine, CT is used primarily to evaluate fracture. When guided by clinical examination and plain films, high-resolution CT can fully characterize fractures and sublux-

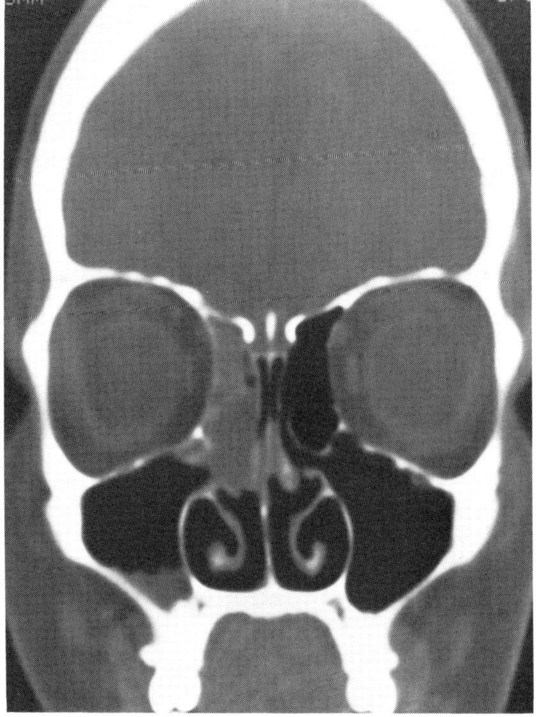

FIGURE 7–5. CT evaluation of the face. Ostiomeatal complex disease. Coronal CT scan at wide window setting shows right frontal sinus opacification in a woman with recurrent sinus obstruction. The focus of abnormality in such patients is the region of the maxillary ostium, where bone deformity, the nasal turbinate, and ethmoid sinus cavities obstruct drainage from the anterior ethmoid, frontal, and maxillary sinuses. Transnasal endoscopic surgery allows removal of bone or soft tissue at the site of obstruction.

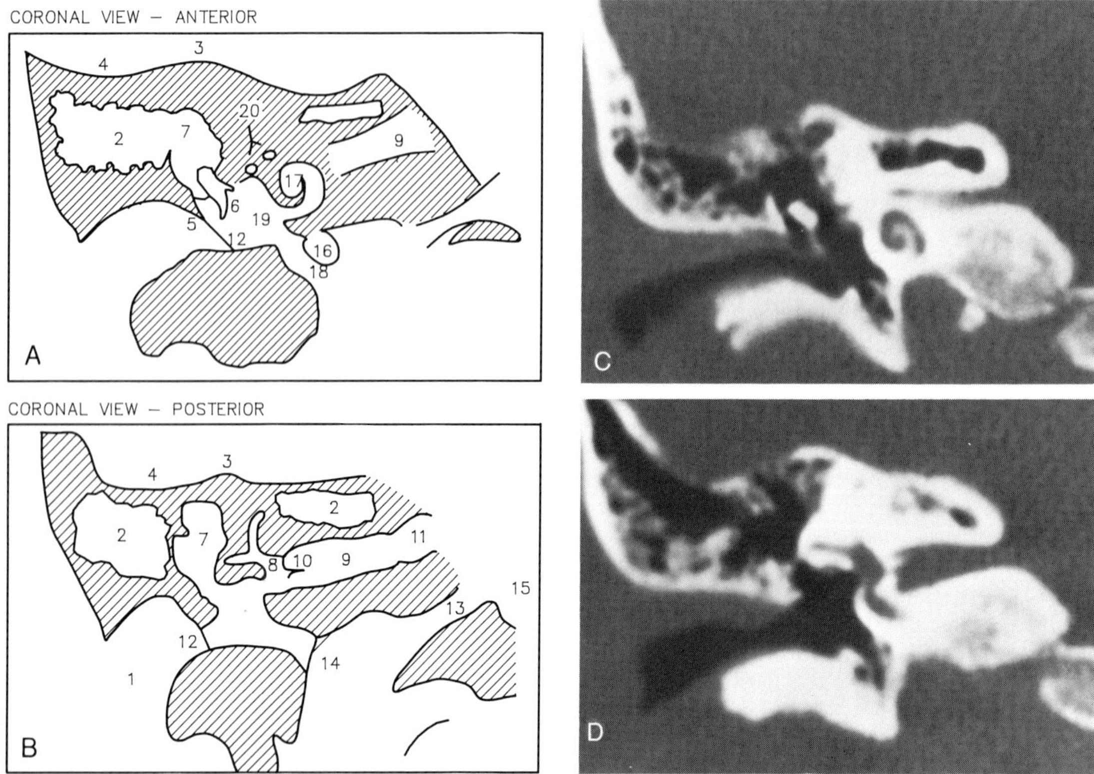

FIGURE 7–6. Temporal bone anatomical structure. Coronal anterior *(A)* and coronal posterior *(B)* diagrams and matching CT scans *(C, D)*.

ation. Degenerative osteophytes are also well shown on CT, but imaging of compression of the spinal cord or the nerve roots by these osteophytes requires myelography or MRI. Tumors, disc diseases, and infections can be shown on CT with the use of thin-slice and contrast enhancement, but these abnormalities are better demonstrated and more fully characterized, and the consequences to the spinal cord are better shown, on MRI or with such complementary studies as conventional myelography and CT myelography.

CT evaluation of cervical spine injury is best performed with the use of thin (1.5 to 2.0 mm) slices and bone algorithms in the axial plane in the area of interest (usually about three vertebral spaces). This method, when guided by plain films, shows two to three times as many fractures as do plain films alone. Sagittal and coronal reformations are especially helpful at the skullbase when subluxation or a burst fracture is suspected. They also assist in the diagnosis of alignment abnormalities. Interpretation requires detection of fractures, assessment of alignment, and identification of the facets and their proper location (Fig. 7–7). Numbering of each bone element on each slice prevents misinterpretation of a posterior element or facet. Degenerative osteophytes, especially those within the canal and the neural foramina, can be precisely located.

CT of the thoracic spine is also primarily used in the evaluation of trauma. Thicker slices (3 to 5 mm) are usually required for adequate coverage of an area of interest. Interpretation requires the same attention to detail and alignment as in the cervical spine.

In the lumbosacral spine, CT is important in the assessment of trauma, infection, disc disease, and for postoperative evaluation. In trauma, after the initial plain film evaluation, CT best identifies and characterizes fractures and abnormalities of alignment. Degenerative disease, including disc herniation and the formation of osteophytes, is well demonstrated by CT because the different densities of bones, discs, the thecal sac, and epidural fat clearly delineate margins. The effects of the osteophytes and disc herniation on the cauda equina and the nerve roots can often be inferred from

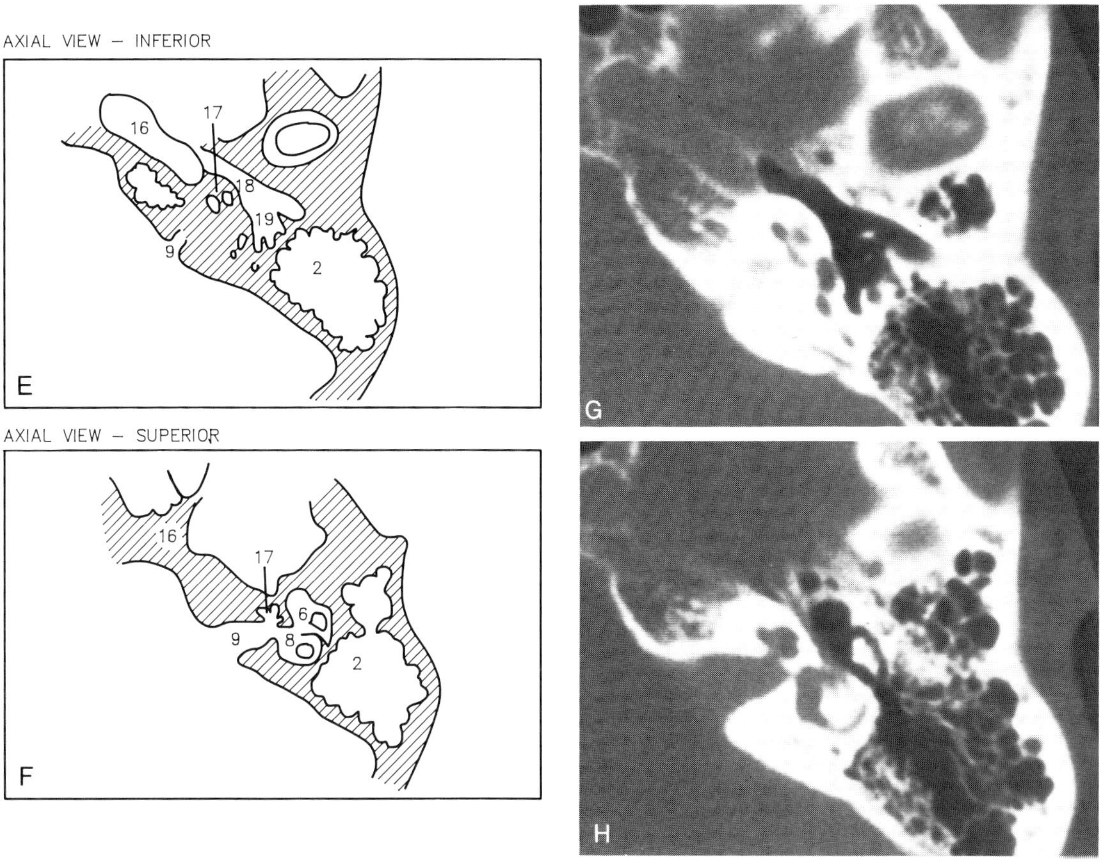

AXIAL VIEW – INFERIOR

16 17 18 19 9 2

E

AXIAL VIEW – SUPERIOR

16 17 6 9 8 2

F

G

H

FIGURE 7–6 *Continued* Axial inferior *(E)* and axial superior *(F)* diagrams and matching CT scans *(G, H)*. 1, external auditory canal; 2, mastoid air cells; 3, arcuate eminence; 4, tegmen tympani; 5, scutum; 6, ossicles; 7, epitympanic cavity; 8, labyrinth and semicircular canals; 9, internal auditory canal; 10, crista falciformis; 11, origin of internal auditory canal; 12, tympanic membrane; 13, canal for superior petrosal sinus; 14, jugular bulb; 15, jugular tubercle; 16, carotid canal; 17, cochlea; 18, eustachian tube; 19, middle ear cavity; 20, facial nerve.

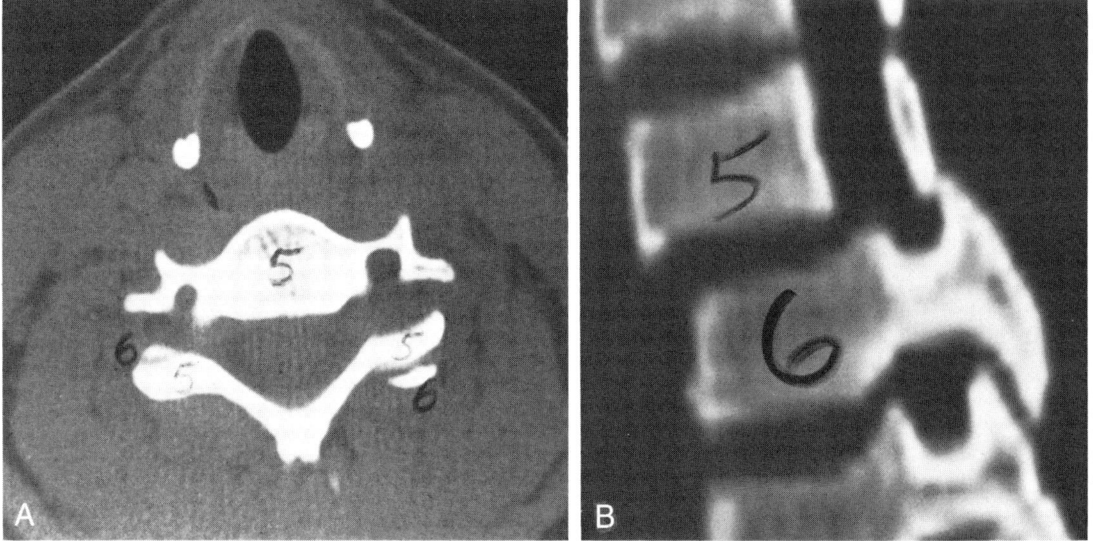

FIGURE 7–7. Facet dislocation. *A.* Axial thin-slice CT shows the left C-6 facet behind the C-5 facet in an 18-year-old motor vehicle accident victim. Numbering of the bones, as shown here, ensures that the subluxation is correctly identified. *B.* Oblique sagittal reformation clearly shows the subluxation.

the location and the size of the abnormalities. Noncontrast CT provides much of the same information as does MRI with the advantage of showing bone detail and osteophytes. Depending on cost and availability, CT may be the first examination in the evaluation of degenerative lumbosacral spine disease.

Evaluation of CT of the lumbosacral spine includes evaluation of bone fracture or alignment abnormality, disc bulging and degeneration, ligamentous prominence, osteophyte formation, and patency and adequacy of the spinal canal and the neural foramina. Cortical fractures are easily identified as sharp, linear interruptions in the dense cortex. Fractures through the trabecular bone (which is of lower density) are more difficult to see. Branching areas of low density without cortical break are vascular channels within the vertebral body. The finding of fracture fragments within the canal or neural foramina indicates the need for intrathecal contrast studies.

The noncontrast CT assessment of degenerative disease is based on the relative compromise of the canal and neural foramina by a disc, osteophytes, ligaments, and a congenitally narrow canal. Usually, it is a combination of these that results in compression of the thecal sac or the nerve roots (Fig. 7–8).

CT of the pelvic bones is commonly employed in the evaluation of trauma because sacral and associated pelvic ring fractures can be more fully demonstrated by CT than by plain films. Such detail is especially important in the assessment of fractures of the sacrum (which can affect sacral nerves) and fractures

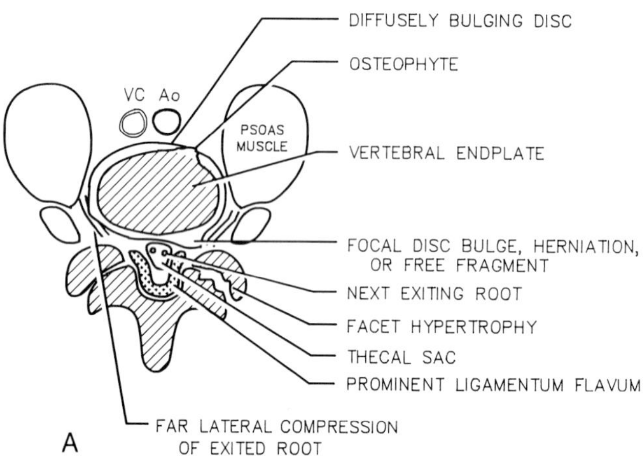

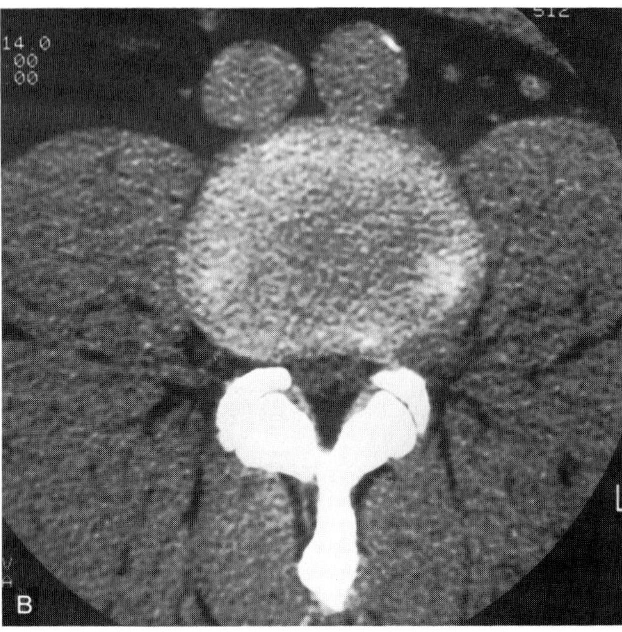

FIGURE 7–8. Disc disease. *A.* Diagram. VC, vena cava; Ao, aorta. *B.* Axial CT scan shows diffuse bulging of the disc in the midline and bilaterally, which effaces the anterior epidural fat, in a 47-year-old man. A small canal further exacerbates the problem. The sciatica on the left was caused by the far lateral compression of the exited L-3 nerve root by the far lateral extent of the bulging disc.

of the acetabulum (which affect the hip joint). For both tumor invasion and traumatic injury, CT can show involvement of pelvic organs and soft tissues in addition to bone abnormalities. These soft tissue abnormalities are usually of great importance in demonstrating a nonspinal cause of symptoms.

Pelvic CT for bone evaluation is performed with the use of axial slices (5- to 10-mm thickness) and bone algorithms. Areas of evaluation include the sacrum, the acetabulum, and the pubic rami. The sacral foramina are difficult to assess because of the curvature of the sacrum. Fractures or tumors involving a neural foramen can be viewed with the use of a curved coronal reformation made from axial images (Fig. 7–9). Fractures and dislocations in the hip joint are best seen on axial CT images. The pubic symphysis and the sacroiliac joints should be carefully evaluated for diastasis. When a fracture or joint diastasis is identified, it should be assumed that a second interruption of the sacral ring is present.

CT of the extremities can be used for specific cases in which medullary involvement, soft-tissue extension, and the location of intra-articular contrast are of interest. In general, however, plain films provide the best views of the cortical margins and the joint surfaces. MRI depicts much higher tissue contrast than does CT and is best for identifying and characterizing lesions within the bones and in the adjacent soft tissues.

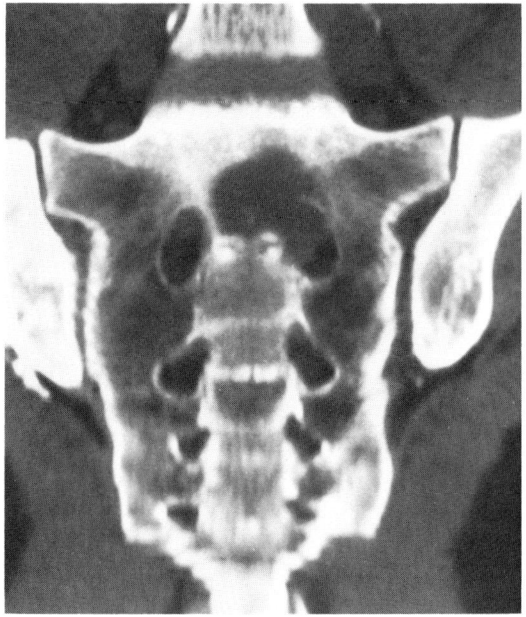

FIGURE 7–9. Sacral tumor. Curved coronal CT reformation shows the curved sacrum as if it were straight, allowing demonstration of all neural foramina in a 50-year-old man with lymphoma. The central marrow at S-1 has been replaced by tumor, which also partially fills the left S-1 foramen.

Magnetic Resonance Imaging

MRI provides both the high tissue contrast and the high spatial resolution necessary for musculoskeletal imaging. MRI can be successfully applied to imaging of soft-tissue masses, bone tumors, joint disease, and bone marrow disorders. For most of these diseases, MRI has completely replaced other diagnostic tests or has become the primary examination. Bone cortex has a weak signal on MRI, and thus it appears black on all types of imaging sequences and is highly contrasted with the marrow cavity, which is composed of fat and blood cells. Normal marrow shows high intensity on T1 spin echo sequences and, when replaced by tumor, infection, or an infiltrative process, shows an absence of the normal fat signal (see Fig. 1–21).

Both T1 spin echo and gradient echo techniques can provide high spatial resolution images that demonstrate anatomical detail in the musculoskeletal system. When coupled with high-contrast images such as short TI inversion recovery (STIR) or T2 spin echo, the examination provides the highest possible sensitivity and excellent characterization of the site and extent of the abnormality. Alterations in the signal in the bone marrow that are caused by trauma, tumor, or metabolic disease are especially well demonstrated by a combination of T1 spin echo and STIR imaging.

Soft-tissue and bone masses are also well shown by T1 spin echo MRI because of the high tissue contrast between marrow fat (high intensity) and cortical bone (low intensity). High-field strength scanners provide the best spatial resolution. Image contrast, especially in the bone marrow, is better on low- and mid-field–strength scans.

In the skull, MRI is effective for evaluating the skullbase (including the temporal bone), usually as a second evaluation after CT. Tumors, infections, and cysts are clearly shown in the skullbase, and information regarding location and extension can be obtained. The MRI signal intensities on different sequences assist in characterization of the lesion (Fig. 7–10).

In the spine, MRI has replaced CT and myelography as the primary method of evalu-

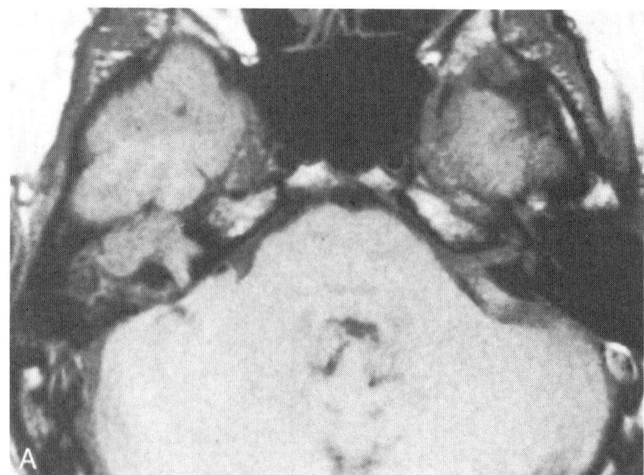

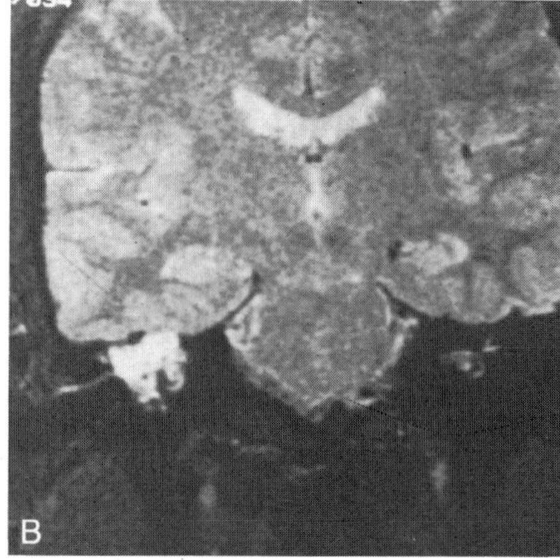

FIGURE 7–10. Cholesteatoma. *A.* Axial T1 spin echo image at the level of the internal auditory canals shows a mass in the right temporal bone. *B.* Coronal T2 spin echo image shows the mass filling the middle ear cavity and extending upward to include the mastoid antrum. Note the comma-shaped cochlea medial and inferior to the mass. The signal intensity characteristics are not sufficient for distinguishing this tumor from infection or for determining the type of tumor.

ation of tumor and degenerative disease. Axial and sagittal T1 spin echo images demonstrate the anatomical appearance with sufficient tissue contrast to show individual structures. A high-contrast sagittal sequence shows the bone marrow and the discs to best advantage. The major limitations of MRI in degenerative spine disease evaluation are the inabilities to show osteophytes (which are best shown on CT) and to fully evaluate the nerve roots (which are best shown on conventional myelography and CT myelography). Artifacts caused by cerebrospinal fluid flow, respiration, and vascular pulsation can sometimes degrade the images, thus limiting their diagnostic value.

Evaluation of degenerative spine disease is similar to that for noncontrast CT (discussed earlier). The sagittal views are first evaluated in order to determine the marrow appearance, alignment, disc integrity, compression of the thecal sac in the midline, and compression of the fat in the neural foramina. Because the central portion of the disc has a higher water content than do the more peripheral portions, disc degeneration as evidenced by loss of this hydration is easily identified on T2 spin echo or STIR images. In the sagittal plane, such images also show compression of the thecal sac as an indentation on the high-intensity cerebrospinal fluid. The T1 spin echo sagittal and axial views clearly show the fat within the marrow and in the neural foramina. When this fat is replaced, a lower intensity is apparent. In addition, the axial views show high spatial detail of the ligaments, the thecal sac, the exiting nerve roots, the cauda equina, and the posterior margin of the disc.

Images of high spatial resolution, best obtained with high- or midfield scanners, are capable of showing the nerve roots and the thecal sac clearly enough to obviate the need for myelography or CT in most cases (Fig. 7–11). In some cases, however, myelography is needed in order to fully identify compression of a nerve root in passage from the thecal sac through the neural foramina, and CT is necessary to clearly define osteophytes. MRI is also the best method of evaluating the postoperative spine by making use of paramagnetic contrast enhancement of scar tissue. In general, recurrent herniated disc material does not enhance, and postoperative scar tissue does enhance. Because there are many exceptions to this generality, the morphological features of the abnormality are the most important elements of diagnosis of recurrent disc disease.

MRI shows excellent detail of the large joints, especially the knee, the hip, and the shoulder and has replaced arthrography as the initial diagnostic procedure in the evaluation of degenerative joint disease. Smaller joints such as the temporomandibular joint, the wrist, and the ankle are also preferentially studied with MRI. The long bones and the soft tissues can be evaluated for tumor, infection, and other mass lesions. The ability to image in any desired plane and the high tissue contrast between fat and muscle allow clear delineation of most soft-tissue and bone masses.

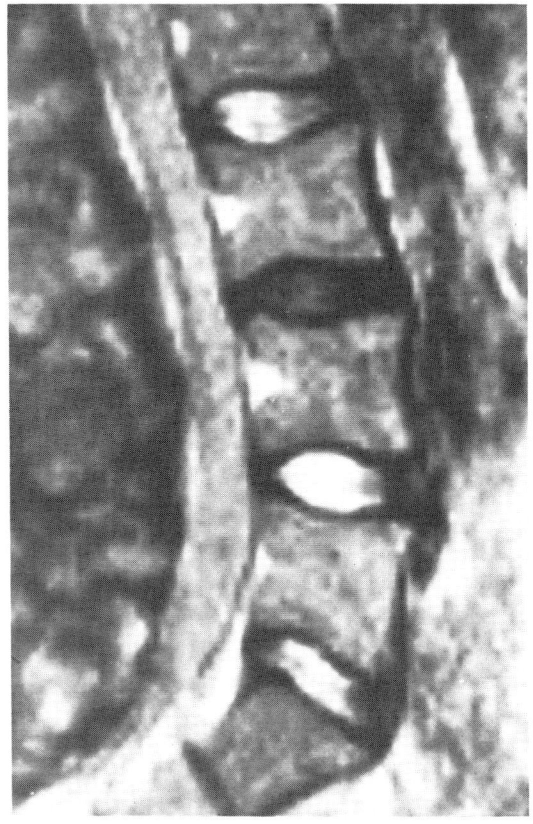

FIGURE 7–11. Degenerative disc disease. Sagittal T2 spin echo image shows high intensity in the central portions of the normal discs. The L3-L4 disc shows central low intensity, no loss of height, and minimal posterior bulging, which indicate partial degeneration in a young man with low back pain. The cerebrospinal fluid is of high intensity, enabling identification of minimal indentation of the thecal sac by the bulging disc.

MRI allows clear characterization of the position of a soft-tissue mass with respect to the bone, and the MRI signal characteristics assist in determining the composition of the mass, especially when fat, blood, or fluid are present.

Evaluation of magnetic resonance images of the joints requires assessment of the many structures, which are more clearly demonstrated on this than on any other imaging examination (Fig. 7–12). As a result, knowledge of the basic anatomical structure of the joint, including the bone and the ligamentous structures, is required. A thorough review includes evaluation of bone alignment and marrow content, the appearance of the articular cartilage (which appears gray on T1 spin echo sequences), the meniscus if present (black), the joint-space fluid (gray), and the presence of fat (white), muscle (gray), and fluid (gray). Degenerative joint disease is best shown on high-resolution T1 spin echo or gradient echo images, and injuries of ligamentous structures appear as interruptions in the contour and intensity pattern. Blood, edema, and tumor are best shown by high-contrast sequences such as STIR and T2 spin echo. Lesions in the soft tissues require both a high-resolution anatomical scan and a high-contrast scan. Evaluation requires attention to the signal intensity of the abnormality, the interruption of fascial planes, and possible extension to the joint space.

Nuclear Medicine

The nuclear medicine bone scan is capable of demonstrating metabolic, infectious, neoplastic, and infiltrative disease. Because it has a high sensitivity for the detection of many bone diseases, especially metastatic tumor, it is widely used for screening and follow-up of patients with known cancer or bone pain. The bone scan allows a survey of the entire body and is therefore much more efficient than any other imaging test in the evaluation of the skeleton. Because results of bone scans can be negative in some destructive tumors, such as myeloma, additional tests are often indicated when there is high clinical suspicion of bone tumor. The high sensitivity of MRI to marrow abnormalities often enables their detection earlier than do nuclear medicine bone scans. Therefore, specific bone symptoms should be further evaluated by MRI with a high-contrast

EVALUATION:

SOFT TISSUES
MARROW
ARTICULAR CARTILAGE
MENISCUS
CRUCIATE LIGAMENTS

JOINT SPACE
COLLATERAL LIGAMENTS
SOFT TISSUES
PATELLA

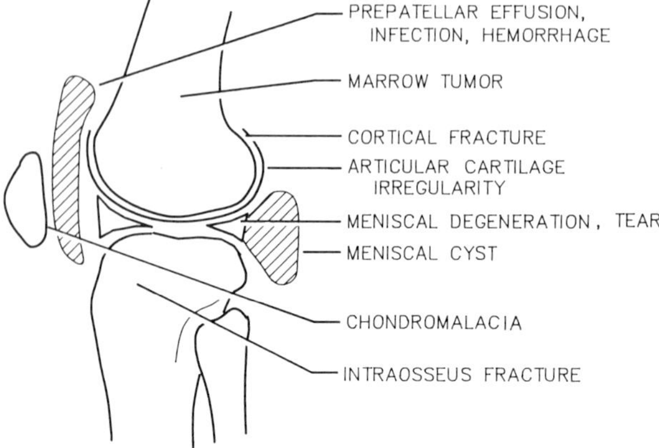

BEST VIEWS

- ARTICULAR CARTILAGE (T1 SAGITTAL)
- MENISCUS (T1 SAGITTAL AND CORONAL)
- CRUCIATE LIGAMENTS (SAGITTAL MIDLINE T1)
- COLLATERAL LIGAMENTS (CORONAL T2/STIR)
- SOFT TISSUE SWELLING, EDEMA, HEMORRHAGE (CORONAL T2/STIR)

A

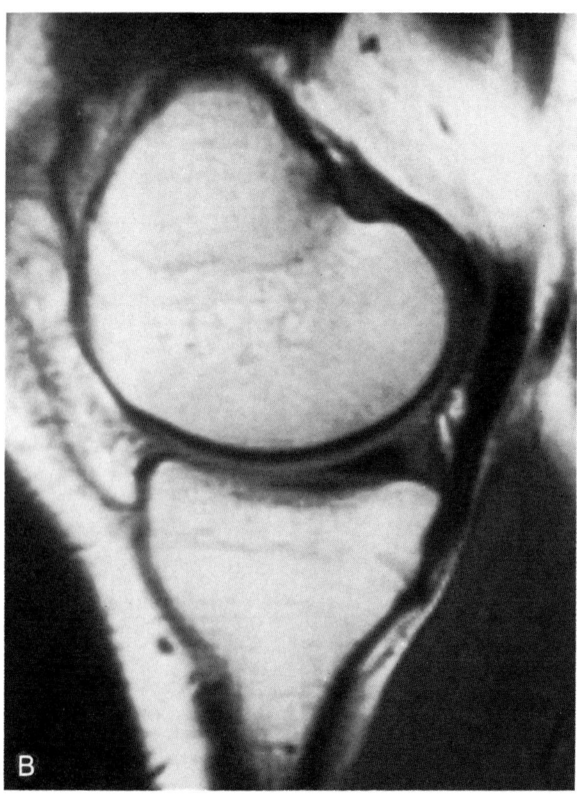

FIGURE 7–12. Magnetic resonance imaging (MRI) evaluation of the knee. *A.* Diagram shows the numerous structures that must be identified on MRI and indicates the locations of various abnormalities. The best views for evaluation of ligamentous and cartilaginous structures are indicated at the bottom. *B.* Sagittal T1 spin echo image of the normal knee. The meniscus is black and bordered by the articular cartilage and (minimal) joint fluid, which are gray. The cortical bone margin is black in contrast to the high-intensity fat and marrow.

technique such as STIR or T2 spin echo sequences when the bone scan is negative. Nuclear medicine bone scintigraphy is discussed in detail in Chapter 9.

TRAUMATIC DISEASES

Traumatic musculoskeletal injuries include fracture, ligamentous injury, and cartilaginous joint space destruction. These injuries can be caused by direct trauma or acute stress or can be the result of chronic degenerative destruction. Because degenerative joint space disease and degenerative bone disease have many characteristics that are similar to those of acute injury, they are discussed together in this section. Arthritis is discussed in a separate section.

Fractures are interruptions of the bone, usually caused by direct trauma. They occur in all parts of the skeleton and may be simple or complex, may occur in multiple bones, and can involve any portion of the bone. Intraosseus fractures—that is, internal crush fractures—are difficult to see on plain radiographs but are well demonstrated by MRI. Many fractures have a characteristic location and appearance and are referred to by the mechanism of injury (e.g., boxer's fracture of the hand; see Fig. 7–3) or by an eponym (e.g., Monteggia's fracture dislocation of the forearm; see Fig. 7–38). Dislocations result when bone fracture or ligamentous injury and subsequent muscle stress cause abnormal alignment.

Skull

Cranial Skull Fractures. Skull fractures of all types commonly result from motor vehicle accidents and blunt trauma to the head. Fractures of the cranium overlying the brain are indicative of severe head trauma. When a skull fracture is present, some degree of brain injury, often microscopic, is likely. Skull fractures are shown with highest resolution on plain films. However, CT best shows the important associated findings of depressed fragment, intracranial hemorrhage, and contusion (Fig. 7–13). Additional examples of skull fractures are shown in Chapter 8, in which head trauma is discussed. MRI, when obtainable, most reliably shows the intracranial injury, including small axonal injuries.

Facial, Orbital, and Sinus Fractures. The face is commonly injured in motor vehicle accidents and high-impact trauma. The many bone surfaces and the complexity of facial fractures limit the usefulness of plain films, although they are usually obtained first. Facial structures are best imaged by CT with thin-slice bone algorithms and in either axial or coronal planes. Various fracture types have been defined according to the pattern, but most fractures are complex and are best described on an individual basis, particularly those caused by high-speed motor vehicle accidents. The Le Fort classification, based on drop-impact of dry skulls, is a simplified description of symmetrical facial fractures through the alveolar ridge (Le Fort I), the maxilla (Le Fort II), and the orbital rims (Le Fort III). The zygomatic complex fracture (formerly called the tripod fracture) is a three-part fracture involving the zygomatic arch, the inferior orbital rim, and the zygomaticofrontal suture (Fig. 7–14).

The orbital blow-out fracture is a compression burst of the floor of the orbit. Tethering of orbital ligaments within the fractured orbital

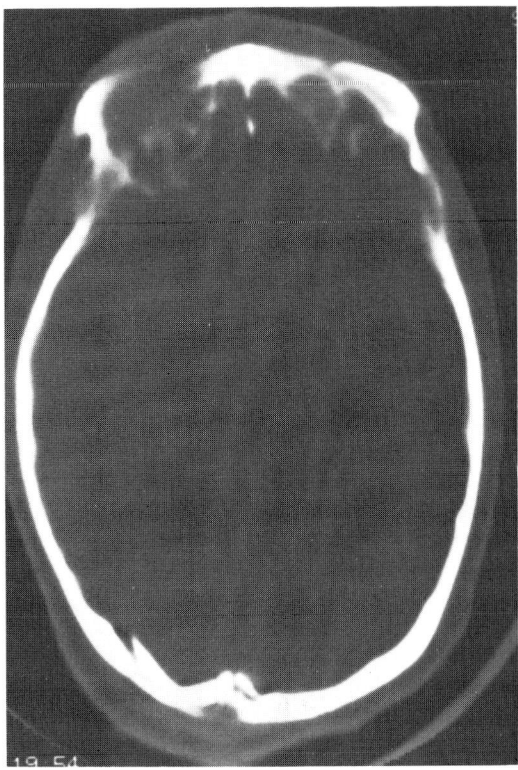

FIGURE 7–13. Depressed skull fracture. CT with bone windows shows a depressed skull fracture in a young woman who was hit in the back of the head with the butt of a gun. Brain windows showed contusion and compression of the sagittal sinus.

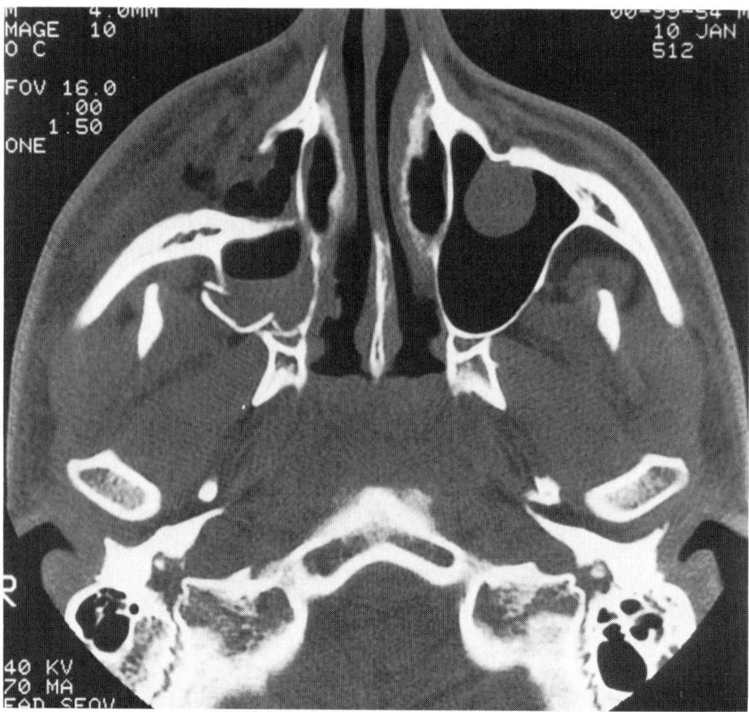

FIGURE 7–14. Zygomatic complex fracture. Axial CT shows a comminuted fracture of the right maxillary sinus. The zygomatic bone is markedly angulated into the sinus cavity. Blood is present posteriorly. This injury was sustained while the patient was working on an automatic garage door. Note a mucous retention cyst in the left maxillary sinus.

floor can constrain the extraocular muscles, resulting in diplopia. Sometimes, the inferior rectus muscle is displaced through and tethered by the fracture.

Fractures of the orbits and sinuses are usually best seen on coronal CT images because of the slope of the orbital floor and the complex orbital roof. CT also clearly demonstrates blood in the orbit or the sinus and extension to the nasal cavity. Intracranial extension of frontal, ethmoid, or sphenoid sinus injury and associated pneumocephalus, adjacent contusion, or developing intracranial infection can also be shown.

Temporal Bone Fracture. Temporal bone fractures, also best seen on CT, can cause disruption of hearing, temporomandibular joint dysfunction, and communication with the cranial cavity, from which brain infection can result. Thin (1.5- or 2.0-mm) slices in the axial and coronal planes may be necessary for showing these fractures (Fig. 7–15; see Fig. 7–6 for normal anatomical structure). Important findings in the temporal bone are ossicle dislocation and the presence of blood in the middle ear, the external auditory canal, and the mastoid air cells. Important associated findings are cranial skull fracture, cranial nerve injury, facial fracture, and intracranial extension.

Jaw Fracture. Jaw fractures occur in all parts of the mandible, the most common sites being the condyle (35%), the angle (20%), and the body (20%). Patients have pain over the area of fracture and have a variety of other signs such as malocclusion, loose teeth, drooling,

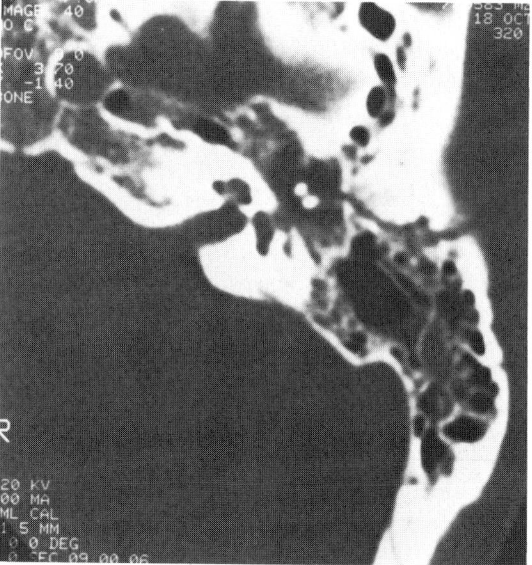

FIGURE 7–15. Temporal bone fracture. Axial thin-slice CT image, magnified to show the left temporal bone, shows a linear fracture extending from the outer skull to the middle ear cavity. Note mastoid and middle ear opacification with blood. The patient, an automobile accident victim, had no function of the left seventh and eighth cranial nerves. The fracture extended near, but not into, the carotid canal.

and, if the mandibular nerve is injured, sensory nerve deficit. Fractures of the jaw are evaluated in the emergency setting with plain films. Angled lateral views show each side of the jaw separately. A Panorex tomographic x-ray, most commonly used by dentists and oral surgeons, shows the entire jaw in profile. CT shows greater detail by means of thin slices and three-dimensional reformations. Important findings in addition to bone fracture include injury to the temporomandibular joint, intracranial extension of the fracture, and injury to the mandibular nerve as it passes through the mandibular canal. Treatment is aimed at stabilization for healing with an acceptable occlusion. Successful stabilization depends on the direction of the fracture lines and the location of the fracture with respect to the muscle attachments.

Cervical Spine

Cervical spine fractures are among the most serious of traumatic injuries because they can result in cord compression or transection. Because of the risk of paraplegia caused by a missed cervical spine fracture, suspected trauma to this region must be carefully evaluated. The clinical consequences and the methods for diagnosing cervical spine fractures depend on the location and the type of fracture. The fractures that are most serious and the most difficult to diagnose are between C-1 and C-3.

Atlanto-Occipital Fractures and Dislocations. Fractures of the occiput are commonly the result of high-speed motor vehicle accidents in which the head is distracted from the spine. Because plain films do not clearly show this area, CT is needed. Small, nondisplaced fractures are often of no consequence. Atlanto-occipital dissociation usually results in fatal brainstem injury. Children show an apparently wide atlantoaxial space on lateral cervical spine plain films as a result of a lesser degree of development of the mastoid bone. Off-midline, sagittal CT reformations can show the normal atlanto-occipital junction in such patients.

C-1 Fractures. Fractures of C-1 (the atlas) can be avulsions or burst fractures. Avulsion fractures usually occur at the attachments of the alar ligament and result when the head is hyperflexed so that the dens pulls the alar ligament posteriorly. These fractures are not serious if the other ligaments are intact. If there is ligamentous instability, the injury is very serious.

Fracture of the complete ring of C-1, called Jefferson's fracture, is a burst injury caused by axial loading, such as that that occurs when a patient sustains a head-first fall. The classic Jefferson's fracture has four interruptions of the bony ring and is easily seen on the open-mouth odontoid view, which shows the lateral displacement of the lateral masses of C-1. Many Jefferson's fractures involve fewer than four interruptions of the ring and do not cause such displacement. This and the frequent difficulty of obtaining a good-quality plain film view make CT the best method for identifying Jefferson's fractures (Fig. 7–16). Coronal reformatted CT images can better demonstrate the findings of the open-mouth view. Jefferson's fractures are unstable and can result in catastrophic cord injury. Many patients become quadriplegic at the time of injury.

C-2 Fractures. Fractures of C-2 (the axis) can involve the odontoid process (dens) or the ring. Both are unstable fractures and can be difficult to diagnose from plain films. Dens fractures are classified in three types by location. Type I (5% of such fractures) is in the upper tip, type II (65%) is in the midportion, and type III (30%) is within the vertebral body. The fractures are best shown on coronal or sagittal CT (Fig. 7–17). Children have a

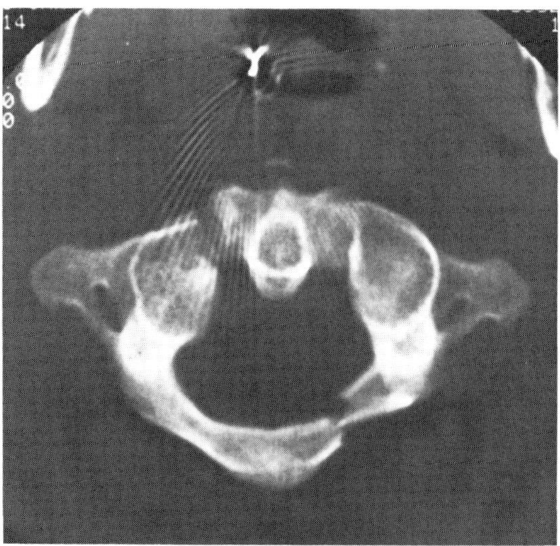

FIGURE 7–16. Jefferson fracture. Axial CT image at the C-1 level shows fractures through the right anterior and left posterior portions of the C-1 ring. The patient, a logger, was hit on the head by a falling tree and driven into the marsh up to his knees, an extreme degree of axial loading. There were only two fractures of the ring, and the odontoid view did not show obvious displacement of the lateral masses.

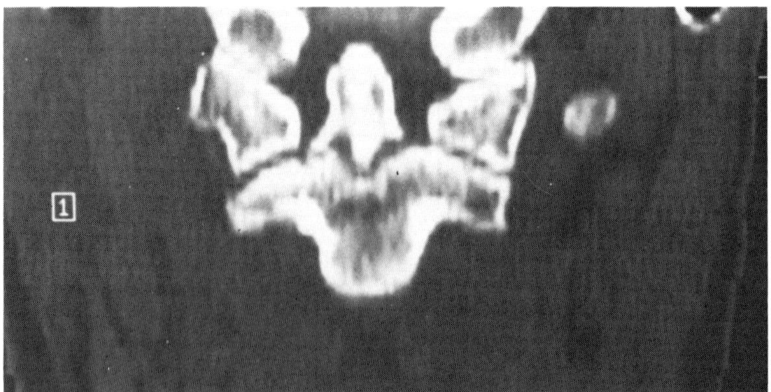

FIGURE 7–17. Dens (odontoid) fracture. Coronal CT reconstruction shows discontinuity of the lower dens and the body of C-2 (type III fracture) in a 16-year-old automobile accident victim. The fracture was less evident on axial views because it was in the plane of section; it was undetectable on routine plain films because of the overlap of structures.

synchondrosis in the middle portion of the dens; fractures of this synchondrosis may not be detected unless the fragments are distracted by traction, flexion, or extension.

Fracture of the ring of C-2, commonly called the hangman's fracture, is a hyperextension fracture of the pars interarticularis or, less commonly, the pedicles. This fracture occurs in judicial hangings from hyperextension of the neck, but it also occurs in motor vehicle accidents (as when the face hits the dashboard). These fractures are best shown on axial CT, which demonstrates the interruption of the bony ring (Fig. 7–18).

Lower Cervical Fractures. Fractures of the C-3 to C-7 vertebrae can have a variety of appearances. These are usually well-shown on the lateral plain film, but axial CT more clearly shows the location of the fracture fragments and compromise of the spinal canal. Sagittal reformations greatly assist in the diagnosis of subluxation and facet dislocation.

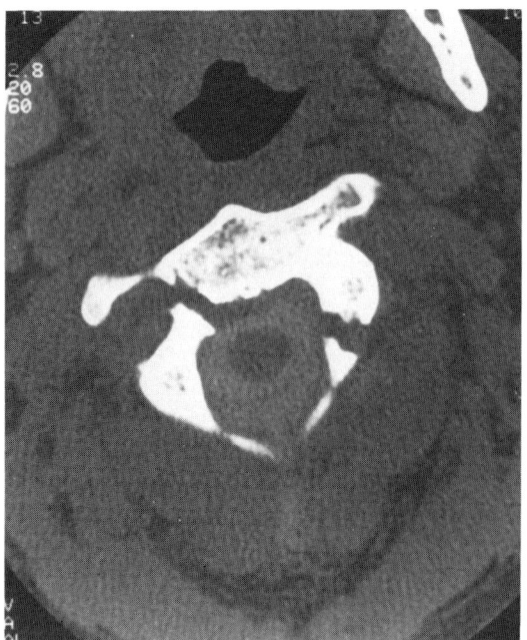

FIGURE 7–18. Hangman's fracture. Axial CT after myelography shows bilateral fractures of the pedicles of C-2. This thin-slice (1.5-mm) examination of 34 slices required only 6 minutes.

The compression-burst fracture (teardrop fracture), the most severe of vertebral fractures, is the result of a hyperflexion-burst injury. The three important components are a teardrop-shaped anterior vertebral body fragment, a sagittal vertebral body fracture, and a retropulsed fragment in the spinal canal. The retropulsed fragment is responsible for the severe spinal cord injury that often results from this fracture.

Other cervical fractures include compression fracture of the vertebral body and fractures of the spinous process and transverse processes. These are, in general, stable fractures. An avulsion fracture of the spinous process is called a clay-shoveler's fracture. Fracture or ligamentous injury near the facets, when associated with rotation or translation, can cause facet dislocation. Facet dislocation can be diagnosed on lateral plain films by focal malalignment of facets and foreshortening of the anteroposterior (AP) diameter of the vertebral body. CT can more fully characterize the fractures and alignment (see Fig. 7–7). Sagittal reformations are especially helpful for demonstrating the abnormal position of the facets. The diagnosis can be difficult on the axial CT slices and is greatly facilitated by careful numbering of each fragment on each slice.

Other injuries and dislocations, including ligamentous disruptions, may not be visible because of return to neutral position at the time of imaging. Patients with a congenitally narrow spinal canal or coexisting degenerative disease may sustain cord or nerve root injury associated with minor trauma or transient subluxation. Children may suffer cord or nerve root injury without ligament rupture or fracture because their ligaments allow hyperextension or hyperflexion.

Penetrating trauma to the cervical spine from bullets, knives, and other implements can result in fracture and direct injury to the cord, the nerve roots, and the soft tissues of the neck. The fractures and foreign bodies are well-shown on CT. The soft-tissue injuries of such trauma may require additional evaluation.

Thoracic Spine

Traumatic injury to the thoracic spine can also cause cord injury. Blunt and penetrating trauma causes a variety of fracture types, especially in high-speed motor vehicle accidents. The most serious injuries are compression-burst fractures and wedge-compression fractures. Facet dislocations and ligamentous injuries are less common in the thoracic spine because of the support of the spinal muscles and the rib cage.

Compression-Burst Fracture. Hyperflexion injuries result in compression of one or more vertebral bodies. Retropulsed fragments, best shown on CT, can compress the spinal cord. CT and CT-myelography are instrumental for evaluatıng surgical stabilization and removal of fracture fragments. Bone algorithms, photographed with wide windows, allow evaluation even in the presence of metallic fixation devices (see Fig. 1–7).

Wedge-Compression Fracture. Abrupt, anterior flexion results in wedge-compression fracture of one or more vertebral bodies. Such injuries are common in the lower thoracic level as the result of seat belt restraint in head-on motor vehicle collisions. Plain films adequately depict these fractures in emergency room evaluation. CT and MRI can more fully characterize the fracture and show compromise of the spinal canal. In many situations, it is important to determine whether a compression abnormality is acute or chronic. Acute injuries may involve distinct fracture lines and hemorrhage, but often it is not possible to make this distinction on radiographic grounds. Other considerations include the possibility of a pathological fracture when there is no history of trauma.

Plain films can show cortical interruptions and widening of the paraspinous soft tissues as evidence of acute fracture and blood in the paraspinous region. CT shows these findings and, in addition, shows the compromise of the spinal canal or neural foramina (Fig. 7–19). MRI is unique in showing edema in the bone marrow; it can also show tumor in the case of pathological fracture. Hemorrhage in the paraspinous region, compression of the thecal sac, and cord injury are also best shown by MRI. The distinction between an old compression fracture and metastatic tumor in the spine can usually be made by MRI.

Lumbar and Sacral Spine

Fractures of the lumbar spine occur most commonly as the result of falls and motor vehicle accidents. The larger size of the vertebral bodies makes fracture less common, and the termination of the spinal cord at approximately L-1 make cord injury less likely. However, injury to the terminal cord (the conus medullaris) can cause serious impairment of lower extremity, bowel, and bladder function. Compression of neural foramina and traumatic disc herniation can compress nerve roots within the canal (the cauda equina) or the peripheral nerves as they exit.

Compression Fracture. A compression fracture, usually the result of a fall or of seat belt restraint in a motor vehicle accident, can cause instability, depending on associated injuries to the ligaments and the posterior elements. Retropulsed fragments produce the same consequences as those seen in the upper spine.

Posterior Element Fracture. Fracture fragments of the pedicles, the facets, and the lamina can project into the canal or the neural foramina, compressing nerve roots. Such fractures are best identified on CT.

Spondylolysis and Spondylolisthesis. Fracture of the pars interarticularis, believed to occur as a result of acute or subacute trauma, causes separation of the posterior column from the middle and anterior support. This fracture, called spondylolysis, usually produces chronic back pain. When the instability allows forward slippage of the upper vertebral body on the lower one (spondylolisthesis), exiting nerve roots or the cauda equina can be compressed. The pars fractures are most easily seen on oblique plain films but are well shown on CT if the posterior elements and disc spaces are carefully labeled. The subluxation is graded by the fraction of the vertebral body offset (Fig. 7–20). CT, myelography, and MRI best demonstrate the compression of nerves.

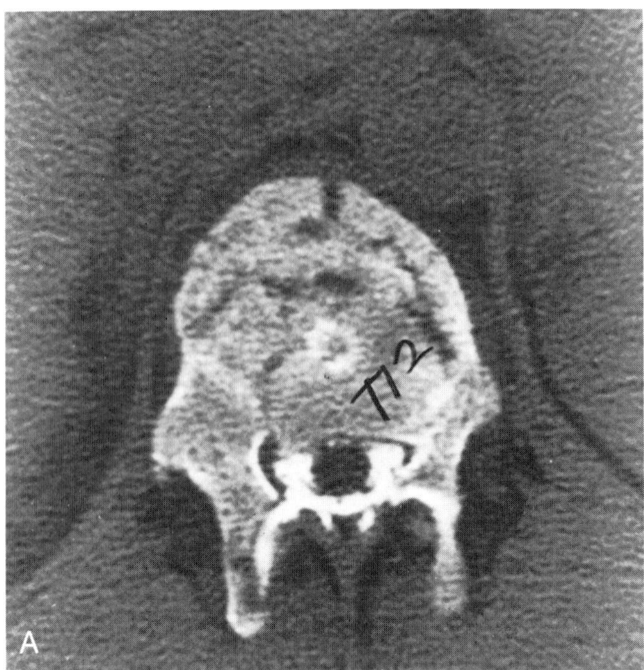

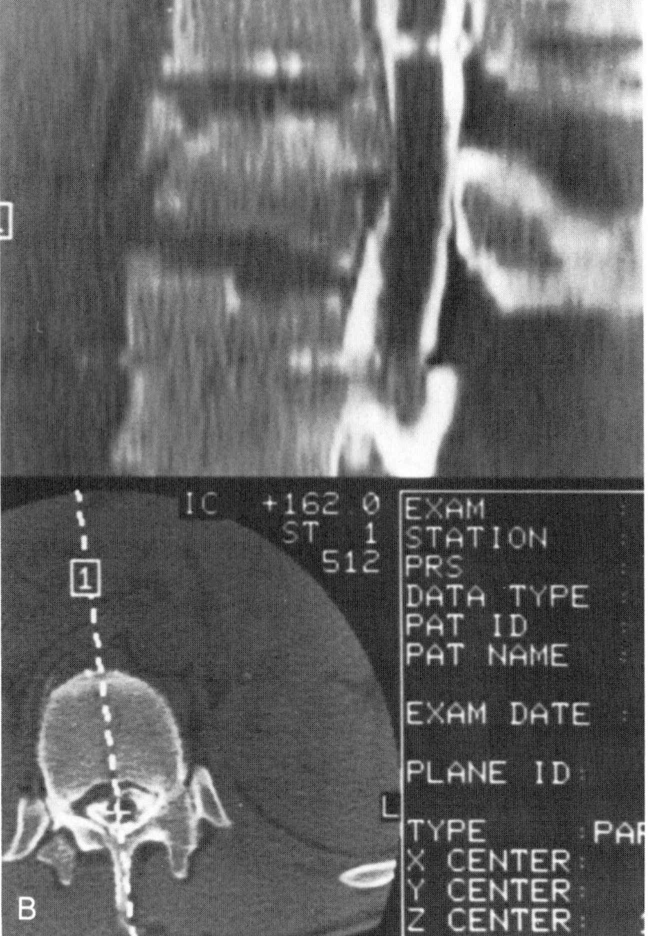

FIGURE 7–19. Wedge-compression fracture. *A.* Axial CT scan, performed after myelography, shows a complex fracture of the T-12 vertebral body and compression of the anterior subarachnoid space. *B.* Midline sagittal reformation shows the wedge-compression fracture and the narrowing of the thecal sac.

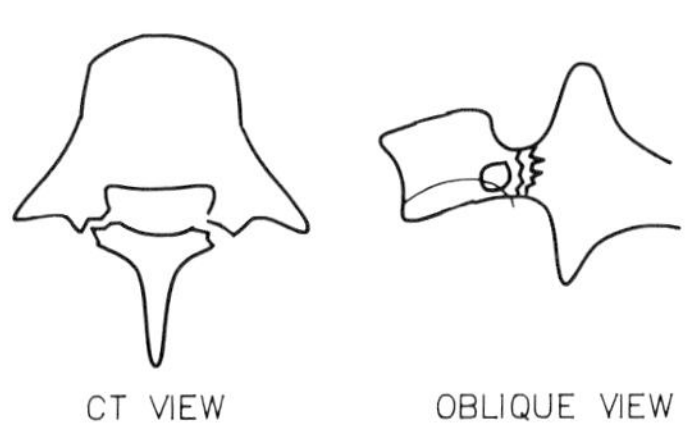

SPONDYLOLISTHESIS
GRADED BY OFFSET
1. 1/4 VERTEBRAL BODY
2. 1/2 VERTEBRAL BODY
3. 3/4 VERTEBRAL BODY
4. COMPLETE OFFSET

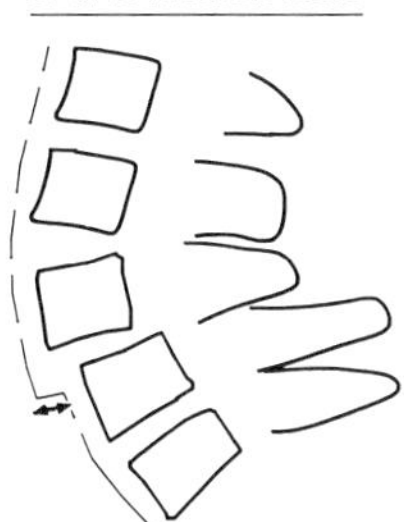

FIGURE 7–20. Characteristics of spondylolysis and spondylolisthesis.

Ligamentous and Disc Injury in the Spine

Ligamentous Injury and Traumatic Disc Rupture. Ligamentous injuries can cause instability of the spine not readily detected on routine films. Such instability is especially serious in the cervical spine. Stress views can show subluxation or distraction of the vertebral bodies. Because of the risk of cord or nerve root injury, these examinations should be conducted under supervision of a clinician, especially in cases of acute injury.

Trauma is frequently a cause of disc injury. The resultant bulging disc or herniated fragments compress the cord, the cauda equina, or the exiting nerve roots. Traumatically herniated discs are generally at a single level and show a focal defect, in contrast to degenerative disease, which is characterized by generalized disc degeneration at multiple levels and diffuse, extended disc herniation.

In injuries of the cervical spine, the typical history includes a slip and fall and a breaking of the fall with an outstretched arm, which thereby places asymmetrical axial loading on the disc space. In the thoracic and lumbar portions of the spine, a motor vehicle accident, a fall, or a lifting injury results in sudden extrusion of a disc fragment. Such herniations occur in lifting accidents because the muscles of the back are capable of sustaining a greater force than are the discs. Traumatic disc rupture is best shown by MRI but is also well-demonstrated by the examinations used to evaluate acute trauma (CT, myelography, and CT-myelography). Disc disease is discussed further with degenerative diseases.

Degenerative Osteophytic and Disc Disease. Chronic trauma, bone hyperostosis, chronic response to mild injuries, and normal aging result in degeneration of discs, formation of osteophytes, and abnormalities of alignment. These abnormalities, collectively termed degenerative disease of the spine, account for a large proportion of medical complaints and therapy. Such disease is frequently the cause of loss of work, disability claims, and personal injury lawsuits. Even when the initial cause is trauma, as might occur in an automobile accident, the long-term consequences are caused by degenerative disease. In addition, people develop degenerative disease as a part of normal aging because of changes in bone mineral content, disc degeneration, and chronic erosion caused by postural or occupational demands. The rate of development of such changes varies among individuals. The severity of symptoms depends on the location of abnormalities and the size of the spinal canal and the neural foramina.

Degenerative spine disease that affects the spinal cord or the nerve roots can be diagnosed with confidence in clinical examination. A variety of radiographic techniques provide confirmation and surgical guidance. MRI, CT, CT-myelography, and conventional myelography are capable of demonstrating disc disease and compression of the cord and the nerve roots by discs and osteophytes (see Fig. 1–15, 8–8, 8–9). Such applications are discussed in Chapter 8. In many cases, it is the combination of abnormalities—disc abnormalities, osteophytes, ligament abnormalities, malalignment, and congenitally narrow canal—that causes the compression of the neural structures (see Figs. 7–8, 7–11).

In many patients, pain is the predominant (or only) symptom, and it is difficult to diagnose and treat the underlying disease. Such pain syndromes, most commonly designated whiplash or strain in the cervical spine and low back pain in the lumbar spine, are caused by ligamentous and soft-tissue injury, degeneration of facet joints, and local irritation of small pain fibers. Radiographic evaluation often shows degenerative disease in such patients but does not provide an explanation of the symptoms. Nevertheless, imaging methods can identify less common causes of disease that are treatable, such as a far lateral disc herniation, ligamentous instability, pseudarthrosis, severe facet disease, and overriding facets that entrap nerves in the foramina.

In the cervical spine, the most common degenerative process involves osteophyte formation and disc herniation, usually between C-4 and T-1, where most of the anterior-to-posterior motion occurs. Early symptoms occur in patients with narrow canals. Evaluation by MRI shows disc degeneration and indentation on the thecal sac and, if severe, of the spinal cord (Fig. 7–21). Osteophytes and neural foramina are more difficult to assess by MRI. These areas are well shown on conventional myelography (best for showing nerve roots) and CT-myelography (best for showing the osteophytes and anatomical structure of the canal).

In the thoracic spine, degenerative disease is less common and less severe. Disc herniation is uncommon (see Fig. 8–101), and osteophytic disease is less severe than elsewhere in the spine. Degenerative collapse is an important consideration in an elderly patient or in a steroid-dependent patient with chronic lung disease.

In the lumbosacral spine, disc degeneration and herniation and osteophytic encroachment on the canal are the most important diagnostic considerations. The discs undergo several changes as they degenerate. MRI can show decreased intensity on T2 spin echo or STIR images (see Fig. 7–8), loss of disc-space height, and posterior extension of the disc against the thecal sac. Because the term "herniation" has many interpretations and has specific consequences in a disability claim, a lawsuit, and a surgical decision, it is important to clearly describe the actual abnormality and suggest its consequences with regard to neurological impairment (Fig. 7–22).

A simplified but logical view of disc degeneration and herniation addresses the specific abnormality, the degree of extension, and the effect on the nervous system. A disc that shows a change in intensity, but not shape, on MRI is at least partially degenerated. Diffuse bulging circumferentially is an early finding of disc degeneration. It can cause symptoms by com-

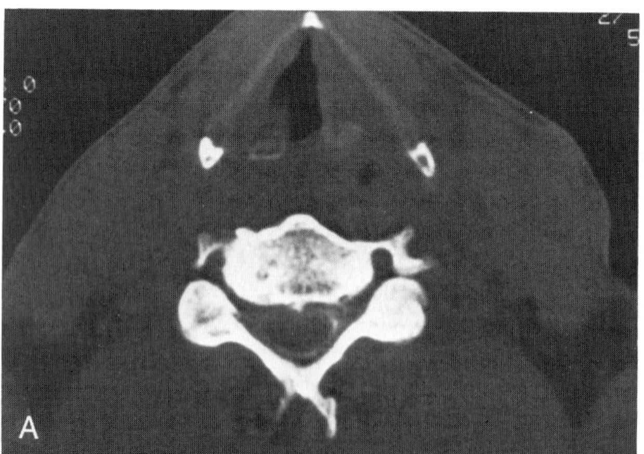

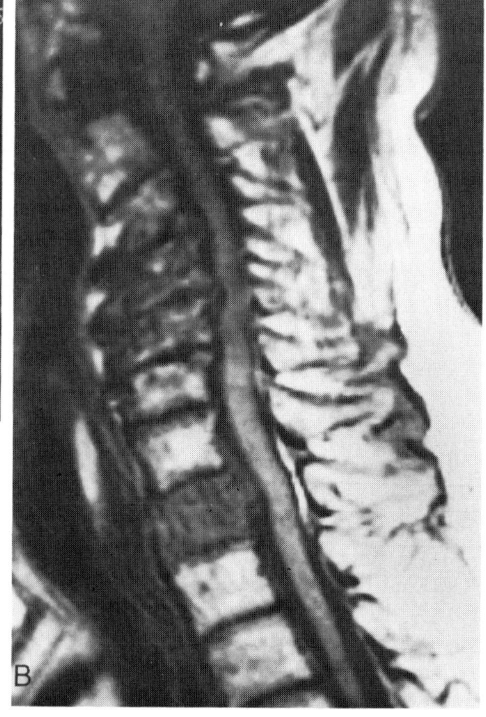

FIGURE 7–21. Cervical degenerative disease. *A.* Axial CT slice at the C-5 level photographed with bone windows shows bilateral encroachment of osteophytes on the neuroforamina, more severe on the right side. Only minimal enhancement of the thecal sac is present on this postmyelogram image because degenerative and congenital narrowing of the canal obstructed flow of the contrast from its injection site at the level of C1-C2. *B.* Sagittal T1 spin echo image in another patient, an 83-year-old woman, shows severe degenerative disease of the entire cervical spine with erosion of the discs and narrowed disc spaces, abnormal alignment, and the formation of osteophytes that compress the thecal sac. The patient also had metastatic involvement of the body of T-1, shown as marrow replacement by breast carcinoma.

FIGURE 7–22. Disc herniation. *A.* Diagram. MR, magnetic resonance. *B.* Parasagittal T2 spin echo images in the midline and slightly to the left of midline show disc disease involving L-3 through S-1. At L3-L4, the disc shows normal height but decreased intensity, indicating partial degeneration. The L4-L5 disc shows herniation, compressing the left anterior thecal sac. The herniated material has a button appearance but is connected to the remainder of the disc. The L5-S1 disc shows degeneration and disc-space narrowing but no compression of the thecal sac.

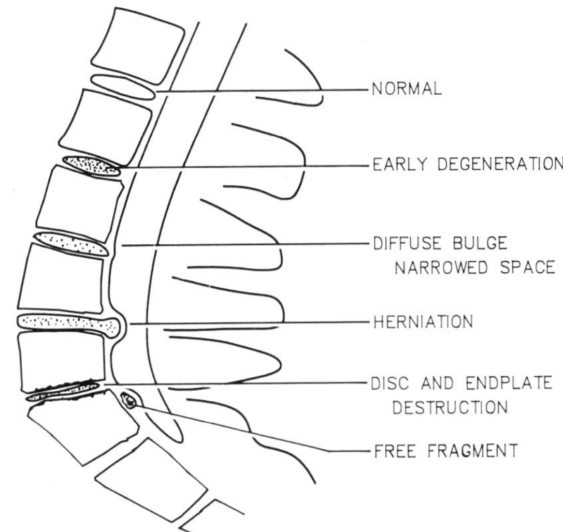

- ABNORMAL MR INTENSITY INDICATES DEGENERATION
- HERNIATION – NUCLEUS THROUGH ANNULUS
  – DISC THROUGH LIGAMENTS
- FRAGMENT – VENTRAL CANAL
  – DORSAL CANAL
  – NEURAL FORAMEN
- NERVE COMPRESSION – CAUDA EQUINA
  – NEURAL FORAMEN
  – FAR LATERAL

A

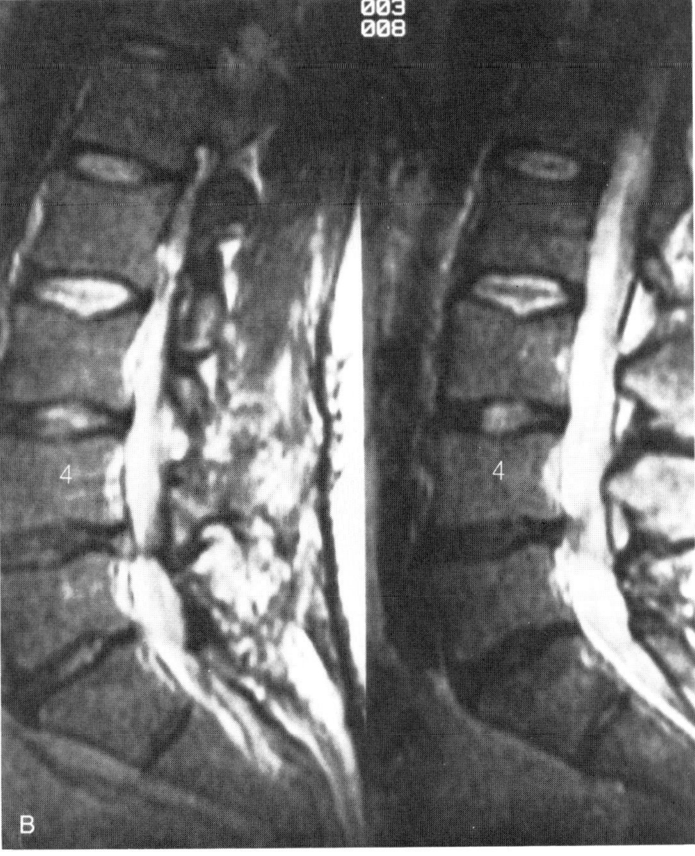

pressing the entire thecal sac, but the actual symptoms may be focal. The loss of disc-space height can result in symptoms from compression of nerve roots as they pass through the neural foramina or from buckling of ligaments within the canal. Such a disc may require surgery, even though it is not herniated. A weakened disc can show focal bulging and result in compression of the cord, the cauda equina, or the exiting nerve roots. Although such a bulge is not a herniation, it may also require therapy.

In more severe degeneration, the inner portion of the disc herniates through the annulus, also causing a focal compression. MRI shows a button shape extending from the degenerated disc. This herniated disc material may or may not pass through the posterior longitudinal ligament (a process that is also called herniation); it may also become separated from the original disc (a process called a free fragment). In some cases, the herniated disc material migrates superiorly, inferiorly, or through a neural foramen. Lateral disc bulging is an important cause of compression of a nerve root that has already exited from the neural foramen. Such abnormalities are seen on CT and MRI scans but not on conventional myelograms (see Fig. 7–8).

Evaluation of the spine after disc surgery is required when symptoms persist or recur or when new symptoms develop. Assessment is performed to determine whether postoperative scar tissue, recurrent disc herniation, or new abnormalities are responsible for the symptoms. The significance of osteophytes, alignment abnormalities, and disc disease at nonoperated levels can usually be determined from CT scans, myelograms and unenhanced MRI scans. The distinction between scar tissue and disc material can often be made with enhanced MRI. In general, disc material does not show enhancement, whereas scar tissue shows prominent enhancement. However, the morphological appearance of the abnormality is important in diagnosing recurrent disease because (1) disc material sometimes enhances, (2) scar tissue sometimes does not enhance, and (3) some amount of scar tissue is usually present even when recurrent disc material is the primary cause of symptoms. Even unoperated discs have some associated scar tissue. A herniated disc fragment is often surrounded by scar tissue (the Beef Wellington sign; Fig. 7–23).

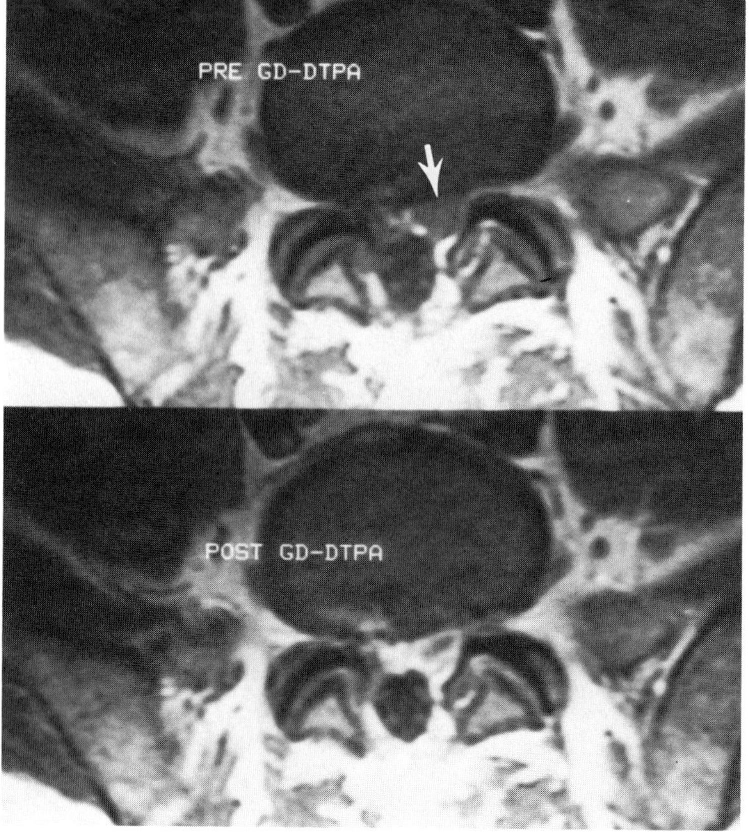

FIGURE 7–23. Recurrent disc herniation. Pre- and post–gadolinium diethylenetriamine-penta-acetic acid (Gd-DTPA) enhanced T1 spin echo images show ring enhancement of a left anterior canal disc fragment *(arrow)* in a 47-year-old man who had previously undergone disc removal. The enhancing material surrounding the disc fragment is scar tissue (the Beef Wellington sign).

Pelvis and Sacrum

Fractures of the pelvis usually involve more than one part because of the complete ring construction. These fractures are common in motor vehicle accidents and other severe trauma and constitute a significant cause of morbidity and mortality. They are especially important in that they cause associated injury to the bladder, the sacral nerves, and the pelvic vessels. Sacral fractures may be isolated or may be associated with other pelvic ring fractures.

Sacral Fractures. Fractures of the sacrum are difficult to detect because of the thin cortex and mostly trabecular structure. Overlying abdominal organs and bowel gas make plain film evaluation difficult. Evaluation with CT and MRI is hampered by the indistinct appearance of the bones and the steep curvature. Nevertheless, full evaluation of sacral fractures is essential in order to diagnose injuries to the sacral plexus and the nerves that control bowel and bladder function. Coronal and oblique coronal MRI scans and CT images provide the optimal view of the neural foramina (see Fig. 7–9). High spatial resolution and thin-slice technique is essential in this area.

Pelvic Ring Fractures. The most common areas of fracture when the pelvic ring is injured are the sacrum and the obturator ring. Diastasis of the pubic symphysis and of the sacroiliac joint is a common finding and should be carefully sought when a single pelvic fracture is identified (Fig. 7–24). The acetabulum is also frequently fractured in pelvic trauma. Sacral injuries are almost always present and include diastasis, lip fracture, shear injury, and comminuted fracture. CT best shows these injuries and, in addition, can show soft-tissue injury in the pelvis. Sacroiliac diastasis and lip fractures can usually be identified on AP plain films, but many are difficult to detect.

Acetabular Fracture and Hip Dislocation. Fractures of the acetabulum can be isolated or can occur with other pelvic fractures. Compression of the acetabulum by the femoral head in a head-on motor vehicle collision is a common mechanism of injury. Although plain films can often show the fracture, CT can demonstrate fracture, integrity of the acetabular margins, and joint dislocation.

Because of the usual mechanism of injury (the knee's hitting the dashboard) and the muscle attachments of the hip joint, dislocations are usually posterior. The displacement of the femoral head is directly posterior with the hip in flexion, adduction, and internal rotation. The diagnosis of posterior hip dislocation is easily made from plain films, but CT is recommended for assessing the possibility of fracture of the acetabulum or the femoral head, which can limit reduction or stability (Fig. 7–25). Complications include sciatic nerve injury (early) and necrosis of the femoral head (late) resulting from injury to its vascular supply. Anterior hip dislocation is less common (about 10% of cases) and results from forced abduction of the hip, which also frequently occurs in motor vehicle accidents. The femoral head lies anterior to the obturator foramen with the hip in extension, abduction, and external rotation.

Lower Extremity Fractures

Fracture of a lower extremity may be isolated or may be one of multiple injuries. Plain films are inexpensive, are easily obtained in multiple projections, and best show fracture lines. Therefore, plain films are used to diagnose and treat the majority of fractures. When intraosseous (marrow cavity), ligamentous, or vascular injury is suspected, additional examinations are required. MRI provides the highest contrast resolution and shows the edema and hemorrhage associated with intraosseous fractures and soft-tissue and ligamentous injury. MRI is also the most informative and least invasive test for evaluating joint injury. Angiography is necessary to evaluate vascular injury from blunt or penetrating trauma.

Femoral Fractures. Fractures occur in all parts of the femur. At the upper end, the head and neck, they are most common in the elderly as a result of osteoporosis and minor trauma or even normal weight-bearing. These fractures involve the area of the joint capsule (subcapital and midcervical portions and base of the neck) and the extracapsular (intertrochanteric) regions. The leg is foreshortened (because of muscle contraction), abducted, and externally rotated. The diagnosis can be made from plain radiographs by identification of fracture lines, indentations of the femoral head, and alteration of the normal alignment. Interruption of Shenton's arch (a normally smooth curve formed by the medial femoral shaft and the upper margin of the obturator canal) is a reliable indicator of fracture. Treatment of femoral neck and head fractures is made difficult by slow and incomplete healing

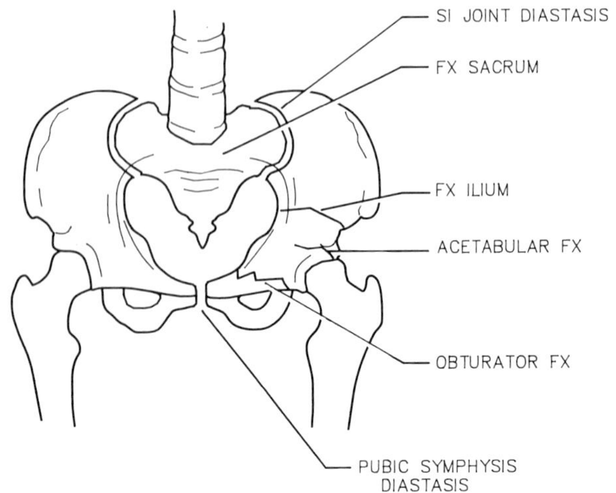

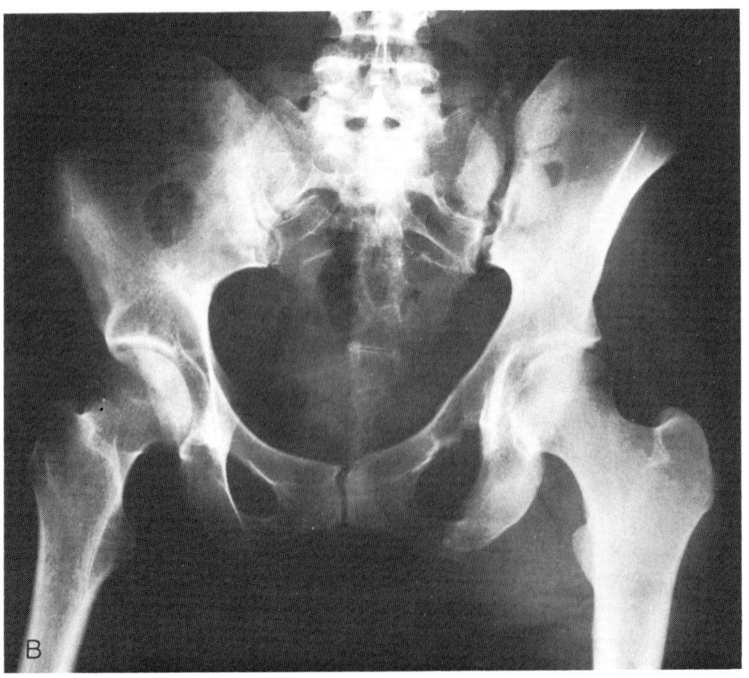

FIGURE 7–24. Pelvic fractures. *A.* Diagram. SI, sacroiliac; FX, fracture. *B.* Pelvic plain film shows left pubic bone fractures evidenced by cortical displacement and overlap of bone density in an automobile accident victim. Marked diastasis of the left sacroiliac joint is also present.

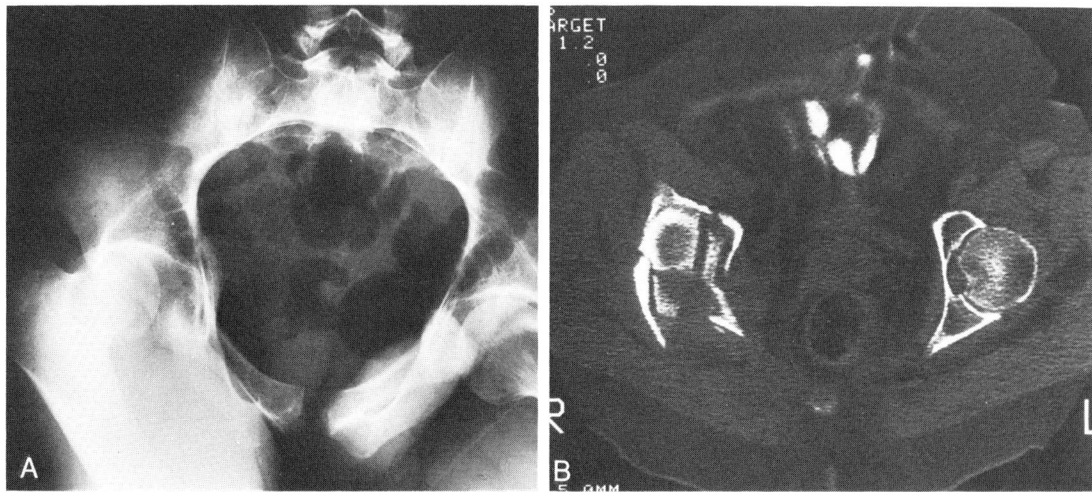

FIGURE 7–25. Hip injury. *A.* Hip dislocation. Anteroposterior (AP) film shows posterior dislocation, adduction, and internal rotation of the right femoral head in a motor vehicle accident victim. Diastasis of the pubic symphysis is also evident. *B.* Acetabular fracture. Axial CT scan at the level of the acetabula in another patient shows a comminuted fracture of the right acetabulum.

in elderly patients and the higher risks associated with surgery and rehabilitation.

Subtrochanteric and femoral shaft fractures occur in all age groups, usually as a result of severe trauma. The proximal fragment is flexed, externally rotated, and abducted. Supracondylar fractures also occur in all age groups. The gastrocnemius muscle generally causes a posterior rotation of the distal fragment, making management difficult. Many such fractures extend to the knee joint. Diagnosis of the fracture is easily made from plain radiographs.

Stress fractures often occur in the femoral neck in elderly patients or as a result of new or excessive forces applied to the leg, such as those that occur in exercise enthusiasts or amateur athletes who undertake a new sport without proper conditioning. The mechanism is osteoporosis, followed by trabecular fatigue fractures and then by mechanical failure. These fractures produce pain in the hip or in the upper leg. Early radiographs may be negative, but eventually (1 to 2 weeks later) sclerosis is shown. In more severe fractures, a lucent fracture line or a displaced fracture may be apparent. Prolonged bed rest is the usual treatment when a fracture line is present; surgical fixation is required in order to avoid collapse of the femoral neck.

Osteonecrosis of the femoral head, also called avascular necrosis (AVN), can be caused by trauma, steroid therapy, and vascular compromise. An initial edematous phase is followed by necrosis and partial collapse of the femoral head. Healing without deformity can occur if the process is identified and treated early. Conservative treatment includes bed rest, use of crutches, and reduction of weight-bearing activity. Severe AVN requires core decompression of the femoral head or surgical fixation. A general discussion of AVN is presented at the end of this section.

Knee Trauma

Trauma to the knee can result in fracture, ligamentous injury, cartilaginous injury, joint-space disease, and soft-tissue injury or hemorrhage. Although the most severe knee injuries are caused by motor vehicle accidents, the more common injuries are sporting and occupational injuries. Skiing, hockey, football, and soccer are the sports most often associated with these injuries, which include meniscal tear, cruciate ligament rupture, collateral ligament distraction, joint effusion, soft-tissue injury, and intraosseous fracture (Fig. 7–26).

The plain film diagnosis of knee injury is limited primarily to fractures by showing displaced fracture lines, regions of hyperdensity caused by overlying fragments or compressed bone, and joint effusions suggestive of intra-articular hematoma. Joint-space effusion, fat, and blood can be detected on lateral plain films from the presence of a fat-fluid level (Fig. 7–27) or from separation of the anterior suprapatellar and prefemoral (posterior suprapatellar) fat and fluid in the suprapatellar

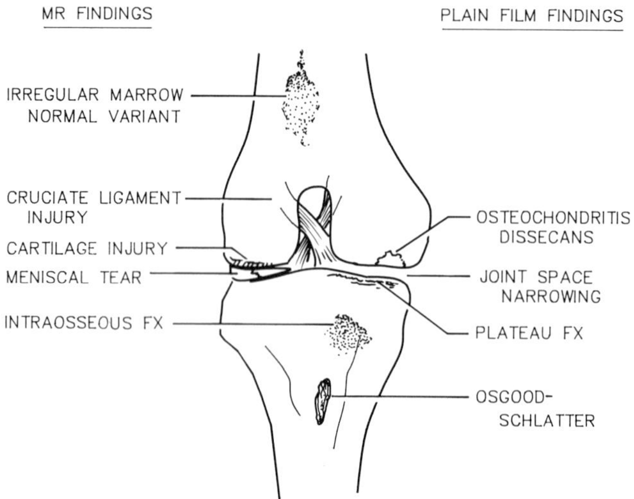

FIGURE 7–26. Traumatic and degenerative disease of the knee. MR, magnetic resonance; FX, fracture.

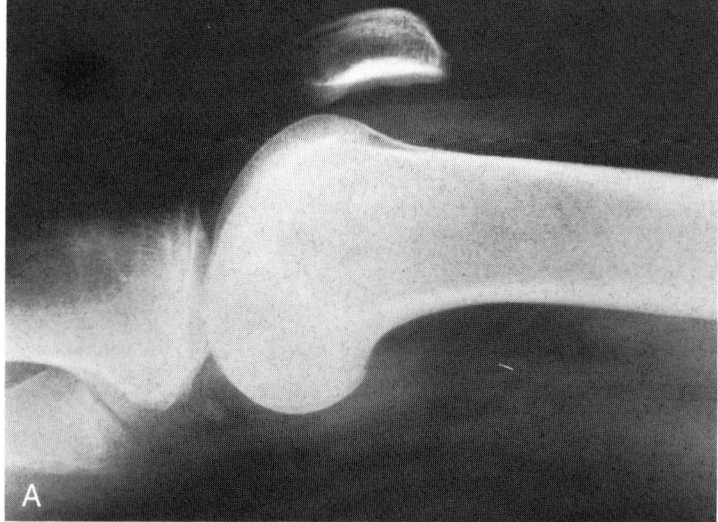

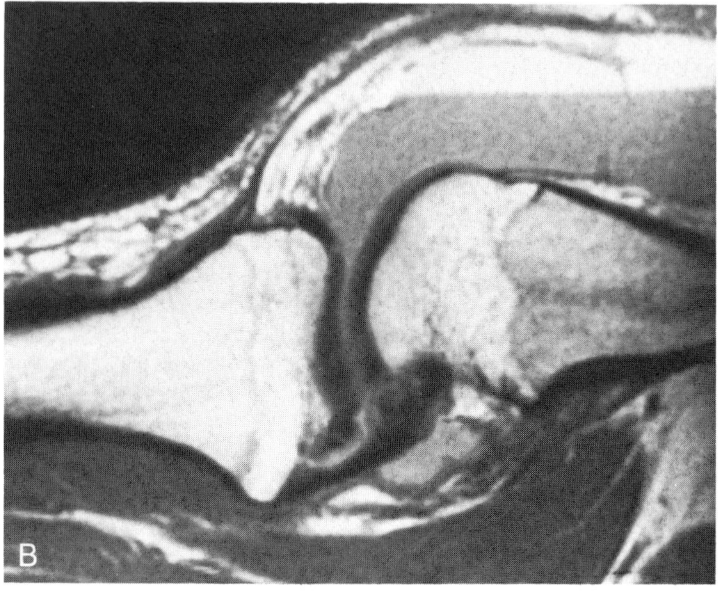

FIGURE 7–27. Lipohemarthrosis. *A.* Cross-table lateral plain film shows fat and fluid in the suprapatellar bursa of an automobile accident victim. The straight horizontal line between the low-density fat above and the medium-density fluid below (fat-fluid level) is indicative of severe trauma and, usually, of the presence of a fracture involving the joint space. *B.* Sagittal T1 spin echo image in a 17-year-old football player shows a fat-fluid level to best advantage. Here, the fat is of high intensity, and the fluid (or blood) is of intermediate intensity.

bursa. MRI is capable of noninvasively demonstrating ligamentous and soft-tissue injury, intraosseous fracture, and joint-space fluid, providing the most comprehensive examination of knee injury (Fig. 7–28; see also Fig. 7–12). Specific injuries, some of which also result from degenerative disease or chronic trauma, are discussed as follows.

Collateral Ligament Injury. The clinical diagnosis of collateral ligament injury is by detection of instability. These injuries are usually caused by varus or valgus stress and are frequently associated with injuries of the meniscus or cruciate ligaments. The bending force on the joint often causes ligamentous distraction (full or partial tear) on one side and compression fracture of the bone on the opposite side. The triad of O'Donoghue—injury to the medial collateral ligament, the medial meniscus, and the anterior cruciate ligament—results from rotation and valgus strain. MRI, with STIR or (less favorable) T2 spin echo sequences, shows edema in adjacent soft tissues, and high-resolution T1 spin echo sequences can sometimes show disruption of the ligaments (see Fig. 7–28). In conjunction with other findings (i.e., meniscal tear, collateral ligament injury, and condylar injury) and clinical examination, a diagnosis can be made and restrictions on activity recommended.

Cruciate Ligament Injury. Cruciate ligament injury commonly occurs in team sports. Rupture of the posterior cruciate ligament is caused either by hyperextension or by a posterior force directed against the flexed knee, as occurs in a motor vehicle accident. The anterior cruciate ligament injury is caused by internal rotation of the femur on the tibia. Both injuries are highly associated with meniscal and collateral ligament injuries.

The normal posterior cruciate ligament has very low intensity on T1 spin echo images and has a curved (boomerang) shape. The injured ligament appears widened and has higher intensity (gray). Hemorrhage, discontinuity, and bone injury may also be evident.

The anterior cruciate ligament is thinner and is not as well seen on MRI. High-resolution images can often show individual linear attachments into the tibia. Injury to the anterior cruciate ligament is similarly demonstrated by interruption, poor visualization, or thickening of the ligament. Chronic or long-term anterior cruciate injuries can have similar appearances but often result in wasting. The ligament can sometimes be reabsorbed entirely and not be visible on MRI. As a consequence, contiguous thin slices are essential for evaluating the anterior cruciate ligament.

Meniscal Tears. The menisci are frequently

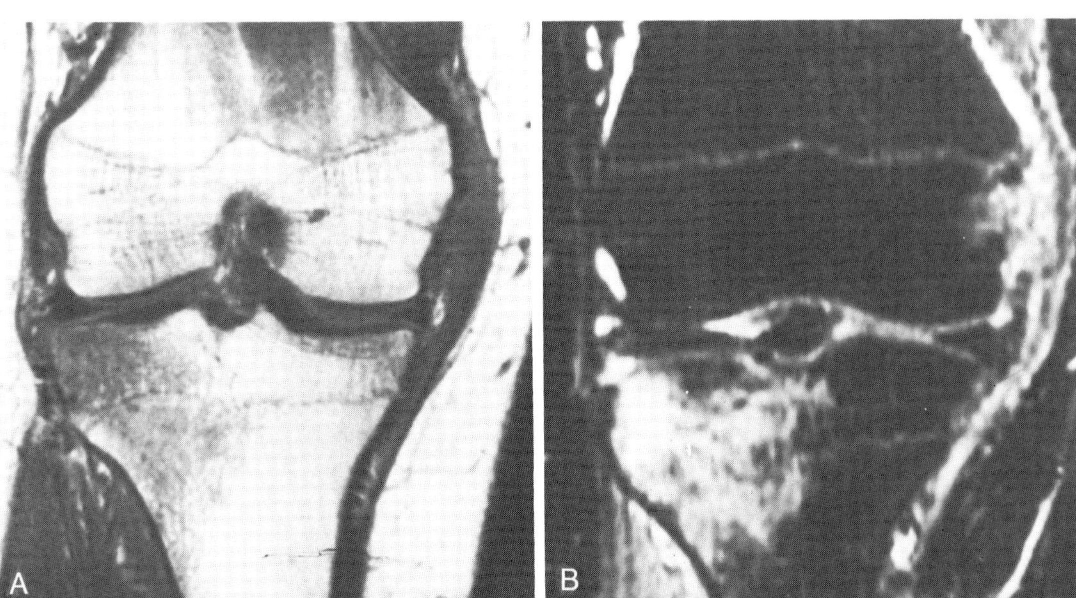

FIGURE 7–28. Knee injury. *A.* Coronal T1 spin echo image of the right knee shows decreased intensity in the lateral tibial marrow, indicating intraosseous fracture. Medial soft-tissue swelling indicates medial collateral ligament injury. The combination is typical of a "clipping" injury, as occurred when the patient, a young pedestrian, was hit in the lateral knee by a car. *B.* Short TI inversion recovery (STIR) image makes the lesions obvious and, in addition, shows medial femoral intraosseous fracture and extension of soft-tissue edema around the medial collateral ligament injury.

injured in knee trauma. MRI allows noninvasive diagnosis of meniscal tears that can be confirmed and treated by arthroscopy. The injury ranges from a simple vertical tear to complex internal derangement and a bucket-handle tear (Fig. 7–29). The meniscus is normally black on T1 spin echo images and is easily seen against the gray-appearing articular

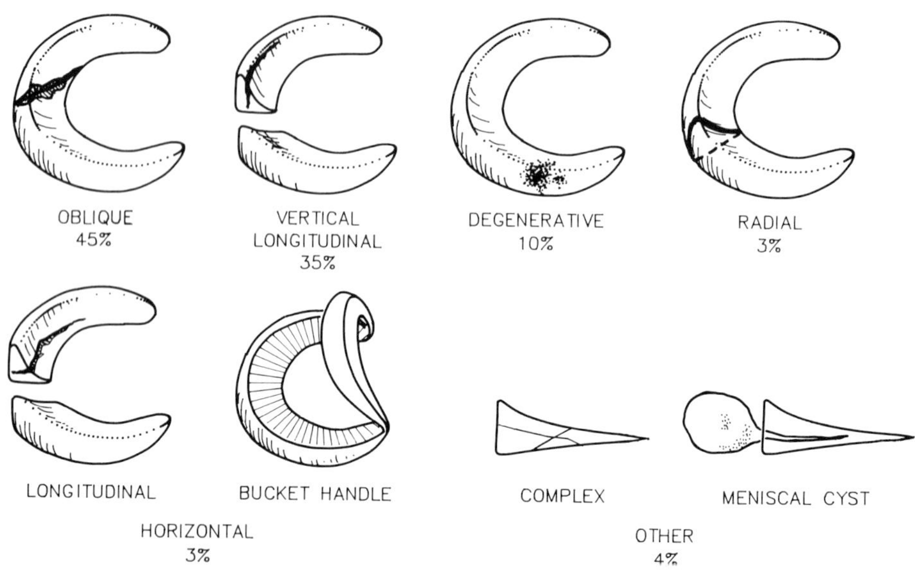

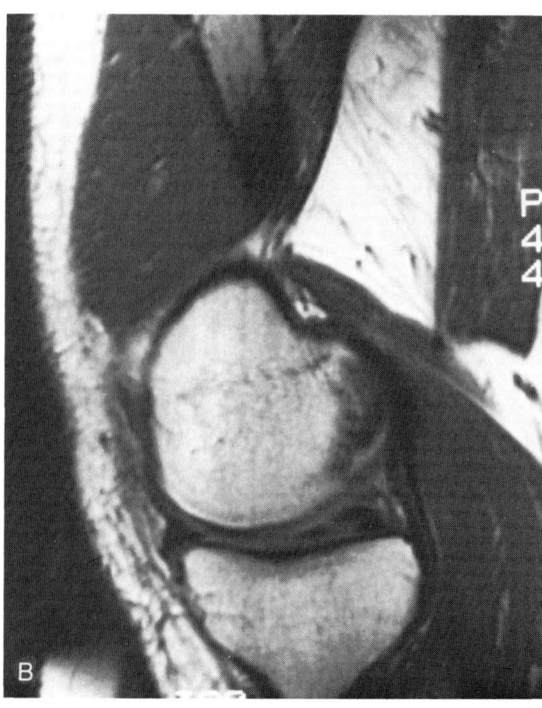

FIGURE 7–29. Meniscal disease. *A.* Diagram. *B.* Sagittal T1 spin echo image of the medial joint space shows a complex tear of the posterior horn that is predominantly horizontal. The tear extends to the superior and inferior margins of the meniscus.

cartilage. Linear or complex areas of increased signal intensity that intersect the margins of the meniscus are diagnostic of meniscal tears. Internal increased signal may also be caused by meniscal injury; however, some degree of internal, increased signal is often present in patients without clinical symptoms. This may represent a normal variation, mild chronic degeneration, or an internal tear that has not become clinically significant. Such internal abnormality is difficult to assess arthroscopically.

Articular Cartilage Injury. The articular cartilage is frequently injured along with the bone and the meniscus. Diagnosis can be made with MRI when irregularity is demonstrated. Arthroscopic examination may be required in order to fully diagnose the injury and to identify loose fragments.

Traumatic Cysts. Trauma to the synovial lining of the joint and tendinous insertions can result in cyst formation. A meniscal cyst communicates with the joint space and is usually associated with a meniscal tear. Cystic lesions can also develop in the femoral condyles and the tibial plateau (and at articular surfaces of other joints) as a result of trauma or degenerative disease.

Popliteal (Baker's) Cyst. The popliteal (Baker's) cyst is a synovial fluid collection in the bursa of the popliteal space. The cyst is painful and is usually the result of trauma or degenerative disease, but it is also seen in rheumatoid arthritis. When it is associated with trauma or degenerative disease, meniscal or cruciate ligament injury must also be suspected.

Degenerative Disease of the Knee

Degeneration of the structures of the knee results from chronic trauma. Bone and ligamentous abnormalities are typically manifested by joint-space narrowing, bone eburnation, and meniscal degeneration. Many of these processes are caused by long-term trauma or exacerbation of an old injury that has led to degenerative and proliferative changes. In general, such abnormalities can be distinguished from acute injury by the symptoms and the clinical history, the lack of well-defined margins, and the proliferative cartilage and bone formation. Several processes that include acute and chronic disease of the knee are discussed as follows.

Joint Bodies. Loose bodies within the knee joint can occur in a variety of processes. These bodies may be composed of articular cartilage, meniscus, bone from the articular surface, and crystal deposition. They are caused by trauma, degenerative disease, arthritis, and metabolic processes. Locked knee, restricted range of motion, and recurrent effusions develop. Radiographic diagnosis is difficult, and arthrography is usually required in order to demonstrate the joint bodies as filling defects within the contrast-enhanced joint space. If the bodies are large enough, they can be seen on thin-slice MRI sequences. Otherwise, they are detected and removed arthroscopically. Arthritic and crystal deposition diseases as causes of joint bodies are discussed in a later section.

Osteonecrosis (Avascular Necrosis). The articular surfaces of the femur and the tibia are affected by several conditions that result in focal bone injury, inflammation, or both. Because of the location, the appearance, and the presumed cause of these conditions, various names are applied to them, even though the mechanism of injury and the development of bone injury are common to all of them. Osteonecrosis, as a general term, indicates a nonspecific bone injury caused by acute or chronic trauma. This term is often used synonymously with AVN, which suggests that interruption of the vascular supply is the cause of the bone necrosis. AVN is discussed in greater detail at the end of this section. Osteonecrosis is usually seen in elderly patients in whom acute symptoms develop when microfractures occur. The most common locations are areas of stress near the knee joint: the medial tibial plateau and the medial femoral condyle.

Osteochondritis Dissecans. Osteochrondritis dissecans is a more focal (i.e., smaller area of involvement) form of osteonecrosis, usually seen in young patients. It generally affects the medial femoral condyle but can also affect the lateral femur or the tibia adjacent to the knee joint. Other areas affected are the talus and the elbow. Onset of symptoms is insidious as intra-articular disease develops, including effusion and loose fragments of bone that break off into the joint. Locking of the knee joint is common. Plain films clearly show the rounded, well-demarcated defects at the articular surface of the femoral condyle. T1 spin echo MRI sequences can clearly demonstrate the lesions as marrow defects on thin-slice sagittal and coronal views (Fig. 7–30) and, at the same time, allow evaluation of other potential causes of disease.

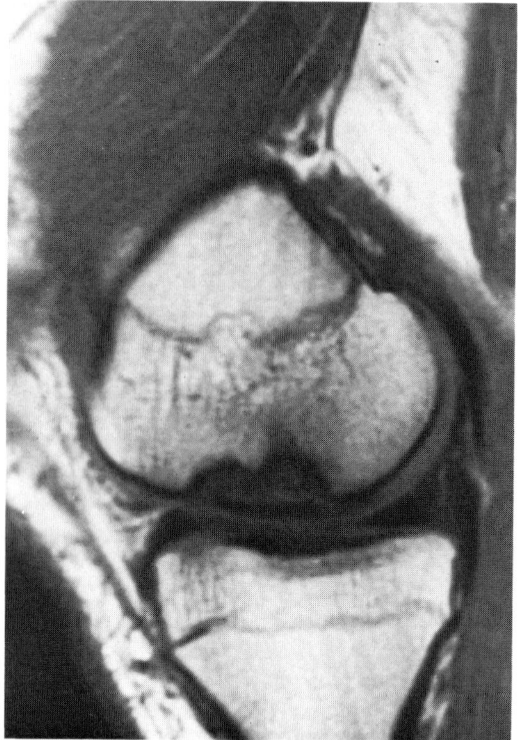

FIGURE 7–30. Osteochondritis dissecans. Sagittal T1 spin echo image shows two adjacent, rounded, defects in the medial femoral condyle of a 19-year-old male with medial knee pain and locking. The abnormality is circumscribed by a low-intensity rim that abuts the articular cartilage.

Osgood-Schlatter Disease. Osgood-Schlatter disease is osteochondrosis of the anterior tibial tubercle involving the bony attachment of the patellar ligament to that of the tibial apophysis. It results from pressure necrosis. Because of the typical mechanisms, it is also called surfer's knee and housemaid's knee.

Lower Leg

Tibia and Fibula Fractures. Fractures of the tibia and the fibula occur most commonly in skiing and motor vehicle accidents. A variety of patterns occur, often with comminuted fracture. Fracture of the tibia is most serious because of its primary function of support. Traumatic fractures of the tibia often involve fracture or dislocation of the less important fibula. Plain radiographs are used exclusively for both diagnosis and treatment (Fig. 7–31). The fractures are usually unstable and require fixation. The distal tibia has a poor blood supply, which often results in delayed union. Other complications include arterial injury (evaluated with angiography) and compartment compression syndrome in which blood and edema compress the neurovascular bundles in the anterior or posterior compartments of the leg.

The tibial fractures most difficult to diagnose are at the joint spaces. Fractures of the tibial plateau are often characterized by impaction, shown on plain films as increased density. The presence of a lipohemarthrosis (see Fig. 7–27) can indicate the severity of the injury and suggests the possibility of tibial plateau fracture. MRI most clearly demonstrates fracture of the tibial plateau and intraosseous fracture (see Fig. 7–28). Intraosseous fractures are nondisplaced microfractures most commonly seen in the articular surfaces of the knee as a result

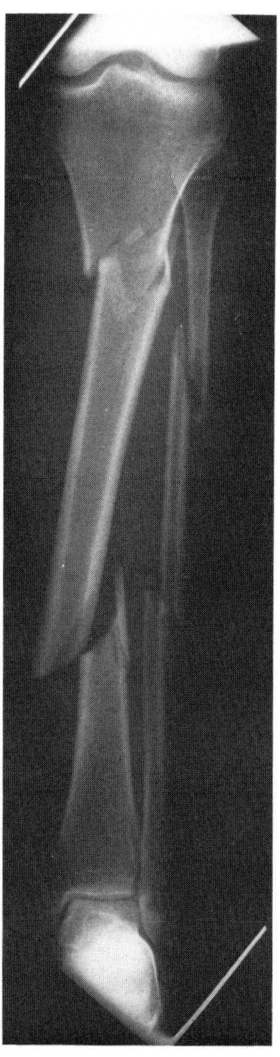

FIGURE 7–31. Comminuted tibia and fibula fracture. AP plain film shows fractures of the tibia and the fibula in two places as a result of a motorcycle accident. Because each bone is broken in two places, the commonly associated fibula dislocation and joint injuries are not present.

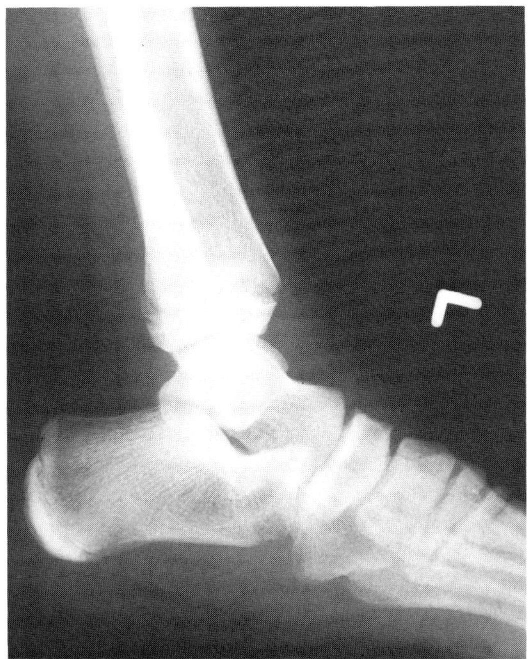

FIGURE 7–32. Posterior malleolar fracture. Off-lateral plain film of the ankle shows a small fracture of the posterior tibia in a girl with a sports injury. In the true lateral view, the fibula was positioned directly over the posterior tibia, obscuring the view of the fracture.

of direct trauma. These fractures do not break through the cortex, as is seen in traumatic cortical fracture or stress fracture. The mechanism of injury is impaction of the marrow spaces, resulting in hemorrhage and edema.

Ankle Injury. At the lower tibia and the fibula (the malleoli), fractures are difficult to repair and can lead to instability of the ankle. Stability depends on the number and the locations of fractures and ligamentous injuries. It is important to identify malleolar (medial and lateral), tibial (anterior and posterior), and fibular shaft fractures and to assess ligamentous separation at the ankle joint. Medial and lateral malleolar fractures are easily diagnosed on the AP radiograph. Posterior malleolar fracture (fracture of the posterior tibia) requires an off-lateral view to best project the fracture away from the fibula (Fig. 7–32).

Foot

Injury to the foot can result in fracture, ligamentous injury, and joint-space derangement. Crush injuries of the talus and the calcaneus occur after a fall (or a jump) from a great height and a landing on the feet. Associated injuries of the spine and the pelvis are often present. The majority of foot fractures are easily seen on plain films. Ligamentous injuries are identified by displacement or abnormal alignment. MRI shows the joint spaces, the ligaments, and the tendons and thus allows noninvasive diagnosis of these injuries. AVN of the talus, a common sequel to talar fracture, is easily demonstrated by high-contrast MRI, especially STIR sequences. The Achilles tendon is normally black on all MRI sequences. Rupture, inflammation, and adjacent bursitis are easily seen on high-contrast sequences such as T2 spin echo and STIR sequences (Fig. 7–33).

Fractures of the tarsals and metatarsals may be caused by direct trauma or by stress. Acute fracture is easily detected in most cases from the presence of cortical disruption and soft-tissue swelling. Fracture dislocation at the tarsal-metatarsal junction (called Lisfranc's fracture) is identified from abnormal alignment. The patient generally can identify the site of trauma and the location of pain, which can greatly assist the radiologist in differentiating a true fracture from a normal variant such as an accessory ossicle, an old injury, or an epiphyseal plate. Stress fractures occur in walking or running and manifest with pain, usually in a metatarsal. Stress fracture of the calcaneus appears as an overlap of density from compacted bone. Radiographs obtained early often do not show the fracture, and so additional films may be required later.

Shoulder (Clavicle, Scapula, Shoulder Joint)

The most important injuries of the shoulder are fracture, dislocation, and joint disease. Such fractures in children result from falls and in adults usually from motor vehicle accidents.

Clavicle Fracture and Separation. Clavicular fractures result from a fall on an outstretched arm and are usually located in the middle or outer third of the bone. The lateral fragment is anteriorly and inferiorly displaced because of the weight of the arm (Fig. 7–34). These fractures usually heal completely if the arm is immobilized in good alignment. Complications from injury to brachiocephalic vessels are rare.

The related injury, acromio-clavicular separation, has a similar mechanism. The injury is made more severe by rupture of the coraco-clavicular ligaments. The clavicle moves upward, and the scapula, under the weight of the

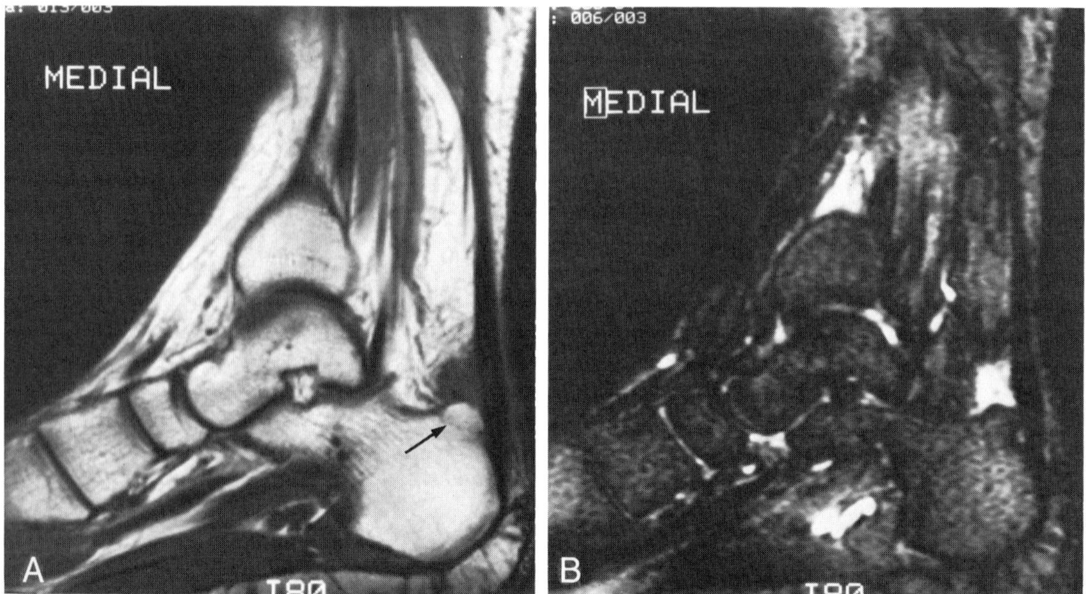

FIGURE 7–33. Retrocalcanear bursitis. *A.* T1 spin echo image shows a normal black intensity of the Achilles tendon in a woman with pain in that area. A bony prominence is present on the superior calcaneus *(arrow)*, and a low-density fluid collection is superior to it. *B.* The fluid collection, caused by retrocalcanear bursitis, is well-shown on the STIR image.

arm, moves down. The separation is clearly shown on AP radiographs. Confirmation can be made from an upright AP film showing both shoulders and made while the patient holds weights in both hands (weight-bearing films). On the injured side, the separation is exaggerated.

Scapula Fracture. Fractures of the scapula are stable because of self-splinting by the muscles that surround it. Stellate fractures of the paper-thin body can be difficult to detect. Fractures of the neck show overriding of the lateral fragment caused by the weight of the arm. Fractures of the coracoid and acromion processes are rare.

Shoulder Dislocation. Dislocation of the shoulder occurs most commonly in sports. Because of the anatomical structure of the joint and the usual mechanism of injury (a fall on an abducted arm), most dislocations (about 95%) are anterior. The anterior, medial, and inferior displacement of the humeral head is easily recognized on AP films (Fig. 7–35). An oblique view along the flat surface of the scapula (transscapular view) shows the humeral head inferior and anterior to the Y formed by the coracoid and acromion processes. An axillary view can show the same displacement, but the positioning is painful for an injured patient. A compression fracture (Hill-Sachs deformity) often occurs on the posterosuperior humeral head, where it impinges on the inferior glenoid fossa. This deformity may be seen in an acute form at the time of

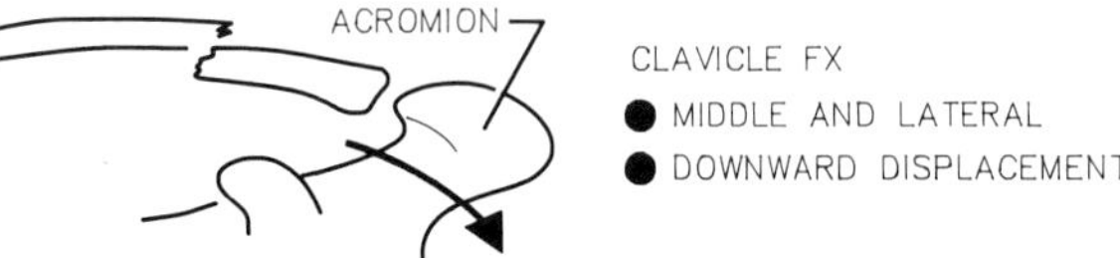

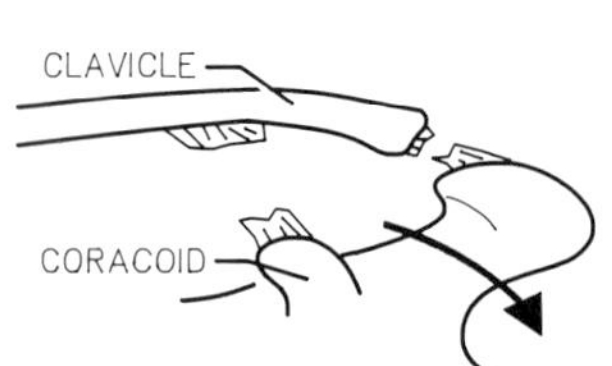

FIGURE 7–34. Characteristics of clavicular injury. FX, fracture.

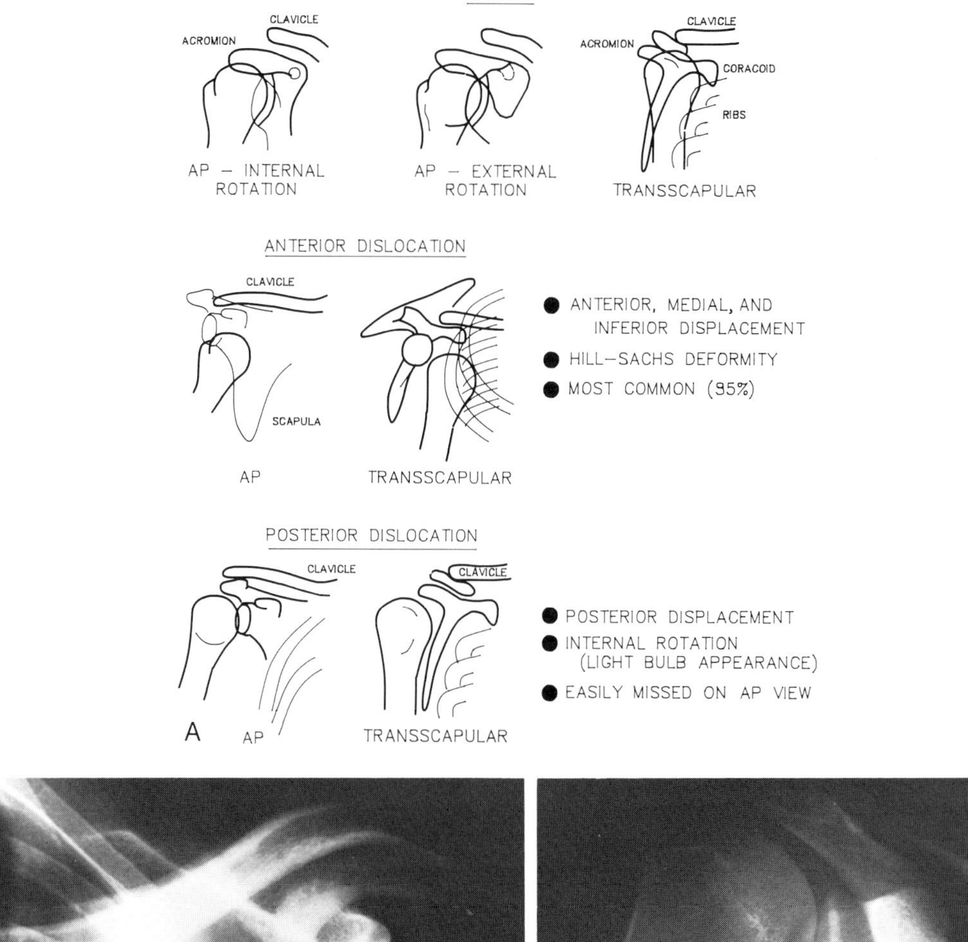

B

C

FIGURE 7–35. Shoulder dislocation. *A.* Diagram. FX, fracture. *B.* Anterior dislocation. AP view of the shoulder shows inferior and medial displacement of the humeral head, caused by anterior shoulder dislocation. Note the flattening of the superolateral humeral head (a Hill-Sachs deformity). *C.* Posterior dislocation. AP view shows apparent normal position of the humeral head. However, the humerus is internally rotated and is not symmetrically placed in the glenoid fossa. Transscapular view showed the humeral head behind the glenoid.

dislocation or later as evidence of previous anterior dislocation. The less common injury to the inferior glenoid fossa is called Bankart's deformity. Complications of anterior dislocation include injuries to the brachial plexus and the axillary nerve.

Posterior dislocation is less common (about 4%, sometimes seen after grand mal seizures) and is more easily missed on radiographs. The head of the humerus becomes internally rotated and is displaced directly posteriorly. On AP films it can appear to be in proper location (Fig. 7–35*C*). However, the internally rotated humerus has a symmetrical appearance (like a light bulb), which should raise suspicion of posterior dislocation. The diagnosis is easily made by means of clinical palpation of the humeral head and, on radiographs, from posterior displacement on the transscapular view. A third type, subglenoid dislocation, is least common (1%) and occurs when the arm is abducted and the humeral head becomes displaced beneath the glenoid fossa. Fractures associated with shoulder dislocation are further evaluated with CT scans.

Degenerative Shoulder Disease. Degenerative disease in the shoulder can involve the joint, the surrounding bursa, and the tendinous and ligamentous attachments. Shoulder pain and reduced mobility result from acute injury or chronic irritation and degeneration. Evaluation depends on an understanding of shoulder joint anatomical structure (see Fig. 7–4). The most common disease involves the rotator cuff, which is composed of the tendinous insertions of four muscles: the supraspinatus, the infraspinatus, the subscapularis, and the teres minor. These fibers join the fibrous joint capsule to rotate the humerus and stabilize the joint. The subacromial-subdeltoid bursa is a cavity separated from the joint space by the rotator cuff. Critical areas are in the supraspinatus tendon (1) as it passes beneath the acromion process and (2) where the cuff attaches to the humerus.

The most frequent cause of degenerative disease of the shoulder is impingement of the supraspinatus tendon as it passes beneath the acromion process. Narrowing of the humeral-acromial space places pressure on the rotator cuff. These tendons become inflamed from chronic rubbing by the bone margins. If untreated, this inflammation progresses to fibrosis, erosion, and degeneration. The most severe progression is a partial- or full-thickness tear of the supraspinatus tendon (rotator cuff tear). Full-thickness tears allow communication between the joint space and the subacromial-subdeltoid bursa. An equally serious tear of the insertion of the tendon into the humerus usually is the result of acute trauma. Endstage shoulder joint disease is the culmination of pain, degenerative disease, and decreased use, which result in smallness and contraction of the joint capsule and limited mobility. It is referred to clinically as adhesive capsulitis or frozen shoulder.

Evaluation of degenerative shoulder joint disease is initially performed with plain films, which can show joint-space narrowing, elevation of the humerus (called a high-riding shoulder), degeneration, and osteophyte formation. Contrast arthrography with plain films and CT can show the size of the joint space and enable diagnosis of a full-thickness tear (see Fig. 7–4), but these examinations are not effective in demonstrating a partial tear or early inflammatory disease. In addition, intra-articular injection of contrast is required. MRI is capable of demonstrating the anatomical structures of the joint in high-resolution T1 spin echo sequences and can show inflammatory tendinitis and abnormal joint and bursal fluid on high-contrast sequences, especially STIR (Fig. 7–36).

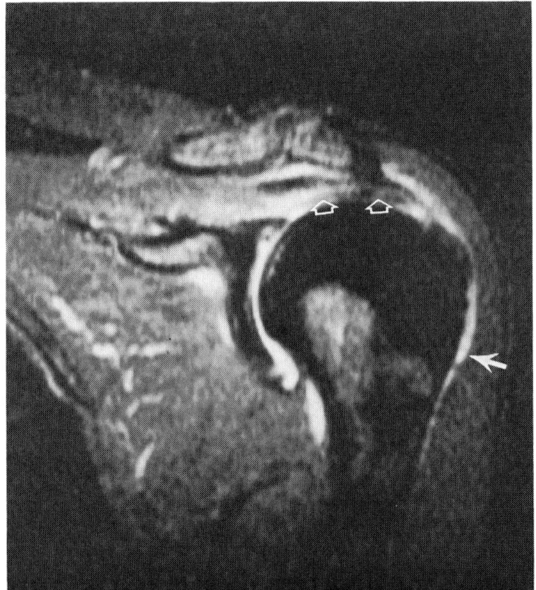

FIGURE 7–36. Rotator cuff tear. Coronal STIR image shows fluid in the subacromial-subdeltoid bursa *(arrow).* Irregularity and edema are present in the supraspinatus tendon insertion *(arrowheads).* This complete tear was also diagnosed on an arthrogram (see Fig. 7–4C).

Upper Extremity Fractures

Humerus Fracture. The most common fractures of the humerus occur at the proximal end and may include shoulder injuries. Fracture in the neck of the humerus is most common in elderly, osteoporotic women who fall on an outstretched arm. Fractures of the midshaft occur in severe trauma and must be suspected of causing injury to the radial nerve or the brachial artery.

Elbow Injury. Fractures at the elbow joint are difficult to diagnose because of the many bony condyles. This evaluation is more complicated in children than in adults because of the presence of growth centers in children. Fractures are detected from the presence of cortical interruption, alignment abnormalities, and displacement of the fat along the distal humerus. This fat is normally within the olecranon fossa posteriorly and is not seen on the lateral radiograph. A small amount of fat is usually seen anteriorly. However, when soft-tissue swelling or joint effusion occurs with fracture, these fat pads are displaced and become visible. Fat displaced posterior to the elbow on a flexed, lateral view (the posterior fat pad sign; Fig. 7–37) is the most reliable indicator of fracture. When this posterior fat is visible in a child, it is most often because of a supracondylar fracture of the humerus caused by a fall on a flexed elbow. In an adult, it usually indicates a fracture of the head of the radius caused by a fall on an outstretched arm. The anteriorly displaced fat (anterior fat pad sign) has a sail shape (the sail sign) and also indicates fracture.

Fractures of the ulna can result from a variety of mechanisms both in children and in adults. They can result from direct impact or avulsion and can occur in conjunction with dislocation. Monteggia's fracture is fracture of the proximal ulna with dislocation of the radial head (Fig. 7–38). These and other fractures at the elbow can be associated with serious complications from injury of the brachial artery; compression of the ulnar, median, and radial nerves; and necrosis of the radial head.

Ligamentous, avulsion, and epiphyseal injuries of the elbow are well-known by their causation. Nursemaid's elbow is the result of upward pull (extension) of the arm, which causes partial dislocation and entrapment of the radial annular ligament. Tennis elbow is tendinitis caused by irritation from repeated stress that affects the lateral humeral condyle. Little League elbow is avulsion of the medial epicondyle ossification center caused by severe valgus stress from throwing a baseball (especially a curve ball).

Forearm Fracture and Dislocation. Central fractures of the forearm occur at all ages. In children the fracture is often of a greenstick type, a break that is incomplete because of the pliability of the bones. It is therefore easily reduced and immobilized; complications are rare. In adults, the fractures are unstable and require internal fixation. Nonunion and cross-union are common in adults and lead to instability and limited function. Either bone can be fractured. The distal radius fracture is often accompanied by distal ulnar dislocation (Galeazzi's fracture). The nightstick fracture occurs when the ulna is used to block a blow by a club, a rod, or a nightstick. Fractures of the distal radius occur in children and in elderly people who fall on an outstretched hand. Frequently, the ulnar styloid is also involved. A distal fracture of both bones with dorsal angulation of the distal fragments is called Colles' fracture.

Wrist

The wrist contains eight bones and has complex function. Fractures are usually easily detected from breaks in the cortical margins. Dislocations and AVN are important considerations in trauma and in follow-up of an injury. The AP view of the wrist normally shows three smooth arcs made by (1) the radius and the ulna, (2) the distal borders of the proximal carpal bones, and (3) the proximal borders of the distal carpal bones. The most common injuries are navicular fracture and subsequent AVN, rotary subluxation of the navicular, lunate dislocation, and perilunate dislocation (Fig. 7–39). Plain films best show the fracture and alignment abnormalities. High-contrast MRI depicts early AVN.

Navicular Fracture. Navicular fracture (see Fig. 7–39*B*) results from a fall on an outstretched hand. Patients have pain in the anatomical snuff box (the space between the extensor pollicis longus and the abductor pollicis longus). The fracture is transverse and may not be immediately evident; repeat examination 1 or 2 weeks later may be required. Because the vascular supply to the navicular bone is retrograde through the distal part, AVN of the proximal fragment is common. AVN or nonunion may require treatment by bone or prosthetic graft.

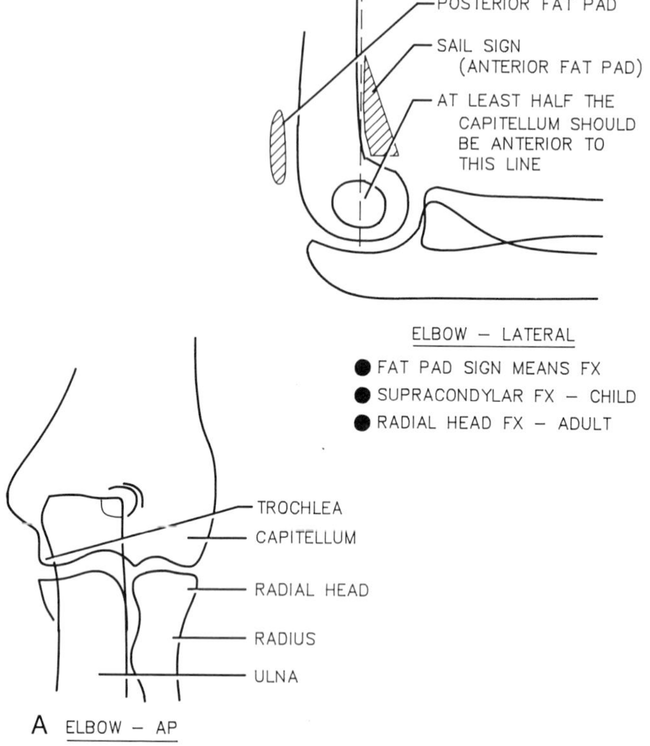

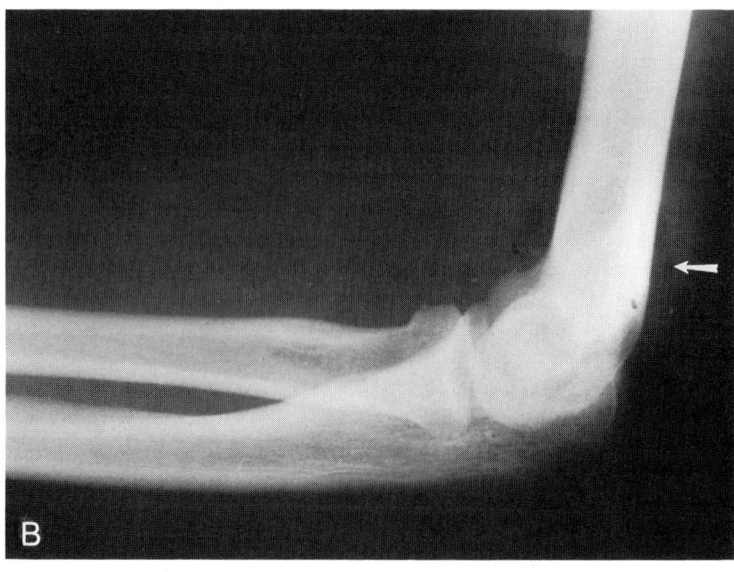

FIGURE 7–37. Elbow fracture (FX). *A.* Diagram. *B.* Lateral plain film of the flexed elbow shows low-density (black) fat directly behind the distal humerus *(arrow),* indicating a fracture, in a young man. The AP view showed a radial head fracture.

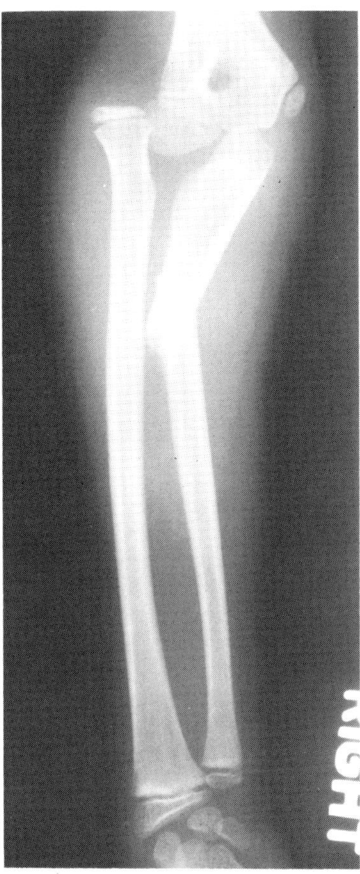

FIGURE 7–38. Monteggia's fracture. AP film of the forearm in a young girl shows a fracture of the proximal ulna and associated dislocation of the radial head.

Lunate Dislocation. Lunate dislocation results from a fall on a severely extended wrist. The crescent-shaped lunate bone rolls forward (volar) from the rest of the carpus (see Fig. 7–39*D*). AP films show interruption of the middle arc and a pie-shaped shadow in the normal location of the lunate bone. The dislocation is obvious on the lateral view. Complications of lunate dislocation include AVN (called Kienböck's malacia; see Fig. 7–40*B*) and median nerve injury from direct compression.

Perilunate Dislocation. Perilunate dislocation is a posterior dislocation of the capitate bone, which normally articulates with the lunate bone. However, in this case, the remainder of the carpus moves with the capitate bone, leaving the lunate and navicular bones in normal articulation with the radius. Navicular fracture is also often present.

Rotary Subluxation of the Navicular Bone. Rotary subluxation of the navicular bone is a dissociation of the navicular and lunate bones caused by distraction and rotation as a result of trauma. It also occurs after reduction of a lunate dislocation and can occur in rheumatoid arthritis. AP radiographs show a widened space between the navicular and lunate bones (see Fig. 7–39*C*).

Hand

Fractures of the hand are easily identified on plain films. Characteristic locations include the distal fourth or fifth metacarpal, broken when a fist hits a solid object (boxer's fracture; see Fig. 7–3); the first carpal-metacarpal joint, fracture dislocation of which results from forced abduction (Bennett's fracture); and the first metacarpal, fracture of which is caused by flexion impact. Fractures and ligamentous injuries of the phalanges have important consequences for normal hand function. Even small avulsions and purely ligamentous injuries may require casting or fixation in order to ensure proper alignment and function.

General Injuries

Avascular Necrosis (Osteonecrosis). AVN as its name implies, is caused by interruption of the blood supply to bone. This can occur in several ways: (1) by a fracture or a dislocation, (2) by compression extrinsic to the blood vessel by local edema or hematoma, (3) by intrinsic thickening of the walls of the vessel by inflammation, or (4) by obliteration of the lumen by thrombus, embolus, or gas. Besides trauma, AVN is associated with alcoholism and steroid therapy. "Osteonecrosis" is a more general term and can be applied to the majority of cases of AVN and infarction.

When the avascular segment of bone is confined to the medullary cavity, it is called a bone infarct. When it involves an articular surface, it is usually called AVN or osteonecrosis. AVN is often seen in the hip and knee. Other characteristic locations are in bones with limited blood supply, such as the talus or carpal bones. Many of these lesions have eponyms: Kienböck's disease of the carpal lunate bone, Freiberg's disease of the head of the second metatarsal, Blount's disease of the proximal medial tibial metaphysis, and Scheuermann's disease in the thoracic spine.

In all forms of AVN, the bone first undergoes an edematous phase during which the patient experiences pain, but no structural

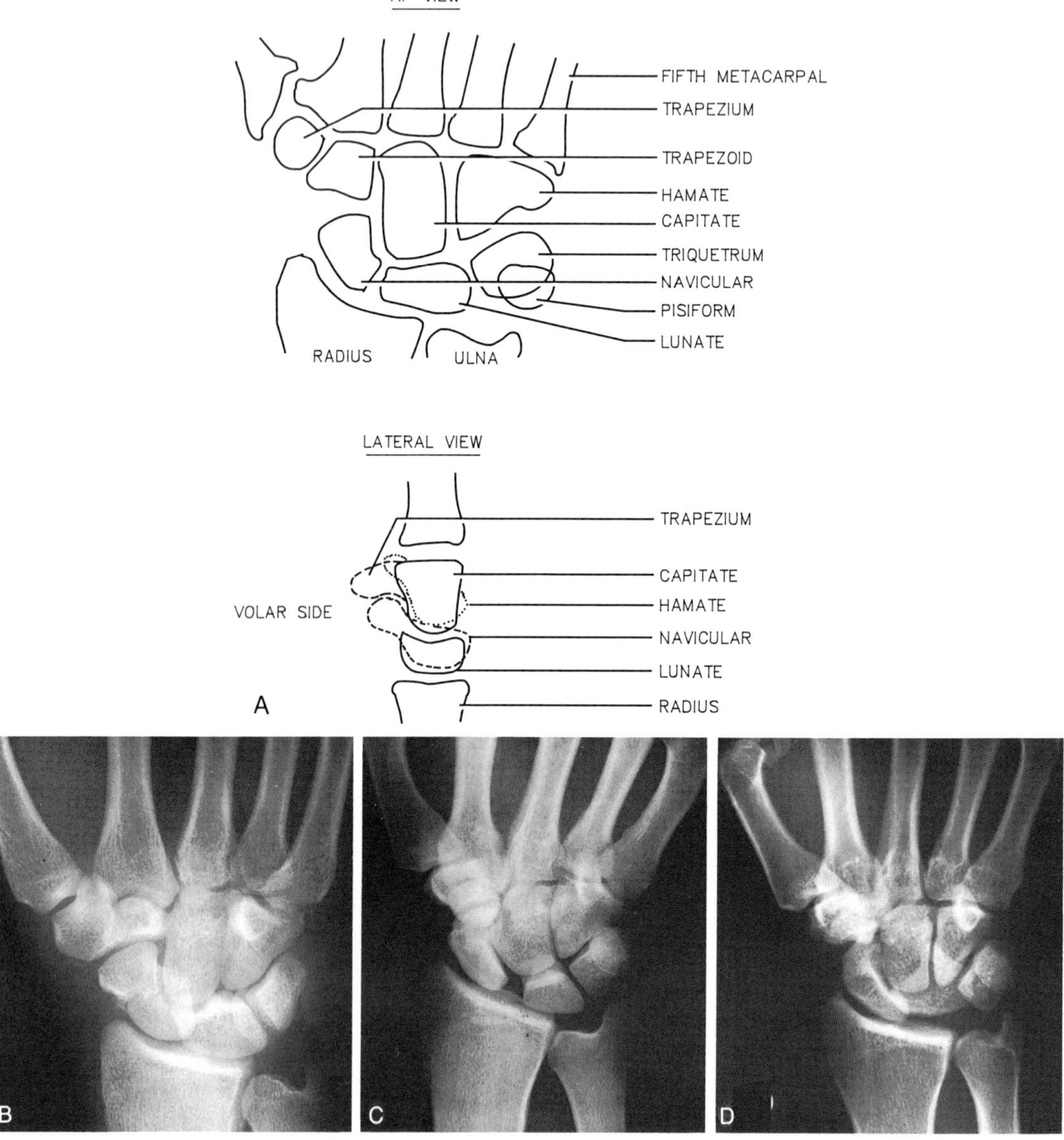

FIGURE 7–39. Carpal injuries. *A.* Diagram. *B.* Navicular fracture. AP hand film shows a transverse break in the navicular bone. The proximal fragment is at high risk for avascular necrosis (AVN). *C.* Rotary subluxation of the navicular. AP film shows a large gap between the navicular and the lunate bones, indicating ligamentous injury in the proximal carpus. *D.* Lunate dislocation. AP film shows loss of the smooth arc of the proximal carpal bones and a triangular appearance of the lunate bone (the pie sign) as a result of anterior subluxation. The patient fell while carrying a heavy box, wedging his wrist between the box and stairs, popping the lunate forward. This was well-shown on the lateral view (not pictured).

damage (apart from the fracture) is evident on plain films. MRI with STIR or T2 spin echo sequences clearly shows the edema in such cases. Nuclear medicine bone scans can show evidence of inflammatory response, but MRI shows such abnormalities earlier in the disease process. Later, the bone shows margin resorption and eventually collapse, well-demonstrated by plain films. Healing of such lesions is difficult to assess. The edema shown on MRI may persist indefinitely.

The MRI appearance is similar in all cases. A T1 spin echo image is most capable of showing the replacement of high-intensity fatty marrow by low-intensity edema (Fig. 7–40). In the carpal navicular bone, the proximal fracture fragment is at risk for AVN because the blood supply enters from the distal portion. In the knee, the most common site for AVN, the lesion is adjacent to the cortical margin of the joint space (Fig. 7–40*A*). In the ankle, the second most common site, AVN occurs in the proximal talus as the result of compression injury or fracture (Fig. 7–40*C*). In the hip (Fig. 7–40*D* and *E*) and the spine, AVN may be caused by fracture or steroid therapy. Initially, edema is present without collapse. At this stage, the MRI appearance is similar to that of tumor. Compression fracture can develop later. A combination of plain films and clinical examination may be required in order to make the distinction between tumor and such compression in both the hip and the spine.

Myositis Ossificans. Myositis ossificans is neither an inflammatory process nor an ossification. It is a calcified residual of trauma or hemorrhage in the soft tissues adjacent to a bone and appears 2 to 8 weeks after trauma. On plain films, it has the appearance of a mass lesion adjacent to the bone. A dense, smoothly marginated rim of calcification surrounds the lesion (Fig. 7–41). The appearance is similar to that of parosteal sarcoma (to be discussed), and a biopsy specimen can appear malignant. In general, these lesions are resorbed over a 6-month period.

Stress Fracture. Stress fractures result from repeated stress, often caused by overuse or new activity. Walking, jogging, sports, and occupational changes are the usual causes. The first symptom is pain. Radiographs are often normal initially. Delayed films a week or so after the onset of pain may show bony sclerosis, a fracture line, or a periosteal reaction. The most common sites are the lower extremities because of their weight-bearing function. Typical sites include the femoral neck (Fig. 7–42), the tibia, and the metatarsals. Stress fracture of the tibia in a young child, called a toddler's fracture, is discussed later with pediatric bone diseases (see Fig. 7–94).

CONGENITAL ABNORMALITIES

Isolated Congenital Anomalies

Isolated congenital anomalies of the osseous system are common and are usually of no concern except when a patient being evaluated for trauma has a normal variant that cannot be definitely distinguished from fracture. In general, these normal variants are caused by additional ossification centers or irregular ossification. They are well-corticated and do not show evidence of acute fracture.

Generalized Bone Dysplasia Syndromes

Many syndromes are associated with bone dysplasia (Fig. 7–43). Some of these syndromes, such as achondroplasia, osteogenesis imperfecta, fibrous dysplasia, and osteopetrosis, involve predominantly the osseous structures. Others, such as neurofibromatosis, Marfan's syndrome, and the hemoglobinopathies are primarily soft-tissue or visceral diseases but have characteristic bone manifestations. These congenital bone diseases are rare. The radiologist's role is usually to suggest a bone dysplasia when a bone anomaly is identified or to describe the complications of the disease in a patient with an established diagnosis. Some typical bone lesions of very rare diseases are listed in Table 7–1.

Achondroplasia. Achondroplasia is the most common syndrome associated with dwarfism. It is caused by defective endochondral bone formation that results in normally formed but short bones of the extremities (see Fig. 7–43). Some cases show autosomally dominant inheritance, but most (90%) are sporadic. A normal-sized trunk, a large head, and short extremities constitute the usual appearance. Serious neurological problems develop as a result of overgrowth of the skull base, which produces a narrow foramen magnum, and as a result of congenital spinal stenosis, which causes lower neurological impairment.

Osteogenesis Imperfecta. Osteogenesis imperfecta is an autosomally dominant inherited disease characterized by a failure of osteoid

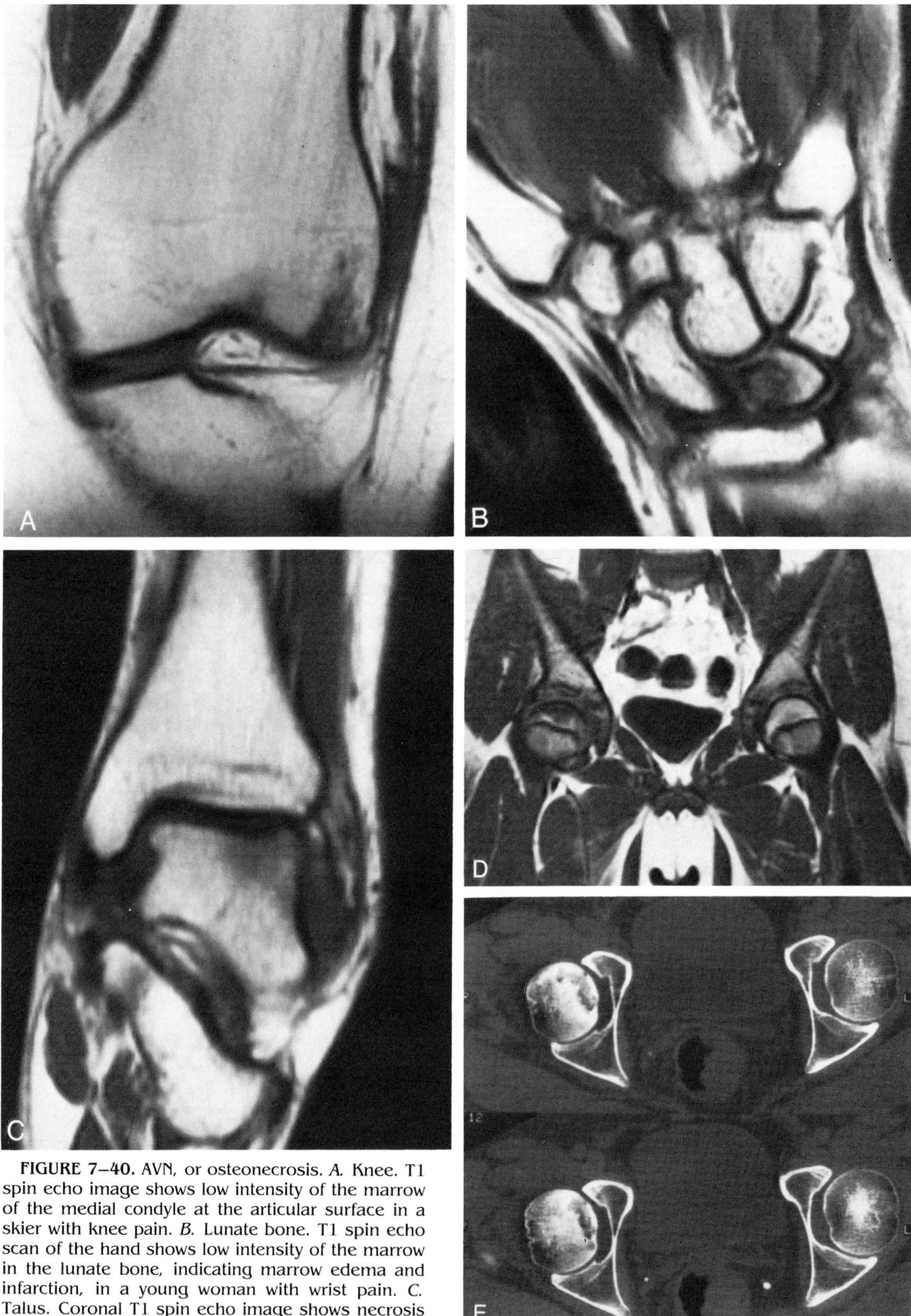

FIGURE 7–40. AVN, or osteonecrosis. *A.* Knee. T1 spin echo image shows low intensity of the marrow of the medial condyle at the articular surface in a skier with knee pain. *B.* Lunate bone. T1 spin echo scan of the hand shows low intensity of the marrow in the lunate bone, indicating marrow edema and infarction, in a young woman with wrist pain. *C.* Talus. Coronal T1 spin echo image shows necrosis of the medial talus in a man who fell from a second story. Low-intensity fluid is present in the medial joint space. *D.* Hip. Coronal T1 spin echo image shows low intensity in the right femoral head in a patient receiving high-dose steroid therapy. The left hip is normal. *E.* Hip. CT in another patient shows low-density necrosis and high-density sclerosis in the right femoral head.

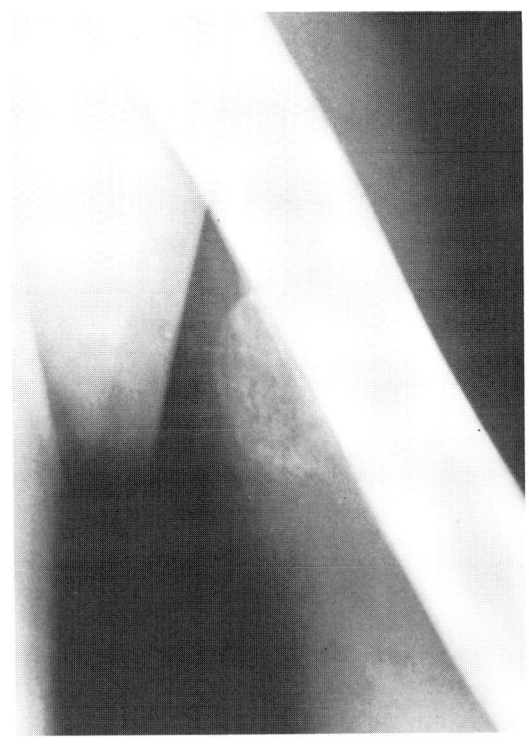

FIGURE 7–41. Myositis ossificans. AP film of the proximal femur shows a calcified lesion extending medially. Associated periosteal elevation is also present. CT scan (not shown) showed the calcification to be in the periphery of the lesion.

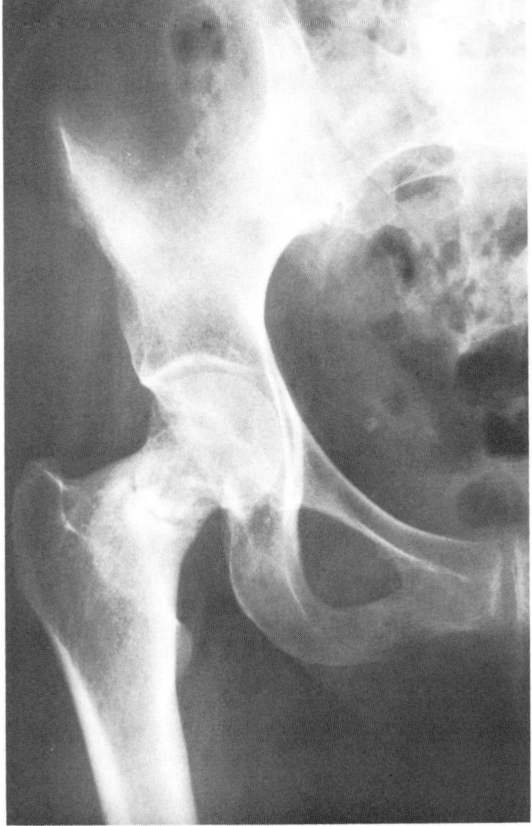

FIGURE 7–42. Stress fracture. AP view of the hip shows a transverse fracture of the femoral neck in a woman who had had pain for 3 weeks. Note also the presence of bone sclerosis.

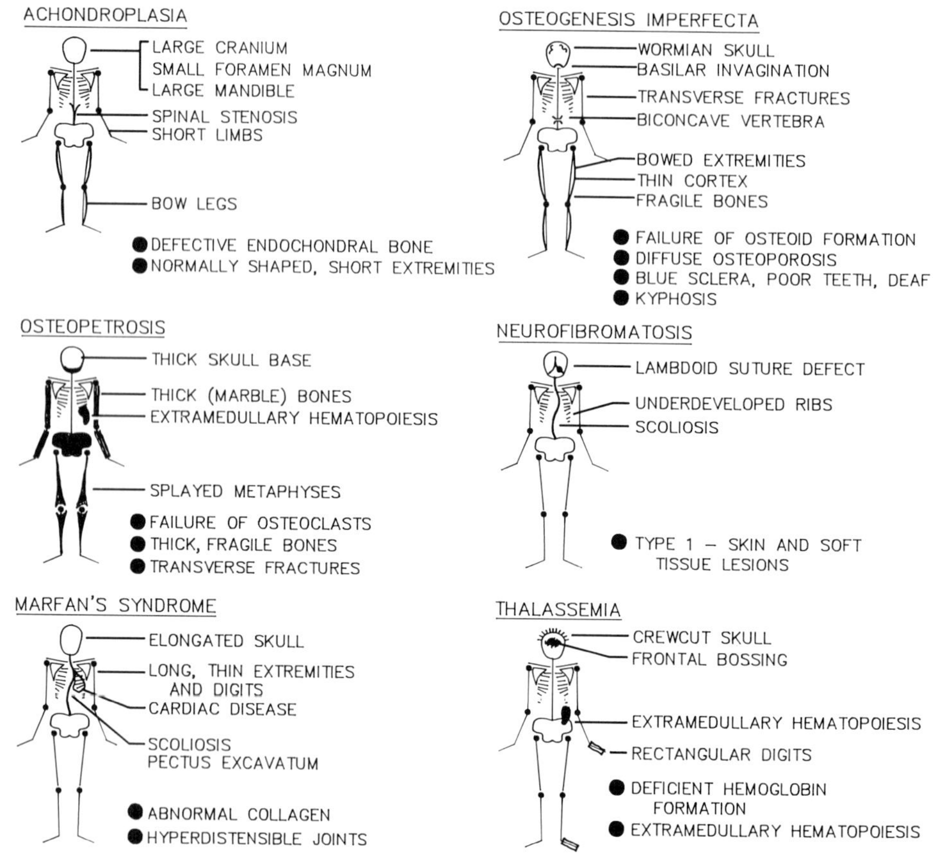

FIGURE 7–43. Types of bone dysplasias.

formation that results in pliable, fragile bones. Bowing of the long bones, concave scalloping of the vertebral bodies, and thin cortex and transverse fractures of the long bones are the most common radiographic findings (see Fig. 7–43). Thin skin, poor dentition, mobile joints, deafness (from otosclerosis), and a bluish color of the sclera are additional clinical findings. The pliability of the bones can lead to severe kyphosis of the spine and invagination of the skullbase (basilar invagination), which in turn lead to serious compression of the spinal cord or the brainstem. Exuberant bone formation can be indistinguishable from osteosarcoma, which is also an important complication of this disease.

Fibrous Dysplasia. Fibrous dysplasia is a congenital lesion of fibrous tissue that causes lysis in one bone (monostotic form) or many bones (polyostotic form). It is uncommon but important because it can have a variety of appearances. The lesions are generally expan-

TABLE 7–1. ABNORMALITIES IN RARE BONE DYSPLASIAS

Cleidocranial dysostosis	Midline defects, including open sagittal suture, cleft sternum, and unfused pubic symphysis; also, absent lateral clavicles
Chondroectodermal dysplasia	Mesectodermal defects, including polydactyly, cone-shaped epiphyses, delayed tooth formation, and congenital heart disease
Diaphyseal sclerosis (Engelman's disease)	Symmetrical, painful thickening of femur, tibia, and skullbase
Hurler's syndrome	Mucopolysaccharide storage disease: early suture closure; thick, flared ribs; short, thick bones of hands and feet; mental retardation
Gaucher's syndrome	Cerebroside storage disease: thickened, rectangular long bones with coarse trabeculae, thin cortex, and decreased density
Turner's syndrome	XO chromosome anomaly: short fourth metacarpal, depressed tibial plateau, abnormal wrist and elbow angulation, webbed neck
Dermatomyositis	Soft tissue calcification, indistinct fat-muscle borders

sile and replace normal cortex and marrow with a disorganized fibrous material. The bones most commonly involved are the pelvis, the proximal femur, the ribs, and the skull.

Patients are usually asymptomatic except when a pathological fracture occurs in a long bone or when thickening of the skullbase compresses the brainstem or the cranial nerves. The lesions are painless. Long bone lesions typically are elongated, well-circumscribed, and of low density on plain films, but the appearance is highly variable (Fig. 7–44). There is no periostitis, as occurs in tumors and infection. T1 spin echo MRI scans show an

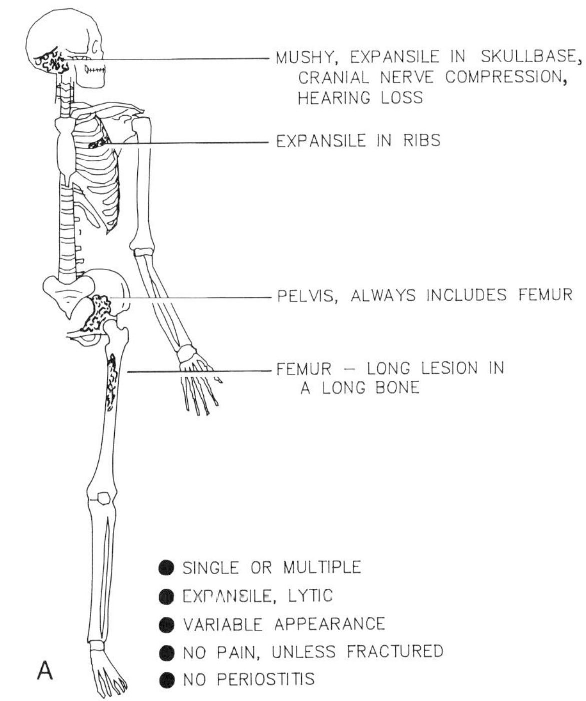

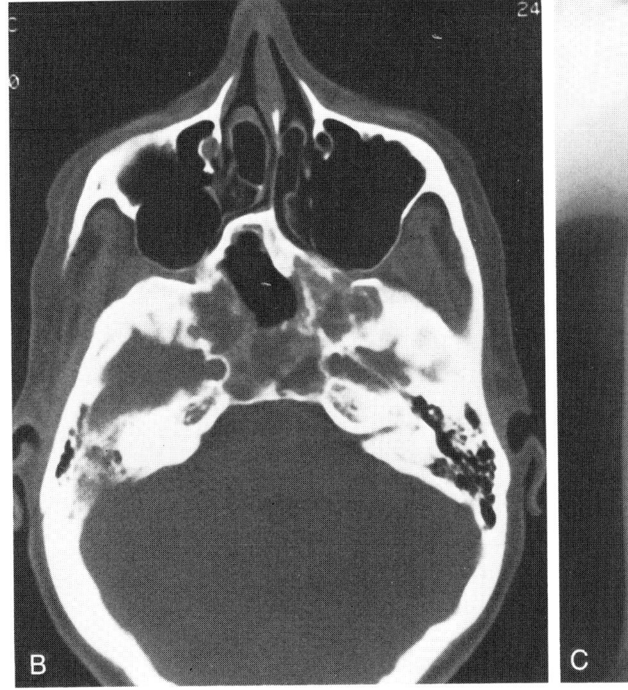

FIGURE 7–44. Fibrous dysplasia. *A.* Diagram. *B.* CT scan shows expansion and low density of the sphenoid bone with distortion of the sphenoid sinus. Surgery was performed in order to rule out skullbase invasion of metastatic disease. The dysplastic, mushy bone was characteristic of fibrous dysplasia. Note also aerated middle turbinates, which are of no clinical consequence unless they cause obstruction to sinus drainage or become obstructed themselves. *C.* The left humerus of a 19-year-old female shows an elongated ovoid osteolytic region with sclerotic margin. The lytic lesion shows a ground-glass matrix characteristic of fibrous dysplasia. The edge of the lesion is well-defined with some areas of scalloping of the endosteal surface of the cortex and other areas of sclerosis. A septum is formed across the medullary cavity, separating the lesion from the normal-appearing distal half of the humerus. (Courtesy of J. F. Garcia, Department of Radiology, University of New Mexico School of Medicine.)

intermediate intensity. A syndrome of cafe au lait spots, precocious puberty, and fibrous dysplasia is called McCune-Albright syndrome. Fibrous dysplasia has no malignant potential.

Osteopetrosis. Osteopetrosis is caused by dysfunction of osteoclasts that results in uniform sclerosis. The entire skeleton contains dense, fragile bones (see Fig. 7–43). The marrow spaces are obliterated and the neural foramina are narrowed, which result in extramedullary hematopoiesis and cranial nerve dysfunction. One of the more common problems is deafness caused by overgrowth of the petrous bones and consequent destruction or obliteration of the internal auditory canals and middle ear structures.

Neurofibromatosis. Neurofibromatosis is the term used to describe two inherited diseases, both of which are characterized by neural tissue tumors. Neurofibromatosis type 1 is associated with cafe au lait skin lesions, neurofibromas, and soft-tissue tumors; it is also termed von Recklinghausen's disease. Bone lesions include low-density lesions in the skull, underdeveloped inferior ribs, scoliosis, spinal dural ectasia, and bone overgrowth (see Fig. 7–43). Other bone abnormalities, such as exophthalmos and widened neural foramina, are caused by adjacent growth of neurofibromas. Neurofibromatosis type 2 is usually limited to neural tissue tumors. Neurofibromatosis is discussed in more detail in Chapters 2 and 8.

Marfan's Syndrome. Marfan's syndrome is caused by abnormal collagen and results in hyperdistensible joints and elongation and thinning of ribs and extremities (see Fig. 7–43). Scoliosis and pectus excavatum are common. Aortic aneurysm, aortic valve insufficiency, and pulmonary artery dilatation are the most serious consequences (discussed in Chapter 5).

Thalassemia. The hemoglobinopathies, of which thalassemia is the most severe, result in bone abnormalities caused by enlargement of the marrow space, a consequence of the accelerated attempt at hematopoiesis. A hair-on-end (crew-cut) appearance of the skull is the result of the expanded diploic space (see Fig. 7–43). Squaring and trabeculation of the bones of the hands and feet are also caused by abnormal marrow expansion. Sickle cell anemia involves similar but less severe changes.

Basal Cell Nevus Syndrome. The basal cell nevus syndrome, inherited by autosomal dominant gene, is characterized by multiple basal cell carcinomas of the skin, seizures, and mental retardation. Rib and vertebral anomalies are common, as are multiple odontogenic cysts of the mandible and maxilla. Lamellar calcification of the falx is seen on CT scans of the brain.

SYSTEMIC DISEASES

Many systemic diseases affect bone formation or mineralization through their effect on calcium metabolism. These diseases are most commonly caused by endocrine or renal dysfunction. The parathyroid glands, the gut, the skin, the liver, and the kidneys affect the use of calcium by bone. Other compounds such as steroids and estrogens also affect bone mineralization. Abnormal bone mineralization is diagnosed and evaluated primarily with plain films, which show the highest resolution and thus easily demonstrate the cortex, the medullary cavity, and the trabecular pattern. For most diagnostic purposes, bone density is adequately assessed from such radiographs. For treatment, quantitative tests are also available through CT and other absorption techniques. MRI best shows the marrow cavity and best addresses pathological fracture caused by tumor. Nuclear medicine bone scintigraphy demonstrates a characteristic pattern of uptake in most metabolic diseases (see Chapter 9).

Osteoporosis. The most common systemic disease of bone is osteoporosis, a generalized demineralization process that is most pervasive among elderly women as a result of age and endocrine factors. Other causes of osteoporosis are disuse, as from immobilization for fracture, and neurogenic atrophy (called Sudeck's atrophy or reflex sympathetic dystrophy), as a result of an injury (Table 7–2). Steroid therapy (to be discussed) also causes osteoporosis. The radiographic appearance is decreased density, thin cortex, and an apparent coarsening of the trabecular pattern. In elderly patients, it is most evident in the spine, the pelvis, and the hips. Compression fractures of the spine and fractures of the femoral neck are common and have serious consequences because they do not heal well.

Hyperparathyroidism. Hyperparathyroidism is the most common cause of abnormalities in calcium metabolism. It exists in three forms: primary, as a result of increased secretion of parathyroid hormone (PTH) by a parathyroid adenoma or hyperplasia; secondary, as a result of renal failure in which the elevated phosphate level stimulates increased production of PTH and, in addition, normal vitamin D me-

TABLE 7–2. CAUSES OF OSTEOPOROSIS

Type	Cause
Disuse	Being bedridden, immobilized fracture
Neurogenic	Distal to an injury after trauma (Sudeck's atrophy)
Postmenopausal	Endocrine change leads to bone resorption
Senile	Disuse or aging leads to decreased mineralization
Corticosteroids	Cushing's disease or steroid therapy causes resorption
Malnutrition	Lack of dietary calcium or vitamin D
Scurvy	Lack of vitamin C, which is essential for bone matrix formation

tabolism is prevented; and tertiary, the result of long-term parathyroid stimulation and chronic renal failure, which cause autonomous PTH secretion.

The effects of PTH stimulation on the bones are the same in all three forms of hyperparathyroidism (Fig. 7–45). They include generalized demineralization, subperiosteal cortical bone erosions, and erosive or cystic changes of the small joints of the hands and wrists. In rare instances, encapsulated cystic lesions filled with a brownish fluid (called brown tumors) are found in the long bones, the jaw, and the pelvis. Later, particularly with renal failure, sclerotic changes occur partly as a result of the relative demineralization in other bones and partly as a result of the complex metabolic process that takes place in long-standing renal failure.

Other problems caused by increased PTH production are attributable to elevated serum calcium levels. The most common problems are metastatic calcification (especially in the arteries, the kidneys, the joints, the pancreas, and the soft tissues) and renal stone formation. In hyperparathyroidism associated with renal failure, the calcium level is generally low because of decreased absorption of serum calcium. Rickets (hypocalcemia caused by decreased vitamin D) and renal osteodystrophy (renal rickets) often result in demineralization, followed by sclerosis.

Corticosteroid-Related Bone Changes. Bone changes caused by elevated corticosteroid levels can result from Cushing's disease or from exogenous steroid therapy for lung disease, cancer therapy, or organ transplantation. The hips and the spine are the most

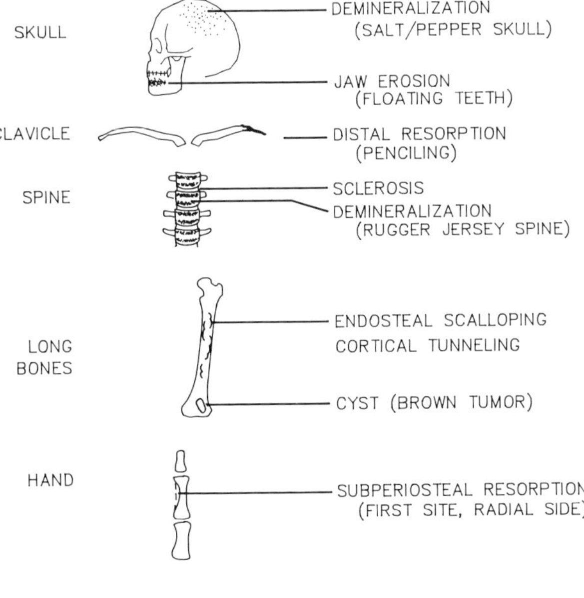

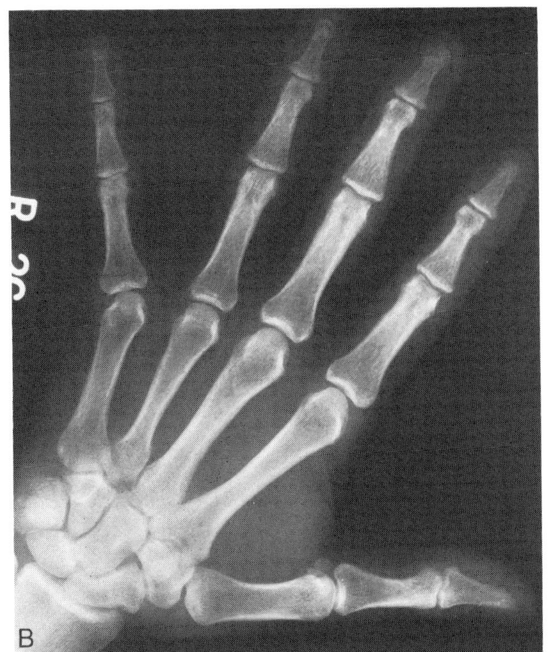

FIGURE 7–45. Demineralization processes in hyperparathyroidism and renal failure. *A.* Diagram. *B.* Plain film of the hand shows erosion of the radial cortex of the middle phalanges in a man with hyperparathyroidism caused by renal failure. The earliest involvement of hyperparathyroidism is often evident in this location.

important areas affected. AVN of the hip (discussed earlier) is best evaluated with MRI, which shows the earliest signs of edema, marrow destruction, and hemorrhage. Hip fracture also occurs as a result of the weakened, demineralized bone.

In addition, the spine becomes demineralized. On plain films, there is apparent accentuation of cortical margins as a result of the internal demineralization (an appearance likened to a picture frame). Vertical striations and compression fractures may also be seen. In patients with lung disease (at risk for lung cancer) or undergoing cancer therapy, a compression fracture of the spine must be distinguished from metastatic tumor involvement. Films of a benign compression fracture show cortical disruption and may show hemorrhage. Films of a pathological fracture show internal tumor, adjacent tumor mass, and tumor in other bones. A pathological fracture generally is of higher intensity on STIR and T2 spin echo images than is a benign fracture. Blood can have a variety of intensities on MRI scans and therefore often provides a confusing appearance. Plain films and CT scans can show fracture margins and a paraspinous soft-tissue mass.

Acromegaly. Acromegaly is caused by excess growth hormone, usually as a result of a growth hormone–secreting tumor. It can also be caused by exogenous growth hormone abuse. The radiographic features are overgrowth of the distal (acral) skeleton. The most obviously affected bones are the digits and the jaw. These changes develop gradually, and so the disease is often not recognized until someone sees the patient for the first time in years or an old photograph is compared with the patient's current appearance. As a result, growth hormone–secreting pituitary adenomas are often large when finally identified. Radiographs of the hands and feet show enlargement of distal digits (Fig. 7–46). Radiographs of the jaw show dense, thickened, elongated bone. Skull films can show sellar erosion, but the diagnosis of pituitary tumor is made from CT and MRI (see Chapter 8).

Other Endocrine Diseases. Other endocrine diseases that affect bone formation or metabolism are thyroid acropachy (which causes thickening of the periosteum of the digits), cretinism (in utero hypothyroidism that causes deformity and delayed maturation), hypophosphatasia (similar to rickets), and hyperphosphatasia (thick diaphyseal cortex, similar to Paget's disease, which is discussed later). These diseases are uncommon, and the diagnosis is usually known or suspected from other signs and symptoms.

Vitamin and Element Excess and Deficiency. Vitamins D, A, and C can affect bone growth and metabolism. Vitamin D is required for calcium metabolism, and so deficiency

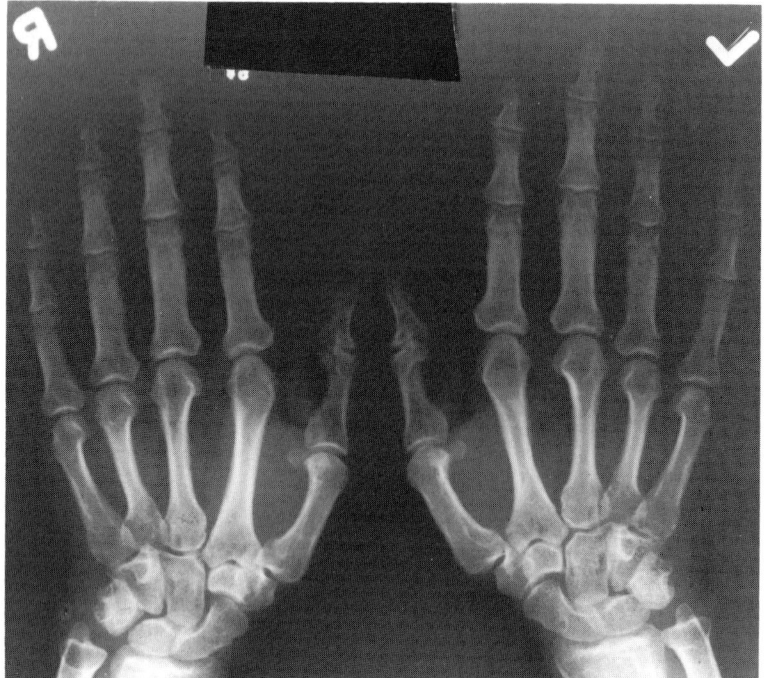

FIGURE 7–46. Acromegaly. Plain film of the hands shows marked enlargement of the phalanges in a man with a pituitary adenoma. Note the size of the phalanges in comparison with that of the metacarpals (see Fig. 7–45 for comparison of normal proportions).

causes rickets in children and osteoporosis in adults. Vitamin D excess causes metastatic calcification, renal stones, and osteosclerosis. Vitamin A excess can cause periostitis, which results in cortical thickening of the long bones. Vitamin C deficiency causes scurvy. The abnormalities are disruption of bone formation and hemorrhage. The effects are most evident in children (see the later section on pediatric bone diseases). Lead poisoning and fluorosis also result in denseness of bone. In lead poisoning, lead-containing bone is laid down in the metaphysis during exposure, forming dense bands in the shaft. Fluorosis results in generalized increased bone density and calcification of ligamentous insertions. The condition is unusual except in areas with high concentrations of fluoride in the drinking water or in patients treated with sodium fluoride for osteoporosis.

Paget's Disease. Paget's disease is a metabolic bone disease characterized by bone breakdown and subsequent replacement by enlarged, thickened bone. This abnormal bone has a coarsened trabecular pattern, and blood flow is greatly increased within it. Patients are usually over the age of 50 and may have a variety of symptoms, including pain, fracture, or the development of a tumor. The most common sites of involvement (in order of frequency) are the pelvis, the femur, the skull, the tibia, the vertebrae, the clavicle, the humerus, and the ribs.

Any part of the pelvis can be involved in Paget's disease. In some cases the entire pelvis is involved, which suggests the presence of a generalized metabolic bone disease. The appearance is often confused with that of blastic metastases. The iliopectineal line is commonly involved in Paget's disease and not in metastatic disease, and this distinction enables differentiation in some cases. In the femur, the lesion typically involves the upper shaft, beginning at the end of the bone and extending inferiorly. The lower margin is often jagged (flame-shaped). The distribution, the bone enlargement, and the thickened trabeculae usually facilitate diagnosis. Paget's disease sometimes originates in the central portion of the tibia but usually begins at the end of a long bone. It is rare for the fibula to be involved.

In the skull, there may be a dense thickening of the calvarium or well-circumscribed areas of low density (called osteoporosis circumscripta). In the spine, cortical thickening and overall enlargement are seen in the vertebral bodies. The trabeculae are large and coarse. This appearance can be similar to that of hemangioma or of metastatic tumor. Differentiation among these lesions can be difficult because all three may show contrast enhancement on CT or MRI.

Diagnosis may be made from plain films, CT, or MRI (Fig. 7–47). The diagnosis is most easily made from plain films, which in most cases show enlargement, cortical thickening, and coarsened trabeculae. The location of the abnormality and the type of bone involved also further assist in diagnosis. CT can show the coarse trabecular pattern, but the generalized enlargement of the bone may not be appreciated. MRI is most useful for ruling out bone disease that has a similar appearance, such as a metastatic tumor. Lesions of Paget's disease show intense uptake on nuclear medicine bone scans (see Chapter 9).

The bone involved in Paget's disease is brittle and can fracture easily. There is also an associated risk of development of osteogenic sarcoma. Osteogenic sarcoma can be detected radiographically from the appearance of bone erosion and the development of a soft-tissue mass.

INFLAMMATORY DISEASES

Osteomyelitis

Osteomyelitis (acute or chronic infection of the bone) is caused by contiguous invasion from a soft-tissue infection or from hematogenous spread in a patient with septicemia.

Local Invasion. Local invasion of infection originates from soft-tissue abscess, cellulitis, and wound infection. The radiographic findings of these infections are effacement of the soft tissue and muscle planes, cortical erosion, and elevation of the adjacent periosteum (Fig. 7–48). These findings are unreliable: they are often not seen in early infection and may be present with other diseases. It is not possible to rule out bone infection from the appearance on radiographs. Delayed or chronic infections often lead to marked reactive bone formation and bone destruction.

Hematogenously Spread Osteomyelitis. Hematogenously spread bone infection is usually caused by *Staphylococcus aureus*. Other infections are caused by gram-negative bacteria in patients with septicemia. The infections usually occur near the metaphysis, the region of maximal blood flow. Cortical destruction, periosteal elevation, and a soft-tissue mass may assist

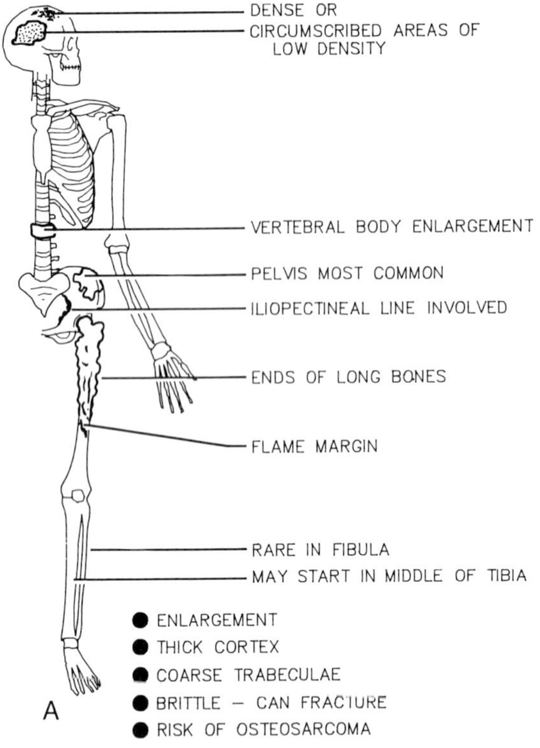

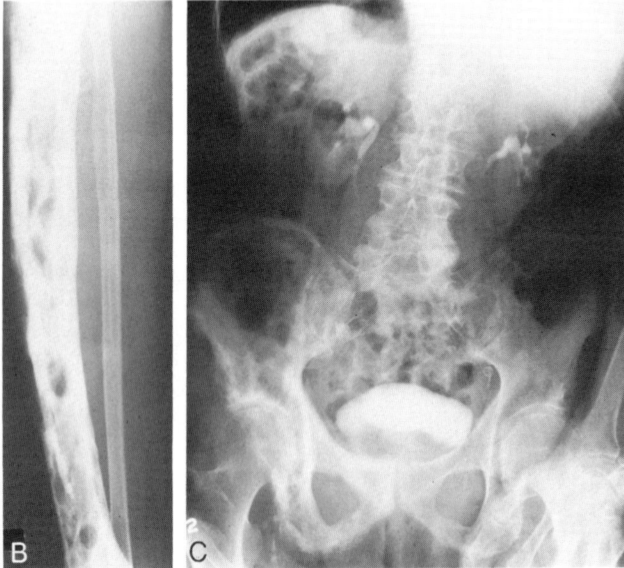

FIGURE 7–47. Paget's disease. *A.* Diagram. *B.* Lateral plain film of the tibia shows tertiary-stage Paget's disease with disorganization of the trabecular cortical pattern, mixed areas of sclerosis and lysis, and anterior bowing and enlargement. *C.* Intravenous urographic film shows Paget's disease of the right innominate bone involving the ischium, the pubis, and the iliac bone. The sacrum is not involved. The ischium and the pubis on the right side are clearly larger than those on the left side, which is not involved. Note involvement of the right iliopectineal line, a characteristic finding of Paget's disease. (Courtesy of J. F. Garcia, Department of Radiology, University of New Mexico School of Medicine.)

in diagnosis but often are not present. These abnormalities do not usually appear until 2 weeks after the infection has begun. Often the infection appears on plain films as a low-density (lytic) lesion similar to many bone tumors and cysts. Bone scintigraphy and MRI are sensitive for evaluation of early osteomyelitis. Bone scintigraphy shows increased uptake as a result of reactive bone formation. MRI shows edema and alteration of the marrow fat. CT can show involvement of the medullary cavity.

Joint Infection. Joint infection is most commonly caused by pyogenic bacteria; infections by atypical organisms and by tuberculosis are less common. Septic arthritis is usually diagnosed clinically and confirmed by joint aspiration (which may be performed by the ra-

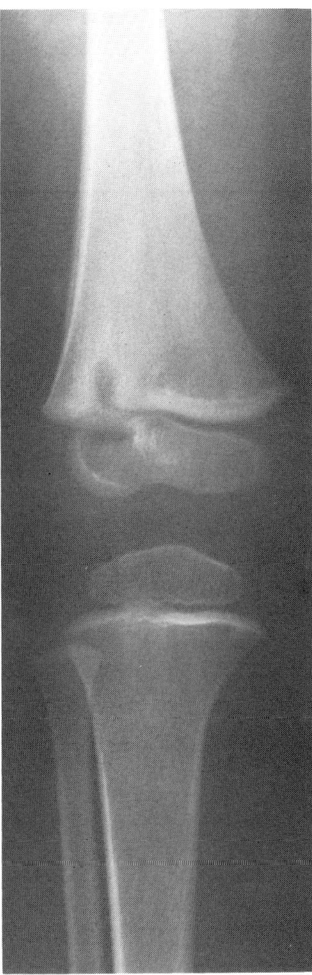

FIGURE 7–48. Osteomyelitis. AP plain film of the right knee of a 2-year-old boy shows lytic changes involving the lateral half of the epiphysis and also extending into the lateral half of the distal metaphysis of the right femur. The lytic defect has a faint sclerotic rim. It contains no matrix. There is also a clear periosteal reaction extending along the lateral aspect of the distal femur from the metaphysis into the shaft. (Courtesy of J. F. Garcia, Department of Radiology, University of New Mexico, Albuquerque.)

diologist). Plain film, arthrogram, or CT may be used to assess bone involvement or the healing phase in a joint infection. Nuclear medicine examination (bone scan, indium-labeled white blood cell scan) is sensitive to early abnormalities (see Chapter 9). Any joint may be involved, and the mechanism of spread to the joint space includes hematogenous and local spread. Early in the course of the disease, an effusion can distend the joint space, but later changes of cartilage destruction and bone demineralization and lysis result in narrowing and deformation of the joint.

Arthritis

Noninfectious inflammatory disease of the joint space occurs in many conditions, most of which are rare. Clinical history and laboratory findings, the location of the abnormalities, and the characteristic radiographic findings are the factors most helpful for establishing a diagnosis. A systematic approach is recommended in the radiographic evaluation of arthritis because atypical characteristics are often present clinically or radiographically. Also, two forms of arthritis may be present at the same time.

A systematic approach to the soft tissues, bone alignment, bone mineralization, and cartilage spaces allows full assessment of arthritis with plain films. MRI is the most effective method for evaluating inflammatory disease involving the tendons, the menisci, and the fluid spaces. Because many forms of arthritis involve the hands, evaluation of the hands is most effective in diagnosis.

Soft-Tissue Evaluation. Important soft-tissue abnormalities include generalized swelling or wasting, localized swelling, the presence of calcification, soft-tissue masses, clubbing of the digits, and nail changes (Fig. 7–49). Generalized changes can indicate a systemic disease such as acromegaly, an edematous process such as Sudeck's atrophy, or disuse atrophy such as that seen in systemic lupus erythematosus (SLE), rheumatoid arthritis (RA), and scleroderma. Localized swelling may be periarticular, which is suggestive of RA, or may involve an entire bone, as in the sausage digit of psoriasis and Reiter's syndrome. Soft tissue calcification may be subcutaneous, as seen in scleroderma, or capsular, as seen in gout, or it may involve the cartilage itself. This calcification of the cartilage, called chondrocalcinosis, has several important causes. Calcific peritendinitis indicates hydroxyapatite deposition disease. Soft-tissue masses may be rheumatoid nodules, granulomas from infection, or metabolic deposits. Clubbing of the digits indicates hypertrophic pulmonary osteoarthropathy. Nail changes are characteristic of psoriasis and, less frequently, Reiter's syndrome.

Alignment Abnormalities. Reducible alignment abnormalities and hyperextension of the thumb are characteristic of SLE (Fig. 7–50). All the digits are deviated to the ulnar side (ulnar deviation). Irreducible alignment abnormalities and boutonniere and swan-neck deformities are seen in rheumatoid arthritis. The boutonniere deformity occurs when the extensor tendons slide off the sides of the

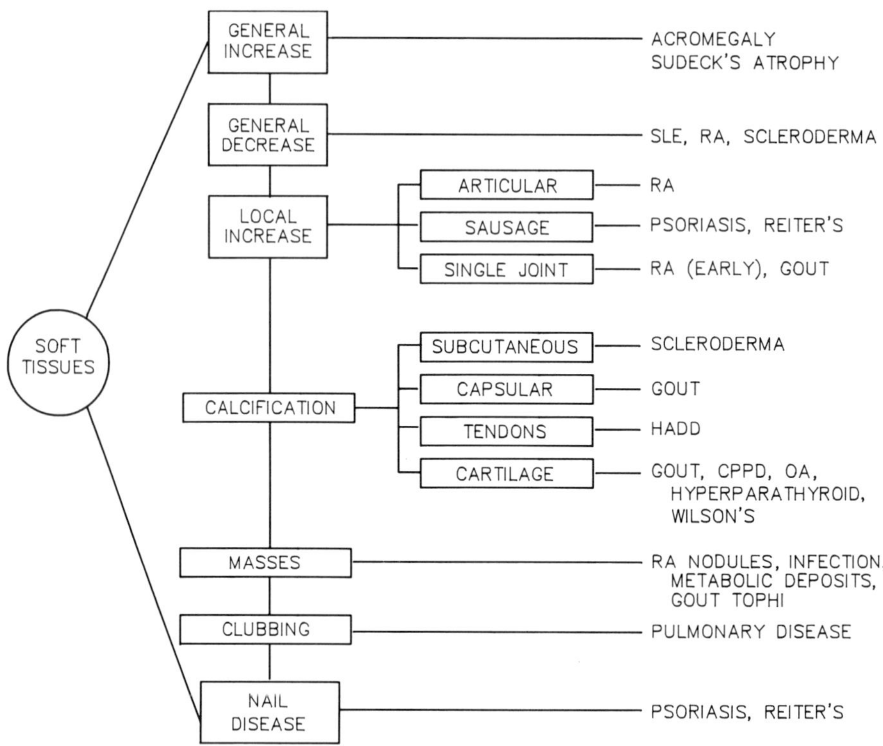

FIGURE 7–49. Soft tissue abnormalities in arthritis. SLE, systemic lupus erythematosus; RA, rheumatoid arthritis; HADD, hydroxyapatite deposition disease; CPPD, calcium pyrophosphate dihydrate deposition disease; OA, osteoarthritis.

proximal interphalangeal joints, causing flexion of the proximal interphalangeal joints and extension at the distal interphalangeal joints. The opposite occurs in the swan-neck deformity.

Bone Mineralization. Bone mineralization is notably normal in most forms of arthritis, including osteoarthritis, psoriasis, Reiter's syndrome, gout, calcium pyrophosphate dihydrate (CPPD) deposition disease, and SLE, except when severe disease is present (Fig. 7–51). Generalized demineralization is present in disuse atrophy, steroid therapy, acromegaly, and Sudeck's atrophy. Decreased juxta-articular

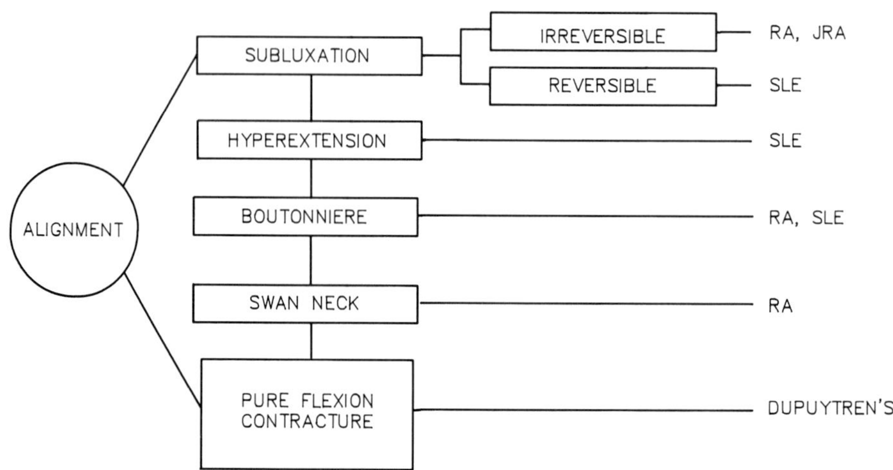

FIGURE 7–50. Alignment abnormalities in arthritis. RA, rheumatoid arthritis; JRA, juvenile RA; SLE, systemic lupus erythematosus.

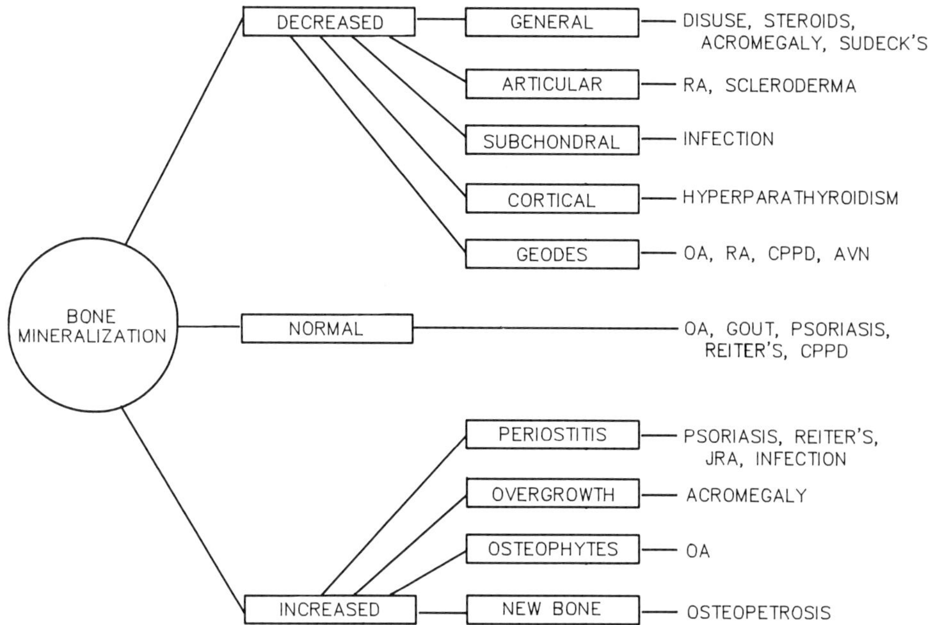

FIGURE 7–51. Bone mineralization abnormalities in arthritis. RA, rheumatoid arthritis; OA, osteoarthritis; CPPD, calcium pyrophosphate dihydrate deposition disease; AVN, avascular necrosis; JRA, juvenile RA.

mineralization is seen in RA and scleroderma. Subperiosteal resorption and cortical tunneling are seen in hyperparathyroid disease.

The presence of subchondral cysts (geodes) is nonspecific, but has a limited differential diagnosis (osteoarthritis, RA, CPPD deposition disease, and AVN). Increase in bone density may be a result of generalized bone overgrowth (as in acromegaly), osteophyte formation (as seen in osteoarthritis), or congenital bone disease (osteopetrosis and pycnodysostosis), or it may be limited to the periosteum. Generalized periostitis is present in hypertrophic pulmonary osteoarthropathy, pachydermoperiostosis, and thyroid acropachy; limited random periostitis is seen in the rheumatoid variants (psoriasis, Reiter's syndrome, and juvenile RA) but not in RA.

Cartilage Space. The most important findings in arthritis are the changes in the cartilage space. By far the most helpful is the anatomical distribution of these abnormalities (Figs. 7–52, 7–53). Large weight-bearing joints develop degenerative changes of osteoarthritis; the majority of the other diseases involve the small joints, particularly of the hand. In the hand, a distal distribution indicates osteoarthritis, psoriasis, and Reiter's syndrome. Proximal disease is the rule in RA, gout, and CPPD deposition disease. Atypical joints (elbow, shoulder, pubis) are involved in CPPD deposition disease. The feet are involved in RA, Reiter's syndrome, gout, and, less frequently, psoriasis. Symmetrical involvement is seen in RA, SLE, and scleroderma, whereas osteoarthritis, gout, and psoriasis are asymmetrical. Erosions of the subchondral line and the bare area with uniform joint space narrowing occurs in RA, whereas proliferative changes with irregular cartilage destruction occur in gout and CPPD deposition disease. Mutilating changes are usually caused by RA and psoriasis.

Systemic Connective Tissue Disease Causing Arthritis

Rheumatoid Arthritis. RA is an autoimmune disease in which antibodies to articular cartilage uniformly destroy the synovial joints. It most commonly occurs in middle aged and older women and involves primarily the hands, wrists, and knees but may involve any joint (Fig. 7–54). Erosions are most severe in areas of motion.

The process is most severe in the hands and wrists and is characterized by symmetrical joint-space narrowing, periarticular demineralization and soft-tissue swelling, bone erosion, and, in advanced disease, joint destruction. In the hand, the disease involves the proximal joints. Erosions often affect the bare area, the lateral joint space in which cartilage is absent.

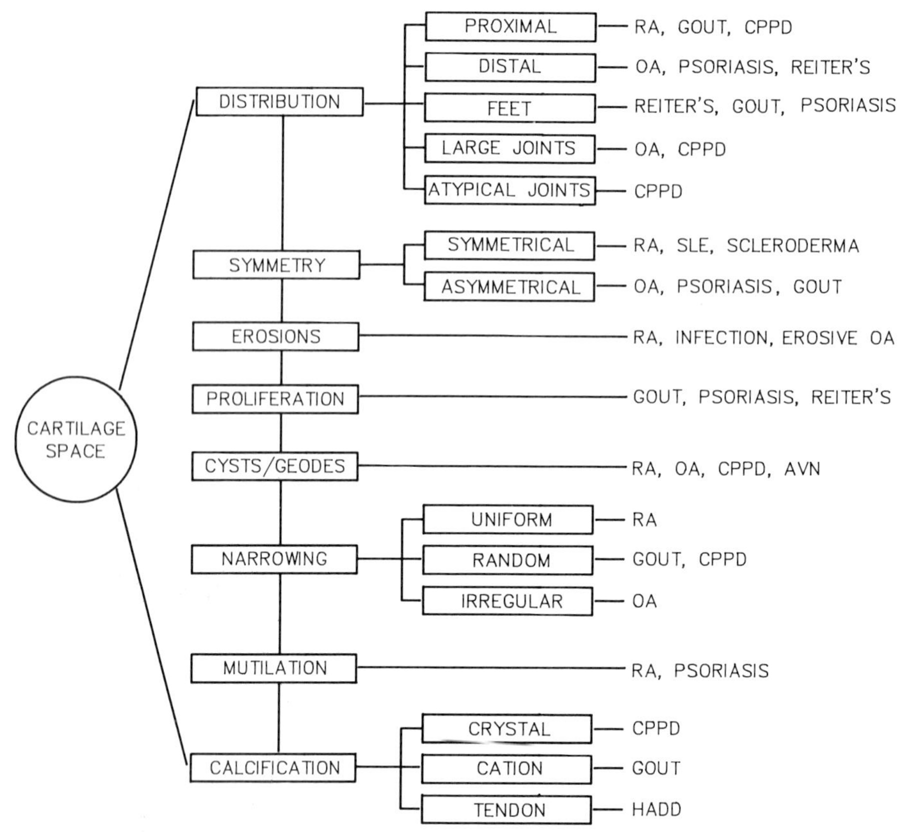

FIGURE 7–52. Cartilage space abnormalities in arthritis. RA, rheumatoid arthritis; CPPD, calcium pyrophosphate dihydrate deposition disease; OA, osteoarthritis; SLE, systemic lupus erythematosus; AVN, avascular necrosis; HADD, hydroxyapatite deposition disease.

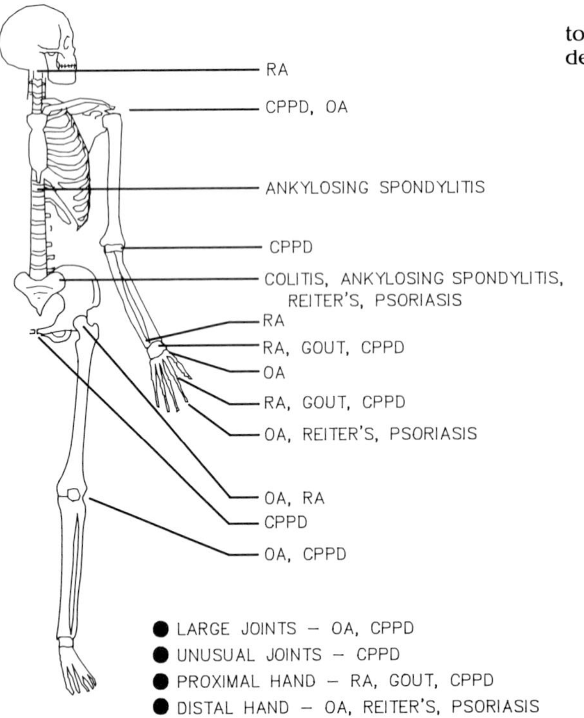

FIGURE 7–53. Distribution of arthritis. RA, rheumatoid arthritis; CPPD, calcium pyrophosphate dihydrate deposition disease; OA, osteoarthritis.

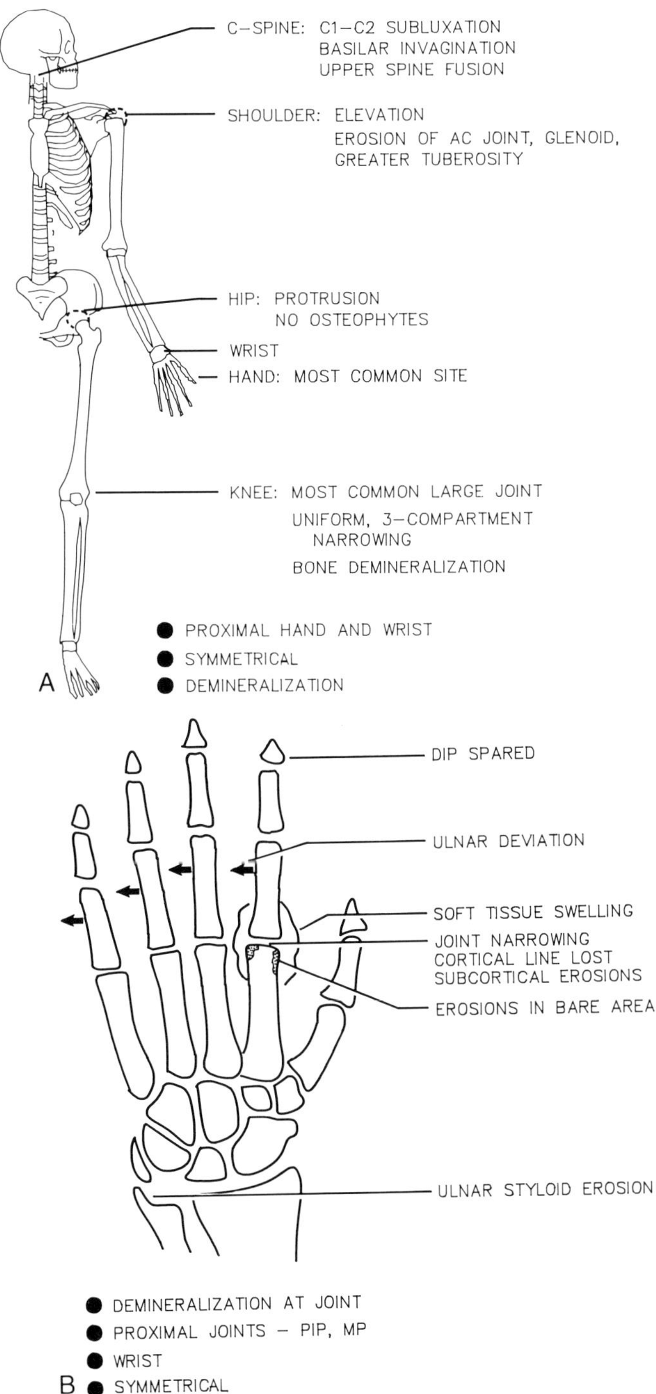

FIGURE 7–54. Rheumatoid arthritis. *A.* Locations of disease. AC, acromio-clavicular. *B.* Disease of the hand and wrist. DIP, distal interphalangeal; PIP, proximal interphalangeal; MP, metacarpophalangeal.

Irreducible ulnar deviation of the digits is also common. Erosion of the ulnar styloid is common in RA and not usually present in degenerative osteoarthritis.

The knee is the most commonly involved large joint; narrowing of all three joint spaces (medial, lateral, patello-femoral) and generalized demineralization occur. In the shoulder, erosion of the joint and ligamentous connections results in elevation of the humerus.

Juvenile Rheumatoid Arthritis. Juvenile rheumatoid arthritis (JRA) is the arthritic com-

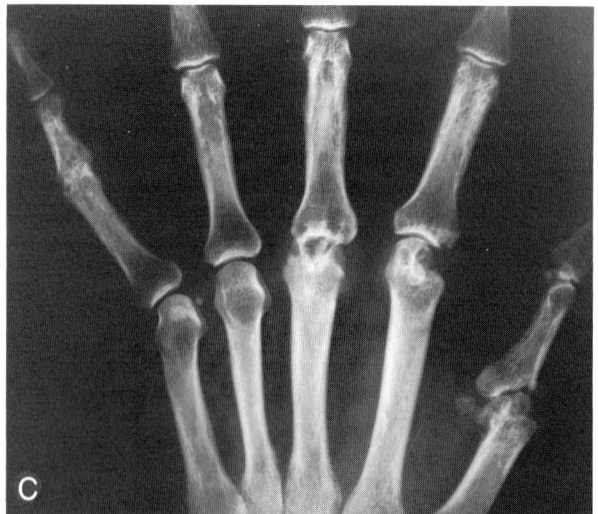

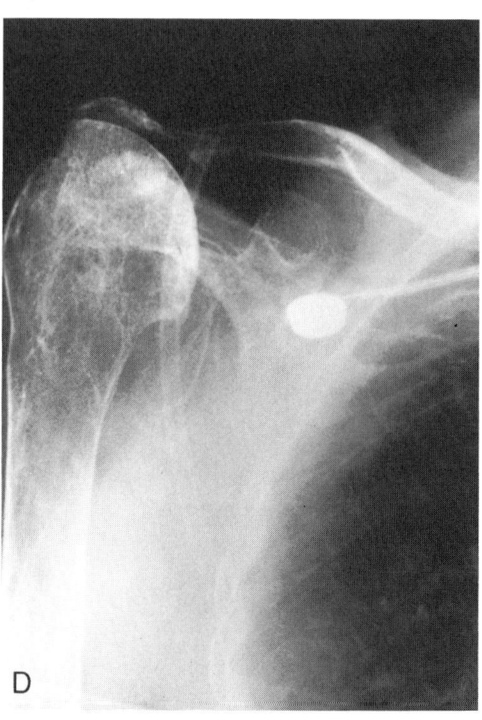

Figure 7–54 *Continued C.* Magnified view of the hand shows erosions at the MP and PIP joints. Note joint-space narrowing and periarticular demineralization. *D.* Coned view of the shoulder shows elevation of the humerus, demineralization, and destruction of the acromio-clavicular joint.

ponent of Still's disease, a systemic seronegative disease of children characterized by fever, rash, splenomegaly, lymphadenopathy, and arthritis. The joint-space abnormalities are similar to those of RA, except that they are less destructive, usually asymmetrical, and often monarticular. The cervical spine is involved more frequently than in RA, and because the disease affects children, growth disturbances often result. In the knee, the changes are indistinguishable from those of hemophilia.

In the hand, JRA affects proximal joints and primarily the wrists (Fig. 7–55). Abnormal maturation results in a squared-off appearance of the bones. Ankylosis of the wrist occurs in advanced disease. Erosion is uncommon. Cervical spine disease is often severe, characterized by fusion of the apophyseal joints, subluxation at C1-C2, and development of osteophytes.

Systemic Lupus Erythematosus. SLE is accompanied by associated arthritis in most patients, but radiographic abnormalities are not seen. The pattern of involvement is similar to that of RA, but joint destruction is rare. Generalized soft tissue swelling and alignment abnormalities are the most common findings. The alignment changes seen in the hand are caused by the predominantly ligamentous involvement and are therefore reducible. Erosion is not present. Other changes, such as mild demineralization and AVN, are probably caused by steroid therapy. Five to ten percent of patients have linear calcification in the soft tissues.

Scleroderma. Scleroderma is a connective tissue disease affecting the skin and smooth muscle of virtually all organ systems. It often includes arthritis (present in 65% of patients), which most commonly involves the distal hands. The radiographic findings are soft-tissue atrophy, bone resorption, flexion contracture, and subcutaneous calcification (calcinosis cutis). Severe soft tissue swelling is often the first abnormality. There is a high association with Raynaud's phenomenon.

HLA-B27 Associated Arthritis

Several forms of arthritis are associated with the HLA-B27 histocompatibility antigen and share common features. These include predominantly axial location, bone proliferation, and ankylosis (fusion of joints). The sacroiliac joint is often involved, and the presence of symmetrical involvement can assist in differential diagnosis (Table 7–3). When there is symmetrical involvement, presence of any of the HLA-B27 diseases is possible (Fig. 7–56). When involvement is asymmetrical, only psoriasis and Reiter's syndrome need be considered; however, both of these diseases have equal likelihood of being symmetrical.

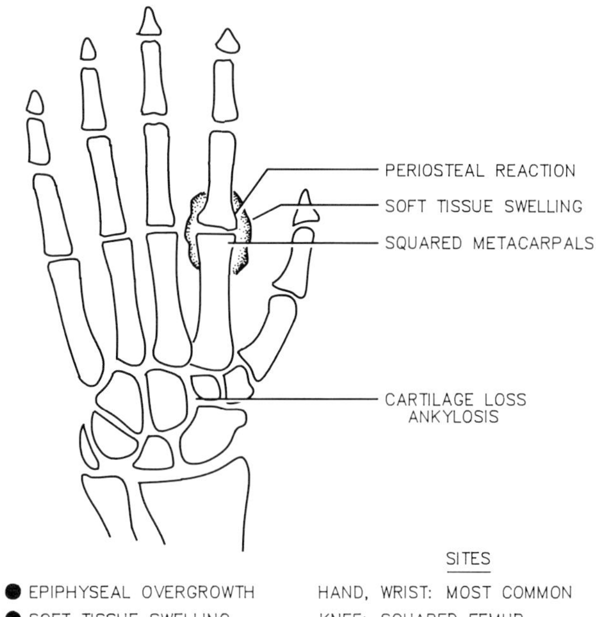

FIGURE 7–55. Characteristics of juvenile rheumatoid arthritis.

Ankylosing Spondylitis. Ankylosing spondylitis involves predominantly the sacroiliac joints and the spine and occurs most commonly in young men. Most patients (90%) carry the HLA-B27 antigen. The arthritis begins in the sacroiliac joints, in which it is always symmetrical and is characterized by erosion and reactive sclerosis. The arthritis progresses up the spine in a continuous fashion, characterized by symmetrical syndesmophytes (osteophytes that bridge adjacent vertebral bodies). Apophyseal joint ankylosis, ligamentous ossification, and squaring of the vertebral bodies give the spine a bamboo appearance (see Fig. 2–42). When the upper thoracic spine is involved, inspiration is impaired, and upper lung disease results. One third of patients have peripheral joint involvement similar to that of RA.

Inflammatory Bowel Disease. Inflammatory bowel disease (ulcerative colitis and regional

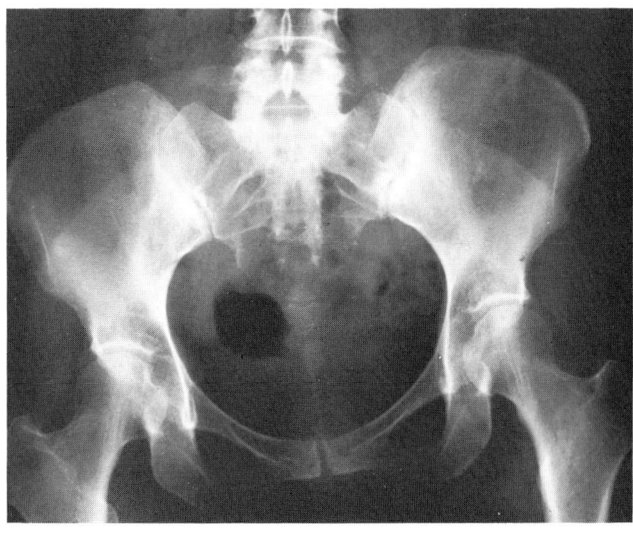

FIGURE 7–56. Arthritis of the sacroiliac joint. Pelvic plain film shows sclerosis of both sides of the sacroiliac joints bilaterally in a patient with the HLA-B27 antigen and colitis. (Courtesy of C. Helms, Department of Radiology, University of California, San Francisco.)

TABLE 7–3. SYMMETRY OF SACROILIAC JOINT ABNORMALITIES

Symmetric
Ankylosing spondylitis*
Colitis*
Psoriasis (50%)*
Reiter's syndrome (50%)*
Osteitis condensans ilii
Asymmetric
Psoriasis (50%)*
Reiter's syndrome (50%)*
Infection
Trauma
Degenerative disease

*Arthritis associated with the HLA-B27 histocompatibility antigen.

enteritis) is associated with arthritis in 5% to 20% of patients. Migratory, transient peripheral arthritis is the usual involvement. This peripheral involvement of the knees, the ankles, or the wrists parallels the activity of the bowel disease. Symmetrical sacroiliitis and spondylitis are usually independent of the course of the colitis. The sacroiliac involvement is identical to that of ankylosing spondylitis except that it is milder.

Psoriasis. Some patients (7%) with psoriasis develop arthritis, either in the axial skeleton or peripherally. The disease is characterized by skin lesions on the extensor surfaces, by nail changes, and by arthritis. In the axial skeleton, sacroiliac joint disease is the most common form of arthritis, where bone sclerosis and ankylosis occur. Asymmetrical involvement is present in the sacroiliac joints and in the spine in half of patients. This asymmetry is in contrast to the symmetrical involvement of ankylosing spondylitis and colitis arthritis. The location of spine disease is random in psoriasis, and skip areas are common (Fig. 7–57); the disease may be limited to the cervical spine. Peripherally, psoriasis involves the hands and, to a lesser extent, the feet; distal asymmetrical joint erosion is similar to that of RA except that proliferative and periosteal reaction is often seen. Psoriasis may cause a severe, mutilating arthritis. The arthritis is not usually correlated with the course of the skin lesions.

Reiter's Syndrome. Reiter's syndrome is diagnosed clinically from the findings of urethritis, balanitis, uveitis, skin rash, and arthritis. The arthritis involves primarily the feet, knees, ankles, and lower spine. It may also involve the hands, but foot involvement is always more advanced and helps to differentiate Reiter's syndrome from psoriasis and RA. Involvement of the sacroiliac joint is asymmetrical in 50% of patients.

Degenerative Arthritis

Diffuse Idiopathic Skeletal Hyperostosis. Diffuse idiopathic skeletal hyperostosis (called DISH, ankylosing hyperostosis, or Forestier's disease) is a disease of older men that is characterized by degenerative changes and hyperostosis. Patients are usually asymptomatic, and the disease must not be confused with arthritis. The spine shows osteophytes bridging the vertebrae (Fig. 7–58). The disc spaces are preserved, and there is no ankylosis.

Degenerative Joint Disease. Osteoarthritis, also called degenerative joint disease, is a noninflammatory destruction of the joint that may be primary (idiopathic) or secondary to trauma, infection, inflammation, or metabolic disease. It involves all joints in the body (Fig. 7–59) but affects predominantly the large, weight-bearing joints. Whatever the cause, the cartilage becomes damaged, leading to narrowing of the joint space, subchondral sclerosis, development of osteophytes, cyst formation, and joint deformity. Bone mineralization is normal, and soft-tissue swelling is minimal. The affected area of the joint is the weight-bearing portion.

In the hip, disease is often related to AVN or trauma (Table 7–4). The process affects the superior joint space (the weight-bearing portion) with narrowing, sclerosis, flattening, and subchondral cyst formation in the femoral head. The acetabular roof may become flattened and sclerotic. The subchondral cysts may fracture. The superior acetabular involvement can often be distinguished from the axial (superomedial) involvement of RA. Reactive bone forms in the femur to provide additional support.

In the knees, osteoarthritis affects the me-

FIGURE 7–57. Psoriasis. *A.* Diagram. *B.* Plain film of the hand shows advanced erosions of the distal interphalangeal joints in a woman with psoriasis. *C.* Plain film of the thoracolumbar spine shows broad-based, bridging osteophytes in another patient. The asymmetrical involvement and the presence of skip areas are common.

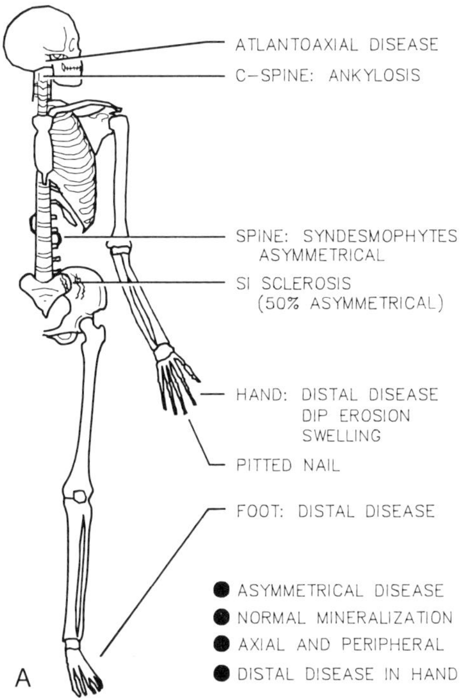

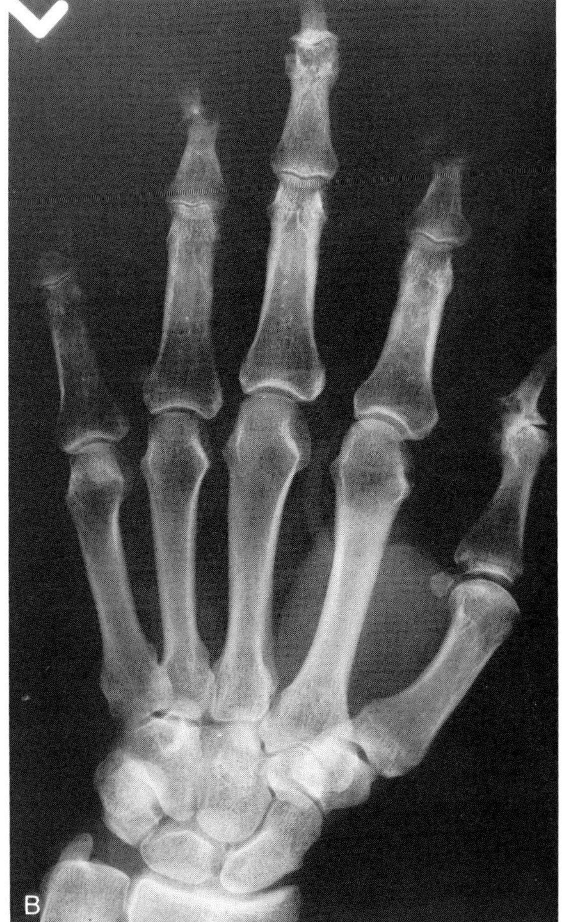

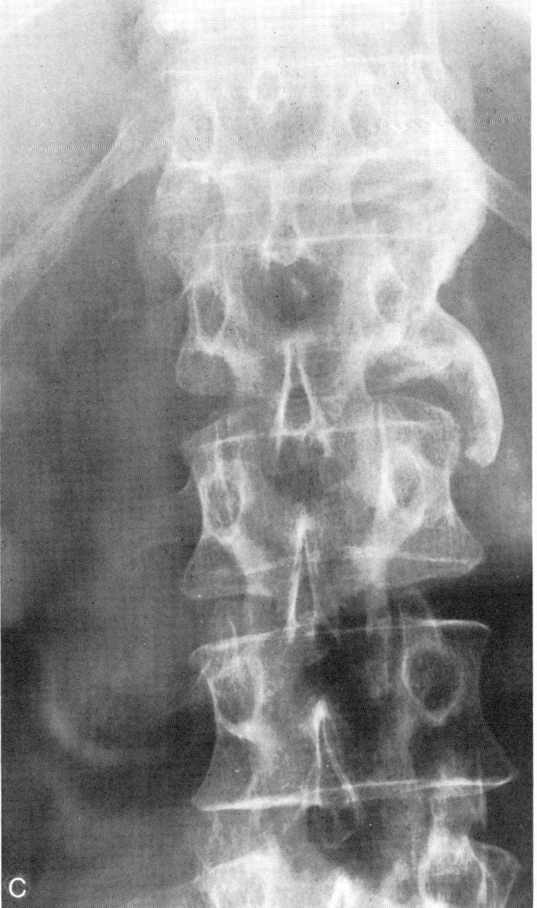

FIGURE 7–57 Psoriasis. *See legend on opposite page*

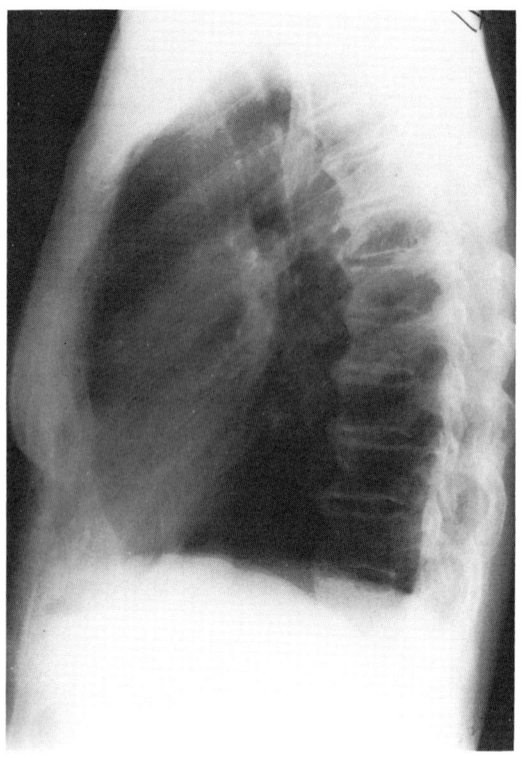

FIGURE 7–58. Diffuse, idiopathic skeletal hyperostosis (DISH) in an asymptomatic man. Lateral chest film shows undulating hyperostosis on the anterior margins of the vertebral bodies. Note the normal disc spaces.

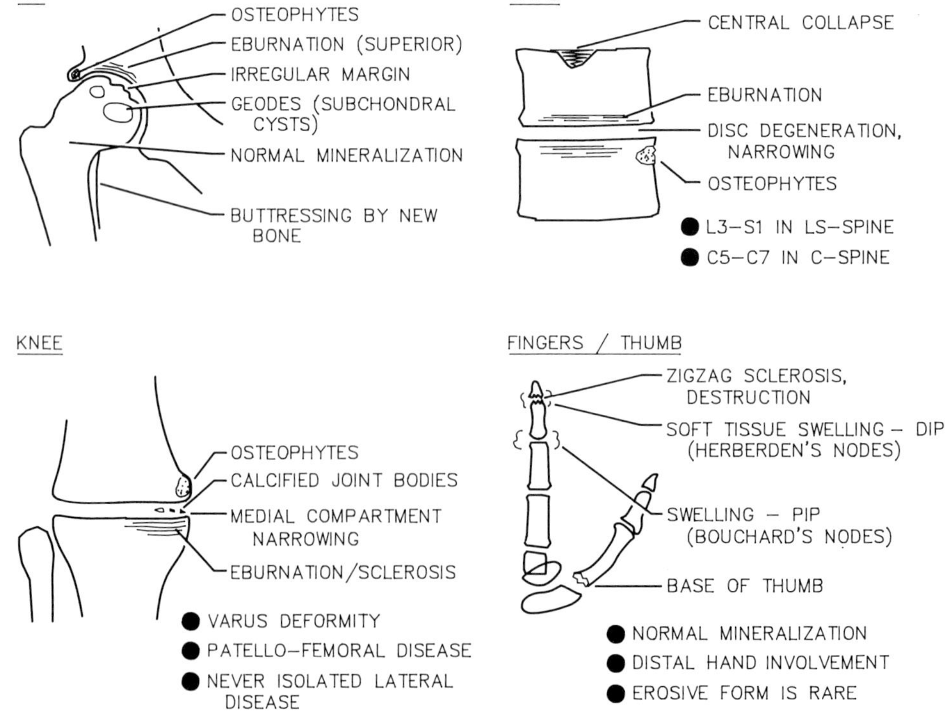

FIGURE 7–59. Characteristics of osteoarthritis. PIP, proximal interphalangeal.

TABLE 7–4. CAUSES OF DEGENERATIVE HIP DISEASE

Trauma
Osteonecrosis
Hip dislocation
Infection
Joint disease (CPPD)
Neuropathy
Epiphyseal dysplasia
Wilson's disease
Acromegaly

CPPD, calcium pyrophosphate dihydrate deposition.

dial or patellar joint space or both. The lateral compartment is affected only in conjunction with the other two compartments. This distribution and the irregularity of involvement distinguish osteoarthritis from RA, which usually entails smooth narrowing of all three compartments. Additional findings include subchondral sclerosis, osteophyte formation, and remodeling.

The hands are frequently involved by osteoarthritis (Fig. 7–60). The distal joint involvement, the normal mineralization, and the lack of soft tissue swelling enable osteoarthritis to be differentiated from inflammatory arthritis. The distal and proximal interphalangeal, first carpal-metacarpal, and naviculomultangular joints are most commonly affected. Irregular joint destruction results in a ragged joint margin. Eburnation, subchondral cysts, and articular swelling are present. In some cases (primary generalized osteoarthritis), patients develop swelling of the distal and proximal interphalangeal joints, called Heberden's and Bouchard's nodes, respectively. A severe form, (erosive osteoarthritis) is limited to the hands, in which destructive degenerative or inflammatory changes occur.

In the spine, disease is most common in the lumbar and cervical regions, where osteophyte formation, disc degeneration and herniation, apophyseal joint sclerosis, and encroachment of neural foramina occurs. In the lumbar spine, the disease is almost always between L-3 and S-1. The best method of evaluation of spinal osteophytes is CT. Normal structures are well outlined by fat and variable soft-tissue density, and the diagnosis can be made with confidence (see Figs. 7–20, 7–21, 7–22). When CT is equivocal, myelography (followed by CT) can be performed. MRI does not show osteophytes but does show the consequences of compression of nerves and spinal cord.

In the cervical spine, plain radiographs demonstrate proliferative changes at the levels of C4-C7 (as opposed to higher levels seen in RA and related arthritis). Oblique views show osteophytic encroachment of the neural foramina. Further evaluation can be performed with the use of intravenous or intrathecal contrast.

Neuropathic Joint Destruction. Neuropathic joint destruction (Charcot's joint) is associated with repeated trauma to weight-bearing joints as a result of neuropathy of any cause, including diabetes, syringomyelia, congenital insensitivity to pain, meningomyelocele, syphilis, and leprosy. Severe joint destruction with effusion, subluxation, sclerosis, and fracture occurs. Destruction, debris, dislocation, disorganization, and distension are the usual findings in advanced disease. The midfeet, ankles, and knees are most commonly involved. Similar findings may also occur with CPPD deposition disease (to be described).

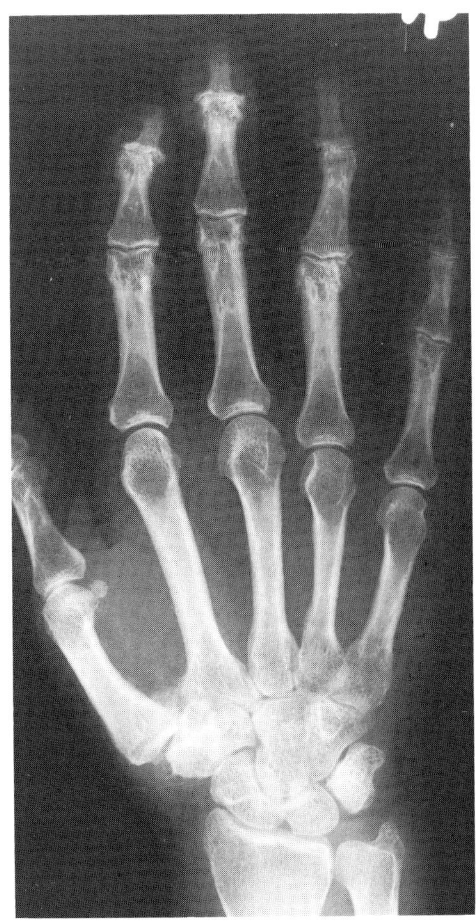

FIGURE 7–60. Osteoarthritis. Plain film of the hand shows destruction of the distal interphalangeal joints. Less severe disease is present in the proximal interphalangeal joints. The first carpal metacarpal joint is also involved, which is characteristic of osteoarthritis.

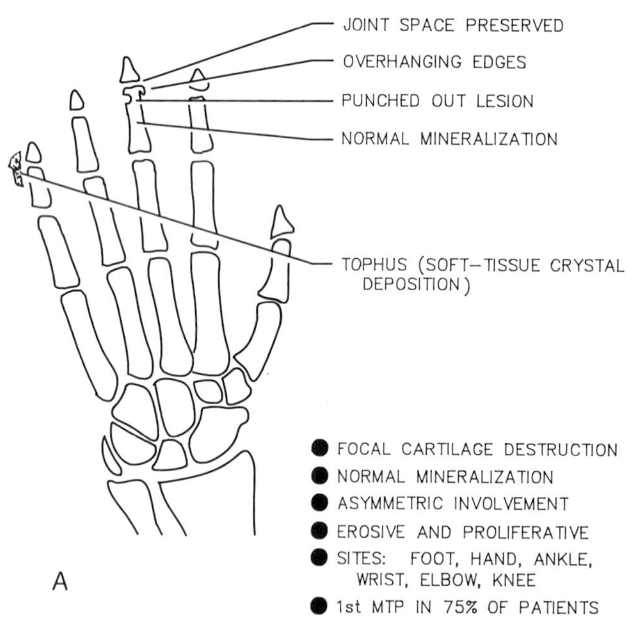

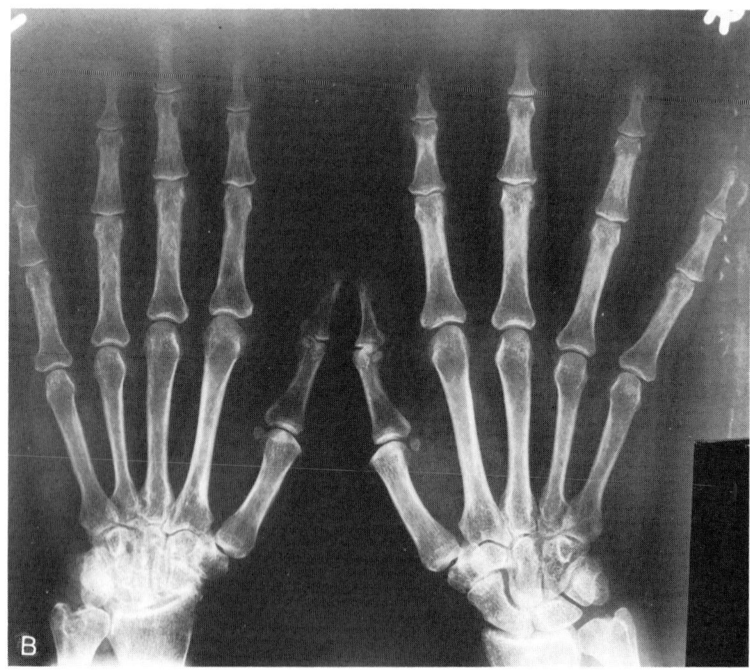

FIGURE 7–61. Gout. *A.* Diagram. MTP, metatarsophalangeal. *B.* Plain film of the hands shows a punched-out erosion of the left third middle phalanx, tophaceous deposits of the right fifth digit, and destruction of the left wrist. (Courtesy of C. Helms, Department of Radiology, University of California, San Francisco.)

Crystal Deposition Diseases

Gout. Gout is a urate crystal–induced arthritis of the feet, hands, wrists, and ankles (Fig. 7–61). It initially is limited only to soft tissue swelling. In advanced disease there may be proliferative bony erosions in the juxta-articular region. The erosions have a punched-out appearance and may have overhanging margins. The joint space is preserved because the cartilage destruction is focal. Bone mineralization is normal except in advanced disease. In most (75%) patients with arthropathy of gout, the first metatarsal phalangeal joint is involved. Most cases are diagnosed from the presence of disease in this location. Tophi (urate crystals formed in the periarticular areas) occur in the feet, ankles, elbows, and knees. They appear as mottled areas of increased density on radiographs.

Calcium Pyrophosphate Dihydrate Deposition Disease. CPPD deposition disease is arthritis caused by deposition of crystals in the articular cartilage. The involvement of the hyaline cartilage and fibrocartilage produces a linear, marginal appearance on radiographs. Calcification of the synovium may accompany the crystal deposition. The degenerative arthropathy that develops with CPPD deposition disease is similar in form to that of osteoarthritis (discussed earlier), being characterized by eburnation, osteophyte formation, subchondral cysts, and joint-space narrowing (Fig. 7–62). Many of the same joints are involved. However, CPPD deposition disease occurs in sites that are not involved in osteoarthritis (Table 7–5), such as the patellofemoral, talonavicular, and radiocarpal joints, and in locations that are less common sites for osteoarthritis (the shoulders, elbows, and wrists).

Severe joint destruction occurs rapidly, especially in the knees, shoulders, hips, and wrists. The knees are the most common sites of involvement (95%). The meniscus is most often involved, but the hyaline articular cartilage may also become calcified. Additional areas of calcification in the knees are the cruciate ligaments, the quadriceps tendon, and the synovial lining. Loose bodies are also present within the joint. As the disease progresses, the degenerative changes become more evident, obscuring the cartilage calcification in many cases.

The wrists and hands are also commonly involved. The distal radioulnar joint is usually the first site. Disease is proximal in the hands and usually involves the wrists. In contrast with osteoarthritis, the first carpometacarpal joint is spared in CPPD deposition disease. Also the proximal involvement of the metacarpophalangeal joints is unusual in osteoarthritis.

Calcification of the symphysis pubis is common, appearing as a vertical calcified line between the pelvic bones. In the hips and shoulders, calcification of the hyaline cartilage produces a curved margin next to the bone. In the spine, the annulus of the disc becomes calcified. When the disc is destroyed, the appearance is similar to that of degenerative disc disease. Elbow involvement includes calcification of the cartilage and the tendons, which eventually leads to joint destruction. Involvement of the elbow is seldom seen in osteoarthritis. The feet and ankles are not commonly involved in CPPD deposition disease. Unlike gout, the first metatarsophalangeal joint is not involved.

TABLE 7–5. JOINT INVOLVEMENT OF CPPD AND OA

Joint	CPPD	OA
Talonavicular	Yes	No
Patellofemoral	Yes	Not isolated
Radiocarpal	Yes	No
Shoulder	Yes	Rare
Elbow	Yes	Rare
Wrist	Yes	Rare
Ulnar styloid	Common	Unusual
Symphysis pubis	Common	Unusual

CPPD, calcium pyrophosphate dihydrate deposition; OA, osteoarthritis.

Hereditary Diseases That Affect the Joints

Hemophilia. Hemophilia is an abnormality of one or more elements of the blood clotting cascade that results in a bleeding diathesis. The most common types are hemophilia A (deficiency of factor VIII), hemophilia B (deficiency of factor IX), and von Willebrand's disease (deficiency of platelets and factor VIII). Repeated hemorrhage into the joint space causes severe destruction and bone overgrowth (Fig. 7–63). The findings are indistinguishable from those of JRA. The knees are the most common sites of hemophilia-induced arthritis, but the elbows, ankles, hips, shoulders, and wrists are also involved.

Hemochromatosis. Hemochromatosis is characterized by deposition of iron in the liver and the spleen (see Chapter 3). In 25% to 50% of patients, CPPD deposition disease is associated. In these cases, the chondrocalcinosis is a result of the CPPD deposition disease. The arthropathy is limited to the metacarpophalangeal joints, in which central collapse and lateral bone proliferation cause a squared-off appearance of the distal metacarpals.

Wilson's Disease. Wilson's disease only rarely causes joint disease. It affects the metacarpophalangeal joints with erosive and proliferative changes. The distal metacarpal heads have an appearance similar to that of hemochromatosis.

Ochronosis. Ochronosis is a metabolic, hereditary defect. A severe, premature arthritis develops and results in marked calcification of articular cartilage and intervertebral discs.

Diabetes. Diabetes involves the joint spaces, usually because of a decrease in blood supply or because of neuropathy. The feet are most commonly involved, and demineralization, joint destruction, and calcification are seen.

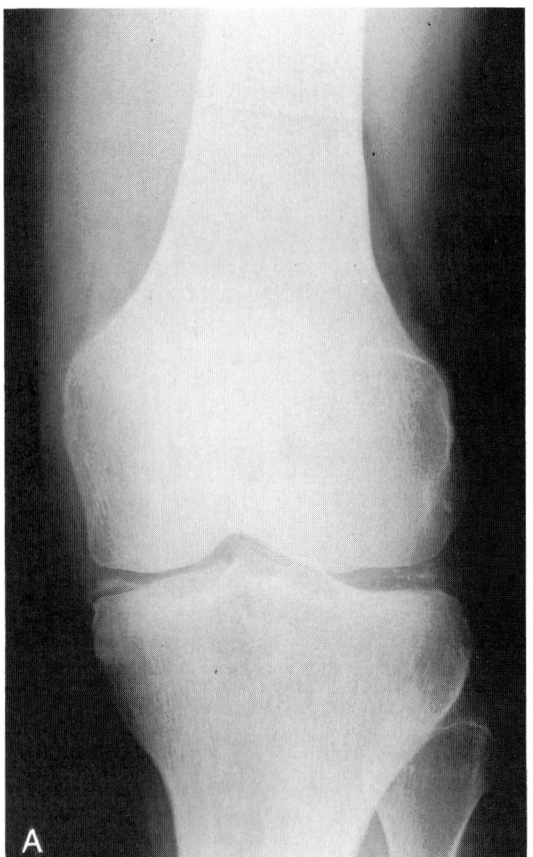

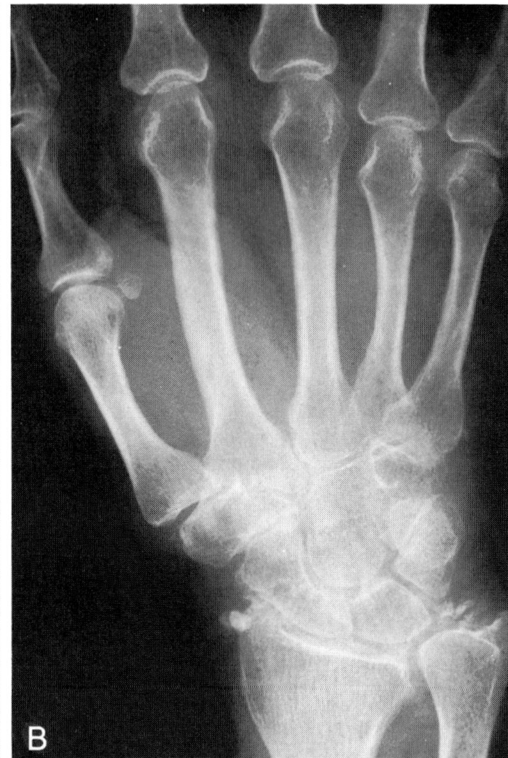

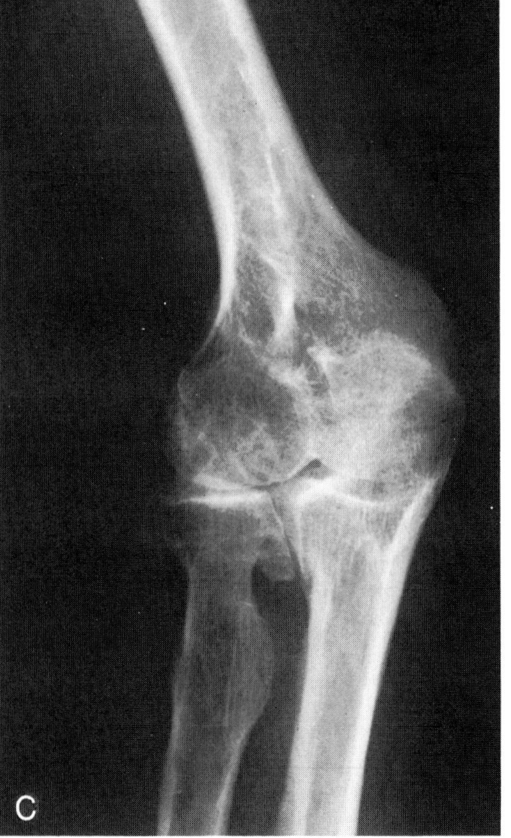

FIGURE 7–62. Calcium pyrophosphate dihydrate (CPPD) deposition disease. *A.* Knee involvement. AP plain film shows calcification of the outer parts of the menisci. *B.* Hand. AP film shows severe destructive disease of the entire carpus. Calcification of the ulnar styloid is very common in CPPD deposition disease. The radiocarpal joint is involved, a finding not present in osteoarthritis. The first metacarpal joint is not involved; this joint, commonly involved in osteoarthritis, is seldom involved in CPPD deposition disease. *C.* Elbow. AP film shows tendon calcification, joint-space narrowing, and radial head degeneration. The elbow is seldom involved in osteoarthritis.

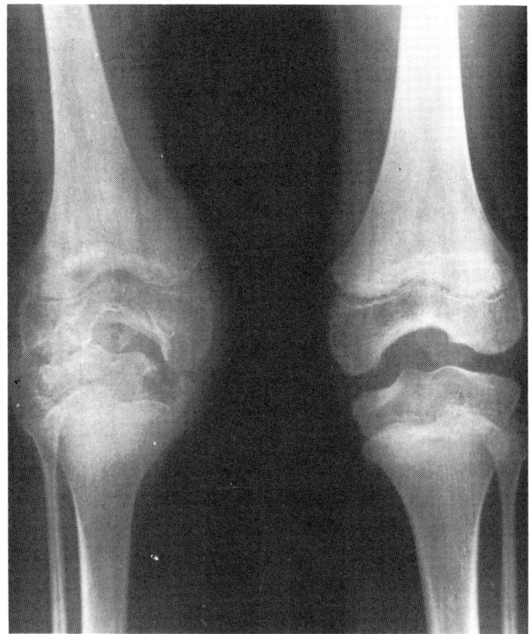

FIGURE 7–63. Hemophilia. AP film of the knees shows severe joint destruction on the right in a teenager with hemophilia. The intracondylar notch is widened in both knees, and the bones show overgrowth and squaring. (Courtesy of C. Helms, Department of Radiology, University of California, San Francisco.)

Neoplastic Diseases of the Joint Space

Pigmented Villonodular Synovitis. Pigmented villonodular synovitis is a benign proliferative joint disease of young adults that involves the knees (the most common sites), hips, ankles, and shoulders. Usually only one joint is involved. The primary abnormality is hyperplasia of the synovium, which becomes infiltrated by hemosiderin-laden macrophages. Pressure erosion causes destructive lesions in the adjacent bone. The joint contains a brownish fluid. Symptoms occur over a period of years. There is minimal disability unless the joint is destroyed.

Plain films often show no abnormality. In more advanced disease, subchondral cystic changes are demonstrated. There is neither associated osteoporosis nor calcification. Arthrography and MRI demonstrate nodular proliferative lesions in the joint space (Fig. 7–64). The hemosiderin causes low intensity on T1- and T2-weighted images because of a paramagnetic effect. The lesions have an appearance similar to that of synovial osteochondromatosis.

Synovial Osteochondromatosis. Synovial osteochondromatosis is a proliferative metaplasia of the synovium. It produces cartilaginous bodies that are first attached to and later separated from the synovium. It occurs at any age but usually in about the fifth decade. The most commonly affected joints are the knees. When the loose bodies are not calcified, they are not apparent on radiographs. The differential diagnosis of joint bodies includes osteoarthritis, osteochondritis dissecans, neuropathic joint, and pigmented villonodular synovitis.

NEOPLASTIC DISEASES

Primary tumors of bones are rare. Nevertheless, correct radiological diagnosis is extremely important because histological characteristics are often ambiguous. Some benign lesions appear histologically malignant. In most cases, the age of the patient, the location of the lesion, and the appearance of the lesion allow an accurate diagnosis or a limited differential diagnosis (see Table 7–6).

Bone tumors are usually first seen on plain films obtained to evaluate trauma or bone pain. These films may show a lytic (low-density) or a blastic (high-density) lesion. The position within the bone and the margins of the lesion enable primary characterization of the lesion in most cases. CT is not usually helpful. MRI can demonstrate the composition

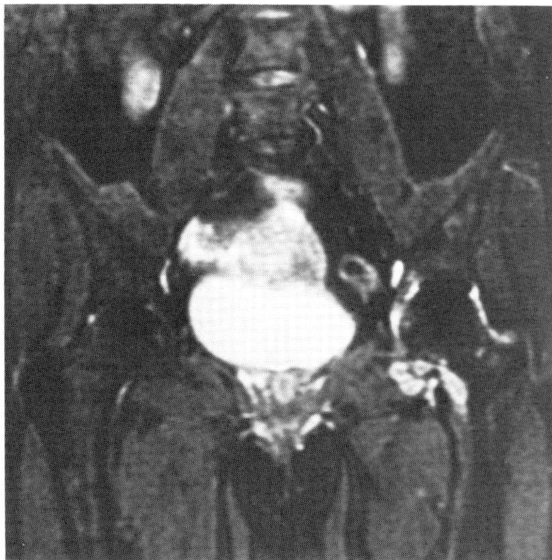

FIGURE 7–64. Pigmented villonodular synovitis. Coronal STIR image shows proliferative changes of the medial joint space of the left hip. High-intensity fluid is also present. Paramagnetic changes of hemosiderin were not observed.

of the lesion and an associated soft-tissue component.

The evaluation of a bone lesion is most reliably done by systematic assessment of radiographic and clinical characteristics (Fig. 7–65). First, the aggressiveness of the lesion is determined. A benign lesion has well-defined borders and a narrow zone of transition between normal and abnormal bone, and a periosteal reaction is absent. An aggressive lesion demonstrates ill-defined borders, a wide zone of transition, periosteal reaction, and bone destruction. An aggressive lesion may be a malignant tumor or an area of infection (the most common bone lesion).

Next, the density of the lesion helps narrow the list of possibilities. Primary malignant bone tumors and certain metastatic lesions are typically blastic, whereas benign tumors are usually lytic. Important lytic malignant lesions are myeloma and most metastases. Several reliable, easily remembered differential diagnostic lists can be consulted at this point in order to eliminate or confirm various diagnoses on the basis of the specific characteristics of each lesion. These characteristics include the age of the patient, the location of the lesion, radiographic caracteristics, and clinical symptoms.

Bone lesions in children are usually infections but also include Ewing's sarcoma, leukemia, benign cystic lesions, and fibrous lesions. Bone lesions in patients over 50 years of age are usually metastatic tumor or myeloma. Lytic lesions in teenagers or young adults are usually benign. The location of the lesion within the bone can limit the differential diagnosis. For example, an epiphyseal lesion is a chondroblastoma if the growth plate is open and a giant-cell tumor after epiphyseal closure. The round-cell tumors (Ewing's sarcoma, reticulum cell sarcoma, myeloma, leukemia, and lymphoma) occur in the marrow cavity. Osteogenic sarcoma occurs in the cortical margin. Important radiographic findings are soft tissue swelling, calcification, periosteal elevation, and sequestered bone. The clinical history can be misleading. Trauma is often the reason for radiographic evaluation but is often not related to the lesion.

Lytic Bone Lesions

Except for metastatic cancer and myeloma, most lytic bone lesions are benign. Although the number of such lesions is large, they are easily remembered with a simple mnemonic (Table 7–6). Knowledge of specific characteristics of the various lesions allows easy inclusion in or exclusion from the final differential diagnostic list. If the lesions are multiple, the list is automatically further limited (Table 7–7).

Fibrous Dysplasia. Fibrous dysplasia is a congenital lesion of fibrous tissue that causes bone lysis. It may affect one bone (monostotic form) or many bones (polyostotic form). The typical lesion is elongated, well-circumscribed,

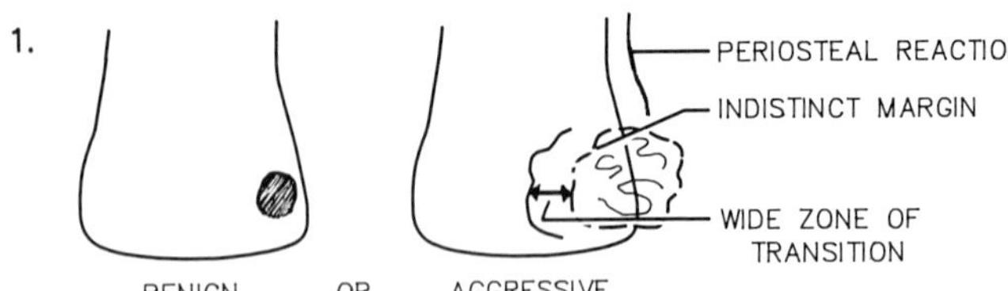

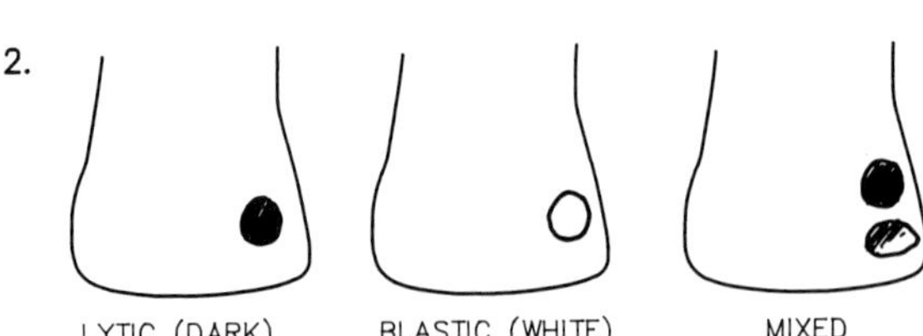

3. AGE (CHILD, ADULT, ELDERLY)
LOCATION (WHICH BONE, WHICH PART OF THE BONE, SINGLE OR MULTIPLE)
SYMPTOMS (PAIN, TRAUMA, FEVER)

FIGURE 7–65. Approach to bone lesion diagnosis.

TABLE 7–6. LYTIC BONE LESIONS*

Lesion	Age	Bone Involved	Bone Area	Benign (B) or Malignant (M)	Radiographic Appearance	Histological Characteristics	Comments
Fibrous dysplasia	Child	Pelvis, femur, skull, ribs; any bone	Shaft	B	Low density; no periostitis; variable appearance; long lesion in a long bone	Loose fibrous tissue	With cafe au lait spots and precocious puberty, called McCune-Albright syndrome
Osteoblastoma	10 to 20	Spine	Arch, pedicle	B	Lytic or sclerotic; lytic lesion looks like aneurysmal bone cyst; half are calcified	Variable	Very painful; hot on bone scan
Giant cell tumor	20 to 35	Femur, tibia, radius, ulna, pelvis, jaw, rib	Epiphysis after closure	B, 85%; M, 15%	Sharp, nonsclerotic margin; abuts joint; eccentric placement	Stromal cells; hard to determine whether malignant or benign	Dull pain, pathologic, fracture; often recurs
Metastasis	Over 40	Axial skeleton, especially spine, pelvis	Marrow cavity	M	Lytic, blastic, mixed; replaces marrow, destroys cortex; soft tissue mass	Tumor cells	Most common bone tumor
Myeloma	40 to 60	Spine, ribs, pelvis, skull, femur, humerus	Marrow cavity	M	Primarily destructive; well-marginated (punched-out appearance)	Malignant plasma cells	Bone pain, hypercalcemia; abnormal serum protein level
Aneurysmal bone cyst	Under 30	Long bone, pelvis, vertebra	Shaft	B	Expansile, lytic, cystic lesion; may have septations, fluid, blood; may have mass; sclerotic margin; rapid growth; soap-bubble appearance	Blood, giant cells, connective tissue; looks malignant	Pain and swelling; like osteoblastoma in spine
Angioma	Any age	Long bones, spine, skull	Any part	B	Multilocular, soap-bubble lesions; low density; cortical holes; phleboliths	Hemangioma	Can mimic Ewing's sarcoma
Chondromyxoid fibroma	Early adulthood	Tibia (50%), femur, fibula, calcaneus	Diametaphyseal	B	Sharply marginated oval low-density lesion; sclerotic rim	Chondroid and fibrous tissue	Similar to nonossifying fibroma; may cause pain; can be aggressive lesion
Chondroblastoma	Childhood	Femur, tibia, humerus	Epiphysis	B	Well-defined, low-density, sclerotic margin; half show calcification	Immature cartilage	Begins in epiphysis before closure
Histiocytosis X	Childhood	Skull, pelvis, femur, ribs	Usually metaphysis	B	Solitary or multiple low-density areas; scalloped margins; may or may not have a sclerotic margin; may have soft tissue mass	Reticuloendothelial cell proliferation	Similar to infection and Ewing's sarcoma

Table continued on following page

TABLE 7–6. LYTIC BONE LESIONS* *Continued*

Lesion	Age	Bone Involved	Bone Area	Benign (B) or Malignant (M)	Radiographic Appearance	Histological Characteristics	Comments
Hyperparathyroid (brown tumor)	35 to 60	Any bone; jaw, pelvis, femur	Anywhere	B	Focal destruction, cystic lesion; called a brown tumor	Fibrous tissue, giant cells, hemosiderin	Associated demineralization, renal osteodystrophy
Infection	Any age	Any bone	Metaphysis	B	Low density, moth-eaten–looking lesion; may have soft tissue swelling, periostitis, sequestrum	Infected material, reactive bone	May have any appearance
Nonossifying fibroma	Childhood	Long bone; most common in medial distal femur	Metaphysis	B	Low density with sclerotic margin	Whorled connective tissue	Small lesion is called fibrous cortical defect; most regress by age 20
Enchondroma	Childhood, early adulthood	Hands and feet. Also long bones	Medullary cavity	B (15% M)	Low-density expansile lesion; scalloped margin; speckled calcification (except in hand); no periostitis	Chondroid tissue	Most common tumor of the hand
Simple cyst	Childhood	Humerus, femur, calcaneus, tibia, fibula, rib	Metaphysis	B	Low density; well circumscribed with thin sclerotic rim	Fluid-filled cyst; connective tissue wall	May fracture

*Mnemonic: FOG *MACH*INES make bubbles (bubbly, low-density lesions). The letters *MACH* represent two diseases each.

and of low density. It is typically a long lesion in a long bone. However, it can have almost any appearance and involve any bone. In the skull, it appears dense on skull films because of increased thickness, but CT shows it to be low-density, fibrous tissue. When cafe au lait spots are present and the patient exhibits precocious puberty, the disease is called McCune-Albright syndrome. Fibrous dysplasia is discussed earlier with congenital diseases (see Fig. 7–44).

Osteoblastoma. Osteoblastoma is a rare lytic or blastic lesion of the neural arch or the spinous process. The most common manifestation is severe pain. The blastic form resembles the osteoid osteoma (to be discussed).

TABLE 7–7. MULTIPLE LYTIC LESIONS*

*M*etastasis and myeloma
*H*emangioma, *h*yperparathyroidism
*I*nfection
*A*neurysmal bone cyst
*E*nchondroma
*F*ibrous dysplasia

*Mnemonic: *M*ultiple *H*ollow *I*nvasions *A*re *E*asy *F*ossils.

The lytic form has a low-density, bubbly appearance. It is expansile, well-corticated, and often in the form of a soft-tissue mass (Fig. 7–66). The expansile nature of this lesion resembles an aneurysmal bone cyst (to be described),

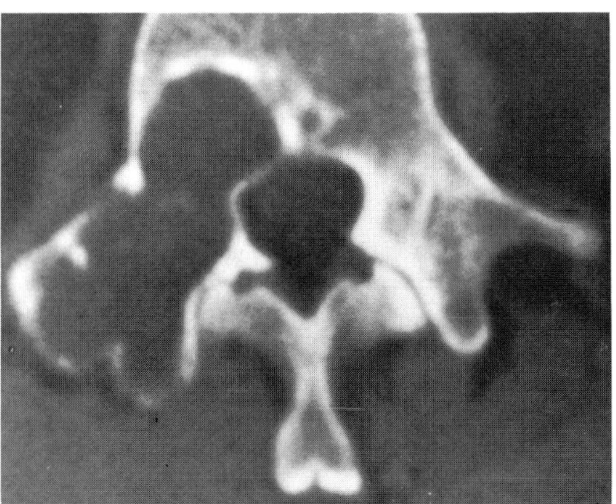

FIGURE 7–66. Osteoblastoma. CT of the spine shows a low-density, expansile lesion involving the vertebral body and lateral masses at the S-1 level. There is no paraspinous soft-tissue mass.

but it can be differentiated from the latter if calcification or ossification is present (seen in 50% of osteoblastomas). Osteoblastomas are benign, but up to 15% can recur and invade locally. Eighty percent manifest before the age of 30 with tenderness, soft-tissue swelling, and pain that is not relieved by aspirin.

Giant-Cell Tumor. Giant-cell tumors constitute 5% of all bone tumors and are expansile lesions of the epiphysis. They occur after physeal plate closure. They are eccentrically located and always abut the joint surface. About 15% of these tumors are malignant, but the distinction cannot be made on radiographs or on histological examination. The radiographic appearance, best shown on plain films, is of a low-density lesion, which abuts the joint space and is eccentrically located at the end of the bone (Fig. 7–67). The tumor has a well-defined but nonsclerotic border. The MRI appearance is similar to that of fluid (i.e., intermediate intensity on T1 spin echo and high intensity on T2 spin echo) but may be complicated by hemorrhage, liquefaction, and necrosis. Some pathologists believe that the intraosseous aneurysmal bone cyst is a giant-cell tumor. Treatment is curettage and packing with plastic. Recurrence requires further curettage and may indicate malignancy.

Metastasis to Bone. Metastatic bone involvement occurs in virtually all tumors but most commonly in those from the breasts, the lungs, the prostate, the thyroid, and the kidneys. Prostate metastases are virtually always blastic. Breast cancer, lung cancer, and lymphoma cause lesions that are usually lytic but may be blastic or mixed. Other metastatic bone lesions are lytic. On plain films, lytic metastases are typically multiple, poorly circumscribed, low-density lesions of varying size. An associated soft-tissue mass may be present, and the lesions often show cortical destruction. Although any bone can be involved, the axial skeleton, especially the spine, is the site of most metastatic lesions. Most patients are over 40 years of age and have known disease. Symptoms range from bone pain to pathological fracture to cord compression.

Plain films show lytic, sclerotic, or mixed density with cortical erosion. Such lesions show intense uptake on bone scans (see Chapter 9); therefore, general screening is performed by means of bone scanning. MRI is highly sensitive for evaluation of bone metastases and bone marrow tumor (such as leukemia and lymphoma) because the tumor is strikingly different from marrow fat on both T1 spin echo and STIR images (Fig. 7–68). T2 spin echo sequences are less effective for diagnosing tumor metastases

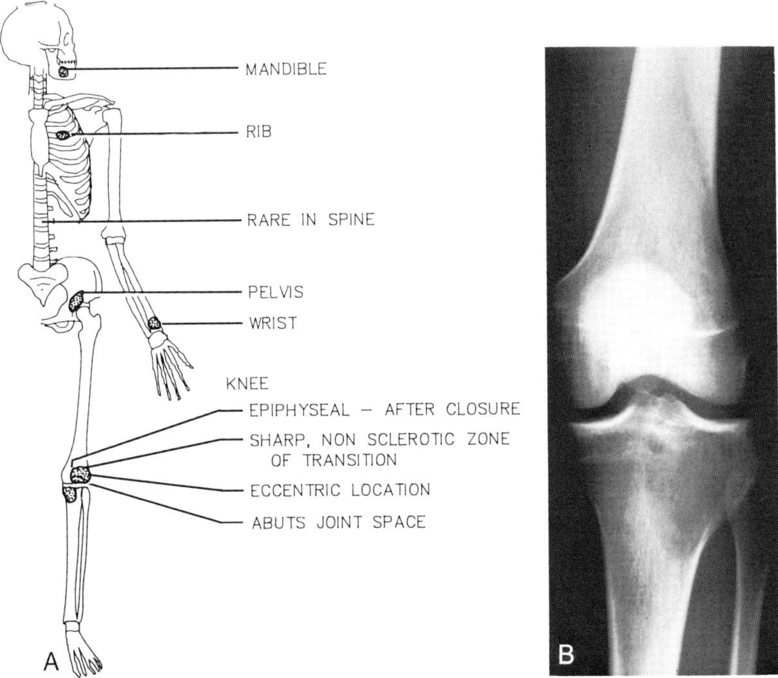

FIGURE 7–67. Giant-cell tumor. *A.* Diagram. *B.* Plain film of the knee shows an eccentrically placed low-density lesion in the proximal tibia that abuts the joint margin. Note also the closed epiphyses and the sharp margins. (Courtesy of C. Helms, Department of Radiology, University of California, San Francisco.)

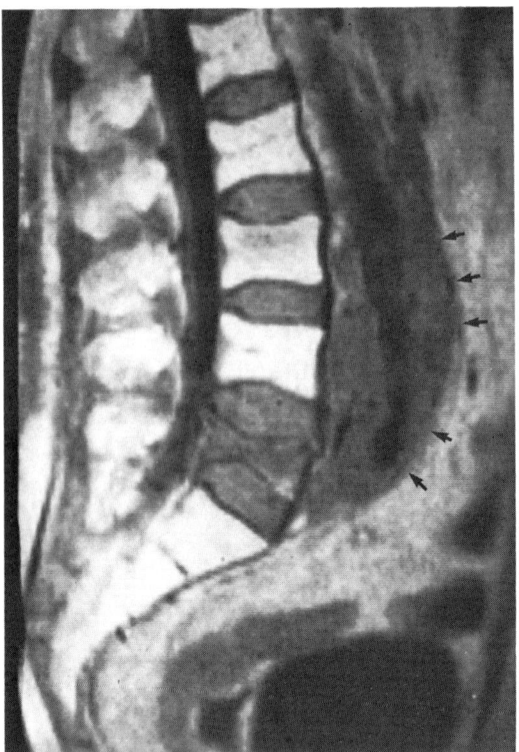

FIGURE 7–68. Metastatic tumor. Sagittal T1 spin echo image shows loss of normal marrow-fat signal and compression of the L-5 vertebral body. This vertebral body was infiltrated by metastatic tumor from prostate carcinoma. Note also the prominent adenopathy surrounding the aorta *(arrows)*. (From Stimac GK, Porter BA, Olson DO, et al: Gadolinium-DTPA-enhanced MR imaging of spinal neoplasms: preliminary investigation and comparison with unenhanced spin-echo and STIR techniques. AJR 1988, 151: 1185–1192.)

The distinction between bone metastasis and degenerative disease can be difficult, especially if a pathological fracture occurs. Usually, however, degenerative disease shows reactive change and bony proliferation. The MRI signal is often high on T1 spin echo images (as opposed to the low intensity of tumors) and is intermediate on STIR images (as opposed to the very high intensity of tumors). Paramagnetic contrast is less effective for evaluation of marrow tumors than, for example, spinal cord tumors, because it enhances the tumor to the point of appearing similar to normal marrow (see Fig. 7–69).

Myeloma. Myeloma is the most common primary bone malignancy. It is characterized by multiple, round, punched-out lesions in all bones. The lesion is predominantly destructive, and so there is no reactive sclerosis and it sometimes does not enhance on bone scans. The diagnosis is often made by the presence of serum protein abnormalities, but in many patients, bone pain is the first symptom. In some patients, central nervous system abnormalities from hypercalcemia are the first manifestations of disease (see Fig. 7–1). Myelomatosis is diffuse marrow involvement with plasma cells that results in demineralization without discrete bone lesions. Solitary plasmacytoma is a local, destructive, expansile lesion caused by malignant plasma cells in the marrow. The MRI appearance of myeloma is similar to that of metastatic bone tumor (Fig. 7–69).

Aneurysmal Bone Cyst. Aneurysmal bone cyst is a low-density, cystic, expansile lesion of uncertain origin. Possible causes include trauma (myositis ossificans) and evolution of a giant-cell tumor. All such patients are under the age of 30. The lesion may be intra- or extraosseous. It is usually eccentric in position and metaphyseal. It has sclerotic margins, in contrast to the giant-cell tumor. The shaft of the long bones, the hips, and the posterior elements of the vertebrae are the most common sites (Fig. 7–70). In the spine, the lesion is indistinguishable from osteoblastoma.

Angiomatous Lesions. Angiomatous lesions of bone include hemangioma, lymphangioma, and, in rare instances, lesions of neurofibromatosis. These lesions occur primarily in the calvarium and the axial skeleton, and the appearance depends on the size and the type of lesion. Well-circumscribed osteolytic cystic lesions are typically seen in the long bones. The appearance is often like that of soap bubbles (Fig. 7–71). Demineralization with prominence of vertical trabeculae is seen in the vertebral bodies. Rounded low-density lesions are seen in the calvarium.

A related vascular tumor, the malignant angioblastoma (adamantinoma), is a rare tumor of the tibia, originally named for its histological similarity to adamantinoma of the jaw. The tumor is of low-grade malignancy and may metastasize to the lungs, lymph nodes, and bones.

Chondromyxoid Fibroma. Chondromyxoid fibroma is a very rare metaphyseal chondroid tumor. The lesion can manifest with pain. Most patients are young adults. It is a trabeculated, oval, low-density lesion with a sclerotic outer margin (Fig. 7–72). The appearance is similar to that of a nonossifying fibroma. The presence of stippled calcification can reveal the chondroid composition.

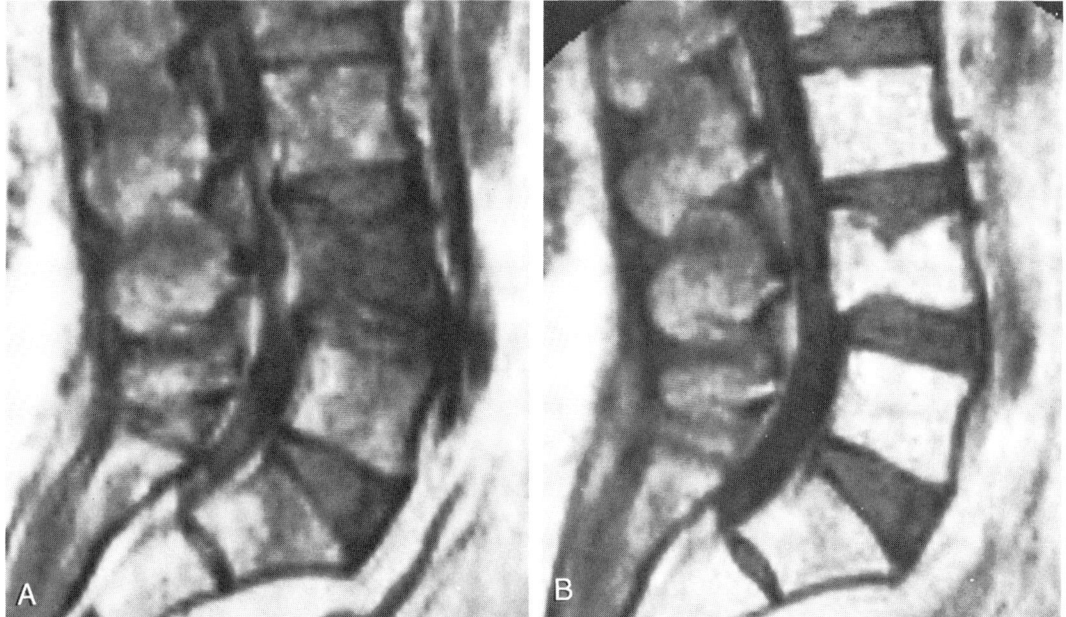

FIGURE 7–69. Myeloma. *A.* Sagittal T1 spin echo image of the spine shows marked abnormality of the vertebral body marrow. The L-4 vertebral body shows partial collapse. *B.* After Gd-DTPA enhancement, an identical T1 spin echo view shows enhancement of the vertebral bodies to an appearance that is virtually identical to that of normal marrow. Only the compression abnormality of the L-4 vertebral body reveals a pathological abnormality. (From Stimac GK, Porter BA, Olson DO, et al: Gadolinium-DTPA-enhanced MR imaging of spinal neoplasms: preliminary investigation and comparison with unenhanced spin-echo and STIR techniques. AJR 1988, 151: 1185–1192.)

Chondroblastoma. The chondroblastoma is a tumor of cartilage that occurs in the epiphyses, always before closure of the physeal plate. The lesion has well-defined, sclerotic margins and a low-density center (Fig. 7–73). Calcification is present in half of cases. The most common sites of involvement are the femur, the tibia, and the humerus. It may be indistinguishable from ischemic necrosis and other lesions that involve the epiphyses.

Histiocytosis X. The bone lesions of histiocytosis X are called eosinophilic granulomas. The lesions can occur in almost any bone and can have a variety of appearances. A single bone is usually involved, but polyostotic disease is common. A common site is the skullbase, in which the associated soft tissue component causes central nervous system symptoms (see Chapter 8). The bone lesions elsewhere can have an appearance suggestive of infection and Ewing's sarcoma and therefore usually require biopsy.

Hyperparathyroid Brown Tumors. Brown tumors, cystic collections of brownish, bloody fluid, are often associated with hyperparathyroidism (discussed earlier). These tumors occur in the long bones, the pelvis, and the jaw and appear as low-density, well-circumscribed lesions. Associated findings of hyperparathyroid disease are present (see Fig. 7–45). On radiographs, the lesion is low density and destructive.

Infection. Infection (discussed earlier) can have a variety of appearances and can affect any bone. Many lesions are of low density and have an appearance similar to that of lytic bone tumors (see Fig. 7–48). Soft-tissue swelling may occur with infection but also occurs with some tumors and eosinophilic granuloma. A bony sequestrum is strongly suggestive of infection but can also occur with eosinophilic granuloma and fibrosarcoma.

Fibrous Cortical Defect and Nonossifying Fibroma. Fibrous cortical defect and nonossifying fibroma represent the early and late appearances of a metaphyseal, well-marginated fibrous mass. Many children (20% to 30%) have a fibrous cortical defect that usually regresses spontaneously. If it progresses and enlarges, it is called a nonossifying fibroma. It usually occurs in the distal medial cortical surface of the femur but also occurs in other long bones. The lesion is of low density and is expansile, with scalloped sclerotic margins

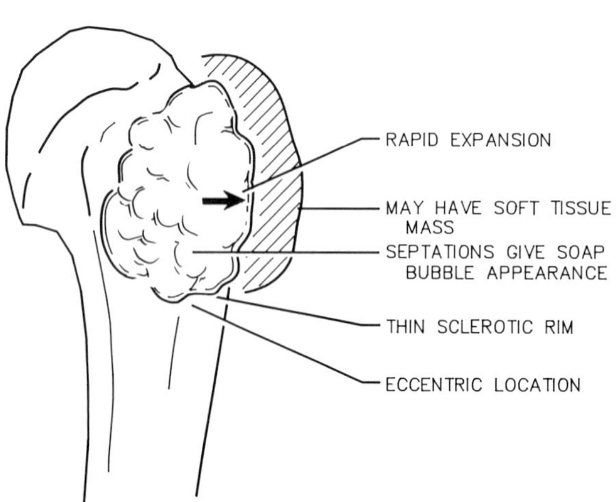

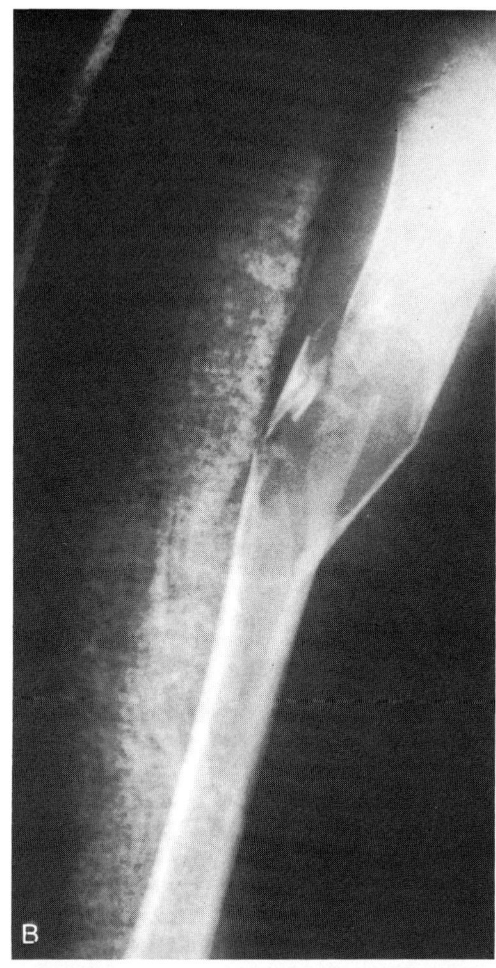

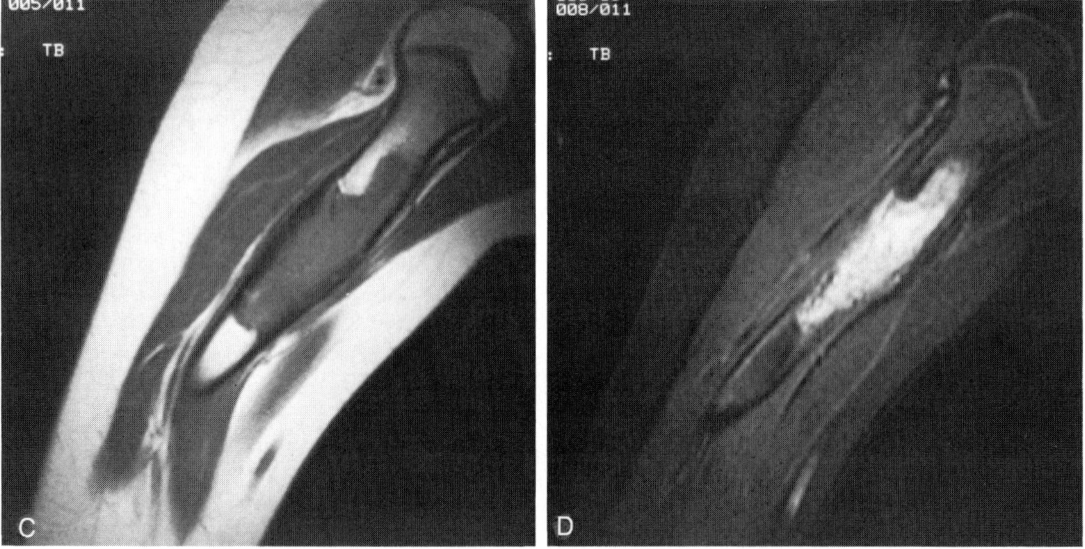

FIGURE 7–70. Aneurysmal bone cyst. *A.* Diagram. *B.* Plain film shows a large, expansile cystic lesion of the proximal humerus. Pathological fracture has occurred through the lesion, which has been radiographed in the cast. *C.* T1 spin echo image shows the expansile nature of the lesion and replacement of the normal marrow fat by low-intensity fluid and debris. *D.* STIR image shows very high intensity of fluid and debris. There is no evidence of periostitis, soft-tissue edema, or extension of the lesion.

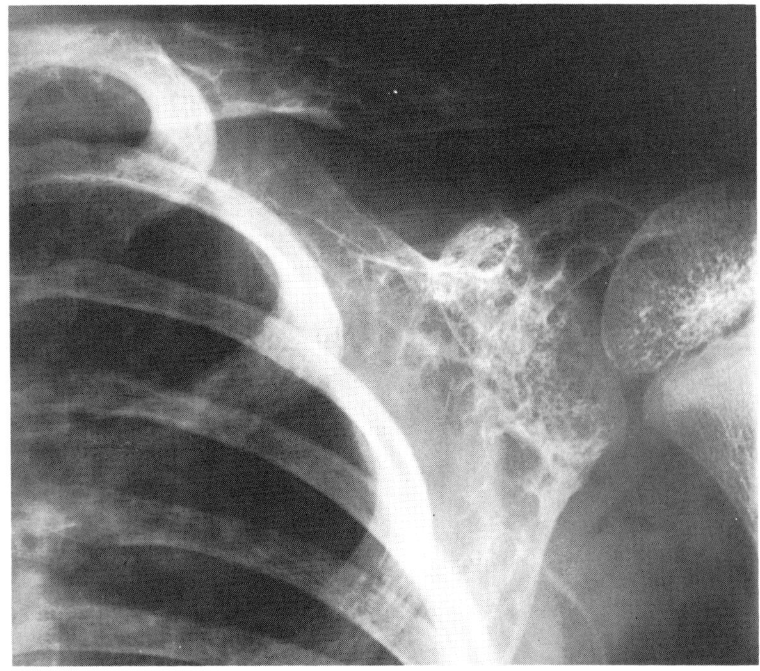

FIGURE 7–71. Angiomatosis. AP view of the shoulder shows multiple lytic lesions throughout the scapula and clavicle in a child with cystic angiomatosis. (Courtesy of C. Helms, Department of Radiology, University of California, San Francisco.)

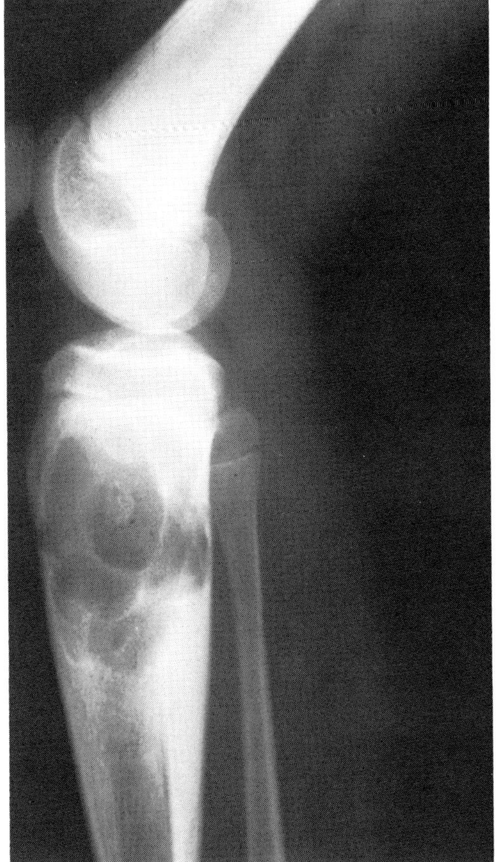

FIGURE 7–72. Chondromyxoid fibroma. Lateral view of the knee shows a low-density, bubbly lesion in the proximal tibia. Note the sclerotic margins and the central calcification. (Courtesy of C. Helms, Department of Radiology, University of California, San Francisco.)

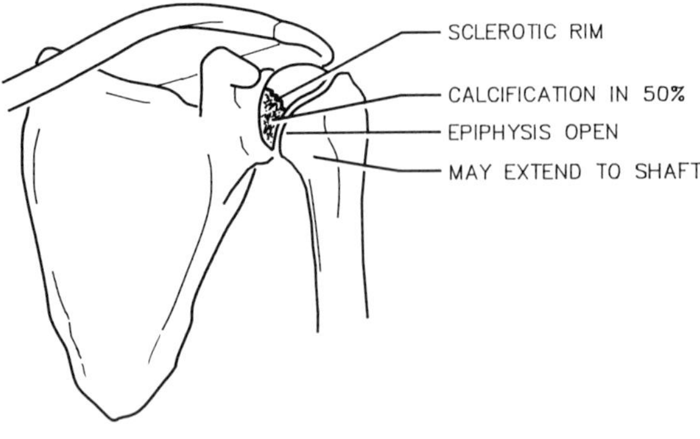

FIGURE 7–73. Characteristics of chondroblastoma. DDX, differential diagnosis; AVN, avascular necrosis.

(Fig. 7–74). The lesions produce no symptoms and there is no reactive periostitis. During the healing phase, the lesions become sclerotic. They then usually disappear.

A similar lesion, cortical desmoid, is also seen in the distal femur and probably represents an avulsion injury to the medial metaphyseal cortex.

Enchondroma. The enchondroma is a common benign medullary cartilaginous tumor. The hands and feet are the most common sites of involvement, but these tumors also occur in the long bones. It is the most common tumor of the hands.

The lesions are expansile and, except in the hands, always contain calcified chondroid,

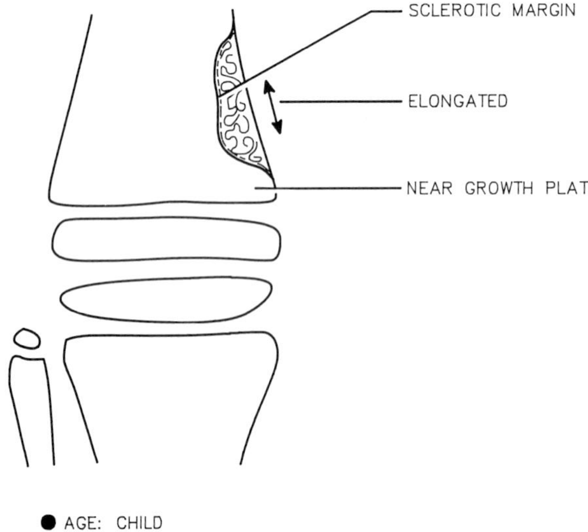

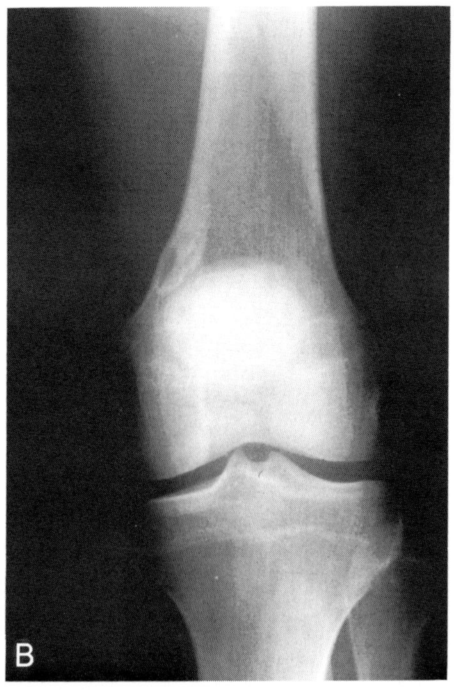

FIGURE 7–74. Nonossifying fibroma. *A.* Diagram. *B.* AP view of the knee shows a low-density lesion in the medial distal femur with sclerotic margins. The central area is becoming more sclerotic as this lesion heals.

which produces a speckled pattern of calcification (Figs. 7–75, 7–76). The margins show endosteal scalloping, in contrast to the bone infarct, which has a serpiginous margin. There is no soft-tissue mass or periostitis, in contrast to chondrosarcoma. Both infarct and chondrosarcoma otherwise have an appearance similar to that of enchondroma. In the hands, the lesions are also expansile and often do not show calcification.

A syndrome of multiple enchondromas is called Ollier's disease. Multiple enchondromas with soft-tissue hemangiomas is termed Maffucci's syndrome. Neither of these syndromes is hereditary. Some enchondromas (about 15%) degenerate to become malignant chondrosarcomas.

A chondroma is a cartilaginous tumor arising from outside the bone.

Simple Cyst. Simple cysts (unicameral bone cysts) are cystic lesions of the central shaft, usually of a long bone. Most are in the humerus and the femur. Such a cyst begins at the metaphysis and, because of bone growth at the epiphysis, migrates toward the center of the bone shaft. The etiological process of simple cysts is unknown, but trauma, healed giant-cell tumor, intramedullary hemorrhage, and circulatory obstruction are possible causes. Bone cysts are best diagnosed on plain films, which show a thin sclerotic margin and central low density (Fig. 7–77). The lesion is round or oval. If fracture through the cyst occurs, there may be irregular margins, central hemorrhage, and central chips of bone (fallen fragments). Simple cysts have no malignant potential. Because of the risk of fracture, large cysts are curetted and packed with bone.

Malignant Lytic Tumors

Fibrosarcoma of Bone. Fibrosarcoma of bone is a tumor of fibroblastic tissue and occurs primarily in the metaphyseal region of the femur and tibia. It is a purely lytic lesion and does not produce bone or cartilage. The lesion has a moth-eaten or permeative appearance, which is suggestive of malignancy. The most common sites are the pelvis, the scapula, the ribs, and the tibia. The tumor is usually of low-grade malignancy. The mass eventually expands into adjacent soft tissue. The differential diagnosis includes giant-cell tumor,

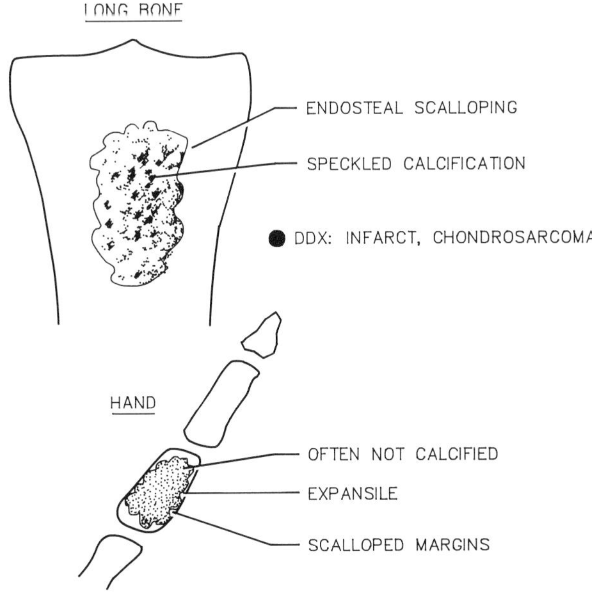

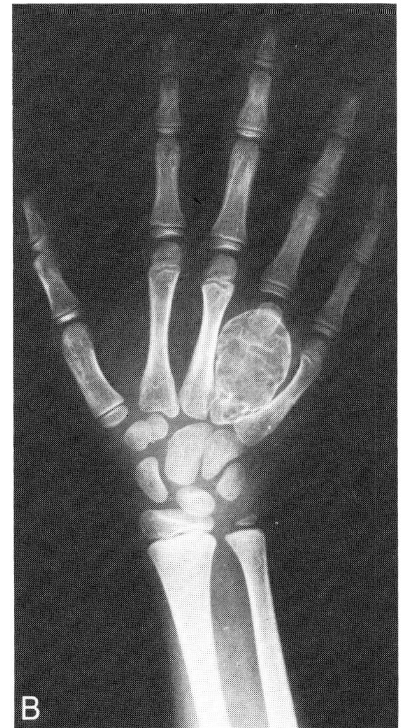

FIGURE 7–75. Enchondroma. *A.* Diagram. DDX, differential diagnosis. *B.* Plain film of the hand shows an expansile lesion of the fourth metacarpal. This has a smooth, gray texture (likened to ground glass) and expands the cortical surface of the bone. (Courtesy of C. Helms, Department of Radiology, University of California, San Francisco.)

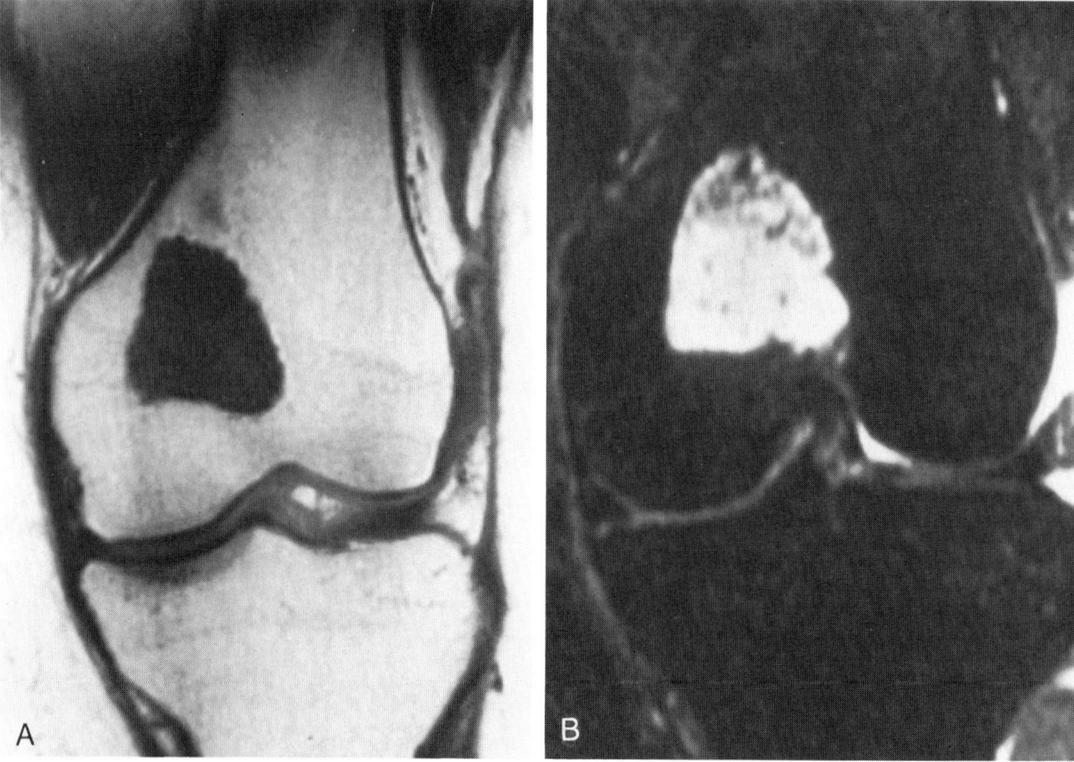

FIGURE 7–76. *A.* Enchondroma. A T1 spin echo image shows a lesion in the distal femur. The scalloped margins and flocculent central appearance are typical. *B.* The STIR image shows very high intensity of the lesion, in contrast to the suppressed fatty marrow.

aneurysmal bone cyst, and noncalcified forms of chondrosarcoma and osteosarcoma.

Round-Cell Tumors

Several tumors arise from bone marrow stem cells. These tumors therefore are called round-cell tumors. They are intramedullary, usually in the diaphysis. The age of the patient is the best aid for distinguishing these tumors from each other (Table 7–8). These tumors are usually lytic, and all are malignant.

Leukemia. Leukemia causes diffuse infiltrates in the bone marrow. Therefore, bone marrow biopsy is very effective for diagnosis. However, imaging assessment of involvement greatly assists therapy in patients with known disease. MRI techniques for imaging the marrow, notably T1 spin echo and STIR sequences, enable evaluation of the response to therapy with accuracy that parallels bone marrow biopsy, and they detect complications such as AVN. Because the marrow is uniformly involved in leukemia, a coronal MRI showing the spine, the pelvis, and the hips provides a comprehensive assessment (Fig. 7–78).

TABLE 7–8. ROUND-CELL TUMORS

Tumors	Age
Leukemia	Any age
Lymphoma	Any age
Reticulum cell sarcoma	30 to 50 years
Ewing's sarcoma	5 to 15 years
Myeloma	50 to 70 years
Neuroblastoma	0–2 months

Permeative bone lesions also result from bone destruction in patients with leukemia. These lesions are particularly evident in growing children. Plain films in such cases show mottled low density in the metaphysis and a lucent band in the epiphyseal margin (see Fig. 7–95).

Lymphoma. Lymphoma causes patchy involvement of the bone marrow. MRI is ideal for detection of bone metastases in generalized lymphoma of either the Hodgkin's or the non-Hodgkin's type by showing replacement of the normal marrow. The bone scan provides a general bone survey, but MRI, especially T1 spin echo and STIR sequences, often shows abnormalities much earlier in the course of the disease (Fig. 7–79). MRI is essential in the evaluation of lymphomatous involvement of

FIGURE 7–77. Simple bone cyst. AP view of the lower leg shows a cystic lesion in the proximal tibia inferior to the epiphyseal plate. A pathological fracture has occurred through the cyst. (Courtesy of C. Helms, Department of Radiology, University of California, San Francisco.)

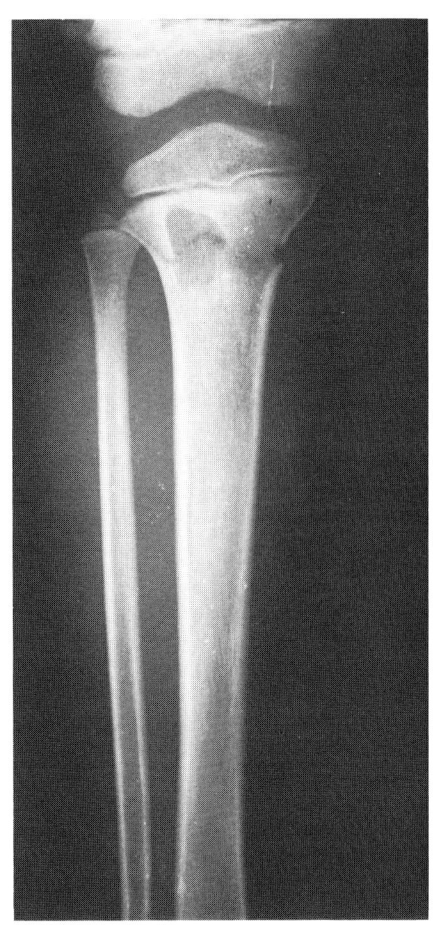

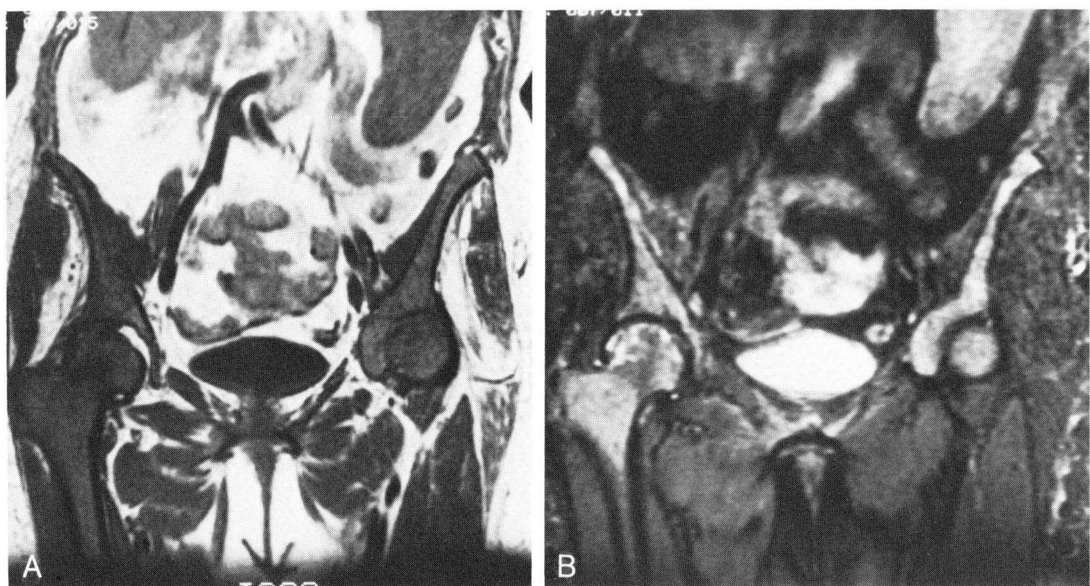

FIGURE 7–78. Leukemia. *A.* T1 spin echo image shows diffuse involvement of the marrow of the iliac bones and femurs in a 73-year-old woman with chronic myelogenous leukemia. The marrow in these regions is normally of high intensity on T1 spin echo images. This diffuse pattern of involvement is typical for leukemia. In addition, the patient had right hip pain. AVN is difficult to identify in the presence of leukemic infiltration. *B.* Matching STIR image shows edema in the proximal femur, indicating AVN. Note also the high intensity throughout the iliac bones and femurs, as opposed to the normally suppressed (black) appearance of marrow fat.

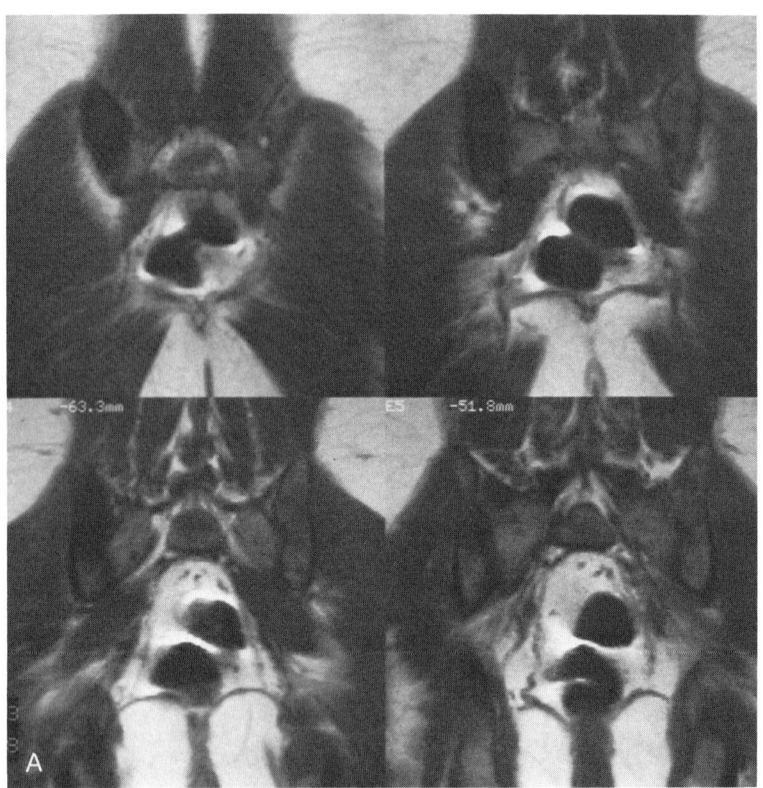

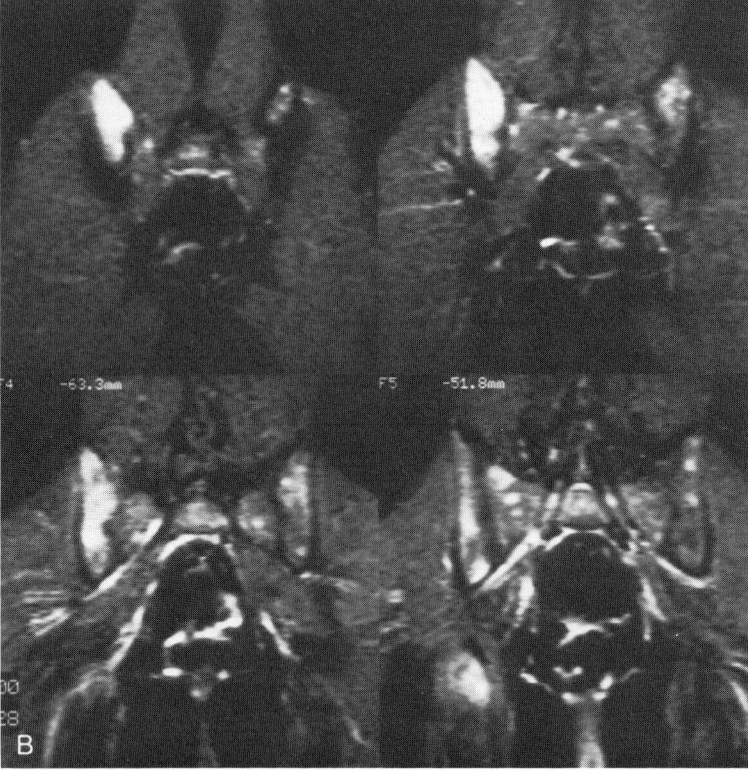

FIGURE 7–79. Lymphoma. *A.* Composite view of coronal T1 spin echo images of the sacrum show low intensity of the right iliac wing in a woman with Hodgkin's lymphoma. The sacrum and the left iliac wing are relatively normal. Mottled intensity in the upper left iliac wing was the site of a negative biopsy procedure. *B.* Matching STIR images show very high intensity in the right iliac wing, demonstrating the asymmetrical, patchy nature of involvement.

the marrow because bone marrow biopsy results can be falsely negative.

When lymphoma involves the bone as a primary tumor, called reticulum cell sarcoma, it has a permeative pattern of cortical destruction similar to that of Ewing's sarcoma. Reticulum cell sarcoma occurs in an older age group (30 to 50 years). The most common areas of involvement are the long bones (usually near the knees), the pelvis, the scapula, the ribs, and the vertebrae. Patients have only mild pain. The permeative pattern of destruction shown on plain films is indistinguishable from myeloma, infection, Ewing's sarcoma, and histiocytosis X.

Ewing's Sarcoma. Ewing's sarcoma is a tumor that occurs in children and young adults. It is the second most common primary malignant bone tumor (after osteogenic sarcoma) in children. It usually involves the long bones, but many of these tumors occur in the flat bones. The tumor is highly malignant and is composed of packed round cells. The lesion is primarily lytic, but reactive changes can produce a mixed or sclerotic appearance. The bone is destroyed centrally. A periosteal reaction produces layers of periosteum, giving the cortex an onion skin appearance. Aggressive growth can also cause a sunburst margin, Codman's triangle, and cortical destruction. There may be an associated soft-tissue mass. Patients have severe pain and fever.

The plain film appearance is highly suggestive of a malignant tumor, but infection, eosinophilic granuloma, and osteogenic sarcoma can have a similar appearance (Fig. 7–80). MRI shows the medullary mass, the periosteal reaction, and the soft-tissue extension. The tumor has extremely high intensity on STIR images.

Among patients with nonmetastatic disease, the 5-year survival rate is between 50% and 70% with radiation and chemotherapy. Most patients who present with or develop metastases die of the disease. Metastases are to bones and the lungs.

Myeloma. Myeloma causes purely destructive lytic bone lesions. Any bone can be involved, but the spine, the ribs, the pelvis, and the skull are most common sites. Myeloma is discussed in earlier sections (see Fig. 7–69 and Table 7–6).

Neuroblastoma. Neuroblastoma is a tumor that occurs in infants. It arises from neural cells along the sympathetic chain or in the adrenal gland. The usual site of metastasis is the bones. Neuroblastoma is discussed in Chapter 4.

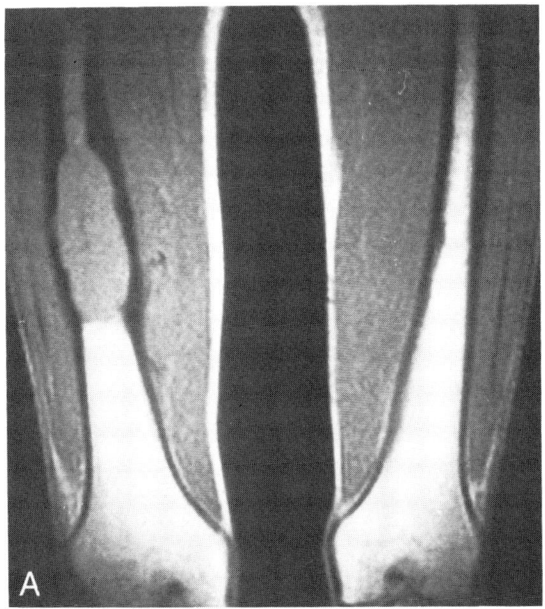

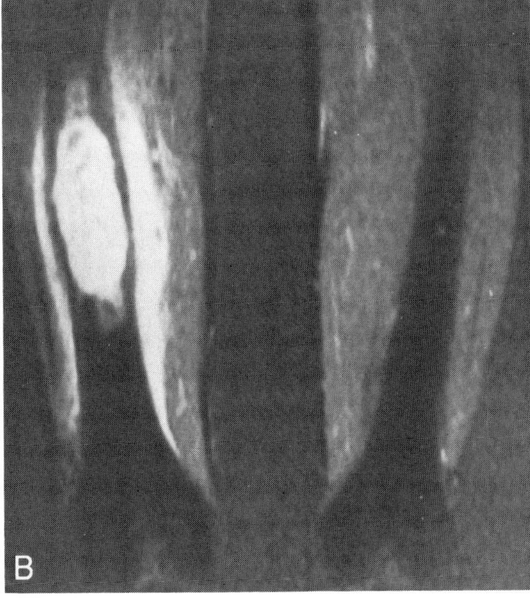

FIGURE 7–80. Ewing's sarcoma. *A.* Coronal T1 spin echo image shows an intramedullary, expansile lesion of the right femur. The marrow has been replaced by low-intensity tumor. *B.* Matching STIR image shows the high-intensity intramedullary tumor mass. In addition, periostitis and reactive soft-tissue edema is well demonstrated. Ewing's sarcoma is typically depicted with extremely high intensity on STIR images, as in this case. (Courtesy of B. Porter, First Hill Diagnostic Imaging Center, Seattle.)

Blastic Bone Lesions

Most blastic bone lesions are benign. They include osteoid osteoma, osteochondroma, and bone island. However, most malignant bone tumors are blastic; they are easily differentiated from benign dense lesions because of the destruction, the aggressive growth, and the soft-tissue mass.

Benign Blastic Lesions

Osteoid Osteoma. Osteoid osteoma is a benign lesion that occurs in children and young adults. The cause is unknown. The most common sites are the tibia and the femur, but it also occurs in the pelvis and the vertebrae. In the femoral neck, the lesion may be similar to a stress fracture. The lesion may be cortical, cancellous, or subperiosteal. Patients often have pain at night, which is relieved by aspirin. The usual lesion is a bony nidus, which forms connective tissue and dense bony sclerosis (Fig. 7–81). The appearance of the central nidus is variable, and tomography or nuclear medicine bone scan may be required for confirmation. The differential diagnosis includes infection, stress fracture, and osteoblastoma. Treatment is excision of the nidus.

Osteoma. Osteoma is a benign tumor of the calvarium or the paranasal sinuses. It manifests in adults. Clinical symptoms are headache and sinus obstruction. The radiographic appearance is dense bone in the skull or sinus.

Osteochondroma. Osteochondroma (also called an exostosis, or an osteocartilaginous exostosis) is a deformity of the ends of the long bones. It originates as a disturbance of the cartilaginous growth plate. Deformation (expansion) of the epiphyseal region and bony protuberances directed along the shaft (away from the end of the bone) constitute the characteristic appearance (Fig. 7–82). Growth of the exostosis ceases when the epiphyseal plate closes. Therefore, growth or pain in an exostosis after epiphyseal fusion suggests malignant degeneration (to chondrosarcoma and, in rare instances, osteosarcoma). Such degeneration occurs in 15% of patients.

Myositis Ossificans. Myositis ossificans is neither an inflammatory process nor an ossification. It appears to be the calcified residue of trauma or hemorrhage in the soft tissues adjacent to the bone. It develops 2 to 8 weeks

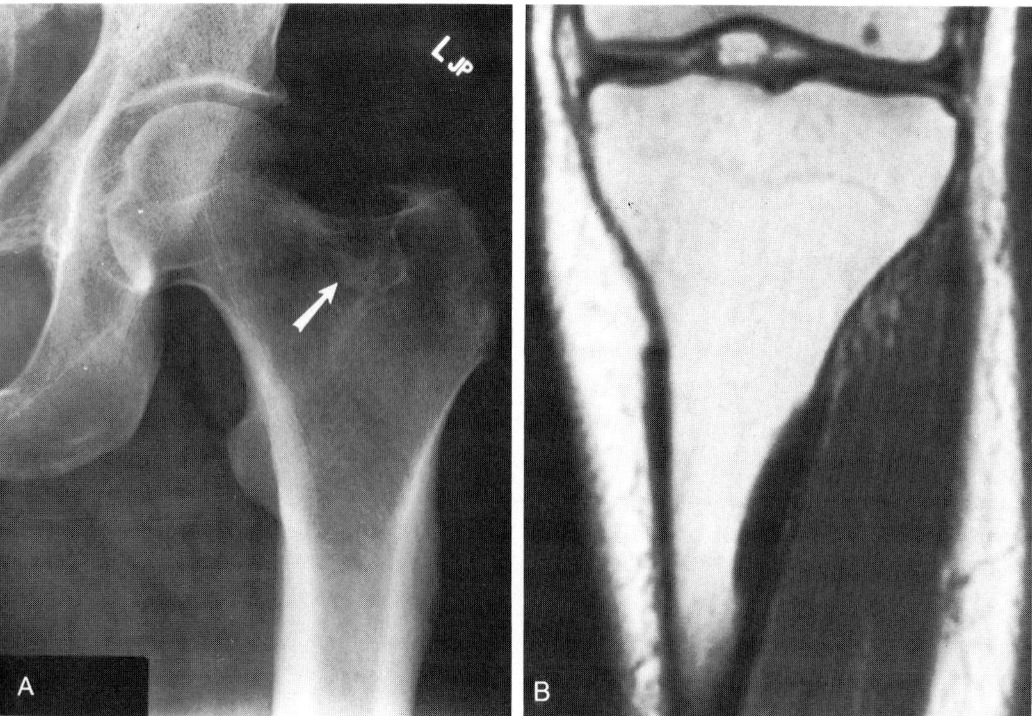

FIGURE 7–81. Osteoid osteoma. *A.* AP film of the hip shows a dense lesion in the femoral neck *(arrow).* A nidus is not identified. *B.* T1 spin echo image in another patient shows dense sclerosis of the lateral tibial shaft in reaction to a small nidus seen on plain films.

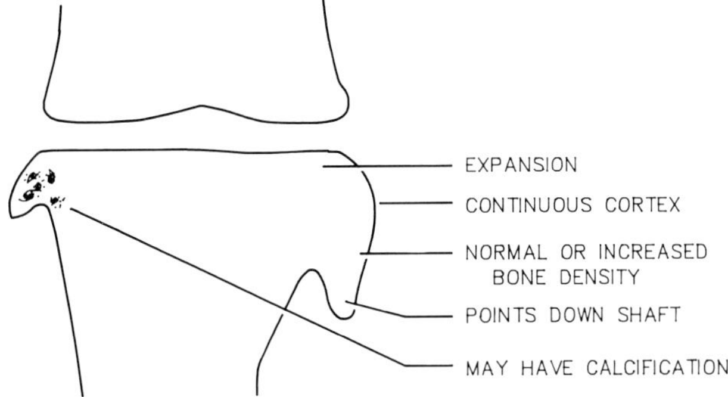

FIGURE 7–82. Characteristics of osteochondroma.

after trauma and regresses within 6 months. The plain film appearance of a smooth, dense peripheral margin of calcification (see Fig. 7–41) distinguishes this lesion from the flocculent calcification of parosteal sarcoma (see Fig. 7–85), which otherwise has a similar appearance. Because this lesion looks malignant histologically, such lesions should be followed radiographically. A false-positive biopsy will cause needless radical therapy.

Bone Island. A bone island is a benign, well-defined area of normal but densely packed trabecular bone. It has no malignant potential and produces no symptoms. It may occur in any bone and may be seen at any age. The differential diagnosis includes osteoid osteoma and metastatic tumor. A bone island has low intensity on T2 spin echo and STIR images and usually does not take up the bone scanning agent.

Osteitis Condensans Ilii. Osteitis condensans ilii is a benign, bony sclerosis limited to the iliac side of the sacroiliac joint. Involvement is bilateral and symmetrical. This lesion is easily differentiated from inflammatory and degenerative conditions, all of which involve both sides of the joint.

Malignant Blastic Lesions

Osteogenic Sarcoma. Osteogenic sarcoma is the second most common primary bone tumor (after myeloma). It most commonly occurs in teenagers, but a second period of increased incidence is in the sixth decade. Many of these sarcomas in older patients arise from a preexisting lesion (Table 7–9). The lesions are usually in the metaphysis of the long bones. The distal femur and the proximal tibia and humerus are the most common sites. The tumor destroys bone and is usually densely sclerotic. The epiphysis may be invaded, and the periosteum is often elevated, producing Codman's triangle. A soft-tissue mass may be present.

Variations of the usually dense osteosarcoma are the osteolytic osteosarcoma and the multicentric osteosarcoma (also called osteosarcomatosis). Osteosarcoma may also arise de novo from the soft tissues. Two additional types of osteosarcoma, the parosteal and the periosteal sarcomas, are discussed below.

Plain films show dense sclerosis (Fig. 7–83), bone destruction, and periosteal elevation. The presence of bone spicules at right angles to the medullary cavity indicates rapid expansion. Radiographs of the osteolytic form show a low-density lesion with ragged margins. There may be a calcified or an ossified soft-tissue mass. MRI best shows the soft-tissue mass and the extent of marrow invasion (Fig. 7–84). Sclerotic lesions are of low intensity on all imaging sequences. However, the presence of dystrophic calcification, hemorrhage, abnor-

TABLE 7–9. LESIONS THAT DEGENERATE TO OSTEOGENIC SARCOMA

Paget's disease
Radiation therapy
Enchondroma
Osteochondroma (exostosis)
Fibrous dysplasia

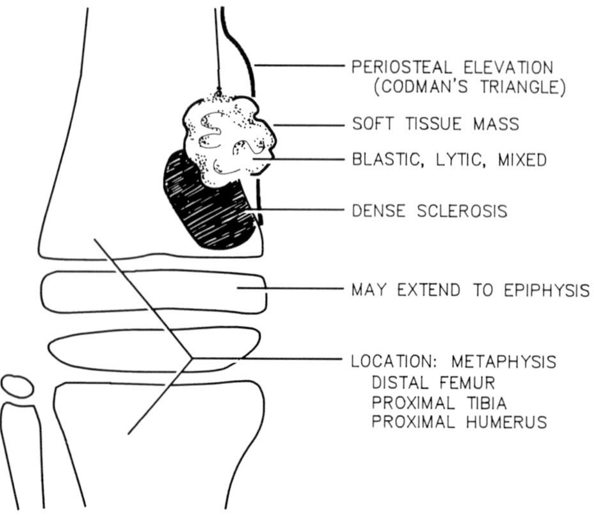

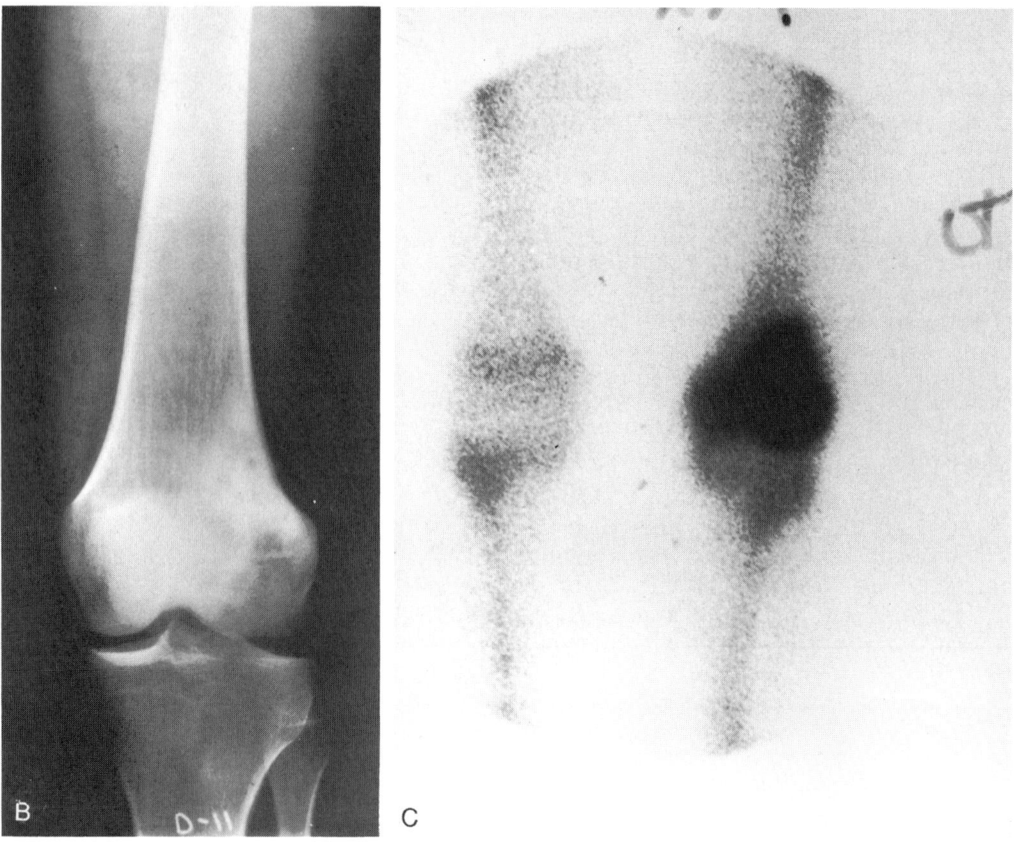

FIGURE 7–83. Osteogenic sarcoma. *A.* Diagram. *B.* AP film shows dense sclerosis in the distal lateral femur. The sclerosis extends into the (closed) epiphyseal region. Periostitis is not evident in this relatively early but painful lesion. *C.* Bone scan of the knees shows extensive uptake, extending to the joint margin. (Courtesy of C. Helms, Department of Radiology, University of California, San Francisco.)

FIGURE 7–84. Osteogenic sarcoma. Coronal spin echo image of the femur shows marked increased intensity caused by the aggressive tumor in the left distal femur of an 8-year-old girl. The marrow has been replaced by dense tumor. (Courtesy of S. Williamson, Department of Radiology, University of New Mexico School of Medicine.)

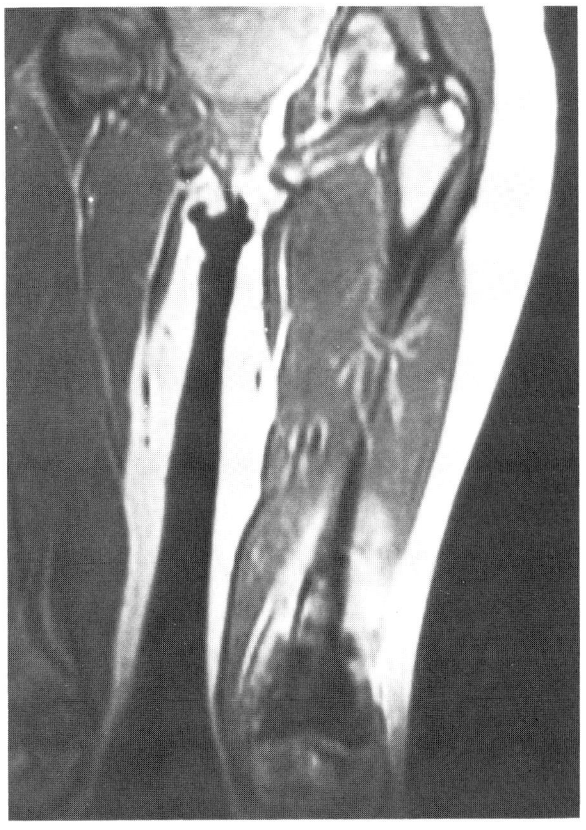

mal vascularity, and necrosis can produce a complex appearance. The tumor shows dense uptake on nuclear medicine bone scans.

Treatment requires early resection and chemotherapy. Pulmonary metastases occur early and appear as single or multiple round lesions. These can be resected individually with good results. Osteosarcomatosis is rapidly fatal.

Parosteal sarcoma (also called juxtacortical osteosarcoma) arises in the periosteum of the long bones and usually grows outward. Much of the tumor is therefore outside the bone. This lesion occurs in an age group (30 to 40 years) older than that in which intramedullary osteosarcoma occurs. The lesion is not aggressive unless it grows into the medullary cavity. Therefore, imaging is directed toward assessing cortical invasion. The lesion most commonly occurs in the posterior distal femur (Fig. 7–85). It may have a stalk connecting the extraosseous mass to the bone. The mass is exophytic. The lesion is sometimes difficult to distinguish from myositis ossificans (see earlier discussion and Fig. 7–41) and cortical desmoid (an avulsion injury).

Periosteal sarcoma is a rare (approximately 50 reported cases) tumor of bone characterized by short bony spicules perpendicular to a long periosteal lesion in the shaft of a long bone. There is a wide base of attachment. The cortex is thickened without destruction. There is no invasion of the medullary canal. This lesion is a high-grade malignancy, but if it is resected, the prognosis for the patient is good.

Chondrosarcoma. Among primary malignant bone tumors, chondrosarcoma is third only to myeloma and osteogenic sarcoma in incidence. Central chondrosarcomas arise in the metaphysis or shaft of the long bones and the trunk, especially the pelvis, and are characteristically expansile, low-density lesions with sclerotic margins and speckled calcification (Fig. 7–86). Peripheral chondrosarcomas appear as bulky soft-tissue masses attached to the ends of bones; they contain chondroid calcification. These peripheral lesions most likely arise from degeneration of exostoses. They appear most commonly in the pelvis, the scapula, and the sternum. The lesion is a low-grade chondroid malignancy and is often indis-

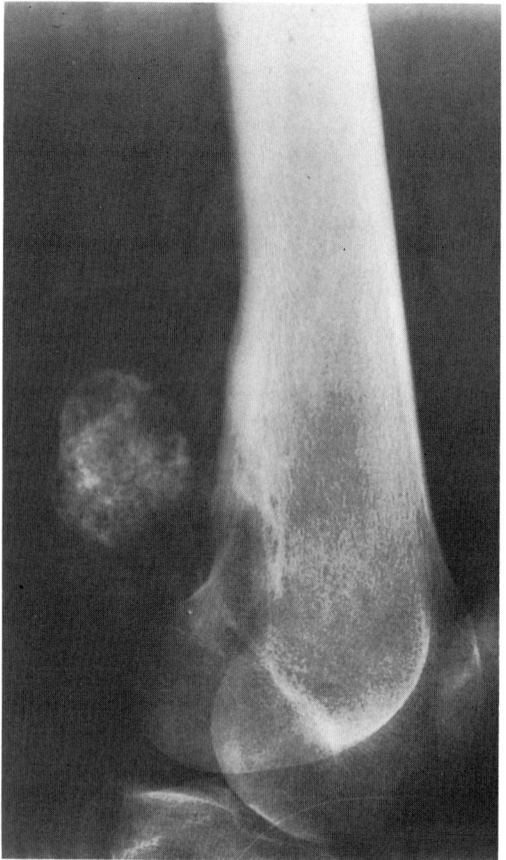

FIGURE 7–85. Parosteal sarcoma. Lateral plain film of the knee shows a calcified lesion at the posterior aspect of the femur. Note also cortical thickening and permeative appearance of the bone. The lesion is connected to the bone (not well demonstrated). The lesion has an appearance similar to that of myositis ossificans. However, parosteal sarcoma shows internal calcification, as opposed to outer shell calcification.

tinguishable from enchondroma. Patients are usually over age 40 and have pain.

Radiographs show an expansile lesion with irregular chondroid calcification. The lesion is poorly marginated and may cause endosteal cortical thickening. The MRI appearance is complex because of the presence of calcification and tumor elements. When the tumor is not calcified, it may be similar in appearance to any of the lytic lesions described earlier.

Synovial Sarcoma. Synovial sarcoma is a rare malignant tumor of the joint space or (more commonly) a tendon sheath. It manifests as a soft-tissue mass near, but not within, the joint (Fig. 7–87). The tumor is often (in 30% of patients) associated with amorphous flocculent calcification.

Blastic Metastases. Blastic metastases to bone occur most often with cancer of the prostate, the breasts, and the lungs and with carcinoid. They occur more rarely with colon cancer and lymphoma. The most common sites are the vertebrae and the pelvis.

Soft-Tissue Tumors

Soft-tissue tumors include a wide variety of tissue types. The majority are sarcomas and fibrous tumors. Some of these tumors invade the bone; others are confined predominantly to the soft tissues. The most obvious finding is a mass, detected clinically. Imaging tests are performed in order to further evaluate the lesion by showing the tissue of origin, local invasion, bone involvement, and the relationship to vascular structures. Plain films (Fig. 7–87) generally show a soft-tissue mass and distortion of soft-tissue planes. These films are most helpful in evaluation of bone invasion.

CT and MRI are the most successful imaging techniques for soft tissue masses. MRI has the added advantage of providing tissue characterization through the use of different sequences, and it better demonstrates the relationship of the mass to other structures through the use of coronal (Figs. 7–88, 7–89) and sagittal planes. Paramagnetic contrast enhancement

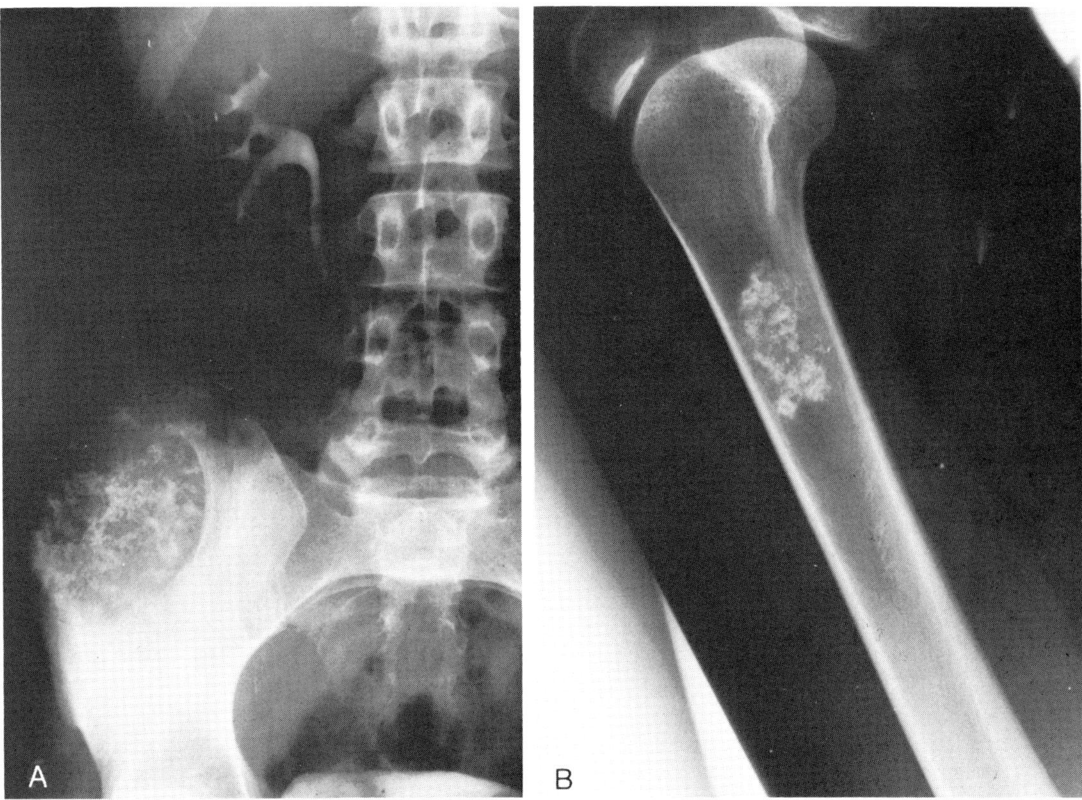

FIGURE 7–86. *A.* Chondroblastic osteosarcoma. AP abdominal film shows a large, destructive, predominantly lytic lesion in the right iliac bone. Central flocculent areas of calcification are indicative of the chondroid character of this tumor. The lesion also has a soft-tissue component superiorly where it has extended through the bone. *B.* Chondrosarcoma. Lateral view of the tibia shows a flocculent area of chondroid calcification in the proximal metaphysis. The margins are irregular. This tumor developed from an enchondroma.

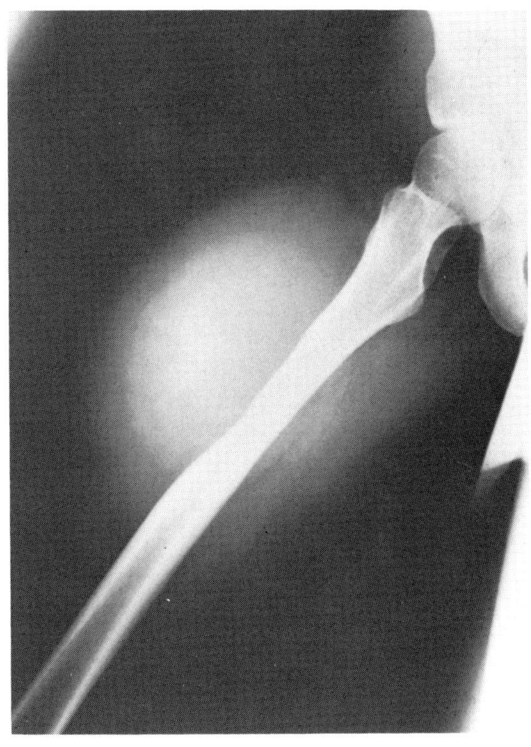

FIGURE 7–87. Synovial sarcoma. Plain film of the hip shows a large soft-tissue mass surrounding the proximal femur. The cortex is eroded, and the bone is thinned. Synovial sarcomas generally arise separately from the joint space, as seen here. They do not primarily involve the bone. (Courtesy of C. Helms, Department of Radiology, University of California, San Francisco.)

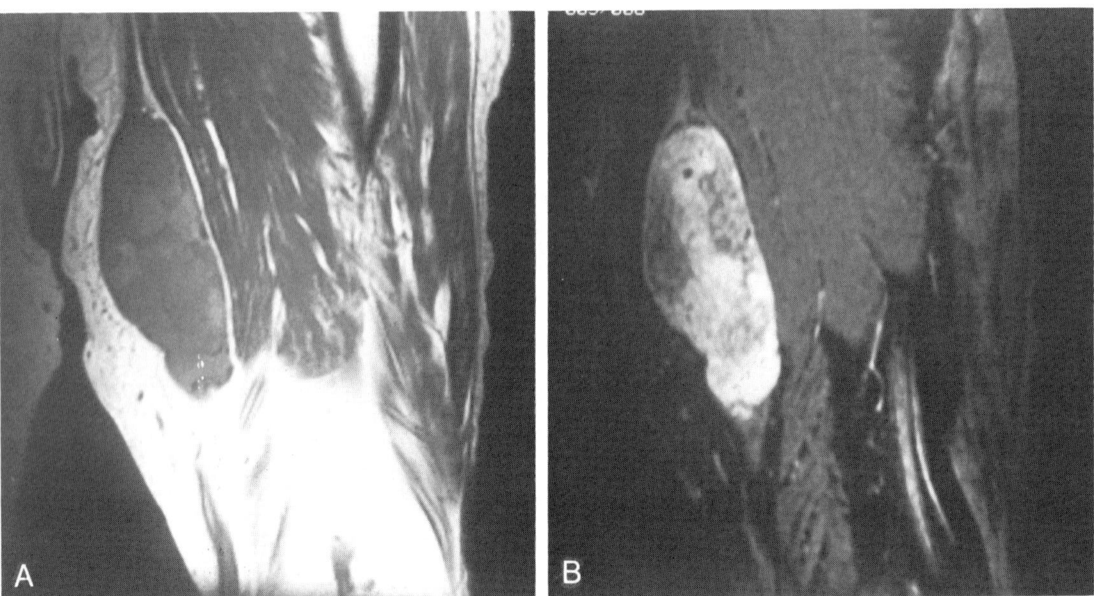

FIGURE 7–88. Liposarcoma. *A.* Coronal T1 spin echo image of the upper leg shows a complex, low-intensity lesion in the medial thigh, between the muscles and the fat. *B.* Matching STIR image shows the intensity of the lesion to be higher than that of fat but not as high as those of many tumors, fluid, and blood. In this case, the liposarcomatous tissue does not have the obvious appearance of fat. It is not of as high intensity as other types of tumor.

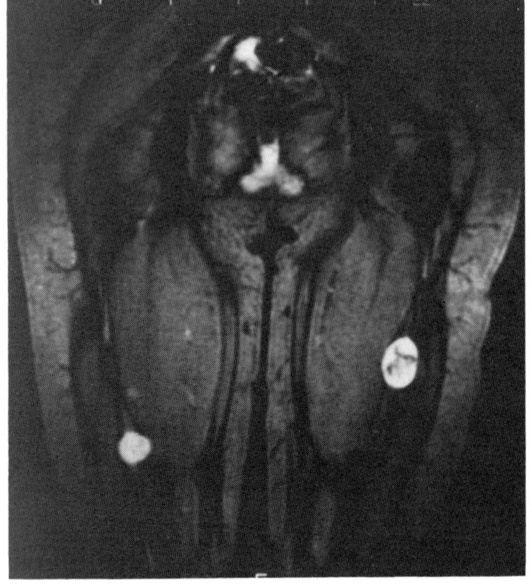

FIGURE 7–89. Neurofibromas. Coronal STIR image in a patient with bilateral thigh masses shows high-intensity lesions in the soft tissue adjacent to the muscles. The very high intensity of these neurofibromas on STIR images is typical. The patient has neurofibromatosis.

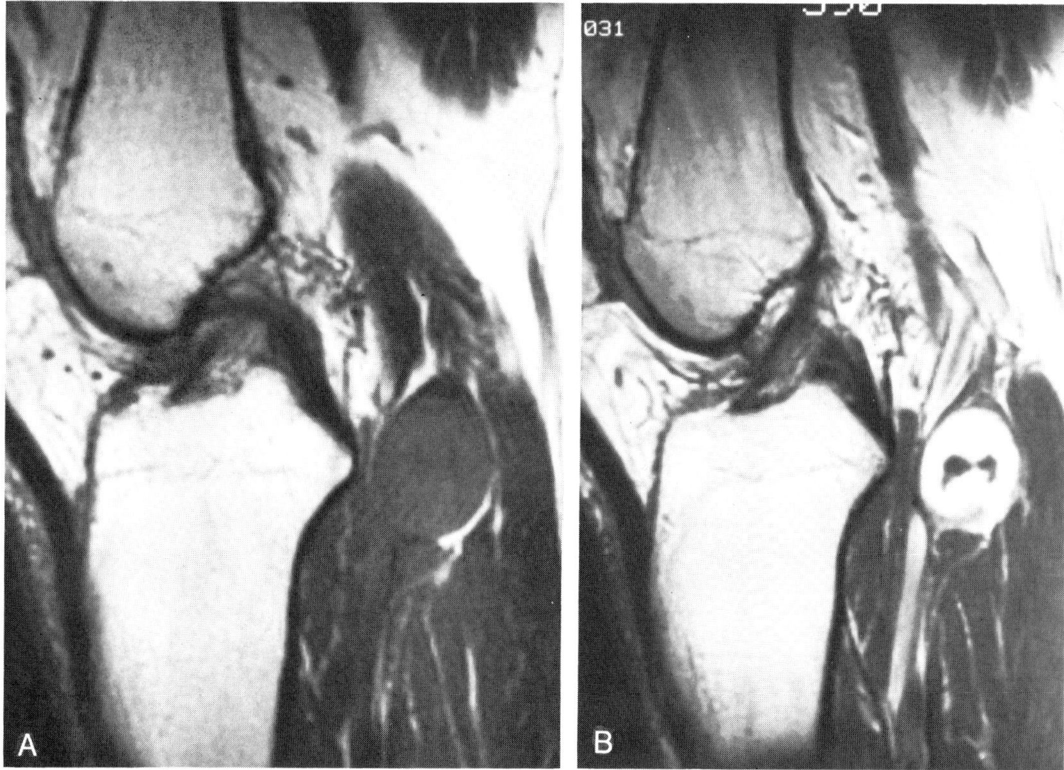

FIGURE 7–90. Neurofibroma. *A.* T1 spin echo image shows a mass in the posterior knee. *B.* Post–Gd-DTPA image shows enhancement with central irregularity.

can demonstrate important properties of the tumor (Fig. 7–90).

SPECIAL TOPICS IN PEDIATRIC MUSCULOSKELETAL RADIOLOGY

Fractures

Growth Plate Fractures. Fractures at the ends of long bones in children are complex because the physeal (growth) plate is open. They are among the most common musculoskeletal injuries in children and are serious because the blood supply to the physeal plate is through the epiphysis. A poor treatment result can therefore affect continued growth and proper alignment. Epiphyseal fractures are classified according to the location and the number of fractures (Salter-Harris classification; Fig. 7–91). The most common ones involve the growth plate and either the epiphysis or the metaphysis (not both) and carry a good prognosis. Fractures that extend through both the epiphysis and the metaphysis or that result in a crush injury to the growth plate carry a poor prognosis. Fractures through the bone are easily seen on radiographs. Fractures through the plate may not be visible. Because the ligaments in children are stronger than the growth plate, a fracture through this plate is more likely to occur than is a ligamentous strain or sprain, and this possibility should be considered when the clinical diagnosis is ligamentous strain or sprain.

Greenstick Fracture. Fractures of the forearm in children are often incomplete breaks because of the elasticity of the bone. In such a fracture, the break may be clean through half the bone and may be a smooth bend on the remainder, which is similar to a break in a green sapling (Fig. 7–92). The fracture is therefore called a greenstick fracture.

Torus Fracture. An impaction fracture, called a torus fracture, occurs in young children, usually in the distal radius or the distal tibia. The bone does not show a fracture line because the thick periosteum holds the bone in place. The radiograph shows a concentric bulge in the region of the impacted bone. The term "torus" is derived from the appearance of a Greek column (Fig. 7–93).

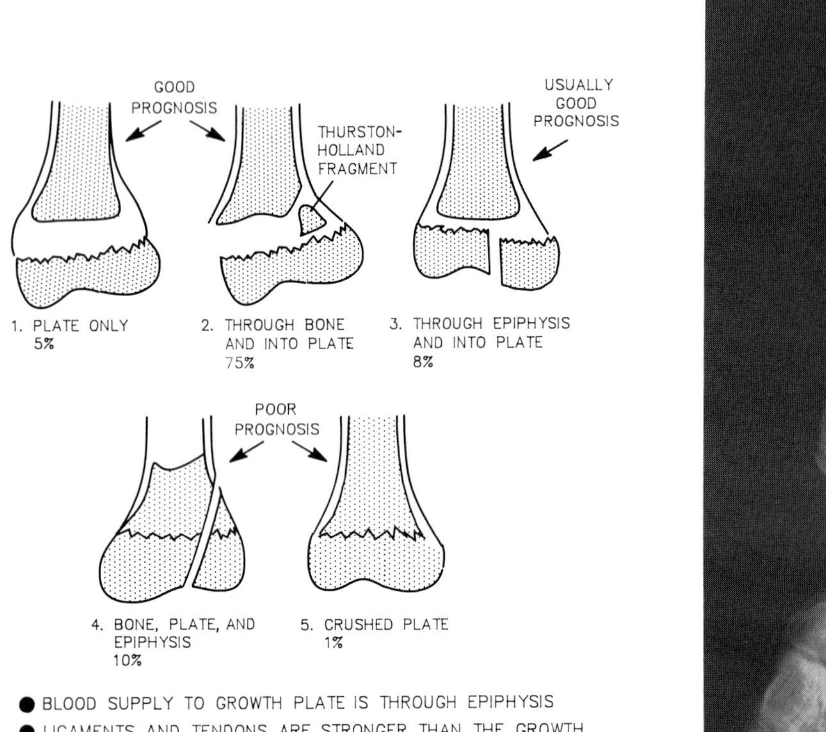

FIGURE 7–91. Epiphyseal fractures. *A.* Diagram. *B.* AP view of the ankle shows a Salter II fracture of the distal tibia in addition to a fracture of the distal fibula. Note the overlying fracture fragments of the distal tibial shaft and the offset at the epiphyseal plate. (Courtesy of C. Helms, Department of Radiology, University of California, San Francisco.)

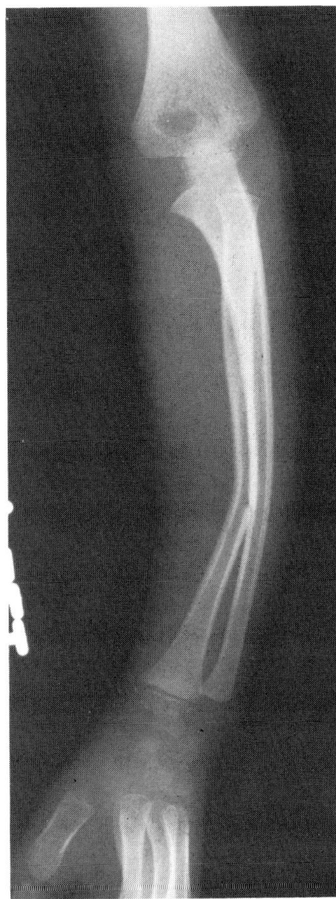

FIGURE 7–92. Greenstick fracture. Forearm film in a young child shows bowing and angulation of the radius and ulna. The inner side of the radius shows smooth bowing. The outer radius shows a fracture line.

Stress (Toddler's) Fracture. Stress fracture of the distal tibia occurs in toddlers who have just begun walking. The fracture, called a toddler's fracture, is usually at the distal end of the bone (Fig. 7–94). The fracture is manifested clinically by the patient's extreme fussiness and a refusal to walk.

Pediatric Diseases Involving the Knee

Many diseases of childhood affect the long bones or the joint spaces and are often identified on plain films of the knees, which are obtained to evaluate difficulty in walking. These disorders include diseases from all disease categories (summarized later and in Fig. 7–95). The normal knee has smooth margins of the ends of the shafts and the epiphyses, uniform mineralization, and a smooth cortical margin along the shaft. Abnormalities attributable to these diseases are caused by fracture and healing, hemorrhage, deposition of toxic elements, arrested or altered bone formation, or inflammation.

The battered child has multiple fractures and normal mineralization. Corner fractures (avulsion injuries) and bucket-handle fractures are characteristic. Soft-tissue hematomas can calcify, and fractures of the shaft may show periosteal elevation as a result of blood or the healing process. The epiphyses have a normal appearance.

Hemophilia results in hemorrhage and joint destruction and, later, bone overgrowth. Characteristic findings are enlargement and squaring of the epiphyses; squaring of the intracondylar notch; cyst (geode) formation at the ends of the femur, the tibia, and the epiphyses; a

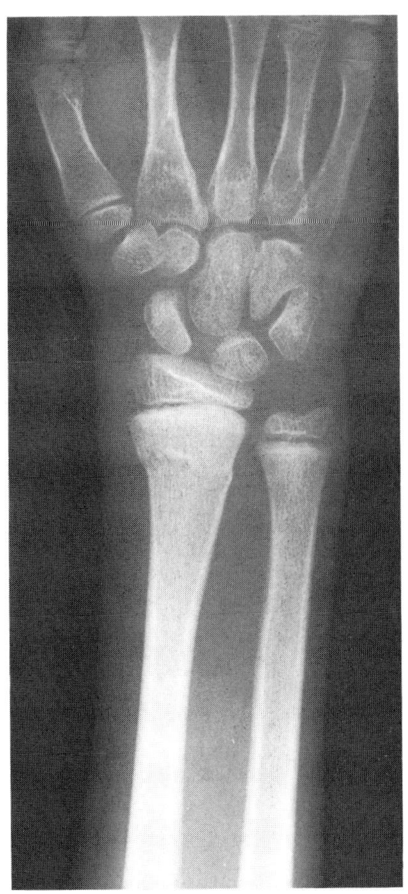

FIGURE 7–93. Torus fracture. Wrist film shows discontinuity, bone overlap, and lateral bulges of the distal radius of a child. This fracture occurred when the child fell on an outstretched hand.

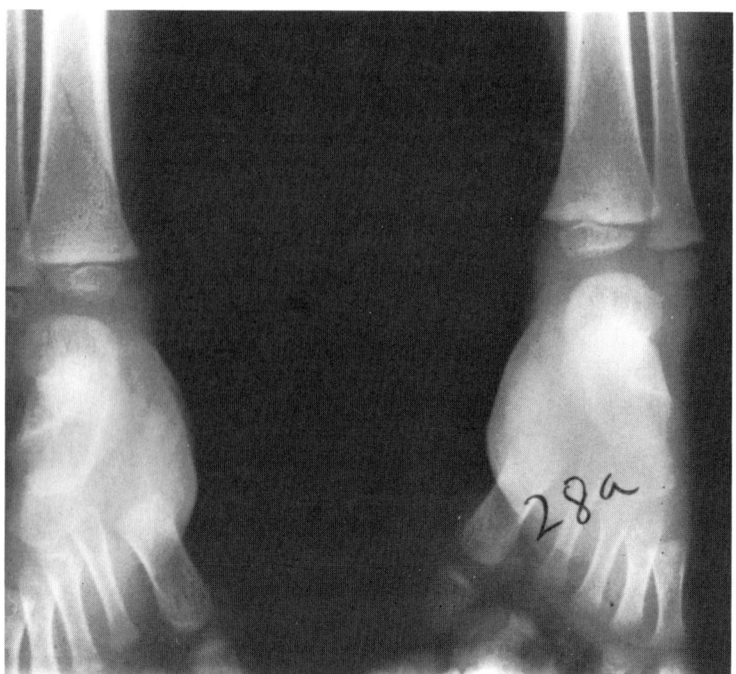

FIGURE 7–94. Toddler's fracture. AP view of the ankles shows a diagonal fracture line through the distal right tibia of an active child who had just begun walking. (Courtesy of C. Helms, Department of Radiology, University of California, San Francisco.)

narrow joint space; and generalized demineralization (see also earlier discussion with arthritis and Fig. 7–63).

Rickets produces a wide growth space, fraying and cupping of the ends of the femur and the tibia, and fraying of the epiphyses. Generalized demineralization is also present.

The abnormalities of scurvy are caused by defective bone matrix formation and hemorrhage. The growth plate has a thick, jagged margin and an adjacent lucent line. The shaft has decreased mineralization and a ground-glass appearance. Corner fractures result from weakness of bone, and periosteal elevation and calcification result from hemorrhage. A dense margin around the epiphyses is called Wimberger's sign.

Lead poisoning results in dense bands of lead deposited at the growth plate at the time of ingestion (usually in the form of lead-based paint). These bands migrate down toward the midshaft as the bone grows.

Osteomyelitis can produce a variety of abnormalities, including periosteal elevation and break (leaving a triangular edge called Codman's triangle), local demineralization and patchy destruction, and a sequestered area of calcified infection (sequestrum). These findings are especially pronounced in syphilis with new bone formation, cupping of the ends of the femur and the tibia, and, sometimes, a notch in the tibia (also named after Wimberger).

Congenital rubella produces a celery stick appearance as a result of vertical striations. There is no cupping of the ends of the femur and the tibia, and there is no periosteal reaction.

Leukemia causes permeative destruction of the bone and subperiosteal bone formation. A lucent line apparent at the growth plate is caused by interrupted growth.

RADIOGRAPHIC DIFFERENTIAL DIAGNOSIS

Frequently, a single radiographic finding or pattern suggests a limited list of diagnoses. Additional findings and clinical history then assist in further limiting the list or in making a firm diagnosis. The following approaches to evaluation of radiographic findings can provide assistance in differential diagnosis. Diseases are listed in order of importance.

DENSE BONES

Generalized increased density of the bones has a limited differential diagnostic list. The diseases can be grouped as congenital, metabolic or systemic, neoplastic, and vascular.

Congenital
- Osteopetrosis
- Pyknodysostosis

Metabolic or systemic
- Renal osteodystrophy

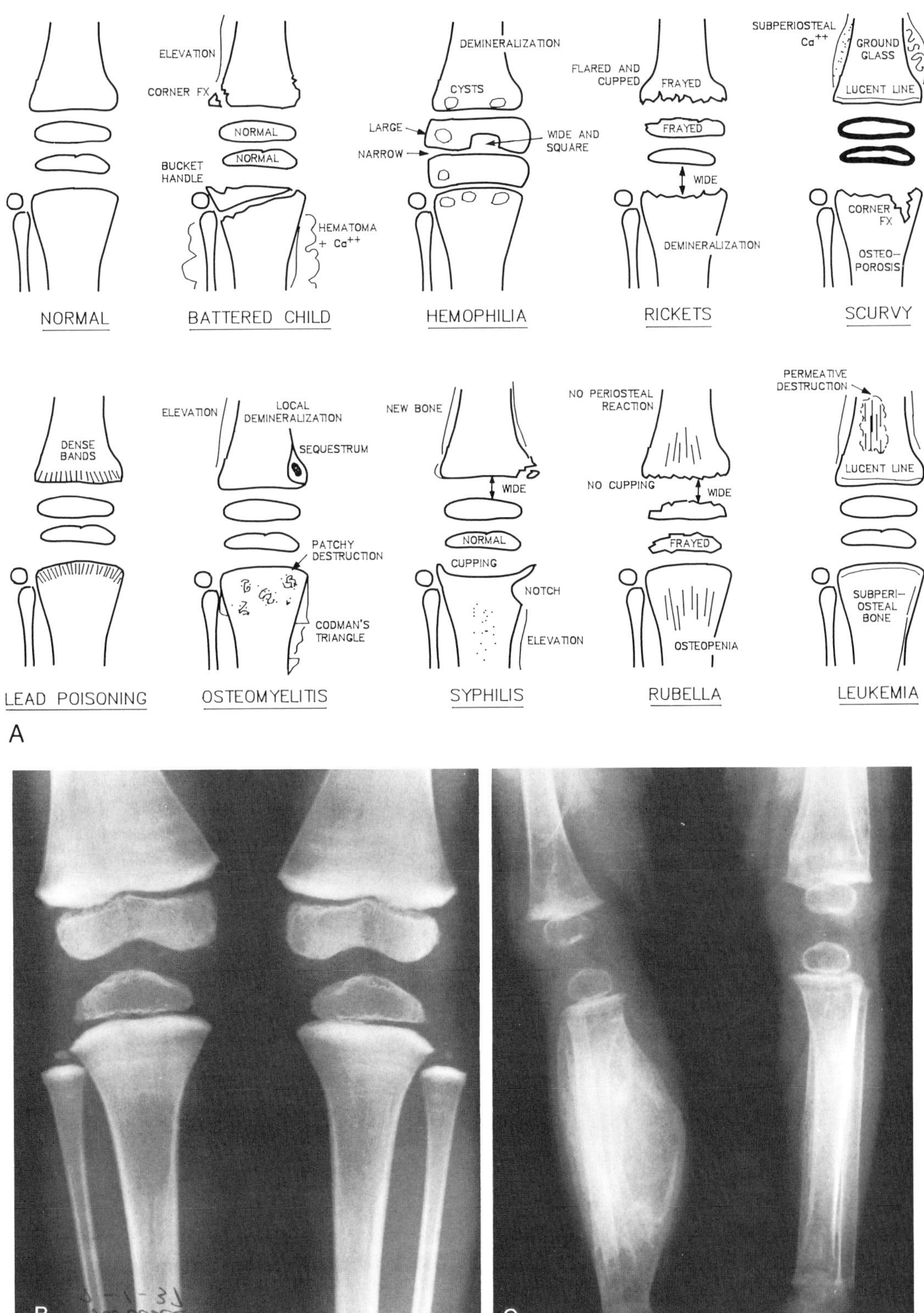

FIGURE 7–95. Pediatric disease involving the knee. *A.* Diagram. FX, fracture. *B.* Lead poisoning. Plain film of a child who ingested paint shows a dense metaphyseal band from lead deposition. Note also the alternating bands in the shaft, which correspond to previous periods of lead ingestion. *C.* Scurvy. Plain film of a toddler with vitamin C–deficient diet shows the results of osteoporosis, hemorrhage, and deficient bone formation. The mass in the right calf is caused by hemorrhage and residual calcification.

Paget's disease
Hypervitaminosis D
Fluorosis
Neoplastic
Metastasis from breast and prostate cancer; also lung cancer, lymphoma, and carcinoid
Vascular
Sickle cell anemia
Myelofibrosis
Mastocytosis

LYTIC BONE LESIONS

Many conditions cause lytic lesions in the bones. Except for metastatic disease and myeloma, these lesions are usually benign. Most of them are rare. A mnemonic for remembering these lesions is FOG MACHINES. This allows a systematic listing of the possible diseases. The annotations listed assist in further reducing the differential diagnosis.

*F*ibrous dysplasia: almost any appearance
*O*steoblastoma: occurs in vertebrae
*G*iant-cell tumor: eccentric, up to the joint, occurs after epiphyseal closure
*M*etastases: old age
*M*yeloma: any appearance; old age; also solitary plasmacytoma
*A*neurysmal bone cyst: expansile lesion in young patients
*A*ngioma: include hemangioma, lymphangioma, and neurofibroma
*C*hondromyxoid fibroma: like fibrous cortical defect
*C*hondroblastoma: only in epiphysis before closure
*H*istiocytosis X: characteristic lesions in skull, pelvis and femur
*H*yperparathyroidism: brown tumors
*I*nfection: any age, any appearance
*N*onossifying fibroma (fibrous cortical defect): long bones
*E*nchondroma: scalloped inner surface
*S*imple cyst (unicameral bone cyst): central in metaphysis

PERMEATIVE LESION IN A CHILD

In a child, a permeative lesion could indicate a benign solitary bone tumor, an aggressive infection, or malignancy. Three lesions have a common appearance and should be listed together.

Ewing's tumor
Infection
Eosinophilic granuloma

BONY SEQUESTRUM (NIDUS)

A sequestered fragment of dense material within a lesion could indicate isolated bone or central calcification. The most common cause of sequestrum is infection.

Infection
Eosinophilic granuloma
Osteoid osteoma
Fibrosarcoma

JOINT BODIES

Loose bodies in the joints can be caused by trauma and degeneration, proliferative diseases, arthritis, and deposition diseases. The joint bodies may be composed of cartilage, calcium, bony debris, or crystals.

Traumatic injury to bone, cartilage, or meniscus
Degenerative joint disease
Osteoarthritis
Chondromalacia
Osteonecrosis (AVN)
Osteochondritis dissecans
Proliferative disease
Synovial chondromatosis
Pigmented villondular synovitis
Arthritis and deposition diseases
CPPD deposition disease
Gout
RA

MARROW EDEMA ON MRI

A high intensity in the bone marrow shown on STIR images and on T2 spin echo images indicates increased water content. This may be caused by cellular tumor, edema, or blood. The finding is nonspecific and may require additional information such as the appearance of T1 spin echo images, CT scanning, plain film evaluation, and nuclear medicine scans.

AVN
Intraosseous fracture
Stress fracture
Osteochondritis dissecans
Osteoid osteoma
Tumor metastasis
Primary osteosarcoma

CORTICAL HOLES IN THE SKULL

Low-density lesions in the skull can be caused by metabolic, infectious, or neoplastic disorders. The skull film or CT appearance alone is often insufficient for diagnosis of the cause of the lesions.

Osteoporosis
Radiation
Renal osteodystrophy
Hemangioma
Infection
Metastasis
Paget's disease (osteoporosis circumscripta)

DENSE BASE OF THE SKULL

Increased density in the skull base usually has a benign cause. CT and MRI can often distinguish the development of dense bone, as occurs in osteopetrosis, from soft-tissue proliferation, as occurs in meningioma or fibrous dysplasia.

Fibrous dysplasia
Paget's disease
Meningioma
Pyknodysostosis
Osteopetrosis
Englemann's disease
van Buchem's disease

ATLANTOAXIAL DISEASE

Laxity of the joints at the atlantoaxial junction can result in marked instability and subluxation of the atlantoaxial joint. It occurs most commonly in various arthritides. Compression of the spinal cord may be life-threatening.

RA
JRA
Down's syndrome
Ankylosing spondylitis
Psoriasis

RIB LESIONS

Only a few diseases commonly affect the ribs. The most well-known rib lesions can be remembered with the acronym FAME (*fame*ous rib lesions).

*F*ibrous dysplasia
*A*neurysmal bone cyst
*M*etastasis and myeloma
*E*nchondroma

ELEVATED HUMERAL HEAD

Elevation of the humeral head (called a high-riding shoulder) is usually a result of an underlying rotator cuff injury with associated retraction. The most common causes are trauma and arthritis.

Trauma
RA
CPPD deposition disease
Hyperparathyroidism

SPINAL POSTERIOR-ELEMENT LESION

Lesions confined to the posterior elements of the spine are rare. Although several primary tumors occur in this location, they are rare. Metastases and myeloma are the most common causes of a lesion in the posterior elements.

Metastases and myeloma
Osteoblastoma
Osteoid osteoma
Fibrosarcoma

WIDENED HIP JOINT SPACE

Enlargement of the hip joint space indicates the presence of fluid or proliferative material. The most common causes are infection and osteonecrosis (AVN). Less common proliferative joint diseases fill the joint space with tissue. MRI can usually identify such joint-space abnormalities clearly and can usually enable a diagnosis to be made.

Infection
Osteonecrosis (AVN)
Pigmented villonodular synovitis
Synovial osteochondromatosis

HIP AND PROXIMAL FEMUR LESIONS

MRI is highly capable of diagnosing osteonecrosis (AVN) in the hip by demonstrating marrow edema. However, a number of other disease processes can also involve the hip. Most of them show either sclerosis or low density on plain radiographs.

Osteonecrosis (AVN)
Stress fracture
Osteoid osteoma
Transient osteoporosis
Lymphoma and leukemia
Metastasis
Fracture

SITES OF STRESS FRACTURE

Stress fractures usually occur when a new, strenuous activity places a repeated load on the bone. The location of the injury depends on the type of activity.

Femoral neck
Femoral shaft
Tibial plateau
Middle or distal tibia
Fibula (rare)
Calcaneus
Tarsal bones

SUBCHONDRAL CYSTS

Subchondral cysts (geodes) are seen in many conditions, usually as a result of degenerative disease or arthritis. Epiphyseal tumors and infection can have a similar appearance.

Degenerative joint disease
Osteonecrosis (AVN)

Arthritis: CPPD deposition disease, RA
Infection
Epiphyseal tumor: chondroblastoma, giant-cell tumor, aneurysmal bone cyst, eosinophilic granuloma, metastases, myeloma

CAUSES OF ARTICULAR CALCIFICATION

Articular calcification (called chondrocalcinosis) results from joint injury and precipitation of calcium crystals. In the early stages, radiographs generally show smooth calcium deposition in the cartilage. Advanced disease results in more complex joint destruction. Many hereditary diseases are accompanied by associated CPPD deposition disease.

CPPD deposition disease
Degenerative joint disease
Hyperparathyroidism
Hemochromatosis
Wilson's disease
Gout
Ochronosis

APPENDIX 7–1

The evaluation of the traumatized patient requires radiographic examinations that can be obtained quickly without moving the patient. Views that reliably show the most common injuries, show associated injuries, and demonstrate the need for additional views or examinations are of the highest priority.

GENERAL CONSIDERATIONS

1. Films should be targeted to the specific area of pain, deformity, or limitation.
2. Comparison views are usually not necessary.
3. A discussion between the radiologist and the clinician assists in provision of the best examination.
4. History and precise mechanism of injury are essential for determining the appropriate radiographs and for identifying injuries. Complex or compound injuries should be evaluated by a physician before the patient is referred for x-rays.

Skull. Most severe head injuries are indications for CT or MRI rather than for plain skull series. Plain film series of the face, the sinuses, the mastoids, and the mandible should be reserved for correlation of specific clinical findings.

Cervical Spine. AP, lateral, and odontoid views should be obtained before the patient is moved or before removal of cervical collars. Flexion-extension views or any movement of a patient with possible cervical spine injury should be supervised by a physician.

Thoracic and Lumbosacral Spine. The AP view of the spine is often evident on chest and abdominal films, although these films are not properly exposed for bone evaluation. Compression fractures and dislocations are best evaluated on lateral views.

Clavicle. The clavicle is usually seen on the posteroanterior (PA) chest film, but it appears as a straight line. To demonstrate its curved structure and thus better identify possible fracture, an angled clavicular view is necessary. When a fracture is seen, the clinician should be alerted to the possibility of vascular injury.

Scapula. Because the scapula is well-protected, injury to it is often associated with injuries to adjacent bones. The shape, the position, and the thin central portion of the scapula make evaluation difficult.

Shoulders. The PA chest film often shows the shoulders, but clinically obvious fractures or dislocations can be missed on this view. AP and transscapular views are required if there is clinical suspicion of shoulder dislocation or fracture.

Ribs. Rib fracture is a clinical diagnosis. If pneumothorax is suspected, a chest radiograph, not a rib detail examination, is indicated.

Humerus. When fracture of the shaft of the humerus is suspected, the joints above and below should be included in the examination. Pulses and extensor function should be tested bilaterally by the clinician in order to assess possible vascular or nerve injury.

Elbows. A true 90-degree flexion lateral film and an AP film are usually sufficient. In children, the mechanism of injury is important because dislocations are often difficult to see radiographically.

Radius and Ulna. It is important to include in the evaluation the joints above and below the radius and the ulna because fracture at one end often results in dislocation at the other. The mechanism of injury and the location of pain are particularly helpful for interpretation.

Wrists. Three views of the wrist are standard. Tenderness in the anatomical snuff box suggests navicular injury, which can be further evaluated by navicular views. Navicular fracture may not be evident early on, and repeated radiographs may be required at a later time.

Hands and Fingers. Only the injured areas should be examined.

Pelvis and Hips. The AP view of the pelvis usually demonstrates the hip joint well. It may be seen on a plain film of the abdomen or on bone films of the pelvis obtained in order to show possible pelvic fracture. The anatomical manifestation (such as internal rotation, foreshortening) is particularly helpful clinical information for evaluating a possible hip dislocation.

Femur. Two views usually suffice. If the patient has pain or loss of function, the joints above and below the femur must be included in the evaluation.

Knees. AP and cross-table lateral (partial flexion) views are adequate.

Tibia and Fibula. Two views usually suffice.

Ankle. Ankle films alone suffice for evaluation of ankle injury; foot films are not usually necessary. Evaluation of posterior malleolar fracture requires a slightly off-lateral view. If calcaneal fracture is suspected (as in a jumping injury), a calcaneal view should be requested.

Foot. The precise point of pain and swelling should be examined, not the entire foot.

Suggested Readings

Forrester DM, Messon J: The Radiology of Joint Disease, 3rd ed. Philadelphia: WB Saunders, 1978.

Greenspan A. Orthopedic Radiology: A Practical Approach. New York: Gower Medical, 1988.

Helms CA. Fundamentals of Skeletal Radiology. Philadelphia: WB Saunders, 1989.

Resnick D, Niwayama G. Diagnosis of Bone and Joint Disorders, 2nd ed. Philadelphia: WB Saunders, 1988.

Stoller DW, Genant HK, Helms CA (eds): Magnetic Resonance Imaging in Orthopaedics and Rheumatology. Philadelphia: JB Lippincott, 1989.

8

Neuroimaging

Gary K. Stimac
William W. Orrison, Jr.

BASIC EVALUATION

Plain Film Interpretation

Plain films of the skull and spine assist in the evaluation of bone tumors (including metastases), changes in bone density caused by metabolic disease, congenital bone abnormalities, and fractures. Other imaging methods, mainly computed tomography (CT) and magnetic resonance imaging (MRI), are far superior to plain radiographs for most central nervous system (CNS) abnormalities because they provide information about the brain, the spinal cord, and the soft tissues in addition to the bone. In traumatic head injuries, skull films can show fractures but are of limited value in the assessment of intracranial injury. A patient suspected of having a serious head injury should have immediate CT or MRI examination. Interpretation of plain films of the skull is discussed in Chapter 7.

In the spine, plain radiographs are useful for demonstrating bone injury or expansile lesions that can compress the spinal cord. The spatial detail of these radiographs may demonstrate metastatic tumor or infectious involvement of bone in patients with neurological abnormalities. The primary use of plain spine films is in the evaluation of trauma. These examinations also assist in the performance and interpretation of myelography, CT, and MRI for both trauma and other diseases. Decreased or increased bone mineralization in the spine (and the skull), such as that seen in Paget's disease, renal failure, and metastatic disease, can be detected on plain radiographs. Congenital CNS abnormalities such as meningomyelocele and achondroplasia are accompanied by spine abnormalities.

In spine injuries, plain radiography of the spine is the first examination because it can be done in the emergency room and can demonstrate fracture and abnormal alignment. If a fracture is present or if the patient has signs of neurological impairment, CT, MRI, or myelography may be indicated. When plain films fail to show a suspected fracture, high-resolution CT is frequently successful. The evaluation of plain films of the spine (discussed in Chapter 7) requires attention to the soft tissues, the bone alignment, and the intervertebral spaces; assessment of the size of the spinal canal and bone mineralization; and identification of fractures.

Angiography

Angiography demonstrates vascular lesions in the brain. Diagnostic angiography is now used primarily to provide additional information about abnormalities demonstrated by CT and MRI. It is used to evaluate atherosclerotic disease, intracranial aneurysm, vascular tumors and vascular malformations, and in the planning of surgical procedures. Interventional angiography techniques are used to dilate or occlude vessels in and around the brain, both as therapy and as an adjunct to surgery for brain tumors, vascular malformations, and vessel injuries.

The traditional radiographic angiographic technique with film-screen combinations provides the excellent spatial resolution necessary in the evaluation of some vascular malformations and small aneurysms and in the detection of vasculitis. However, for most applications, film-screen technique has been replaced by digital-subtraction angiography. This technique has superior contrast resolution, instant image subtraction, and continually improving spatial resolution. Such examinations require less contrast material and can be performed more rapidly and at lower cost than film screen examinations. In patients at high risk for complications from arterial injections, venous injections may be sufficient for diagnosis of some vascular abnormalities. In general, however, venous injections are less often used because they yield poor image contrast and require a large amount of contrast material.

Evaluation of the Extracranial Carotid and Vertebral Arteries

An understanding of the extracranial cephalic circulation is important in the evaluation of atherosclerotic and other vascular disease and in the selective catheterization of these vessels (Fig. 8–1*A*). The origins of these vessels are best examined by means of an aortic arch injection. Although most patients have a left-sided aortic arch with right brachioce-

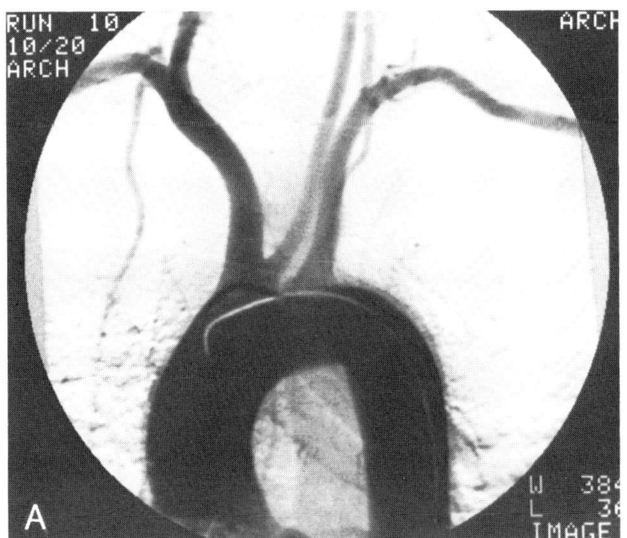

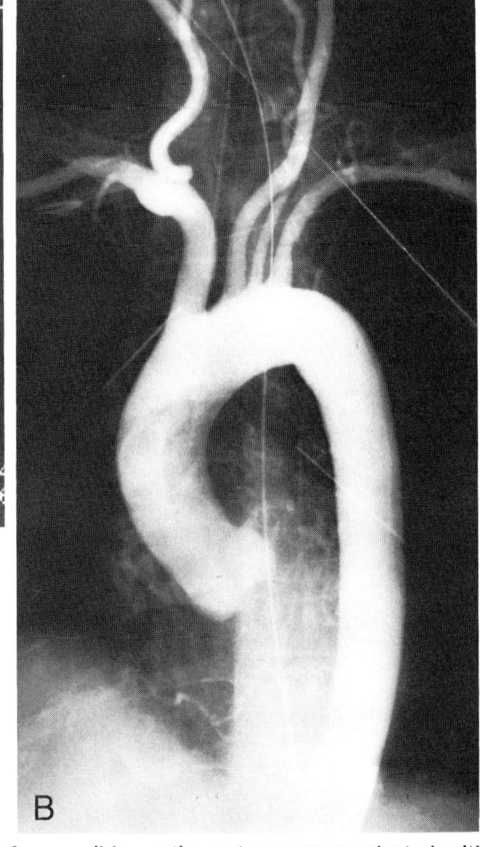

FIGURE 8–1. Aortic arch and brachiocephalic vessels. *A.* Only a small amount of contrast was needed for this digital-subtraction angiogram, in which an aortic arch injection demonstrates the normal origins of the brachiocephalic vessels. The first artery (right brachiocephalic) divides into the right common carotid and subclavian arteries. The right vertebral artery arises from the subclavian artery and, in this projection, overlaps the right carotid artery. The left common carotid artery is the second artery, arising just distal to the right brachiocephalic or, as shown here, as a common trunk with it. The left subclavian artery originates more distally; from its genu arises the left vertebral artery. *B.* Variant of the brachiocephalic vessels in a trauma patient. Evaluation for possible aortic rupture was conducted with conventional film angiography, which shows origin of the left vertebral artery from the aorta between the left carotid and subclavian arteries.

phalic, left carotid, and left subclavian arteries originating in sequence, variations are not unusual. Often the left carotid artery arises from the brachiocephalic artery; sometimes the vertebral arteries arise from the aortic arch (Fig. 8–1*B*); and, in rare instances, the vessels arise in a different order (see Chapter 5).

Atherosclerotic disease affects most severely the bifurcations of the carotid arteries in the neck, apparently because of turbulence at this site. This area can be examined through the use of digital-subtraction angiography after arterial or, under ideal conditions, intravenous injection. The large amount of contrast material required, the frequent overlapping of vessels, and the creation of artifacts by the patient's motion (many patients swallow involuntarily during the examination) often render intravenous examinations inadequate for presurgical diagnosis. Most neuroradiologists and vascular surgeons prefer arterial-injection digital-subtraction angiography or arterial injection and conventional filming for the evaluation of carotid bifurcation disease. Venous digital-subtraction angiography is a preferred alternative for patients in whom

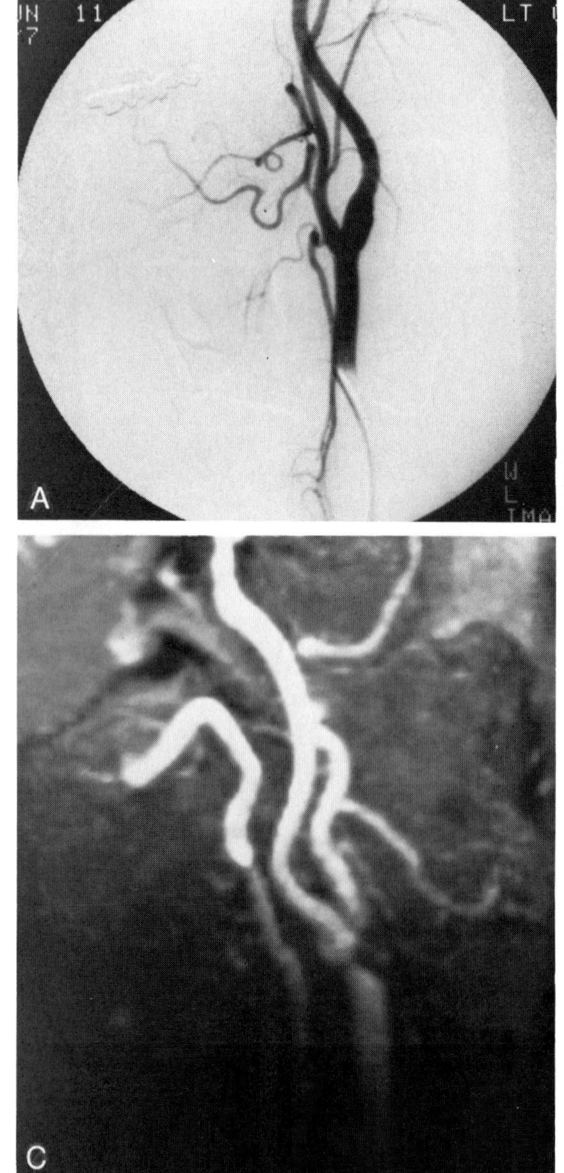

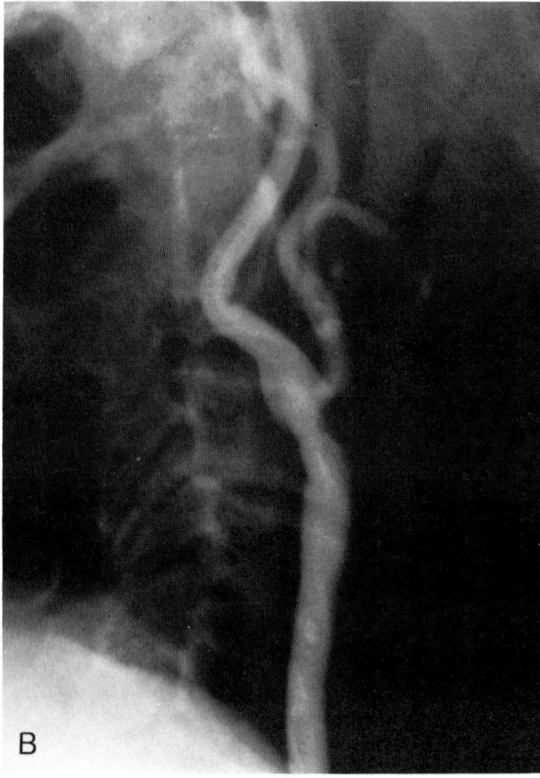

FIGURE 8–2. Carotid bifurcation. *A.* Common carotid arterial digital-subtraction angiogram shows smooth contour of the carotid bulb and the normal origin of the external carotid branches. *B.* Carotid arteriogram demonstrates stenosis at the carotid bifurcation with ulcerated plaque. *C.* MRA with time-of-flight technique in the patient of part *B* shows stenosis at the carotid bifurcation with ulcerated plaque.

TABLE 8–1. BRANCHES OF THE EXTERNAL CAROTID ARTERY

Branch	Importance
Ascending pharyngeal	Supply to glomus tumors of the skullbase (chemodectomas)
Superior thyroid	Supply to thyroid tumors
Lingual	Can usually be safely embolized*
Facial (external maxillary)	Can usually be safely embolized*
Occipital	Can communicate with vertebral artery; embolization is a risk
Posterior auricular	Can usually be safely embolized*
Internal maxillary	Origin of the middle meningeal artery; may anastomose with the ophthalmic artery
Superficial temporal	Used for external carotid to internal carotid bypass; can be safely embolized*

*Refers to therapeutic embolization with the use of small particles. Occlusion with liquid agents (glue) can occlude small branches to intracranial structures and cranial nerves. Embolization should not be undertaken without careful review of anastomotic channels.

there is high risk of complications from arterial injections. Carotid Doppler ultrasonography or magnetic resonance angiography (MRA) are the preferred methods for initial evaluation and follow-up of carotid artery disease.

The carotid bifurcation, generally located near the angle of the jaw, normally has a smooth, rounded contour without filling defects or indentations (Fig. 8–2). Calcified plaques (which appear as filling defects) and ulcers (seen as cavities in the diseased vessel wall that fill with contrast) predispose the patient to embolic disease.

Evaluation of the External Carotid Arteries

The external carotid artery usually passes anteromedially from the bifurcation and has important branches to the nasopharynx, the face, the skullbase, the occiput, the meninges, and the scalp (Table 8–1). An understanding of the course, the anatomical variations, and the anastomotic channels of these vessels is essential for adequate diagnosis of vascular tumors and for embolization procedures (Fig. 8–3). For example, most peripheral meningi-

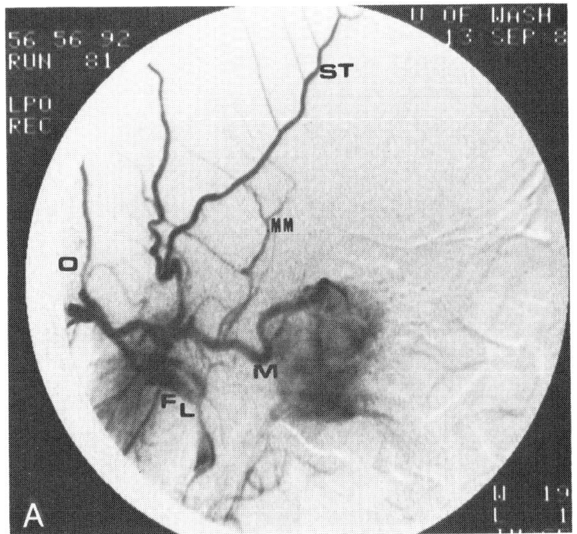

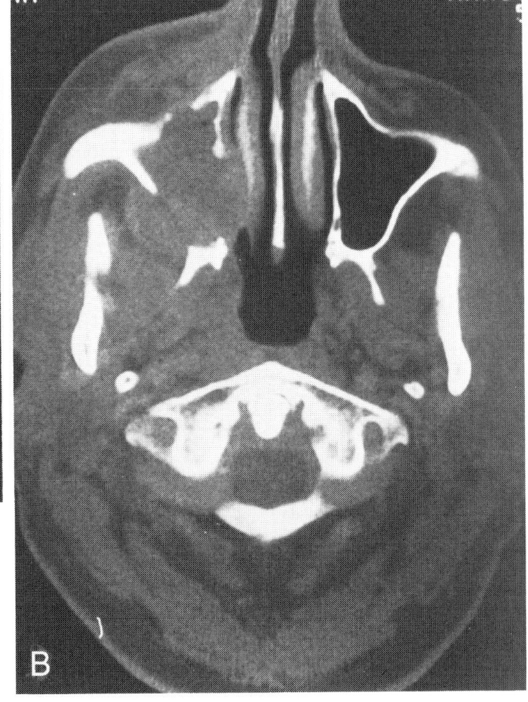

FIGURE 8–3. External carotid arterial circulation. *A.* Lateral view of a right external carotid digital-subtraction angiogram (the face is on the viewer's right) shows the branches of the external carotid artery. The maxillary artery feeds a squamous cell carcinoma of the maxillary sinus, evident from an intense vascular blush. The maxillary artery was used to infuse chemotherapy directly into the tumor. ST, superficial temporal; M, maxillary; MM, middle meningeal; O, occipital; F, facial; L, lingual. *B.* Computed tomogram (CT) shows the mass filling and extending from the right maxillary sinus with bone erosion.

omas have predominantly external carotid supply, usually from the middle meningeal arteries, and can be diagnosed and embolized by external carotid angiography. External carotid embolization is generally safe. However, vascular anastomoses, such as those between the occipital and vertebral arteries and between the maxillary and ophthalmic arteries, must be considered before embolization of these vessels is undertaken.

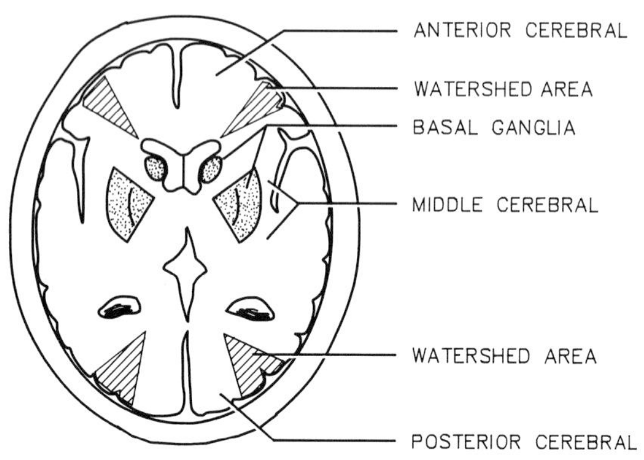

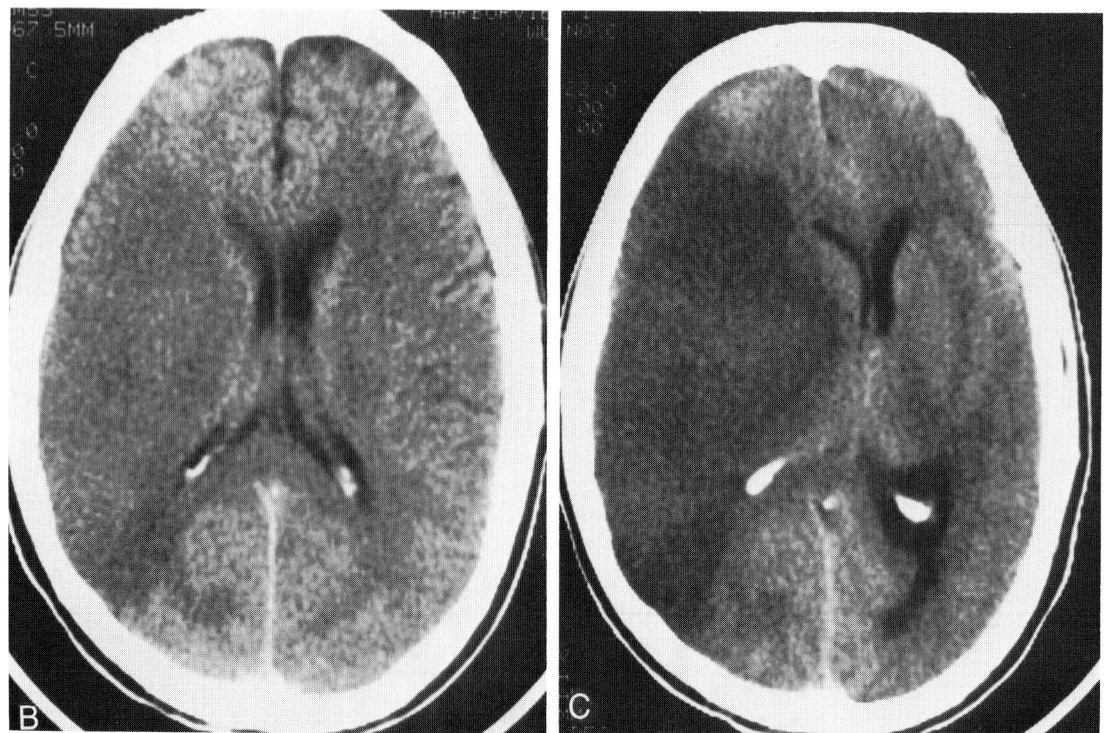

FIGURE 8–4. Vascular territories of the brain. *A.* Diagram. Knowledge of the vascular territories of the intracranial arteries allows determination of the origins of infarcts caused by embolic occlusion, hypoperfusion (watershed infarcts), and anoxia. *B.* Early appearance of an infarct demonstrating the territory supplied by the right middle cerebral artery (6 hours old). The findings—loss of differentiation of gray and white matter, effacement of cerebral sulci, and low density in the brain—are subtle but unmistakable. The anterior cerebral and posterior cerebral artery circulations are spared. *C.* Three days later, interstitial edema has developed, resulting in massive swelling, displacement of the midline, and entrapment of the left lateral ventricle.

Evaluation of the Intracranial Circulation

The intracranial circulation is best evaluated by means of selective internal carotid and vertebral artery injections. In nearly all cases, digital-subtraction techniques are recommended over direct film-screen techniques because they can be performed more rapidly and require less contrast material. Evaluation of the internal carotid circulation requires inspection of the petrous, intracavernous, and supraclinoid segments of the carotid artery and of the intracranial branches. Important branches of the internal carotid artery are the ophthalmic artery, the posterior communicating artery, the anterior choroidal artery, and the anterior and middle cerebral arteries. The anterior and middle cerebral arteries supply the frontal, temporal, and parietal lobes. Knowledge of these distributions is also helpful for assessing the cause of cerebral infarction (Fig. 8–4). The anterior communicating artery joins the two anterior cerebral arteries and is the most common site of aneurysm. Displacement of vessels, vascular malformation, vascular occlusion, aneurysm, and the presence of tumor vessels, tumor "blush," abnormal draining veins, and early shunting to the venous system are important angiographic abnormalities.

The posterior circulation is most commonly supplied by the vertebral arteries, which normally arise from the subclavian arteries, pass through the foramina transversaria in the cervical spine, and enter the skull through the foramen magnum. After giving off the posterior inferior cerebellar arteries, they join to form the basilar artery, which lies along the ventral brainstem. Important branches of the basilar artery are the anterior inferior cerebellar arteries and the superior cerebellar arteries. The basilar artery bifurcates at the level of the midbrain to form the posterior cerebral arteries, which supply the posterior temporal lobes and the occipital lobes. Knowledge of the vascular supply to the posterior fossa is important for evaluation of tumors and vascular malformations (Fig. 8–5).

The circle of Willis, an anastomotic system at the base of the brain, generally allows cross-filling of vessels that are diseased proximally (Fig. 8–6). The size of the various communicating vessels varies from patient to patient, and so the response of a given patient to a vascular stenosis or occlusion is not predictable. Some patients have persistence of the fetal

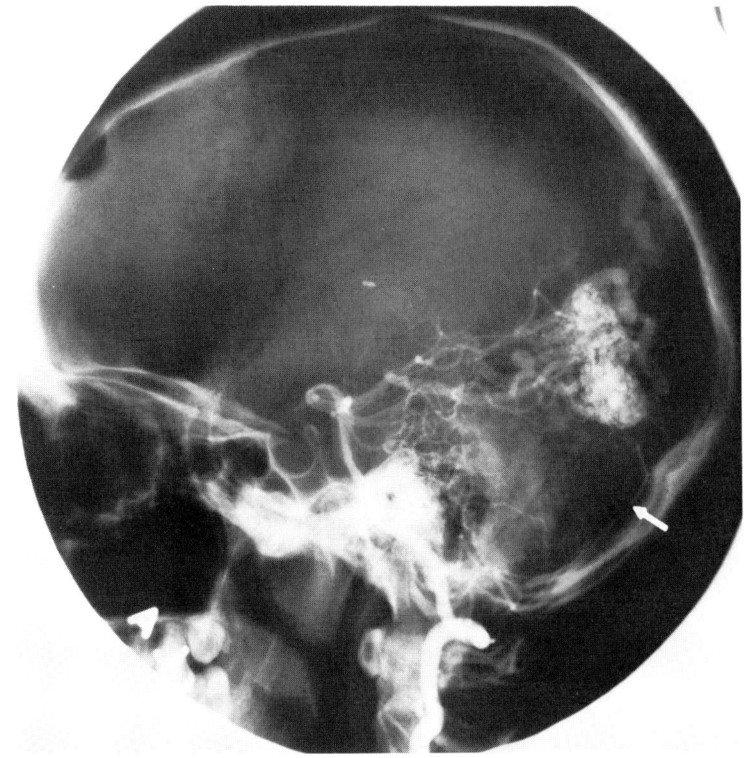

FIGURE 8–5. Posterior fossa circulation. Conventional lateral vertebral angiogram of a patient with an arteriovenous malformation (AVM) that is fed predominantly by the posterior cerebral arteries. Many additional feeding vessels include the posterior inferior cerebellar artery and muscular branches of the vertebral arteries *(arrow)*. The appearance of the dense tangle of abnormal vessels is typical of AVM, as is the early shunting into the venous system superiorly.

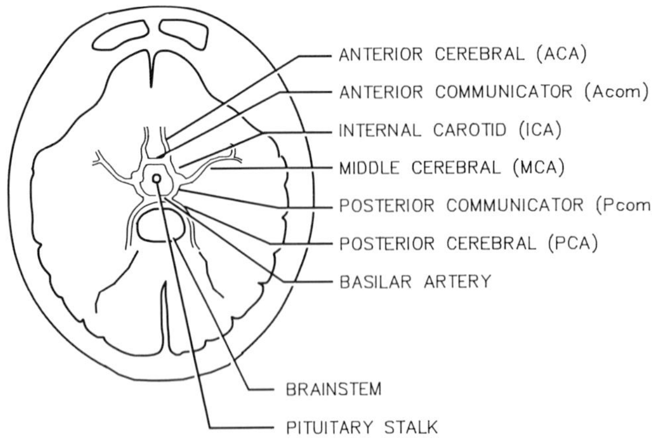

CONGENITAL ANEURYSMS ARISE:
40% FROM Acom
30% FROM ICA AND Pcom
20% FROM MCA TRIFURCATION
10% FROM BASILAR AND VERTEBRAL ARTERIES
CIRCLE OF WILLIS AND MCA TRIFURCATION ARE EASILY SHOWN ON CT AND MR
A

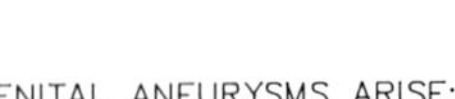

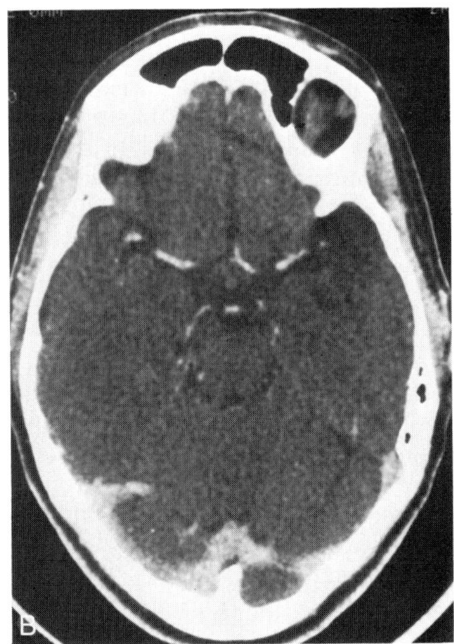

FIGURE 8–6. Circle of Willis. *A.* Diagram of an enhanced CT shows the vessels, landmarks, and locations of aneurysms. *B.* Thin-slice CT during contrast infusion can demonstrate cerebral aneurysms, most of which occur in the plane of the circle of Willis (see Fig. 8–81*A*).

circulation to the occipital lobes, in which the posterior communicating artery remains the predominant supply to the posterior cerebral artery. A common variation, supply of both anterior cerebral arteries from only one side, can have important consequences if aneurysm or surgery obstructs the side of the supply.

The venous drainage of the brain is somewhat variable but is predominantly by way of the dural sinuses to the jugular venous system (Fig. 8–7). Additional small but numerous anastomotic venous channels to the face and through the skullbase to the vertebral veins are also present.

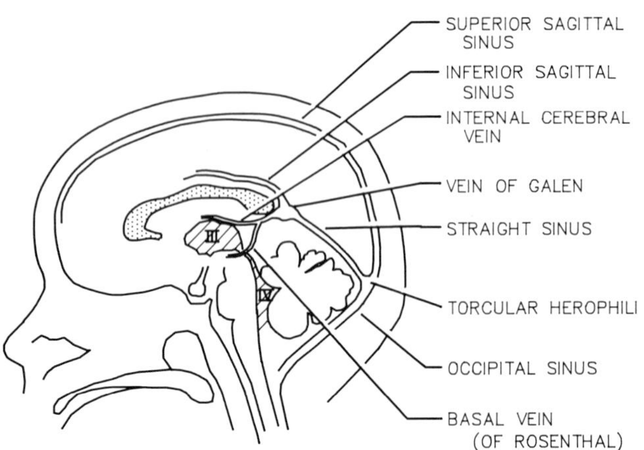

FIGURE 8–7. Venous drainage of the brain.

Myelography

Conventional myelography is being replaced by CT-myelography (to be described) and MRI, but it still provides unique information about the spinal cord and nerve roots and the relationships of these structures to surrounding bone and soft tissue. It is most often used in conjunction with CT or MRI in the evaluation of degenerative disease affecting the spinal cord or nerve roots. CT after the administration of intrathecal contrast provides information complementary to that of myelography and is usually performed shortly after conventional myelography.

Myelography has been safer, more accurate, easier to perform, and better tolerated by patients since the development of water-soluble intrathecal contrast agents (e.g., metrizamide, iopamidol, and iohexol). The lower density and the lower viscosity of these materials in comparison with the lipid-soluble agents (iophendylate) enable visualization of individual nerves, filling of nerve root sleeves (Fig. 8–8), and passage through a nearly totally obliterated subarachnoid space. Furthermore, the lower attenuation of these contrast materials enables CT (CT-myelography) to provide exceptional internal detail of the thecal sac that is complementary to that provided by the myelogram. Because these contrast agents are water soluble and not highly viscous, they can be injected by small (22- or 25-gauge) needles, thereby eliminating postpuncture headaches. They are absorbed into the blood stream via the cerebrospinal fluid (CSF) pathways, and so the needle can be removed after the contrast material has been injected. Most important, these agents do not cause inflammation of the meninges (arachnoiditis), as oil-based agents commonly do.

Side effects occur with the water-soluble agents in many patients, usually 4 to 6 hours after the injection, when brain absorption is maximal. Patients may have headache, nausea, vomiting, disorientation, and, in rare instances, seizure. Such side effects are minimized by adequate hydration and upright positioning after the procedure.

Cervical myelography can be performed with either lumbar or cervical injection. Cervical injection, by puncture at the C1-C2 interspace posteriorly, can be performed by a neuroradiologist with the use of lateral fluoroscopy and enables optimal placement of the contrast material and real-time fluoroscopic monitoring (Fig. 8–9). Because of the potential for serious cord injury, cervical puncture is usually performed when a lumbar injection is not possible or is not successful (as in obstruction of the cervical subarachnoid space) or when postmyelography CT is unavailable. Cer-

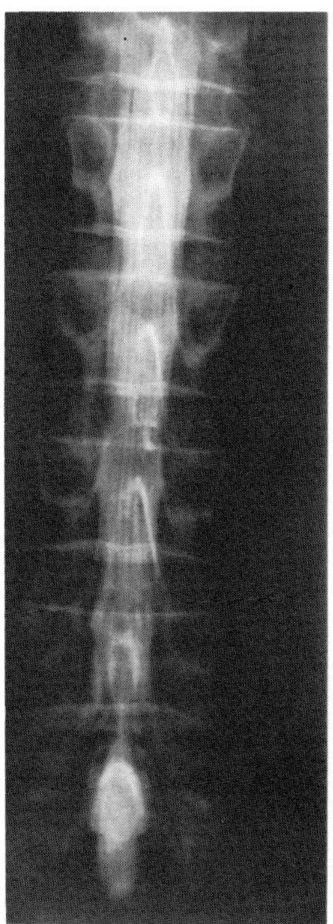

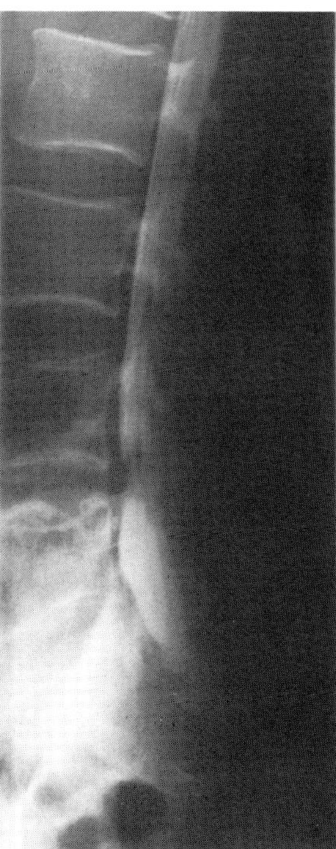

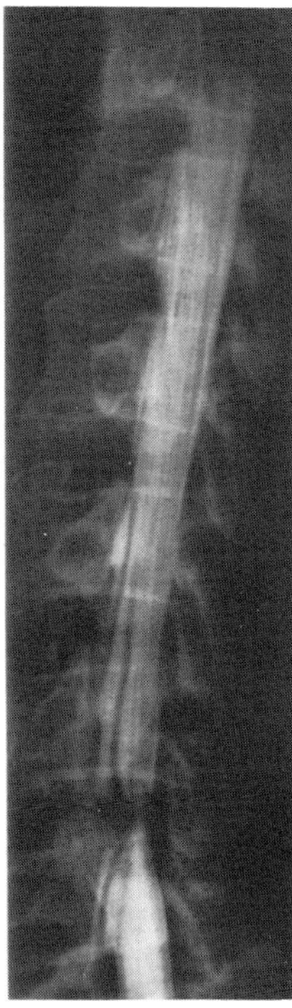

FIGURE 8–8. Iopamidol lumbar myelogram in anteroposterior, lateral, and oblique projections. Nerve roots appear as linear filling defects passing through the thecal sac. Disc herniation at the L4-L5 level causes compression, displacement, and edematous thickening of the lower roots as they pass through the disc space.

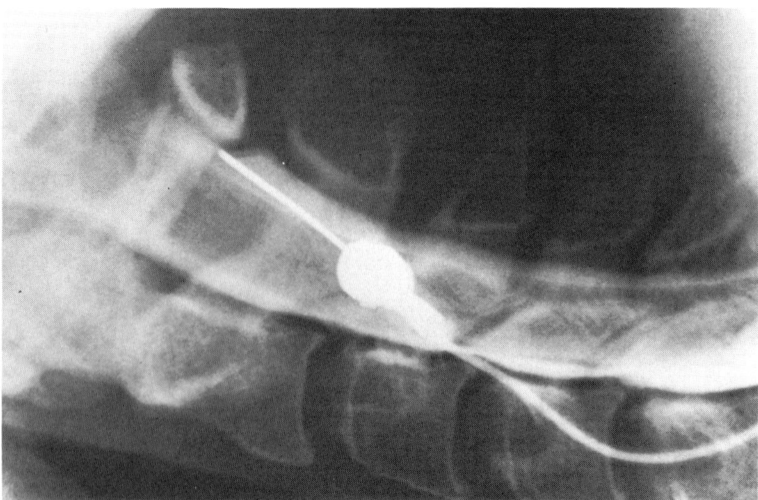

FIGURE 8–9. Cervical myelogram performed by lateral puncture at the level of C1-C2. Under fluoroscopic guidance, the needle is placed into the posterior subarachnoid space, and contrast is injected. The needle is then removed, and films are obtained.

vical puncture must be conducted only by highly skilled radiologists or neurosurgeons trained in the performance of the examination.

Films are obtained with anteroposterior, lateral, and oblique projections. Important abnormalities are obstruction to filling of the subarachnoid space, large or narrow size of the cervical cord, indentations on or filling defects of the subarachnoid space, and truncation of nerve root sleeves.

Performance of thoracic myelography is difficult because the thoracic kyphosis prevents optimal placement of the contrast material, x-ray penetration of the spine in the lateral projection varies from poor in the shoulders and hips to excessive in the midthorax, and the contrast material becomes diluted when it moves from the point of injection (cervical or lumbar level) to the thoracic region. Clinical examination of thoracic cord abnormalities is also difficult, and so less information about the type and the location of the lesion is available to the radiologist. The most serious abnormalities seen on thoracic myelography are obstruction to flow of contrast material and widening or effacement of the subarachnoid space (Fig. 8–10). The caudal end of the spinal cord (conus medullaris), usually located between T-12 and L-2, should always be evaluated when thoracic or lumbar myelography is performed because a lesion in this area can simulate a peripheral radicular lesion.

Lumbosacral myelography in conjunction with CT provides excellent evaluation of neural abnormalities in the lumbar and sacral portions of the spine. A neurologist, a neurosurgeon, or an orthopedic surgeon can usually locate the level of the abnormality clinically, which is of much assistance for obtaining good radiological views of the lesion. The contrast is injected at a midlumbar interspace with the use of fluoroscopy.

The most important abnormalities seen on lumbosacral myelography are degenerative changes and disc protrusions that compress the thecal sac or nerve roots, truncation of nerve root sleeves, swelling of nerve roots, filling defects, and obstruction to flow of contrast material (see Fig. 8–8).

Total myelography, or examination of the entire spine, is occasionally necessary when several levels of neurological dysfunction are present, when it is clinically not possible to locate the level of abnormality, or in the evaluation of spinal metastatic disease. The examination of one or more areas is usually suboptimal because the contrast material becomes rapidly diffused during filming and during movement from one part of the spine to another. Usually, it is best to obtain a high-quality examination of the area of most interest. Other areas can be evaluated with CT after the myelogram or even with a second myelogram.

Computed Tomography

CT has greatly expanded the role of radiologists in the evaluation of CNS disease. In the brain, tumors, vascular malformations, hemorrhage, infarction, infection, and large aneurysms can be demonstrated and characterized. In addition to axial scanning, such techniques as coronal scanning, reformatting, contrast enhancement, and high-contrast resolution algo-

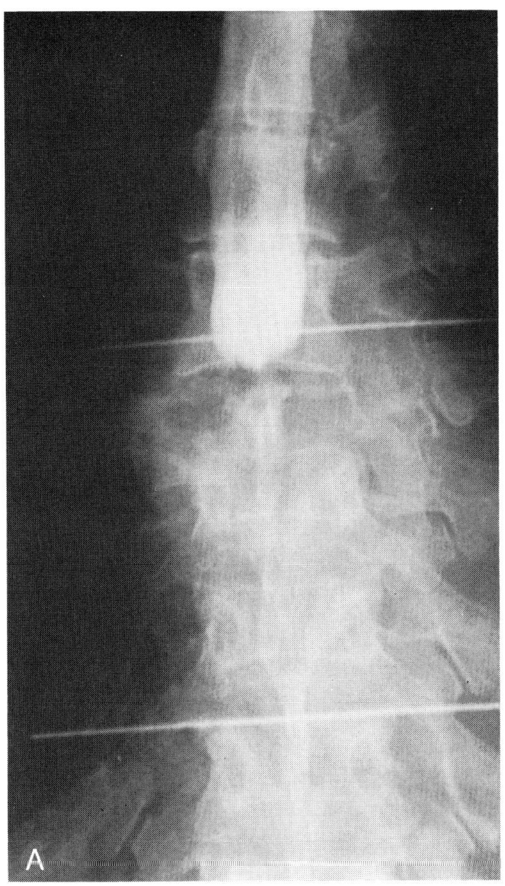

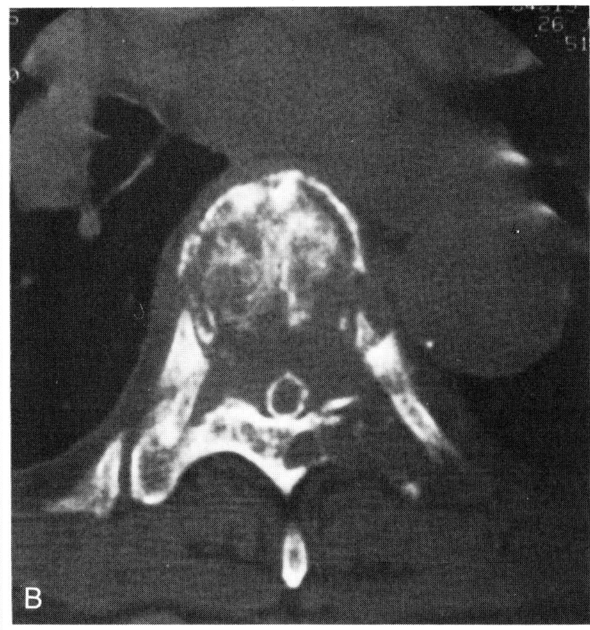

FIGURE 8–10. Emergency myelogram in a patient with T-6 cord compression caused by metastatic lung cancer. *A.* Complete obstruction to flow of intrathecal contrast necessitated myelography with lumbar and cervical injections. The upper and lower extent of the obstruction are marked on the patient and the film for radiation therapy. *B.* CT after myelography shows contrast in the compressed thecal sac and demonstrates the surrounding destructive soft-tissue mass. MRI can provide similar information noninvasively and more rapidly.

rithms provide excellent images. Although MRI is recommended as the first examination in detecting and characterizing most intracranial abnormalities, CT continues to be an essential brain imaging technique in most hospitals because of its greater availability, lower cost, and superior ability to show bone and acute hemorrhage. It also continues to be important for the evaluation of emergency patients and for examination of the temporal bone, the orbits, and the skullbase because it can be obtained easily, has excellent spatial resolution, and demonstrates bone, fat, acute hemorrhage, and fluid well. In many cases, CT and MRI provide complementary information, and both tests should be obtained.

Initial CT brain evaluation in most cases is performed with the use of contiguous axial images of 1-cm thickness, either with or without contrast, depending on the clinical circumstances. In most acute diseases in which the primary concerns are infarction and hemorrhage, a noncontrast examination is most informative. When a vascular tumor, an aneurysm, or an infection is suspected, contrast is administered after a noncontrast examination. Narrow slices (5 mm or less) can be obtained in areas of question. Coronal scanning can be helpful for evaluating lesions that are adjacent to bone, near the tentorium, or in the skullbase. Bone window views should be obtained and recorded in any patient suspected of having head trauma, metastatic disease, or bone erosion.

Interpretation of brain CT includes evaluation of the bones, the extracranial soft tissues, the orbits, the paranasal sinuses, the pituitary fossa, and the brain. Fractures (see Figs. 7–13, 7–14, 7–15, and 8–18*B*), infection, and tumor involvement are the most important bone abnormalities. Sutures and synostoses must not be confused with fractures, and venous grooves, particularly over the superior portion of the skull, should not be mistaken for metastatic tumor. Many fractures of the cranium and most metabolic or metastatic bone diseases are well-defined by plain films. CT is the most informative examination for facial bone fractures.

Evaluation of the soft tissues includes examination of the orbits, the paranasal sinuses, the mastoid air cells, the nasopharynx, and the pituitary fossa. Although the thick-slice axial technique is suboptimal for full evaluation of these areas, important abnormalities can be detected, which can contribute to the diagnosis of intracranial abnormalities. A mass in the orbit can be suggestive of infection, tumor, or a vascular abnormality. Soft-tissue density and, in particular, air-fluid levels in the paranasal sinuses are suggestive of sinusitis. Opacification and bone sclerosis of the mastoid air cells are indicative of mastoiditis. Prominent soft tissue in the nasopharynx in an adult can represent tumor but in a child is usually adenoid tissue. Enlargement of the pituitary fossa is suggestive of tumor in this area, and the need for a high-resolution pituitary CT or MRI examination should be considered.

After the areas outside the brain have been reviewed, examination of the brain is performed most efficiently from the base upward. The lowest levels (Fig. 8–11, slices 1 to 3) show the foramen magnum and the cerebellar hemispheres. The fourth ventricle appears as a low-density horseshoe shape at the level of the petrous ridges (slice 4). If it is not well seen or if it is asymmetrical, mass effect caused by tumor or another space-occupying lesion should be suspected. The next higher slices include the cerebellar vermis and the midbrain (slices 5 and 6). The quadrigeminal plate cistern appears as a low-density W shape behind the midbrain (slice 6). Effacement of this cistern can be caused by compression from a space-occupying lesion, by blood, or by infection in the subarachnoid space (see Fig. 8–44).

Higher slices (6 and 7 of Fig. 8–11) show the thalami, the third ventricle, and the temporal lobes. Slightly higher are the lateral ventricles, the basal ganglia, and the internal capsules (slices 7 to 9). A nonhemorrhagic infarct (which appears as low density) and acute hemorrhage (which appears as high density) are common in the basal ganglia. The highest slices show the deep white matter tracts and the cerebral cortex. Masses, blood, sulcal effacement, poor differentiation of gray and white matter, decreased brain density, and midline shift are serious abnormal findings at these levels.

CT of the spine can be performed with or without intrathecal contrast. Noncontrast CT of the lumbar spine can be used to evaluate disease of the discs, facet joints, and lateral recesses, but it provides little information about the nerve roots, the cord, or the thecal sac. Intravenous contrast has been used to identify scar tissue in the lumbar spine, but enhanced MRI is more successful in this assessment. In the cervical and thoracic spine, noncontrast scanning is of less value for cord and nerve root evaluation. The vertebral bodies are small, the disc spaces are narrow, and the thecal sac is not outlined by fat as in the lumbar spine. Enhanced, high-resolution CT can show a cervical disc indenting the thecal sac and the cord because of the enhancement of the venous plexus and the disc margin. In some cases, this technique is preferable to MRI, which cannot show osteophytes and may be degraded by artifact.

Depending on the findings, CT with intrathecal water-soluble contrast (frequently after myelography) may be indicated. Myelography and CT are complementary. Myelography provides an overview of the spine and is usually followed by narrow (3-mm) axial CT slices through the area of interest, which is determined either from clinical signs or from myelographic abnormalities. The initially high concentration of the intrathecal contrast can cause CT artifacts, and so patients are often scanned 1 to 3 hours after myelography. If myelography is not required or is contraindicated, a small amount of low-concentration contrast material can be injected, and CT can be performed immediately; this technique is known as CT-myelography.

Interpretation of spine CT with intrathecal contrast begins with evaluation of the soft tissues outside the bone so that a lymphoma, a meningomyelocele, or another mass lesion is not missed. Then the bones are assessed for adequacy of the spinal canal and of the lateral recesses and for whether degenerative bony overgrowth of the facets or vertebral bodies encroaches upon the canal. Next, the soft tissues within the canal are evaluated for prominence of the ligamentum flavum, bulging of the discs, and the presence of normal epidural fat and epidural veins. Finally, the thecal sac and the spinal cord or the cauda equina are examined for the presence of syrinx, tumor, asymmetry, or clumping of nerve roots.

Ultrasonography

Ultrasonography is used for intraoperative evaluation of spinal and brain tumors. After the skull or a vertebra has been opened, the ultrasonographic transducer can be placed directly on the brain or the spinal cord to locate

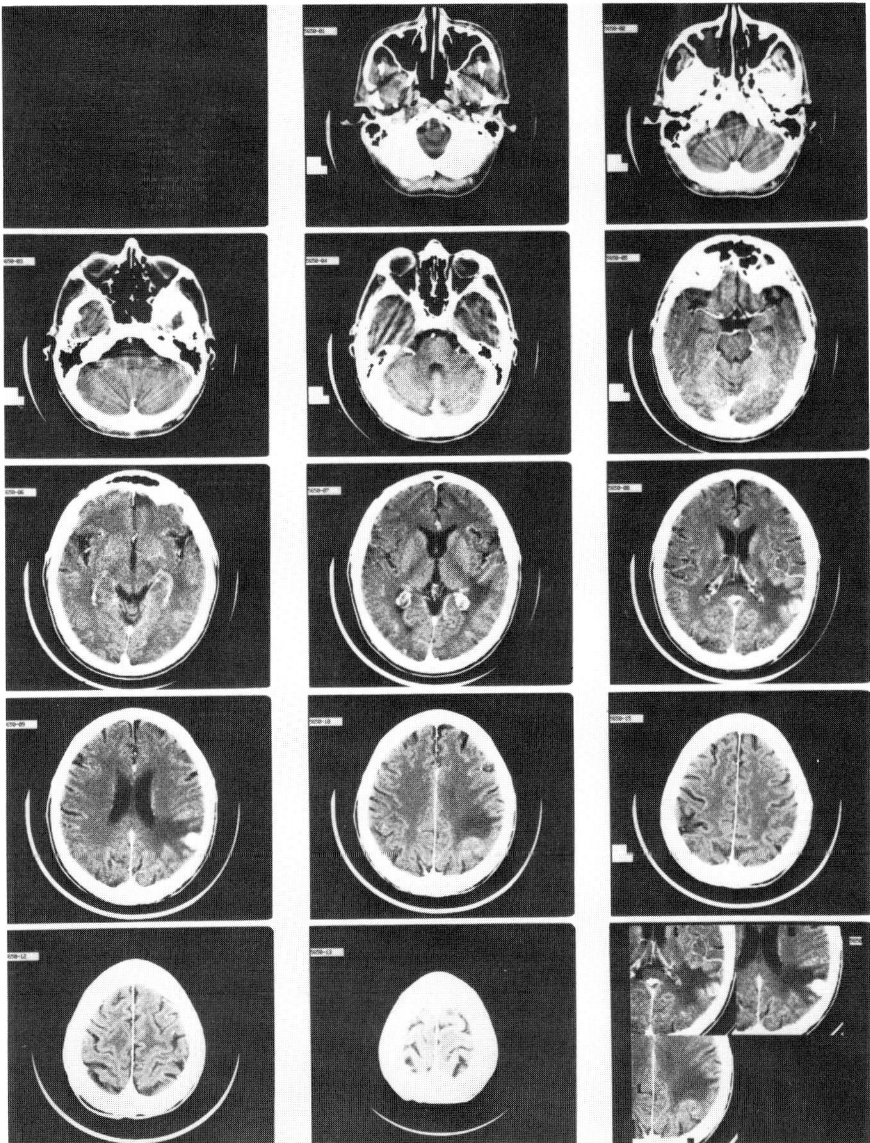

FIGURE 8–11. Axial contrast-enhanced CT of the brain. Slice numbers are the last two digits of the number in the upper left. Note especially the clear definition of the fourth ventricle (slice 4) and the quadrigeminal plate cistern (slice 6, always visible in a normal scan) and the slightly higher density of the ribbon of gray matter in the outer cortex. Slice 9 shows a metastatic focus of renal cell carcinoma. The lesion shows central enhancement and marked surrounding edema, which are typical of such tumors. Also typical is the location peripherally at the gray-white matter junction, a result of the hematogenous spread.

masses for biopsy or excision. In utero ultrasonography is performed in order to determine fetal age and to identify possible congenital anomalies. The anterior or posterior fontanelles and the sutures are used as windows through the skull in neonatal ultrasonography to evaluate for congenital anomalies, hydrocephalus, and subependymal hemorrhages (Fig. 8–12; see also Fig. 4–5). Ultrasonography is also useful in the evaluation of abnormalities of the globe, but these examinations are usually conducted by an ophthalmologist. Doppler ultrasonography is the primary method for evaluating carotid artery disease.

Magnetic Resonance Imaging

MRI is, in most cases, superior to other imaging methods in the evaluation of the brain and the spinal cord. As a result, it is recommended as the first method of examination for

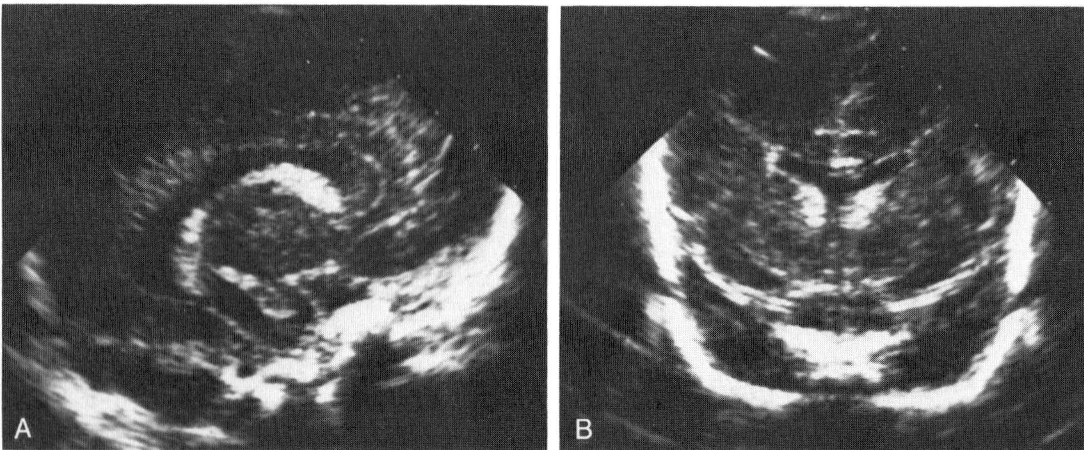

FIGURE 8–12. Neonatal subependymal hemorrhage. Sagittal *(A)* and coronal *(B)* cranial ultrasonographic examinations demonstrating abnormal increased echogenicity in the subependymal region of a premature infant with germinal matrix hemorrhage. (Courtesy of S. Williamson, Department of Radiology, University of New Mexico, Albuquerque.)

most diseases of the brain and the spine. Because most pathological lesions in the CNS are characterized by increased water content, nearly all have prolonged relaxation times (T1 and T2) in comparison with adjacent or contralateral structures. Tumor, infarction, and demyelinating diseases are well-demonstrated on MRI by the identification of a prolonged T2 with spin echo sequences or prolonged T1 on inversion recovery techniques (Fig. 8–13). Hemorrhages have complex appearances but, except for subarachnoid hemorrhage, are most clearly shown on MRI. In addition, MRI usually demonstrates more foci or a larger focus

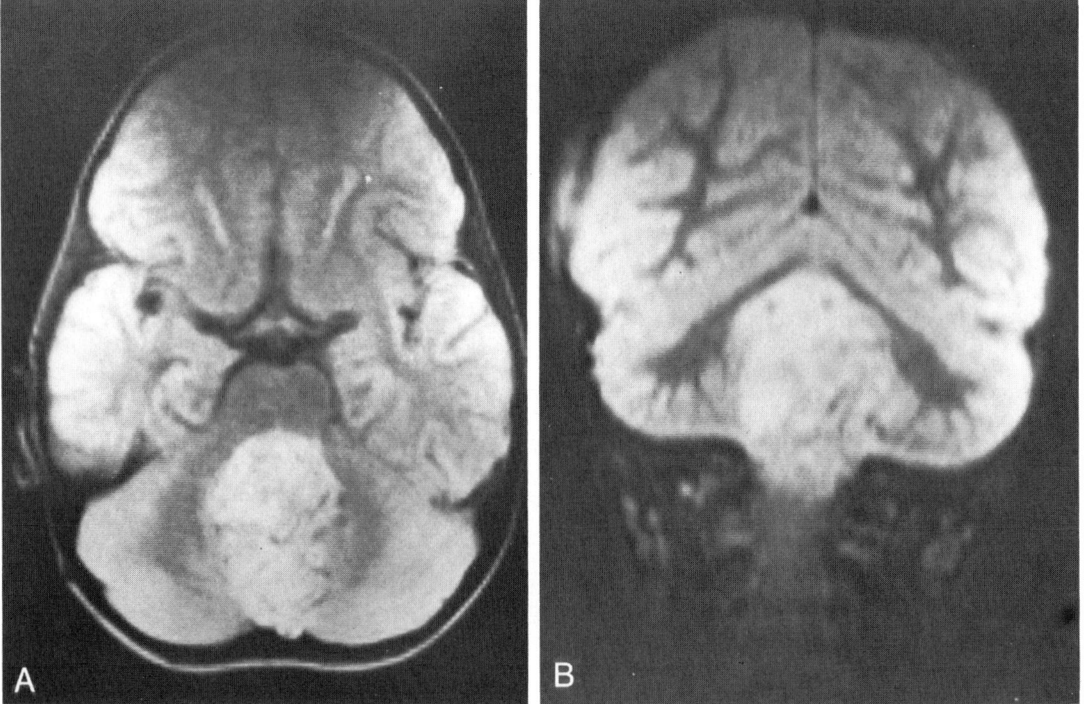

FIGURE 8–13. Medulloblastoma in a 5-year-old boy. *A.* Low-field (0.15 T) axial T2 spin echo image shows the midline cerebellar tumor obliterating the fourth ventricle and compressing the brainstem cisterns (image acquisition time was 34 minutes). *B.* Additional planes were obtained with short TI inversion recovery (STIR) sequences to demonstrate the extent of the tumor. This high-contrast image was obtained in only 10 minutes.

of abnormality than does CT and is more comprehensive for evaluating white matter disease, posterior fossa lesions, and most types of hemorrhage.

In many disorders, such as multiple sclerosis, the MRI findings are positive when CT usually shows no abnormality at all. Although several imaging techniques can be used, T2-weighted spin echo and short TI inversion recovery (STIR) techniques provide the high tissue contrast required for general screening and for the evaluation of specific lesions. Because many options are available, the examination must be conducted, monitored, and interpreted by a radiologist with substantial training in MRI and in neuroradiology.

MRA can be used to evaluate intracranial aneurysms and arteriovenous malformations (AVMs), to assess extracranial carotid stenosis, and, outside the CNS, detect abdominal venous thrombosis and abdominal aortic aneurysm. Images appear similar to those of conventional arteriography (see Fig. 8–2). Time-of-flight MRA (also referred to as flow-related enhancement) is a common method for cerebral examinations. A two- or three-dimensional gradient echo pulse sequence typically causes flowing blood to appear bright. The longitudinal magnetization of stationary tissues is reduced by the repeated application of radio frequency pulses, whereas the flowing blood continually produces a stronger signal. Problems inherent in MRA include a tendency to exaggerate the extent of vascular stenosis because of flow-related dephasing, a result of chaotic flow distal to a stenosis. Any lesion that has extremely slow flow or continually recirculating blood, such as a giant aneurysm, may also be incorrectly or incompletely visualized. However, in many instances the appearances of routine angiograms and MRA are strikingly similar.

MRI evaluation requires anatomical knowledge more precise than that required for CT evaluation. The superior definition by MRI between tissue types shows structures that are not visible with other techniques. The variation in intensity (displayed as shades of gray) among soft-tissue lesions attained by MRI is 20 times that of CT. Tissue planes are often defined by connective tissue, which provides a weak MRI signal, or by fat, which on T1-weighted spin echo images provides an intense signal. The intensity of a lesion on various imaging sequences enables characterization of an abnormality. The considerations for interpretation of brain and spine MRI are the same as for CT, but more extensive knowledge of coronal and sagittal anatomical structure is required.

Injectable paramagnetic contrast materials (such as gadolinium-diethylenetriaminepenta-acetic acid [Gd-DTPA] dimeglumine) are effective in enhancing tumors, vascular lesions, infarction, and demyelinating disease. These agents are generally safe and do not cause significant adverse effects. In the spine, Gd-DTPA is effective in enhancing areas of infection or tumor and in differentiating recurrent disc disease from scar tissue (see Fig. 7–23).

Positron Emission Tomography, Single-Photon Emission Tomography, and Xenon-Enhanced CT

Several continually developing techniques are applied to neuroradiology. Positron emission tomography, single photon emission computed tomography, and xenon-enhanced CT can demonstrate metabolic and physiological changes in the CNS. Many biologically active molecules can be labeled with radioisotopes and can provide unique functional and anatomical information about the brain. Important areas of investigation include the quantification of blood flow in ischemia, the anatomical mapping of brain functions, determination of sites of injury in diseases such as multiple sclerosis and Alzheimer's disease, and the identification of chemical mediators of CNS function and disease. These techniques are best suited to evaluation of the brain, in which imaging is not complicated by such factors as respiratory motion, cardiac pulsation, and peristalsis. Much of the application of these techniques remains experimental because of the cost of examinations and the need for special equipment.

Part I
The Brain

TRAUMATIC DISEASES

Acute Injury

Brain injury is the most common cause of morbidity and mortality in traumatic insults. Evaluation of head trauma must be rapid and comprehensive in order to detect treatable injuries, and it is best accomplished by CT and MRI. The indications for emergency brain evaluation (Table 8–2) after trauma should be used as guidelines, but the clinical examination and the history of the injury are the deciding factors for ordering emergency scans.

The most important findings affecting management of patients after head trauma are parenchymal injury and compression of the brain by hematoma or edema. The appearance of hemorrhage depends on the time delay before the examination and on the location, the vascular supply, and the type of bleeding (arterial or venous) (Fig. 8–14). On CT, acute hemorrhage appears dense because of its high protein content. As the protein is broken down over 1 to 2 weeks, the blood becomes isodense with brain tissue and can be difficult to detect. Thereafter, the disintegrating blood is of low density. In patients in whom the hematocrit content is low, even new hemorrhage may appear as intermediate or low density. On MRI, blood can have a confusing appearance because it depends on the time and the composition of the hemorrhage, the magnetic field strength, and the imaging sequence. In low-field sequences, acute hemorrhage is generally of high intensity on all types of images (T1 and T2 spin echo, STIR, and gradient echo).

TABLE 8–2. INDICATIONS FOR EMERGENCY BRAIN EVALUATION

Depressed skull fracture
Palpable foreign body
Unconsciousness
Documented mental deterioration
Unexplained focal neurological signs
Hemotympanum or mastoid ecchymosis
Cerebrospinal fluid rhinorrhea
Bilateral orbital ecchymosis

These indications should serve as guidelines. Computed tomography or magnetic resonance imaging is recommended whenever clinical findings suggest intracranial injury, particularly in children.

In high-field sequences, blood is initially black on T2 spin echo images because of paramagnetic effect; as the blood degenerates, it changes to a higher intensity. Low-field images show less dramatic low intensity of acute hematomas in the first 48 hours after hemorrhage.

Mass effect on the brain by blood or internal swelling can be detected from a shift of the midline, compression of ventricles, effacement of sulci, and obliteration of the Sylvian and brainstem cisterns. Compression of the brain can cause direct injury, or it can cause ischemia by compressing arteries and veins and thereby interfering with normal perfusion of blood. A mass effect can also occur when the brain swells as a result of increased perfusion when autoregulation of blood flow is disturbed by trauma. Loss of autoregulation, which is common in children, can lead to arterial blood flow that exceeds the venous capacity, resulting in an intravascular leakage through capillaries (called vasogenic edema).

Either a mass effect or generalized edema can cause the brain (confined by the skull) to herniate through the tentorial incisura and the foramen magnum. The most easily recognized finding of impending transtentorial herniation is effacement of the pontine and quadrigeminal

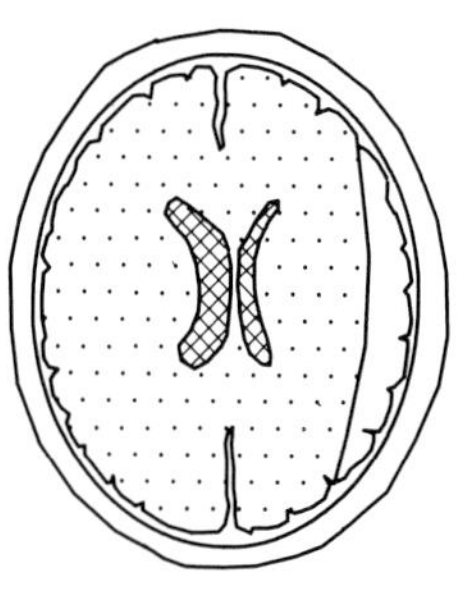

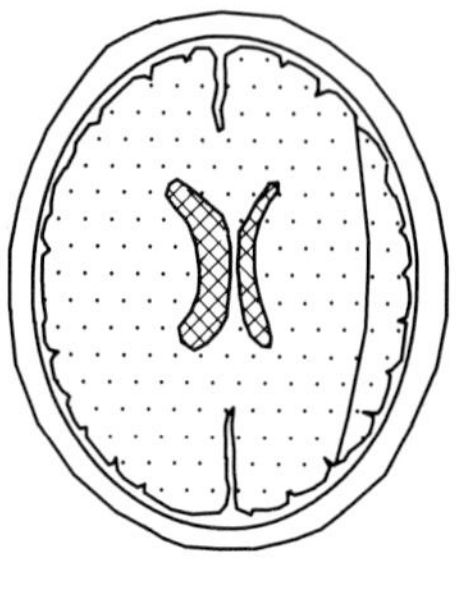

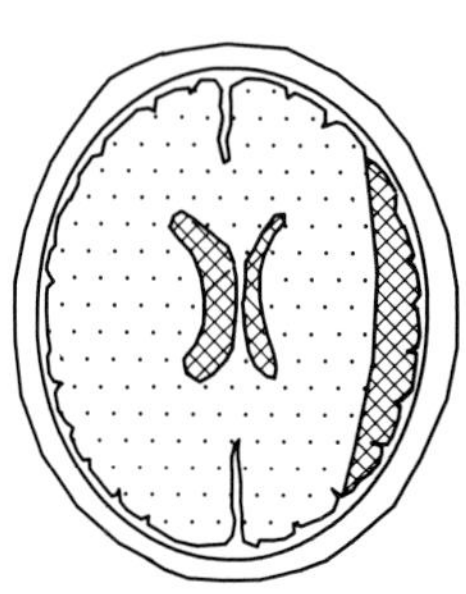

FIGURE 8–14. Time course of appearance of blood on CT. The subdural hematoma depicted here initially shows high density (white). After about 1 week, it becomes isodense with the brain. After 2 weeks, the blood is low density (dark gray).

cisterns. The finding of brain compression is especially important because effective cerebral perfusion ceases when the intracranial pressure becomes elevated above that of venous pressure.

Serious lesions in the head caused directly by trauma are diffuse axonal injury, concussion, epidural and subdural hematoma, traumatic subarachnoid hemorrhage, brain contusion and hematoma, penetrating injury, and vascular injury. Secondary complications are discussed in the "Delayed Injury" section.

Diffuse Axonal Injury. Rotational forces or abrupt deceleration can induce shearing forces that stretch or tear the axons and cause rupture of small vessels in the brain. Although patients with this damage may be comatose, it is not unusual for a CT scan to appear normal. In such cases, MRI often and CT sometimes show punctate areas of hemorrhage or edema in the deep white matter, the corpus callosum, and the brainstem (Fig. 8–15). Histological postmortem examinations of these patients show that the lesions represent diffuse axonal injury and associated hemorrhage. The axonal injury results in disconnection of the cerebral hemispheres from the rest of the CNS. This disconnection and the often associated brainstem injury imply a poor prognosis.

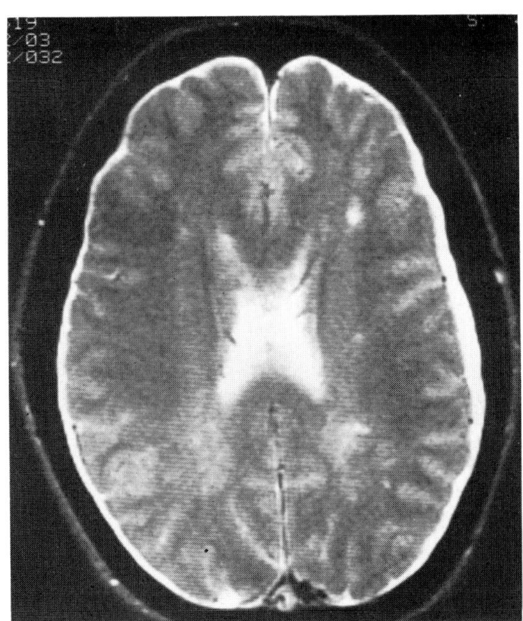

FIGURE 8–15. Diffuse axonal injury. Axial T2 spin echo image shows punctate lesions bilaterally in the deep white matter in a 48-year-old motor vehicle accident victim. Note also the bilateral subdural hematomas.

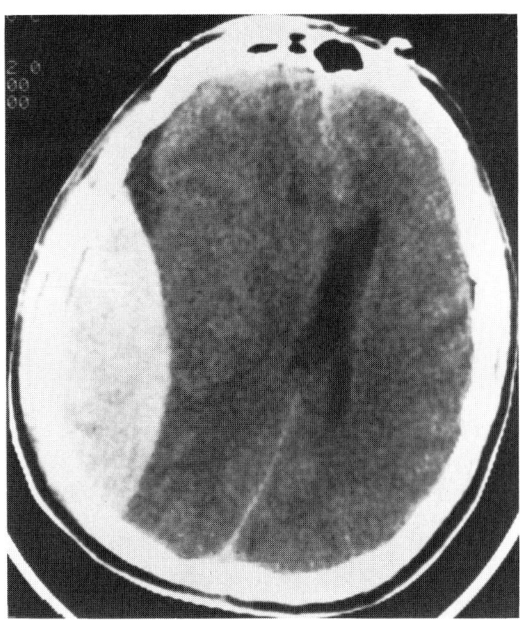

FIGURE 8–16. Epidural hematoma. Brain windows show a large lens-shaped, dense mass of blood. The brain is compressed, and the midline is shifted to the left.

Concussion. Concussion is by definition a transient loss of consciousness as a result of head trauma without an identifiable lesion. The process probably involves the brainstem reticular formation. MRI, by showing small hemorrhages, indicates that brain injury occurs in some patients previously classified as having concussion injuries. The identification of brain injury in patients with transient loss of consciousness has important consequences in the treatment and follow-up of closed-head injuries.

Epidural Hematoma. An epidural hematoma is found in 20% of all fatal head injuries. It results from bleeding, usually from the middle meningeal artery and occasionally from epidural veins or other meningeal arteries, into the extradural space. The dura, normally tightly apposed to the inner skull, is dissected locally by the expanding hematoma, which in this location appears as a dense, lens-shaped mass on CT (Fig. 8–16). Epidural hematoma is often limited by the sutures, but it can strip the falcine attachment from the inner table of the skull and cross the midline; this characteristic differentiates a midline epidural from subdural hematoma, which is limited by the superior sagittal sinus. When bleeding is arterial, the mass expands rapidly and can cause herniation in minutes to hours. When brain compression or displacement is present or herniation is impending, the hematoma requires immediate surgical evacuation.

Subdural Hematoma. A subdural hematoma is usually caused by hemorrhage when bridging veins or dural sinuses are torn, but it can also be caused by rupture of small arteries. Acute subdural hematomas appear as crescent-shaped, dense collections that follow the contour of the subdural space, separating the arachnoid layer from the dura (Fig. 8–17). Symptoms may be acute or delayed and insidious. The hematoma does not cross the midline because it is limited by the falx, but it can enter the interhemispheric subdural space adjacent to the falx. Marked mass effect may result from the circumferential extent of the blood. Bilateral subdural hematomas compress brain parenchyma and efface cisterns and sulci but may not shift the midline. Bilateral subdural hematomas may be extremely difficult to diagnose, particularly when isodense with brain tissue.

A subdural hematoma can also occur or become clinically significant long after trauma or even in the absence of known trauma. A delayed subdural hemorrhage may appear several days or much later after injury. A chronic subdural hematoma is isodense with brain tissue or of low density. It can develop without obvious symptoms in older patients or in alcoholics because the extra space inside the skulls of these patients accommodates the collection of blood. Hyperemia of the outer membrane of the resolving hematoma predisposes a patient to hemorrhage. Young children can develop subdural hematomas as a result of vigorous shaking or other types of abuse.

Diagnosis of a subdural hematoma is best made on CT or MRI. CT has the advantage of more readily showing bone fracture and may be more clinically practical for a confused or comatose patient. Because the crescent-shaped, subdural blood is adjacent to the dense skull, CT identification may require intermediate window settings in which blood appears gray but the adjacent bone is white. If the hemorrhage is old (1 to 2 weeks), the blood may be isodense or hypodense in comparison with brain tissue, and contrast enhancement of the brain may be helpful (see Fig. 8–14). Contrast can also enhance the hyperemic outer membrane associated with a chronic subdural hematoma.

MRI can more clearly show subacute and chronic blood and provides better detail of brain compression. T1 spin echo images are

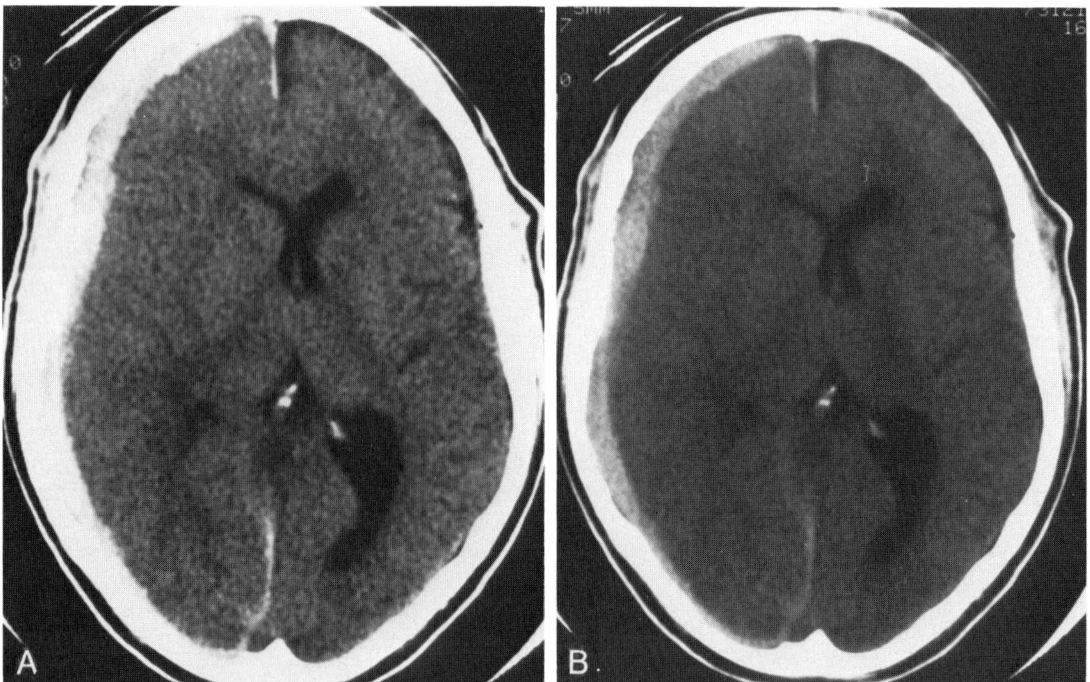

FIGURE 8–17. Subdural hematoma. *A.* CT shows a large crescentic hematoma in the right subdural space causes brain compression, shift of the midline, and early entrapment of the left lateral ventricle. *B.* Intermediate windows show bone as white, blood as light gray, and brain tissue as dark gray, which makes the blood more visible. These window settings are especially advantageous in identifying small subdural blood collections.

generally sufficient for diagnosis of hemorrhage. Because blood can have a complex appearance at high-field strength, T2 spin echo or other high-contrast images are also indicated. MRI shows bilateral subdural hematomas well (see Fig. 8–15).

Traumatic Subarachnoid Hemorrhage. Traumatic subarachnoid hemorrhage frequently accompanies all forms of indirect trauma (Fig. 8–18). It is commonly a venous hemorrhage and rarely causes focal compression. In general, other injuries are more significant than subarachnoid hemorrhage. It is not uncommon in newborns, apparently because of venous injury during childbirth. The presence of such hemorrhage does not seem to be clinically significant. Subarachnoid hemorrhage can result in hydrocephalus or in an arachnoid cyst or subdural hydroma from focal fibrosis.

Contusion and Hematoma. Parenchymal contusion and hematoma are focal brain injuries that result from compression or tearing of brain tissue or from hemorrhage into brain parenchyma. They are usually caused by blunt trauma to the head and occur adjacent to (coup) or opposite (contrecoup) the blow (Fig. 8–19), depending on the relative motion of the skull and its contents at the moment of impact. Most injuries, including a direct blow, a head-on collision, and a free fall, produce predominant injury at the site of impact. A fall with a rotational component, such as falling backwards during ice skating, usually produces a more severe contrecoup contusion because the brain, falling more slowly than the accelerating skull, is pressed against the part of the skull opposite the site of impact. Complex injuries, such as those from motor vehicle accidents, have a rotational component that results in coup, contrecoup, and additional internal shearing injuries.

Contusions often can be recognized by their location. The most common sites are the anterior temporal poles, the temporal lobes overlying the petrous pyramids, and the inferior frontal lobes (Fig. 8–20). The brain is easily injured at these locations by adjacent bony prominences. Contusions of the occipital lobes are less common because the cranial vault is smooth in this location. On CT, a parenchymal contusion appears as a focal lesion of inhomogeneous high density (from blood) and low density (from edema and necrotic brain tissue). MRI in T2 spin echo sequences shows high intensity of hemorrhage and edema (see Fig. 8–15). MRI also shows small contusions more effectively than does CT.

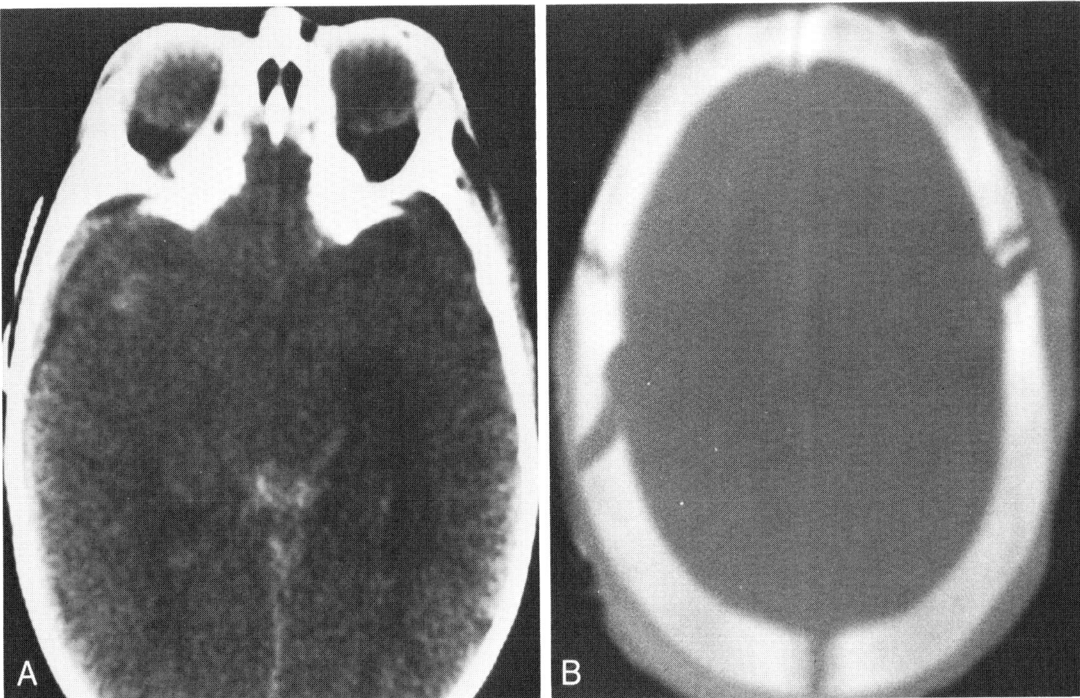

FIGURE 8–18. Traumatic subarachnoid hemorrhage in an infant who suffered severe head injury after a fall down a flight of stairs. *A.* In addition to right subdural hematoma and right temporal contusion, there is subarachnoid blood around the brainstem. *B.* Skull fracture demonstrates the severity of the head injury.

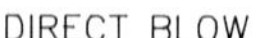

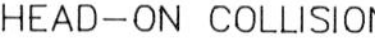

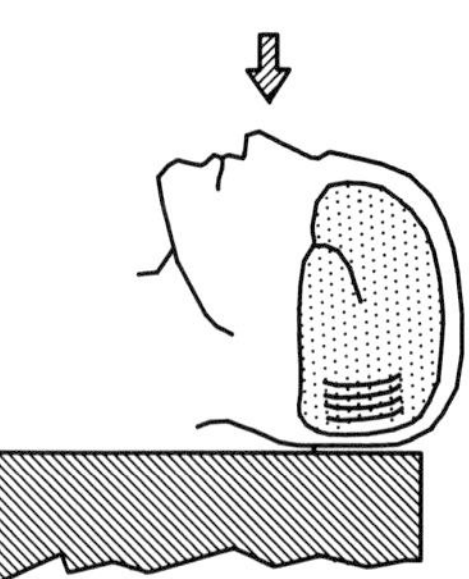

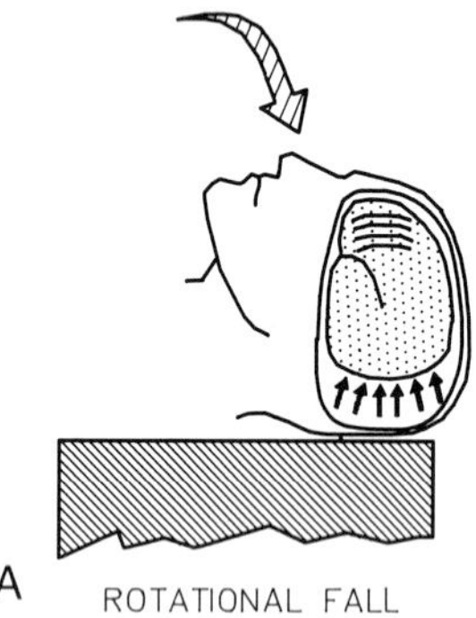

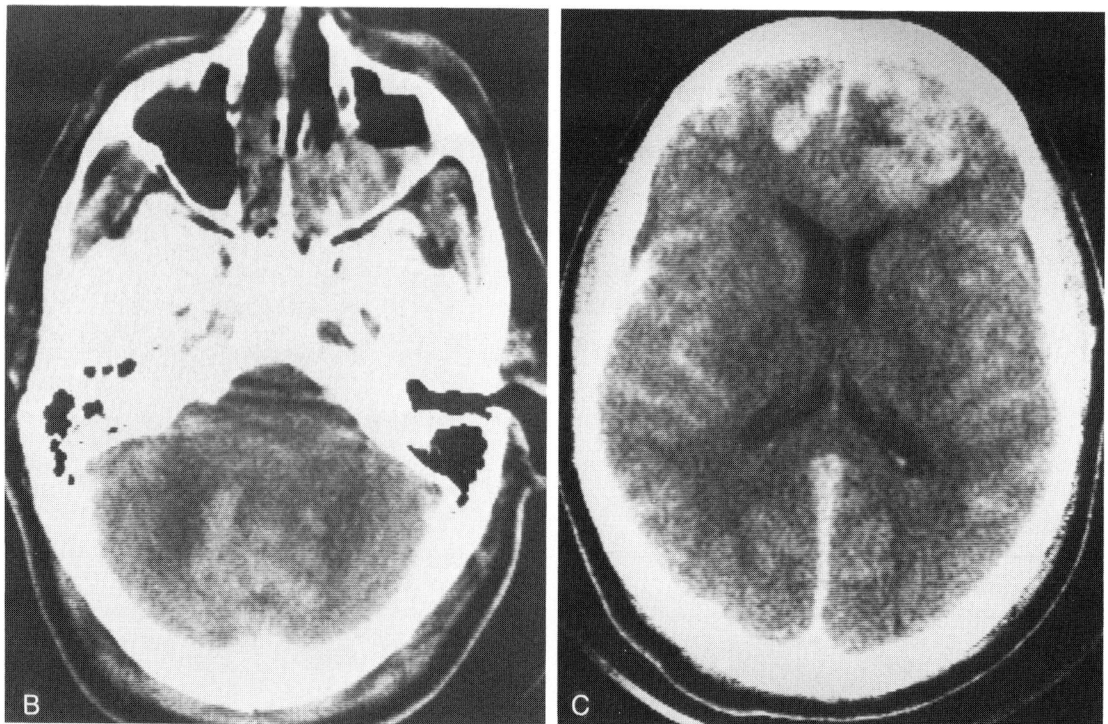

FIGURE 8–19. Coup and contrecoup injury. *A.* Diagram shows the mechanism of coup and contrecoup injury (see text). CSF, cerebrospinal fluid. *B.* Image at the posterior fossa level in a man who fell backwards on stairs and sustained a coup injury at the site of impact, and (C) a contrecoup injury in the frontal lobes.

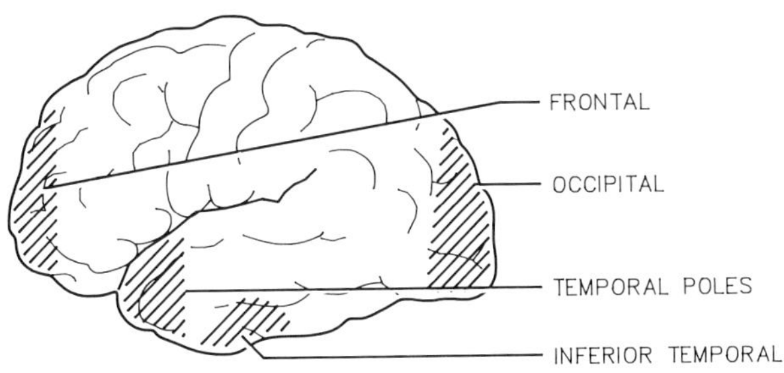

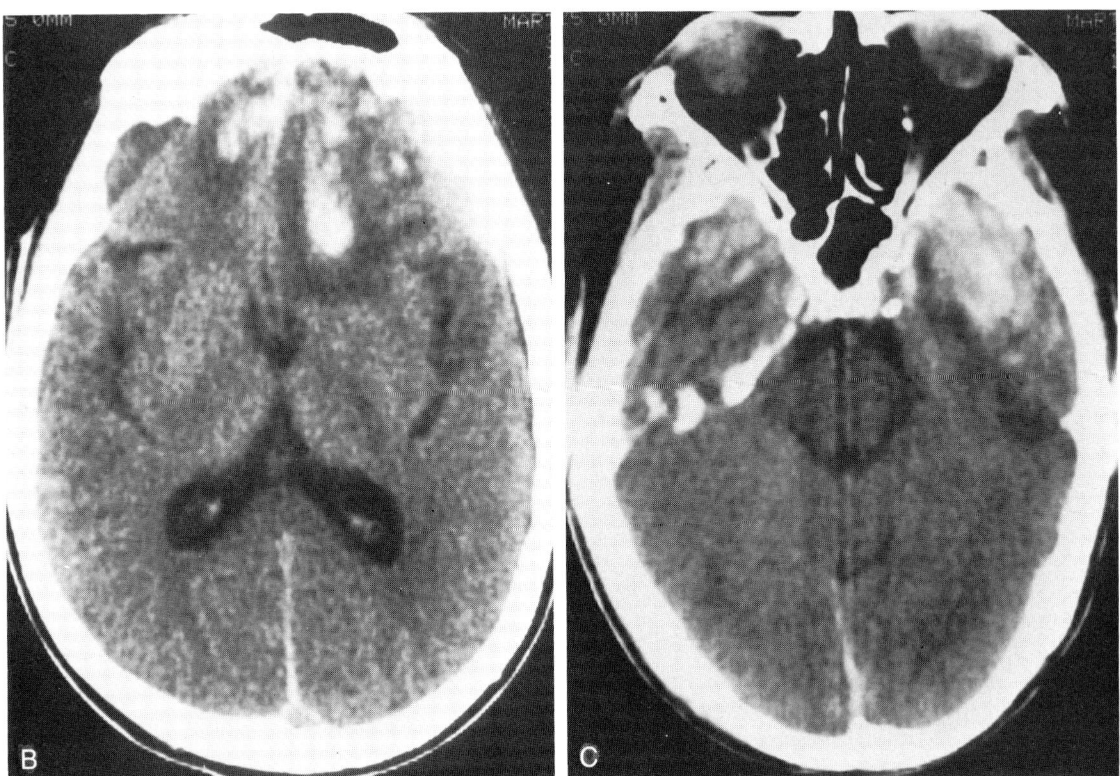

FIGURE 8–20. Sites of contusion. *A.* Diagram shows most common sites of contusion where the brain is injured by irregular bone. *B, C.* Bifrontal and bitemporal contusions in an alcoholic with head trauma. The multiple blood collections in typical locations allowed exclusion of other diagnoses.

A hematoma is a focal and circumscribed blood collection in the brain, easily shown as high density on CT. On MRI, the abnormality is well-demonstrated, but the variable appearance of blood, especially in high-field sequences, can make contusion and hematoma difficult to distinguish (Fig. 8–21).

Small contusions or hemorrhages are sometimes seen on high-quality CT or MRI images, especially in children (Fig. 8–22). These lesions, often seen on delayed images (1 to 3 days after trauma) may represent small contusions or lesions of diffuse axonal injury (described earlier). It is important to identify such lesions in order to ensure adequate hospital management and to interpret later developments, such as seizures.

Penetrating Injury. Foreign objects can penetrate the brain and damage the parenchyma and blood vessels, resulting in subarachnoid

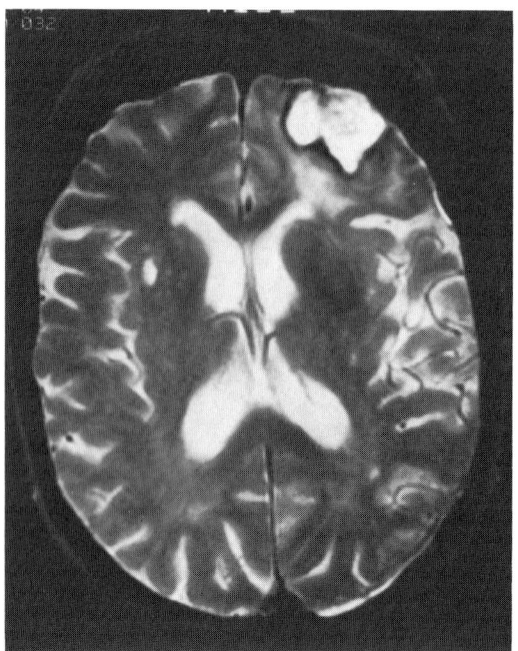

FIGURE 8–21. Cerebral hematoma. Contrecoup frontal injury caused a hematoma in an 80-year-old woman who fell backwards. Clot on this high-field T2 spin echo image shows high intensity centrally and a peripheral paramagnetic rim. The center was of low intensity on the T1 spin echo image. Note also edema in the brain posterior to the hematoma.

and parenchymal bleeding and necrosis of brain tissue. Edema often accompanies the injury. A bullet traveling at low velocity is slowed considerably by the skull and causes destruction only along its path. A bullet traveling at high velocity causes a conical shock wave whose axis is along the path of the bullet. The shock wave temporarily compresses the brain and can result in herniation into the foramen magnum. The direction of the bullet can be determined from the conical hole in the skull, the apex of the cone being the site of entry.

Vascular Injury. Fracture of the skullbase can cause carotid artery rupture or pseudoaneurysm that can result in communication between the carotid artery and the cavernous or sphenoid sinus. Affected patients may have pulsatile exophthalmos or persistent nasal bleeding. CT (often requiring coronal images) best identifies the fracture and can indicate the site of injury in the cavernous sinus and the carotid artery. A palsy of the sixth cranial nerve may be the first sign of a communication between the carotid artery and the cavernous sinus because this nerve travels through the sinus. Delayed hemorrhage from these lesions is common, and so even asymptomatic patients in whom there is CT evidence of basilar fracture near the carotid artery should undergo angiography.

Delayed Injury

Delayed effects of head trauma occur frequently and must be suspected when a patient's clinical condition deteriorates. Serious secondary lesions of head trauma are delayed hemorrhage, increased intracranial pressure and cerebral ischemia, development of hydrocephalus, and infection. Posttraumatic leptomeningeal cyst formation is discussed later in the section on cystic brain lesions.

Delayed Hemorrhage. Delayed hemorrhage can occur when compression of damaged arteries is alleviated by a decrease in edema or by surgical evacuation of a hematoma. These damaged arteries, initially tamponaded by the mass effect of edema or blood, reperfuse and bleed (Fig. 8–23). Delayed hemorrhage usually occurs within 1 to 2 days of injury but may occur even later. Other factors, such as clotting abnormalities and hypertension, can also contribute to delayed hemorrhage.

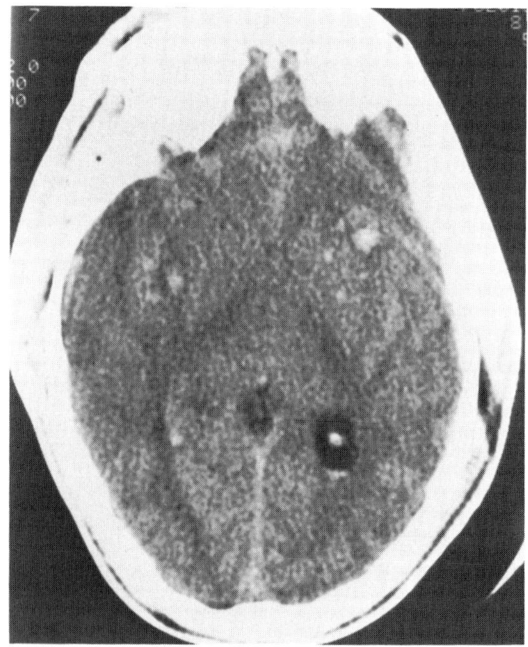

FIGURE 8–22. Punctate contusions. Multiple small contusions are present in addition to diffuse brain swelling in a 17-year-old male injured in a motor vehicle accident. These lesions, representing small hemorrhages or contusions, may not be evident until brain swelling is reduced, usually about 24 hours after the injury.

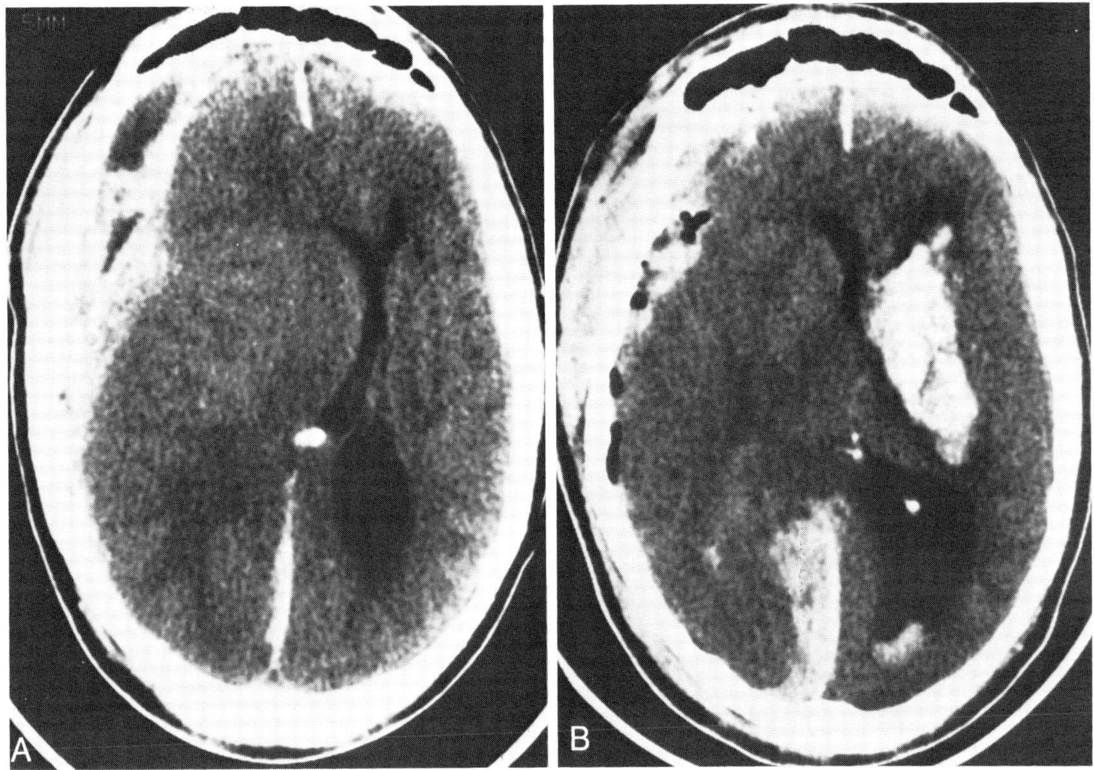

FIGURE 8–23. Delayed hematoma. *A.* Initial image shows massive right subdural hematoma with a hematocrit effect (layering of the cells in the serum), massive brain swelling, shift of the midline, and entrapment of the left lateral ventricle. *B.* Five hours later, after surgical decompression, a large left basal ganglia hemorrhage occurred.

Increased Intracranial Pressure and Cerebral Ischemia. Generalized or local elevation of intracranial pressure can compress the veins and capillaries, obstructing the drainage from the brain. The result is decreased perfusion and, consequently, ischemia. Hemorrhage, generalized edema, and loss of autoregulation of blood flow are common causes of increases in intracranial pressure. Hemorrhage may be immediate or delayed. Cerebral edema often develops immediately from closed-head trauma and can increase if infarction occurs. In children, head trauma can cause loss of autoregulation of blood flow, which leads to increased intravascular volume. Whatever the cause of the increased brain volume, the result is compression of the brain and obstruction of blood flow in the small veins and capillaries. MRI and CT in patients with elevated intracranial pressure show small ventricles, sulci, and cisterns. However, correlation of this appearance with actual measurements of intracranial pressure is only fairly accurate, and most patients with elevation of intracranial pressure need intracranial monitors. The final outcome is often infarction, which progresses from the least collateralized area of the brain to the better perfused areas.

Delayed infarction of brain can result from severe ischemia caused by edema or brain swelling, from compression of the brain by hematoma, from spasm of cerebral vessels, or from compression of large arteries in the brain. Such compression of the posterior cerebral arteries (as they cross the incisura) or of the anterior cerebral arteries (as they pass beneath the falx) can lead to large infarcts in those arterial distributions.

Development of Obstructive Hydrocephalus. Obstructive hydrocephalus—enlargement of the ventricular system of the brain from obstruction of CSF flow—can develop and become acute as a result of either obstructing clot or compression of the CSF pathways. Increased intracranial pressure and its complications result. Hemorrhage can extend into the ventricles with obstruction to the normal flow of CSF at the foramina of Monro, the cerebral aqueduct (of Sylvius), the foramina of Luschka and Magendie, the basal subarachnoid cisterns, or the arachnoid granulations. The type and location of ventricular dilatation determines the CT appearance. Hydrocephalus is discussed later in the section on congenital abnormalities.

Infection. Infection is a potential and serious complication in all penetrating injuries, open fractures, and facial fractures that communicate with the brain. Patients may develop meningitis or brain abscess. Antibiotic therapy has significantly reduced the incidence of these complications.

Other Brain Injury

Radiation and Chemotherapy Injury. Radiation and chemotherapy injury cause gliosis and demyelination, vascular damage, and injury at the gray-white matter junction. The effects generally occur many months after therapy. On histological examination the white matter areas show vascular thickening, demyelination, gliosis, and necrosis. The gray matter is relatively normal. The cortical U-fibers are less susceptible to the effects of edema because they are compressed rather than stretched.

CT shows low intensity in the white matter that is indistinguishable from that of recurrent tumor. MRI also does not distinguish between recurrent tumor and therapeutic changes. However, when the abnormality is substantial, it appears as high intensity on T2 spin echo scans, extending to the peripheral margins of the gyral white matter but sparing the cortical U-fibers (Fig. 8–24). The high intensity represents gliosis, demyelination, and increased water content in the altered myelin or in the interstitial space. Contrast CT or MRI may be of benefit for distinguishing between recurrent tumor and therapeutic changes, particularly when there is an increase in the size of an enhancing lesion in comparison with its size on earlier scans.

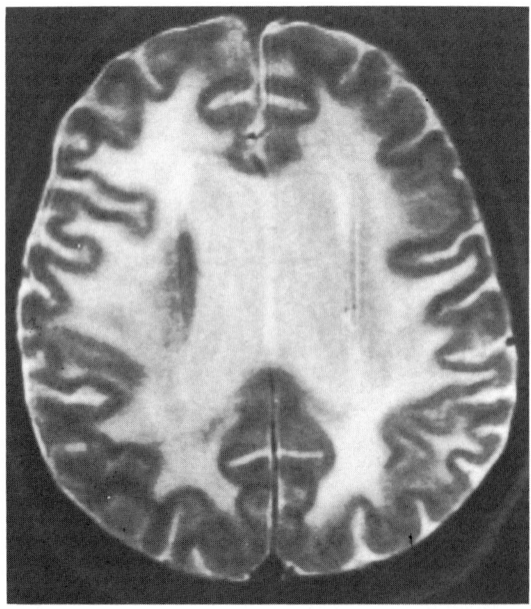

FIGURE 8–24. Radiation injury in a woman who had undergone surgical resection and radiation therapy for a brain tumor 2 years before this examination. T2 spin echo images show high intensity throughout the white matter extending into the gyri but sparing the cortical U-fibers. There were no clinical signs of recurrent tumor.

CONGENITAL ABNORMALITIES

Congenital abnormalities of the CNS are common because of the duration and the complexity of development of these structures. They may be caused by genetic abnormalities or intrauterine insults. The most important congenital abnormalities are cysts, hydrocephalus, fusion abnormalities, and lesions associated with congenital and genetic syndromes.

Cysts

Cysts in the brain are primarily congenital and developmental, but traumatic cysts have a similar appearance. On CT, a cyst appears as a low-density, circumscribed lesion with curved margins and usually exhibits a mass effect on adjacent brain tissue. MRI sequences can demonstrate intensity similar to that of CSF in the ventricles, showing that the cyst contains simple fluid. Normally, no enhancement occurs. If an adjacent soft-tissue mass or contrast enhancement is present, the possibility of a tumor or an infectious cyst should be considered. Many types of cysts occur in specific locations as a result of their mechanism of formation (Fig. 8–25).

Porencephalic Cyst. A porencephalic cyst is, literally, a hole in the brain. Although this term has various meanings, it is used here to represent a cyst that is the result of early brain injury. The cyst is actually a local area of encephalomalacia that results from infarction, infection, trauma, or subependymal hemorrhage. When the insult occurs early, the developing brain envelops the area of encephalomalacia, producing a cyst within the brain. When near the ventricle, the cyst appears as a

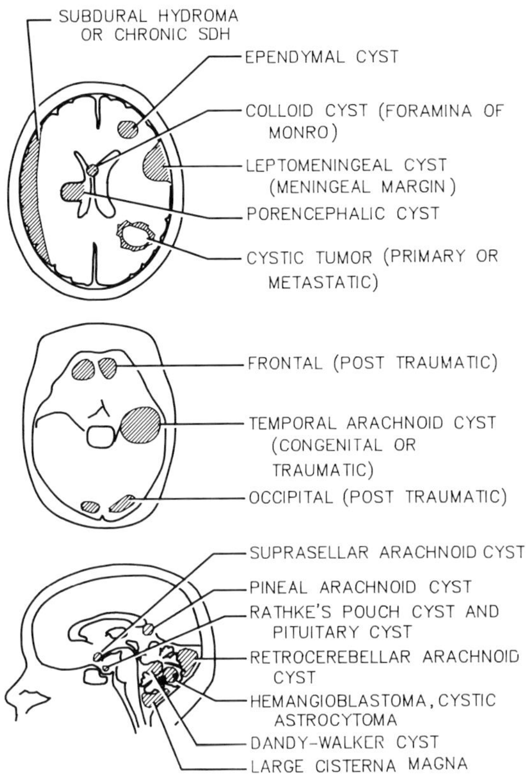

FIGURE 8–25. Locations and appearance of cystic lesions in the brain. SDH, subdural hematoma.

focal ex vacuo dilatation of the ventricle (Fig. 8–26). CT and MRI both show a focal area of fluid. Lesions deep in the brain are surrounded by the gray matter of the developing brain. Lesions adjacent to the ventricle are usually located posteriorly, reflecting the watershed area (the area of poorest perfusion) in the developing fetus. This is the predominant site of periventricular leukomalacia in preterm infants who suffer hypotension or asphyxia (discussed later in the section on vascular diseases).

Arachnoid Cyst. Arachnoid cysts are fluid collections in the subarachnoid space confined by the arachnoid layer. Most are congenital, but some are secondary to trauma. The intact cysts do not communicate with the ventricular system (Fig. 8–27). Many cysts eventually break down and then communicate with the subarachnoid space. In infants, these collections can be so large and symmetrical that they simulate brain atrophy or bilateral chronic subdural hematomas. In the posterior fossa, they can conform to the shape of the tentorium and may appear to be congenitally large subarachnoid spaces. The most common sites are the middle cranial fossa, the posterior fossa, and the suprasellar region. Arachnoid cysts can cause a mass effect and symptoms, most commonly seizures.

In the posterior fossa, cysts may be related to congenital dysgenesis of the cerebellum, and there may be associated anomalies of the cerebellar vermis, the fourth ventricle, or the brainstem. A large cisterna magna can be distinguished from a cerebellar arachnoid cyst by instillation of contrast into the subarachnoid space. Suprasellar cyst is a common cause of precocious puberty (as is hamartoma of the tuber cinereum).

Ependymal Cyst. Ependymal cells occasionally become separated from the ventricular system during formation or as a result of injury. These cells may form an ependymal cyst, which is usually near but separate from the ventricles and does not communicate with them. It can enlarge by means of either a one-way valve phenomenon or CSF secretion by the ependymal cells. An ependymal cyst may cause symptoms through mass effect. On CT or MRI, the cyst appears as a well-circumscribed mass that contains simple fluid. The appearance is indistinguishable from that of an

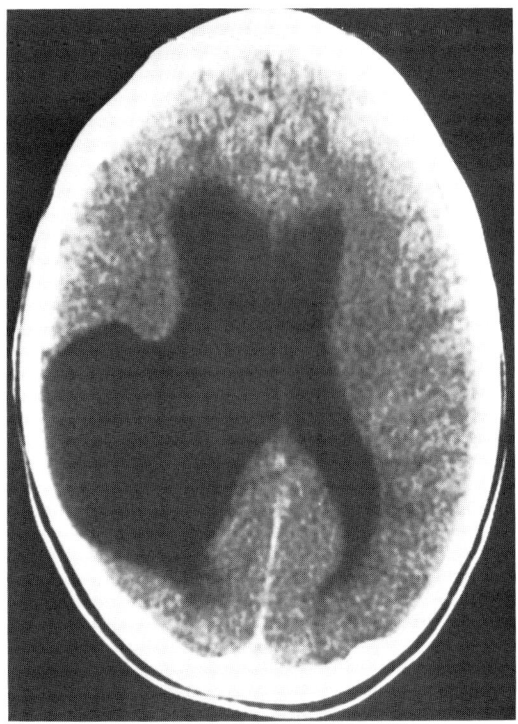

FIGURE 8–26. Porencephalic cyst. CT in an 8-year-old child who suffered asphyxia at birth shows a large right parietal area of encephalomalacia, indicating resorption of infarcted brain in the periventricular watershed area.

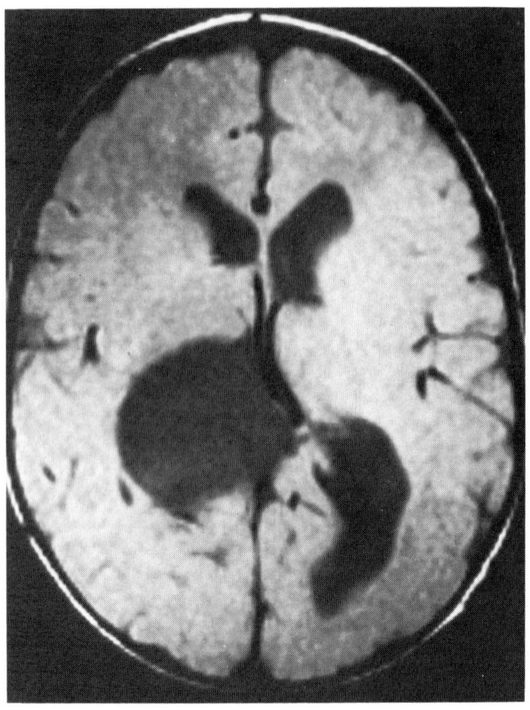

FIGURE 8–27. Arachnoid cyst. T1 spin echo image in a 6-day-old asymptomatic boy shows a well-circumscribed cyst posterior to the right thalamus. The MRI characteristics on several sequences were identical to those of cerebrospinal fluid (CSF). Note the lack of differentiation between gray and white matter, which is typical for a newborn on this high-field image (TR = 3000 msec).

arachnoid cyst except by its more common location near the midline.

Leptomeningeal Cyst. Skull fractures usually heal with minimal residual sclerosis. In children, the cleft along the fracture margin occasionally contains leptomeningeal tissue, which enlarges into a cyst (growing fracture). These cysts can reach considerable size and compress brain tissue (Fig. 8–28). They do not communicate with the subarachnoid space.

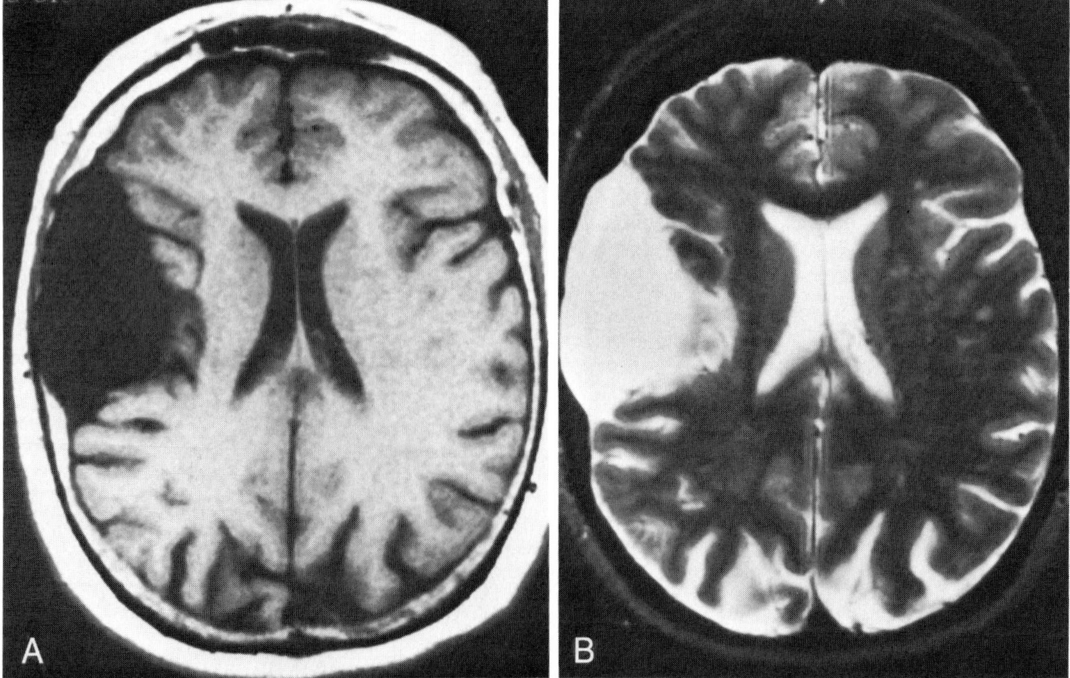

FIGURE 8–28. Leptomeningeal cyst. *A.* T1 spin echo image shows a large peripheral simple fluid collection with associated encephalomalacia and skull thinning in a middle-aged woman who suffered a skull fracture in childhood. *B.* T2 spin echo image also shows simple fluid characteristics.

Membranous encapsulation of subdural blood collections frequently occurs, especially in infants. The blood is resorbed, leaving a thin-walled cyst containing clear watery fluid. These cysts are called subdural hydromas.

Congenital Diseases That Cause Hydrocephalus

Hydrocephalus, enlargement of the ventricular system as a result of obstruction of CSF flow, can be acquired (caused by trauma, tumor, or infection) or congenital. The radiographic appearance depends on the site of obstruction (Fig. 8–29). CSF flows from the lateral ventricles through the third and fourth ventricles out to the basal cisterns and through the arachnoid granulations into the venous (mostly sagittal) sinuses. In general, the portions of the ventricles upstream from the obstruction become dilated. However, obstruction of the arachnoid granulations or sagittal sinus can cause generalized brain swelling and ventricle compression because fluid cannot exit the cranium. Enlargement of ventricles as a result of brain atrophy or encephalomalacia (called ex vacuo dilatation) is not obstructive hydrocephalus.

The most common cause of congenital hydrocephalus is stenosis of the cerebral aqueduct (the aqueduct of Sylvius). Patients who have the Chiari type II malformation (to be described) or Dandy-Walker syndrome develop hydrocephalus as a result of different abnormalities in the region of the fourth ventricle: in the former, the fourth ventricle is small; in the latter, it is large. Subarachnoid hemorrhage, meningitis, and meningeal carcinomatosis can also result in obstruction of the basal cisterns or arachnoid granulations.

Aqueductal Stenosis. Stenosis of the cerebral aqueduct accounts for most cases of congenital hydrocephalus. Atresia of the aqueduct or overgrowth of the subependymal glial tissue results in obstruction to flow of CSF from the third to the fourth ventricle. Usually, the abnormality is isolated. Symptoms depend on the degree of obstruction. Patients with only partial obstruction may not be identified until adulthood. The CT and MRI findings are dilatation of the third and lateral ventricles and a normal-sized fourth ventricle (Fig. 8–30). MRI can show the narrowed aqueduct and

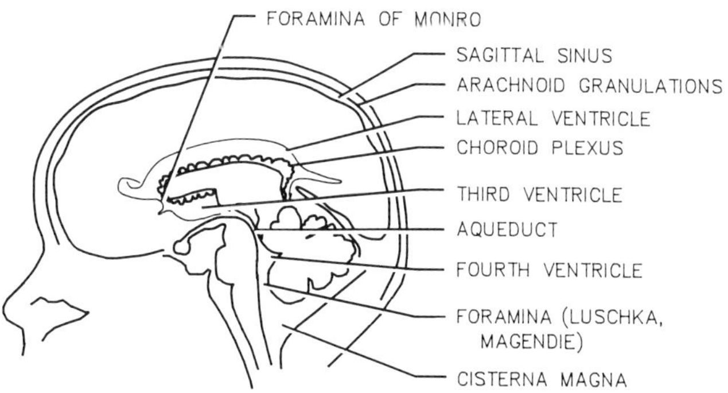

LATERAL VENTRICLE – CHOROID PLEXUS TUMOR (EXCESS CSF)

FORAMINA OF MONRO – COLLOID CYST, CLOT, MASS COMPRESSION

THIRD VENTRICLE – CYST, TUMOR

AQUEDUCT (OF SYLVIUS) – ATRESIA, CLOT

FOURTH VENTRICLE – TUMOR, DANDY–WALKER CYST, CHIARI

FORAMINA (LUSCHKA, MAGENDIE) – CHIARI, DANDY–WALKER, VERMIAN AGENESIS, CYST, CLOT

BASAL CISTERNS – INFECTION, CYST

ARACHNOID GRANULATIONS – BLOOD, MENINGITIS

SAGITTAL SINUS – THROMBOSIS

NOTE: ALL HYDROCEPHALUS IS OBSTRUCTIVE.
TUMOR CAN OBSTRUCT ANYWHERE.
CHOROID PLEXUS TUMORS PRODUCE EXCESS CSF BUT ALSO BLEED.
ATROPHY OR FOCAL BRAIN LOSS CAUSES EX–VACUO VENTRICLE DILATATION – NOT OBSTRUCTIVE HYDROCEPHALUS

FIGURE 8–29. Locations and causes of obstruction in hydrocephalus. CSF, cerebrospinal fluid.

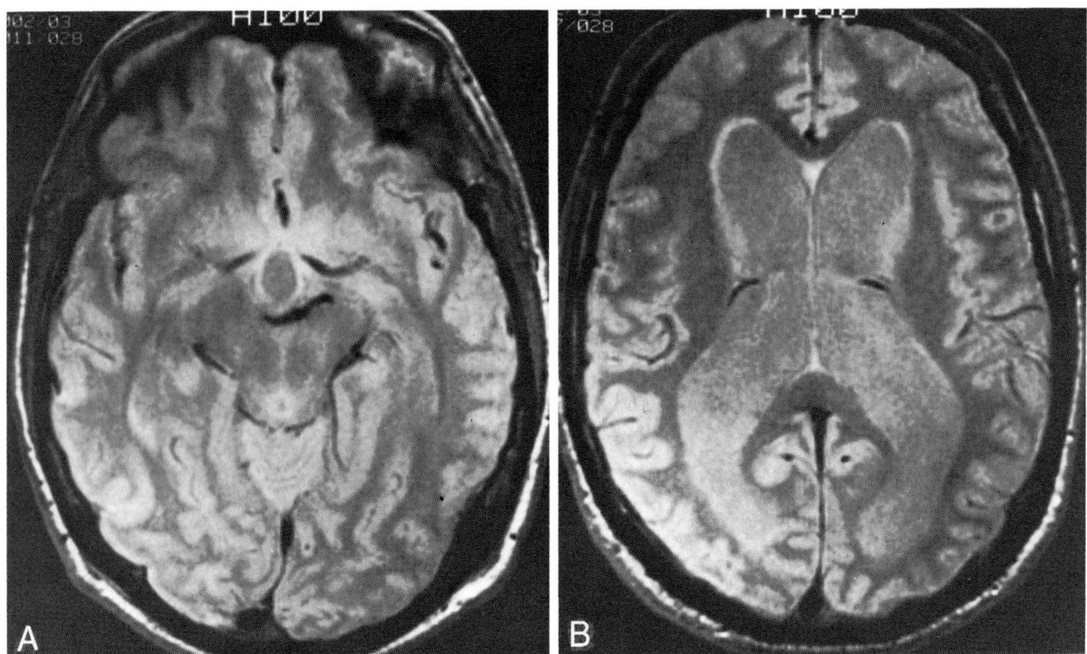

FIGURE 8–30. Aqueductal stenosis. *A.* Axial early echo T2 image at the level of the cerebral aqueduct shows characteristics of static fluid instead of the usual low intensity of flowing CSF. This finding indicates obstruction of flow. *B.* The lateral ventricles show dilatation and subependymal fluid, which indicate obstructive hydrocephalus.

indicate whether flow is adequate by the change in signal that occurs with pulsating CSF. MRI can also show ependymal fluid as a smooth rim of increased intensity, which is caused by transudated fluid from the obstructed ventricle. Patients with aqueductal stenosis generally require ventricular shunting.

Chiari Malformations. Chiari malformations are a spectrum of posterior midline abnormalities involving the skullbase, the brain, the spine, and the spinal cord. The mildest form, Chiari type I, is characterized by caudal position of the cerebellar tonsils into or below the foramen magnum. Patients are usually adults who have nonspecific symptoms such as pain or headache but may have signs of cerebellar disease, compression of the foramen magnum, or central cord syndrome. Associated abnormalities include skullbase and cervical vertebral anomaly, syrinx, and hydrocephalus, but not meningocele. MRI best demonstrates the low position of the tonsils and the associated syrinx (Fig. 8–31). Treatment includes decompression of the foramen magnum and shunting of the syrinx.

Chiari type II (also referred to as Arnold-Chiari) malformation is a more severe form of the disease and involves the entire neural axis. It is detected in infants and young children, usually from symptoms of hydrocephalus and the presence of a meningomyelocele. The most important abnormalities are low position of an abnormal cerebellar vermis below the foramen magnum; low, elongated fourth ventricle; obstructive hydrocephalus; and, in more than 90% of cases, a meningomyelocele (Fig. 8–32). Whereas Chiari type I malformation is characterized by herniation of the cerebellar tonsils, Chiari type II malformation is caused by vermian and posterior medullary velum dysgenesis.

In Chiari type II malformation, the caudal vermis (the nodulus), which normally forms the posterior roof of the fourth ventricle, is abnormally positioned below the foramen magnum. The choroid plexus and posterior medullary velum are elongated and displaced caudal to the fourth ventricle. These distinctions and the other associated abnormalities can be detected best by MRI but are also shown by myelography and CT. Patients who have Chiari type II malformation may require shunting for hydrocephalus, decompression of the cerebellar vermis, and treatment of the associated meningomyelocele, syrinx, and tethered cord.

Chiari type III malformation consists primarily of a cerebellar encephalocele. Chiari

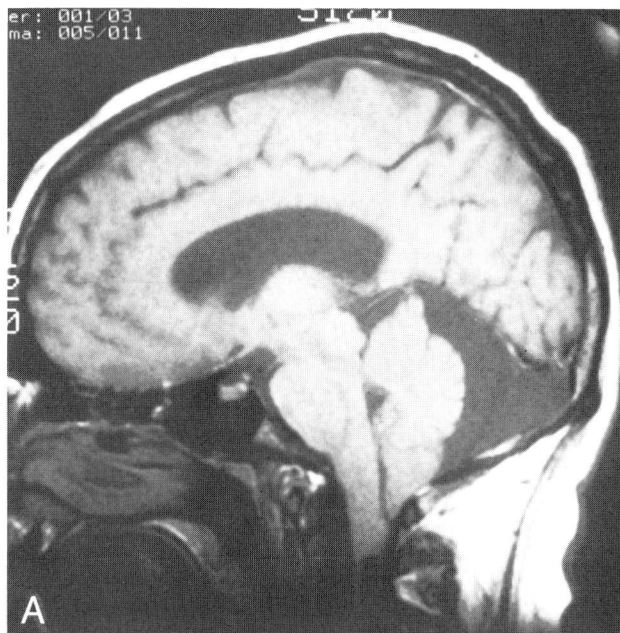

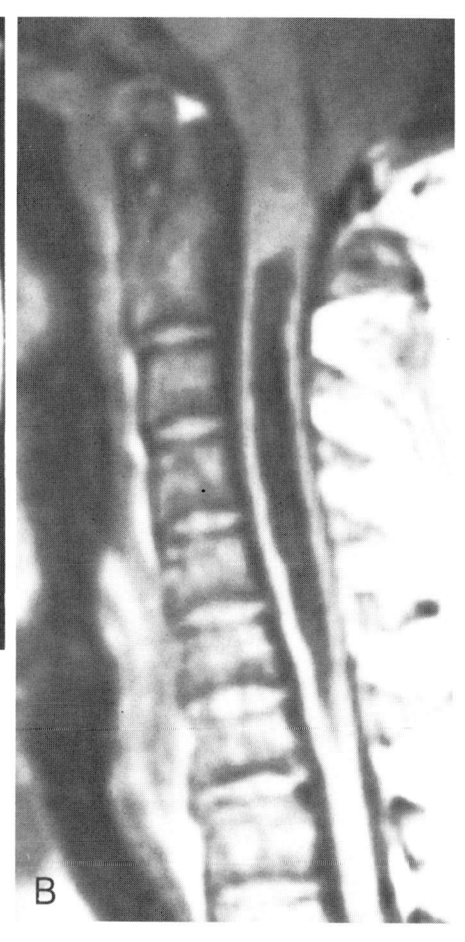

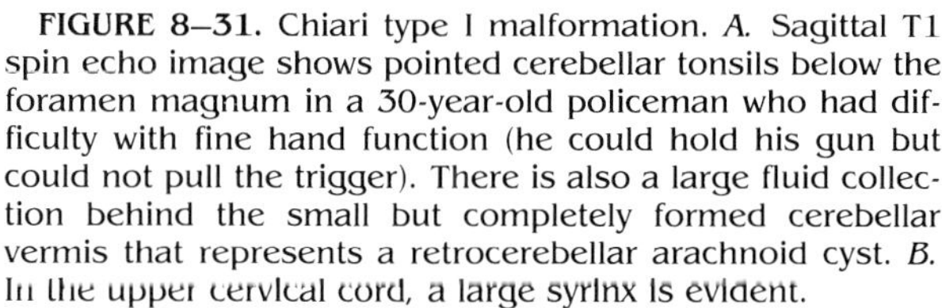
FIGURE 8–31. Chiari type I malformation. *A.* Sagittal T1 spin echo image shows pointed cerebellar tonsils below the foramen magnum in a 30-year-old policeman who had difficulty with fine hand function (he could hold his gun but could not pull the trigger). There is also a large fluid collection behind the small but completely formed cerebellar vermis that represents a retrocerebellar arachnoid cyst. *B.* In the upper cervical cord, a large syrinx is evident.

type IV malformation is a hypoplastic cerebellum. Neither is easily confused with Chiari type I or II malformation.

Dandy-Walker Syndrome. A rare congenital anomaly associated with hydrocephalus is the Dandy-Walker syndrome, a developmental agenesis of the midline posterior fossa. The primary abnormalities are hypoplasia of the cerebellar vermis (absence of the posterior vermis) and atresia of the foramina of Luschka and Magendie, with resultant obstructive hydrocephalus and enlargement of the fourth ventricle. Clinical symptoms are caused by hydrocephalus. Axial MRI and CT show a large fourth ventricle with cystic dilatation, absence of the posterior cerebellar vermis, and hydrocephalus (Fig. 8–33). The enlarged fourth ventricle is often called a Dandy-Walker cyst. Its midline location and continuity with the fourth ventricle differentiate it from arachnoid cyst. Two thirds of patients who have Dandy-Walker syndrome have other CNS and systemic abnormalities.

Fusion Abnormalities

Midline closure abnormalities (called dysraphism or neuroschisis) include cranial and spinal defects of varying severity, and many are incompatible with life. In the head, failures of midline closure range from anencephaly, in which the skull and much of the cerebrum are absent, to cranium bifidum, in which a portion of the midline skull (usually the occipital) is absent. In cranium bifidum, the defect allows the formation of an encephalocele.

Encephalocele. Encephaloceles are herniations of brain tissue through a cleft in the skull; most (80%) are posterior. An anterior encephalocele can be confused with tumor or infection, and coronal or sagittal scans are required in order to demonstrate the continuity with the brain. CT best shows the bone defect in the skullbase. MRI most clearly shows and characterizes the herniated brain tissue. In the subfrontal region, an encephalocele can be confused with nasal or paranasal sinus disease.

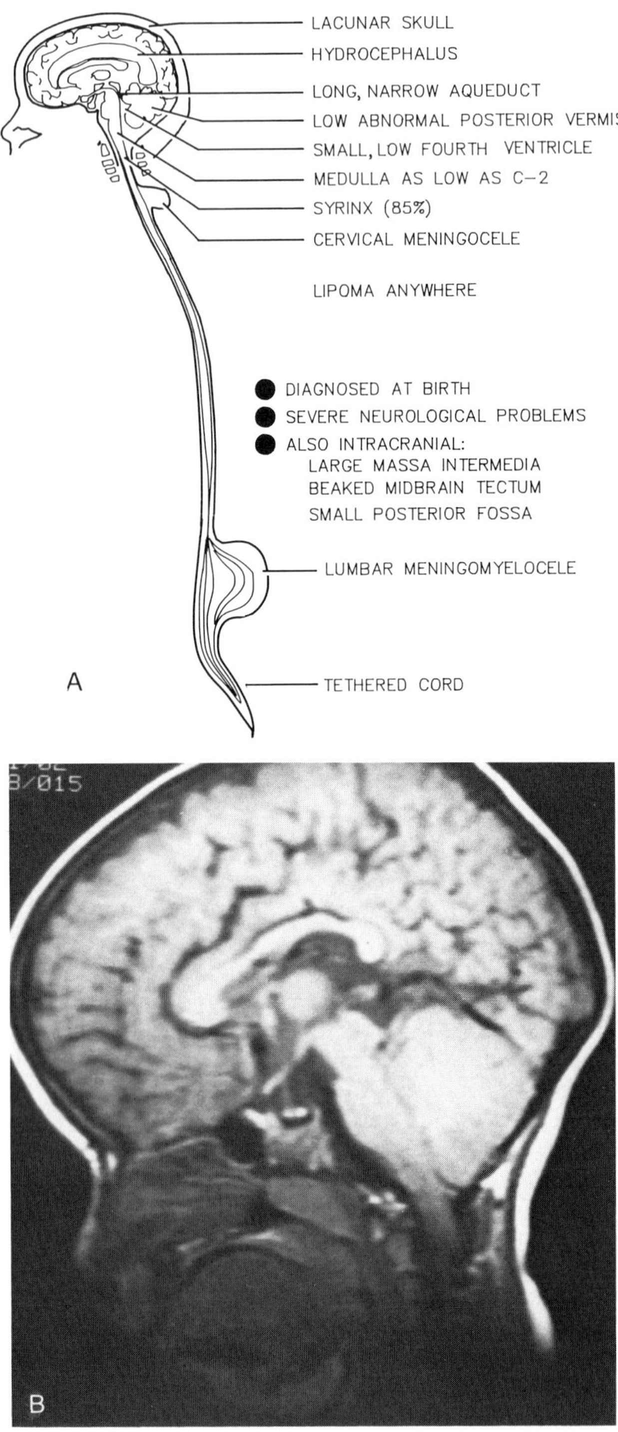

FIGURE 8–32. Chiari type II malformation. *A.* Diagram shows the locations of abnormalities. *B.* Sagittal T1 spin echo image of a child with Chiari type II malformation. Note absence of a well-defined fourth ventricle, beaking of the tectum, and the towering cerebellum with low-lying cerebellar tonsils.

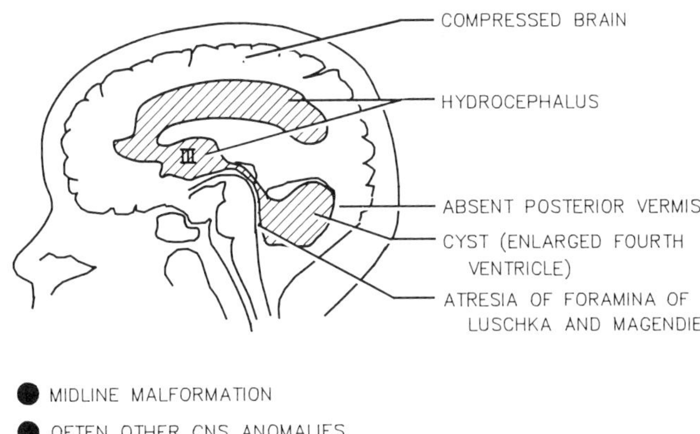

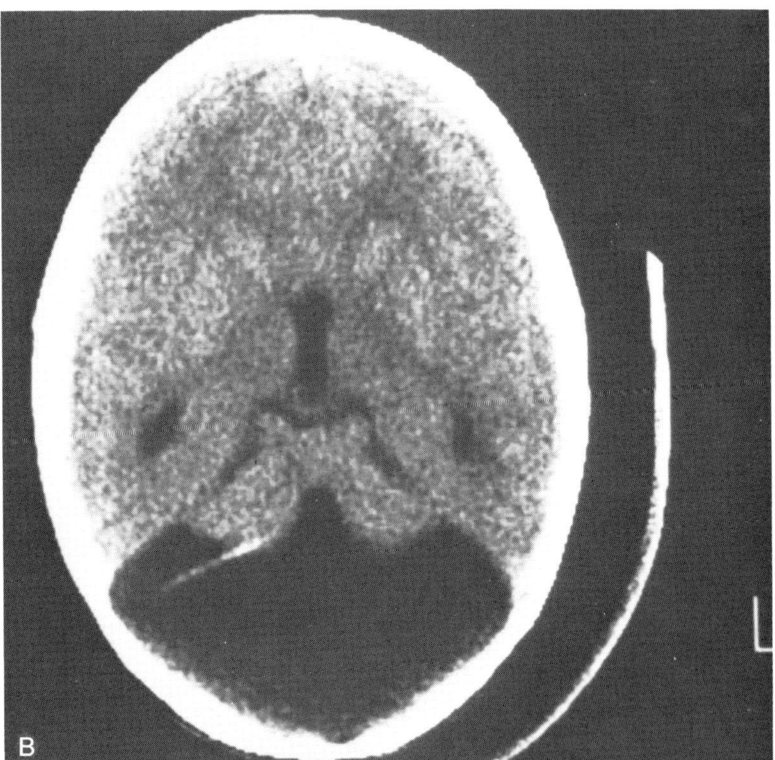

FIGURE 8–33. Dandy-Walker syndrome. *A.* Diagram. *B.* Noncontrast CT shows midline cystic dilatation of the fourth ventricle and absence of the posterior cerebellar vermis.

Such a lesion requires full radiographic evaluation, including coronal scans before biopsy.

Developmental Defects

Cerebral dysgenesis is a spectrum of diseases characterized by absence or abnormalities of parts of the cerebrum, usually frontal or parietal cortex, but with an intact skull. The term "cerebral dysgenesis" is applied to a variety of developmental defects that include the presence of heterotopic gray matter, microcephaly and megalencephaly, schizencephaly, lissencephaly, porencephaly, hydranencephaly, arhinencephaly, holoprosencephaly, and agenesis of the corpus callosum. Heterotopic gray matter is brain tissue in an abnormal location as a result of the arrest of migration from ventricle to cortex. It may vary in size from microscopic to grossly visible. Microcephaly and megalencephaly are defined by brain size and may be correlated with poor function. Schizencephaly is the result of interruption of very early development of the cerebral hemispheres with the formation of a cleft between parts of brain tissue. The cleft may be grossly obliterated by the apposition of the further development of the preserved cerebral cortex. "Lissencephaly" means smooth brain: that is, a brain without gyri; it results from arrest of cerebral development before gyral formation.

Porencephaly and Hydranencephaly. Porencephaly and hydranencephaly result from destruction of cerebral tissue in varying amounts. Hydranencephaly represents complete or nearly complete absence of the cerebral hemispheres, which are then replaced by CSF. The smaller lesions are frequently in the distribution of one of the branches of the middle cerebral artery; the larger lesions are in the distribution of all of the middle and anterior cerebral arteries. These lesions are usually bilateral and almost symmetrical. Small cystic spaces in the brain are termed porencephaly (see earlier description of porencephalic cyst). More substantial involvement produces large CSF spaces and is called hydranencephaly (i.e., water brain). The CT and MRI appearances depend on the distribution of abnormality.

Arhinencephaly and Holoprosencephaly. Arhinencephaly is absence of the olfactory bulbs and tracts. It may occur in isolation or in association with holoprosencephaly, a spectrum of congenital midline fusion abnormalities. These abnormalities range from complete failure of formation of the interhemispheric fissure, which results in a single cerebral sphere, a single ventricle, and a single midline cyst (called holotelencephaly or alobar holoprosencephaly), to various degrees of incomplete formation of the interhemispheric fissure (semilobar holoprosencephaly). The mildest form (lobar holoprosencephaly) is identified from partial fusion of the cerebral hemispheres anteriorly. The abnormalities in such congenital malformations are often complex. It is usually most effective to describe the structural appearance rather than to categorize the findings into a specific syndrome.

Agenesis of the Corpus Callosum. A limited midline defect occurs as a failure of development of the midline telencephalon that results in partial or total agenesis of the corpus callosum. Other associated midline anomalies may be present, including lipoma, meningioma, arachnoid cyst, and the absence of the anterior and hippocampal commissures. The formation of the corpus callosum is complex but basically follows an anterior-to-posterior pattern. When agenesis is partial, the posterior part is absent. The absence of the corpus callosum enables the lateral angles of the lateral ventricles to rise higher than normal, producing a bat-wing appearance on coronal views (Fig. 8–34). Similarly, high axial slices through the lateral ventricles often show only the frontal and occipital poles of the lateral ventricles, which appear as four separate CSF

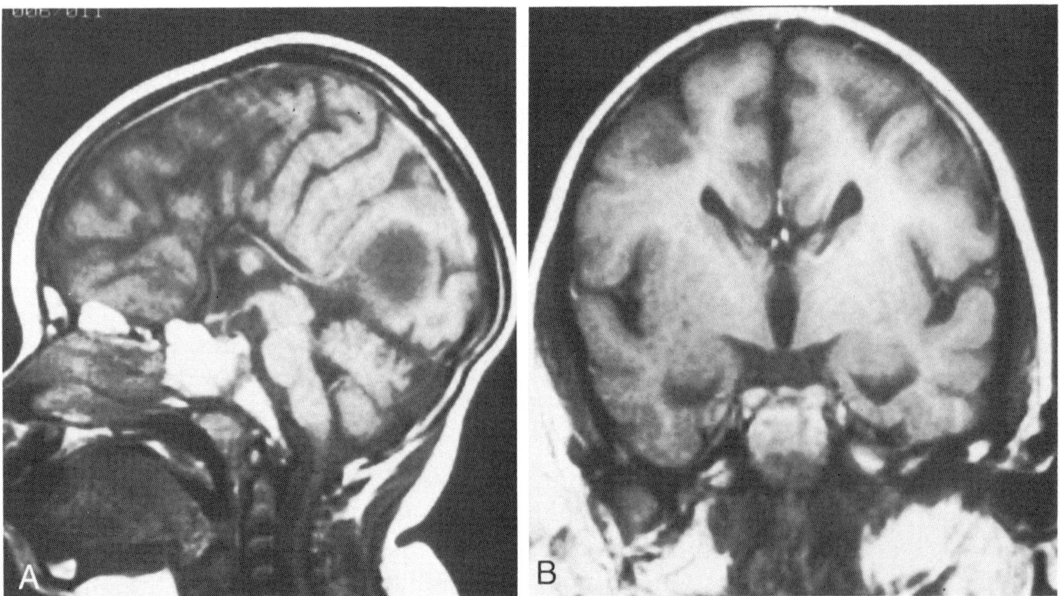

FIGURE 8–34. Agenesis of corpus callosum. *A.* Sagittal T1 spin echo image shows the outline of the third ventricle with the massa intermedia centrally. No corpus callosum is present (see Fig. 8–31 for comparison). *B.* Coronal view at the level of the foramina of Monro shows a complete cleft between the hemispheres.

collections. The third ventricle may extend to the interhemispheric fissure, and the medial cortical gyri tend to radiate from the cingulate gyri.

Genetic Syndromes

Various congenital syndromes severely affect the CNS. Many are storage diseases and enzyme deficiency syndromes, which involve predominantly the white matter. Because of their rarity and nondescript appearance, they are not considered here. Two congenital diseases with characteristic appearances similar to those of several more common diseases are olivopontocerebellar degeneration and Leigh's disease. Another group of diseases are termed the neurocutaneous syndromes or, because they all involve the retina, the phacomatoses. The neurocutaneous syndromes are inherited diseases that affect several organ systems, especially skin, the brain, and the retina, with tumors. Important neurocutaneous syndromes are neurofibromatosis, tuberous sclerosis, encephalotrigeminal angiomatosis (Sturge-Weber syndrome), and retinocerebellar angiomatosis (von Hippel-Lindau disease).

Olivopontocerebellar Degeneration. Olivopontocerebellar degeneration is one of a spectrum of multisystem atrophies with progressive degeneration of the inferior olive, the pons, and the cerebellum. The most common form of the disease begins in the second or third decade and is characterized by ataxia and other signs of cerebellar dysfunction. The cerebellar vermis is atrophic but fully formed, as opposed to cerebellar vermian dysgenesis (Dandy-Walker syndrome). Sagittal MRI best demonstrates the atrophic cerebellum and pons, and T2 spin echo images can show the degenerating fibers of the olivopontocerebellar tracts (Fig. 8–35). Other parts of neural systems may be affected (the retina, the substantia nigra, the basal ganglia) with resultant blindness, parkinsonism, and motor dysfunction.

Several more common diseases produce atrophy in the brainstem and the cerebellum. The late onset, the progression of disability, and the hereditary association distinguish olivopontocerebellar degeneration from acquired disorders such as birth-related injury, brainstem infarction, alcoholism (anterior vermian atrophy), and phenytoin- (Dilantin-) induced diffuse cerebellar atrophy.

Leigh's Disease. Leigh's disease is a rare,

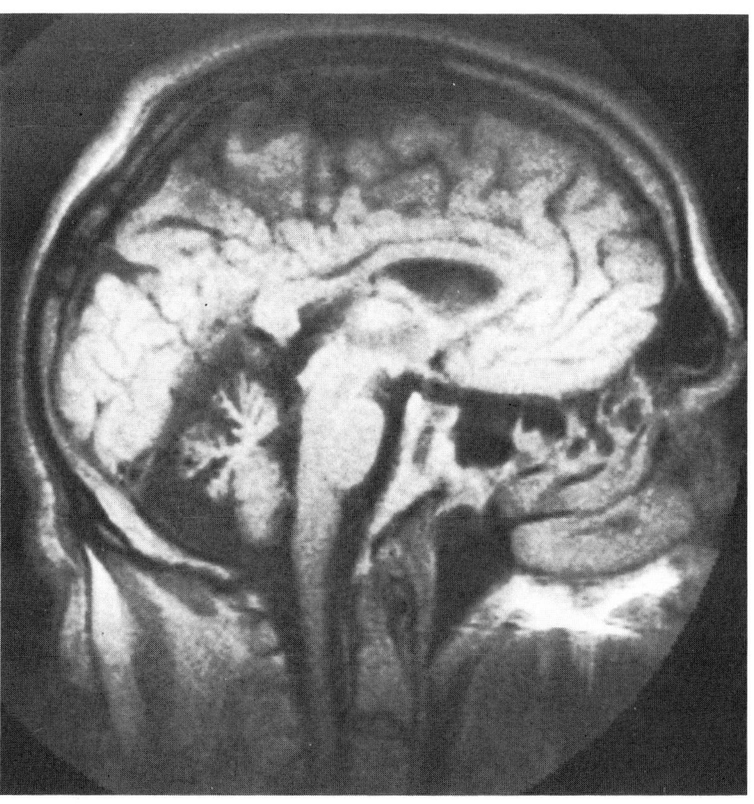

FIGURE 8–35. Olivopontocerebellar degeneration. T1 spin echo low-field image shows marked atrophy of the normally formed cerebellar vermis in a 40-year-old man with ataxia and a strong family history of the disease.

autosomal recessive syndrome that involves the basal ganglia, the brainstem, and the spinal cord as well as white matter tracts and peripheral nerves. The disease is usually evident in infancy and is manifested by failure to thrive, hypotonia, and seizures. CT shows bilateral low density in the putamen (and elsewhere), which indicates basal ganglia degeneration (Fig. 8–36). T2 spin echo images show these areas as high intensity and, in addition, show similar abnormalities throughout the brainstem and the cerebellum.

The pattern of disease in the basal ganglia is important because several more common conditions, including cerebral anoxia and carbon monoxide poisoning, can produce similar bilateral abnormality. Wilson's disease and mitochondrial cytopathy are rare but also produce bilateral basal ganglia abnormality.

Neurofibromatosis. Neurofibromatosis has two distinct forms: types 1 (NF1) and 2 (NF2). NF1 (also called von Recklinghausen's disease) is the better known type and consists of skin and neural tissue lesions. NF2 is characterized

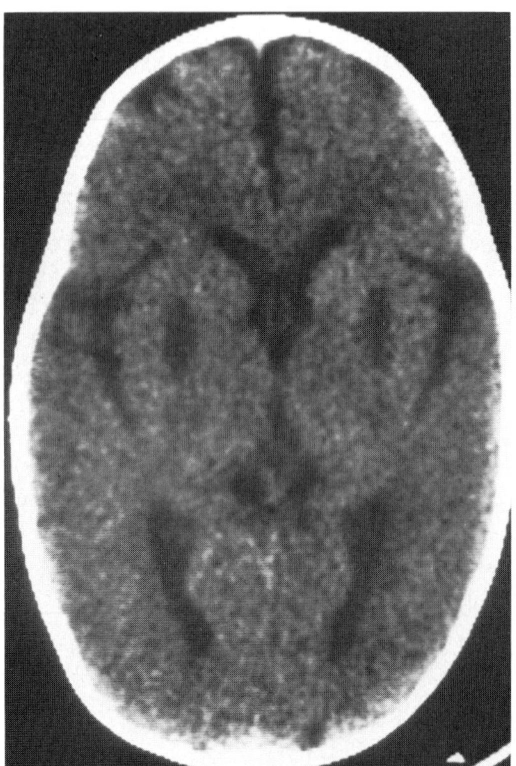

FIGURE 8–36. Leigh's disease. Noncontrast CT shows bilateral low density in the putamen in this 10-month-old girl with progressive weakness and dyskinesia. The patient's twin and a deceased brother also had the disease. The bilateral basal ganglia pattern is seen in several other diseases, notably anoxia.

by bilateral acoustic neurilemmomas (schwannomas). The genes for these two disorders are on chromosomes 17 and 22, respectively. Both show dominant inheritance; NF1 is 10 times more common than NF2.

NF1 is characterized by café au lait spots on the skin, neurofibromas of the skin and in the CNS (Fig. 8–37), and other lesions (bone defects, hamartomas, neurofibromas, gliomas, and meningiomas). Although patients may be severely disfigured, they are of normal intelligence. Skull abnormalities, including sphenoid hypoplasia and lambdoid suture defect, shown on plain skull films or CT, are not clinically significant. The two most serious problems are the development of peripheral disfiguring lesions and CNS tumors, particularly gliomas (especially optic nerve gliomas) in addition to acoustic neurilemmomas.

Patients with NF2 generally develop hearing loss in their teens or twenties from bilateral acoustic neurilemmomas. They may also have signs of cerebellar or brainstem compression. Additional tumors such as meningiomas and cranial nerve tumors occur, but skin lesions are less common and less extensive. Tumors of the neck and spine occur in both types. In these areas, neurofibromas and dural ectasia can compress or distend nerve roots or vessels (see Fig. 8–104).

Tuberous Sclerosis. Tuberous sclerosis is an autosomal dominant inherited syndrome characterized clinically by mental retardation, seizures, and a nasolabial skin lesion (adenoma sebaceum). In the brain, patients develop subependymal and cortical hamartomas (called tubers), which often calcify and do not enhance with intravenous contrast (Fig. 8–38). These tubers, when located near the foramina of Monro, can become large and cause obstructive hydrocephalus. The rate of growth of the tubers is not known, but the subependymal ones tend to become giant-cell astrocytomas, which behave in a less malignant fashion than their histological appearance would suggest.

CT shows the calcified hamartomas, which, when subependymal, bulge into the ventricles (an appearance likened to dripping candle wax). A soft-tissue component, interval enlargement, and contrast enhancement in a previously calcified and quiescent lesion indicates growth, which may represent malignant transformation. MRI can show the uncalcified cortical lesions and cortical heterotopias but may poorly demonstrate the small subependymal calcified tubers. Additional associated lesions include retinal phacoma, renal angiomyoli-

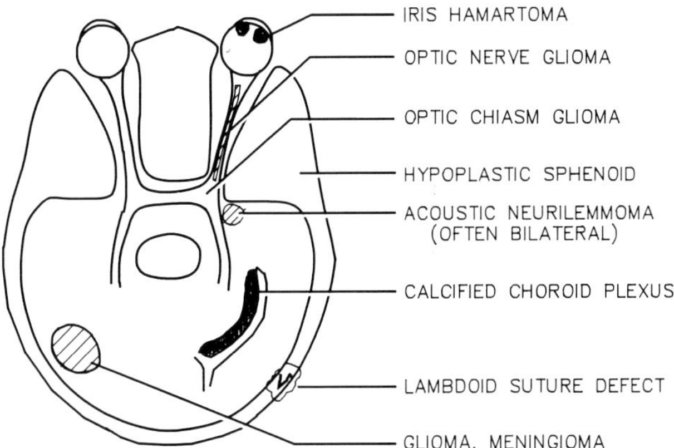

- TYPE 1 – SKIN AND NEURAL TISSUE LESIONS
- TYPE 2 – BILATERAL ACOUSTIC SCHWANNOMAS
- NORMAL INTELLIGENCE
- AUTOSOMAL DOMINANT
- SKIN LESIONS: CUTANEOUS NODULES, AXILLARY FRECKLES
- LUNG: INTERSTITIAL DISEASE
- NECK: NEUROFIBROMAS
- SPINE: DUMBBELL NEUROFIBROMAS, DURAL ECTASIA

A

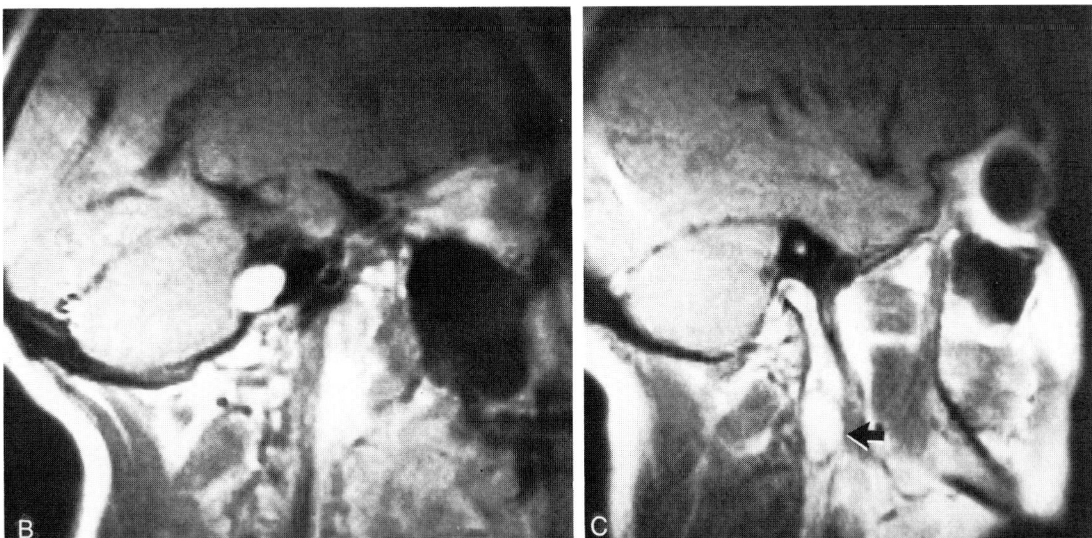

FIGURE 8–37. Neurofibromatosis type 2. *A.* Diagram shows types and locations of abnormalities in the brain and summarizes other findings of the disease. *B.* Gadolinium–diethylenetriaminepenta-acetic acid (Gd-DTPA) enhanced T1 spin echo image shows a left acoustic schwannoma (neurilemmoma) in a man with neurofibromatosis. *C.* A smaller acoustic schwannoma is also present on the right side, as is a schwannoma of the neck *(arrow)* obstructing the jugular vein. The patient had four neural tumors and two meningiomas in the head, the neck, and the spine (see Fig. 8–104C) but no café au lait spots.

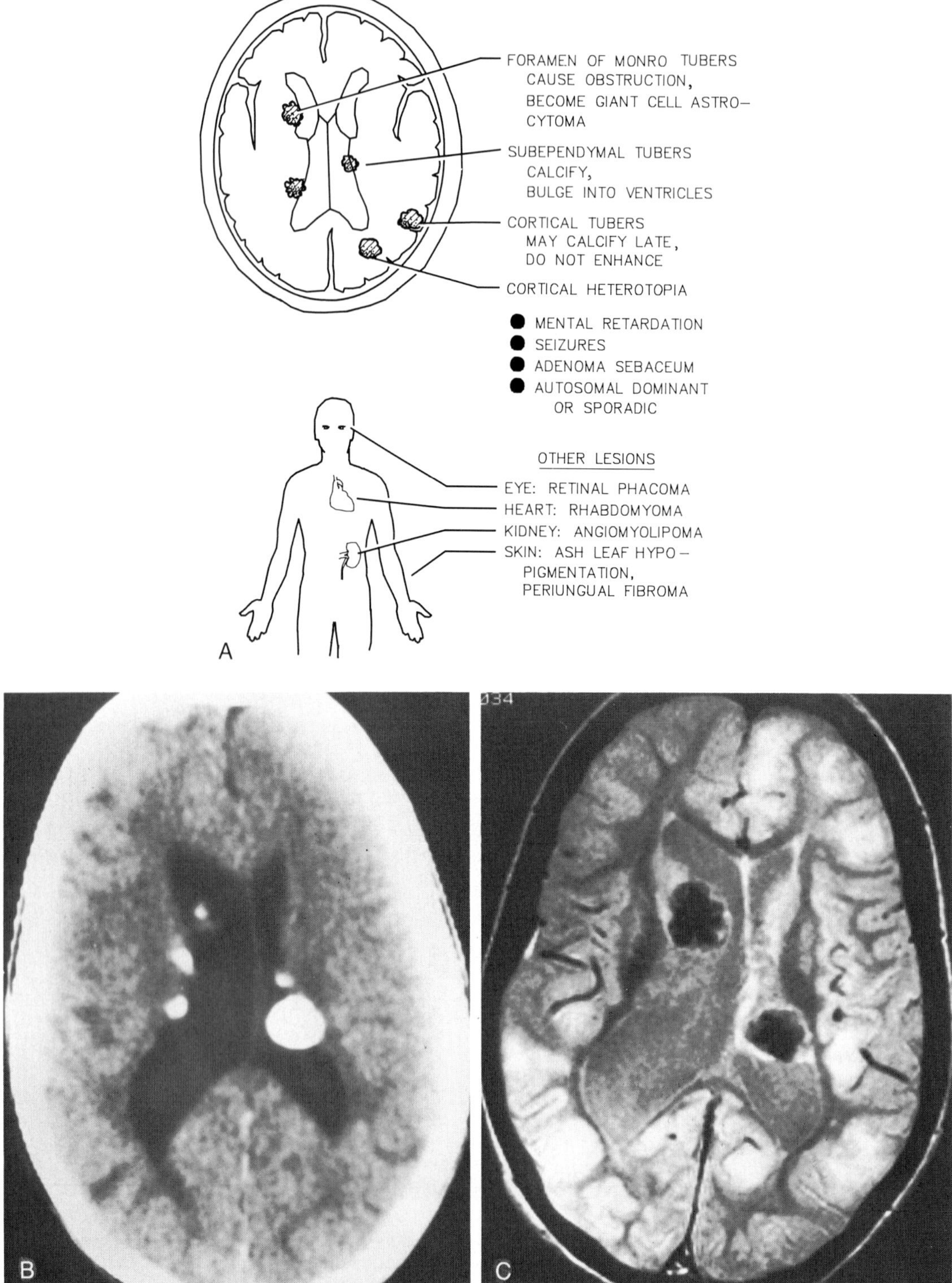

FIGURE 8–38. Tuberous sclerosis. *A.* Diagram. *B.* Noncontrast CT of an 8-year-old boy with tuberous sclerosis shows several densely calcified periventricular lesions that extend into the ventricle. Additional low-density areas, representing noncalcified cortical tubers, were poorly demonstrated on this and other slices. *C.* MRI at a slightly lower level shows high-intensity cortical lesions throughout the brain. The small subependymal lesions are not well-demonstrated. The largest lesions have a black appearance because of dense calcification and possibly paramagnetic effect of blood or deposited minerals. The right-sided large tuber is in the location typical for tubers undergoing malignant degeneration.

poma (discussed in Chapter 4), and cardiac rhabdomyoma (discussed in Chapter 5).

Encephalotrigeminal Angiomatosis. Encephalotrigeminal angiomatosis (Sturge-Weber syndrome) is a rare neurocutaneous syndrome characterized by a port wine stain of the face (nevus flammeus) in a trigeminal nerve distribution and by ipsilateral leptomeningeal angiomatosis or telangiectasia. Calcification is usually not within the abnormal vessels but within the middle layers of the underlying cortex, which is at least partly ischemic. Although most cases are sporadic, some are the result of autosomal dominant or recessive inheritance. The facial and intracranial abnormalities are apparently caused by maldevelopment at the time that the ectoderm and neural tissue are in apposition. Almost all patients have a seizure disorder, and most are mentally retarded. Hemiatrophy of the brain and of the contralateral side of the body, as well as glaucoma, also occur.

CT shows serpiginous, cortical, and gyral calcification beneath an enhancing leptomeningeal angioma on the side of the facial stain (Fig. 8–39). Brain atrophy occurs in the region of the malformation and leads to underdevelopment of the skull. MRI shows similar findings and can provide better definition of anatomical relationships. However, the calcified atrophic brain adjacent to the enhancing leptomeningeal angioma may be better defined on CT. Angiograms show prolongation of venous filling of the angioma and, often, absence of superficial cortical veins. Prognosis is poor when seizures begin; patients often die within 1 year of the development of severe seizures. Hemispherectomy at birth has been successful in eliminating the seizures, and patients compensate well by early childhood.

Retinocerebellar Angiomatosis. Retinocerebellar angiomatosis (von Hippel-Lindau disease) is a neurocutaneous syndrome of predominantly mesodermal elements characterized by hemangioblastomas of the retina, the cerebellum, the medulla, and the spinal cord; angiomas of the kidney and the liver; adenomas of the kidney and the epididymis; renal cell carcinoma; pheochromocytoma; and cysts of the kidneys, the pancreas, and the epididymis (Fig. 8–40). It is inherited through an autosomal dominant gene with incomplete penetrance. Patients usually develop symptoms from cerebellar hemangioblastoma (headaches),

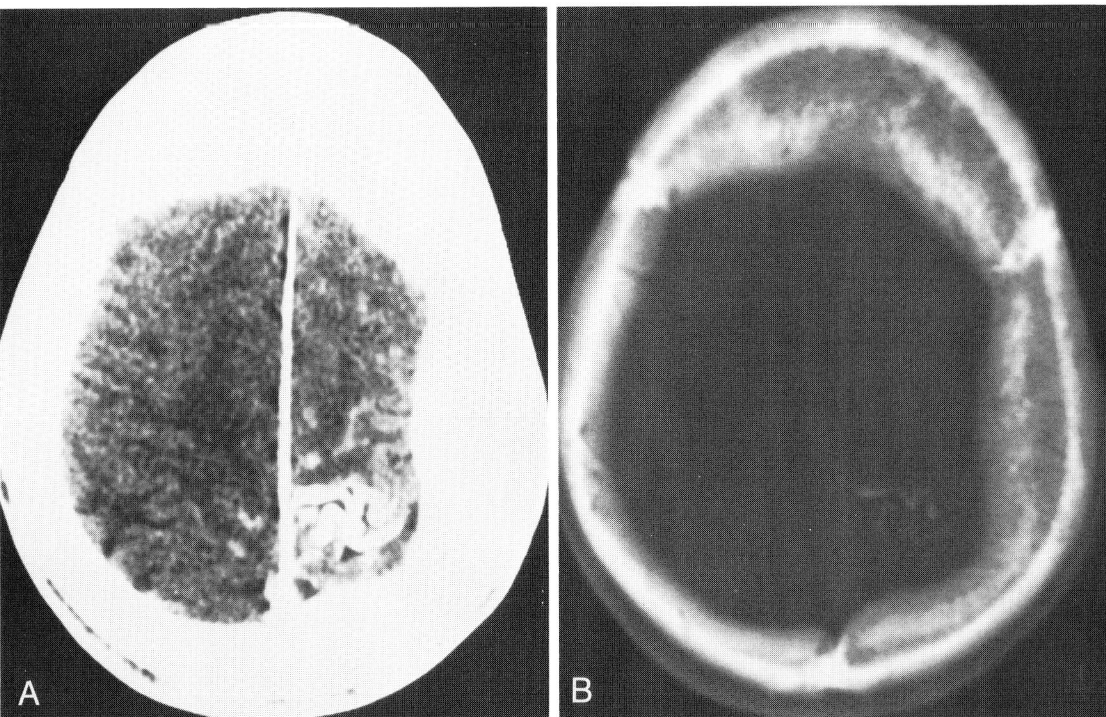

FIGURE 8–39. Encephalotrigeminal angiomatosis (Sturge-Weber) syndrome. *A.* Noncontrast CT scan shows serpiginous calcification along the gyri beneath the leptomeningeal angioma. *B.* Marked widening of the medullary cavity of the skull is present as a result of myelofibrosis associated with the long-term phenytoin (Dilantin) therapy for control of seizures.

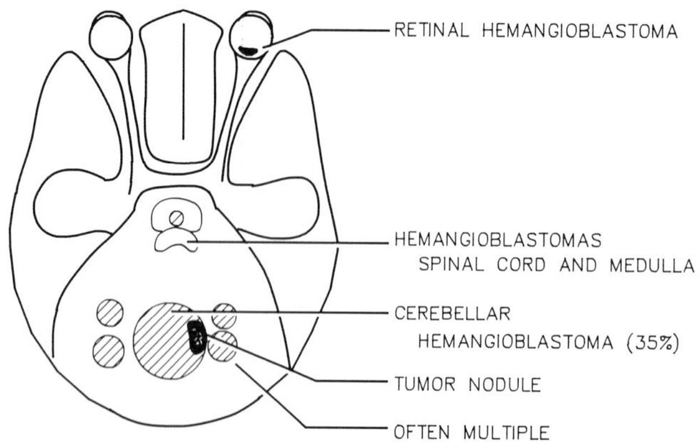

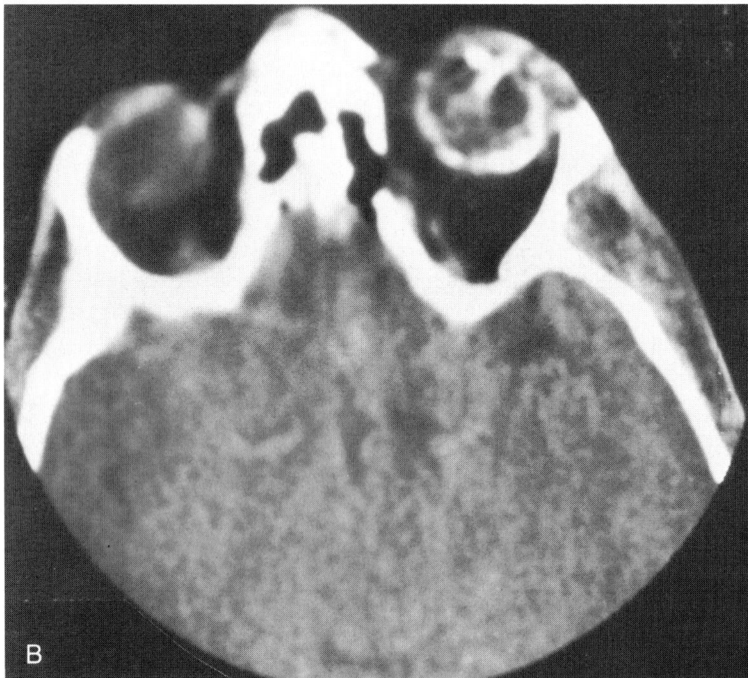

FIGURE 8–40. Retinocerebellar angiomatosis (von Hippel-Lindau disease). *A.* Diagram. *B.* Noncontrast CT shows a left retinal hamartoma in a young girl with multiple cerebellar hemangioblastomas.

cerebellar ataxia, hydrocephalus) or retinal hamartoma (loss of vision) during the second or third decade. The major lesion in this disease is the hemangioblastoma, a slow-growing tumor that usually comprises a large cyst and a highly vascular mural nodule. It is generally considered benign but recurs locally after resection. A solitary hemangioblastoma is a rare occurrence in the general population (see Fig. 8–59), but in retinocerebellar angiomatosis these tumors are often multiple.

CT shows single or multiple cystic masses in the cerebellum with an enhancing mural nodule (80%) or a solid enhancement (20%). It can also show retinal lesions (Fig. 8–40*B*). MRI better demonstrates the cystic tumor in sagittal and coronal planes and more reliably differentiates the lesion from congenital abnormalities, such as Dandy-Walker syndrome, cerebellar dysgenesis, and simple arachnoid cyst. Furthermore, Gd-DTPA enhancement can assist in defining the mural tumor. Angiography shows the enhancing area to be a collection of abnormal vessels resembling an arteriovenous malformation (AVM). The hemangioblastomas are not locally invasive and do not metastasize. Surgical resection may be curative, but the tumors have a tendency to recur. The most serious problem in patients with retinocerebellar angiomatosis is the development of renal cell and pancreatic carcinoma or pheochromocytoma. Patients and family members require careful screening for the many lesions associated with this disease.

SYSTEMIC DISEASES

Endocrine Diseases

Endocrine diseases that cause changes in serum calcium levels can produce extensive calcification in the brain. These diseases include hyperparathyroidism, renal failure, and abnormal levels of vitamin D. Calcification can be demonstrated in the falx, the tentorium, the basal ganglia, and the dentate nucleus of the cerebellum. Excess corticosteroid levels can alter the fluid balance in the brain and result in enlargement of the CSF spaces. Corticosteroids are often used in the therapy for brain tumors and can reduce the swelling and the degree of contrast enhancement on CT and MRI. Therefore, consideration of the patient's steroid therapy is important in the assessment of brain swelling or tumor enhancement. Many pituitary lesions cause endocrine problems. Pituitary conditions are discussed in Part II of this chapter.

Immune Diseases

The collagen vascular diseases may be associated with detectable abnormalities in the CNS. On occasion, in patients with these diseases there is demyelination of the white matter tracts in the brain. These findings are nonspecific. The most obvious manifestation of immune disease in the brain is caused by vasculitis, best seen on angiograms, which reveal multiple focal narrowings of cerebral arterial branches. Although pathological proof of the origins of brain lesions is difficult to obtain, the lesions shown by CT and MRI are most likely caused by infarction or inflammation. MRI shows these lesions best as multiple, high-intensity abnormalities throughout the white matter (Fig. 8–41). Such lesions are most commonly seen in lupus and giant-cell arteritis.

Metabolic Diseases

Alcoholism. Chronic alcoholism is one of the most common causes of CNS disease, affecting cognitive and motor functions and predisposing patients to diffuse brain changes, seizures, hemorrhage, and trauma. The most common finding in alcoholics is diffuse decrease in brain size, often called cerebral atrophy. Reversible factors are related to water content of the brain and may be caused by dehydration, nutritional status, and steroid therapy (e.g., for lung disease). Cessation of alcohol use and proper nutritional and fluid therapy can eliminate the effects of dehydration. Other effects such as the toxic effects of alcohol, abused drugs, and prolonged protein malnutrition result in cell death and therefore cannot be treated. CT and MRI show diffuse

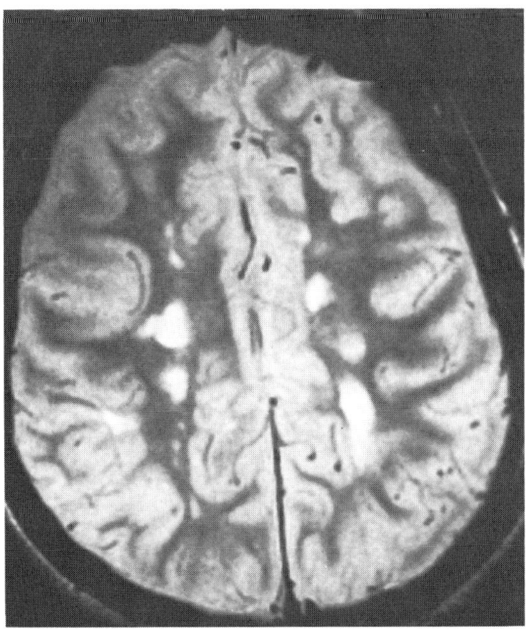

FIGURE 8–41. Lupus vasculitis in the brain. T2 spin echo image shows multiple periventricular and deep, white matter lesions in a 45-year-old woman with lupus. The lesions are similar to those of multiple sclerosis and may represent inflammation, demyelination, or infarction. The patient did not have symptoms of multiple sclerosis and responded to steroid therapy.

shrinkage of the brain and enlargement of the ventricles and the cortical sulci (Fig. 8–42). The effects are often more prominent in the cerebellum, especially the anterior vermis, where histological studies show loss of Purkinje cell bodies.

In addition to mental and motor dysfunction, alcoholics have other complications. Seizures and trauma lead to contusions and hematomas. The shrinkage of the brain causes stretching of dural veins, leading to chronic or repeated bleeding into the subdural space (chronic subdural hematoma). These complications can cause a progressive mass effect and, because of the patient's alcoholic stupor or amnesia, go undetected.

Central Pontine Myelinolysis. Central pontine myelinolysis is a profound demyelination of the central pons commonly associated with electrolyte imbalance. The condition is most frequently seen in alcoholics and people with bizarre dietary habits, such as anorexia nervosa and bulimia, who are treated for dehydration. Patients develop spastic quadriplegia, pseudobulbar signs, and mutism, which can appear clinically as a "locked-in" syndrome. CT and MRI show a central area of demyelination (low density on CT, high intensity on T2 spin echo MRI) that often has an arrowhead configuration (Fig. 8–43). However, many conditions that affect the pons can have a similar appearance and produce brainstem symptoms; these conditions include multiple sclerosis, infarct, tumor, and encephalitis. With supportive care, some patients gradually recover to a variable degree. Others die of respiratory arrest or other complications.

INFLAMMATORY DISEASES

Brain infections may be caused by all types of organisms. Early diagnosis and prompt therapy are required because most cause devastating injury. Intracranial infection can involve the meninges (meningitis), a focal area of parenchyma (brain abscess), or diffuse areas of the brain (cerebritis and encephalitis). Many fungal and parasitic diseases have a characteristic appearance when they affect the brain. Multiple sclerosis and sarcoidosis are listed here as inflammatory diseases of the brain even though they are probably not infectious in origin.

Meningitis

Infectious meningitis is inflammation of the meninges caused by bacteria, viruses, mycobacteria, parasites, or fungi. It can produce acute or chronic signs and symptoms, including

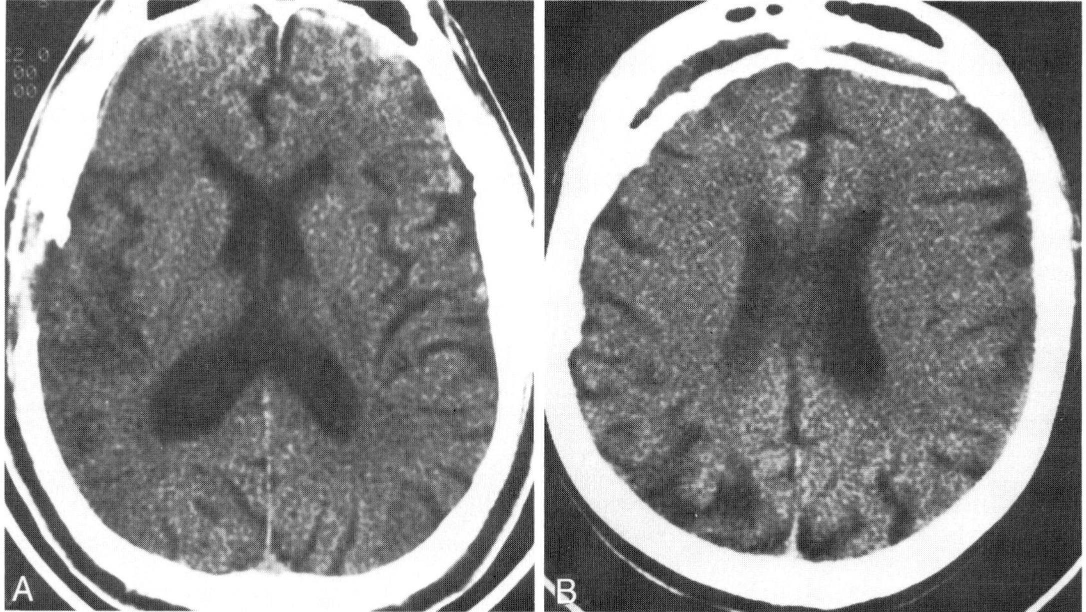

FIGURE 8–42. Chronic alcoholism. *A*. Noncontrast CT shows a diffuse loss of brain volume with compensatory enlargement of the ventricles and cortical sulci in a 30-year-old alcoholic. This appearance is more like that of a normal 60-year-old. Note also the right-sided skull defect from previous trauma. *B*. CT in another alcoholic patient shows a bifrontal chronic subdural hematoma, demarcated from the brain by a thick, calcified membrane.

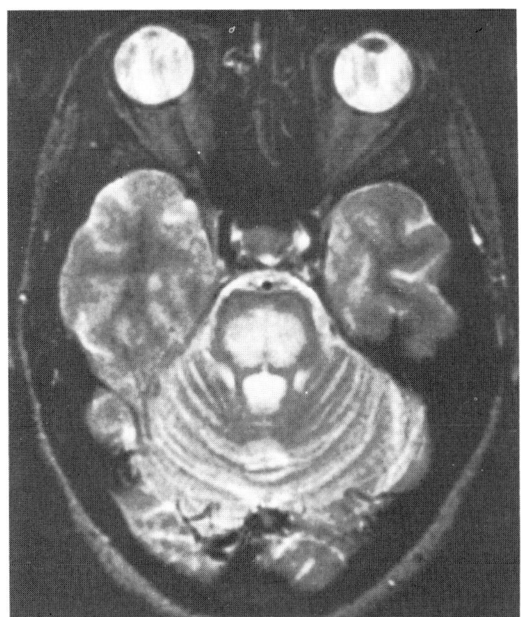

FIGURE 8–43. Central pontine myelinolysis. T2 spin echo image shows symmetrical central increased intensity in the pons of a young woman admitted after excessive diuretic use for weight loss. Because of her bizarre behavior and, later, mutism, the development of quadriparesis was thought to be further evidence of malingering. The diagnosis was made by the radiologist when this MRI scan was obtained.

fever, headache, and nuchal rigidity. A lumbar puncture with CSF examination is the best method for diagnosis in children and, in the absence of focal neurological signs, can precede CT or MRI so that therapy is not delayed. Adults are more likely to have an intracranial mass lesion with such symptoms and should have MRI or CT before lumbar puncture. Infection must also be considered in elderly patients whose immune system is incapable of generating a white cell response. In such patients, the CSF may contain organisms but few inflammatory cells.

Bacterial Meningitis. Bacterial meningitis usually has an acute onset. Although CT and MRI findings are frequently normal, they can show purulent exudates in subarachnoid (and subdural) spaces, meningeal enhancement, and, in rare instances, infarction resulting from vascular inflammation. CT in most cases is normal. However, large amounts of purulent material in the subarachnoid spaces can obliterate the cisterns and subarachnoid spaces, which should normally be visible. When the cisterns become sufficiently inflamed, enhancement with intravenous contrast occurs and produces a CT appearance similar to that of subarachnoid hemorrhage on a noncontrast scan (see Fig. 8–81). A noncontrast scan should be obtained before the contrast-enhanced scan when infection is suspected, because both the enhanced CT and the clinical manifestation of meningitis are similar to those of subarachnoid hemorrhage. MRI is more sensitive to parenchymal abnormalities and enhancement and better demonstrates meningitis and its complications, such as infarction, abscess, and edema.

Viral, Tuberculous, and Fungal Meningitis. Viral meningitis is caused by a variety of organisms. In general, CT and MRI are normal. Tuberculous meningitis preferentially affects the basal cisterns, in which increased density and contrast enhancement of the meninges can be demonstrated. The clinical course of tuberculous meningitis is usually chronic and may be complicated by an intracranial abscess (tuberculoma). Fungal meningitis is rare except in persons with compromised immune systems. The most common causes are histoplasmosis and cryptococcosis. Tuberculous and fungal meningitis produce a thick, chronic exudate and are more likely to produce positive findings on unenhanced and enhanced scans (Fig. 8–44).

Sequelae of Meningitis. Delayed sequelae to meningitis include infarction, development of hydrocephalus, and formation of extra-axial fluid collections. Hydrocephalus, which frequently follows meningitis, is often caused by obstruction of the arachnoid granulations, but in tuberculous meningitis, the obstruction is usually in the basal cisterns. Treatment of purulent meningitis may require ventricular shunting to relieve the life-threatening mass effect from hydrocephalus. Subdural exudates, sterile or purulent, may also be present. Extra-axial empyema may cause a densely enhancing meningeal border as a result of inflammation but is frequently difficult to diagnose. This is especially true in the floor of the temporal or frontal fossa, in which paranasal sinus infection frequently enters the intracranial cavity. Coronal MRI can demonstrate such basal infection.

Parenchymal Infection

Brain Abscess. Brain abscess occurs with generalized sepsis, embolism of septic material, direct spread from infected sinuses, penetration by foreign bodies, or infestation of the brain by parasites. Patients have signs and

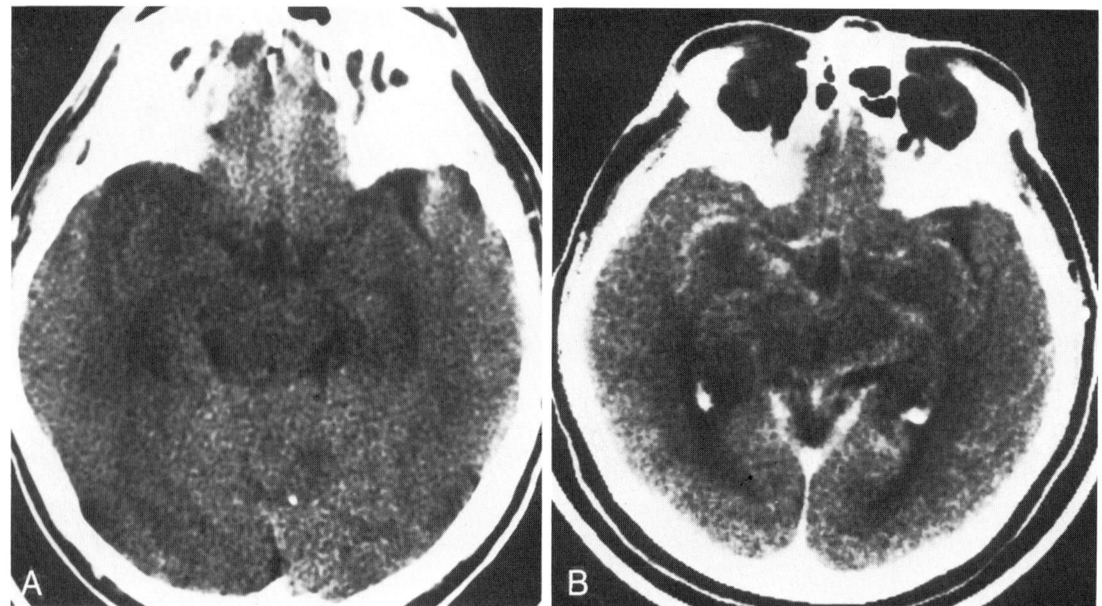

FIGURE 8–44. Tuberculous meningitis. *A.* Noncontrast CT in a 45-year-old man with miliary tuberculosis fails to show the quadrigeminal and ambient cisterns normally seen at this level (see Fig. 8–11, slice 6). *B.* Contrast CT confirms inflammation of the basal cistern meninges and those of the middle cerebral arteries (a location in which such inflammation and subarachnoid blood can often be identified).

symptoms of infection, a neurological defect, or a mass lesion in the brain.

The number or the location of the abscesses frequently indicates the origin of the infection (Fig. 8–45): frontal abscess in the presence of sinus disease indicates contiguous spread; temporal lobe lesions are suggestive of spread from mastoid, middle ear, or paranasal infections; multiple peripheral lesions are usually from a hematogenous source. Most brain abscesses are caused by bacteria, notably staphylococci, that incite an intense inflammatory response that eventually liquifies the infected tissue and surrounds the lesion by a capsule of collagenous and neovascular fibroblastic tissue. The incidences of mixed infections and infestation by unusual microaerophilic organisms appear to be increasing as use of antibiotics becomes more widespread.

The CT appearance of a brain abscess depends on the age of the lesion, the aggressiveness of the organism, and the host's response. The center of the abscess is filled with pus and necrotic debris and appears as low density. By about 3 days after the abscess forms, an outer wall becomes apparent as an irregular hyperemic border on enhanced CT. MRI shows high intensity centrally in an area of edema. The appearance may be complicated by the presence of blood or necrosis. The capsule enhances with paramagnetic contrast.

The cyst wall becomes regular and well-defined in 7 to 10 days, at which time the lesion is more easily resected or aspirated. The smooth, thin margin often enables differentiation from tumor, which usually has a thick and irregular wall. Daughter abscesses and ventriculitis occur when the infection spreads locally. The latter can be diagnosed from the presence of ependymal enhancement. Ventricular pus-CSF levels also indicate intraventricular spread. When the organism is less virulent or when impaired host defenses limit the response, a well-defined abscess cavity may not form. Therapy for brain abscess depends on the location and the number of lesions, as well as the type of organism.

Diffuse Brain Infection

"Cerebritis" and "encephalitis" both refer to inflammation or infection of the brain. Cerebritis is usually more localized. Encephalitis is more diffuse and occurs in severe meningitis or septicemia as a result of bacterial, tuberculous, or fungal infection. The CT findings of local or diffuse enhancement, infarction, and edema are nonspecific. MRI shows multiple areas of high signal intensity. Patients with diffuse infections may die despite vigorous therapy, but more localized infections often

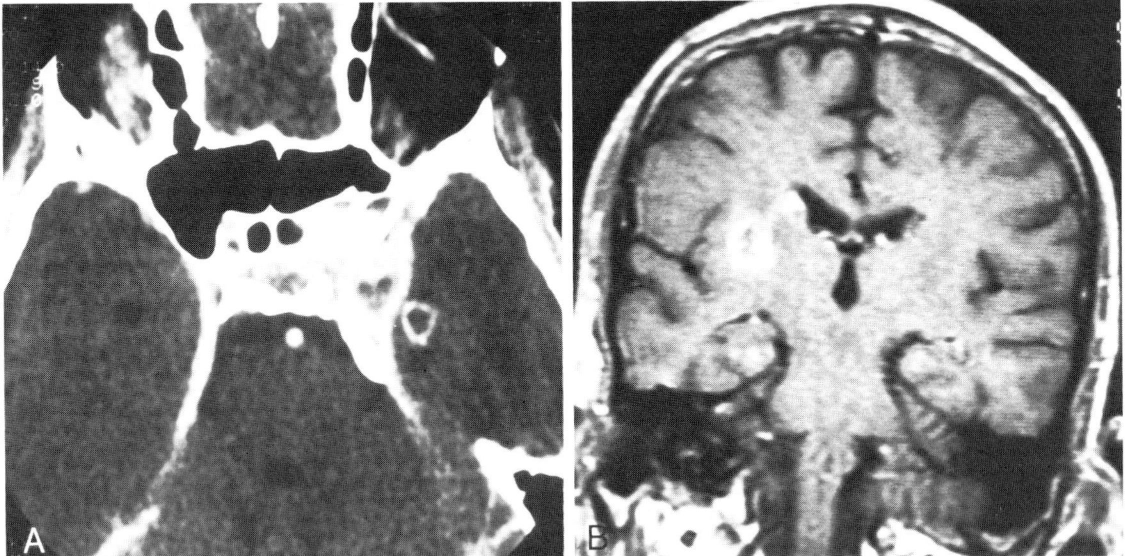

FIGURE 8–45. *A.* Temporal lobe and cavernous sinus infection. Contrast-enhanced CT with narrow slices and magnification shows a ring-enhancing abscess in the left temporal lobe and enlargement of the adjacent cavernous sinus. Dural enhancement of the margins of the sinus is present, and a low-density center indicates thrombosis in a male intravenous drug abuser with ophthalmoplegia and fever. It is not possible from the scan to determine whether the patient had infectious cavernous sinus thrombosis with adjacent spread to the temporal lobe or septic embolus to the brain and adjacent involvement of the cavernous sinus. He responded to antibiotic therapy. *B.* Coronal T1 spin echo image after Gd-DTPA administration demonstrates a ring-enhancing mass in the region of the basal ganglia on the right in a different patient with toxoplasmosis abscess.

progress to abscess or granuloma, at least some of which respond to surgical or antibiotic therapy.

Viral Infection

Viral diseases often affect the brain diffusely, causing encephalitis. Patients have fever, headache, altered mental status, seizures, and coma. Early diagnosis is imperative because some types of encephalitis, such as herpes simplex encephalitis, can be successfully treated. Brain biopsy is necessary for establishing the correct diagnosis, but treatment is often begun before biopsy or culture results are available. In addition to herpes encephalitis, other viral infections are seen in immunocompromised patients who have acquired immunodeficiency syndrome (AIDS), cancer, or immunological disorders. These include progressive multifocal leukoencephalopathy, cytomegalic inclusion virus infection, and subacute sclerosing panencephalopathy, all of which appear as patchy areas of white matter inflammation and edema. Cerebritis caused by the human immunodeficiency virus can have a central or global distribution and is discussed with complications of AIDS.

Herpes Encephalitis. Herpes simplex type I virus can cause a fulminant, necrotizing, hemorrhagic encephalitis. It occurs most commonly in adolescents and young adults. Characteristic initial areas of involvement are the inferior and medial portions of the temporal lobes, the orbital surfaces of the frontal lobes, and the insular and cingulate gyri. The infection is usually bilateral but often is initially more severe on one side, as shown on early scans. Patients frequently have uncontrolled seizures and are difficult to assess clinically; they often must be sedated for radiographic evaluation.

CT diagnosis is best made from narrow (3-mm) slices through the temporal lobes without contrast material. Contrast-enhanced CT can show central or gyral enhancement. Repeated scans may be necessary because the lesions are not always seen early in the course of the disease. MRI is more sensitive to the abnormalities, which appear as high intensity on T2 spin echo or STIR images, but the patient often cannot lie still for scanning. CT and MRI show temporal lobe abnormality (frequently bilateral), which often extends along the outer surface of the putamen. Hemorrhage, necrosis, and a mass effect are present (Fig. 8–46). The temporal lobe location of abnormality is highly suggestive of herpes encephalitis, but brain

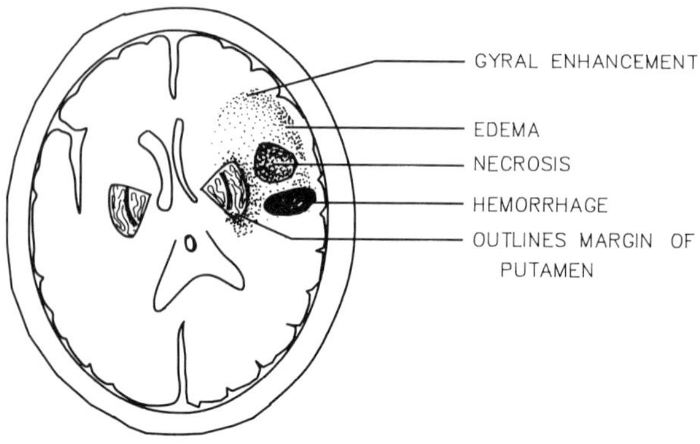

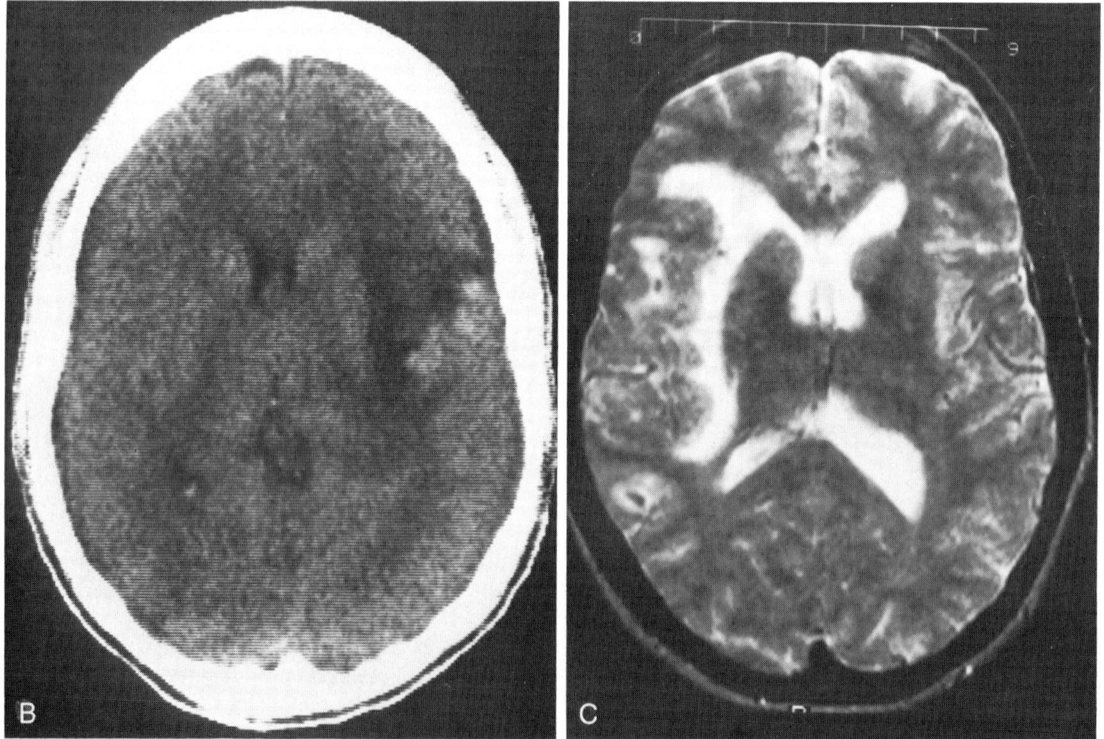

FIGURE 8–46. Herpes type I encephalitis. *A.* Diagram. *B.* Noncontrast CT shows low-density edema in the left temporal and frontal lobes that extends to and outlines the putamen, a typical appearance for herpes cerebritis. Lateral and posterior are foci of hemorrhage in 20-year-old jail inmate whose complaint of headache was ignored for 1 week until seizures and hemiparesis finally led to medical evaluation. *C.* T2 spin echo magnetic resonance image in a different patient shows edema outlining the right putamen.

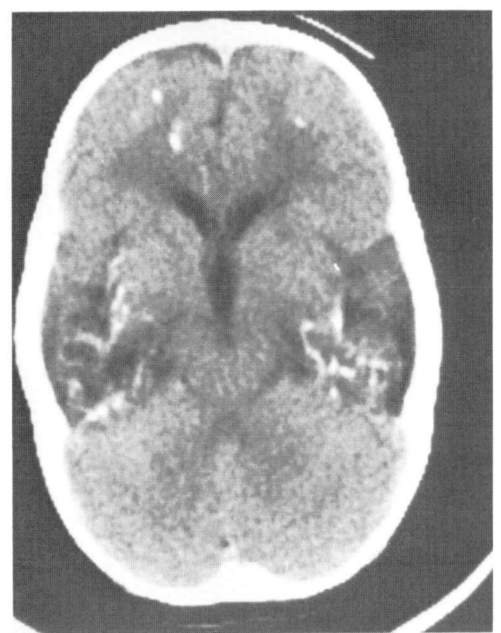

FIGURE 8–47. Congenital herpes simplex type II infection. CT shows loss of temporal lobe tissue and peripheral calcification in a young child who acquired herpes cerebritis from vaginal delivery.

biopsy may be required in order to exclude other treatable infections and tumor. Treatment with acyclovir can be successful, if begun early.

Herpes simplex type II virus can cause disseminated disease in infants and immunocompromised hosts. In infants, the virus is acquired during passage through the birth canal. CNS disease is a severe, multifocal, necrotizing panencephalitis. Diffuse brain injury with consequent mental and motor retardation occur. CT shows cerebral calcification and loss of brain substance (Fig. 8–47). This appearance is similar to that of any of the congenital infections, which include syphilis, toxoplasmosis, rubella, cytomegalovirus, and herpes. Calcification occurs in the neonatal brain as a response to tissue injury.

Fungal Diseases

Fungal infections of the CNS usually cause chronic symptoms. They are more common in immunocompromised patients. Organisms include *Cryptococcus*, *Nocardia*, *Candida*, *Coccidioides*, and *Histoplasma*. These and other fungi can cause a varied appearance of disseminated disease in the brain. Cryptococcal and nocardial infections may have a distinctive appearance.

Cryptococcosis. *Cryptococcus neoformans* is a budding yeast that is found in the soil throughout the world. As a result, CNS infection is relatively common in immunocompromised patients. The usual form of infection is meningitis with extension into the cortex through the Virchow-Robin spaces around blood vessels. This pattern produces a typical fine cystic appearance, from which the original name "torula histolytica" was derived. Large parenchymal subependymal lesions also occur. CSF is an ideal culture medium for cryptococci because of its nutrients and lack of the anticryptococcal factor. As a result, there is a tendency for parenchymal lesions to form near the lateral ventricles and the subependymal spaces (Fig. 8–48). CT and MRI show ill-defined, enhancing lesions in the brain or the ependyma.

Nocardiosis. Nocardial infection also occurs primarily in immunocompromised patients. In the brain it is possible to see multiple small (5-mm) lesions, all the same size. These abscesses show contrast enhancement and are surrounded by edema (Fig. 8–49). Encephalitis is rare.

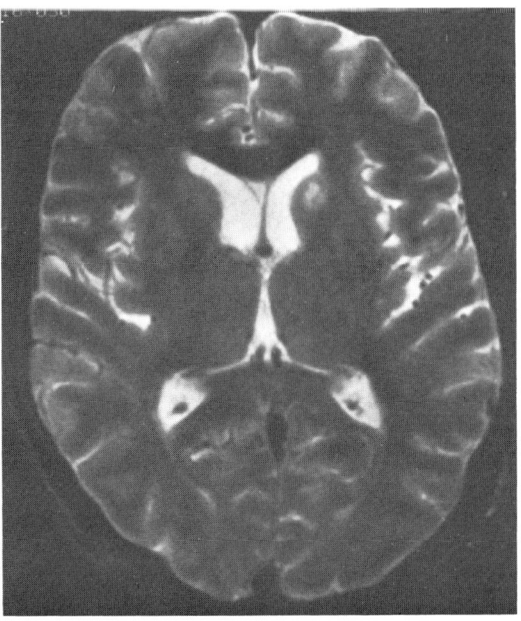

FIGURE 8–48. Cryptococcosis infection. T2 spin echo image shows a focus of high intensity adjacent to the left frontal horn in a 42-year-old man with acquired immunodeficiency syndrome (AIDS) and cryptococci in the CSF. The location adjacent to the anterior part of the lateral ventricles is a common site of cryptococal brain infection. The patient also had lesions near the fourth ventricle.

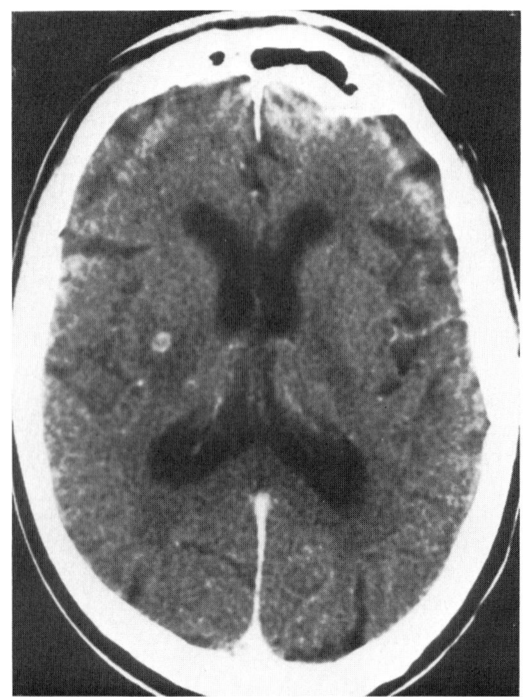

FIGURE 8–49. *Nocardia* abscesses. Contrast CT shows a single, 5-mm enhancing lesion with surrounding edema in a 57-year-old man with chronic myelogenous leukemia and disseminated *Nocardia* infection. Four additional lesions, identical in size, were seen at other levels.

Parasitic Infestation

Parasitic infestation can manifest as an acute change in mental status, as acute or chronic seizures, or as chronic CNS disease. The most common parasitic diseases are cysticercosis, echinococcosis, and toxoplasmosis. Noncontrast CT can demonstrate calcification, edema, and a mass effect. Active lesions may enhance with contrast material. When a parasitic cyst causes ventricular obstruction, CT or MRI demonstrates hydrocephalus.

Cysticercosis. Cysticercosis is a parasitic infestation caused by the intestinal tapeworm *Taenia solium.* It is rare in the United States but is the most common CNS infection in Mexico, affecting 3% of the population. CNS involvement occurs when the tapeworm embryos (oncospheres) enter the blood stream and travel to the brain parenchyma, the meninges, the ventricular system, or, in rare instances, the spinal cord. At these sites, they become encysted and cause an intense glial reaction. After the larvae are destroyed, a noninfectious calcified mass remains. Symptoms appear about 5 years after exposure and include seizure, stroke, or, if the cysts cause obstruction of the ventricular system, symptoms and signs of hydrocephalus. The diagnosis is usually based on clinical history and on CT or MRI findings; serological cultures are positive in fewer than half of cases.

The CT or MRI appearance of cysticercosis depends on the stage of disease and the location of the lesions. Images early in the course of parenchymal disease show one to three focal, 1-cm nonenhancing lesions surrounded by intense edema. Subsequently, the cysts show ring enhancement, followed by a granulomatous stage that appears as a well-defined enhancing nodule. The parenchymal lesions heal and calcify as small, millet seed–shaped densities (Fig. 8–50). Persistent enhancement of the dead scolex is common.

Echinococcosis. Infection of the CNS by *Echinococcus granulosus,* a small tapeworm, is rare. When the larvae are trapped, they produce round cysts filled with infective material. The large cysts often contain daughter cysts attached to the inner wall. The lesions in the brain, similar to those elsewhere in the body, produce a mass effect and ventricular obstruction. CT and MRI show the large cystic mass and the daughter cysts (Fig. 8–51).

Toxoplasmosis. Toxoplasmosis results from infestation by *Toxoplasma gondii,* a protozoan parasite. Humans are infected after ingestion of infested meat. The organism can remain dormant for the life of the host. If the patient becomes immunosuppressed, a fulminant CNS infection can occur.

Toxoplasmosis acquired in utero causes severe encephalitis and resultant brain damage. CT demonstrates periventricular calcification, infarction, and atrophy similar to those produced by other in utero infections (see Fig. 8–47). When toxoplasmosis occurs in healthy adults, it is usually a self-limiting, flu-like syndrome with lymphadenopathy. In immunosuppressed patients, a serious infection of the CNS occurs, probably as a result of reactivation of dormant organisms. These patients develop encephalopathy, meningoencephalitis, or cerebral abscesses. CT shows single or multiple round, low-density lesions in the brain parenchyma, often with an enhancing outer rim. MRI shows high-intensity lesions on T2 spin echo or STIR images. These enhance with paramagnetic contrast (Fig. 8–52). Patients with AIDS are particularly prone to develop CNS toxoplasmosis. CSF titers can establish the diagnosis, but brain biopsy may be neces-

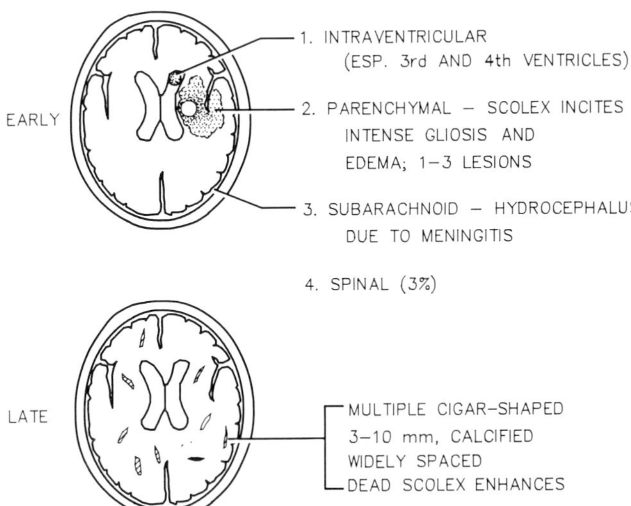

- MOST COMMON INFECTION OF CNS
- PREVALENT IN MEXICO (3% OF POPULATION)
  ALSO IN SOUTH AMERICA AND ASIA
- CAUSE: PORK TAPEWORM (TAENIA SOLIUM)
- PRESENTATION: SEIZURE, HYDROCEPHALUS, STROKE
- ONSET: 5 YRS. AFTER EXPOSURE
- COURSE: MAY HAVE SEIZURES FOR LIFE; OTHERWISE BENIGN

A

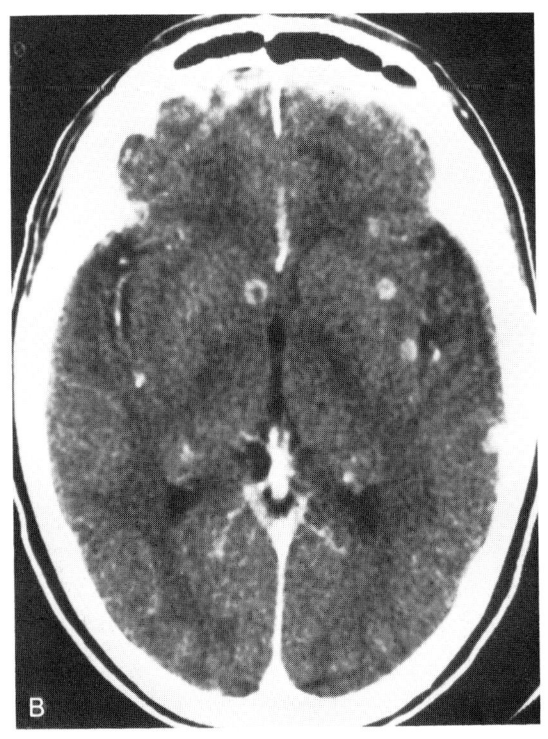

FIGURE 8–50. Cysticercosis. *A.* Diagram. CNS, central nervous system. *B.* Contrast CT shows multiple lesions that enhance but have no surrounding edema in a Cambodian woman with a 2-year history of seizures. The lesions were unchanged from an initial examination 2 years earlier and represent residuals of previous cysticercosis.

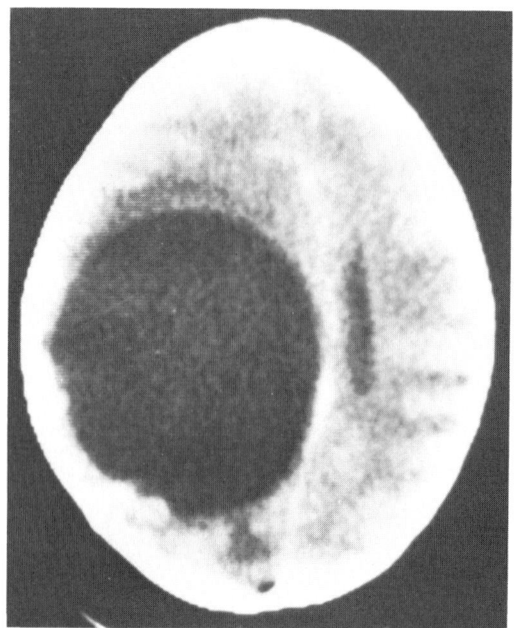

FIGURE 8–51. Echinococcosis. CT shows a large cyst compressing the brain and the ventricles. Posteriorly are daughter cysts on the inner margin.

sary for immediate diagnosis. Treatment with agents such as pyrimethamine and sulfonamide, if instituted early, can be curative.

Other Infections

CNS Infection in Patients With AIDS. Immunosuppressed patients frequently develop compound infections, often caused by unusual organisms. Patients who have AIDS develop CNS infections from *Toxoplasma*, *Cryptococcus,* herpesvirus, cytomegalovirus, *Pneumocystis,* and *Candida.* In addition, a deep infection by the human immunodeficiency virus itself causes periventricular and deep inflammation involving the basal ganglia and the white matter (Fig. 8–53). This infection often coexists with the CNS infections just listed and eventually leads to progressive loss of brain substance and, in parallel, loss of mental function. The loss of brain substance is characterized by ventricular and sulcal enlargement similar to that seen in alcoholics and in many

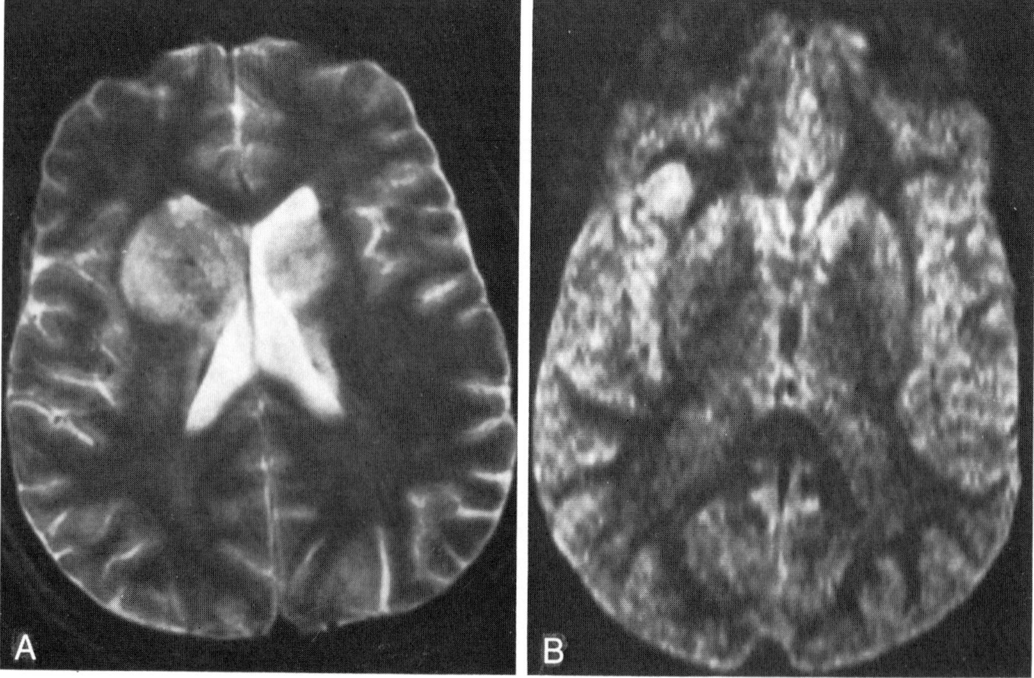

FIGURE 8–52. Toxoplasmosis in two patients with AIDS. *A.* T2 spin echo image shows bilateral basal ganglia abscesses. *B.* STIR images were used to produce high tissue contrast and show a right frontal abscess in a man who, in a state of confusion, set his apartment on fire. Later, he was noted to be febrile, and toxoplasmosis was diagnosed.

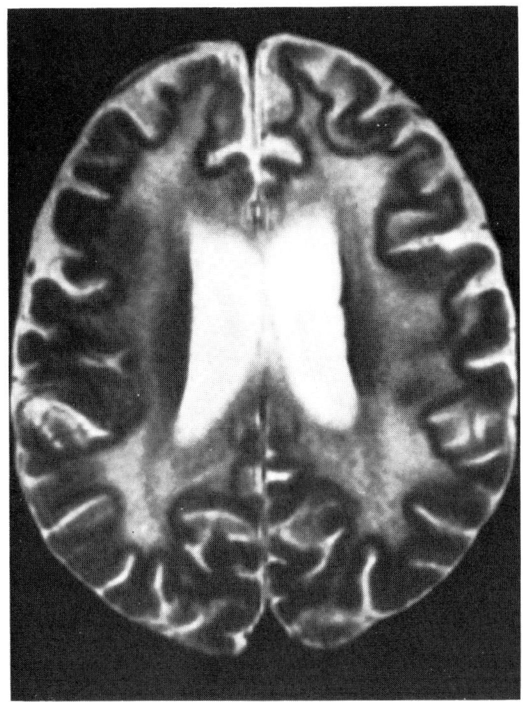

FIGURE 8–53. Human immunodeficiency virus cerebritis. T2 spin echo image shows high intensity throughout the white matter in periventricular, deep, and peripheral areas. Note sparing of the cortical U-fibers (compare similar appearance and sparing of the U-fibers as a result of radiation injury in Fig. 8–24). The patient, a 35-year-old man, died of AIDS virus cerebritis shortly after this examination.

symptomatic or asymptomatic elderly patients (Fig. 8–54; see also Fig. 8–42). Such infections are difficult to treat, primarily because of the impairment of the patient's immune system. Even with early diagnosis, they are often fatal. Patients with AIDS are also prone to develop Kaposi's sarcoma and CNS lymphoma.

Infectious (Mycotic) Aneurysm. Bacteremia can result in infection of the blood vessels in the brain. The weakened vessels undergo aneurysmal dilatation and can rupture, causing fatal hemorrhage. These aneurysms are virtually always bacterial in origin. The term "mycotic aneurysm" does not refer to a fungal cause but describes the mushroom-like appearance of the lesion. These aneurysms are discussed in more detail in the section on vascular diseases.

Inflammatory Brain Disease

Multiple Sclerosis. Multiple sclerosis is a disease of unknown cause characterized by separate abnormalities in both time and location within the CNS. The pathogenesis of the disease is thought to be either viral or autoimmune, but the result is an inflammatory demyelinating process. Multiple sclerosis is more common in women than in men (by a ratio of 2:1), and the onset is usually within the 15- to 45-year age range. The clinical course is that of multiple neurological abnormalities of varying severity and occurring at different times, causing a vast variety of symptoms. The pathological lesions of multiple sclerosis are discrete demyelinated plaques and associated inflammation in the periventricular and deep white matter of the brain and the spinal cord.

The CT appearance of multiple sclerosis ranges from normal to nonspecific abnormalities. The most common is a low-density periventricular plaque. Enhancing lesions are sometimes seen in the white matter on contrast images. MRI is far more effective than CT in demonstrating the lesions of multiple sclerosis. The characteristic plaques appear as high-intensity focal lesions in periventricular and deep white matter locations on T2 spin echo or STIR images. They are often multiple, well-circumscribed, and oval in shape with their long axis along the direction of the white matter tracts (Fig. 8–55*A* and *B*). The brainstem is frequently involved. Because the lesions are similar to those of white matter disease caused by a variety of conditions, including infarction from small vessel disease, normal aging, and other demyelinating processes, they must be interpreted with clinical and CSF findings.

Factors that can be helpful in making the diagnosis are the appearance and the location of the lesions, the age and the clinical symptoms of the patient, the results of other tests, and evidence of previous neurological disease (Table 8–3). Nevertheless, the diagnosis can be difficult to make because of atypical lesions and clinical circumstances. Large lesions are not uncommon and can mimic abscess or tumor (Fig. 8–55*C*). White matter lesions in an older patient can be the result of long-standing multiple sclerosis rather than vascular disease. On MRI, many older patients are found to have lesions that do not represent demyelination or vascular disease and appear to be caused by a change in water content that is associated with aging.

Patients with multiple sclerosis undergo a remission-relapse or chronic course, and most have either remission or minimal disability for

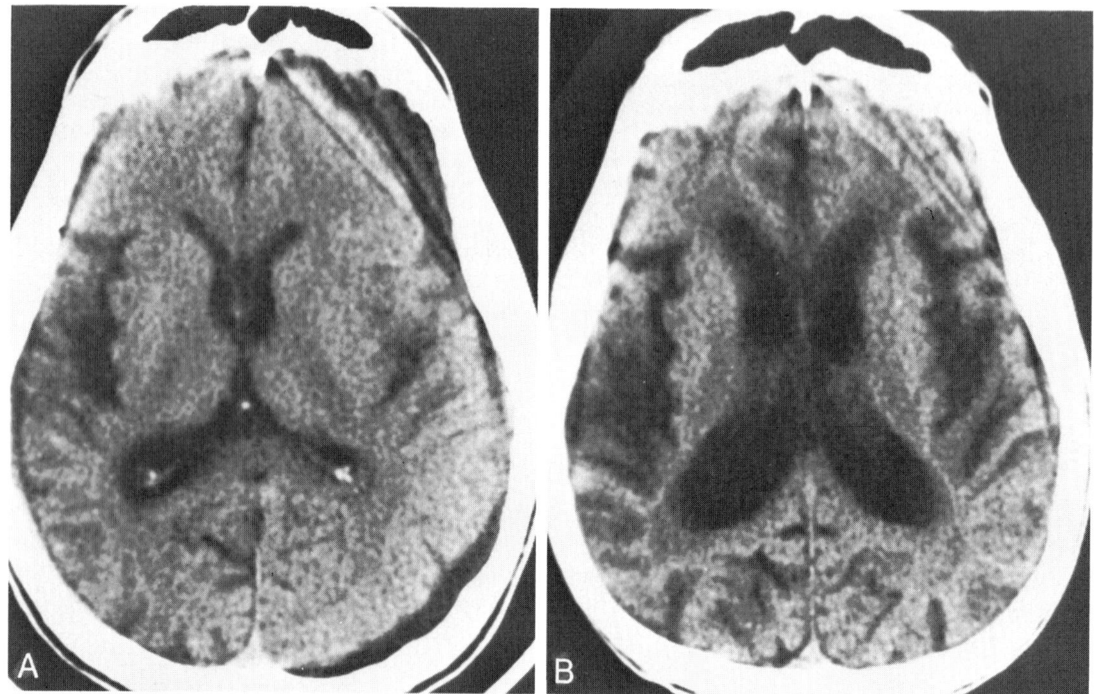

FIGURE 8–54. Brain atrophy in AIDS. *A.* Initial evaluation. Enlargement of the cerebral sulci and, in addition, a left subdural effusion are already evident. *B.* Six months later, the sulci and ventricles are markedly dilated, which indicates substantial loss of brain volume. The patient's mental function and ability to care for himself were severely impaired, and he died shortly after this scan was obtained. The diffuse loss of brain tissue seen in AIDS is probably caused by the diffuse deep infection by the human immunodeficiency virus and by other infections.

many years. Approximately 20% of patients have progressive impairment over a 5- to 20-year period.

Sarcoidosis. Sarcoidosis is a chronic granulomatous disease, most common in young black adults, that predominantly involves the lungs (discussed in Chapter 2). The second most common area of involvement is the CNS, especially the orbit. Patients with orbital disease usually have visual symptoms. CNS disease can have confusing and nonspecific symptoms. The radiographic appearance of CNS lesions is highly variable but is usually one of either a parenchymal mass or a granulomatous basal leptomeningitis in the region of the circle of Willis. Usually there are diffuse enhancing

TABLE 8–3. INTERPRETATION OF WHITE MATTER LESIONS: COMPARISON OF MULTIPLE SCLEROSIS, VASCULAR DISEASE, AND NORMAL AGING

Finding	Multiple Sclerosis	Vascular Disease	"Normal" Aging
Age*†	20 to 40	Older	Older
Clinical multiple sclerosis	Yes	No	No
Laboratory multiple sclerosis	Yes	No	No
Other disease‡	No	Vascular	No
Mental function	Often abnormal	Often abnormal	Normal
Basal ganglia infarct	No	Often	No
Other infarcts§	No	Sometimes	No
Lesion size ‖ ¶	5 to 10 mm	Larger	Larger
Lesion shape¶	Oval	Patchy	Patchy
Lesion margins¶	Sharp	Indistinct	Indistinct
Subependymal lesions¶	Discrete	Diffuse	Diffuse

Cautions: *an elderly patient may have had multiple sclerosis for 40 years; †white matter lesions may occur with "normal" aging; ‡some patients have two or all three of the conditions listed; §dilated vascular spaces are not plaques: ‖ discrete lesions may coalesce to form large diffuse ones; ¶many lesions are atypical.

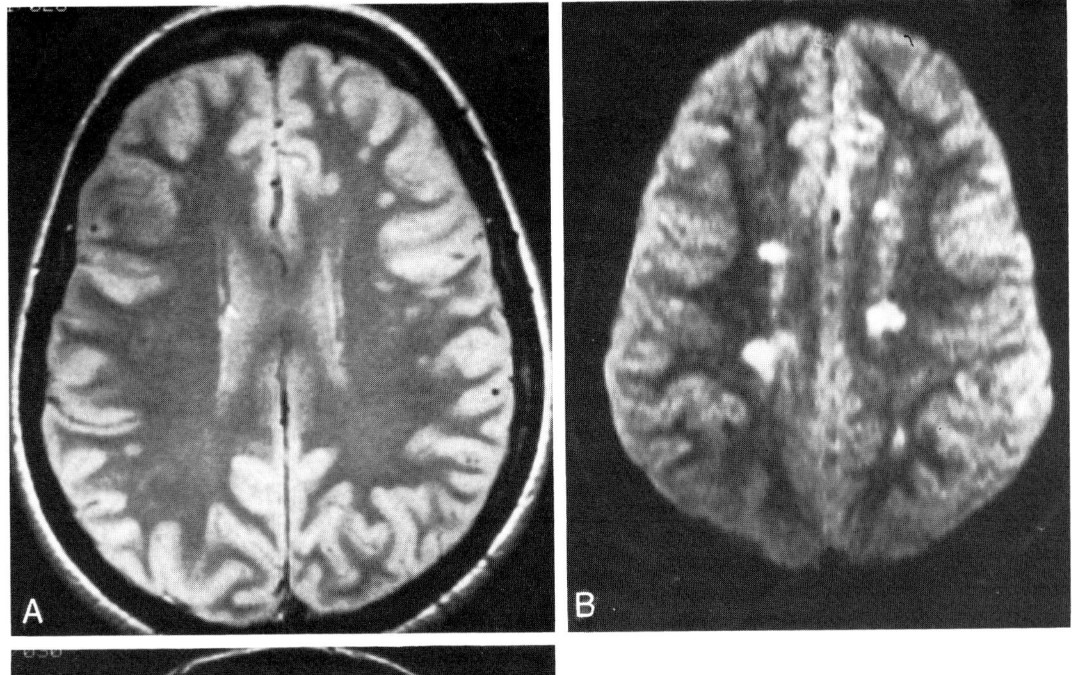

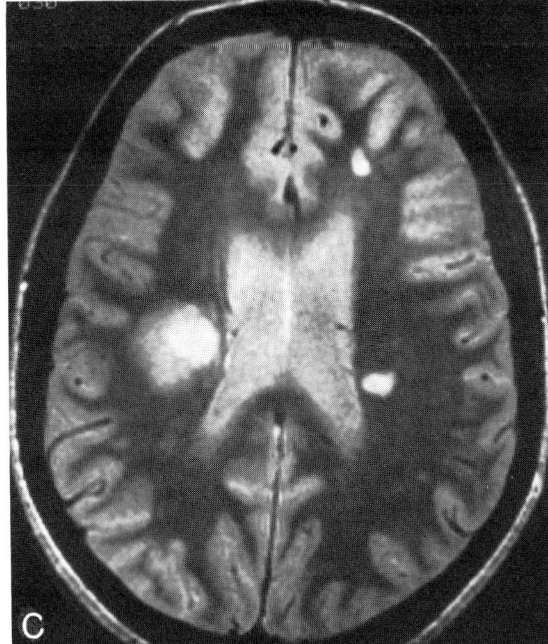

FIGURE 8–55. Plaques of multiple sclerosis. *A.* Oval plaques. high-field T2 spin echo image shows multiple high-intensity plaques. The oval shape whose axis is in the direction of the nerve fiber reflects the distribution of inflammation along the demyelinated segment and can assist in distinguishing multiple sclerosis from other diseases. *B.* Multiple sclerosis in a 55-year-old woman. Low-field STIR image shows typical periventricular plaques with very high tissue contrast, obtained in one third of the imaging time required for spin echo. The patient's age alone might have suggested vascular disease as a likely diagnosis, but she had had clinical multiple sclerosis for at least 17 years. *C.* Large lesions of multiple sclerosis. High-field T2 spin echo image shows a very large lesion adjacent to the right lateral ventricle and two smaller lesions. Large lesions are not uncommon in multiple sclerosis. This one appears to be the coalescence of several smaller ones.

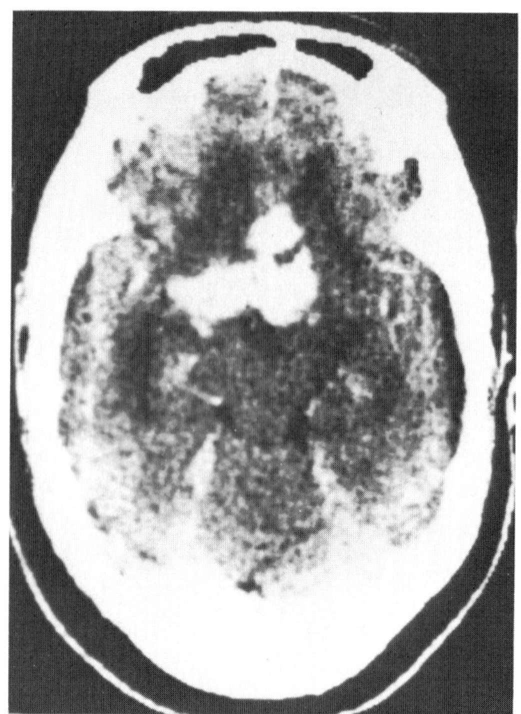

FIGURE 8–56. Sarcoidosis. Contrast CT shows enhancing granulomatous material in the leptomeninges surrounding the circle of Willis, a typical pattern and location for sarcoid.

areas on CT or high-intensity areas on MRI (Fig. 8–56). CNS sarcoidosis often responds to steroid therapy.

NEOPLASTIC DISEASES

Benign Tumors of the Brain and the Meninges

Benign tumors of the brain and the meninges are relatively common and are derived from a large number of cell types. Although these tumors seldom metastasize, they can cause a mass effect and local destruction, recur after resection, and occasionally undergo malignant transformation. Most benign tumors are extra-axial (i.e., they originate outside the brain substance). By far the most common benign intracranial tumor is the meningioma. Many benign tumors, including epidermoid and dermoid tumors, lipomas, craniopharyngiomas, and pineal tumors, are caused by embryonic abnormalities and are therefore located in or near the midline. Other benign tumors include schwannoma, choroid plexus papilloma, and colloid cyst.

Meningioma. The coverings of the brain and the spinal cord, collectively called the meninges, are composed of three layers. The thick outer dura functions as the periosteum of the inner skull and continues into the spinal canal as a separate membrane caudal to the foramen magnum. The middle (arachnoid) layer is a thin, transparent membrane over the outer brain and the spinal cord immediately adjacent to the dura and superficial to the subarachnoid space that contains the CSF. The inner layer (pia) is a thin, transparent membrane that is directly against the brain and the cord, follows the cortical sulci, and is deep to the subarachnoid space. Between the arachnoid layer and the pia are arachnoid trabeculae, numerous fibers that hold the leptomeninges (the pia and the arachnoid layer) together. Leptomeningeal tissue also forms the stroma of the choroid plexus and the tela choroidea.

The meningioma, a tumor of the leptomeninges, accounts for 15% of all primary benign brain tumors and 25% of primary spinal tumors. It is rare in children, and its incidence increases in the third or fourth decades. It is more common in women than in men both in the brain and in the spine. It is typically hemispherical, the base of the tumor being attached to the dura, as it arises from arachnoid villi in the dura or the arachnoid layer and becomes a vascular, space-occupying lesion. The pathogenesis of this tumor is not known, although trauma, radiation to the meninges, and loss of part of chromosome 22 have been suggested as causes.

The most common sites of meningioma are along the sagittal sinus, the lateral convexity, and the sphenoid wing (Fig. 8–57). Other sites are the sellar region (tuberculum sella, olfactory groove, parasellar area, and optic nerve sheath) and the posterior fossa (tentorium cerebelli, sigmoid sinus, and foramen magnum). Intraventricular meningioma occurs in the choroid plexus and the tela choroidea of the lateral ventricles. Its location in the spinal canal is usually thoracic, occasionally cervical, and rarely lumbar. Spinal meningiomas are usually located within the subdural space at the site of nerve root exit.

A meningioma can invade the dura, the venous sinuses, and bone, but it rarely grossly invades the brain. Microscopic invasion of the brain can occur and may account for the fact that 20% of grade 1 (benign) meningiomas recur in 20 years. Symptoms depend on the location of the lesion; they may be minimal

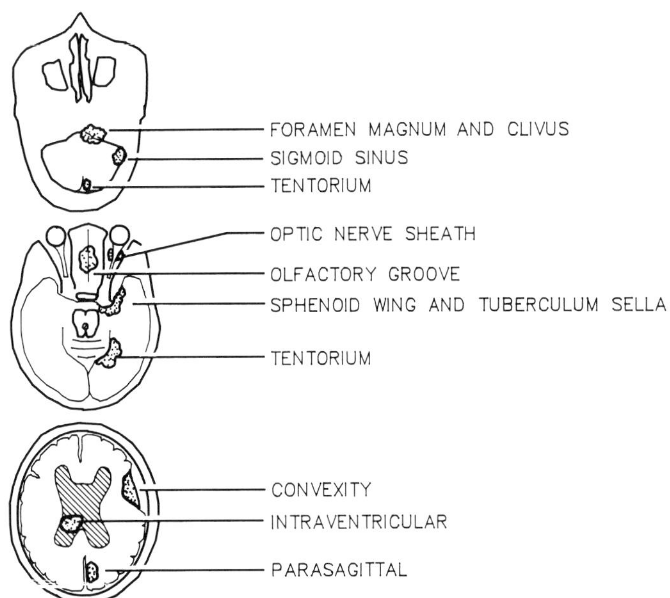

- EXTRA–AXIAL MASS
- 15% OF BENIGN BRAIN TUMORS
- ARISE FROM ARACHNOID VILLAE
- AGE 20–40 YEARS, WOMEN (3:2)
- MULTIPLE IN NEUROFIBROMATOSIS
- CT – CALCIFICATION, ENHANCEMENT
- ANGIOGRAPHY – PROLONGED BLUSH
- MR – SIMILAR TO GRAY MATTER

FIGURE 8–57. Locations and characteristics of meningiomas. MR, magnetic resonance.

even when the tumor is very large. The CT appearance depends on the location but is usually that of an extra-axial, rounded, densely enhancing mass (Fig. 8–58*A*). Associated findings of calcification, hyperostosis of adjacent bone, and brain edema may also be evident. On the sphenoid wing, the tumor may be elongated, conforming to the irregular shape of the bone. Arteriograms show a dense late venous blush but without early venous drainage. In most cases the dominant blood supply is from the external carotid circulation. Unenhanced MRI does not demonstrate meningioma as well as does CT. On most MRI views, a meningioma has an intensity similar to that of normal gray matter and is difficult to detect except by the presence of a mass effect or edema (Fig. 8–58*B*). Enhanced MRI shows dense contrast uptake and may have rapid washout and so images must be obtained immediately after injection (Fig. 8–58*C*).

Surgical resection, often preceded by vascular embolization, is successful for lesions that are separate from the skullbase. In the skullbase, they are difficult to remove entirely because of encasement of important structures. After resection, 20% of grade 1 meningiomas recur within 20 years, presumably from residual cells; about 50% of grade 2 (atypical) meningiomas recur within 12 years; and 100% of grade 3 (anaplastic) meningiomas recur within 6 years. A variety of cell types is seen on histological examination—meningothelial, fibrous, psammomatous, and so forth—but the cell type has no prognostic significance, except for the angioblastic type, which behaves like a grade 2 meningioma.

Hemangioblastoma. Hemangioblastoma is a neoplasm of blood vessels. It is rare (about 1% of all intracranial neoplasms) except among patients with von Hippel-Lindau disease (discussed earlier). Most of these tumors arise in the cerebellum near the midline, where they compress the fourth ventricle or cerebellum. The tumor can also occur in the medulla or the spinal cord. It seldom occurs above the tentorium. In the cerebellum the tumor is cystic, is well-circumscribed, and has a nodular tumor nidus. Patients develop symptoms of hydrocephalus or cerebellar compression. CT and MRI show a large cyst and an enhancing mural nodule (Fig. 8–59). A mass effect com-

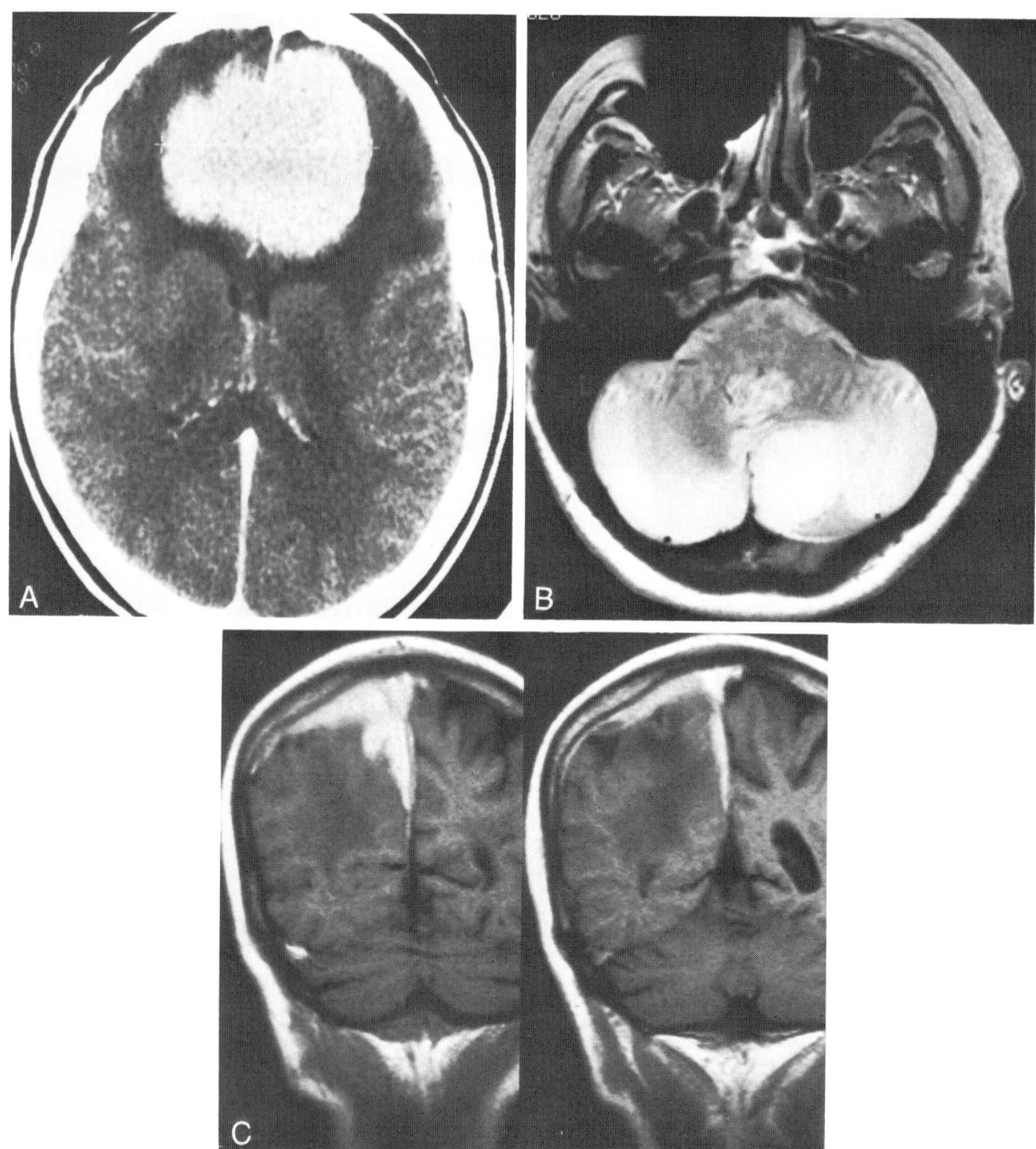

FIGURE 8–58. Appearance of meningiomas. *A.* Contrast CT shows a large, densely enhancing mass arising from the anterior falx in a 51-year-old woman who had intermittent symptoms of leg paralysis, blindness, and anosmia (she was being evaluated as an outpatient). Note mass effect and edema in adjacent brain tissue. Cursor measurement revealed a lateral diameter of 6.3 cm. *B.* Noncontrast magnetic resonance image (early echo of T2 spin echo) in a 60-year-old woman with cerebellar signs shows a round mass of similar intensity to gray matter in the left posterior fossa. A thin, dark margin and expansion of the adjacent CSF space indicates that the lesion is extra-axial. Sagittal and axial T1 spin echo images showed a similar appearance. C. Coronal T1 spin echo image with Gd-DTPA shows densely enhancing superior convexity en plaque meningioma involving the sagittal sinus in a 65-year-old man who had suffered a stroke. These and other views show a large right parietal venous infarct as a result of sinus obstruction. (Courtesy of B. Porter, First Hill Diagnostic Imaging Center, Seattle.)

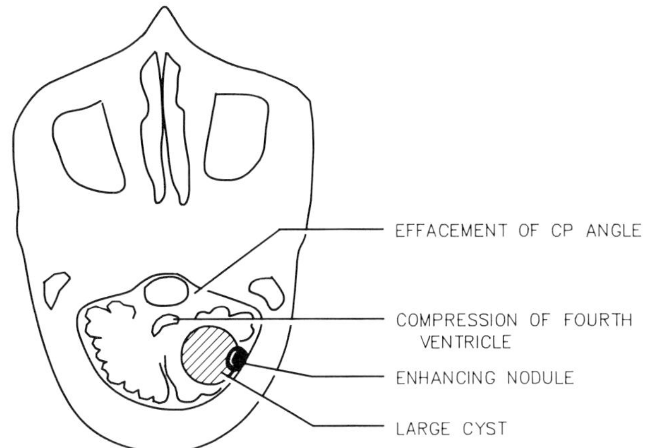

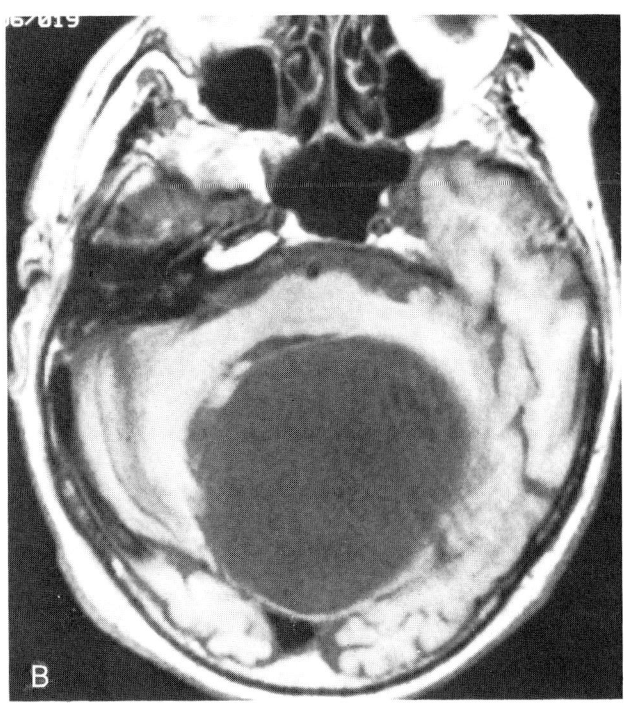

FIGURE 8–59. Hemangioblastoma. *A.* Diagram. CP, cerebellopontine; DDx, differential diagnosis. *B.* T1 spin echo image shows a large cyst that is nearly midline. The fourth ventricle, almost completely compressed, is anterior to the thin, right anterior membrane. More posteriorly on the right, this membrane has a nodular appearance representing the tumor nidus, which enhanced on CT. The patient had long-standing but nonprogressive symptoms and elected not to have surgery.

presses the fourth ventricle. Differential diagnosis includes cystic astrocytoma, Dandy-Walker cyst, and arachnoid cyst. On occasion, the tumor nodule is not found at surgery when the cyst collapses, and the lesion is erroneously called an arachnoid cyst. Therefore, preoperative detection of this nodule is extremely helpful. The tumor is benign, and surgery should be curative, but local recurrence is common.

Congenital Tumors Near the Midline

Many tumors of the CNS result from failures of embryogenesis and are caused by incomplete fusion of the midline structures or by abnormal cell layer migration. Most are found at or near the midline and have a composition that produces a distinctive CT appearance. Some of these lesions occur in characteristic sites, and their position can be determined precisely when anatomical structures such as the optic chiasm, the pituitary stalk, the fornix, and the vein of Galen can be identified (Fig. 8–60; see also Fig. 8–25). Most are benign, but several have a potential for malignancy. The most common of these are epidermoid and dermoid tumors, teratomas, craniopharyngiomas, and tumors of the pineal region.

Epidermoid Tumor. The epidermoid tumor is a rare tumor of ectodermal origin composed only of epidermal elements. It can occur subcutaneously or as an isolated skull lesion confined to the diploic space or within the cranial vault as an extra-axial mass (Fig. 8–61). In rare instances, it occurs within the ventricles or in the internal capsule as a result of the relatively late fusion of the telencephalon around the diencephalon. A derivative of skin, it contains dry keratin, dandruff-like dehydrated cells with no cholesterol. Thus it should not be called a "congenital" cholesteatoma and should not be confused with acquired cholesteatoma of the tympanic membrane. Patients usually have chronic symptoms caused by the mass effect of these slow-growing lesions. The most common CT appearance is a low- (water-) density mass in or near the ventral cerebellopontine angle that displaces the brainstem and the cerebellum medially. MRI almost always shows the tumor as low intensity on T1-weighted images and high intensity on T2-weighted images. An unusual appearance can result from the complexity of material in the tumor. The epidermoid tumor does not enhance with contrast. Surgical resection is curative unless residual cells form a recurrent tumor.

Dermoid Tumor. Dermoid tumor is a rare tumor of ectodermal origin that contains all epidermal elements (hair, sebaceous glands, sweat glands, and squamous cells). This tumor, like the epidermoid tumor, is also a product of abnormal embryogenesis, but it is usually located in the dorsal midline; most dermoid tumors are located in the midline posterior fossa, where they involve the cerebellar vermis or the fourth ventricle. On occasion, they are located at the base of the brain in the frontal lobes and in the lumbosacral spine. Patients, usually between the ages of 5 and 20 years, develop symptoms of increased intracranial pressure or cerebellar mass. If the tumor ruptures and spills the sebaceous and keratinous

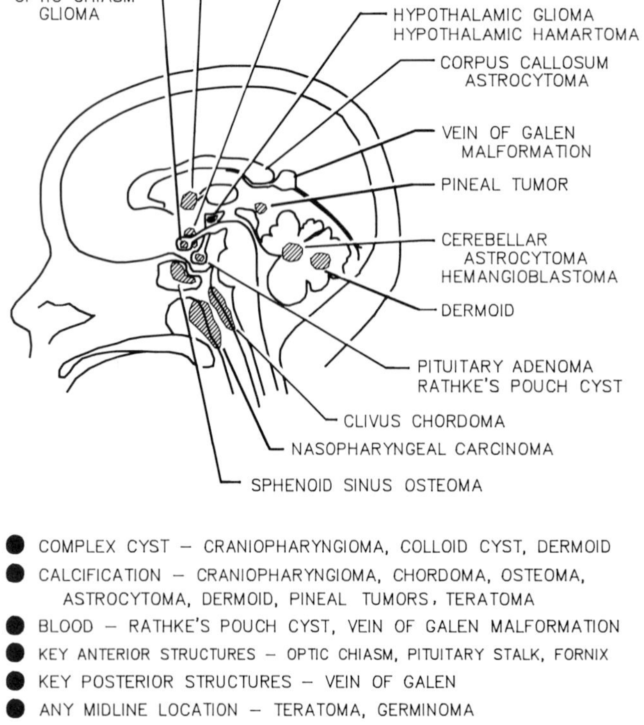

COLLOID CYST
OPTIC CHIASM GLIOMA
CRANIOPHARYNGIOMA
HYPOTHALAMIC GLIOMA
HYPOTHALAMIC HAMARTOMA
CORPUS CALLOSUM ASTROCYTOMA
VEIN OF GALEN MALFORMATION
PINEAL TUMOR
CEREBELLAR ASTROCYTOMA
HEMANGIOBLASTOMA
DERMOID
PITUITARY ADENOMA
RATHKE'S POUCH CYST
CLIVUS CHORDOMA
NASOPHARYNGEAL CARCINOMA
SPHENOID SINUS OSTEOMA

- COMPLEX CYST – CRANIOPHARYNGIOMA, COLLOID CYST, DERMOID
- CALCIFICATION – CRANIOPHARYNGIOMA, CHORDOMA, OSTEOMA, ASTROCYTOMA, DERMOID, PINEAL TUMORS, TERATOMA
- BLOOD – RATHKE'S POUCH CYST, VEIN OF GALEN MALFORMATION
- KEY ANTERIOR STRUCTURES – OPTIC CHIASM, PITUITARY STALK, FORNIX
- KEY POSTERIOR STRUCTURES – VEIN OF GALEN
- ANY MIDLINE LOCATION – TERATOMA, GERMINOMA

FIGURE 8–60. Location and characteristic locations of midline solid and complex cystic lesions.

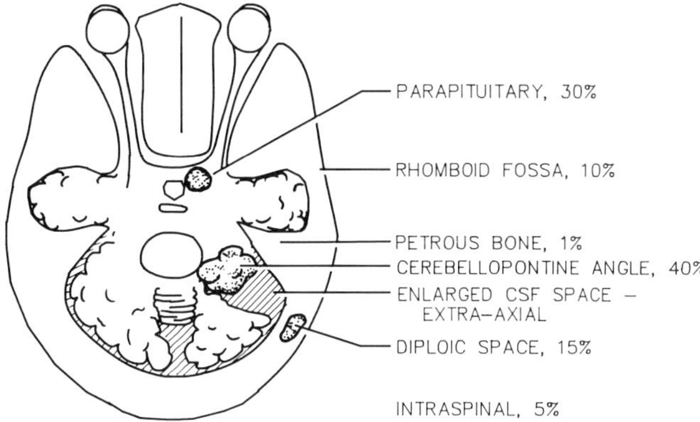

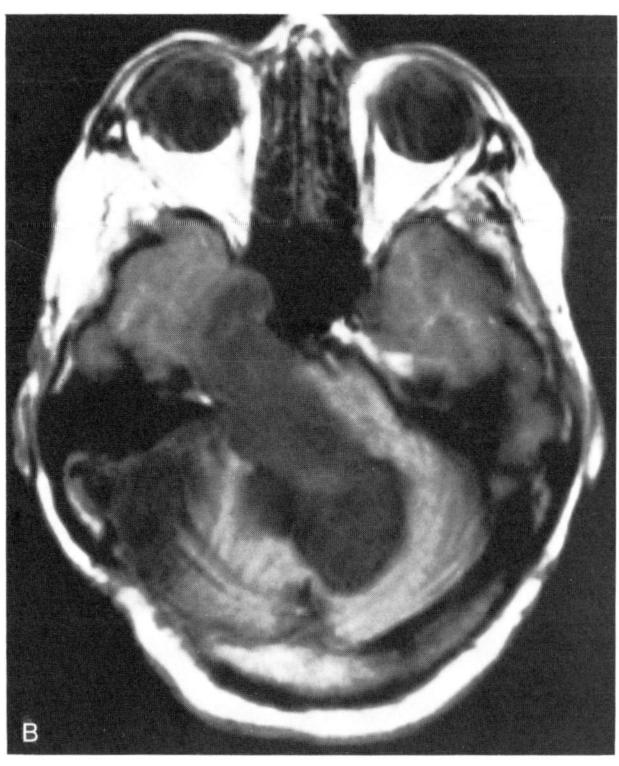

FIGURE 8–61. Epidermoid tumor. *A.* Diagram. CSF, cerebrospinal fluid. *B.* T1 spin echo image shows a massive lesion in the left cerebellopontine angle that is compressing an atrophic brainstem and cerebellum and invading the petrous bone in an elderly woman with previous (poorly documented) surgery for epidermoid tumor. The intensity was similar to but slightly higher than that of CSF on T2 spin echo images. At surgery, a large, flaky epidermoid tumor was resected.

contents into the subarachnoid space or ventricular system, a chronic chemical meningitis can occur.

CT typically shows a round, low-density mass in the midline posterior fossa and often an associated midline bone defect through which a dermal sinus passes to the skin (Fig. 8–62). The tumor may be of water density because of hair and keratin or may have fat density because of cholesterol. Calcification may be present, but ossified structures, such as teeth, are not. CT evaluation with bone windows is important before surgical resection in order to identify a dermal sinus. On MRI the tumor is of variable intensity on both T1- and T2-weighted images. These lesions are

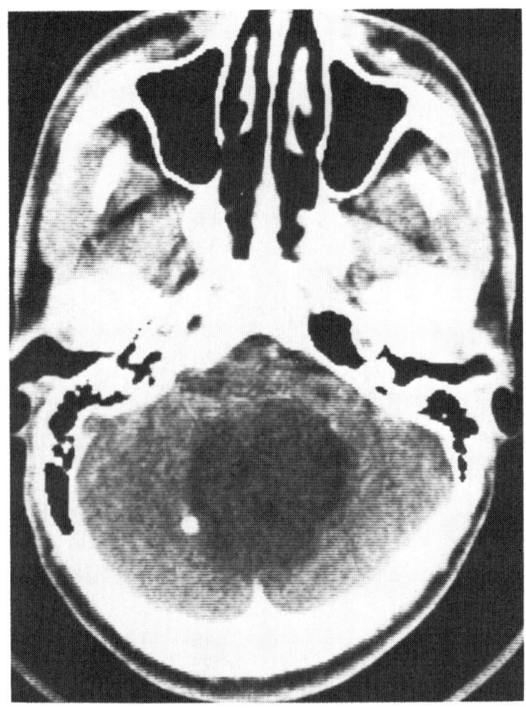

FIGURE 8–62. Dermoid tumor. Contrast CT shows a large midline cerebellar cystic lesion and a focus of calcification in a 30-year-old man with cerebellar ataxia. The low density in this case was attributable to the keratinaceous, cottage cheese–like composition of the mass.

usually of high intensity on T1 spin echo images and low intensity on STIR images, which indicate a lipid component. However, complex binding of water and cholesterol may produce a variable appearance.

Lipoma. CNS lipoma is a rare developmental abnormality of the meninges and the subjacent neural tissue. In the brain, it is found in the midsagittal region, particularly the corpus callosum, the quadrigeminal plate cistern, and the tuber cinereum, and is commonly associated with other midline anomalies (notably agenesis of the corpus callosum). Patients may have seizures, hypothalamic dysfunction, or obstructive hydrocephalus because of the mass. CT shows the fat-density mass in a midline location and the associated abnormalities. MRI clearly shows the fat as high intensity on T1-weighted images (Fig. 8–63). In the spine, a lipoma extends over several segments as a combined intra- and extramedullary mass. It is often associated with spinal dysraphism. CNS lipoma arises in the pia and is difficult to resect because of extension in the Virchow-Robin spaces around blood vessels.

Craniopharyngioma. Craniopharyngioma is a tumor of the suprasellar region; it apparently arises from cell rests derived from the nasopharynx that project into the region of the pituitary stalk where the adenohypophysis joins the neurohypophysis. It is composed of squamous cell epithelium that forms mucosa, and thus it contains "wet" keratin composed of microscopic pearls of swollen cells. It should not be confused with the epidermoid tumor. Craniopharyngiomas are not uncommon; they constitute 3% of all intracranial tumors. They may be detected at any age as a result of mass effect in the suprasellar region (Fig. 8–64).

The composition varies, but there are usually solid, cystic, and calcific components. The cyst contains a thick, gelatinous material that can have low or (rarely) high density on CT and low or high intensity on MRI. CT shows a suprasellar mass with cystic and solid components. These tumors are usually calcified. The tumor occasionally extends into the sella and appears as a dumbbell-shaped mass, narrowed by the sellar diaphragm. MRI scans can demonstrate the cystic component of the tumor and help to confirm its suprasellar location. The tumor is usually of high intensity on both T1 and T2 spin echo scans, which distinguishes it from other cystic tumors. However, because the composition varies, the MRI appearance may be complex. Masses of similar congenital origin include Rathke's pouch cyst (which may occur within the sella) and colloid cyst (of the anterior third ventricle); both are usually distinguished easily from the craniopharyngioma,

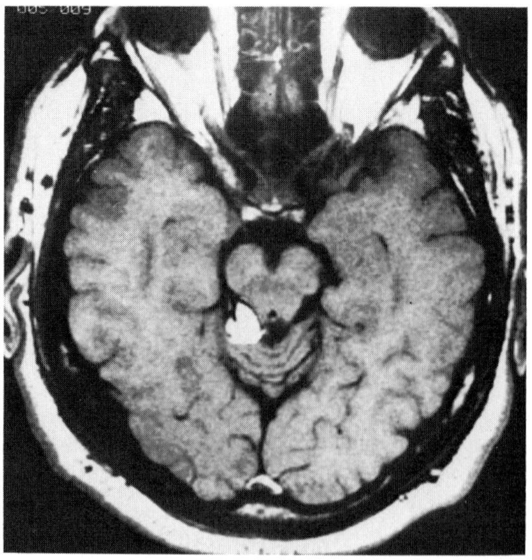

FIGURE 8–63. Lipoma. Thin-slice T1 spin echo image shows a high-intensity mass infiltrated into tissues around the quadrigeminal plate cistern in a 42-year-old man evaluated for visual disturbance.

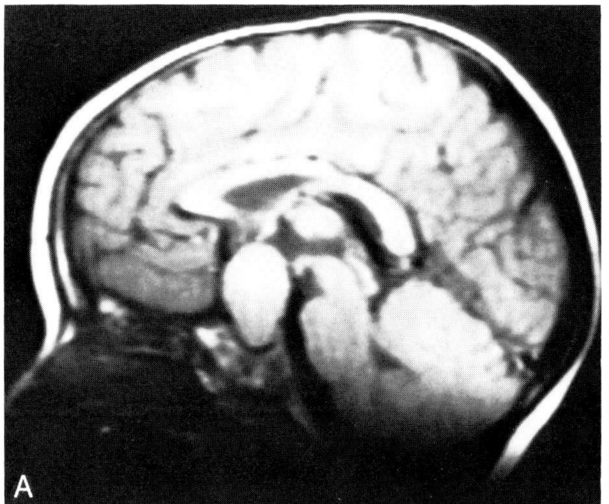

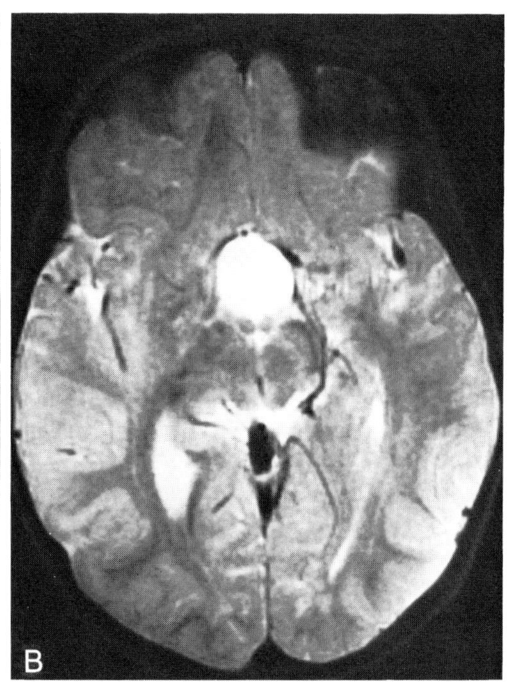

FIGURE 8–64. Cranial craniopharyngioma. *A.* Sagittal T1 spin echo image shows an ovoid high-intensity mass in the suprasellar cistern in a 2-year-old boy with bitemporal hemianopia. *B.* Axial T2 spin echo image shows similar high intensity. CT and plain films showed thin, irregular rim calcification.

which is suprasellar and inferior to the third ventricle.

Pineal Region Tumors. Tumors of the pineal region (sometimes collectively called pinealomas) constitute fewer than 1% of all intracranial tumors. Most are germinomas, teratomas, and various glial tumors; only about one fifth arise from pineal parenchymal cells. The most common manifesting signs of a pineal region mass are increased intracranial pressure caused by obstruction of the cerebral aqueduct and paralysis of upward gaze (Parinaud's syndrome) caused by compression of the superior colliculus. CT shows a mass in the pineal region with necrosis, cyst formation, fat, hemorrhage, or calcification, depending on the tumor type (Fig. 8–65). MRI, because it is especially sensitive to fat, cystic fluid, and the presence of tumor tissue, is of much benefit for identifying and characterizing pineal region masses. Most are of high intensity on T2 spin echo or STIR images.

Pineoblastoma is a tumor of primitive pineal cells and is highly malignant and infiltrative. Cyst formation, hemorrhage, and necrosis are common. The tumor is histologically similar to medulloblastoma. Pineocytoma is a tumor of mature pineal cells and generally becomes evident in teenagers. It grows slowly and is relatively benign.

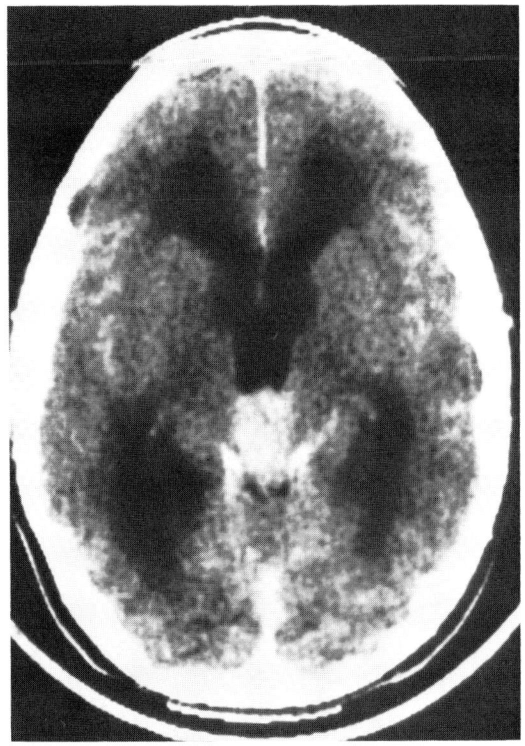

FIGURE 8–65. Pineocytoma. Contrast CT shows a 2.5-cm enhancing pineal mass and associated hydrocephalus caused by compression of the cerebral aqueduct in an 11-year-old boy with paralysis of upward gaze.

Teratoma. Teratomas are tumors of all three embryonic cell layers and constitute 0.5% of all brain tumors. They usually become clinically evident during the first 10 years of life, causing symptoms of a midline intracranial mass lesion. These tumors can be located in the pineal region (40%, usually in boys), the pituitary region (15%), and along the third ventricle and the suprasellar area (45%).

On CT, the tumor appears as a mixed-density mass with cystic, fatty, and ossific components located in the midline of the brain (Fig. 8–66). There is usually no enhancement when intravenous contrast is administered. The tumor's MRI appearance is variable, depending on whether fat is a substantial component. The behavior of the tumor and its response to therapy depends on its composition.

Germinoma. Germinomas are the most common pineal region tumor and can be of any primary germ cell type. These tumors are histologically identical to germ cell tumors of the testes and the ovaries with large epithelioid cells and small lymphocytes. They are thought to arise as a result of aberrant migration of primordial germ cells during early embryogenesis. The degree of malignancy varies with cell type and differentiation, but most of these tumors are malignant. Seminoma, embryonal cell carcinoma, and choriocarcinoma of the pineal region have been described. These tumors are infiltrative and spread to adjacent structures. CT or MRI shows a homogeneous, enhancing mass in the pineal region. Contiguous spread to adjacent structures and the ventricles is helpful for differentiating germinoma from other pineal region tumors. Germinoma and teratoma share a number of common characteristics, and the distinction between these tumors is often not possible to make.

Pineal Region Glioma. Pineal region glioma can arise either from pineal glial tissues or from adjacent brain tissue, particularly the corpus callosum, the midbrain, and the cerebellum. It appears on CT as a minimally enhancing, low-density mass. Glioma is discussed in more detail later.

Neurofibroma and Schwannoma. Peripheral nerve tumors (neurofibromas) and nerve sheath tumors (schwannomas, also called neurilemmomas) are extra-axial tumors that originate from peripheral nerves. The neurofibroma is a fibrous tumor within the nerve characterized by branching (plexiform) disorganized axons separated by a proliferation of fibrous tissue, which forms the bulk of the mass. Because the axons pass continuously through the tumor, there is neither encapsulation nor a proximal or distal margin, and thus resection is difficult or impossible. The schwannoma arises from the neural sheath and forms an eccentric mass surrounding the nerve. It can therefore be dissected from the nerve in most cases. The mass does not contain axons. Patients with neurofibromatosis have both neurofibromas and schwannomas. The term "neuroma" is best used to describe a disorganized mass of regenerating neural tissue that develops as a result of trauma, especially transection, of the nerve root.

Schwannomas most commonly arise from the lower cranial nerves, especially the eighth, but sometimes they arise from spinal roots. Most intradural spinal tumors are schwannomas, rather than neurofibromas. Peripheral tumors are more often neurofibromas. The usual clinical manifestation is a cranial nerve deficit. The tumor can also cause signs of a local mass effect on other nerves, the brainstem, the spinal cord, and vascular structures and can invade and destroy bone.

On CT scans, neurofibromas and schwannomas appear as low-density, extra-axial, rounded masses that enhance with intravenous contrast. CT cisternograms can demonstrate the lesion if it is within the subarachnoid space. Enhanced MRI is the best imaging test because it shows the enhancing tumor surrounded by low-intensity CSF and can provide the optimal imaging plane. Unenhanced MRI can often show large lesions, and STIR imaging is especially valuable in demonstrating spinal neuromas (Fig. 8–67; see also Figs. 8–37, 8–99, and 8–104). Arteriography is usually not helpful except for evaluating invasion of vascular structures, but it can demonstrate a faint tumor

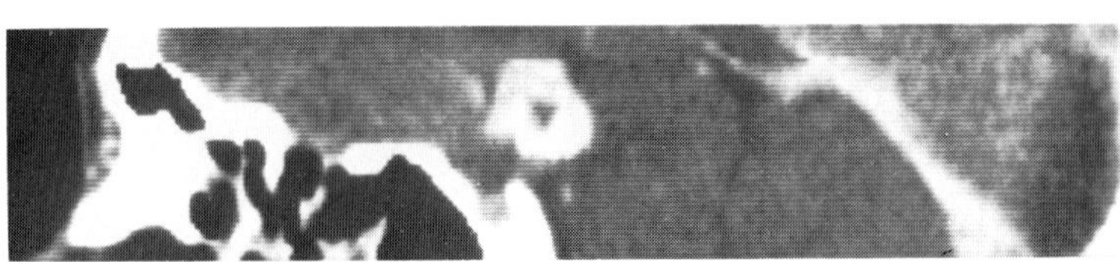

FIGURE 8–66. Teratoma. Midline sagittal CT reformation shows a suprasellar, mixed-density mass with calcification and fat in a 12-year-old boy with visual disturbance. Note the normal pituitary gland inferiorly.

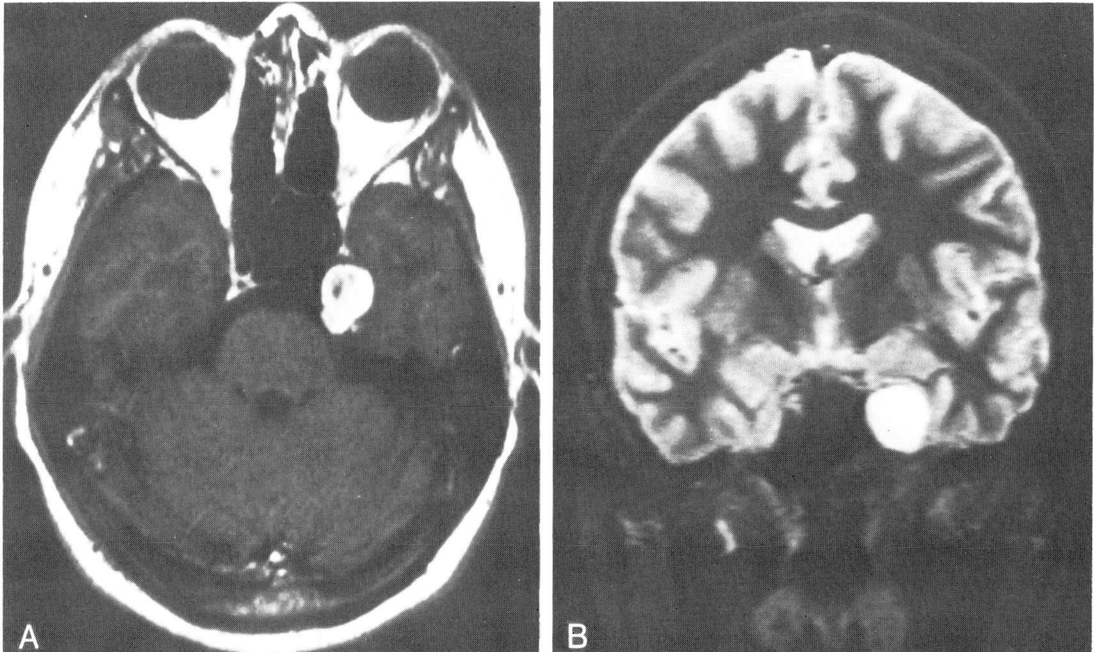

FIGURE 8–67. Schwannoma (neurilemmoma). *A.* Gd-DTPA–enhanced, midfield T1 spin echo image shows a left fifth cranial nerve schwannoma in a 27-year-old woman with left facial numbness. The tumor, including its inhomogeneous center, is well-shown against the low-intensity brain and CSF. *B.* Coronal STIR image, obtained without contrast, shows the tumor to be of distinctly higher intensity than brain tissue, a common finding on STIR images of neuromas. (Courtesy of B. Porter, First Hill Diagnostic Imaging Center, Seattle.)

blush that is attributable to increased blood flow to the tumor. It can also distinguish a tumor from an aneurysm in the cerebellopontine angle. The most common of these tumors, acoustic schwannoma and neurofibroma of the spine, are discussed in the sections on the temporal bone and the spine.

Choroid Plexus Papilloma. Choroid plexus papilloma is a rare, benign tumor of the choroid plexus, usually in children under 10 years of age. The tumor is typically located in the glomus of the choroid plexus in the lateral ventricle. When it occurs in adults, it is usually in the fourth ventricle. Patients have signs and symptoms of increased intracranial pressure and hydrocephalus. The histological appearance of both the cells and stroma mimics that of the normal choroid plexus. On radiographs, the tumor appears as an enlarged, irregular, enhancing mass, locally expanding the ventricle and causing a generalized increase in ventricular size, as a result of either increased production of CSF or hemorrhage that has obstructed normal CSF flow (Fig. 8–68). The tumor is often locally invasive and spreads by seeding throughout the CSF pathways. The rare choroid plexus carcinoma represents the malignant end of the spectrum of choroid plexus papilloma and is characterized by invasion and metastasis, loss of papillary structure, and anaplasia.

Colloid Cyst. Colloid cysts are benign congenital tumors that usually arise from ependymal cells of the roof of the diencephalon. About 20% have nonciliated cells, which suggests that the tumor arises from the paraphysis. These cysts constitute about 1% of all intracranial tumors. They are located in the anterior third ventricle, where they can obstruct the foramina of Monro. Despite the congenital origin of the mass, the first symptoms usually occur in young adults when obstruction causes acute symptoms of hydrocephalus that are frequently intermittent and sometimes change with posture. The cyst has an epithelium-lined collagenous wall, which is attached to the choroid plexus in the roof of the third ventricle, and it contains a homogeneous gelatinous (colloid) material.

On CT, the cyst is of similar or slightly higher density than brain tissue and may enhance slightly when intravenous contrast is administered. The MRI appearance depends on the complex composition of the cyst. Like craniopharyngiomas, colloid cysts often are of high intensity on both T1- and T2-weighted

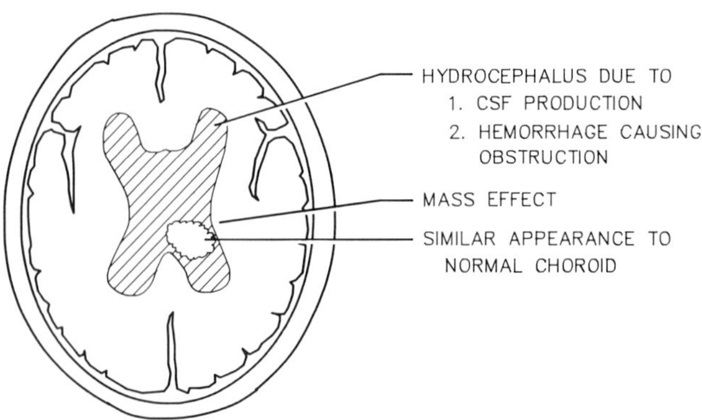

- 0.5% OF INTRACRANIAL TUMORS
- AGE 0–10 YEARS
- SYMPTOMS OF HYDROCEPHALUS
- BENIGN, HYPERPLASIA OF NORMAL CHOROID
- RARELY MALIGNANT CARCINOMA
- DDx: EPENDYMOMA, MENINGIOMA, METASTASIS

A

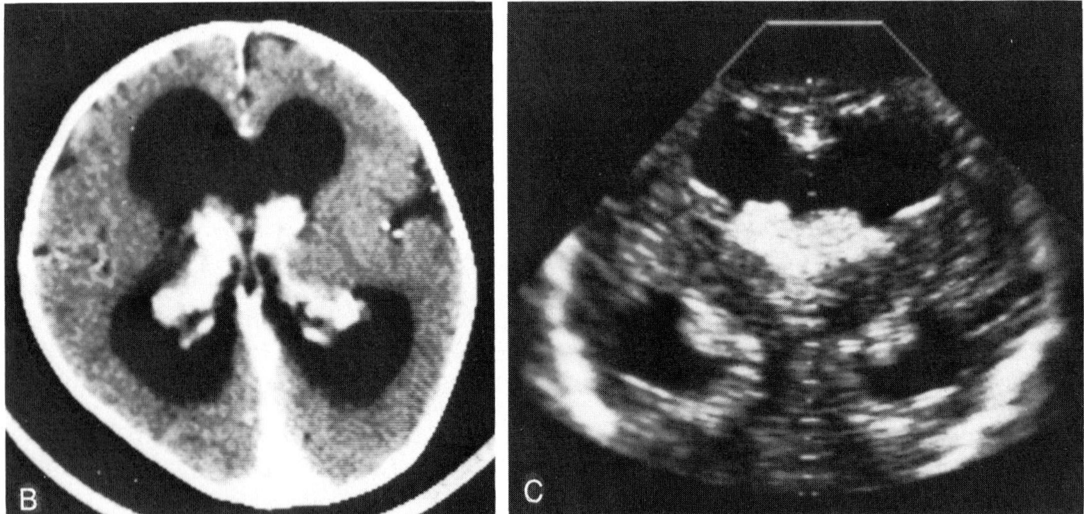

FIGURE 8–68. Choroid plexus papilloma. *A.* Diagram. CSF, cerebrospinal fluid; DDx, differential diagnosis. *B.* Contrast CT shows bilateral enlargement of the choroid plexus and hydrocephalus in an 8-month-old boy. *C.* Coronal ultrasonogram shows similar enlargement of the choroid plexus bilaterally.

images, but many appear similar to fat or cholesterol (Fig. 8–69). The characteristic location at the level of the foramina of Monro, the associated enlargement of the lateral ventricles, and the normal posterior third and fourth ventricles and aqueduct usually enable the diagnosis to be made. Colloid cysts are commonly surgically resected from above, through the hydrocephalic lateral ventricles and foramen of Monro. If untreated, the patient can die when the tumor acutely obstructs flow of CSF from the lateral ventricles.

Malignant Brain Tumors

Most malignant brain tumors are gliomas, which arise from neuroectoderm. The most important of these tumors are astrocytoma, glioblastoma multiforme, ependymoma, oligodendroglioma, medulloblastoma, CNS lym-

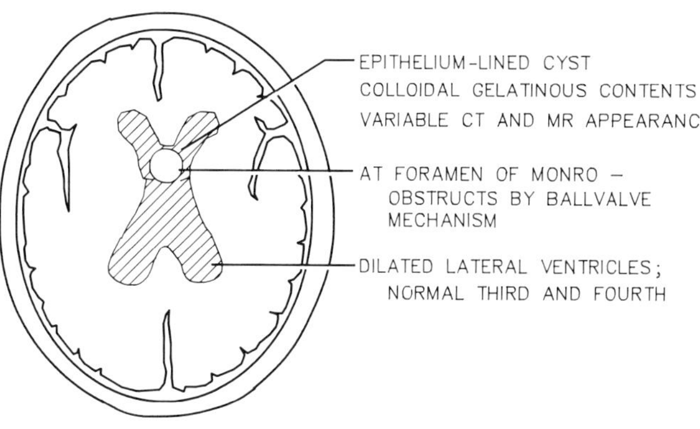

- 0.5% OF BRAIN TUMORS
- FROM DIENCEPHALON EPENDYMA
- SYMPTOMATIC AT AGE 20–55 YEARS
- INTERMITTENT OBSTRUCTION – HEADACHE, VISUAL Sx

A

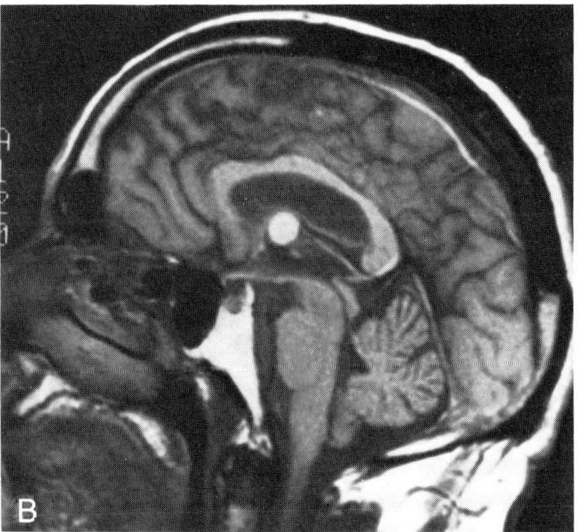

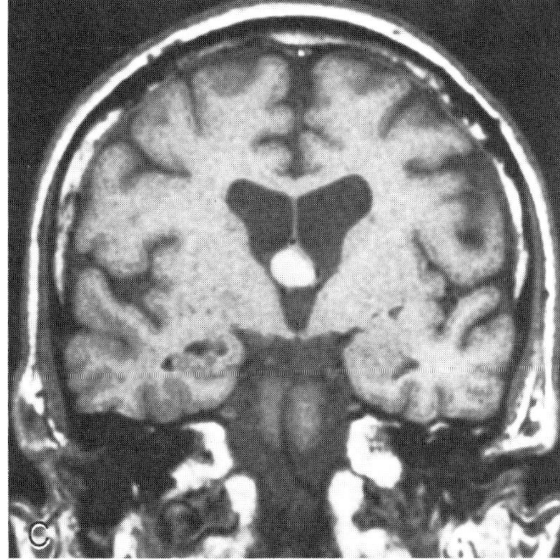

FIGURE 8–69. Colloid cyst. *A.* Diagram. MR, magnetic resonance; Sx, symptoms. *B, C.* Sagittal and coronal T1 spin echo images show a high-intensity mass obstructing the foramina of Monro in a 64-year-old man with intermittent and nonspecific symptoms. *D.* Axial T2 spin echo image shows the cyst as low intensity and also demonstrates hydrocephalus.

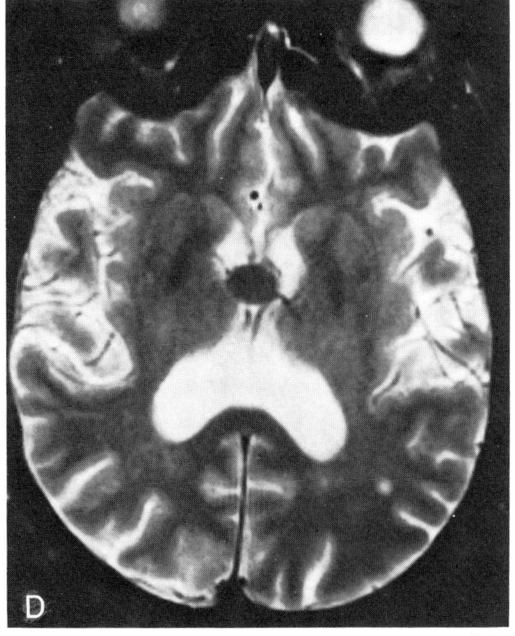

phoma, and metastatic tumors. In many cases, malignant brain tumors comprise more than one cell type, and their classification is controversial: some neuropathologists prefer to classify them by the predominant or the most aggressive cell type, and others term them mixed gliomas. Gliomas constitute 45% of all intracranial tumors. In children, two thirds of intracranial gliomas are in the posterior fossa and are about equally divided among astrocytomas, ependymomas, and medulloblastomas. In adults, two thirds of intracranial gliomas are supratentorial, and the majority of these tumors are astrocytomas, half of which are glioblastomas. In the spinal cord, most intramedullary tumors are gliomas, about 60% of which are ependymomas and 25% astrocytomas.

Most brain tumors manifest with insidious onset of symptoms caused by a gradually enlarging mass. However, both primary and metastatic brain tumors can cause abrupt deterioration of mental status when they bleed, obstruct the ventricular system, or cause herniation. In many patients with large tumors or lesions obstructing the ventricular system, a slight increase in mass effect from edema, ventricular enlargement, or hemorrhage can cause catastrophic clinical deterioration.

Astrocytoma. The astrocytoma is the most common malignant CNS tumor of children and adults. The tumor is composed of astrocytes, which are cells of the CNS supporting structure. The type of astrocyte, the degree of hypercellularity and pleomorphism, the degree of mitotic activity, and the presence of necrosis and endothelial proliferation provide the basis for the histological classification. The gross anatomical location is sometimes more significant in that astrocytomas of the spinal cord, the brainstem, the cerebellum, and the cerebrum have different biological behavior. The age of the patient is also important; astrocytomas in young adults and children grow more slowly. Most astrocytomas contain various amounts of normal tissue and include or are surrounded by reactive cells (astrocytes), and so a limited biopsy may not reflect the true composition of the tumor.

The radiographic appearance of an astrocytoma depends on the location (Table 8–4) and the degree of malignancy. In some locations, the tumor has a distinctive name. When associated with tuberous sclerosis, it is called a giant-cell subependymal astrocytoma because of the presence of giant cells and the location in the wall of the ventricle. In the posterior fossa (and elsewhere) in children, it is often cystic and is called a cystic astrocytoma. When it is adjacent to the ventricle (beneath the ependyma), it is called a subependymal astrocytoma or a subependymoma. These terms suggest the origin of the subependymoma from subependymal astrocytes; the tendency of this tumor to recur locally after x-irradiation suggests an important relationship with ependymoma.

An astrocytoma is generally of low density on CT, and if it is an aggressive tumor, it shows irregular rim enhancement. Calcification is not unusual in astrocytomas but is more typical of oligodendrogliomas. A moderate amount of edema is associated with astrocytomas and is indistinguishable from the tumor on imaging tests.

T2 spin echo MRI shows a high-intensity mass (representing tumor and edema) (Fig. 8–70). Further definition of the tumor can often be made with the use of enhanced MRI, which can distinguish a highly vascular portion from a less aggressive portion. However, low-grade astrocytomas show only minimal contrast enhancement on CT or MRI. In addition, non-

TABLE 8–4. CHARACTERISTICS OF ASTROCYTOMAS BY LOCATION

Location	Usual Age	Characteristics
Cerebrum	Adult	Deep white location; spread across corpus callosum; solid tumor, sometimes cystic; usually gliobastoma in patients over 45
Periventricular	Child	Malignant degeneration of periventricular cells of frontal horns of the lateral ventricles in patients with tuberous sclerosis
Diffuse	Any	Multicentric astrocytoma; separate, primary foci or diffuse cerebral tumor
Third ventricle	Child	Infiltrate optic tracts, chiasm, and hypothalamus
Brainstem	Child	Symmetrical mass in the pons and (rarely) the medulla and the midbrain; about half are glioblastomas
Cerebellum	Child	Circumscribed solid cystic tumors
Spinal cord	Any	Rare, intramedullary tumors, usually cervical; symmetrical cord enlargement, often with syrinx

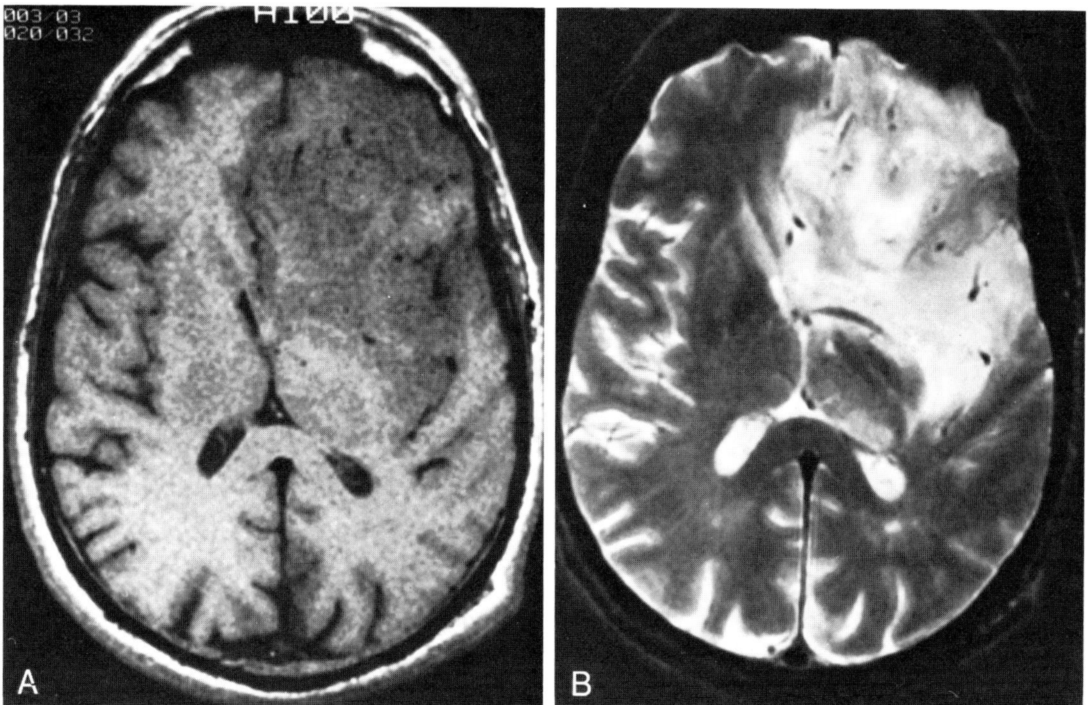

FIGURE 8–70. Astrocytoma. *A.* T1 spin echo image shows a large left frontal mass that crosses the midline and displaces vessels in a 67-year-old man with seizures and a sensation of pressure in the head. *B.* T2 spin echo image shows a large inhomogeneous area of abnormality. The distinction between tumor and edema cannot be made.

enhancing areas cannot be presumed to represent edema (Fig. 8–71). Other findings of hydrocephalus, compression of normal structures, cysts, multiple foci, or hemorrhage also depend on the location and the type of tumor. CT and MRI are reliable examinations for identifying and following CNS tumors, but they cannot distinguish among different tumor types.

The prognosis for children with astrocytoma is relatively good because the tumors in this age group are generally of low-grade malignancy, but x-irradiation does not prevent local recurrence. In adults the tumors are more aggressive, and despite vigorous therapy, patients with highly malignant neoplasms live only 1 or 2 years after diagnosis.

Glioblastoma Multiforme. Glioblastoma multiforme is the most malignant of the gliomas. Sometimes it appears to be a primary malignancy, other times a malignant form of astrocytoma. Both types are highly malignant and rapidly fatal, and they are histologically indistinguishable. The tumor almost always occurs in the cerebrum, arising in the deep white matter or the basal ganglia. On histological examination, the tumor shows infiltration of normal adjacent tissue, marked hypercellularity, and pleomorphism with many giant cells and abnormal mitoses, necrosis, and vascular proliferation. A variety of cell types, including sarcomatous degeneration of vessels and fibroblasts, can be present. It is highly invasive and spreads to the meninges and the ventricular system. Patients have rapidly progressive neurological deficits and symptoms of an intracranial mass.

On CT and MRI, glioblastoma multiforme appears as an enhancing cerebral mass surrounded by edema (Fig. 8–72). Extension laterally to the meninges, medially to the ventricles, and across the corpus callosum is common and causes enhancement of these structures. MRI shows the tumor and edema as high intensity on T2-weighted spin echo or STIR scans and also shows contrast enhancement, especially at the rim. Necrosis, cyst formation, hemorrhage, and edema are well-demonstrated, although tumor and edema cannot be reliably differentiated. Approximately 5% of glioblastomas have more than one focus. The prognosis of patients with glioblastoma is poor; most patients die within 1 year of the diagnosis despite vigorous treatment.

Ependymoma. Ependymomas arise from ependymal cells that line the ventricular system

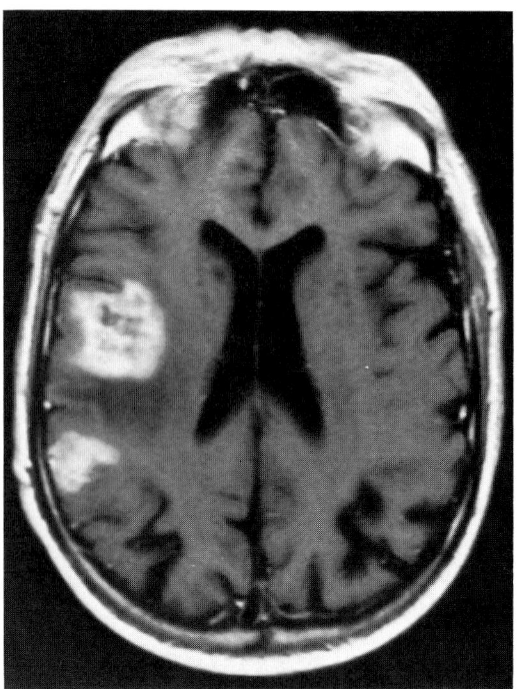

FIGURE 8–71. Astrocytoma. Gd-DTPA–enhanced T1 spin echo image shows two areas of enhancement in the right frontoparietal region in an elderly man with sudden left hemiparesis. The nonenhancing region between these two areas was thought to represent edema, but continuity of tumor in the entire region was found at surgery. (Courtesy of E. Dienes, Venice MRI Center, Venice Hospital, Venice, Florida.)

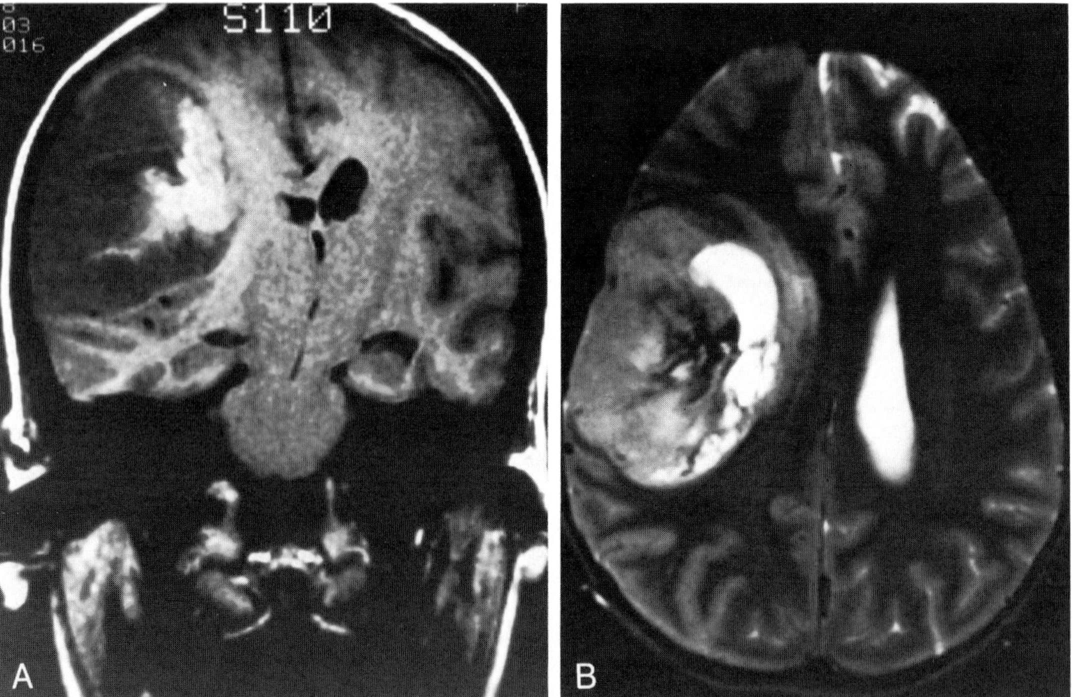

FIGURE 8–72. Glioblastoma multiforme. *A.* Coronal T1 spin echo image shows a large right parietal mass with medial hemorrhage in a young woman with severe headache and left-sided face and body weakness. The right lateral ventricle is compressed. *B.* Axial T2 spin echo image shows solid and hemorrhagic components; note that this sequence shows the main bulk of the tumor to be solid (similar to gray matter) as opposed to the possibly cystic appearance on the T1 spin echo image. This was interpreted as glioblastoma multiforme at one institution, but the highly malignant character of this tumor was suggestive of primitive neuroectodermal tumor, according to neuropathologists at another center.

of the brain and the central canal of the spinal cord. They constitute 6% of all intracranial gliomas (most involve the fourth ventricle) and 60% of gliomas of the spinal cord, in which they usually involve the cauda equina and the filum terminale. Children and adolescents are most often affected, but there is a second peak incidence among young adults. Symptoms are hydrocephalus, cerebellar signs, or cord compression, depending on the site of involvement. In the brain, the tumor is slow-growing and infiltrative, often with exophytic components. CT or MRI shows a mass adjacent to the ventricular system, particularly at the fourth ventricle (Fig. 8–73). In the spinal cord, the cauda equina, and the filum terminale, the tumor is elongated and relatively smooth (see also Figs. 8–108, 8–109).

Most ependymomas appear benign on histological examination, but their location adjacent to vital structures and their infiltrative growth causes serious neurological problems and makes surgical removal difficult. When the tumor does not infiltrate other structures, it is easily removed at surgery with minimal injury to adjacent tissue, but even in these cases, local postoperative x-irradiation may be required in order to prevent recurrence. More aggressive (malignant) forms of ependymoma also occur in rare instances, and whole neuraxis x-irradiation is required in order to eradicate seeding of tumor along the ventricular system or the central canal, as also occurs with medulloblastoma. Distant metastases to the lung are very rare.

Oligodendroglioma. Oligodendrogliomas constitute 5% of intracranial gliomas. They occur in adults between the ages of 20 and 60 (peak age is 40) and are usually located supratentorially in the deep white matter of the centrum semiovale, although one gross characteristic is an anaplastoid appearance resembling hypertrophic cortex. They are occasionally in the cerebellum, in the spinal cord, or adjacent to the third ventricle. The tumor is generally of low- to medium-grade malignancy, and even when necrosis and extreme hypercellularity are present, patients do not die as rapidly as those with glioblastoma multiforme. Symptoms may be present for years before diagnosis.

On CT, oligodendroglioma appears as a deep, white matter mass with minimal contrast enhancement. Calcification is common. The location of the tumor, the chronicity of symptoms, and the presence of calcification suggest the diagnosis (Fig. 8–74). However, as discussed earlier, astrocytoma (which is more common) must also be considered when these findings are present. MRI is more sensitive to the presence of the tumor than CT but does not identify the calcific component. More aggressive tumors may also contain sufficient numbers of malignant oligodendrocytes to be called malignant oligodendrogliomas. Survival of patients depends on the aggressiveness and invasiveness of the tumor, which is difficult to predict from the histological examination. Unlike glioblastomas, which can be differentiated from astrocytomas by the presence of necrosis, oligodendrogliomas carry the same prognosis whether necrosis is present or not.

Medulloblastoma. Medulloblastomas constitute 8% of all intracranial tumors and generally occur in children. They probably arise from primitive neuronal cell rests of the posterior midline cerebellum (the nodulus) and frequently the fourth ventricle and cerebellum. They are the most common of a group of tumors classified as primitive neuroectodermal tumors. Thirty percent of medulloblastomas occur in young adults, in whom they may be in the lateral cerebellum (40% of the time) and are more sclerotic (called a desmoplastic medulloblastoma). The tumor is highly malignant and infiltrative. It spreads via the CSF to the third and lateral ventricles and to the leptomeninges of the cerebral convexities and the spinal subarachnoid space. Patients have signs of hydrocephalus and a cerebellar mass.

CT shows a mass in the cerebellum that is of slightly higher density than brain tissue and that enhances with intravenous contrast. Enhancement of the leptomeninges can be seen if subarachnoid spread has occurred. MRI shows the mass (see Fig. 8–13) and, after administration of paramagnetic contrast, most clearly demonstrates subarachnoid spread (Fig. 8–75). Surgery, chemotherapy, and radiation therapy have improved the prognosis of patients with medulloblastoma. Many live 5 years or more. Tumors in adults are rare, usually are better differentiated, and may carry a better prognosis.

CNS Lymphoma. Lymphoma can affect the CNS by metastatic spread or as a primary tumor. Primary lymphoma of the brain may arise from reticulum cells (hence the alternative term "reticulum cell sarcoma") and contains a mixture of lymphocytes and microglia, but most CNS lymphomas are composed predominantly of B cells. T cell lymphomas are rare. The tumor is characteristically located in the periventricular white matter but also occurs

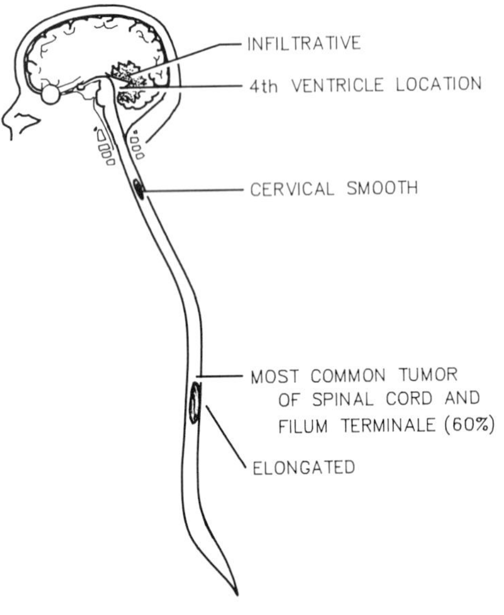

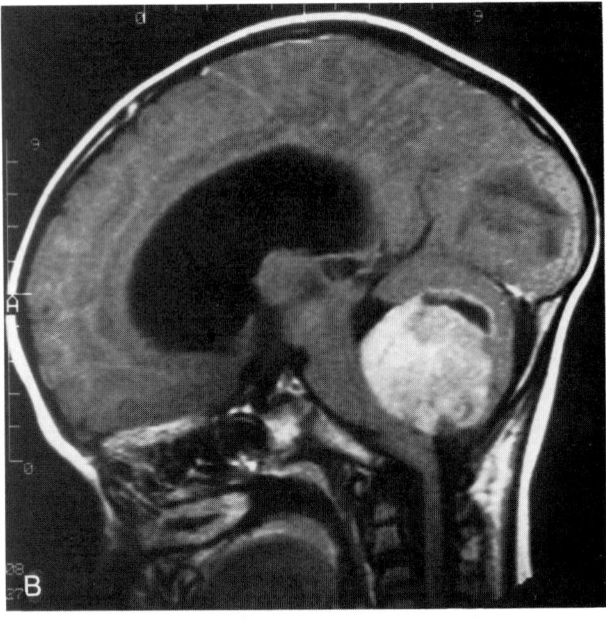

FIGURE 8–73. Ependymoma. *A.* Diagram. *B.* Sagittal T1-weighted MRI after administration of Gd-DTPA shows a large mass lesion in the posterior fossa. The mass abuts the fourth ventricle. It shows a cystic area posteriorly. The lesion is clearly separate from the brainstem. This tumor arose from the ependyma of the fourth ventricle.

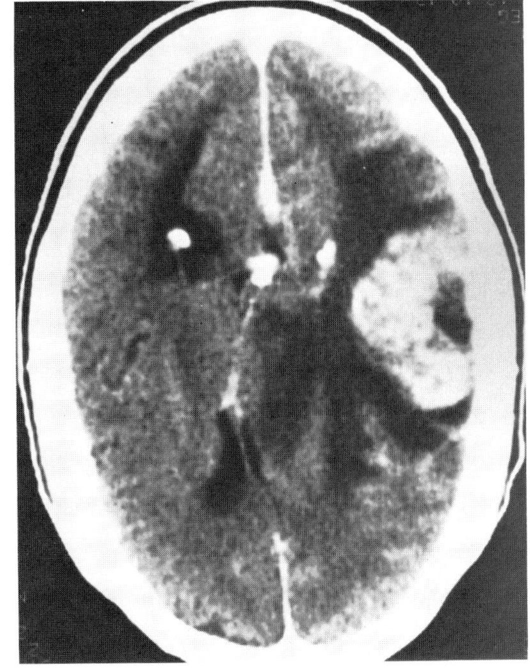

FIGURE 8–74. Oligodendroglioma. Contrast CT shows a densely enhancing right frontoparietal mass with marked surrounding edema. The patient's bizarre behavior—he was a drug user who thought that people with ray guns were chasing him—first led to his arrest. Neurological examination and subsequent CT revealed a brain mass of highly malignant character that proved to be a malignant oligodendroglioma.

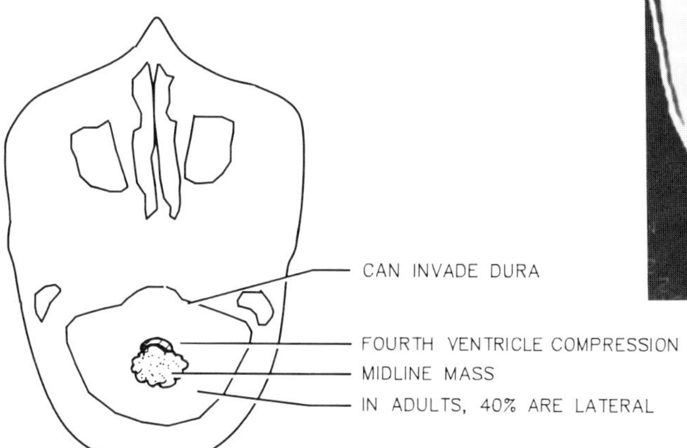

- 8% OF INTRACRANIAL TUMORS
- USUALLY CHILDREN AGE 5–10 YEARS
- ALWAYS IN CEREBELLUM – FROM MIDLINE CELL RESTS
- NO CALCIFICATION
- LATERAL TUMORS ARE BETTER DIFFERENTIATED
- LOCAL SPREAD BY CSF
- DISTANT SPREAD TO BONE

A

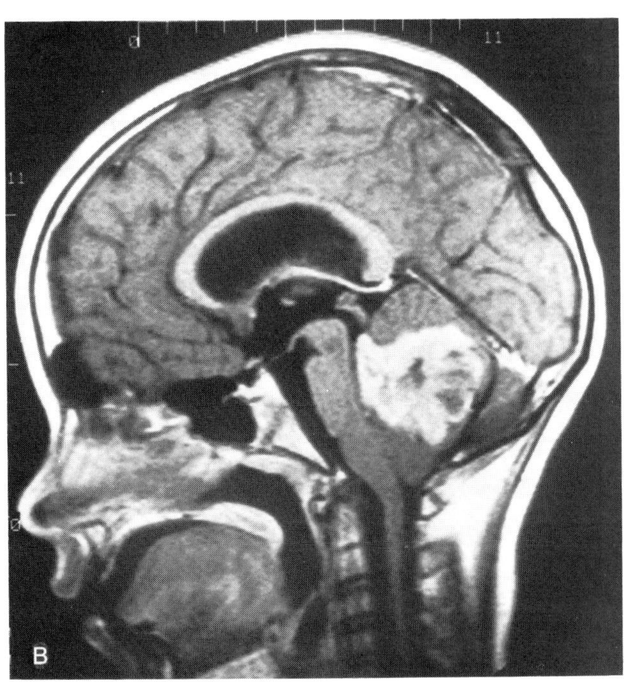

FIGURE 8–75. Medulloblastoma. *A.* Diagram. *B.* Sagittal T1 spin echo scan after administration of Gd-DTPA shows a large enhancing mass in the cerebellum that compresses the fourth ventricle. The lesion is predominantly in the midline, involving the vermis. A large medulloblastoma has a similar appearance to the ependymoma (compare with Fig. 8–73*B*).

in the basal ganglia, the thalamus, the corpus callosum (Fig. 8–76), and the cerebellar vermis. Patients are often immunosuppressed as a result of cancer, AIDS, drug therapy, or primary immunodisorder. CT or MRI shows an enhancing lesion that in many cases has an appearance that is atypical for a primary glioma. The lesion may share similarities (and coexist) with infection, hemorrhage, and other tumors. The appearance and location of the mass, in conjunction with a clinical history of immunocompromise, should raise suspicion of CNS lymphoma.

Metastatic Tumors. In older patients, the most common brain tumors are metastases, most from the lungs and breasts. A common metastatic tumor to the brain is the melanoma. This and other vascular tumors, such as renal cell carcinoma, thyroid carcinoma, and choriocarcinoma, show a predilection for the brain. Because these tumors are blood-borne, involvement is usually at the gray-white junction. Most metastatic tumors exhibit intense surrounding edema and contrast enhancement on either CT or MRI (see Figs. 8–11, 1–23). The lesions can be shown on unenhanced MRI, but small ones may be difficult to differentiate from other white matter lesions in elderly patients.

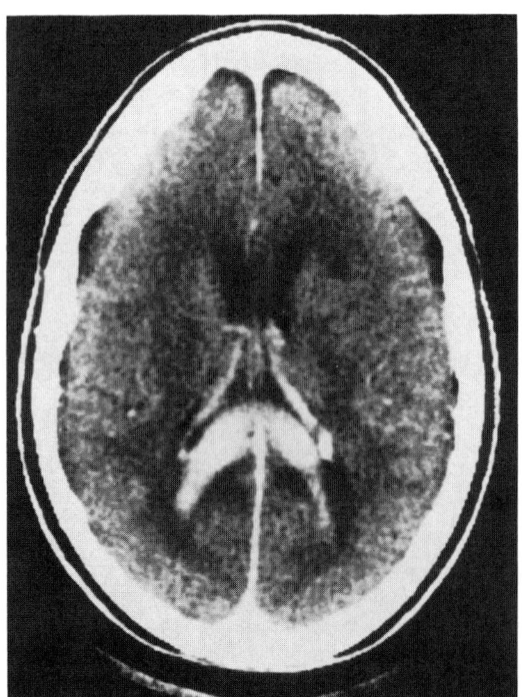

FIGURE 8–76. CNS lymphoma. Contrast-enhanced CT shows tumor involvement of the splenium of the corpus callosum in a 50-year-old man with confusion and dissociation of the right and left cerebral hemispheres. The patient was immunosuppressed as a result of chemotherapy for lung carcinoma.

Lung carcinomas of all cell types (but notably oat-cell carcinoma and adenocarcinoma) spread early to the brain. The brain lesion identified on CT or MRI is solitary in 30% of patients and is detected before the primary lung tumor in 30% of patients. Treatment by radiation or chemotherapy is temporarily successful, but many patients die of the brain lesions. Metastases from breast carcinomas generally appear years after the initial diagnosis and treatment. Multiple small enhancing lesions are the most common appearance, in addition to skull metastases. Intense edema is usually present. Treatment of breast metastases is limited because patients usually have disseminated disease throughout the body. Melanomas commonly metastasize to the brain, often without symptoms from the primary lesion. Because of their vascularity, they often hemorrhage and appear on scans to be high-grade primary malignant tumors. The presence of paramagnetic material can produce a decreased intensity on MRI. Metastasis from melanoma or carcinomas of the lungs, the breasts, the kidneys, or other sites is frequently solitary and therefore can be treated surgically.

VASCULAR DISEASES

Vascular diseases of the brain can be congenital, atherosclerotic, or acquired as a result of trauma, infection, tumor, or vascular insufficiency. These diseases usually manifest acutely as stroke (defined as the sudden development of a permanent neurological deficit). The most important causes of stroke are infarction and hemorrhage. Infarction can be caused by cerebral embolism, hypoperfusion, spasm, and hypoxemia. Hemorrhage can be caused by hypertension, ruptured aneurysm, AVM, anticoagulation, tumor, and amyloid angiopathy. Transient neurological deficit is usually caused by atherosclerotic disease. The clinical evaluation of patients with possible stroke who fall should be correlated with the radiographic findings in order to distinguish primary traumatic brain injuries (sometimes the patients show little external evidence of trauma as the result of a fall after losing consciousness) from primary vascular disease or a combination of both traumatic and vascular injury (see Fig. 8–80).

Ischemia and Infarction

Necrosis of neurons occurs when brain or spinal cord tissue receives insufficient blood (ischemia), insufficient oxygen (hypoxemia), or insufficient glucose (hypoglycemia). Hypoglycemia rarely produces visible areas of necrosis, whereas hyperglycemia appears to potentiate hypoxemia to produce large areas of necrosis (infarction). The sequential changes in the gray and white matter determine the CT appearance. In the first few hours of infarction, production of adenosine triphosphate in the gray matter ceases, resulting in failure of the sodium-potassium pump and consequent swelling of the cells. At this time, usually 6 to 12 hours after infarction, CT can show loss of density in the gray matter and, as a result, loss of the differentiation of gray from white matter. Slight mass effect (seen as effacement of adjacent CSF spaces) is often present in the affected area (see Fig. 8–4*B*). The blood-brain barrier is intact in the early stages of infarction, and so no enhancement occurs.

As the breakdown of the blood-brain barrier progresses (by 24 to 48 hours after the infarction), fluid fills the interstitium. CT shows more pronounced edema (manifested by low density), a mass effect, and loss of gray-white matter differentiation (Fig. 8–4*C*). Increased perfusion (so-called luxury perfusion) and incompetence of the blood-brain barrier cause contrast enhancement of many infarcts after 48 to 72 hours. Watershed infarcts enhance early because of the many contiguous vessels that supply the area. Embolic and thrombotic strokes usually require more time to recruit vessels from separate territories to supply the injured area, although congenital anastomotic channels may persist in some people.

The mass effect caused by edema persists for 3 to 4 weeks; contrast enhancement may last 3 months or longer. When the edema subsides and the infarcted brain tissue is absorbed, CT shows a focal, low-density area of encephalomalacia, often associated with ex vacuo dilatation of adjacent sulci and ventricles. This appearance is typical for old infarction, but a new area of infarction could be present within part of the same region and may not be detectable. The clinical findings are usually helpful in the evaluation of a new stroke in a patient who has had previous infarction.

Small infarcts occur in the basal ganglia and the deep white matter, particularly in hypertensive patients, as a result of atherosclerotic small vessel disease (lacunar infarcts). They appear on CT as focal areas of low density and on MRI as similar punctate areas of high intensity (T2-weighted images). Infarcts of the brainstem can be devastating; spinal infarcts are rare. Both are low density on nonenhanced CT but are better shown on MRI.

Evaluation of infarction depends on the time of the stroke. A patient who has had signs or symptoms of an infarction for less than 48 hours should undergo noncontrast CT or MRI to document the infarction and rule out hemorrhage. Beyond 48 hours, if no infarct is demonstrated, contrast may be helpful. Infarcts may enhance for 3 months or more, and high intensity has been shown on MRI for as long as 40 years after the injury. Persistent (especially progressive) mass effect beyond 2 weeks is suggestive of an alternative diagnosis, such as tumor or infection. MRI with T2 spin echo sequences shows a generalized high-intensity abnormality in early infarction. This appearance can clearly delineate the vascular distribution of the infarct (Fig. 8–77), but the high intensity can be confused with tumor or infection. Paramagnetic contrast may be helpful for studying the early stages of infarction because no enhancement occurs in regions of ischemia.

Cerebral Embolism. Emboli can reach the brain from the venous circulation in patients with right-to-left cardiac shunts; from cardiac sources; or, most commonly, from the carotid,

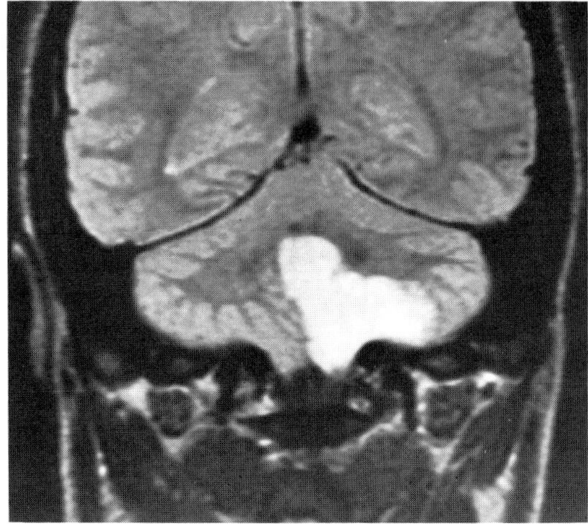

FIGURE 8–77. Acute infarction. Coronal T2 spin echo image shows well-circumscribed increased intensity in the posterior inferior cerebellar artery distribution in a 47-year-old man with a 3-day history of left sided weakness, nausea, and vomiting.

TABLE 8–5. SOURCES OF CEREBRAL EMBOLI

Source	Type of Emboli
Noncranial veins	Thromboembolus via cardiac shunt
	Tumor metastases
Heart	Mural thrombus from infarct or aneurysm
	Atrial clot in mitral disease or atrial fibrillation
	Myxoma
	Valve vegetations in endocarditis or from prosthetic valve
Extracranial arteries	Atherosclerotic plaque at the carotid bifurcation
	Trauma to the carotid or vertebral arteries

vertebral, or basilar arteries in patients with atherosclerotic disease (Table 8–5). The emboli comprise thrombi (platelets, fibrin or both), calcified plaque, or microorganisms. When these emboli reach cerebral vessels, they obstruct blood flow and can cause infarction of a portion of the brain. Infarction is most common in areas perfused by the middle cerebral arteries, in which blood flow is greatest. Emboli from the heart find the most direct route to the right middle cerebral artery. Both the gray matter and the white matter supplied by the occluded vessel are affected. When a vascular-distribution infarction occurs, evaluation is directed at determining the site of occlusion or the source of the embolus. The carotid artery bifurcations can be evaluated with angiography and ultrasonography (discussed in the "Basic Evaluation" section). The intracranial carotid artery can be evaluated with routine MRI, MRA, or both in order to qualitatively assess flow in the vessels. MRA can demonstrate many of the findings of conventional angiography noninvasively.

Hypoperfusion. Transient hypotension, cardiac arrest, and arrhythmia are the most common causes of hypoperfusion infarction. Vasculitis, spasm, AVM, and diffuse atherosclerosis are less common causes of hypoperfusion. Hypoperfusion first affects the parts of the brain with a high metabolic rate (the middle cortical layers and some of the basal ganglia, especially the putamen) and those with least collateral flow (the so-called watershed areas between the middle and anterior cerebral distributions and between the middle and posterior cerebral distributions) (see Fig. 8–4*A*). CT shows low density in the infarcted area as a result of the infarcted and edematous brain tissue.

Hypoxemia. Hypoxemia can cause edema and infarction when the supply of oxygen is insufficient to meet the demands of the cells. Hypoxemia can be caused by lung disease (acute and chronic), suffocation, near drowning, narcotic overdose, and carbon monoxide poisoning. The region of the basal ganglia (especially the globus pallidus) is most seriously affected by hypoxemia and appears as bilaterally symmetrical areas of low density on noncontrast CT or as areas of high intensity on MRI (Fig. 8–78).

Perinatal Hypoxemia and Ischemia. Anoxia, asphyxia, and ischemia can have a devastating effect on the developing brain, depending on the severity, the duration, and the presence of underlying conditions. When ischemia causes infarction in a full-term infant, the location and the appearance are highly variable (cerebral cortex and deep cerebral nuclei) and frequently asymmetrical. Ultimately, large areas of the brain become infarcted, and encephalomalacia, cyst formation, and decreased brain development become evident later. The deep cerebral nuclei frequently show status marmoratus and gliosis of partially necrotic foci. Premature infants show hemorrhage or necrosis in periventricular tissue: germinal matrix hemorrhage and periventricular leukomalacia. These insults can occur in utero but most, perhaps as many as 95%, occur hours to days after premature birth.

Periventricular Leukomalacia. Hypoperfusion or anoxia in the premature infant or in utero results in infarction in the watershed distribution of the developing fetus. The infarction involves the periventricular area, predominantly the posterior region near the trigone of the lateral ventricles. At birth, the lesions can be diagnosed on ultrasonograms but MRI most clearly shows the subsequent findings of the process: enlargement of the posterior ventricles and deepened sulci, as a result of loss of white matter, and periventricular patches of high intensity, which indicates infarction (Fig. 8–79). Similar infarction may also be the cause of some porencephalic cysts (see Fig. 8–26), but most porencephalic cysts appear in the distribution of one or more branches of the middle cerebral arteries, usually bilaterally and symmetrically, apparently caused by a transient episode of hypotensive hypoperfusion early in utero.

Vascular Occlusive Disease. Other causes of infarction include immune-mediated and congenital vascular occlusion. Moya Moya disease is a progressive occlusion of the supraclinoid

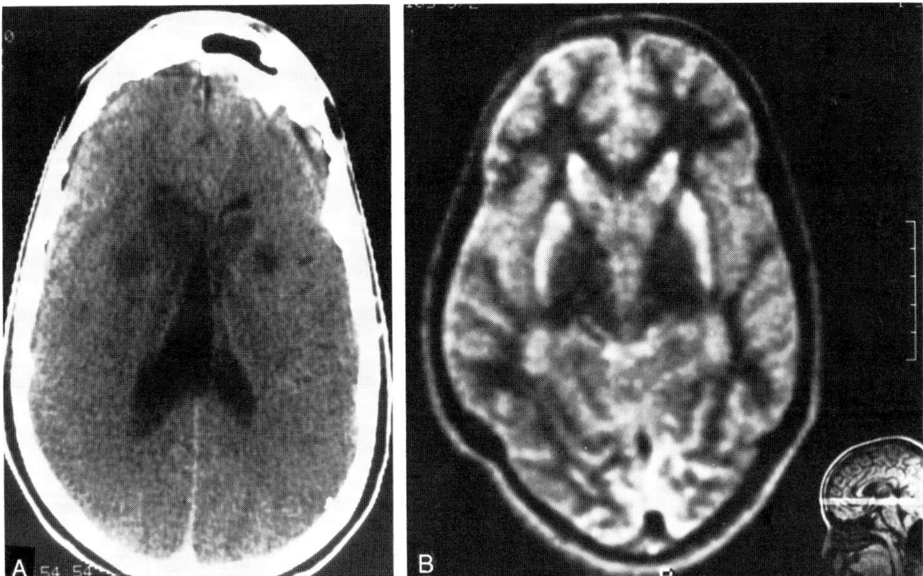

FIGURE 8–78. Hypoxemia infarct. *A.* Noncontrast CT shows bilateral low density with swelling and near effacement of the frontal horns in a young man who drove his car into a lake and nearly drowned. *B.* T2 spin echo image shows bilateral, symmetrically increased intensity in the putamen in a 12-year-old boy who suffered a neck injury. During resuscitation, he sustained an approximately 10-minute period of hypotension from brainstem compression, which resulted in the putamen injury.

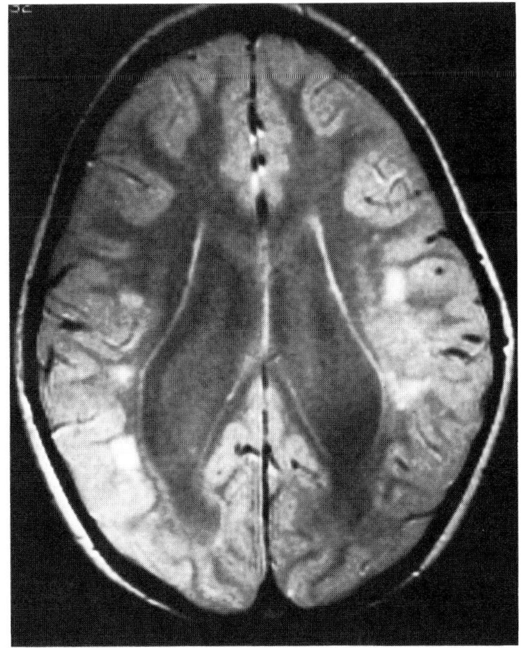

FIGURE 8–79. Periventricular leukomalacia. Early echo T2 spin echo image shows bilateral loss of posterior deep white matter with resultant deepening of the cerebral sulci and enlargement of the trigones of the lateral ventricles. The patient, now 4 years old, had language delay and hearing loss. He was born prematurely and suffered asphyxia at birth. Deep, patchy areas of periventricular infarction are also noted.

part of the internal carotid artery and its branches. Resulting collateral formation fills the base of the brain with small vessels, which can be seen on CT, MRI, or angiograms. Patients with Moya Moya disease are usually less than 15 years of age, and the female-to-male ratio is two to one. Adults more often present with hemorrhage, and ischemia is most common in children. Other causes of vascular occlusive disease are Takayasu's arteritis, herpes zoster arteritis, granulomatous (giant-cell) arteritis, and lupus.

Hemorrhage

Nontraumatic hemorrhage is caused by hypertension, rupture of an aneurysm or an AVM, anticoagulation, tumor, and amyloid angiopathy. Sagittal sinus thrombosis and vasculitis can also cause infarction or hemorrhage. Diagnosis is best made through detection of blood on noncontrast CT or unenhanced MRI. The blood may be parenchymal, subarachnoid, subdural, or intraventricular and is often in more than one of these spaces. The location of the blood greatly assists in determining the cause of the hemorrhage. In general, blood in the basal ganglia indicates hypertensive hemorrhage, blood in the subarachnoid region indicates aneurysm rupture, and blood in the deep white matter suggests AVM rupture. Small, repeated, subcortical hemorrhages suggest amyloid angiopathy. The location of blood in subarachnoid and AVM hemorrhage can often be used to identify the location of the lesion but is not totally reliable. Hemorrhage caused by a coagulation disorder can have any appearance on CT and MRI scans.

Hypertensive Hemorrhage. Prolonged pressure effects of hypertension affect primarily the small vessels at the base of the brain: those that supply the basal ganglia, the deep white matter, the cerebellum, and the brainstem. Microaneurysmal dilatation of these vessels can occur (so-called Charcot-Bouchard aneurysms). Complications include secondary dissections along small vessels; hemorrhage, which is often massive, results when they rupture. Alternatively, they may heal by thrombosis, producing small, punctate lacunar infarcts. Patients exhibit acute onset of severe neurological deficit; the symptoms depend on the location and size of the hemorrhage. Large hemorrhages are identified on CT by the presence of parenchymal blood in the region of the putamen (the site of more than half of hypertensive hemorrhages), the thalamus, the cerebellum, and the brainstem (Fig. 8–80). Varying amounts of subarachnoid and intraventricular blood are seen, but the parenchymal hemorrhage predominates.

Aneurysmal Hemorrhage. Rupture of an intracranial aneurysm is the most common cause of nontraumatic subarachnoid hemorrhage. Most "congenital" saccular aneurysms are really caused by a combination or a superimposition of factors: congenital absence of the media, acquired degeneration of the internal elastica as a result of atherosclerosis, and hypertension. The acquired factors are usually the most important because medial defects are present in 80% of bifurcations, and aneurysms develop in only about 1%. Aneurysms occur in the crotch of branches of the circle of Willis (see Fig. 8–6). Therefore, the most common and the most important CT or MRI finding in aneurysmal hemorrhage is blood in the basal cisterns. The correlation between the presence of subarachnoid blood from spinal puncture and CT abnormality is high (about 90%). The distribution of the blood suggests the anatomical origin of the aneurysm but not accurately enough for determining the vessel of origin for angiography or emergency surgery. High-resolution CT of the circle of Willis during contrast infusion or MRA can often identify the aneurysm and assist in the performance of angiography (see Fig. 8–6*B*). When aneurysm is suspected, angiography should be performed, beginning with the suspected artery. All four vessels should be studied because more than one aneurysm is present in 15% of patients.

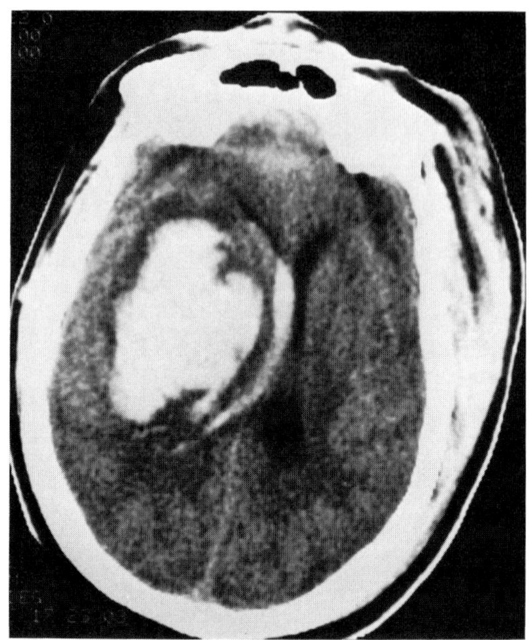

FIGURE 8–80. Hypertensive hemorrhage. Noncontrast CT shows a massive right putaminal hemorrhage in an elderly woman with severe diabetes and uncontrolled hypertension. Her car went off the road when she lost consciousness. The injuries from the accident were initially suggestive of a traumatic cause of the brain hemorrhage.

The anterior communicating artery is the most common site of aneurysm (40%). Hemorrhage from such an aneurysm can be suspected from the presence of blood in the basal cisterns and the interhemispheric fissure (Fig. 8–81).

The second most common site of intracranial aneurysm is the distal internal carotid artery (30%), just distal to the origin of the posterior communicating artery, but also at the origin of the ophthalmic artery and in the intracavernous portion of the internal carotid artery. Rupture of one of these aneurysms appears as blood, symmetrically distributed in the basal cisterns. About 20% of intracranial aneurysms are located at the middle cerebral artery "trifurcation" (usually a double bifurcation), where rupture causes leakage of blood into the subarachnoid region, especially in the ipsilateral Sylvian fissure, and parenchymal leakage of blood in the temporal lobe. The remaining

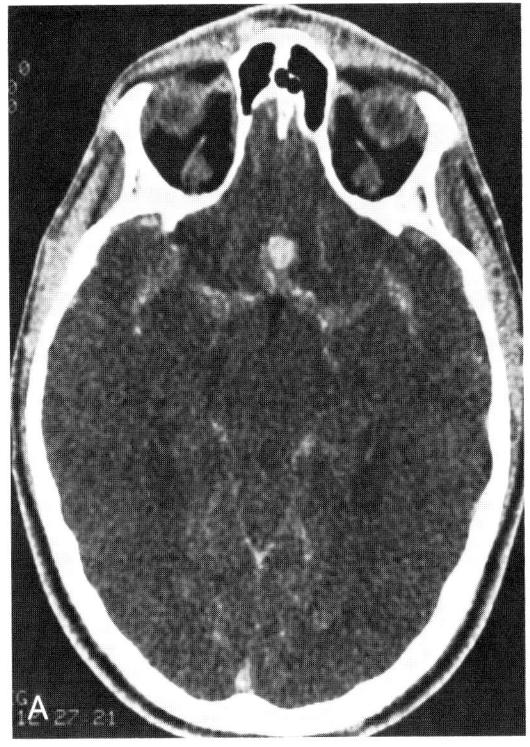

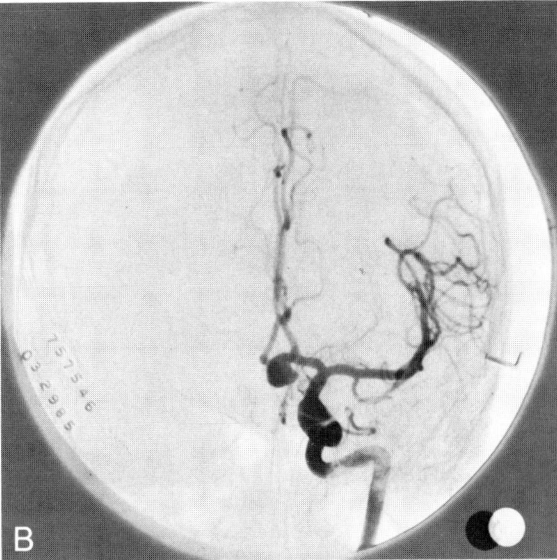

FIGURE 8–81. Aneurysm hemorrhage. Initial noncontrast CT showed blood throughout the subarachnoid spaces. *A.* Thin-slice CT image obtained during infusion of contrast and photographed at intermediate windows shows the subarachnoid blood as light gray and the anterior communicating artery aneurysm as high density (white). *B.* Conventional subtraction angiogram shows the aneurysm.

10% occur in the posterior fossa (at the tip of the basilar artery and near the posterior inferior cerebellar artery), in which the rupture produces prepontine or parenchymal (brainstem) leakage of blood. Saccular aneurysms of peripheral branches of cerebral arteries are rare (fewer than 1% of all aneurysms); they are usually infectious (called mycotic aneurysms) or, occasionally, traumatic. Parenchymal and, on occasion, subdural hematomas may be associated with the subarachnoid hemorrhage of an aneurysm.

Other Aneurysms. Aneurysms that occur outside the circle of Willis or outside the branches of the vertibral-basilar arteries are rare, constituting fewer than 1% of all intracranial aneurysms. They occur in a more peripheral location, usually in distal middle cerebral or pericallosal branches. Aneurysms of the distal middle cerebral arteries are most often infectious (mycotic) aneurysms caused by septic emboli, whereas pericallosal aneurysms are usually caused by trauma when the artery is injured by compression against the falx. The list of differential diagnoses of peripheral aneurysms is limited (Table 8–6). They can be caused by infection, tumor, trauma, and vascular disease.

The most serious of these aneurysms are those caused by infection (mycotic aneurysms). They are virtually always associated with subacute bacterial endocarditis that has caused seeding of the vessels and resultant weakening of vessel walls. Patients usually have hemorrhage. The effective treatment of subacute bacterial endocarditis has markedly decreased the incidence of mycotic aneurysms and the severity of hemorrhage from rupture. CT or MRI shows subarachnoid blood; angiograms can demonstrate one or more peripheral aneurysms. Management of patients who survive the first hemorrhage is controversial. Early surgery is difficult because the vessel is infected and friable, and the aneurysm is not at a bifurcation and lacks a clearly definable neck. The alternative treatment, conservative antibiotic therapy, carries the risk of fatal rupture.

Arteriovenous Malformation. AVM is a congenital collection of abnormal, arterial and

TABLE 8–6. CAUSES OF PERIPHERAL ANEURYSMS

Type	Cause
Infection	Subacute bacterial endocarditis *(Streptococcus viridans, Staphylococcus aureus)*
Tumor	Left atrial myxoma, choriocarcinoma
Trauma	Intimal injury against falx or bone
Vasculitis	Moya Moya disease, immune vasculitis

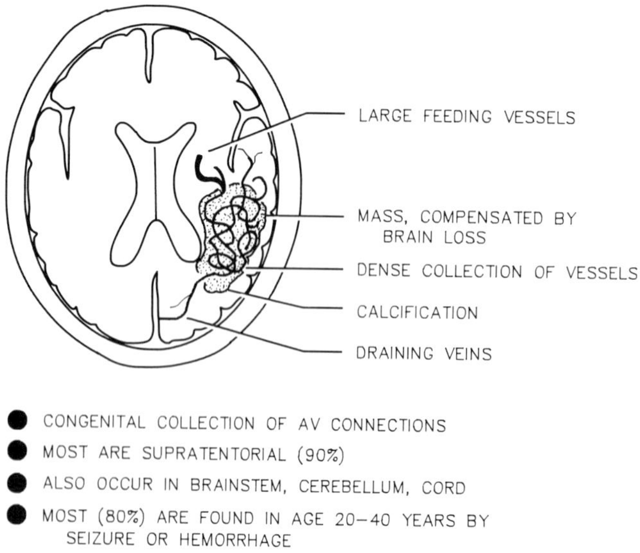

LARGE FEEDING VESSELS

MASS, COMPENSATED BY BRAIN LOSS

DENSE COLLECTION OF VESSELS

CALCIFICATION

DRAINING VEINS

- CONGENITAL COLLECTION OF AV CONNECTIONS
- MOST ARE SUPRATENTORIAL (90%)
- ALSO OCCUR IN BRAINSTEM, CEREBELLUM, CORD
- MOST (80%) ARE FOUND IN AGE 20–40 YEARS BY SEIZURE OR HEMORRHAGE

FIGURE 8–82. Characteristics of arteriovenous malformation. AV, arteriovenous.

venous, and sometimes sinusoidal or capillary connections. It is usually detected in patients 20 to 40 years old, when it causes hemorrhage or seizure. Some 20% of AVMs are discovered in patients older than 40. AVM hemorrhage can be intraventricular or subarachnoid, but most of the blood is adjacent to the lesion and therefore is almost always intra-axial. The proliferation of vessels is accompanied by brain atrophy in the region of the lesion, and so mass effect is minimal.

Contrast CT shows a densely enhancing lesion that exhibits a minimal mass effect (Figs. 8–82, 8–83, 8–84; see also Fig. 8–5). This lack of a mass effect is helpful for distinguishing between an AVM and a malignant tumor. One or more large feeding arteries supply the tumor at the expense of portions of brain normally supplied by these vessels. Draining veins are often visible, as is calcification. The angiogram shows a characteristic dense collection of vessels and early venous shunting of blood.

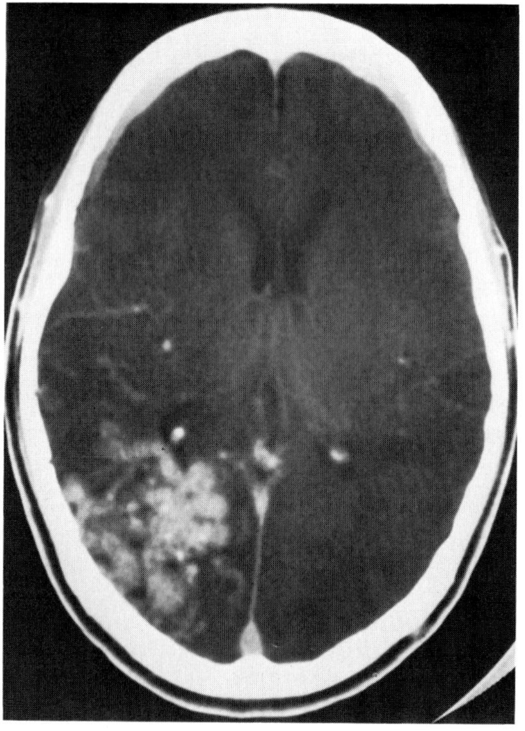

FIGURE 8–83. AVM. Contrast CT at intermediate window settings shows a dense tangle of enhanced vessels in a 49-year-old man who had his first seizure while cramming for an employment examination. The draining veins were shown on lower slices (and angiograms) to be lateral. Note the lack of mass effect as a result of brain tissue atrophy in the area of the AVM. When hemorrhage has occurred, intermediate windows can show blood as medium gray and enhanced vessels as white.

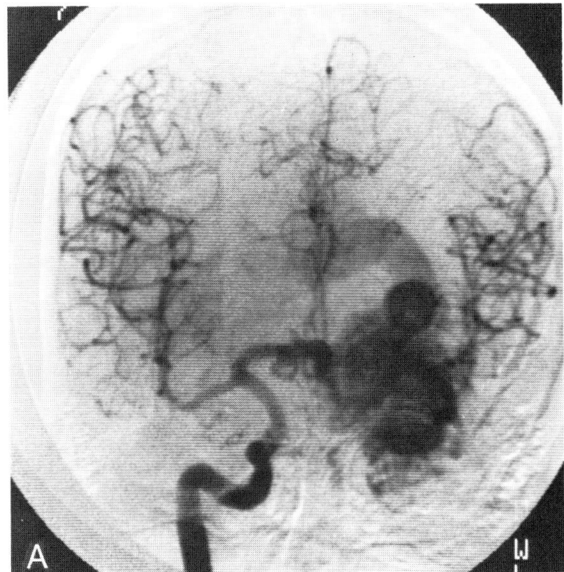

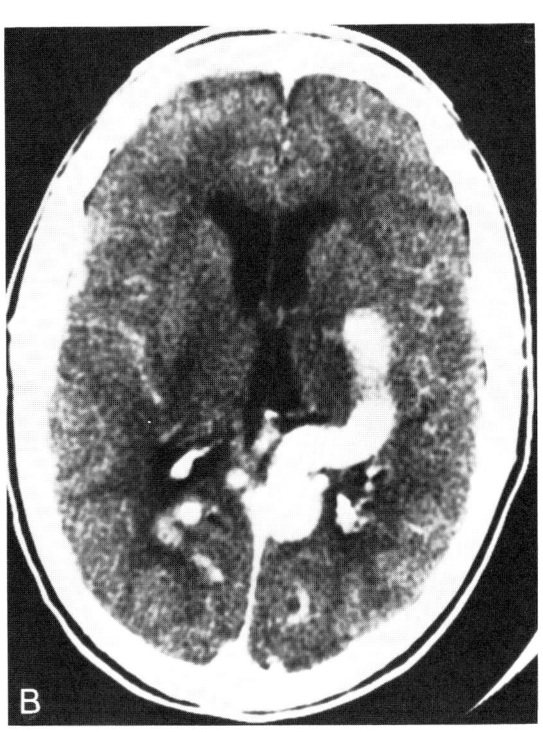

FIGURE 8–84. AVM. *A.* Right carotid angiogram shows dramatic cross-filling of the left cranial circulation caused by a high-flow arteriovenous connection in a 35-year-old woman with seizures and left homonymous hemianopia. The massive vein draining to the vein of Galen is shown here and on CT *(B)*.

MRI can show both the malformation and the vessels supplying and draining it. MRI is especially advantageous in that it provides both the CT and angiographic findings simultaneously. AVMs can be treated by angiographic embolization, surgery, or, less invasively, by radiation therapy.

Occult Arteriovenous Malformation. Some AVMS are not demonstrated on angiograms. Such angiographically occult (cryptic) AVMs are seen on CT as deep hemispheric or brainstem lesions with varying amounts of calcification and enhancement. MRI shows a small focus of high intensity with a rim of paramagnetic low intensity that is attributable to earlier hemorrhage (Fig. 8–85). The lesions may enhance slightly.

Hemorrhage Caused by Coagulopathy. Parenchymal or extra-axial hemorrhage can occur spontaneously or as a result of minor trauma in patients whose coagulation factors are altered. Causes of coagulation disorders include trauma, anticoagulation therapy, alteration of clotting factors caused by tumor or liver disease, hemophilia, and platelet deficiency diseases. Disseminated intravascular coagulation as a result of bleeding elsewhere in the body can deplete clotting factors and lead to hemorrhage. The clinical history is the most important factor for making the diagnosis. The CT appearance of such a hemorrhage varies and can appear similar to any of the hemorrhages described previously. Usually there is parenchymal and subarachnoid blood.

Tumor Hemorrhage. Parenchymal hemor-

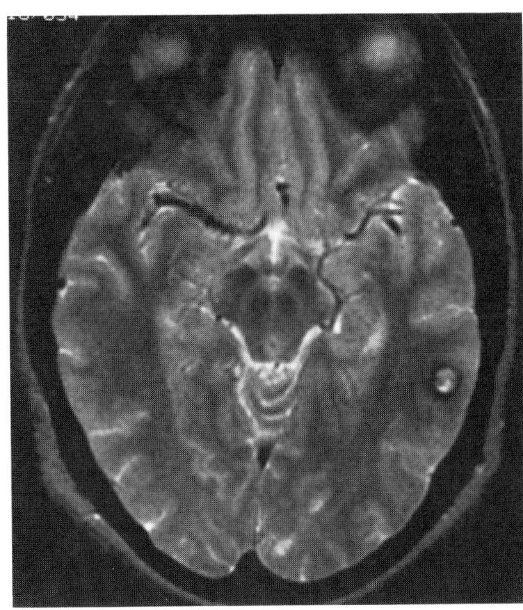

FIGURE 8–85. Occult AVM. Axial T2 spin echo image shows a small lesion with central high intensity in a 33-year-old woman with seizures. The central high intensity, present on both T1 and T2 images, indicates blood. The peripheral low intensity represents paramagnetic material.

rhage can occur with necrosis of a tumor and rupture of its vascular supply. A contrast image does not reliably differentiate among hemorrhage, enhancing tumor, and infarct, and so a noncontrast image should be done first when a patient with a brain tumor suffers acute deterioration. Primary brain tumors, such as glioblastoma, occasionally bleed, but metastatic tumors are more often hemorrhagic in the brain (especially melanoma, renal cell carcinoma, thyroid carcinoma, and choriocarcinoma). Although lung and breast metastases to the brain rarely bleed, they are so common that they cause a large number of hemorrhagic lesions.

Amyloid Angiopathy Hemorrhage. Many cerebral hemorrhages in elderly patients are considered to be caused by amyloid angiopathy. This disease, characterized by the deposition of amyloid protein in the meningeal and parenchymal vessels of the brain, is associated with multiple, small, severe hemorrhages, usually in subcortical sites in elderly patients. Because of amyloid staining by Congo red, the disease is also called congophilic angiopathy. CT shows parenchymal hemorrhage.

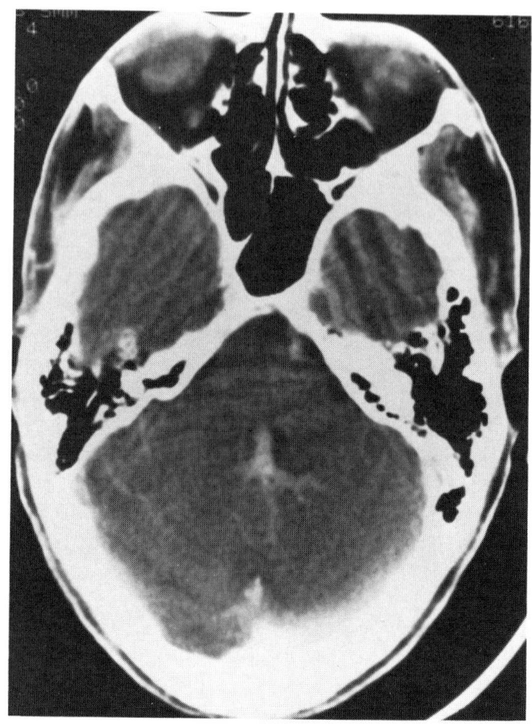

FIGURE 8–86. Venous angioma. Contrast-enhanced CT shows a spoke-like collection of vessels entering a large draining vein in a 47-year-old man with right hypesthesia. Higher slices and angiogram showed drainage superiorly into the vein of Galen.

Venous Abnormalities

Venous abnormalities in the brain and the spinal cord are generally of lesser importance than arterial abnormalities because they are at low pressure and seldom cause hemorrhage. Venous obstruction can cause seizures or necrosis. The most serious lesions are venous angioma, dural arteriovenous communication, and sagittal and cavernous sinus thrombosis.

Venous Angioma. The venous angioma is relatively common (found in 2% of all autopsies) but clinically silent. It is a spider-like collection of veins that drain via a single vein into a large vein or a dural sinus. In rare instances, these tumors cause hemorrhage or seizure. Most are noted incidentally on CT or MRI either as a nodular area of enhancement (the focus of the venous angioma) or as a linear enhancement (the draining vein) (Fig. 8–86). Angiography shows a normal arterial phase and a spoke-like collection of veins draining into a large vein. No therapy is indicated unless the patient has had hemorrhage or seizure.

Dural Arteriovenous Communication. Dural arteriovenous communication (also called dural AVM) is an abnormal communication between meningeal vessels and a dural sinus. This communication occurs either spontaneously or as a result of trauma and appears to be the result of rupture of the small meningeal vessels that supply the walls of the dural sinus. It is most common in the cavernous sinus. Most spontaneous cases occur in middle-aged women. Symptoms depend on the location and the amount of blood flow. They include headache, double vision, proptosis, and cranial nerve deficit.

Angiography demonstrates communication of external or internal carotid meningeal branches with the dural sinus. CT and MRI may show enlarged vessels, particularly an obstructed superior ophthalmic vein. Many dural arteriovenous communications close spontaneously. Various interventional techniques, including manual compression and vascular embolization, are successful in most cases.

Sagittal Sinus Thrombosis. Sagittal sinus thrombosis is an important cause of morbidity and mortality in patients who have cancer, coagulation disorders, cerebral infections, and congenital CNS abnormalities. Important contributing factors include dehydration and, possibly, steroid therapy and birth control pills.

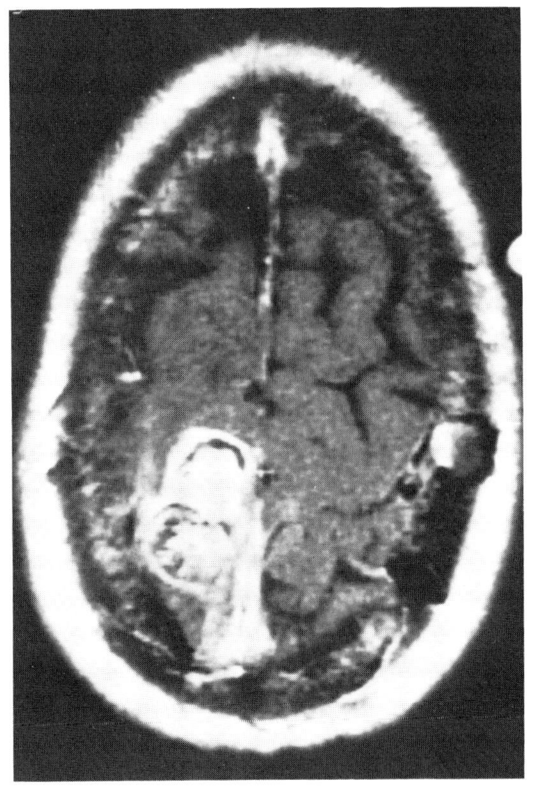

FIGURE 8–87. Sagittal sinus thrombosis. Axial T1 spin echo image that followed Gd-DTPA administration shows dense enhancement of the sagittal sinus and rim enhancement of a hemorrhagic infarct. Higher slices revealed an extracranial sarcoma that apparently arose from radiation to a previously treated temporal lobe glioma (which enhanced on lower slices). Angiography and surgical findings showed that the sarcoma invaded the dura (but not the brain) and occluded the sinus, causing the venous infarction.

When the sinus becomes obstructed, there may not be sufficient collateral veins to prevent brain necrosis. The drainage of CSF from the subarachnoid space is usually impaired, resulting in increased intracranial pressure. The back pressure from obstructed veins results in venous infarction at a superficial (cortical) level or deep in the cerebral hemispheres, depending on which sinus is obstructed. Such infarctions are often hemorrhagic. The clinical signs and symptoms include seizure, headache, nausea, respiratory dysfunction, and neurological deficit, all of which are nonspecific.

CT can show cortical hemorrhage, white matter venous infarction, decreased enhancement of the lumen of the sinus, and small ventricles. Angiograms, which can be obtained quickly with the use of digital arterial or venous injections, show absence of blood flow in the thrombosed sinus. MRI shows the clotted blood in the sinus, which appears as high intensity on T1 and T2 spin echo images and on STIR images. MRI also demonstrates venous infarcts, including a hemorrhagic component. Contrast MRI shows dense enhancement of the clotted blood in the sinus (Fig. 8–87). Magnetic resonance angiography can also show the absence of flow in the sinus.

Cavernous Sinus Thrombosis. The cavernous sinus can become thrombosed when invaded by tumor or infection. Less common causes are trauma and clotting disorders. The most obvious sign of cavernous sinus thrombosis is proptosis resulting from the obstructed and engorged superior ophthalmic vein. The diagnosis is best made on CT or MRI, both of which can show the abnormality in and near the cavernous sinus (see Fig. 8–45). The enlarged superior ophthalmic vein is easily identified by its S-shaped course from medial to lateral, just superior to the optic nerve.

Part II
Orbits, Pituitary Region, and Temporal Bone

DISEASES OF THE ORBITS

Disease in the orbits is caused primarily by tumor, infection, and vascular abnormality. The lesions are divided into those that are outside the cone formed by the extraocular muscles (extraconal), those inside this cone (intraconal), and those within the globe (intraocular).

CT with thin (3-mm) contiguous slices in the axial and coronal planes demonstrates the bones, the soft tissues of the face, the extraocular muscles, the optic nerves, and the globes. Reformatted views in parasagittal planes provide vertical slices along the optic nerve. Slices thinner than 3 mm are not recommended because of the high radiation dose to the lens. Tilting the head back slightly positions the optic nerves in the axial plane. The orbit contains structures of markedly different densities (i.e. fat, vitreous, bone, muscle), and so intravenous contrast is usually not necessary for the demonstration of abnormalities. At present, CT is the best method for the evaluation of most orbital diseases. The orbital fat provides a very intense signal on MRI, which dominates T1 spin echo images. STIR and fat-suppression techniques provide high tissue contrast and excellent spatial resolution and enable imaging in any desired plane.

Extraconal Abnormalities

Extraconal abnormalities are most often caused by infection, inflammatory disease, and tumor. Disease can involve the bone, the adjacent sinuses, and the soft tissues of the orbit. Several systemic and immune inflammatory diseases involve the orbit, including histiocytosis X, midline granulomatous disease, and multisystem lymphoid diseases.

Orbit Infection. Although any infection of the face, the sinuses, or the brain can spread to involve the orbit, the most serious are the opportunistic infections, such as mucormycosis and aspergillosis, because they occur primarily in diabetic or immunosuppressed patients and are difficult to treat (Fig. 8–88). When they extend through the optic canal to the brain, they are rapidly fatal. Many infections arise initially in the paranasal sinuses.

Histiocytosis X. Histiocytosis X includes a group of at least three diseases of young people with characteristics of both immune and neoplastic disease. In very young patients (0 to 3 years of age), it is a systemic disease (Letterer-Siwe disease) that involves the skin and viscera but not the bone. This disease is often fatal with a diffuse encephalitis. In young children (3 to 10 years of age), it involves the sphenoid bone with histiocytic soft tissue mass accompanying bone destruction (Hand-Schüller-Christian disease). These patients often have proptosis and diabetes insipidus as a result of involvement of the orbit, the hypothalamus, and the sella by eosinophilic granulomas. Hand-Schüller-Christian disease responds well to low-dose radiation. Older patients (and those with Hand-Schüller-Christian disease) develop lytic bone lesions called eosinophilic granulomas. These lesions are benign and are

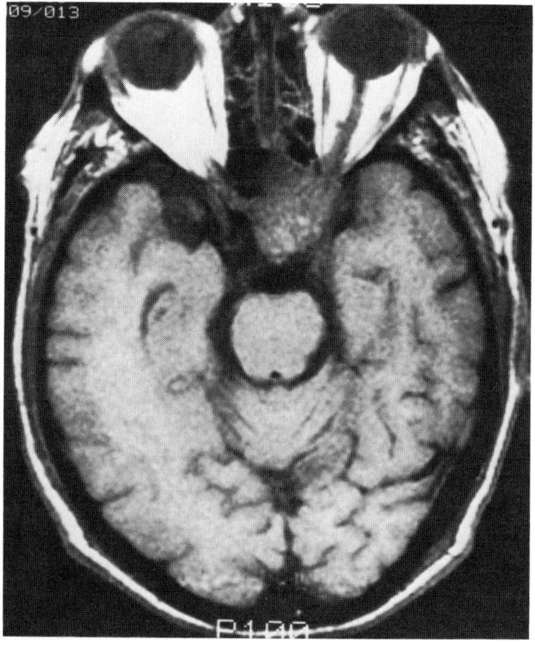

FIGURE 8–88. Aspergillosis. Axial T1 spin echo image shows extensive abnormality involving the optic canal, the sphenoid sinus, the pituitary region, and the cavernous sinus in a 73-year-old man with steroid-induced immunosuppression. Additional slices and coronal views showed extension to the left maxillary, ethmoid, and sphenoid sinuses. Note high intensity of normal fat in the orbits.

of no consequence unless fracture occurs as a result of the weakened bone cortex.

Tumors. The most common extraconal orbital tumor is the benign dermoid. Other primary tumors, such as meningioma, lacrimal gland neoplasms, and osteogenic sarcoma, can also occur in this region. Metastatic tumors to the orbit include those from the common primary tumors (of the lungs, the breasts, and the gastrointestinal tract), those that spread to the bone (such as neuroblastoma), and tumors that arise near and extend into the orbit (such as head and neck tumors, intracranial brain tumors, and lymphoma). Metastatic tumors can be extraconal, intraconal, and intraocular.

Intraconal Abnormalities

Intraconal abnormalities usually arise from the extraocular muscles, optic nerves, or ophthalmic vessels. Inflammatory diseases include Graves' disease, orbital pseudotumor, sarcoidosis, and optic neuritis. A variety of tumors occur in the orbit, the most important of which are meningioma, glioma, and lymphoma. Vascular abnormalities in the orbit include hemangioma, orbital venous varix, ophthalmic artery aneurysm, and distension of the superior ophthalmic vein.

Graves' Disease. The ophthalmopathy of Graves' disease is caused by infiltration of the extraocular muscles by lymphocytes, plasma cells, edema, and mucopolysaccharides, which results in enlargement and consequently proptosis. CT demonstrates enlargement of one or more of the extraocular muscles, most commonly the medial and inferior ones (Fig. 8–89). Because Graves' disease usually affects the belly of the muscles, the optic nerve is rarely compressed except in severe involvement. This pattern differs from that of orbital pseudotumor and orbital lymphoma in most cases.

Orbital Pseudotumor. Orbital pseudotumor is an inflammatory disease of the orbit that most affects the uvea (the rim around the globe) and the insertions of the extraocular muscles. It is the most common intraorbital mass in the 10- to 40-year age group and manifests with proptosis, pain and swelling, and visual loss. CT or MRI shows contrast enhancement, usually around the muscle insertions of the globe, but the inflammation can involve all orbital structures (Fig. 8–90). The appearance and the enhancement, as well as the dramatic response to steroids, enable the correct diagnosis.

Other Inflammatory Diseases. Sarcoidosis of the orbit is a granulomatous involvement of the optic nerve. It often extends intracranially to involve the basal meninges. It is best imaged by contrast CT. Optic neuritis is an inflammation, usually with demyelination of the optic nerve. It is probably an allergic reaction to various infections. It is best shown on coronal STIR MRI.

Optic Nerve Meningioma. The most com-

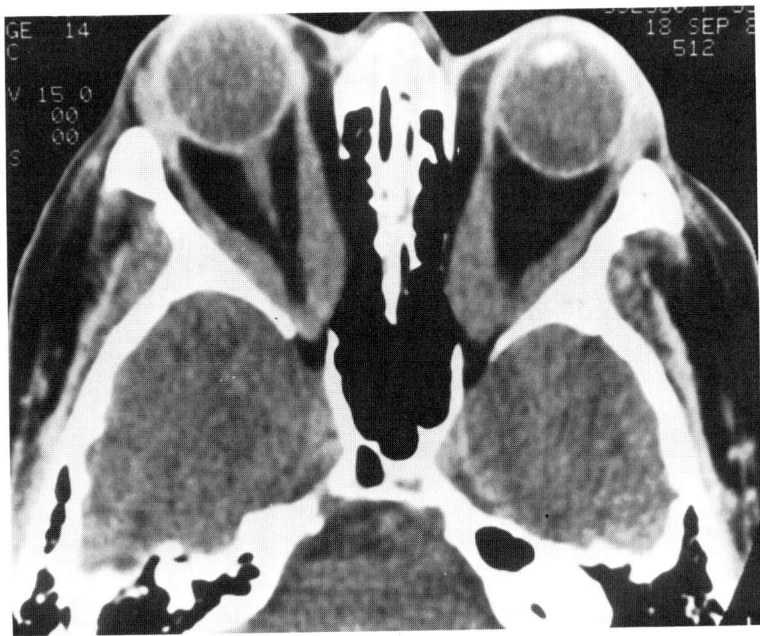

FIGURE 8–89. Graves' disease. Magnified thin-section axial CT of the orbits shows enlargement of the bellies of the medial and lateral rectus muscles bilaterally in a 35-year-old woman with Graves' disease.

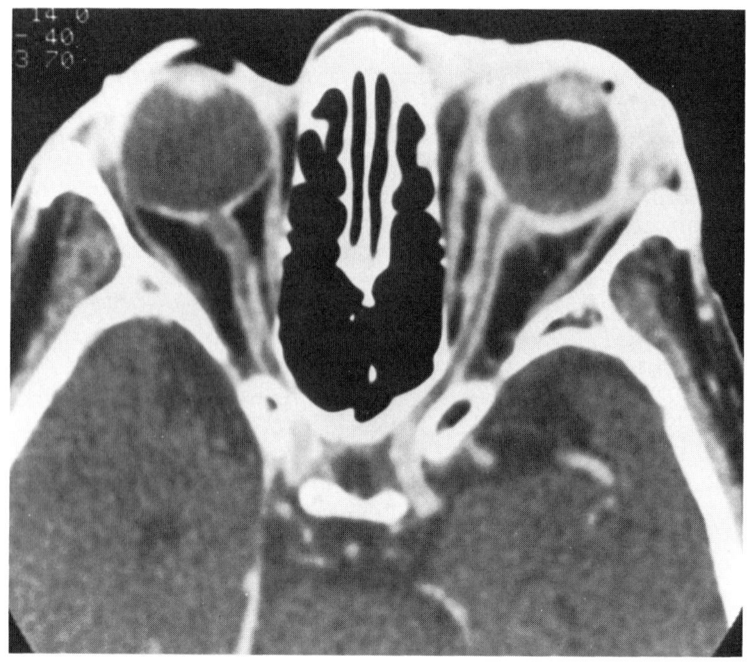

FIGURE 8–90. Orbital pseudotumor. Contrast CT shows dense left-sided enhancement of the uveoscleral rim, the periorbital soft tissues, and the optic nerve sheath in a 42-year-old woman with acute left orbital pain. Enhancement within the orbital fat and consequent proptosis is evident. The enhancement on the right side is much less prominent but is also abnormal (compare with Fig. 8–91, which shows normal enhancement).

mon intraconal tumor is the optic nerve meningioma. It arises from the leptomeninges of the optic nerve and is usually a circumferential mass. The tumor can cause proptosis and blindness when it compresses the optic nerve. CT shows a high-density enhancing mass with the low-density optic nerve traveling through it, a so-called tram-track appearance that shows that the tumor is separate from the nerve (Fig. 8–91). Unenhanced MRI with T2 spin echo sequences shows low-intensity fat, high-intensity tumor, and intermediate-intensity optic nerve. It is difficult to resect the tumor and preserve the patient's vision because of the attachment of the tumor to the optic nerve.

Optic Nerve Glioma. The optic nerve glioma is an astrocytoma of the optic nerve that can extend intracranially or anteriorly to the globe. The low-grade histological appearance of these tumors is not an accurate predictor of the behavior, which can vary from rapid to slow expansion. Most appear to decelerate in growth over time. Patients develop vision loss

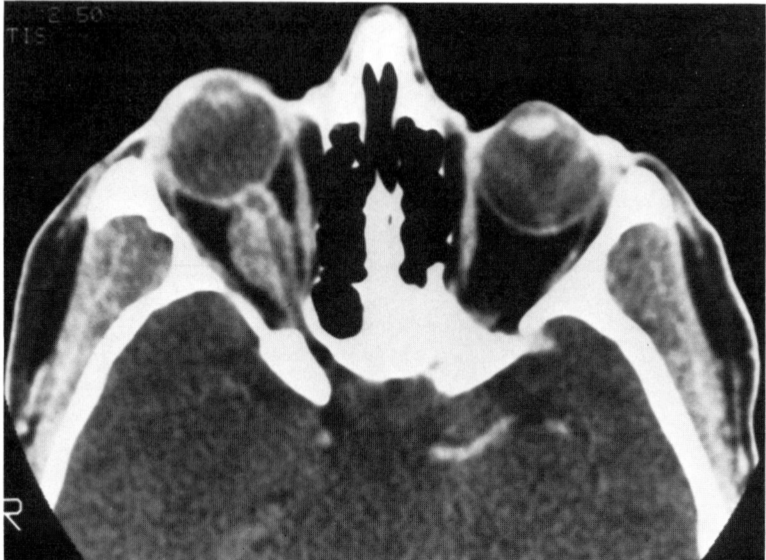

FIGURE 8–91. Optic nerve meningioma. Contrast CT shows a circumferential mass surrounding the low-density optic nerve.

and proptosis, usually without pain. Images show a fusiform or bulbous expansion of the optic nerve and can show extension into the brain along the visual pathways (Fig. 8–92). Prognosis is good, and vision is spared, if the tumor is confined to the orbit, because it can be excised or can be arrested by x-irradiation. In neurofibromatosis, the tumor is usually bilateral and intracranial. Chiasmal gliomas usually occur in the absence of optic nerve gliomas or of neurofibromatosis.

Other Tumors. Other intraconal tumors include orbital lymphoma, neurofibroma, and rhabdomyosarcoma. Primary orbital lymphoma is composed of benign lymphoid tissue, in contrast to secondary lymphoma from elsewhere in the body. It manifests as a painless mass that causes proptosis. The tumor can involve the extraocular muscles, the inner cone, and the lacrimal region. Neurofibroma can arise from any of the orbital nerves, but these are rare. Rhabdomyosarcoma is a rare tumor of the extraocular muscles in children.

Orbital Cavernous Hemangioma. Orbital cavernous hemangioma is the most common primary mass lesion in the orbit. Histological examination shows that it is an encapsulated collection of large vascular spaces in the orbit. It causes proptosis and diplopia. The tumor enhances with intravenous contrast and often fills the orbit, without bone erosion. Calcification is usually present. The tumor is benign and is easily removed at surgery.

Other Lesions. Orbital venous varix is a distensible, redundant venous system in the orbit that fills by gravity or venous backpressure, causing proptosis. CT without and with the Valsalva maneuver can demonstrate the varix, which may be distinguished by calcified phleboliths. Aneurysms of the ophthalmic artery are usually near its origin from the carotid artery. Distention of the superior ophthalmic vein occurs when obstruction or arteriovenous communication causes slowing or reversal of blood flow. Orbital pain, proptosis, and pulsatile sensation are the most common symptoms. CT can demonstrate the enlarged vein and often suggests an abnormality in the cavernous sinus.

Intraocular Abnormalities

The most important intraocular abnormalities are caused by trauma, infection, tumor, and vascular lesions. Traumatic disease of the bony orbit is discussed in Chapter 7. Many congenital syndromes (the neurocutaneous

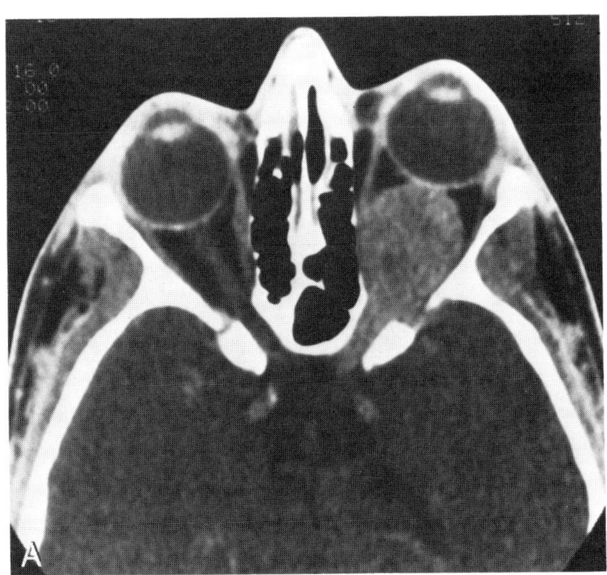

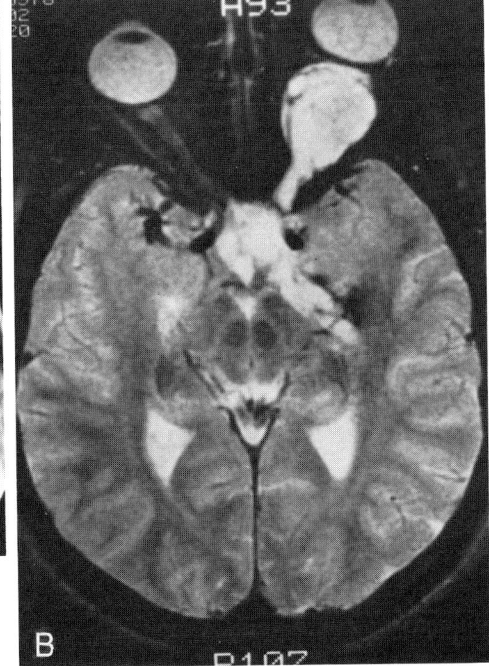

FIGURE 8–92. Optic nerve glioma. *A.* Contrast CT shows a bulbous mass in the left orbit that is causing marked exophthalmus, enlargement of the posterior orbit, and extension through the optic canal in a 15-year-old boy who developed painless visual loss and proptosis. The lesion cannot be separated from the optic nerve on any slices. *B.* MRI 6 months later shows interval enlargement of the orbital mass and intracranial extension involving the optic chiasm and the left optic tracts. Note low intensity of fat in the orbits on this high-field T2 spin echo image.

syndromes) involve the retina and are discussed in the section on congenital brain diseases.

Blunt or penetrating trauma to the globe usually produces obvious abnormalities of fracture, orbital emphysema, and globe displacement. Hemorrhage into the globe is uncommon even in severe blunt facial trauma. Infection of the globe is very rare. The most common infection is toxocariasis, a parasitic disease caused by *Toxocara canis.* The most important tumors are retinoblastoma and choroidal melanoma.

Vascular disease in the globe is usually telangiectasia, most commonly caused by Coats' disease. Pseudotumor cerebri is a syndrome of intracranial hypertension that causes papilledema.

Retinoblastoma. Retinoblastoma is the most common tumor of the globe. It usually occurs by the age of 3 years, can be bilateral (25%), and is usually inherited by autosomal dominant gene. The tumor, composed of malignant retinal cells, causes strabismus and leukokoria. CT shows high density in the globe and, in nearly all cases (95%), calcification (Fig. 8–93). Metastases are to the sclera, the optic nerve, and the brain and CSF pathways. CT or MRI evaluation of patients with retinoblastoma therefore requires careful review of the orbits and the brain.

Choroidal Melanoma. Choroidal melanoma is a primary melanoma of the globe, arising from the choroid and forming an intraocular mass. It is the most common malignant orbital tumor in adults. Patients are asymptomatic until vitreous opacification or retinal detachment occurs. A choroidal melanoma is well-demonstrated on CT as a high-density, noncalcified intraocular mass. The density on MRI is variable, depending on the presence of hemorrhage or pigment, which can cause paramagnetic effects. The tumor may be of the benign nevus type or may be malignant, showing invasion and early metastasis.

Coats' Disease. Coats' disease is a condition of abnormal telangiectatic retinal vessels that result in a hemorrhagic retinitis. Eighty percent of patients are male; the peak age is about 10 years, well above the maximal age for retinoblastoma. Symptoms are painless loss of vision and strabismus. CT shows increased density in the vitreous and retinal detachment, but no calcification. Despite photocoagulation treatment, the disease is progressive.

Pseudotumor Cerebri. Pseudotumor cerebri is a condition of increased intracranial pressure originally defined as idiopathic (i.e., not caused by a mass lesion). It usually occurs in women who are obese or pregnant or who have venous obstruction. Papilledema (100%), headache (90%), and visual symptoms (50%) develop. CT or MRI is required in order to rule out an intracranial mass lesion. These scans also show small ventricles and sulci and swelling of the optic nerve sheaths. Other causes of venous obstruction, such as sagittal sinus thrombosis, may also be demonstrated.

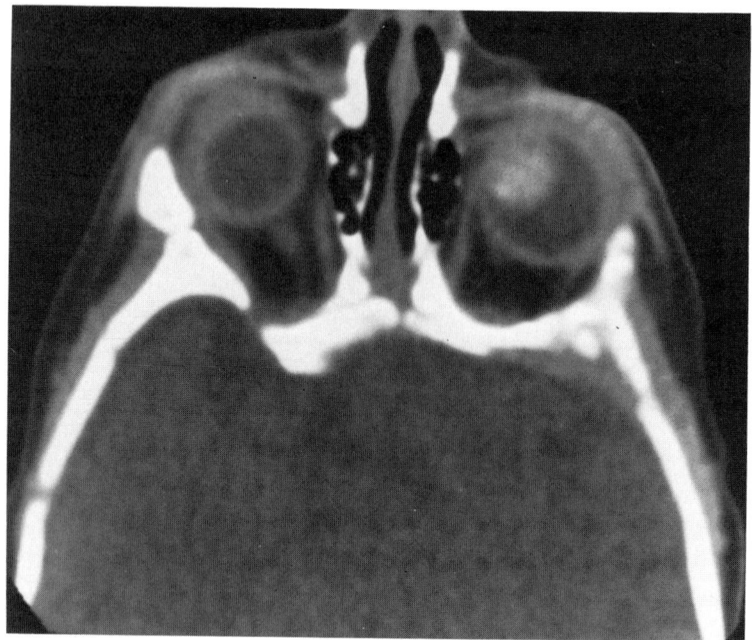

FIGURE 8–93. Retinoblastoma. Noncontrast CT shows a dense lesion in the left eye of a 2-month-old boy with leukokoria. A small fleck of calcium is visible posteromedially.

Treatment may include weight loss, fluid and sodium restriction, steroids, hyperosmotic agents, acetazolamide, and ventricular shunting. The elevated intracranial pressure persists after symptoms subside, and 25% of patients have permanent loss of vision.

DISEASES OF THE PITUITARY REGION

Abnormalities of the pituitary region include bone and cavernous sinus abnormalities and pituitary tumors. Large suprasellar abnormalities (discussed earlier) can be confused with pituitary tumors. The most important suprasellar lesions are aneurysm, meningioma, craniopharyngioma, and optic nerve or chiasm glioma.

Both CT and MRI are effective in imaging the pituitary region. The best technique for demonstrating the pituitary gland is MRI with narrow, contiguous slices in the sagittal and coronal planes. The gland has no blood-brain barrier and enhances more with intravenous contrast than does the normal brain tissue. The evaluation of the pituitary region includes assessment of the clivus, sella, and paranasal sinuses for bone erosion and associated soft-tissue masses and assessment of the pituitary gland for abnormal size and contour and for the presence of focal masses. Most abnormalities of the pituitary gland are of low density on CT and low intensity on T1 spin echo images. They generally enhance less than the normal gland.

Abnormalities of the Bones and the Paranasal Sinuses

Pituitary CT provides excellent detail of the sella turcica, the clivus, and the adjacent sphenoid and ethmoid sinuses. Expansion or erosion of the sella is usually caused by a pituitary mass. Tumors affecting the sella, the petrous apex, and the clivus include meningioma and chordoma. Opacification of the sinuses indicates the presence of sinusitis, tumor invasion, hematoma, or previous surgical resection.

Parasellar Meningioma. Between 10% and 20% of meningiomas occur in the parasellar region. These tumors arise from the dura of the sphenoid wing, the petrous apex, or the dorsum sella. The extra-axial location of the mass can usually be deduced from dural attachment and widening of adjacent cisterns. Bone erosion and dense confluent enhancement are typical of meningioma. The clinical manifestation of parasellar meningioma depends on the structures involved. Symptoms include headache, visual disturbance, and cranial nerve deficits. Meningiomas in this location have the same histological and radiographic appearance as those elsewhere in the cranium. Because they invade the petrous and sphenoid bones, they are difficult to resect.

Chordoma. The chordoma is a rare, slow-growing tumor of notochordal origin that arises in the sacrum (50%), the clivus (35%), and the cervical vertebral bodies (15%). When it occurs in the clivus, it causes symptoms of brainstem compression, including headache, ocular muscle palsy, visual field defect, and long tract signs. It can extend superiorly to involve the sella turcica, the optic chiasm, the cavernous sinus, and the sphenoid sinus. The tumor is a highly vascular, fungating mass that invades locally.

CT demonstrates a predominantly midline, mildly enhancing mass associated with and destroying the clivus (Fig. 8–94). The bone destruction and calcification are most clearly shown on CT. The expansile mass displaces the brainstem. MRI demonstrates the mass as high intensity on T2 spin echo and STIR sequences. It also demonstrates skullbase invasion and displacement of the brainstem. The tumor is difficult to resect and responds poorly to radiation therapy.

Pituitary Tumors

Pituitary Adenoma. Pituitary adenomas can arise from all types of pituitary cells. The classical definition of acidophilic, basophilic, and chromophobic cells is inadequate for defining the many types of adenomas. Many of the functional tumors are chromophobic because they do not possess enough storage granules to take up the appropriate dye, but they can be identified immunocytochemically with specific antibodies to the hormones. Nonfunctional tumors are also chromophobic, but some can be recognized as oncocytomas by the excessive content of mitochondria.

The most common adenomas secrete hormones and cause clinical symptoms as a result of end-organ response (Table 8–7). Nonsecreting tumors do not cause symptoms until they become very large and compress suprasellar or cavernous sinus structures. The pro-

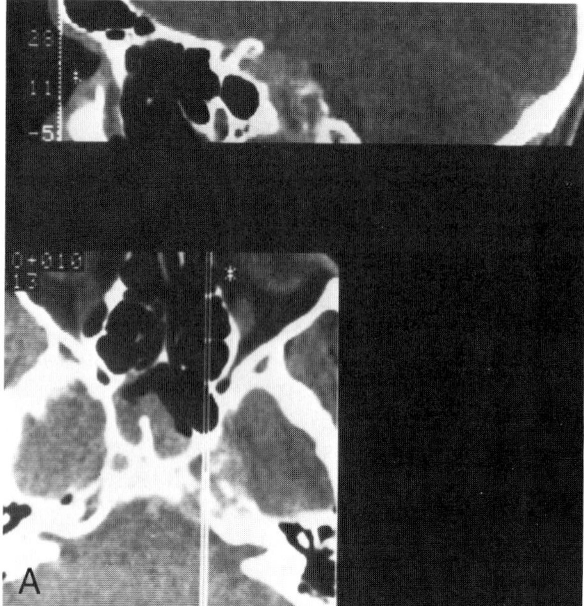

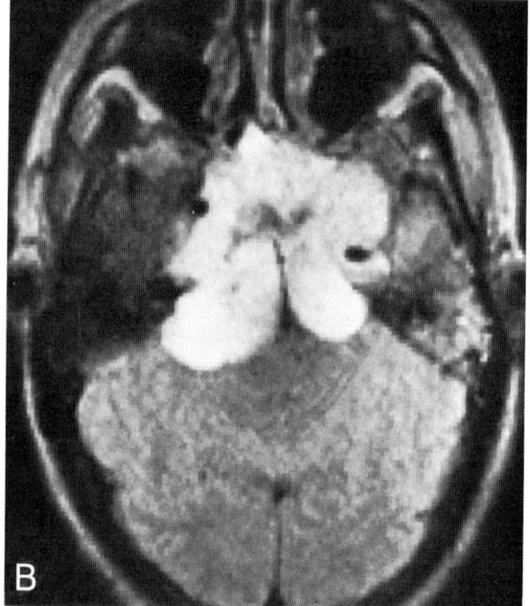

FIGURE 8–94. Clivus chordoma. *A.* Axial and reformatted sagittal CT views show a destructive, calcified lesion in the clivus extending upward to the pituitary fossa in a 41-year-old man with left sixth cranial nerve palsy. The mass involves the left cavernous sinus and carotid canal. *B.* Low-field T2 spin echo image shows tumor invasion of the clivus, parasellar area, and petrous apices in another patient, a physicist with visual impairment and brainstem symptoms. The carotid arteries are patent (the flow void gives them a black appearance) but laterally displaced. The brainstem is posteriorly displaced and merges with the cerebellum because the cisterns are compressed.

lactinoma is the most common pituitary tumor. It usually occurs in young women and causes galactorrhea or amenorrhea; when the tumor occurs in men, it causes impotence. Adrenocorticotropic hormone (ACTH) producing tumors are small (often not visible on images) and cause excessive adrenal gland stimulation with Cushing's syndrome. Growth hormone–secreting tumors often go unnoticed until a friend or a relative of the patient notes the long-term changes of acromegaly or gigantism.

The radiographic appearance of pituitary adenoma depends on the size of the lesion and whether extrasellar extension has occurred. Small endocrine-secreting tumors can be seen as round lesions within the gland. They are of low density on CT and low intensity on MRI and do not enhance as much as the normal gland on immediate postcontrast imaging. Chromophobic adenomas usually enhance. Superior extension causes a convex upper border of the gland, most clearly seen on sagittal views (Fig. 8–95). Such upward convexity of the gland is present in some young women as a normal variation, and so this finding must be interpreted in conjunction with clinical examination. Lateral extension of pituitary adenomas can also be demonstrated by displacement

TABLE 8–7. TYPES OF PITUITARY TUMORS

Type of Secretion	Symptoms	Size of Tumor at Diagnosis	CT/MRI Appearance
ACTH	Cushing's syndrome	Small	Undetectable
Prolactin	Women: galactorrhea, amenorrhea Men: impotence	Small	Low density/intensity
Growth hormone	Acromegaly	Small or large	Low density/intensity
Nonsecreting	Headache, visual abnormalities	Very large	Mass extending up to optic chiasm

CT, computed tomography: MRI, magnetic resonance imaging; ACTH, adrenocorticotropic hormone.

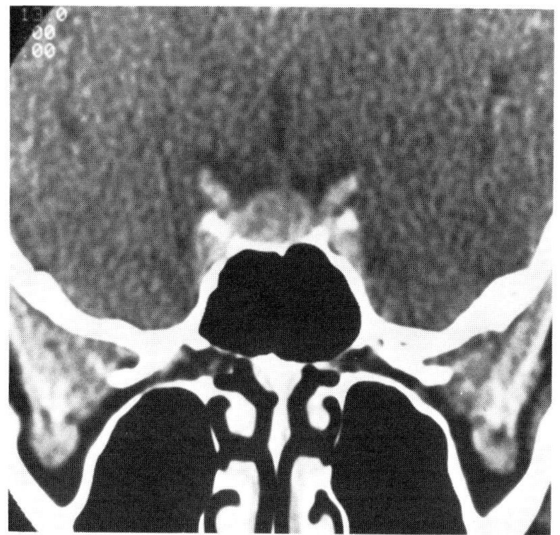

FIGURE 8–95. Chromophobe pituitary adenoma. Direct coronal contrast CT shows enlargement and enhancement of the gland, including a convex superior border, in a 23-year-old woman with Cushing's syndrome. Venous sampling showed an increased adrenocorticotropic hormone (ACTH) gradient, and resection demonstrated an ACTH-producing adenoma. Note the enhanced internal carotid arteries and cavernous sinuses on either side of the mass.

of the cavernous sinus. Large lesions extend superiorly to compress the optic chiasm and hypothalamus and displace the pituitary stalk posteriorly.

In general, adenomas are diagnosed by clinical endocrine signs and symptoms and by biochemical tests. CT or MRI is performed to evaluate the size of the lesion, its location within the gland, and whether it extends outside the sella. Diagnosis of small lesions must be made conservatively because many people have small asymptomatic cysts in the pituitary gland.

ACTH-secreting tumors can be evaluated further on CT of the adrenal glands (see Fig. 4–50) and by means of sampling of the venous system with angiographic catheters. Comparison of the ACTH levels in the inferior petrosal sinus, the jugular bulb, the jugular vein, and the innominate vein bilaterally enables assessment of the likelihood of a pituitary tumor (as opposed to a peripheral endocrine-secreting tumor, such as oat-cell carcinoma). The side on which the tumor occurs can also be predicted. Surgical removal of the pituitary adenoma, usually performed through a transsphenoidal approach, is curative and is associated with low morbidity rates if the lesion is localized within the sella. Bromocriptine, which reduces the size and amount of secretions of prolactinomas, is sometimes used with or instead of surgery.

Other Pituitary Lesions

Other important considerations in the diagnosis of a pituitary mass include empty sella, pituitary apoplexy, arachnoid cyst, Rathke's pouch cyst, granular cell tumor, and lymphocytic adenohypophysitis.

Empty Sella. Empty sella and partially empty sella occur when the sellar diaphragm weakens and the CSF-filled subarachnoid space extends down into the sella and displaces and compresses the pituitary gland (Fig. 8–96). At least 30% of normal persons have a partially empty sella, and so such a finding represents a normal variant rather than a significant lesion. CT or MRI shows CSF in the sella with posterior, midline displacement or flattening of the pituitary gland. The pituitary

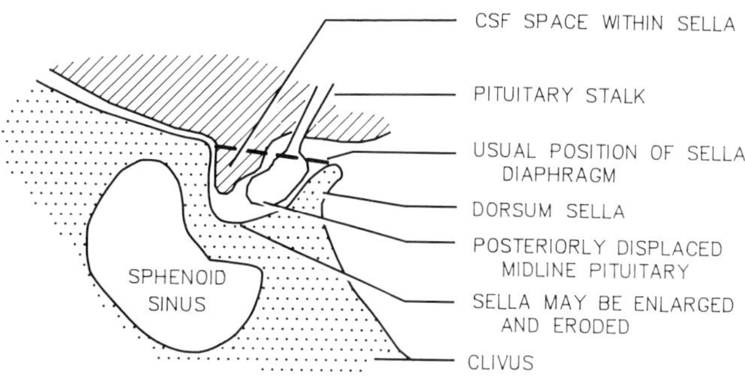

FIGURE 8–96. Characteristics of empty sella. CSF, cerebrospinal fluid; DDx, differential diagnosis.

stalk is in the midline. The condition, when long-standing, can result in enlargement and erosion of the sella. The appearance can be indistinguishable from that of a midline cystic pituitary mass.

Pituitary Apoplexy. Pituitary apoplexy is the spectrum of clinical symptoms associated with stroke in the pituitary gland. The most common manifestation is hemorrhage into a pituitary adenoma. The same symptoms can occur with hemorrhage or infarction of the normal pituitary gland. Patients experience acute onset of symptoms of subarachnoid hemorrhage and hypopituitarism. CT or MRI shows a large sella with blood or tumor. Causes include anticoagulation, Sheehan's syndrome, angiography, and possibly bromocriptine therapy.

Cysts. Arachnoid cysts can occur in the sella and the suprasellar region, resulting in a cystic mass lesion. Most of these cysts cause no symptoms unless they cause ventricular obstruction. CT and MRI show simple fluid, an appearance that is indistinguishable from that of empty sella unless the pituitary stalk is displaced laterally.

Other cysts in the sella may be lined by simple cuboidal epithelium (cyst of the pars intermedia with colloid), columnar nonciliated epithelium (Rathke's pouch cyst), columnar ciliated epithelium, squamous epithelium (craniopharyngioma if it is mucosal; epidermoid tumor if it is epidermal epithelium), or arachnoid epithelium (arachnoid cyst).

Rathke's Pouch Cyst. Rathke's pouch cyst, a cyst of the pituitary gland or stalk, is generally midline within the pituitary fossa. Rathke's pouch cyst is often classified with craniopharyngioma because of its similar embryonic origin, but it is identified on CT and MRI within the sella. Hemorrhage or complex fluid fills the cyst, giving it an unusual signal intensity on MRI, usually high intensity on T1 spin echo images, and low intensity on T2 spin echo images (Fig. 8–97). This appearance, similar to that of fat, is caused by the complex composition and binding of water. Treatment of Rathke's pouch cyst is surgical resection.

Granular Cell Tumor. Granular cell tumor (myoblastoma or choristoma) is a benign tumor of unknown origin. When it occurs in the brain, it is usually in the suprasellar region, separate from the pituitary. The tumor is an amorphous mass composed of polyhedral, granular-appearing cells. Symptoms are produced by the mass effect on the optic chiasm, the pituitary gland, or the hypothalamus. CT shows a homogeneous, enhancing mass in the suprasellar region. The tumor does not metastasize.

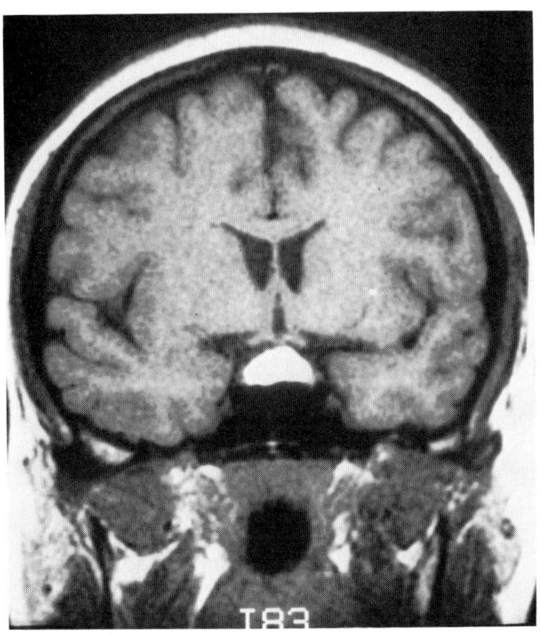

FIGURE 8–97. Rathke's pouch cyst. Coronal T1 spin echo image shows a high-intensity mass that looks like a bag of fluid in the sella in a 23-year-old woman with galactorrhea and mild prolactin elevation. A T2 spin echo sequence showed low intensity, similar to that of fat. At surgery, this cyst was found to contain a dark, thick fluid.

Lymphocytic Adenohypophysitis. Lymphocytic adenohypophysitis is an autoimmune lymphocytic proliferation in the pituitary gland that occurs during pregnancy. It causes hypopituitarism and can result in a large pituitary mass that compresses the optic chiasm. The disease is usually self-limiting, but surgical decompression of the optic chiasm may be necessary.

TEMPORAL BONE DISEASE

Temporal bone disease is usually inflammatory or neoplastic. The most serious inflammatory diseases are external otitis, otitis media, and mastoiditis. The most important tumors are cholesteatoma, epidermoid tumor, cholesterol cyst, and acoustic schwannoma.

Radiographic examination of the temporal bone is directed by the clinical question. CT is generally the preferred examination when bone or middle ear abnormality is suspected because it shows high detail of the osseous structures (see Fig. 7–6). MRI is best for acoustic schwannomas and for invasive soft-tissue masses. When an infection or tumor (particularly cholesteatoma) of the external canal or the middle ear is considered, thin-slice CT (1.5 mm) in the coronal plane without intravenous contrast most clearly shows the area near the tympanic membrane. This technique provides excellent anatomical detail and most clearly displays the abnormalities. Bone and soft-tissue level settings can show the vascular channels, middle ear structures, and nerve canals. For patients who cannot tolerate the neck-extended position required for coronal imaging, axial imaging can be performed and coronal reformations obtained, but structures are not as easily identified. MRI can also demonstrate these lesions, but the lack of bony landmarks and the uniformly high intensity of most abnormalities limit the diagnostic value.

Evaluation of patients who have symptoms of sensorineural hearing loss requires images of the internal auditory canal and the brainstem. For this examination, T1 spin echo axial MRI is recommended, without and with contrast enhancement, of the internal auditory canals and routine imaging of the posterior fossa. Schwannomas show excellent contrast enhancement and are easily seen against the low-intensity CSF on T1 spin echo images (see Fig. 8–99). Because of its good spatial resolution and thin slice capability, CT can also be used to evaluate the internal auditory canals. However, abnormalities in the brainstem and the posterior fossa are difficult to detect on CT because of artifact from adjacent bone.

External Otitis. Infection of the external auditory canal (external otitis) is usually easily detected clinically. Scans are obtained in order to evaluate internal spread. A particularly fulminant infection, malignant external otitis, occurs primarily in diabetic patients. The disease is caused by *Pseudomonas* species and is difficult to treat because of the patient's immune incompetence. CT scans can show fluid and pus in the external ear canal, erosion of adjacent bone, opacification of the mastoid air cells, and spread to the middle ear (Fig. 8–98).

Otitis Media and Mastoiditis. Otitis media and mastoiditis may be acute or chronic and are caused by a variety of bacterial organisms. The normal mastoid air cells and septations are clearly shown on MRI and CT. When the mastoid air cells are opacified as a result of fluid or sclerosis, the cause is usually infection. Otitis media is an infection, usually acute, involving the middle ear and causing opacification of the middle ear cavity. Normal structures, such as the ossicles, are then difficult to identify (see Fig. 8–98).

Cholesteatoma. Acquired cholesteatoma (sometimes called secondary cholesteatoma) is the most common tumor of the temporal bone. It is composed of epidermal squamous cell epithelium and granulation tissue. It arises from the tympanic membrane as a result of chronic inflammation or trauma. Although its cell type is similar to that of epidermoid tumor, cholesteatoma occurs only in the middle ear, and these terms should not be interchanged. Cholesteatomas grow medially and superiorly from the superior border of the tympanic membrane and erode the scutum and ossicles, filling the inner ear.

Coronal CT best demonstrates the erosion of the scutum and the extension into the middle ear and the epitympanum (see Fig. 7–6). MRI shows the mass as high intensity on T2 spin echo and STIR but does not show the bone erosion and the precise location of origin. The cholesteatoma does not metastasize but is locally invasive, and so surgical resection is necessary.

Epidermoid Tumor. The epidermoid tumor, sometimes called a congenital or primary cholesteatoma, is discussed in an earlier section with tumors of the brain. It usually occurs in

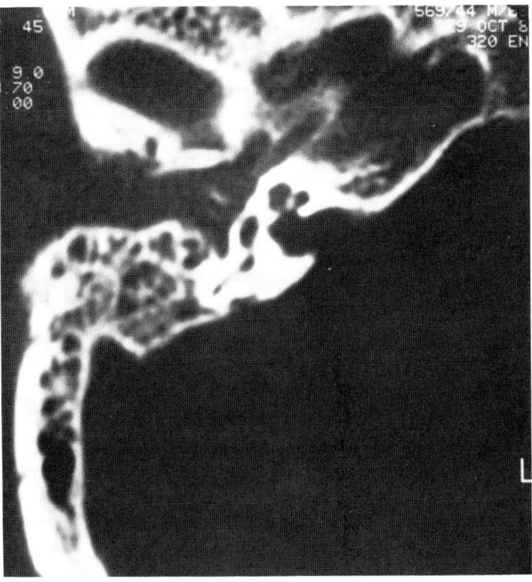

FIGURE 8–98. External otitis. Magnified axial CT of the right temporal bone with the use of bone settings shows fluid within the external auditory canal and anterior bone erosion in a 68-year-old man with purulent drainage. The infection has entered the middle ear cavity and the mastoid antrum, and the mastoid air cells are mostly opacified (these airspaces are normally black on CT).

the ventral subarachnoid space, often in the cerebellopontine angle. It can also occur near the tympanic membrane, and this causes confusion of nomenclature. The tumor has a low-density, nonenhancing appearance on CT. MRI shows the tumor to have characteristics similar to those of water (see Fig. 8–61).

Cholesterol Cyst. The cholesterol cyst, a benign cyst of the paranasal sinuses or the cerebellopontine angle, develops when air-spaces (sinus or mastoid and petrous air cells) become obstructed. The cholesterol contents of the cyst result in a CT appearance similar to that of arachnoid cyst or epidermoid tumor. However, the MRI appearance is of high intensity on T1 spin echo images and low intensity on T2 spin echo images. Treatment is surgical drainage, but it is important not to expel the cholesterol contents into the subarachnoid space.

Acoustic Schwannoma. The most important tumor of the temporal bone is the acoustic schwannoma, a Schwann-cell tumor of the vestibular nerve. Patients usually have sensorineural hearing loss (as a result of compression of the cochlear nerve), tinnitus, or facial pain. Schwannoma of the cochlear or facial nerves also occurs but is less common. The tumor may be in the cerebellopontine angle or within the internal auditory canal.

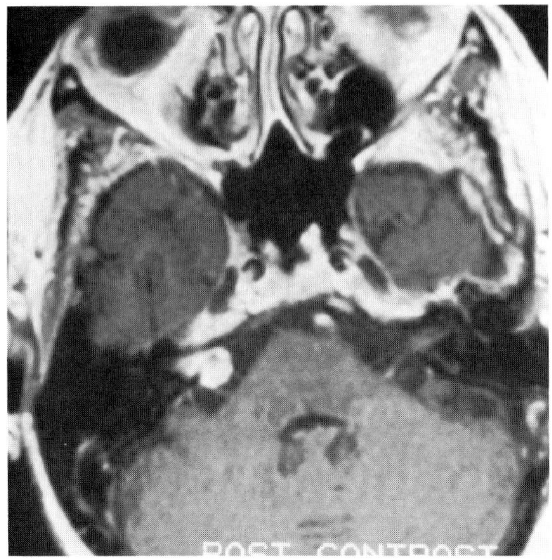

FIGURE 8–99. Acoustic schwannoma. Gd-DTPA enhanced T1 spin echo image shows a left, internal auditory canal mass that is causing the facial nerve to splay anteriorly and the superior vestibular nerve to splay posteriorly in a 68-year-old woman with sensorineural hearing loss. The next lower slice confirmed that the origin of the tumor was the inferior vestibular nerve. Note the intracanalicular extension of the tumor and the normal appearance of the nerves on the left side.

Initial evaluation is best performed with axial T1 spin echo sequences to show the anatomical structures in the optimal plane (Fig. 8–99). The tumor is of intermediate intensity in comparison with low-intensity CSF and cortical bone. Contrast T1 spin echo images show densely enhanced tumor against the low-intensity surrounding structures. Because intracranial lesions can also cause similar symptoms, a routine brain scan is also indicated. Additional evaluation can be performed with coronal MRI and high-resolution CT with intravenous contrast or intrathecal air. The tumor is benign but must be surgically removed in order to prevent permanent impairment.

Vascular Lesions. It is important to recognize vascular lesions of the temporal bone because they can rupture spontaneously or as a result of surgery and because they are often treatable angiographically. CT shows enhancement of the lesion and demonstrates the location of the mass within the bone. MRI can show a variety of appearances as a result of flow phenomena. The most important vascular lesions of the temporal region are glomus tumor, anomalous jugular bulb, and aberrant carotid artery.

Part III
Spinal Disease

Neurological disease of the spine can result from mechanical compression caused by trauma, from congenital disease, from infection, from tumor, and from vascular disease. The extraneural aspects of these diseases are discussed in Chapter 7. Intrinsic lesions, such as infection and tumor, directly involve the cord and the nerve roots.

TRAUMA

Trauma to the spine can result in contusion or transection of the spinal cord or avulsion of nerve roots. Causes include fracture, dislocation, penetrating injuries, and hemorrhage. Most of these causes can injure the cord or the nerve roots directly or can produce delayed mass effect from hemorrhage or edema.

Additional factors that contribute to the severity of spinal cord trauma are a congenitally narrow canal, disc herniation, pre-existing degenerative disease, and the presence of fracture fragments in the canal. Transection of the cord at the cervical level can be obvious when marked spondylolisthesis is present. However, when such a traumatic injury is followed by realignment of the vertebral bodies, the cord may appear normal on myelograms or CT, even if the patient is paraplegic. MRI can show hemorrhage or contusion of the cord. The most serious nervous system injuries are contusion, myelomalacia and syrinx, and cord or nerve root compression.

Contusion. Cord contusion, like similar lesions in the brain, is the result of traumatic compression of tissue. In the spinal cord, however, the lesion is small and more difficult to detect. It is not well shown on CT or myelograms unless there is obvious swelling of the cord. On MRI with T2 spin echo or STIR sequences, the edematous area of compression or hemorrhage is of high signal intensity. The prognosis of cord contusion depends on the severity of the initial clinical symptoms. Delayed swelling can cause catastrophic progression of symptoms if there is inadequate room for expansion. Improvement in neurological function, if it occurs, is usually within the first week after the injury. Later effects of cord contusion are myelomalacia (resorption of infarcted tissue) and syrinx (Fig. 8–100).

Myelomalacia and Syrinx. Traumatic injury to the cord can cause infarction of tissue with subsequent resorption, leaving cystic cavities called myelomalacia (see Fig. 1–15). A large cavity, which is often not in the center, may be called a posttraumatic syrinx. In addition, a syrinx can form as a result of obstruction of the central canal and can have an appearance similar to that of congenital syrinx (see Fig. 8–31). The posttraumatic syrinx may communicate with the subarachnoid CSF space and the central canal of the cord and can become evident days to months after injury. The CSF collection within the cord compresses nerve tracts and leads to neurological dysfunction. Although a syrinx can be demonstrated on CT after injection of intrathecal contrast, it is most clearly and most easily demonstrated on sagittal MRI.

The most common thoracic cord injury is a compression fracture caused either by a fall or by an automobile accident when the seat belt

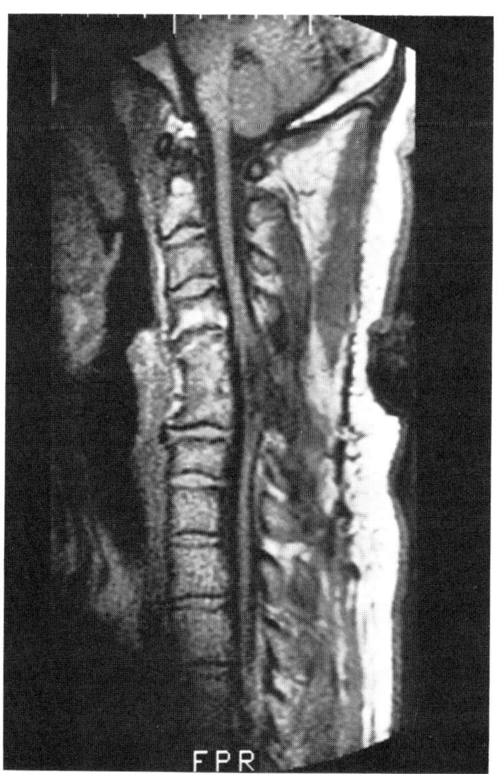

FIGURE 8–100. Posttraumatic myelomalacia. Sagittal T1 spin echo MRI shows fusion at the level of C5-C6, which was necessitated by a football injury. The spinal cord was damaged at the time of the injury and shows marked myelomalacia and posttraumatic syrinx. The distal cord is atrophied.

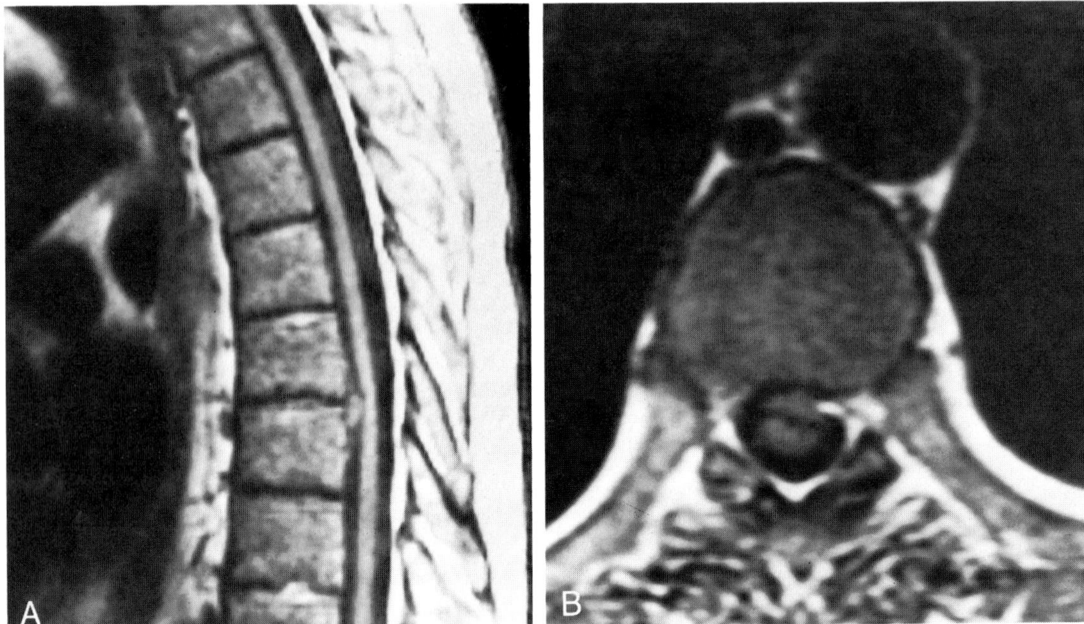

FIGURE 8–101. Thoracic disk herniation. *A.* Sagittal T1 spin echo image shows a soft-tissue mass at the disc space between T-8 and T-9 in a man who developed a T-5 sensory level after a fall. *B.* Axial T1 spin echo image shows the herniated disc material compressing and flattening the cord.

holds the body steady and the spine bends rapidly forward. MRI is ideal for noninvasive evaluation of thoracic cord injury, hematoma, or herniated disk (Fig. 8–101). Evaluation of nerve roots and identification of bone fragments requires CT or myelography.

Lumbar spine injuries that involve the spinal cord and the nerve roots include traumatic disc herniation, fracture, and dislocation. Because of the strength and orientation of the lumbar vertebral bodies, injuries of the lower back do not affect the cord or the roots as frequently as do injuries of the cervical and thoracic spine. Because the posterior elements are large, facet fractures and dislocations are uncommon. Traumatic disc rupture typically results from a fall from an awkward position. Neurological deficit is localized to the distribution of the compressed nerve root (see Fig. 8–8).

CONGENITAL DISEASES

Congenital spinal abnormalities are often associated with brain anomalies. The most commonly encountered congenital spinal abnormalities are part of the spinal dysraphic syndromes, especially Chiari malformations (see the "Congenital Diseases" section in Part I). These lesions, which can also occur separately, include meningocele, syrinx, tethered cord, and lipoma.

Meningocele. Fusion defects of the vertebrae can allow bulging of nervous tissue outside the spinal canal (Fig. 8–102). The least severe fusion defect, spina bifida occulta, is a failure of closure of the posterior elements of the spine, usually in the lumbar region, without bulging of the thecal sac. The bone defect is well shown on plain films, CT, and MRI. A myelogram demonstrates the normal thecal sac. These patients are at risk for nerve root trauma at the location of the defect and may have other occult congenital malformations.

A meningocele, a bulging of the thecal sac but not of the nerve roots into a spina bifida defect, is usually apparent clinically as a visible mass. Myelograms demonstrate the bulging CSF-containing thecal sac and the normal position of nerve roots. A meningomyelocele is a bulging thecal sac that contains nerve roots, the spinal cord, or both. Meningomyeloceles are highly associated with Chiari type II malformation, especially when they occur as weeping, open lesions (not covered by skin) in the lumbar region, but not when they occur in the sacral region as skin-covered masses. In addition to an obvious mass in the lower back noted at birth, infants usually have lower extremity, bowel, and bladder dysfunction. Children with meningomyeloceles are prone to

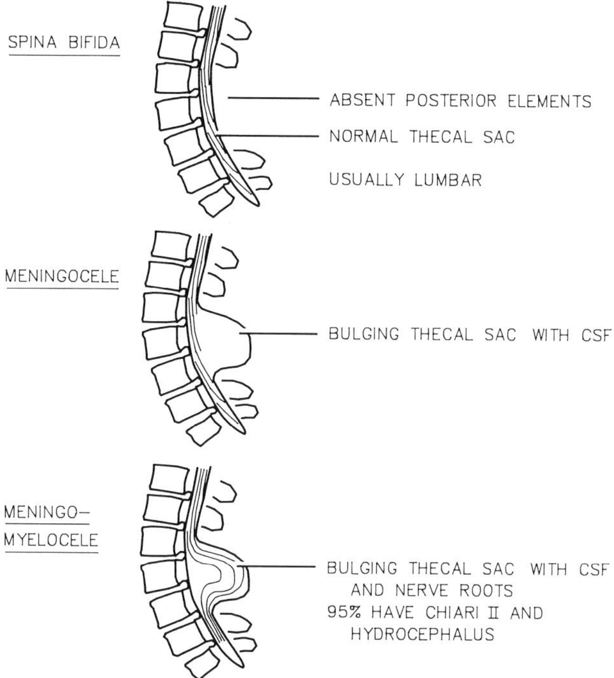

FIGURE 8–102. Characteristics of spinal fusion defects. CSF, cerebrospinal fluid.

injury and infection. Modern therapy, including surgical closure on the day of birth and shunting of the accompanying hydrocephalus, has resulted in nearly normal lifestyles for many patients with meningomyelocele.

Syrinx. A syrinx may be seen in patients with Chiari type II malformation, and most patients with congenital syrinx have additional midline CNS abnormalities. The most important mechanism in the causation of cervical syrinx is postulated to be obstruction of the foramina that drain the fourth ventricle and persistence of the central canal from the obex into the spinal cord. The pulsation of the ventricular CSF then causes the ependyma of the central canal of the spinal cord to break, which in turn causes CSF to dissect into the subependymal gray matter and to form the syrinx (see Fig. 8–31).

Tethered Cord. The spinal cord is normally attached at its sacral end by the filum terminale as a result of atrophy of most of the embryonic coccygeal segments. The distal end of the cord, the conus medullaris, is normally at about the L-1 level. In midline fusion anomalies, the end of the cord can become tethered lower. A syrinx, a meningocele, or a lipoma is often associated with the low position of the cord (Fig. 8–103). Thickening of the filum terminale, sacral agenesis, and clear attachment of the low-lying cord are additional radiographic findings. The term "tethered" should be used carefully for two reasons: (1) sometimes the cord is low in position but not tensely tethered, and (2) the term can also refer to scarring of the surgically released cord to the healed wound site. Surgical release of a tethered cord results in symptomatic improvement, but in general the cord remains in the low position.

Duplication of the spinal cord, diastematomyelia, is a midline fusion defect with splaying or doubling of the spinal cord. A bony spur often separates the cords. Tethering of the cord at the sacrum, lipoma, dermoid tumor, and epidermoid tumor are commonly associated as part of the spectrum of spinal fusion defects. Patients usually develop bladder or lower extremity dysfunction in early childhood.

Neurofibromatosis. Neurofibromatosis (discussed with congenital brain lesions earlier) also affects the spine with neural tissue tumors (either schwannomas or neurofibromas) and meningiomas. These tumors are usually extramedullary and intradural, and as such they compress the cord or cauda equina (Fig. 8–104). Neurofibromas often arise at the neural foramina, causing compression of the nerve and enlargement of the foramen. They are often partially intradural and partially extradural, and thus they have a bilobed shape (called dumbbell neurofibromas). Dural ecta-

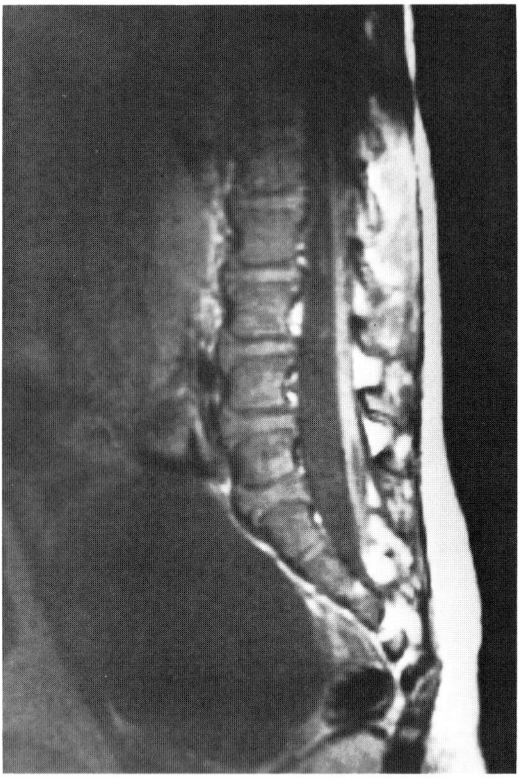

FIGURE 8–103. Tethered cord. Sagittal T1 spin echo image shows a low-lying cord with a central syrinx (low intensity) and ending in a lipoma (high intensity). The cord has a taut appearance and is clearly posteriorly constrained, and so it can be described as being tethered. Note also absence of lower posterior elements, the dilated dural sac, sacral agenesis, and the enlarged, neurogenic bladder.

sia, a developmental enlargement of the thecal sac, can cause distention of nerve roots.

INFECTION

Infection of the spinal cord or nerve roots usually occurs in conjunction with osteomyelitis or a paraspinous abscess. Osteomyelitis of the spine is usually a hematogeneously spread infection from the genitourinary tract, the skin, or the lungs. Paraspinous abscess with resultant spinal cord involvement can occur in retropharyngeal abscess, pleural empyema, psoas abscess, infected aortic aneurysm, rectal abscess, decubitus ulcer, or a congenital dermal sinus tract. Neurological symptoms develop when the infection spreads to the subdural space or when an epidural abscess compresses the cord or the nerve roots. Infections can be caused by bacteria, tuberculosis, and fungal infections.

Bacterial Infection. Bacterial infection of the spine, the spinal cord, and the nerve roots is most commonly caused by staphylococci, streptococci, and gram-negative rods. It can affect any portion of the spine. Hematogeneously spread bacterial infection most often involves the lumbar and thoracic levels. Patients have fever and general malaise, back pain, and, in particular, point tenderness. These symptoms assist in locating the level of the infection. Such infections usually involve one disc and the adjacent vertebral body endplates. When the infection spreads to the epidural space (about 20% of cases), neurological signs of cord or nerve root compression develop.

Spine plain films and CT show irregular destruction of the endplates of the vertebral bodies, narrowing of the disc space, and, in advanced disease, a paraspinous mass. Myelograms and enhanced CT shows cord or nerve root compression and effacement of fat in addition to the aforementioned findings (Fig. 8–105). When the infection is from a paraspinous source, such as pleural empyema or retropharyngeal abscess, MRI is most informative for evaluating the involvement of the spine, the paraspinous soft tissues, the spinal cord, and the nerve roots. High-contrast sequences, such as STIR and T2 spin echo, are necessary for demonstrating the abscess against the normal tissues. Use of intravenous paramagnetic contrast is particularly advantageous because it shows the high-intensity enhanced infection

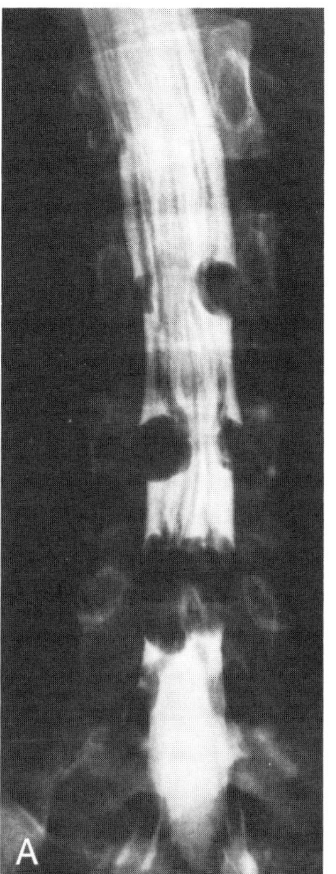

FIGURE 8–104. Neurofibroma. *A.* Myelogram, performed with water-soluble contrast, best demonstrates the numerous intradural neurofibromas in a young woman with neurofibromatosis. Thirteen tumors that caused symptoms had been resected previously. *B.* Extradural tumors are best detected by means of MRI. A Gd-DTPA enhanced T1 spin echo image barely shows this extraforaminal lesion in another patient (the one described in Fig. 8–37) with multiple lesions. *C.* The STIR sequence, by suppressing fat and showing very high contrast of the tumor, provides easy diagnosis.

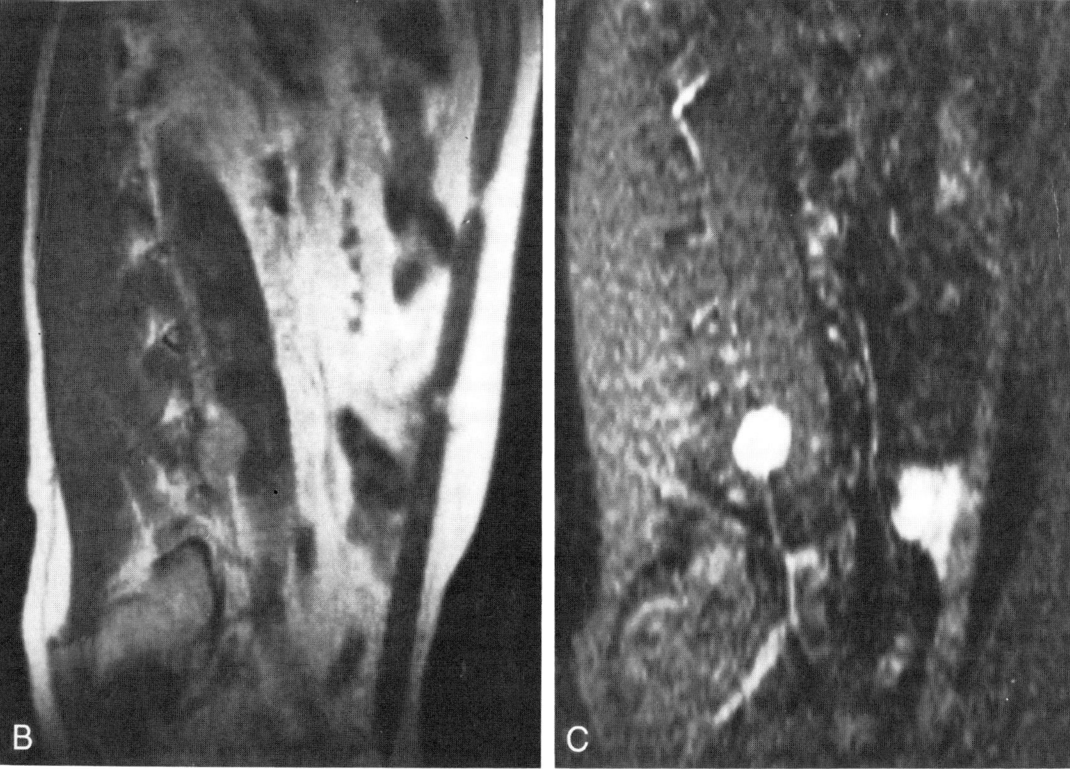

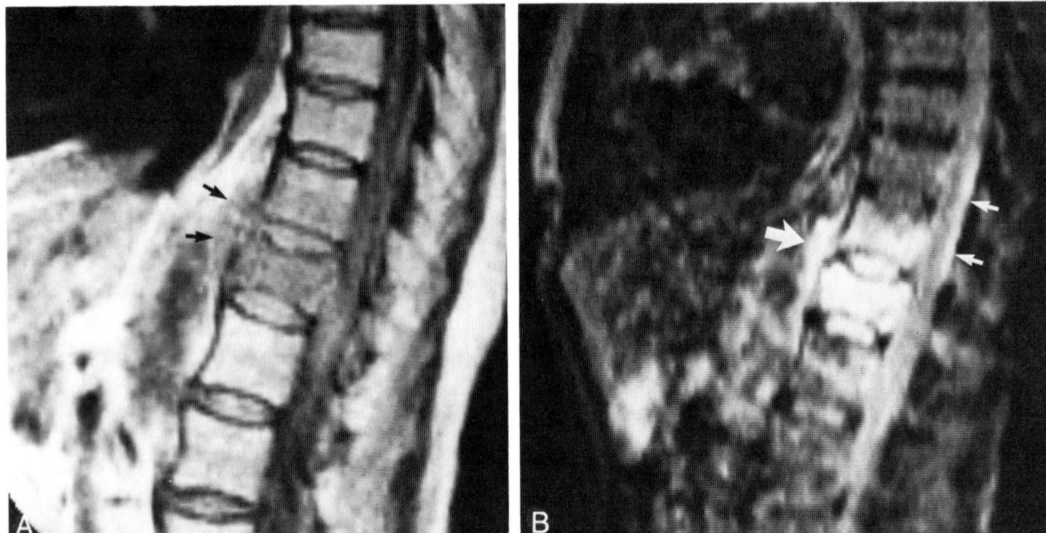

FIGURE 8–105. Spinal epidural abscess. *A.* T1 spin echo image shows decreased marrow intensity in the T-11 and T-12 vertebral bodies, a paraspinous mass *(arrows)*, and compression of the thecal sac in an elderly woman with *Klebsiella* sepsis. *B.* STIR image provides very high contrast, showing involvement of T-11, T-12, and L-1. A linear zone, posterior to the thecal sac (*small arrows*), shows an epidural abscess. The paraspinous mass (*large arrow*) is also well shown. This examination was performed in less than an hour and provided all the findings of CT, myelography, and bone scan. (From Bertino RE, Porter BA, Stimac GK, Tepper SJ: Imaging spinal osteomyelitis and epidural abscess with short TI inversion recovery (STIR). Am J Neuroradiol 1988, 9:563–564.)

against the low-intensity CSF on T1 spin echo images.

Tuberculosis. Tuberculosis of the spine is now rare in the United States because of the availability of antibiotic therapy, but it is still common in underdeveloped countries. Symptoms of back or abdominal pain, general malaise, and fever are nonspecific, and the infection often goes undiagnosed for years. The infection involves the vertebral bodies and spreads through disc spaces. A paraspinous abscess (Fig. 8–106) and abrupt angulation of the diseased spine (gibbous deformity) can be demonstrated by plain radiographs and CT. MRI shows all aspects of the disease noninvasively and should be the first examination when symptoms and signs of cord compression develop. Further evaluation with myelography or contrast CT may assist in surgical drainage or follow-up of therapy.

Fungal Infection. Fungal infections of the spine are rare. They can be caused by hematogenous involvement in septicemia or, rarely, by contiguous spread from a local process. The most common organisms are *Coccidioides immitis* and *Blastomyces dermatitidis*. Other organisms are occasionally seen in immunosuppressed patients. Usually, fungal infections involve the spine diffusely and cause a variety of nonspecific symptoms. MRI most clearly demonstrates destructive lesions in the bone, paravertebral abscess, and spinal cord or nerve root compression.

NEOPLASTIC DISEASE

The most important factor in the assessment of spinal tumors is the location (Fig. 8–107). Intramedullary tumors generally cause a diffuse widening of the cord and symmetrical effacement of the CSF space. Most intramedullary tumors are ependymomas (60%) and astrocytomas (25%). Intradural (extramedullary) lesions displace the cord to one side and cause enlargement of the CSF space above and below the mass. The most common of these lesions are schwannomas, neurofibromas, and meningiomas. Extradural lesions cause asymmetrical compression of the thecal sac and bone destruction. The most common causative tumors are metastases. However, degenerative disease and disc herniation are the most common causes of extradural lesions.

Schwannoma and Neurofibroma. The schwannoma, a tumor of Schwann's cells of the neural sheath, is the most common spinal canal tumor. It most often occurs as an isolated

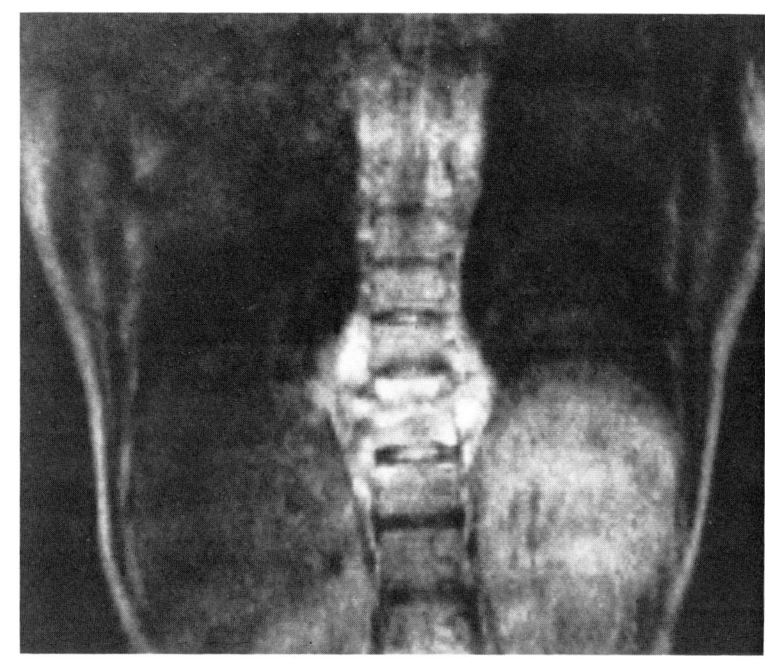

FIGURE 8–106. Spinal tuberculosis. Coronal T2 spin echo image shows the infection in the bone and the paraspinous abscess. Tissue contrast is not as high as that provided by STIR sequences, but it is acceptable. Image detail is good and respiratory artifact does not interfere with the appearance of the spine in this low-field image (0.15 T).

INTRAMEDULLARY

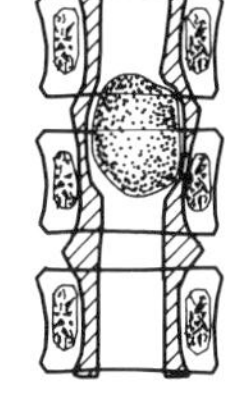

TUMOR	OTHER
EPENDYMOMA	SYRINX
GLIOMA	CONTUSION
METASTASIS	MYELITIS
LIPOMA	HEMORRHAGE
HEMANGIOBLASTOMA	

EXTRAMEDULLARY

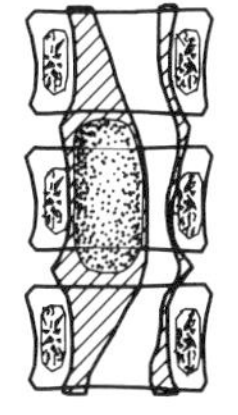

TUMOR	OTHER
MENINGIOMA	AV MALFORMATION
NEUROFIBROMA	ARACHNOID CYST
METASTASIS	ARACHNOIDITIS
LIPOMA	
DERMOID	

EXTRADURAL

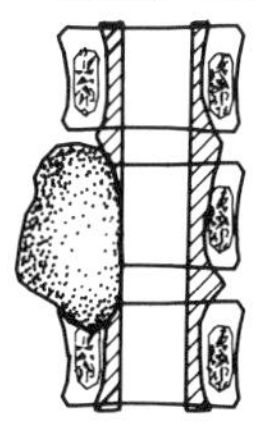

TUMOR	OTHER
METASTASIS	HERNIATED DISK
LYMPHOMA	FRACTURE FRAGMENT
NEUROFIBROMA	SURGICAL SCAR
MENINGIOMA	HEMATOMA

FIGURE 8–107. Locations of spinal tumors. AV, arteriovenous.

lesion but is frequently seen in patients with neurofibromatosis. The tumor is usually eccentric and encapsulated. The usual manifesting sign is nerve root compression. When the tumor is in the dural space, it is well-demonstrated by myelograms and enhanced MRI. In the paraspinous area, STIR images provide the best tissue contrast (see Fig. 8–99, 8–104).

Neurofibromas are usually multiple and diffusely enlarge the nerve root; thus they are not encapsulated proximally or distally. In the spine they are often peripheral in location. Like schwannomas, they are of very high intensity on STIR images and enhance intensely with paramagnetic contrast.

Meningioma. The spinal meningioma is the second most common spinal canal tumor. It is difficult to detect in the spine because it is often a plaque conforming to the shape of the canal. Dense enhancement with contrast is essential for CT or MRI diagnosis. The same difficulties with unenhanced MRI in the detection of meningiomas encountered in the brain are present in the spine.

Ependymoma. Ependymomas arise from the ependymal cells that line the ventricular system of the brain (see also discussion in Part I) and the central canal of the spinal cord. They constitute 60% of gliomas of the spinal cord, in which they usually involve the cauda equina and the filum terminale (Fig. 8–108). Children and adolescents are affected most often and develop symptoms of central cord compression, conus syndrome, or cauda equina syndrome, depending on the location of the tumor. Although the tumor is infiltrative in the brain, it is usually elongated and relatively smooth in the spinal cord, the cauda equina, and the filum terminale. Most spinal ependymomas are histologically benign, but the compression of the cord can cause serious neurological problems. When the tumor does not infiltrate the normal cord, it is easily removed at surgery with minimal injury to adjacent tissue (Fig. 8–109), but local x-irradiation is still essential in order to prevent recurrence. More aggressive forms of ependymoma also occur in rare instances in the spinal region,

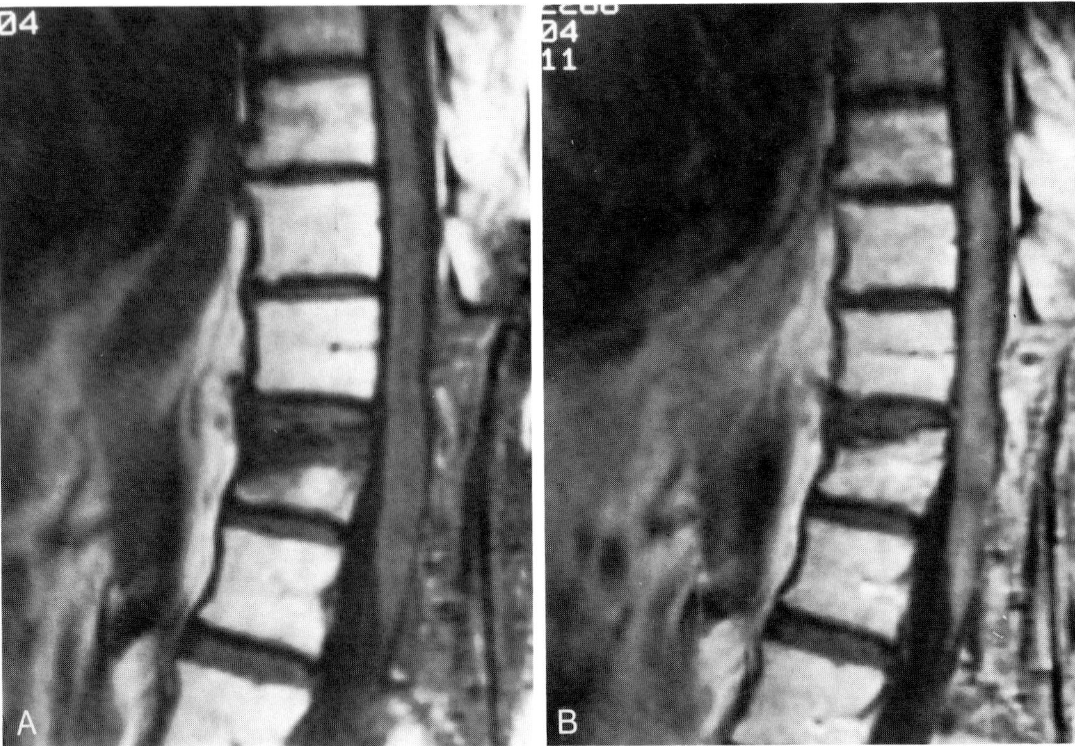

FIGURE 8–108. Recurrent conus medullaris ependymoma. *A.* Precontrast T1 spin echo image shows enlargement and inhomogeneity in the conus medullaris in this previously operated low-grade malignant ependymoma. Postoperative changes are noted in the soft tissues, and there is partial collapse of the T-12 vertebral body. *B.* After Gd-DTPA administration, the terminal cord and the conus enhance markedly as a result of diffuse involvement with recurrent tumor. Note the Gd-DTPA enhancement of tumor in the collapsed vertebral body and the posterior postsurgical scarring. The normal cord does not enhance because of the blood-cord barrier.

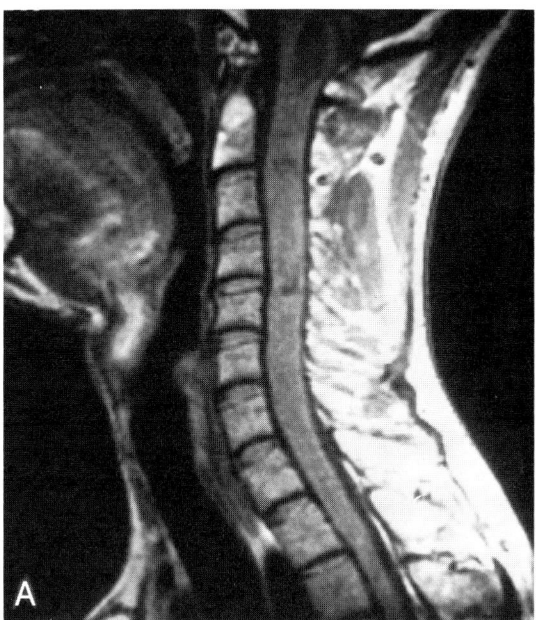

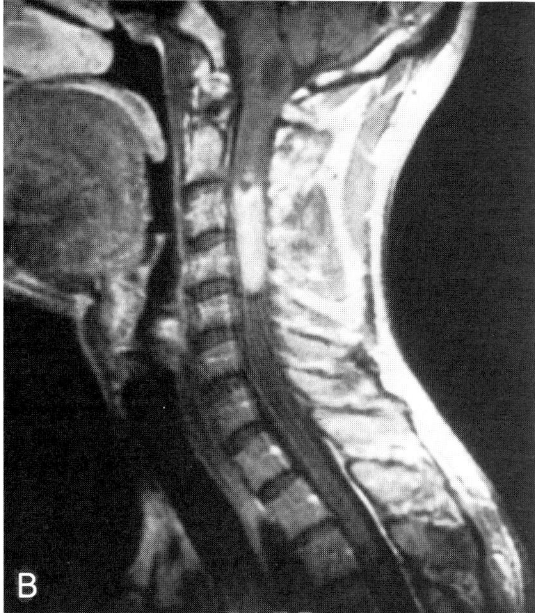

FIGURE 8–109. Ependymoma of the cervical cord. *A.* Precontrast T1 spin echo image shows expansion of the cervical cord, central encephalomalacia or syrinx, and enlargement of the central canal near the obex. The patient, an automobile accident victim, had complained of tightness in the chest when he bent over, a symptom that began before the accident. *B.* Gd-DTPA enhanced T1 spin echo scan shows an enhancing mass lesion within the cord at the C-3 and C-4 levels. This ependymoma was completely resected at surgery with little residual deficit because the tumor was easily shelled out from the surrounding cord.

and metastasis can occur by means of seeding along the ventricular system or the central canal, but this is uncommon.

Other Gliomas. About 20% of cord tumors are other gliomas. These tumors are usually astrocytomas of low-grade malignancy and occasionally oligodendrogliomas, and they cause diffuse enlargement of the cord. Clinical symptoms are those of central cord impairment. MRI is the most effective form of screening and can show the abnormal cord contour in the sagittal plane. T2 spin echo and STIR images show high-intensity tumor. Myelograms and CT can show the abnormal contour but do not show the tumor well. Most gliomas in the cord, being low-grade, show minimal enhancement. More aggressive tumors (anaplastic astrocytoma, glioblastoma multiforme) show areas of necrosis, cysts, and syrinx. Treatment is difficult because of diffuse involvement of normal structures.

Metastatic Tumor. Compression of the cord and nerve roots by metastatic tumor to the spine (especially from lung and breast cancer) is the most common cause of neurological deficit in older patients. Metastasis directly to the cord or the dural sac can also occur (Fig. 8–110). Spinal metastases are discussed in Chapter 7.

VASCULAR DISEASES

Spinal Infarction. Spinal infarctions are rare because the blood supply to the spinal cord is generally adequate to compensate for decreases in perfusion. Embolism to the cord is also rare. Many spinal cord infarctions are traumatic and result from direct cord injury, from occlusion of the anterior spinal artery (which supplies all of the gray matter and most of the white matter of the cord), or from injury to branches of intercostal and lumbar arteries that supply the cord. The lower cord in the anterior spinal artery distribution is the most common site of infarction because this area is supplied by a single artery, the artery of Adamkiewicz.

Spinal infarction is difficult to diagnose on radiographs because the lesion is small. MRI with T2 spin echo or STIR sequences provides the spatial and contrast resolution necessary for identifying the lesion. The appearance of high intensity is not specific; it is also seen in multiple sclerosis, infection, and tumor.

Spinal Arteriovenous Malformation. AVM in the spine is rare. The lesions are similar to AVM lesions in the brain. Usually they are fed by intercostal or lumbar arteries. Symptoms can be confused with those of tumors

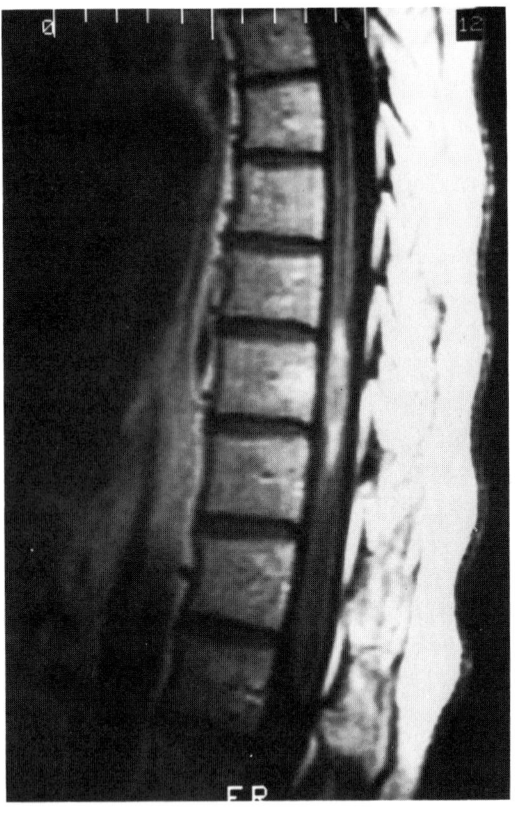

FIGURE 8–110. Spinal cord metastasis. Gd-DTPA enhanced sagittal T1 spin echo image shows a focal abnormality within the spinal cord at approximately the T-10 level. The more inferior portion of the cord shows low intensity and possibly syrinx. This tumor represented metastatic lung carcinoma.

and spinal inflammatory disease. Diagnosis can often be made with MRI by showing multiple flow voids in the dural space; however, flow-related artifacts are common in the thoracic spine, and the diagnosis often requires angiography. Most of these lesions can be treated angiographically.

RADIOGRAPHIC DIFFERENTIAL DIAGNOSIS

Frequently, single radiographic findings or patterns suggest a limited list of diagnoses. Additional findings and clinical history can then assist in further limiting the list or in making a firm diagnosis. The following approaches to evaluation of radiographic findings provide assistance in differential diagnosis. Diseases are listed in order of importance.

CHARACTERISTICS OF EXTRA-AXIAL LESIONS

One of the first and most important observations to be made in the diagnosis of an intracranial lesion is whether the abnormality is intra-axial (within the brain substance) or extra-axial (the meninges, the subarachnoid space, or the bone). Except for metastases, extra-axial lesions are usually benign and often have a characteristic appearance in addition to radiographic findings that place them outside the brain substance.

Adjacent to bone or a dural surface
Sharp delineation by CSF
Widening of adjacent CSF spaces
Vascular displacement
Bone destruction
Involvement of more than one anatomical space

POSTERIOR FOSSA LESIONS

Lesions in the posterior fossa can usually be diagnosed by their CT or MRI appearance and their location. The location limits the differential list.

Location	Intra-Axial	Mass	Comment
Anterior: brainstem	Yes	Brainstem glioma	Noncalcified
	No	Chordoma	Clivus
	No	Meningioma	Sphenoid wing
Middle: fourth ventricle and cerebellopontine angle	Yes	Ependymoma	May calcify
	No	Acoustic schwannoma (neurilemmoma)	Enhances
	No	Meningioma	Vascular

	No	Epidermoid	Water density
Posterior:	Yes	Astrocytoma	Often cystic
cerebellum	Yes	Hemangioblastoma	Cystic with mural nodule
	Yes	Medulloblastoma	Posterior vermis; may be lateral in an adult

SUPRASELLAR MASSES

A mass in the suprasellar region has a long differential diagnostic list because there are many structures in this area. Many lesions have a characteristic appearance and can be easily identified; frequently the entire differential list must be considered. A helpful mnemonic is "SATCHMO on the sella."

*S*ellar tumor (pituitary adenoma), *s*chwannoma
*A*neurysm
*T*eratoma (and germinoma), *t*hird ventricle tumor
*C*raniopharyngioma, *c*hordoma
*H*ypothalamic glioma or *h*amartoma, *h*istiocytosis X
*M*eningioma
*O*ptic chiasm glioma

PINEAL REGION MASSES

Masses in the pineal region are usually tumors and usually are identified in children. Paralysis of upward gaze is a common manifesting sign caused by compression of the midbrain. When an AVM drains directly into the vein of Galen, aneurysmal dilatation results.

Pineal tumors (pineocytoma, pineoblastoma)
Teratoma
Germinoma
Glioma
Vein of Galen malformation
Meningioma

RETROPHARYNGEAL MASS

Masses in the retropharyngeal space are usually caused by tumor: benign in children, malignant in adults. CT, MRI, and angiographic characteristics can often enable differentiation of the various lesions.

Nasopharyngeal carcinoma
Squamous cell carcinoma
Lymphoma
Retropharyngeal abscess
Juvenile angiofibroma
Teratoma
Chordoma
Inverting papilloma

SUPERIOR NASAL MASSES

Masses in the superior nasal cavity may originate in the brain, the nasal cavity, or the ethmoid sinuses. Radiographic evaluation in the coronal plane is essential for diagnosis before biopsy. The most common tumor to cross the cribriform plate is the esthesioneuroblastoma.

Esthesioneuroblastoma
Encephalocele
Olfactory groove meningioma
Ethmoid sinus disease or mucocele

HEMORRHAGIC BRAIN TUMORS

In most primary brain tumors, hemorrhage is not the manifesting sign. Metastatic tumors more commonly manifest with hemorrhage. Although lung and breast metastases do not usually bleed, they are the most common hemorrhagic tumors because they occur frequently.

Glioblastoma multiforme
High-grade astrocytoma
Lung and breast carcinoma
Melanoma
Renal cell and thyroid carcinoma
Choriocarcinoma

MULTIPLE ENHANCING BRAIN LESIONS

When enhancing brain lesions are multiple, the diagnosis is usually a diffuse hematogenous process. Multicentric primary brain tumor must also be considered.

Metastases
Lymphoma, reticulum cell sarcoma
Septic emboli
Nocardiosis, cysticercosis
Multiple sclerosis
Multicentric glioma

CENTRAL BRAINSTEM LESIONS

Most brainstem lesions are caused by vascular disease, including infarction and hemorrhage. Tumor and, in a patient with electrolyte imbalance, central pontine myelinolysis are additional important considerations.

Infarction
Hemorrhage
Brainstem glioma
Metastatic tumor
Lymphoma
Multiple sclerosis
Central pontine myelinolysis
Brainstem encephalitis

SUBEPENDYMAL CALCIFICATION

Calcification along the ventricles can be caused by tumor, infection, or hamartoma. The appearance of the calcification assists in the diagnosis.

Tuberous sclerosis (calcified hamartomas or gliomas project into the ventricles)
Toxoplasmosis (periventricular calcification)
Cytomegalovirus (periventricular calcification)
Ependymoma (enhancing periventricular tumor associated with the calcification)
Heterotopic gray matter

CEREBELLAR ATROPHY

Isolated or predominant atrophy of the cerebellum is usually caused by phenytoin (Dilantin) therapy (diffuse atrophy) or alcohol ingestion (anterior vermian atrophy). Congenital malformations of the vermis show abnormal architecture and are easily distinguished from atrophy.

Alcoholism
Phenytoin (Dilantin) therapy
Paraneoplastic syndrome (associated with lung and breast carcinoma)
Olivopontocerebellar degeneration
Friedreich's ataxia

BILATERAL BASAL GANGLIA LESIONS

Bilateral abnormality of the basal ganglia implies either a systemic process or a global insult. Because the basal ganglia require high amounts of oxygen and glucose, they are particularly susceptible to asphyxia, hypoxia, and hypoperfusion.

Anoxic infarction
Carbon monoxide poisoning
Lead poisoning
Leigh's disease
Wilson's disease
Mitochondrial cytopathy
Therapeutic radiation
Methotrexate therapy
Cytomegalic inclusion disease
Toxoplasmosis
Cysticercosis
Encephalitis

BASAL GANGLIA MINERALIZATION

The basal ganglia calcify or become mineralized as part of a normal aging process. Calcium excess and injury also result in such calcification.

Normal aging
Hyperparathyroidism
Renal failure
Infarction
Radiation injury

CEREBRAL HEMORRHAGE IN AN OLDER PATIENT

Cerebral hemorrhage in a patient over age 40 has a limited differential diagnostic list. Usually, the CT appearance is characteristic.

Hypertensive hemorrhage
Congenital aneurysm
Infectious or embolic aneurysms
AVM (20% occur after age 40)
Tumor hemorrhage
Congophilic angiopathy (amyloidosis)
Coagulopathy hemorrhage

CAUSES OF SEIZURE

The age of the patient is important in the evaluation of the cause of seizure. This and the CT or MRI appearance narrow the differential diagnosis considerably. MRI is more sensitive than CT and can show low-grade tumors and gliosis.

Age (years)	Cause	Image Abnormality
0 to 20	Idiopathic	None
20 to 40	Tumor	Low-density mass with rim enhancement
	AVM	Confluent enhancing mass
40 +	Alcoholism	Diffuse atrophy
	Trauma	Contusion
	Metastatic tumor	Enhancing mass with edema
	Primary tumor	Enhancing mass, edema, necrosis

DEMYELINATING DISEASE

Distinguishing among the demyelinating diseases is usually not possible on scans. Clinical history and other tests are often required for establishing the diagnosis. Multiple sclerosis has a characteristic pattern on MRI scans—multiple, focal lesions in the deep and periventricular white matter—but the lesions are indistinguishable from white matter infarcts and changes in myelin that are associated with aging.

Multiple sclerosis
Progressive multifocal leukoencephalopathy
Subacute sclerosing panencephalitis
Acute hemorrhagic leukoencephalopathy
Diffuse gliomatosis
Allergic demyelinating syndromes
Genetic demyelinating syndromes

ABNORMAL SELLA ON MRI

Fluid intensity in the sella is usually caused by herniation of the subarachnoid space into the sella (called empty sella). At least 30% of all people have empty or partially empty sella, a benign condition. MRI can identify CSF, fat, tumor, or blood.

Condition	MRI Appearance
Empty sella	CSF
Pituitary adenoma	Tumor
Pituitary apoplexy	Tumor, blood
Arachnoid cyst	CSF
Rathke's pouch cyst	CSF, blood

CALCIFIED LESIONS IN THE GLOBE

Many lesions in the globe have similar appearances. One method of distinguishing them is by the presence of calcification. Except for retinoblastoma, calcified lesions are benign.

Calcified	Noncalcified
Retinoblastoma	Choroidal melanoma
Meningioma	Coats' disease
Tuberous sclerosis	Toxocariasis
Drusen	
Phthisic globe	
Choroidal osteoma	

INTRACONAL LESIONS OF THE ORBIT

Intraconal lesions of the orbit, those confined to the cone defined by the attachment of the extraocular muscles, usually arise from the optic nerve, orbital fat, or vessels.

Optic nerve glioma
Optic nerve meningioma
Ectopic meningioma
Orbital hemangioma
Dermatolipoma
Orbital pseudotumor

PULSATILE TINNITUS

Pulsatile tinnitus indicates the presence of a vascular lesion. Angiography should be performed before surgical exploration of such lesions.

Aberrant carotid artery
Glomus jugulare or vagale tumor
Intrapetrous carotid aneurysm
Jugular bulb dehiscence
Dural AVM

Suggested Readings

Atlas SW (ed): Magnetic Resonance Imaging of the Brain and Spine. New York: Raven Press, 1991.
Barkovich JA: Pediatric Neuroimaging, vol 1. New York: Raven Press, 1990.
Orrison WW: Introduction to Neuroimaging. Boston: Little, Brown, 1989.
Osborn AG, Maack JG: Introduction to Cerebral Angiography. Philadelphia: Harper & Row, 1980.
Som P, Bergeron RT, Curtin HD (eds): Head and Neck Imaging, 2nd ed. St Louis: Mosby Year Book, 1981.

9

Nuclear Medicine

Michael F. Hartshorne
Gary K. Stimac

BASIC EVALUATION

Nuclear medicine techniques are used to image most organs and to provide diagnostic information that is complementary to that obtained through other radiological techniques. In some cases, these examinations provide unique information because uptake of the radionuclide occurs only in a specific disease. Nuclear medicine examinations are important in the screening for the presence of disease and in follow-up, evaluation of physiological function, and, often, establishing a definite diagnosis. They are, in general, highly sensitive to the presence of disease but not highly specific as to a particular diagnosis.

Nuclear medicine examinations involve the use of a radioactive element (the radionuclide) attached to a molecule or a compound chosen for its ability to map a physiological or pathophysiological process. The radionuclide, in combination with the molecule or compound, is called a radiopharmaceutical. Sometimes the free radionuclide (e.g., iodine 131 [^{131}I] or 123 [^{123}I], thallium 201 [^{201}Tl], or gallium 67 [^{67}Ga]) is ingested or injected, and it acts as a physiological analog to an element in the body.

The radionuclides (Table 9–1) are chosen for their radiative properties (decay life, types of emission, and gamma ray energy), availability (cost and half-life), and ability to be attached to the desired compound. Many compounds are labeled with technetium 99m (^{99m}Tc) because of its short half-life (6 hours), nearly ideal gamma ray energy (140 keV), absence of particle emissions, availability (it is produced by a molybdenum generator), and ease in labeling many compounds.

The physical and chemical properties of the compound, rather than of the radioisotope, cause the radiopharmaceutical to become isolated in a particular body compartment (e.g., a blood pool, the liver, bone marrow, the thyroid) or to pass through the body by a particular mode of excretion (renal, biliary). The most commonly used radiopharmaceuticals are described in Tables 9–2 and 9–3.

Images are obtained with the use of a large gamma ray detector (gamma camera) placed over the patient's body in order to quantify and determine the distribution of the radioactivity. Because the gamma rays come from various depths within the body, the total number of counts, corrected for background and self-absorption, provides a volume distribution

TABLE 9–1. RADIONUCLIDES USED IN NUCLEAR MEDICINE

Radionuclide	Half-Life	Source	Energy (keV)	Particle Emission	Comments
$^{99m}_{43}$Tc	6 Hours	Molybdenum generator	140	None	Used in majority of radiopharmaceutical agents
$^{131}_{53}$I	8.1 Days	Fission	364	β^-	High radiation dose; used in thyroid therapy and renal function studies
$^{123}_{53}$I	13.3 Hours	Accelerator	159	None	Best iodine for thyroid imaging
$^{67}_{31}$Ga	78 Hours	Accelerator	93 (38%) 185 (23%) 300 (16%) 393 (4%)	Minimal	Free gallium binds transferrin in the body and goes to inflammatory and tumor cells
$^{111}_{49}$In	68 Hours	Accelerator	172 (90%) 247 (90%)	None	Best for labeling white blood cells
$^{201}_{81}$Tl	73 Hours	Accelerator	69 to 83 from mercury x-rays	None	Used in cardiac perfusion imaging
$^{133}_{54}$Xe	5.4 days	Fission	80	β^-	Used in lung ventilation scans
$^{81m}_{36}$Kr	13 Seconds	$^{81}_{37}$Sr decay	191	None	Used in lung ventilation scans; expensive, limited availability

Tc, technetium; I, iodine; Ga, gallium; In, indium; Tl, thallium; Xe, xenon; Kr, krypton; Sr, strontium.

of the radioisotope. This is of use particularly in cardiac examinations.

The best spatial resolution available for conventional gamma cameras is approximately 0.5 cm, measured at the body surface; deeper in the body, resolution decreases. Poorer resolution also occurs with gamma energies that are higher or lower than ^{99m}Tc. A typical detector arrangement is shown in Figure 9–1. Portable cameras and computers allow any examination to be conducted anywhere in a hospital.

LUNG EXAMINATION

Lung scanning is used primarily to exclude the diagnosis of (and, to a lesser degree, detect) pulmonary embolus. The examination carries few risks and should be performed before pulmonary angiography. Lung ventilation and perfusion (V/Q) scans should be obtained even when it is highly likely that angiography will be performed because

1. V/Q scans can rule out embolus (significant pulmonary embolus is present in only a small percentage of patients with a normal perfusion scan).
2. V/Q scans can unequivocally demonstrate a massive perfusion defect and thus render angiography unnecessary.
3. V/Q scans can guide the angiographer to the suspicious lung or segment.

Lung scanning is also valuable for evaluating regional lung function, particularly before surgery.

Although the perfusion scan is the most informative part of the lung examination, the ventilation scan is usually done first so that the ^{99m}Tc radioisotope used for the perfusion scan does not visually interfere with the xenon 133 (^{133}Xe) used for ventilation imaging. Such interference occurs because Compton-scattered radiation from ^{99m}Tc is approximately the same energy as the ^{133}Xe gamma rays. Therefore, if the ^{99m}Tc scan is performed first, Compton scatter is superimposed on the ^{133}Xe images. The two scans are interpreted in conjunction with the chest radiograph.

Ventilation Lung Scan

For ventilation lung scanning, the patient inhales ^{133}Xe. First-breath, equilibration, and washout images are obtained. Smooth inflation of both lungs distributes gas symmetrically to both lungs. The most sensitive detection of airway disease is made in the washout phase, in which gas trapping is visible after the normally ventilated lung clears (Fig. 9–2). Rapid clearance in the washout images reflects nor-

Text continued on page 554

TABLE 9–2. ADMINISTRATION AND PHARMACOKINETICS OF RADIOPHARMACEUTICALS USED IN NUCLEAR MEDICINE

Organ	Agent	Dose (mCi)	Mechanism	Excretion	Biological Half-Life
Lung	^{133}Xe	15 Inhaled	Gas enters alveoli as an aerosol and washes out	Lung	30 Seconds
	^{99m}Tc–MAA	5 IV	Albumin is trapped by alveolar arterioles	Reticulo-endothelial system	4 Hours
Liver, spleen	^{99m}Tc–sulfur colloid	5 IV	Colloid particles trapped in liver, spleen, bone marrow	Reticulo-endothelial system	6 Hours
Biliary	^{99m}Tc–HIDA	5 IV	Binds to protein; uptake and secretion by liver	Liver	2 to 6 Hours
Kidney	^{99m}Tc–DTPA	15 IV	Renal excretion by glomerular filtration	Kidney	45 Minutes
	^{99m}Tc–glucoheptonate or ^{99m}Tc–DMSA	15 IV	20% to 50% is bound by proximal and distal tubule cells of the renal cortex	Kidney	4 Hours
	Iodine I 131–labeled hippurate	0.1 to 0.3 IV	Filtered (20%) and secreted (80%) by kidneys	Kidney	30 Minutes
Bone	^{99m}Tc–MDP	20 IV	Pyrophosphate analog that binds hydroxyapatite	Kidney	6 Hours
Heart					
Infarct	^{99m}Tc–pyrophosphate	15 IV	Phosphate binds to calcium in infarcted myocardium	Kidney	6 Hours
Ischemia	^{201}Tl	2 IV	K^+ analog; 3% goes to heart where 90% is extracted	Kidney, bowel	3 Days
Wall motion	^{99m}Tc–labeled red blood cells	20 IV W/Sn	Gated study shows passage of red blood cells through heart	None	6 Hours
Central nervous system	^{99m}Tc–DTPA	15 IV	Large molecule remains in blood except at blood-brain barrier defect	Kidney	45 Minutes
	^{99m}Tc–albumin colloid or ^{111}In–DTPA	0.5 to 1.0 Intrathecal	Large molecule remains in subarachnoid space	Kidney	6–24 Hours
Inflammation	^{67}Ga	5 IV	Binds transferrin; uptake by inflammatory and tumor cells	Kidney, bowel	36 Hours
	^{111}In-labeled white blood cells	0.5 IV	Accumulate in acute infection; less uptake by chronic or sterile processes	Spleen	3 Days
Vascular bleeding	^{99m}Tc–labeled red blood cells or ^{99m}Tc–sulfur colloid	20 IV 10 IV	Isotope leaves vascular space at bleeding site	None None	6 Hours 6 Hours
Vascular flow	Pertechnetate Tc 99m	5 IV/Leg	Dynamic scanning demonstrates venous flow	Kidney, bowel	4 Hours
Thyroid	Pertechnetate Tc 99m	15 IV	2% Trapped by thyroid, but not organified	Bowel, kidney	4 Hours
	^{123}I	0.2 PO	10% to 35% Trapped and organified by thyroid	Kidney	10 Hours
	^{131}I	0.1 PO	Same as ^{123}I	Kidney	16 Hours
Adrenal cortex	^{131}I–NP59	1.0 IV	Steroid hormone precursor analog	NA	NA
Adrenal medulla	^{131}I–MIBG	0.5 IV	Presynaptic sympathetic analog	NA	NA

Xe, xenon; Tc, technetium; MAA, macroaggregated albumin; IV, intravenous; HIDA, hippuran imino diacetate; DTPA, diethylenetriaminepenta-acetic acid, DMSA, dimercaptosuccinic acid; MDP, methylene diphosphonate; Tl, thallium; K^+, potassium; In, indium; Ga, gallium; PO, per orum; MIBG metaiodobenzyl guanide; W/Sn, with tin.

TABLE 9–3. APPLICATIONS AND TECHNIQUES FOR RADIOPHARMACEUTICALS USED IN NUCLEAR MEDICINE

Organ/ Condition	Agent	Radiation Dose: Organ (Gy)	Radiation Dose: Body (mGy)	Scanning Technique: Projection	Comments
Lung	^{133}Xe (ventilation)	0.005	0.08	First breath, equilibration, then every 30 seconds for 3 minutes: posterior	Defects are usually pneumonia, tumor, airway disease; the ventilation in pulmonary embolus is normal
	^{99m}Tc–MAA (perfusion)	0.005	0.50	Immediately: anterior, posterior, right and left posterior oblique, right and left lateral	Reduce dose in patients with pulmonary hypertension
Liver, spleen	^{99m}Tc–sulfur colloid	0.03	0.70	Wait 15 minutes to clear blood: anterior, posterior, right and left lateral, left posterior oblique	Metastases show low uptake; compare liver, spleen, marrow
Biliary system	^{99m}Tc–HIDA	0.05	1.00	Every 10 minutes until gallbladder is seen; then right lateral, right posterior oblique; may need another scan at 4 hours	Patient fasts 3 hours before test; test works if bilirubin below 20 mg/dL
Kidney	^{99m}Tc–DTPA	0.005 kidney, 0.02 bladder	3.00	Flow study every 3 seconds for 1 minute; then static scan	Show blood flow; often follow with a renal function study
	^{99m}Tc–glucoheptonate or ^{99m}Tc–DMSA	0.03 kidney, 0.02 bladder	1.00	At 1 and 3 hours (glucoheptonate); at 5 and 24 hours (DMSA)	Kidney dose is large because agent binds to the cortex
	Iodine I 131–labeled hippurate	0.0003 kidney, 0.001 bladder	0.30	Every 4 minutes, 7 times; then scan postvoid bladder or urine bag	Shows blood flow, tubule uptake, and excretion; thyroid must be protected with free iodine
Bone	^{99m}Tc–MDP	0.005 bone, 0.02 bladder	1.00	Scan in 3 hours to allow renal and vascular labeling to diminish	Calcification processes show uptake; myeloma may not
Heart					
Infarct	^{99m}Tc–pyrophosphate	0.006	1.50	At 2 to 4 hours postinjection: anteroposterior, right posterior oblique, lateral	Positive at 18 to 48 hours postinfarct; may be positive up to 5 days
Ischemia	^{201}Tl	0.008	5.00	Immediately and at 4 hours: anterior; left anterior oblique 30 to 40 degrees, 70 degrees if planar; SPECT preferred	Ischemic area is not perfused by ^{201}Tl, but it fills in when patient is at rest
Wall motion	^{99m}Tc-labeled red blood cells	0.0015 body	1.50	First-pass scan, then gated studies: anteroposterior, left anterior oblique, lateral	Measures ejection fraction, rates of emptying and filling; shows ventricular wall motion
Central nervous system	^{99m}Tc–DTPA	0.005 kidney	1.00	Flow images at 3, 6, 9, 24 seconds; static scan at 30 seconds, 2 hours	Images vascular flow and blood-brain barrier defects
	^{99m}Tc–albumin colloid or ^{111}In–DTPA	0.005 spine, brain	1.00	Scan for expected flow; for cisterns at 0, 4, 24, 48, 72 hours: anterior, posterior, right and left lateral	Shows shunt patency, cisterns; use indium if slow flow is expected
Inflammation	^{67}Ga	0.05 kidney, bowel	2.00	At 6, 24, 48, 72 hours for inflammation, at 72 hours for tumor	Taken up by neoplastic and inflammatory cells
	^{111}In–labeled white blood cells	0.1 spleen	3.00	Scan whole body at 24 hours	Large radiation dose to spleen

Table continued on following page

TABLE 9–3. APPLICATIONS AND TECHNIQUES FOR RADIOPHARMACEUTICALS USED IN NUCLEAR MEDICINE *Continued*

Organ/ Condition	Agent	Radiation Dose: *Organ (Gy)*	Radiation Dose: *Body (mGy)*	Scanning Technique: Projection	Comments
Vascular flow	^{99m}Tc–labeled red blood cells	0.001 spleen	1.50	Immediately	Detects active bleeding of 1.0 ml/minute or more
	^{99m}Tc–sulfur colloid	0.05 liver	1.50	During 0 to 15 minutes	Detects acute gastrointestinal bleeding only; rates of more than 1.0 ml/minute
	Pertechnetate Tc 99m	0.01	1.50	Immediately, with or without tourniquet: pelvis, leg, knee	Useless in the calf; shows only venous patency
Thyroid	Pertechnetate Tc 99m	0.02 thyroid, colon	2.00	At 15 minutes with pinhole camera	Demonstrates entire gland; rarely fails to show a hot nodule
	^{123}I	0.03	2.00	At 6 hours, with pinhole camera	Long-distance shipping may mean inconvenience, but half-life and gamma energy are ideal
	^{131}I	1.00	2.00	At 24 hours	High radiation dose, used for therapy

Xe, xenon; Tc, technetium; MAA, macroaggregated albumin; HIDA, hippuran imino diacetate; DTPA, diethylenetriaminepenta-acetic acid; DMSA, dimercaptosuccinic acid; MDP, methylene diphosphonate; Tl, thallium; SPECT, single photon emission computed tomography; In, indium; Ga, gallium; I, iodine.

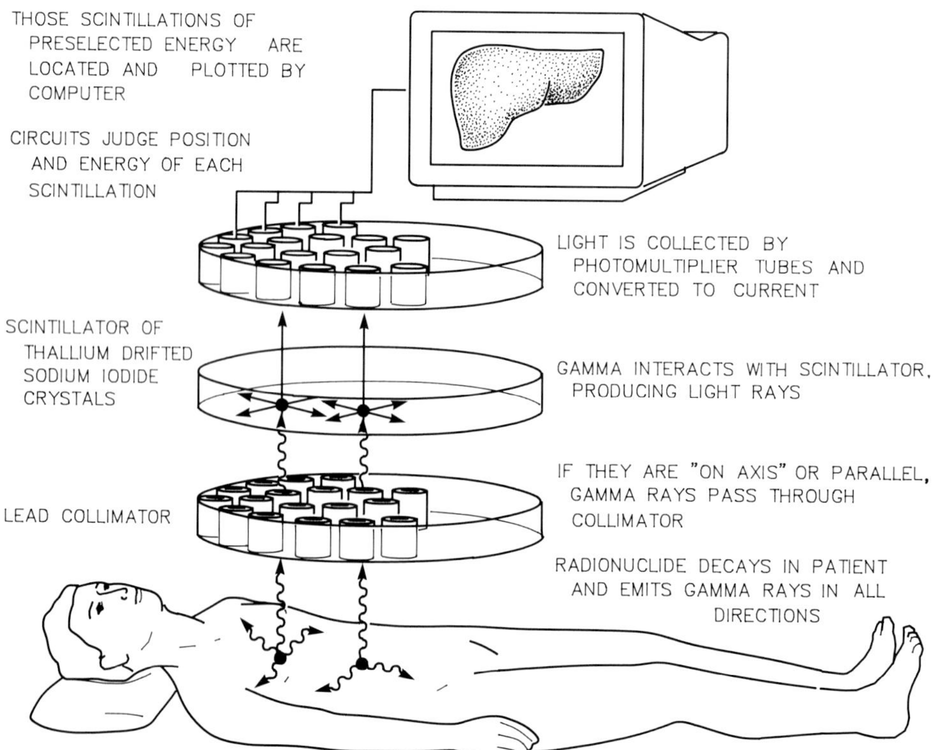

FIGURE 9–1. Gamma ray detection system.

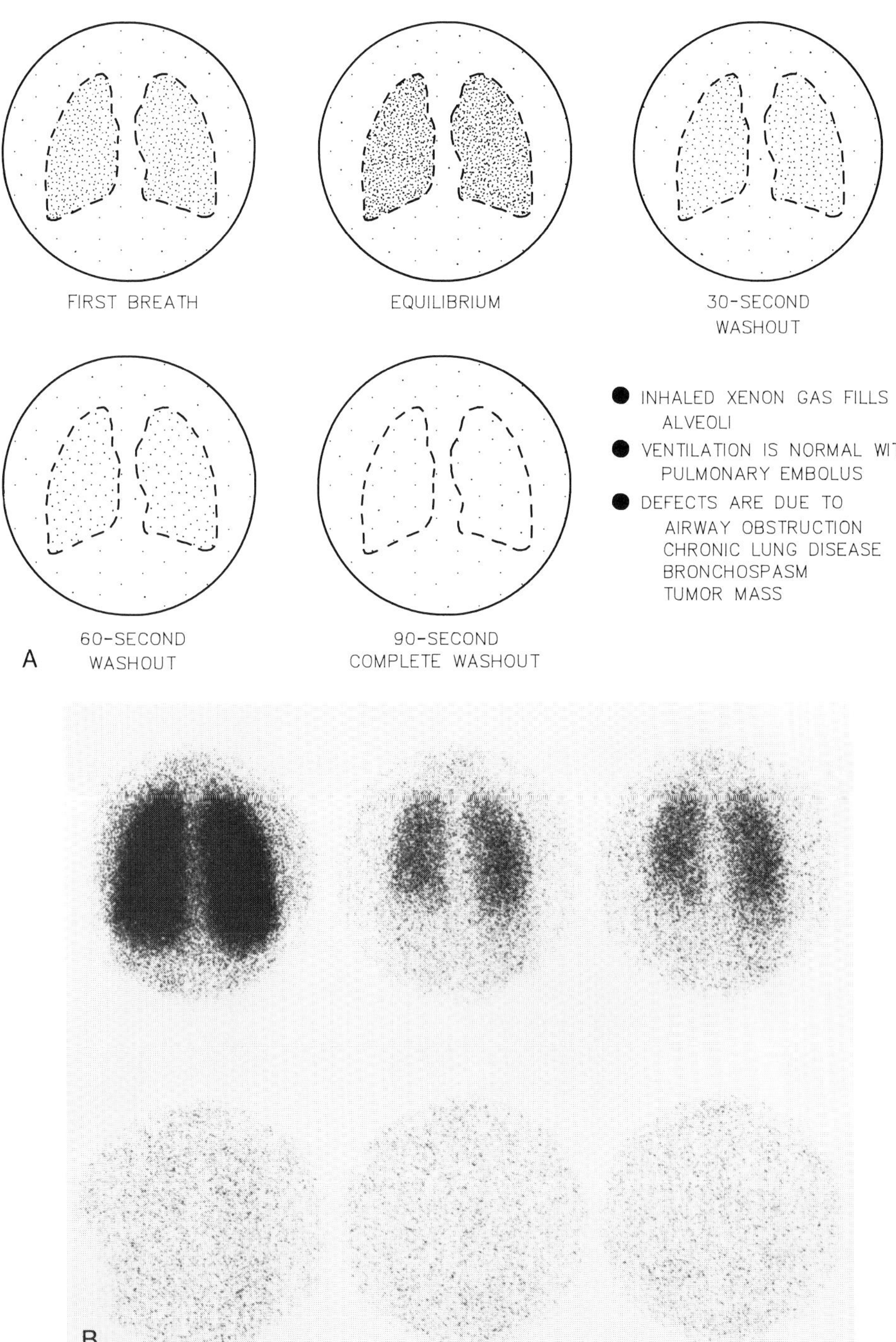

FIGURE 9–2. Normal ventilation scan. *A.* Diagram. *B.* Xenon 133 (^{133}Xe) scan in the posterior projection shows the distribution of a single breath (upper left). The next two images show the distribution of gas during equilibrium breathing. The bottom three images were taken as the patient exhaled into a charcoal trap after inhaling fresh air. This washout phase documents prompt clearance of the ^{133}Xe, without trapping of gas behind obstructed airways.

mal ventilation. The ventilation scan is extremely sensitive to the presence of airway abnormalities. Diseases that obstruct the airways, such as hilar adenopathy and bronchial disease, can cause lobar ventilation defects that may or may not match perfusion abnormalities. Most ventilation scan abnormalities are caused by airway obstruction, chronic lung disease, bronchospasm, or tumor. Ventilation usually remains normal when pulmonary embolus is present.

Abnormally ventilated areas frequently show evidence of abnormal perfusion as well. Without the ventilation scan, such perfusion can be confused with abnormal perfusion caused by pulmonary emboli. To be convinced that a perfusion scan abnormality represents a pulmonary embolus, the interpreting physician must know that the same area is normally ventilated. The improved certainty of diagnosis of pulmonary embolus more than justifies the concomitant use of V/Q scans.

Some centers use krypton 81m (^{81m}Kr) for ventilation scanning. The parent isotope, rubidium 81, has a short half-life (4 hours), and ^{81m}Kr has an extremely short half-life (13 seconds). The generator is expensive and short-lived and, in a given hospital, may be available on only certain days of the week. Images produced with ^{81m}Kr are roughly equivalent to first-breath images of a ^{133}Xe scan as decay occurs before washout can be observed. The

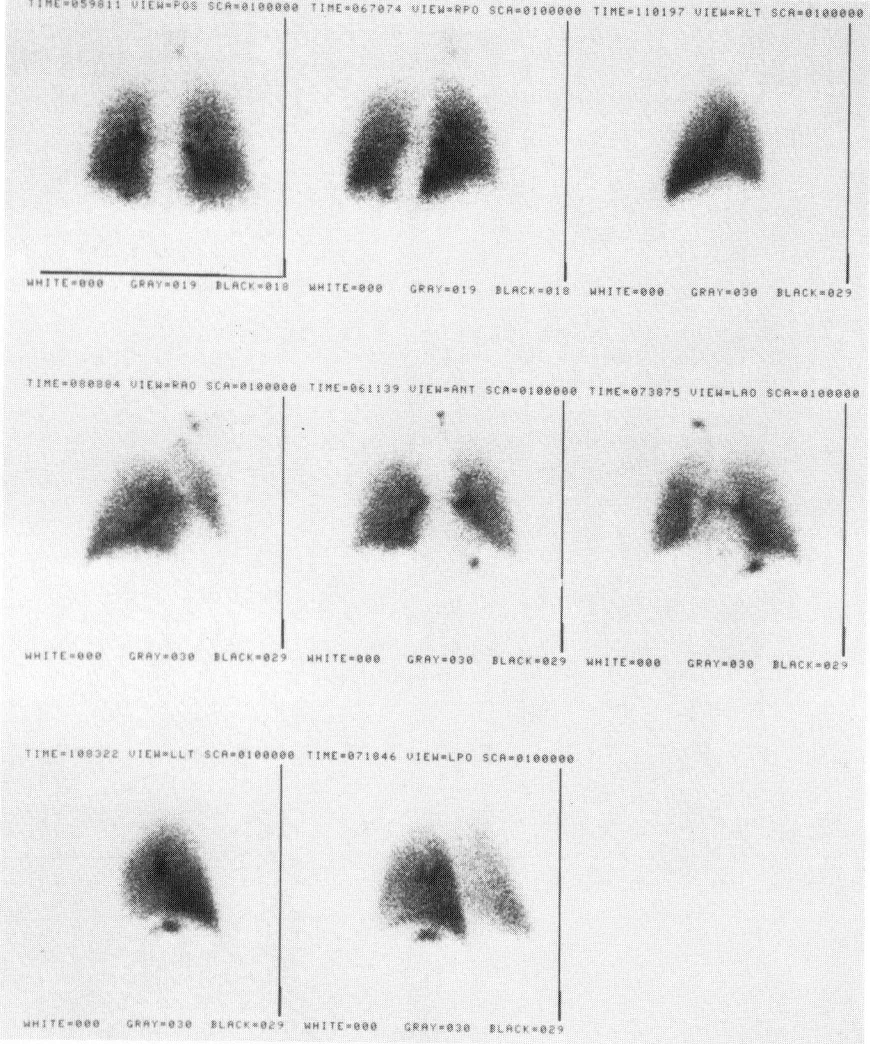

FIGURE 9–3. Normal aerosol scan. Nebulized technetium 99m–labeled diethylenetriaminepenta-acetic acid (^{99m}Tc–DTPA) aerosol is smoothly distributed during quiet breathing and is imaged in as many projections as desired. Some activity is normally seen in the upper airways (right and left main bronchi) as well as in the mouth (above the lungs) and in the stomach (just below the left lung).

quality of a krypton scan is equal to or better than that of a ^{133}Xe scan because it is possible to obtain a high-count rate with a low dose. Because of the higher energy of the ^{81m}Kr (191 keV), the lungs can be imaged when ^{99m}Tc is present. Multiple ^{81m}Kr scans can be done in exactly the same projections as the ^{99m}Tc images, which greatly assists in the comparison of ventilation and perfusion data.

Technetium-labeled diethylenetriamine-penta-acetic acid (^{99m}Tc–DTPA) aerosol scans have been substituted for ^{133}Xe gas scans in some hospitals. The nebulized droplets of ^{99m}Tc–DTPA, in a dose of a few hundred microcuries, follow laminar airflow to the peripheral airways, in which they are deposited in terminal bronchioles and alveoli and are slowly absorbed into capillary blood. Excretion is by the kidney, and so it is not necessary to vent exhaled isotope (as occurs with ^{133}Xe). As with the ^{81m}Kr scan, the information obtained is similar to the first-breath images with ^{133}Xe. Images of the lungs may be obtained in each projection used for the subsequent perfusion scan (Fig. 9–3).

There is, however, a disadvantage to this technique. Extensive airway disease can cause turbulent flow in the main airways and, consequently, central disposition of the aerosol, which makes interpretation difficult. As discussed earlier, such a scan does document the airway disease, reducing the likelihood that a perfusion scan abnormality represents a pulmonary embolus. Technetium 99m–DTPA aerosol scans are widely used in clinics or remote sites that are not authorized to handle a radioactive gas. Aerosol ^{99m}Tc scans provide reasonable diagnostic accuracy, produce a low radiation dose to the patient and the technologist, and are less expensive than ^{81m}Kr scans.

Lung Perfusion Scan

Lung perfusion scanning is performed by intravenous injection of technetium 99m–labeled macroaggregated albumin (^{99m}Tc–MAA) or technetium–labeled albumin microspheres. These particles (20 to 50 microns in size) are trapped by pulmonary precapillary arterioles, which enables imaging of regional blood flow to the lungs (Fig. 9–4). The particles are broken down by circulating proteases in 4 to 8 hours. The fraction of vessels occluded is small (1 per 1000 arterioles), and so there is very little chance of causing pulmonary problems. This is, however, the one nuclear medicine examination in which serious deterioration in lung perfusion has occurred. A few deaths have been reported among patients with severe pulmonary hypertension who received routine doses of ^{99m}Tc–MAA. In patients with right-to-left cardiac shunts, the embolic particles pass to the systemic circulation. A cardiac shunt is, therefore, a relative contraindication to ^{99m}Tc–MAA injection. In many cases, a scan with a lung perfusion agent can be used to diagnose and quantify an intracardiac shunt. Small doses that may arrive at the brain and other organs after crossing the right-to-left shunt do not produce symptoms. The shunt is quantified by the radioactivity in the lungs in comparison with that in the rest of the body.

Abnormal ventilation and perfusion scans are always interpreted in conjunction with the chest radiograph (which often shows no abnormality). The combination of radiographic, clinical, and nuclear medicine findings enables predictions of the probability of pulmonary embolus. In general, a pulmonary embolus is suspected if a perfusion defect is seen in an area of normal ventilation and is not accounted for by a similar abnormality on a chest radiograph (Fig. 9–5). A probability of pulmonary embolus is assigned according to the algorithm depicted in Figure 9–6. The presence of lung disease makes detection of pulmonary embolus difficult and frequently results in an intermediate probability of pulmonary embolus. A normal perfusion scan rules out pulmonary embolus in the vast majority of patients.

Inflammatory Lung Disease Scan

Inflammatory lung disease can be evaluated with the use of agents that are taken up by inflammatory cells. Gallium 67 citrate (^{67}Ga citrate) is used to evaluate the severity and the response to therapy of various inflammatory lung diseases such as sarcoidosis, *Pneumocystis carinii* pneumonia, and amiodarone toxicity. This scan is discussed later in the section on whole-body examination for inflammation.

GASTROINTESTINAL EXAMINATION

Because of uptake in the liver, the spleen, and the gastric mucosa and excretion by the

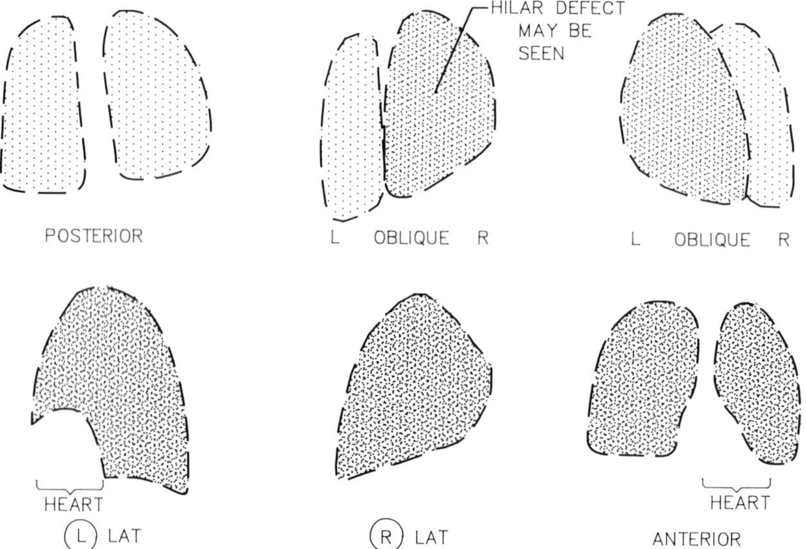

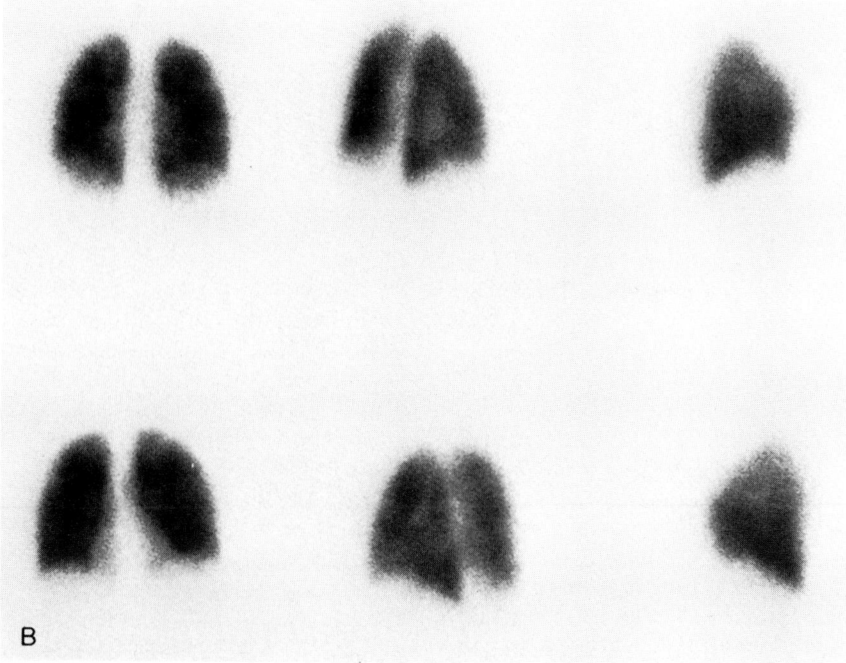

FIGURE 9–4. Normal perfusion scan. *A*. Diagram. L, left; R, right; RES, reticuloendothelial system. *B*. Technetium 99m–labeled macroaggregated albumin (^{99m}Tc-MAA) perfusion scan shows homogeneous perfusion of both lungs. Beginning at the top left, the projections are posterior, right posterior oblique, right lateral, anterior, left posterior oblique, and left lateral. Note that normal hilar structures indent the lungs centrally and that the two oblique projections show these as vague defects in the midlung.

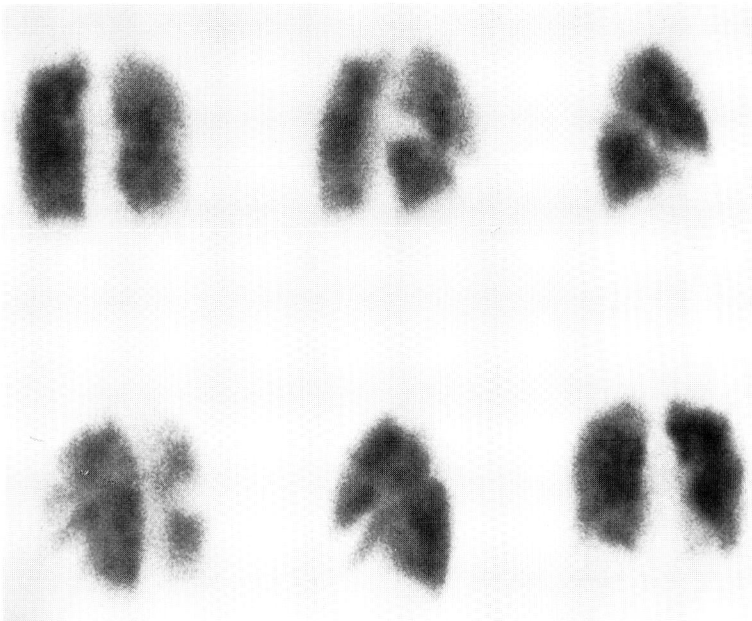

FIGURE 9–5. Pulmonary emboli (abnormal perfusion scan). The distribution of ^{99m}Tc–MAA is interrupted by multiple emboli obstructing branches of the pulmonary arteries. The sequence of images is from, left to right (top row), posterior, right posterior oblique, and right lateral and (bottom row) left posterior oblique, left lateral, and anterior. Multiple, wedge-shaped, pleura-based, segmental- and subsegmental-sized defects are seen in these various projections. The ventilation scan and the chest radiograph were normal.

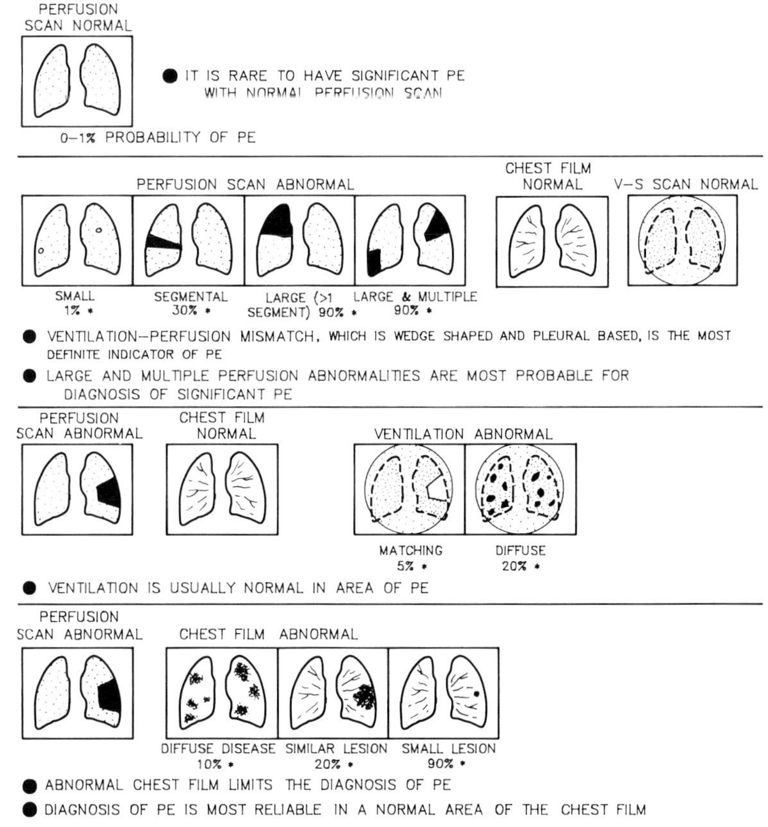

FIGURE 9–6. Lung scan interpretation. PE, pulmonary embolus. The probability of PE is listed beneath each scan.

alimentary tract and the biliary system, nuclear medicine examinations of the gastrointestinal tract can show structure and function. The primary applications are evaluation of the liver and the biliary system, assessment of gastroesophageal reflux and gastric emptying, and detection of ectopic gastric mucosa.

Liver-Spleen Scan

The liver and the spleen are evaluated with the use of an intravenous injection of technetium 99m–labeled sulfur colloid particles (^{99m}Tc–sulfur colloid) or technetium 99m–labeled albumin colloid particles (^{99m}Tc–albumin colloid), which are small enough to pass through the lungs but large enough to be trapped by the reticuloendothelial system of the liver (Kupffer's cells), the spleen, and the bone marrow. In normal patients, 85% of particles 0.3 micron in diameter are taken up by the liver, 10% by the bone marrow, and 5% by the spleen. Because most liver diseases affect Kupffer's cells and hepatocytes equally, they are demonstrated by the liver-spleen scan, even though the hepatocytes do not take up the isotope (Fig. 9–7).

Interpretation of the liver-spleen scan requires evaluation of relative uptake in the liver, the bone marrow, and the spleen; identification of focal or diffuse areas of decreased uptake; and identification of possible artifacts (breast shadow, kidney impression, gallbladder impression, and technically produced irregularities).

A so-called cold lesion (a focal area that does not take up the radiopharmaceutical) is usually demonstrated if it is larger than 2 cm in diameter. Such an abnormality is seen in liver abscesses, primary tumors, metastatic disease, focal nodular hyperplasia, liver cysts, and hemangiomas. The pattern of uptake can show hepatosplenomegaly and identify splenic tissue. Because the finding of a cold lesion is often nonspecific, comparison of liver-spleen scan findings with those of CT and ultrasonography is helpful. When the liver function is normal or nearly normal, all the ^{99m}Tc–sulfur colloid is taken up, and there is very little activity in the bone marrow. Increased uptake by the bone marrow indicates severe liver dysfunction.

The liver-spleen scan has been largely displaced by ultrasonography and computed tomography (CT) for most clinical purposes. It is used to confirm the presence of accessory spleens or splenosis and to determine whether a right diaphragmatic mass represents functioning liver tissue. Because it is less expensive than CT, the liver-spleen scan is often used to follow known liver metastases.

The liver-spleen scan is an excellent measure of the severity of cirrhosis. It is also effective in conjunction with ^{67}Ga and indium 111–(^{111}In–) labeled white blood cell scans of the abdomen for distinguishing physiological uptake of ^{67}Ga- or ^{111}In–labeled white blood cells in the liver and the spleen from a pathological accumulation of these agents adjacent to the liver and the spleen.

Biliary System Scan

The biliary system, including the gallbladder, is imaged with the use of a technetium 99m–labeled iminodiacetate (^{99m}Tc–IDA). These scans therefore are called by names such as ^{99m}Tc–IDA, ^{99m}Tc–HIDA (H, hydroxy), and ^{99m}Tc–DISIDA (DIS, diisopropyl). Technetium 99m–IDA radiopharmaceuticals are administered intravenously. They bind to blood protein, are rapidly extracted by the liver, and are secreted unconjugated into the biliary system. The liver, the gallbladder, the common bile duct, and the duodenum normally fill in sequence.

Indications for ^{99m}Tc–IDA scans are detection of acute cholecystitis, biliary tract obstruction, biliary leaks, and biliary atresia and evaluation of biliary surgery and hepatic function. Both ^{99m}Tc–IDA scanning and ultrasonography are excellent examinations for detecting acute cholecystitis. Technetium 99m–IDA scans are superior to ultrasonography in that they show the abnormal function that accompanies acute cholecystitis.

Interpretation of the ^{99m}Tc–IDA scan consists of assessments of the hepatic phase, the filling of the gallbladder and common bile duct, and the excretion into the duodenum after 1 or 2 hours (Fig. 9–8). If the ^{99m}Tc–IDA fills the gallbladder, acute cholecystitis can be virtually ruled out. Failure to fill the gallbladder may be a result of liver disease (with failure to extract and excrete the isotope), biliary obstruction, intravenous alimentation or recent ingestion of a meal (both of which cause the gallbladder to contract), or acute or chronic cholecystitis. In the patient who has not eaten for days, the gallbladder may be

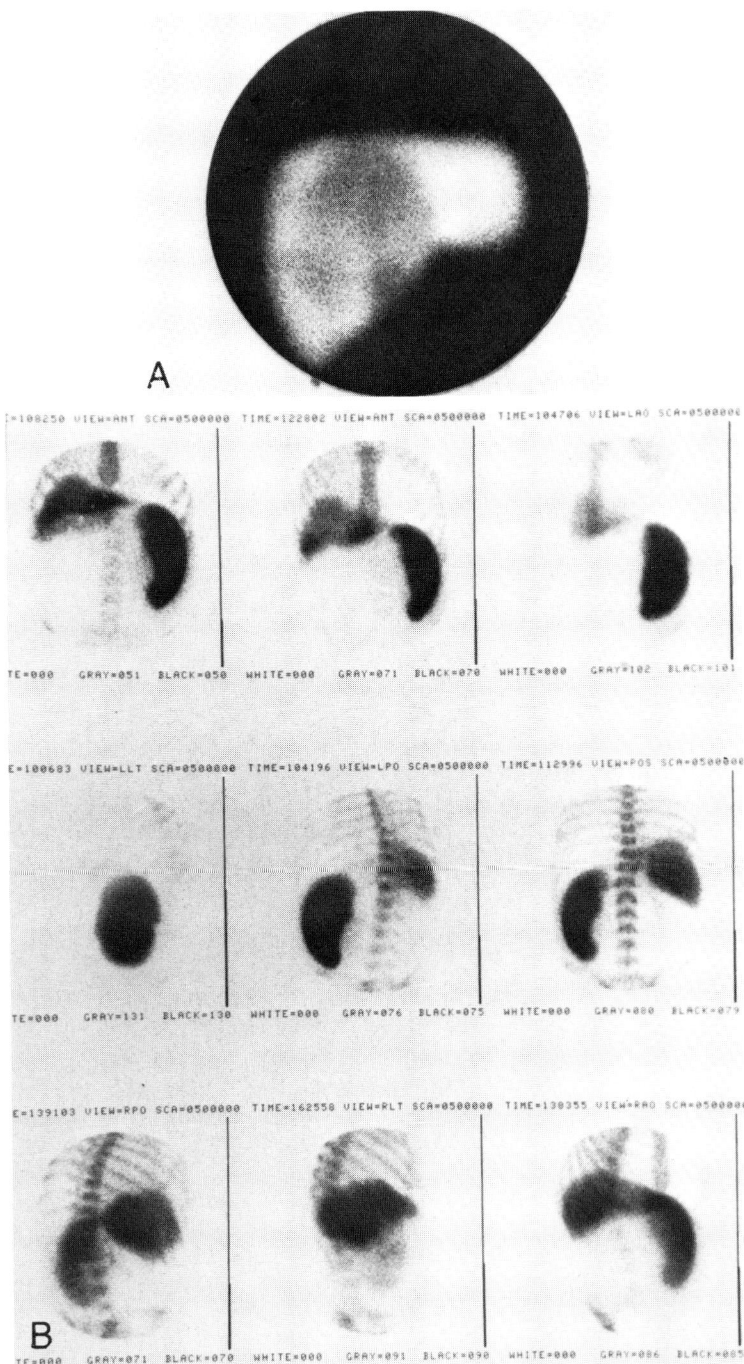

FIGURE 9–7. Liver-spleen scan. *A.* Hepatoma. Image of the liver from a ^{99m}Tc–sulfur colloid scan shows a large spherical defect in the right lobe of the liver. *B.* Cirrhosis of the liver. Multiple images of the liver and spleen from a ^{99m}Tc–sulfur colloid scan show a small liver, an enlarged spleen, and extensive bone marrow labeling in a patient with advanced cirrhosis. The reversal of flow in the portal vein contributes to the expansion and increased radioisotope uptake in the spleen. Because the reticuloendothelial (RE) cells in the liver do not accumulate much ^{99m}Tc–sulfur colloid, there is greater than normal uptake in the RE system associated with the erythropoietic bone marrow.

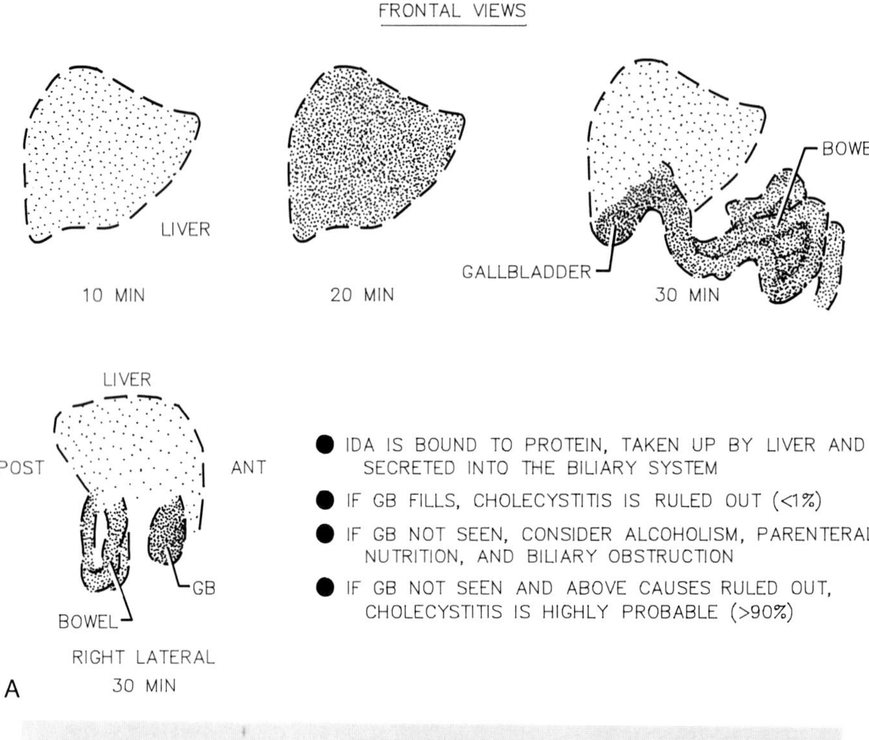

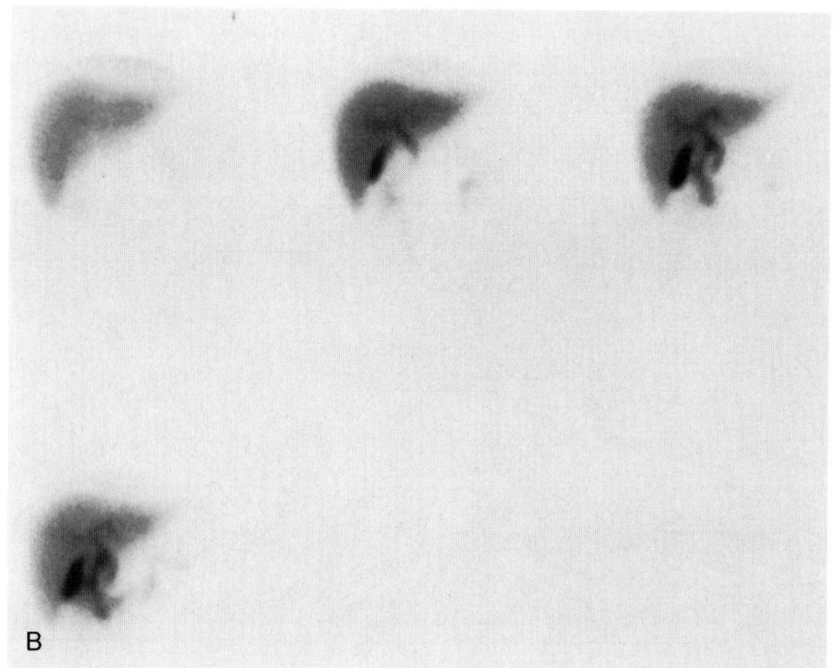

FIGURE 9–8. Biliary Scan. *A.* Diagram. POST, posterior; ANT, anterior; GB, gallbladder; IDA, iminodiacetate. *B.* Normal pattern of ^{99m}Tc–labeled iminodiacetate (IDA) radiopharmaceutical is shown in the anterior projection 5, 15, 30, and 45 minutes after injection. There is prompt accumulation of the radiopharmaceutical by the hepatocytes. A small amount is excreted by the kidneys. The gallbladder fills quickly and is seen paralleling the inferior margin of the right lobe of the liver. The common bile duct is also seen as it exits the porta hepatis in the second image. The midportion of the duodenum is seen as an accumulation of radiopharmaceutical between the intensely enhanced gallbladder and the distal common bile duct in the third image. Activity appears in the proximal jejunum in the fourth image.

maximally distended, preventing further storage of bile. In such circumstances, the radioactive bile does not accumulate in the gallbladder. Liver abnormalities incidentally detected during the hepatic phase of the biliary scan should be followed by other examinations such as liver-spleen scan or CT.

Gastroesophageal Reflux and Gastric Emptying Scan

In order to detect gastroesophageal reflux, the patient swallows 0.5 mCi (18.5 MBq) of ^{99m}Tc–sulfur colloid, and images of the esophagus are obtained during the next 30 minutes. Persistent presence of the radioisotope in the esophagus suggests gastroesophageal obstruction, and recurrent retrograde appearance of activity in the esophagus is diagnostic of reflux. Delayed images centered over the lungs can be used to diagnose occult tracheoesophageal fistula or aspiration, a condition often encountered in pediatric patients with recurrent pneumonia. More sophisticated esophageal transit studies performed during swallowing are available in some nuclear medicine laboratories, and the results correlate well with results of manometry studies of motility disorders.

The rate of disappearance of the radioisotope from the stomach can be quantified to provide a description of the kinetics of gastric emptying. Solid-phase (such as ^{99m}Tc–sulfur colloid scrambled in eggs) or liquid-phase (e.g., dissolved in juice) emptying values are calculated as half-life emptying times. It is important to standardize this measurement by beginning when the patient's stomach is empty.

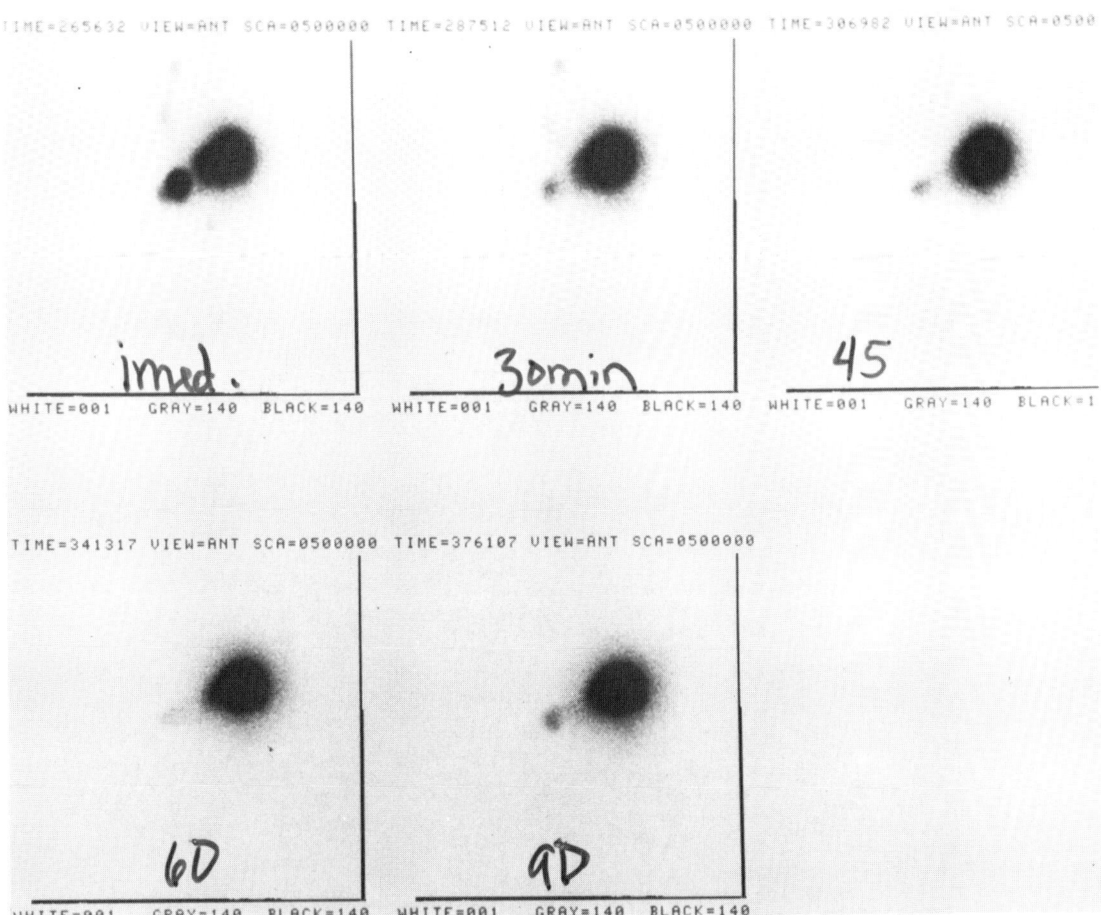

FIGURE 9–9. Diabetic gastroparesis. Gastric emptying study with images taken immediately and 30, 45, 60, and 90 minutes after the ingestion of ^{99m}Tc–sulfur colloid mixed in scrambled eggs shows a grossly abnormal, aperistaltic stomach in a diabetic male. The half-time of emptying is extremely prolonged with no apparent emptying of the stomach. The first two images show traces of activity in the esophagus, which could indicate reduced esophageal peristalsis or reflux.

The use of the supine position avoids confusion with the effects of gravity. The adynamic stomach in patients with diabetes mellitus, neuromuscular disorders, or gastric outlet obstruction and in association with the effects of drugs such as metoclopramide hydrochloride (Reglan) also can be evaluated (Fig. 9–9).

Meckel's Diverticulum Scan

In order to assess Meckel's diverticulum, 15 mCi (555 MBq) of sodium pertechnetate Tc 99m is intravenously administered after 24 hours of cimetidine administration, and then the abdomen is imaged every 5 minutes for 30 minutes. The radiopharmaceutical is concentrated in normal gastric mucosa. Meckel's diverticula that contain ectopic gastric mucosa (found in 15% of Meckel's diverticula) also take up the radiopharmaceutical. Other sites of ectopic gastric mucosa, such as Barrett's esophagus and duplication cysts of the gut, may also be found with this technique.

GENITOURINARY EXAMINATION

Three types of renal imaging examinations are used in nuclear medicine: blood-flow (perfusion), cortex, and function scans. These examinations are valuable for examining patients with allergy to intravenous contrast material, with poor renal function, and with renal transplants, as well as for quantitatively following renal function. Renal scans can be used to determine whether a solid mass contains functioning renal tissue. This technique has also been used for detection of wedge-shaped areas of pyelonephritis in children. The renal cortical agents are also effective in conjunction with ^{67}Ga, ^{111}In–labeled white blood cells, and ^{131}I–NP59 adrenal cortical scans and iodine I 131–metaiodobenzyl guanide (^{131}I–MIBG) adrenal medullary scans to clarify the position of retroperitoneal abnormalities. Ultrasonography, CT, and magnetic resonance imaging (MRI) have rendered the anatomical images of cortical agents obsolete for most applications.

Renal Perfusion Scan

Renal perfusion and glomerular filtration rate can be evaluated with ^{99m}Tc–DTPA. This agent remains in the blood vessels and in the extracellular space and is rapidly cleared from the kidneys by means of glomerular filtration.

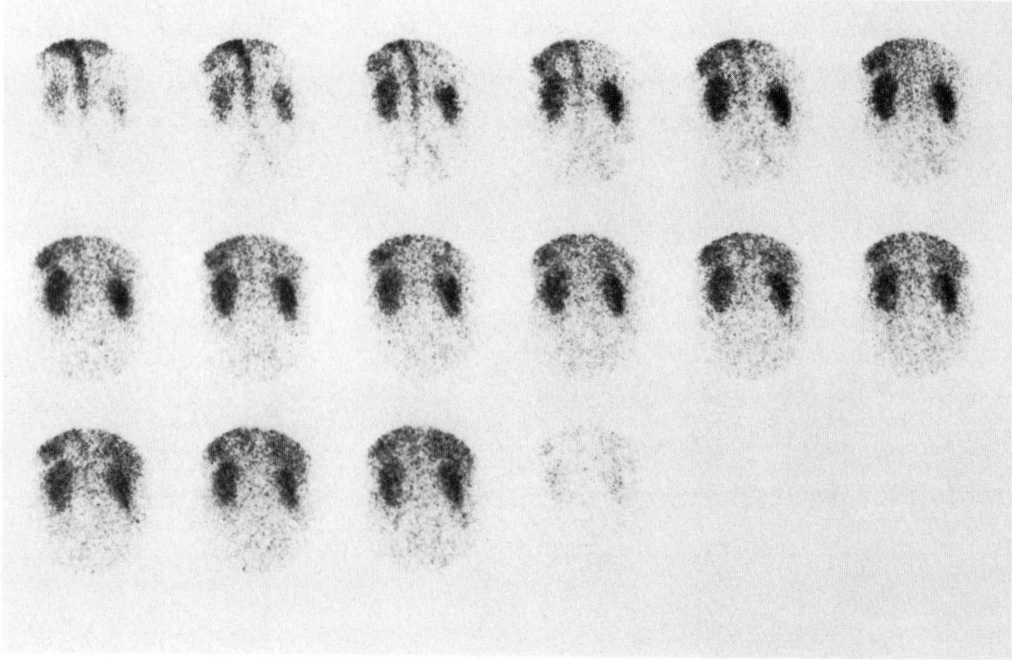

FIGURE 9–10. Normal renal perfusion scan. Posterior projection images obtained at 1-second intervals after the bolus injection of ^{99m}Tc–DTPA are displayed from left to right and top to bottom. The bolus starts down the abdominal aorta and is promptly seen in the kidneys. Above and lateral to the left kidney there is also an immediate blush of radioactivity in the spleen. Blood arriving later through the portal system begins to fill in the liver above the right kidney.

Perfusion scans are usually requested in order to evaluate renal artery blood flow in patients with suspected renovascular hypertension, trauma, or other vascular occlusion. Renal perfusion is assessed by the timing and the symmetry of function. Normally, there is prompt symmetrical perfusion of both kidneys (Fig. 9–10). The glomerular filtration rate can be quantified through a variety of methods by which to measure the clearance of the ^{99m}Tc–DTPA. These methods, which are complex, have varying degrees of accuracy.

Renal Cortex Scan

The renal cortex is best evaluated with technetium 99m–labeled glucoheptonate (^{99m}Tc–glucoheptonate) or technetium 99m–labeled dimercaptosuccinic acid (^{99m}Tc–DMSA). Both agents bind to the proximal and distal tubule cells of the kidney and enable imaging of the functioning renal cortex. Indications are findings of renal cortical dysfunction and focal renal abnormalities such as infection, infarction, and tumor. The patient with an allergy to intravenous contrast can also be studied with a renal cortical scan. Sometimes intravenous pyelography, CT, or ultrasonography of the kidney identifies a column of Bertin that simulates a tumor. Demonstration of a normally functioning column of Bertin by cortical function imaging eliminates the question of tumor.

Interpretation of the renal cortex scan is based on identification of focal areas of decreased uptake or of diffuse areas of decreased uptake in relation to the opposite kidney or to normal kidneys. Because the agent is bound to the renal cortex, the radiation dose to the kidney is higher than for other renal examinations (0.02 Gy).

Renal Function Scan

Renal function, measured by the effective renal plasma flow (ERPF), is determined with I 123– or I 131–labeled hippurate (Hippuran I 123 or I 131). Hippurate is a variation of para-aminohippuranic acid, which is used for physiological studies of the kidneys because of its rapid clearance by means of both glomerular filtration (20%) and tubular secretion (80%). A technetium-labeled radiopharmaceutical, mercaptoacetyl triglycine, is also available as an ERPF agent. Because of the high image quality of ^{99m}Tc images and ease of preparation, ^{99m}Tc–mercaptoacetyl triglycine has obvious advantages over Hippuran I 131; however, Hippuran I 131 is widely used.

Each aspect of renal function (blood flow, uptake, filtration, and secretion) influences the duration and the intensity of uptake; therefore, of the three types of renal scans, the renal function scan yields the most information. It is used to evaluate overall renal function, to follow the course of acute tubular necrosis, and to assess renal transplant function. These studies have an extra advantage for patients who are allergic to radiographic contrast or patients who must have frequent examinations, such as those with renal transplants. A renal function examination cannot definitively distinguish between acute tubular necrosis and chronic rejection of a transplanted kidney. However, the clinical context and particularly the clinical time course often assist in making this distinction. Acute rejection is characterized by a marked decrease in perfusion shortly (hours) after transplantation and is easily distinguished from acute tubular necrosis.

Interpretation of the renal function scan is based on uptake of the radiopharmaceutical by the renal cortex (usually by 4 to 8 minutes after administration) and excretion by the kidneys over the subsequent 20 to 30 minutes. A plot of renal uptake over time (renogram curve) can be used to compare function with that from previous examinations (Fig. 9–11). It is important to ensure that the bladder has been drained, either by voiding or with a Foley catheter, in order to prevent the bladder from receiving an unnecessary dose of radiation.

The use of furosemide (Lasix) with a renal function study enables evaluation of a kidney with a dilated collecting system or ureter or both. Congenital caliectasis, megaureter, or relieved obstruction of the collecting system have an appearance similar to that of truly obstructed ureters. A dilated collecting system visible on standard renograms (without furosemide), ultrasonograms, CT scans, and intravenous urograms may be suggestive of obstruction, indicating the need for a renal function examination. The characteristic renogram curve after furosemide administration shows continued accumulation of radioactivity in the truly obstructed kidney. There is a rapid washout from the unobstructed, normal kidney when collecting system dilation is not obstructive (Fig. 9–12).

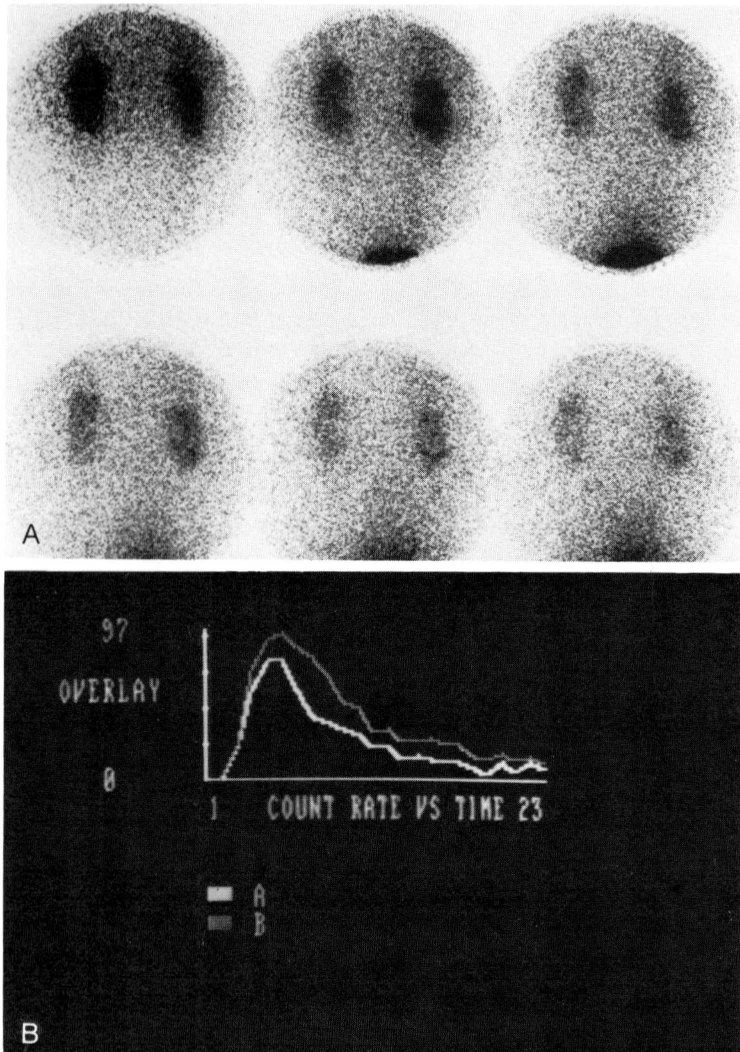

FIGURE 9–11. Renal function scan. *A.* Normal renogram. Normal Hippuran I 131 renal function study in the posterior projection was filmed every 4 minutes after injection. The grainy, low-resolution images are characteristic of ^{131}I radiopharmaceuticals. The kidneys promptly and symmetrically extract and excrete this agent, which passes rapidly to the bladder. *B.* The time course of uptake and excretion (renogram curves) are plotted for each kidney. There is a rapid rise to a peak in 4 to 6 minutes with an exponential decrease in kidney radioactivity thereafter as the urine passes to the bladder.

Captopril Renogram

In a small subset of patients with hypertension, the cause is renal artery stenosis. The renal arterial flow study is fairly specific for this but grossly insensitive. Not all renal artery stenosis causes hypertension. When it does, the postcapillary renal arteriole constricts under the influence of angiotensin II to keep filtration pressure up. Thus glomerular filtration continues, even with low input pressure from the perirenal arteriole. Under the acute influence of an angiotensin-converting enzyme inhibitor (such as captopril), the postcapillary sphincter pressure drops, and a renal scan demonstrates the failure of the affected kidney to produce urine. This physiological test can be used to detect a curable cause of hypertension (Fig. 9–13).

Cystography

Cystographic examinations of the bladder are performed with the use of radiopharmaceuticals that are not absorbed by the bladder mucosa, such as ^{99m}Tc–sulfur colloid. The presence of ureteral reflux during filling or emptying is much more sensitively detected with isotopes than with intravenous contrast technique. The radiation dose from a nuclear medicine cystogram is lower than that from an x-ray cystogram. If the volume of agent administered and the pressure in the urinary bladder are measured, a cystometrogram can be conveniently combined with this study in order to determine the volume and the pressure at which the reflux occurs.

Renal Scans With Iodine 131 Metaiodobenzyl Guanide and NP59

Two radiopharmaceuticals are used for imaging tumors in the adrenal gland. Iodine 131–MIBG is relatively specific for both intra- and extra-adrenal pheochromocytoma and neuroblastoma. Imaging with ^{131}I–MIBG carries no associated risk of hypertensive crisis as does iodinated contrast in patients with pheochromocytoma (Fig. 9–14). In large doses, ^{131}I–

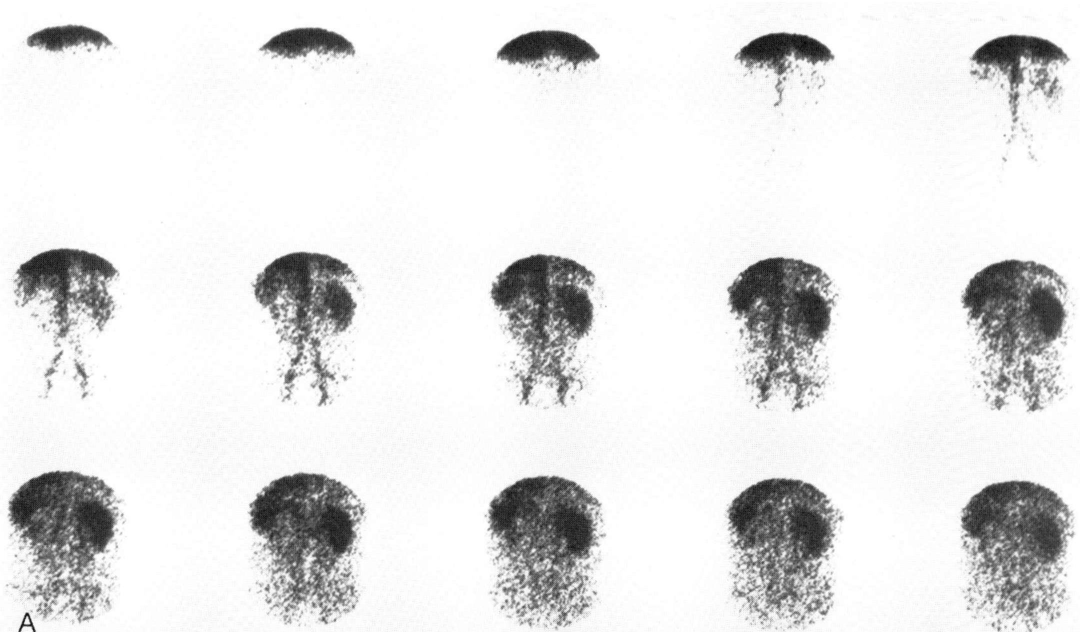

FIGURE 9–12. Renal function scan for hydronephrosis. *A.* Renal perfusion scan with ^{99m}Tc–DTPA (posterior projections at one-second intervals) shows from left to right and top to bottom a bolus of radioactivity in the lungs and the heart and then in the descending aorta (fourth image), rapidly perfusing the right kidney and the spleen, which is just below the base of the left lung. As the study progressed, there was gradual but poor perfusion of the left kidney.

Illustration continued on following page

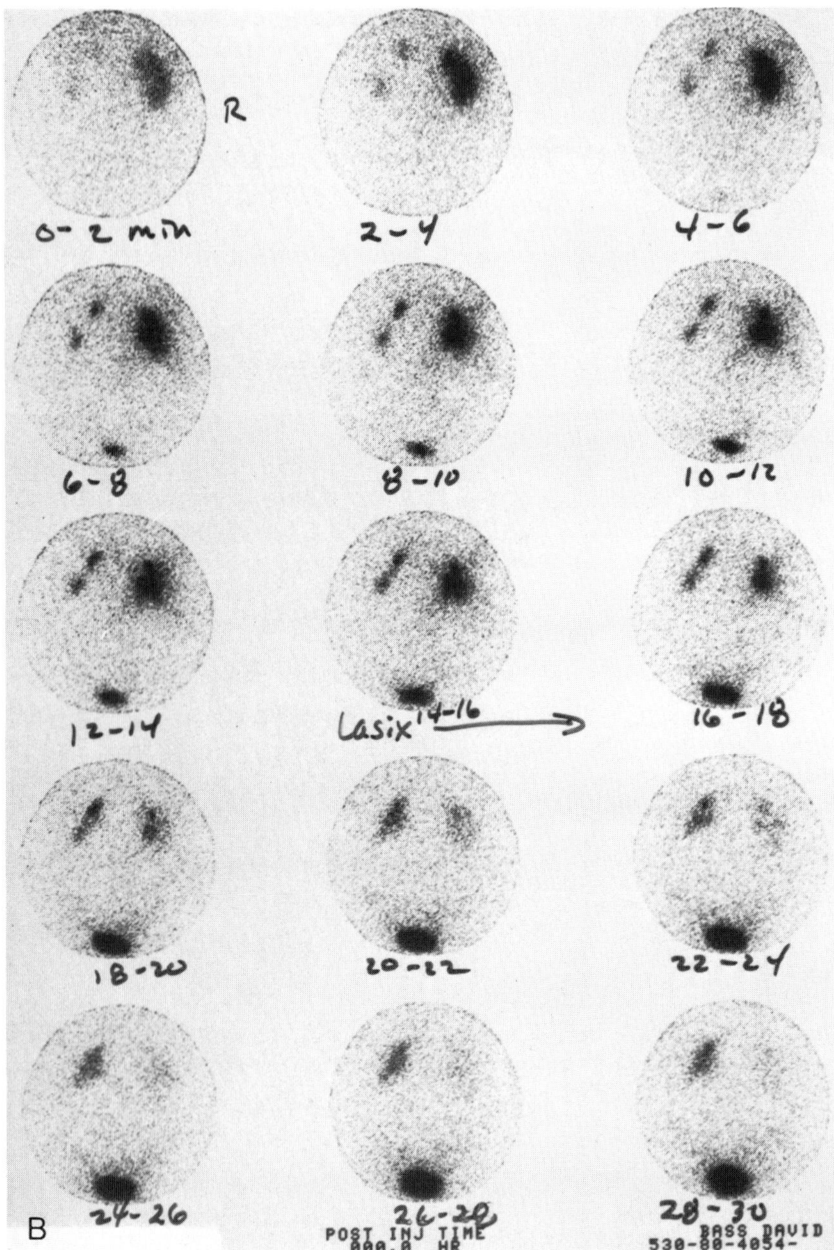

FIGURE 9–12 *Continued B.* Immediately after the perfusion study, the renogram is continued at 2-minute intervals for 30 minutes. Initially, the right kidney extracts ^{99m}Tc–DTPA normally. By 6 to 8 minutes, the right kidney showed dense uptake, which raised the question of hydronephrosis with an obstructed upper collecting system. Furosemide (Lasix) was administered at 15 minutes, and the radioactivity of the right kidney diminished quickly, indicating that the dense uptake was attributable to a dilated extrarenal pelvis, with a reservoir of urine that quickly drained with diuresis. The left kidney slowly accumulated ^{99m}Tc–DTPA at the beginning of the study and continued to do so even after furosemide was administered. This accumulation reached maximal radioactivity at the end of the study. This represented a complete obstruction at the level of the ureteropelvic junction.

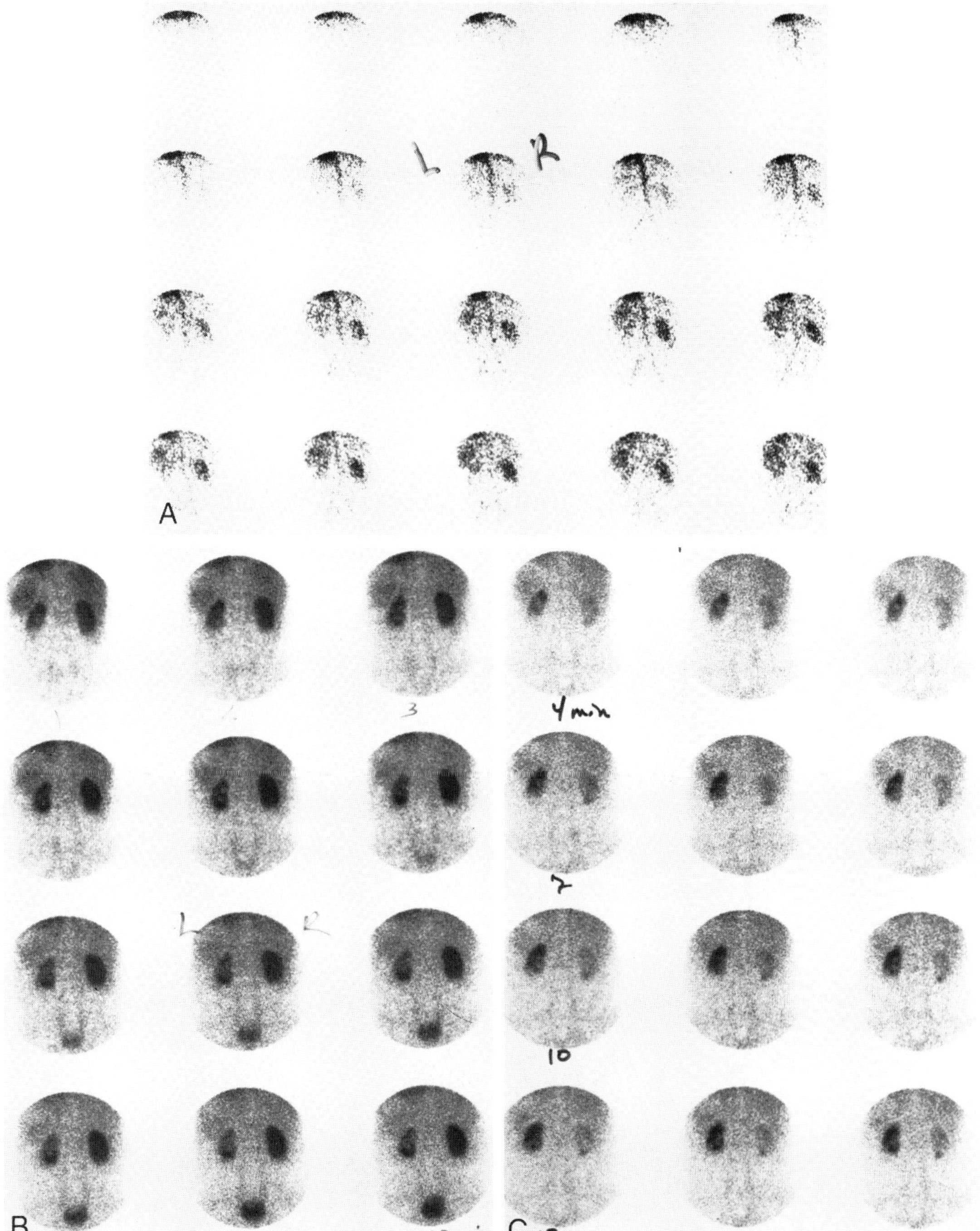

FIGURE 9–13. Captopril renography for renal artery hypertension. *A.* Renal perfusion study with ^{99m}Tc–DTPA (in the posterior projections at 1-second intervals) shows delayed perfusion to both kidneys. The left kidney (inferior to the spleen) is more poorly perfused than the right. One or both renal artery stenoses could be the cause of this pattern and the patient's hypertension. *B.* Continuation of the renogram, pursued for the next 12 minutes, shows the left kidney to be smaller than the right. Both make urine at a reduced rate. Normally, there is peak activity at 4 to 6 minutes and more rapid washout. *C.* A second renogram 1 hour after the oral administration of 50 mg of captopril is shown from 4 to 15 minutes after the injection of ^{99m}Tc–DTPA. There is now a marked reduction of urine formation in the right kidney. The small left kidney functions as before. The glomerular filtration rate in the right kidney decreased when angiotensin II was no longer present to increase postcapillary pressure in the right kidney. This study is predictive of normalization of blood pressure after correction of the right renal artery stenosis.

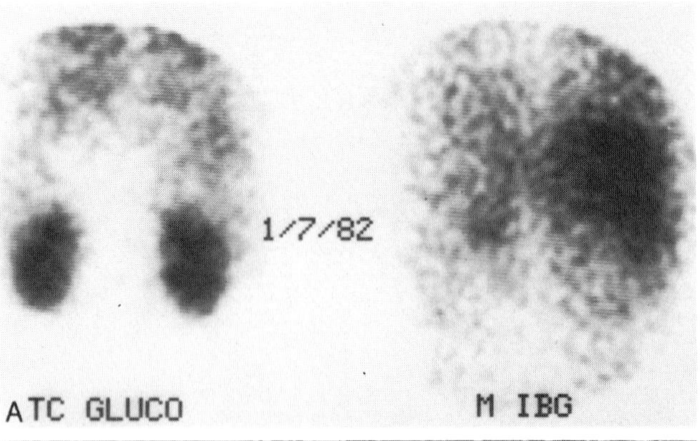

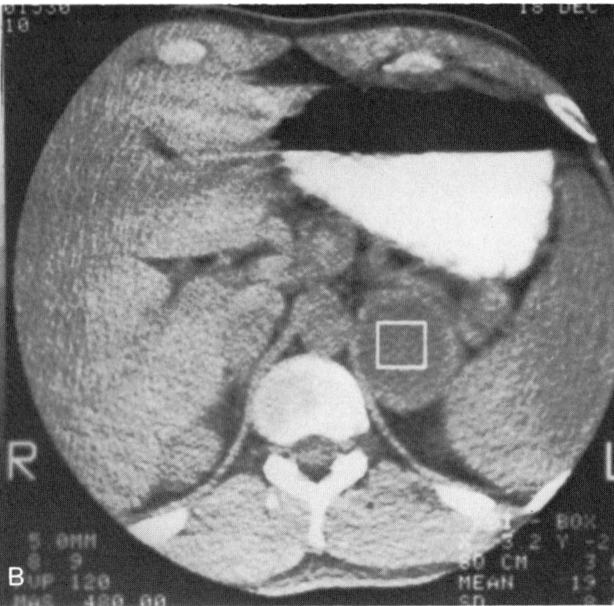

FIGURE 9–14. Pheochromocytoma. *A.* Two scans were performed simultaneously in the posterior projection. The ^{99m}Tc–glucoheptonate scan (on the left) shows the locations of the kidneys. The iodine 131–metaiodobenzyl guanide (^{131}I–MIBG) scan (on the right) shows normal liver uptake and an abnormal area of uptake superior to the left kidney. *B.* The square region of interest on the computed tomogram (CT) marks the round, left adrenal pheochromocytoma located between the spleen and vertebral column. The nuclear medicine study is important for confirming the location of the tumor and any additional pheochromocytomas before surgery.

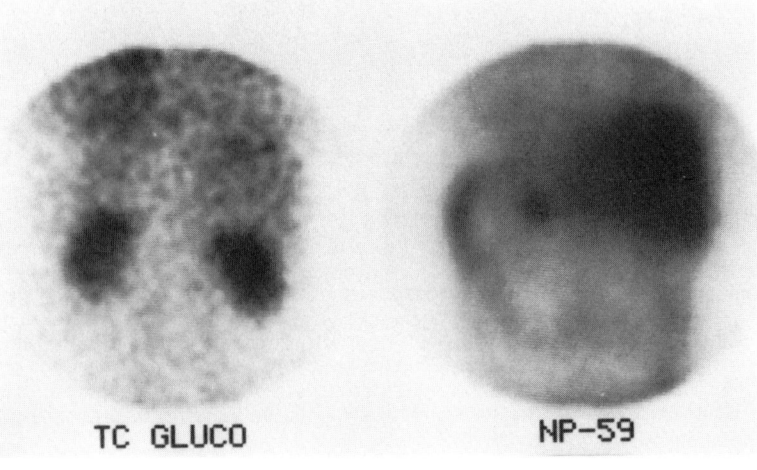

FIGURE 9–15. Left adrenal cortical adenoma. In a manner similar to that in Figures 9–14*A* and 9–14*B*, a ^{99m}Tc–glucoheptonate scan locates the kidneys for reference to the ^{131}I–labeled NP59 scan that shows physiological uptake in the liver and colon and abnormal uptake in the left adrenal. Iodine 131 NP59 accumulates only in the autonomous cortical tissue because normal adrenal uptake of this radionuclide is blocked by the administration of dexamethasone.

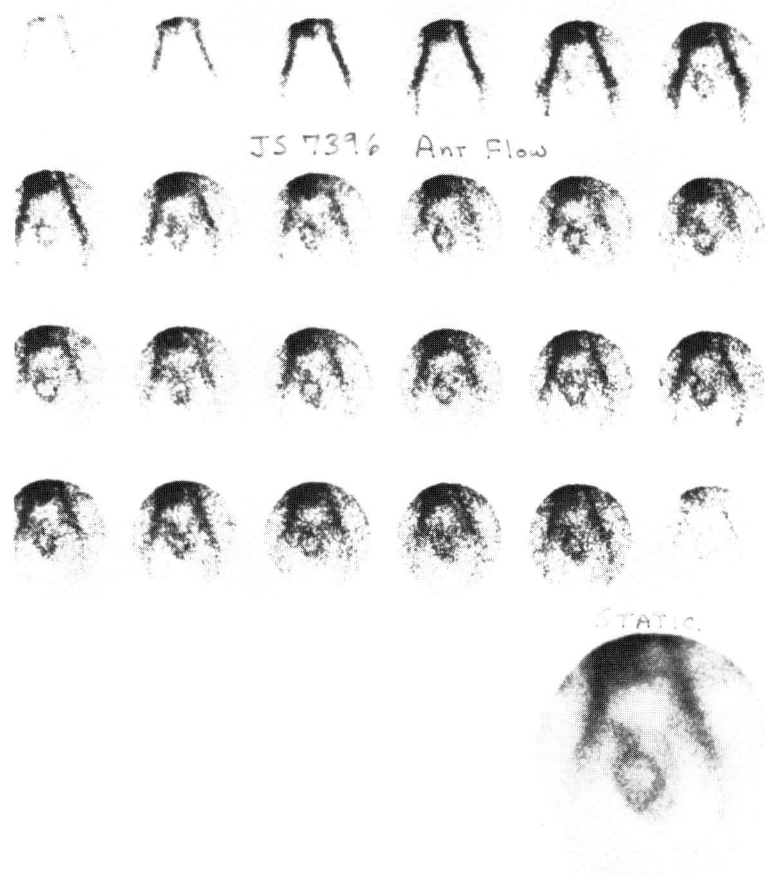

FIGURE 9–16. "Missed" testicular torsion. Twenty-four hours after the onset of testicular pain, flow-study images document early and abnormally intense perfusion to the right hemiscrotum. The immediate static image shows a "hot" (high-uptake) ring around the right testicle, which has a "cold" (low-uptake) center. These findings correspond to reactive hyperemia around a torsed, infarcted testicle. It is too late for surgery to save this testicle. Surgery may be performed to prevent the development of torsion of the other testicle.

MIBG has been used with partial success as a therapeutic agent in the treatment of pheochromocytoma. The experimental radiopharmaceutical ^{131}I–NP59 localizes autonomous adrenal cortical adenomas after suppression by dexamethasone of normal adrenal tissue. Examinations with this agent can determine that an expanded adrenal found on CT is functioning normally and is not a metastatic deposit (Fig. 9–15). The low frequency of these adrenal problems has delayed approval of these agents by the United States Food and Drug Administration because there is very little market to induce a drug manufacturer to complete expensive clinical trials. These two radiopharmaceuticals will therefore probably remain investigational indefinitely.

Testicular Scan

Epididymitis and "missed" testicular torsion (said to be missed if it is too late for surgical salvage of a viable testicle) can be efficiently differentiated on a testicular scan. A simple dynamic perfusion study with pertechnetate Tc 99m or ^{99m}Tc–DTPA generally shows an increased arterial supply to the affected hemiscrotum. A static image demonstrates hyperemia along the curved epididymis when it is inflamed. The hyperemia of a late torsion encircles the entire testicle, which is itself nonperfused and appears cold on the scan (Fig. 9–16).

SKELETAL EXAMINATION

A variety of radiopharmaceuticals are taken up by bone or bone marrow. Many of these agents are used primarily for imaging other organs such as the heart (with technetium 99m–labeled pyrophosphate [^{99m}Tc–pyrophosphate]), the liver and the spleen (with ^{99m}Tc–sulfur colloid), or the distribution of leukocytes (with ^{111}In–labeled white blood cells). In addition to focal areas of abnormal uptake, the uptake by bones in comparison with other

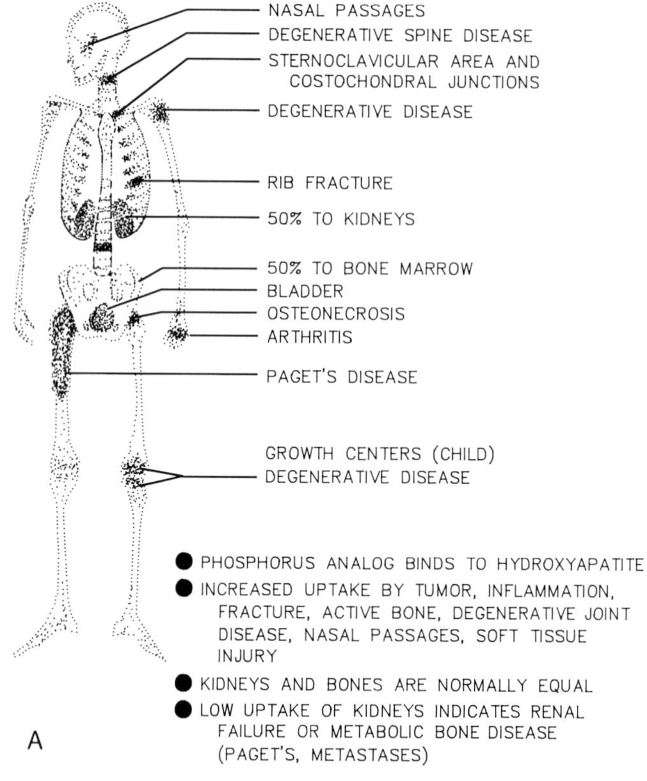

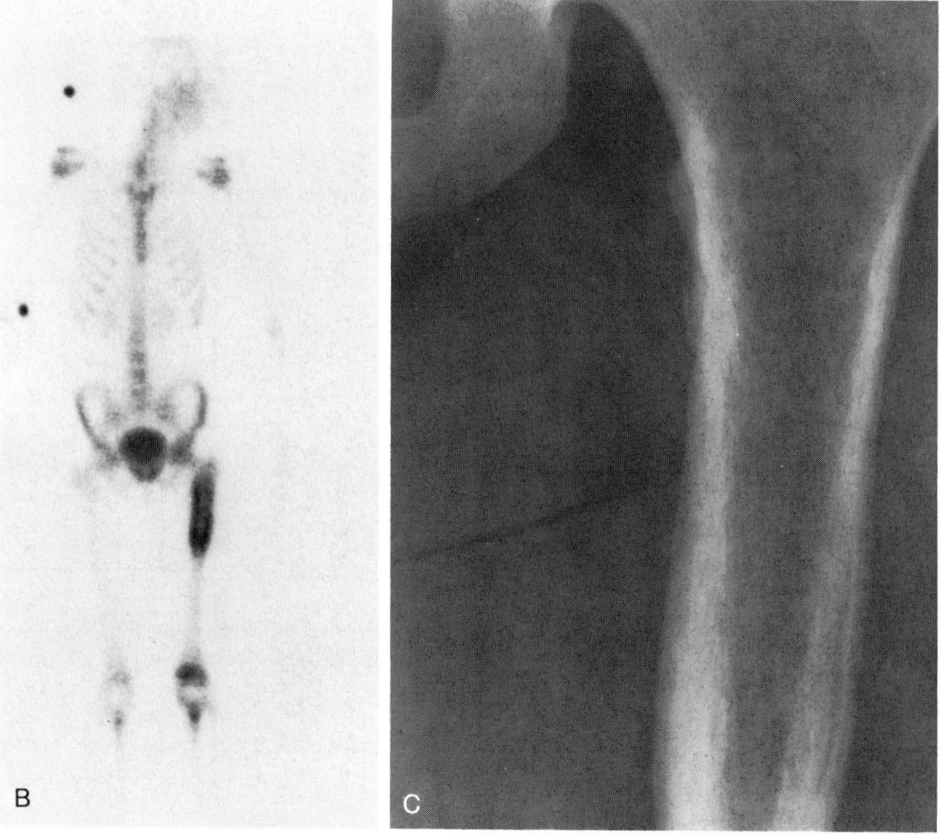

FIGURE 9–17 *See legend on opposite page*

organs often provides important diagnostic information about generalized bone disease.

Bone Scan

Bone imaging is performed with technetium 99m–labeled methylene diphosphonate (^{99m}Tc–MDP), a phosphate analog that osteoblasts incorporate into hydroxyapatite (Fig. 9–17). Bone reacting to tumor, infection, or fracture shows increased uptake with ^{99m}Tc–MDP and similar agents (Fig. 9–18). Metabolic and degenerative disease can also lead to increased uptake (Figs. 9–19, 9–20). Myeloma inconsistently produces areas of increased, decreased, or normal ^{99m}Tc–MDP accumulation. However, the likelihood of a completely normal scan in a patient with myeloma is low.

A bone scan is the most informative test for general screening for metastatic bone lesions and is helpful for further evaluating known bone lesions. MRI, particularly with short TI inversion recovery (STIR) sequences, is the most sensitive test for detecting marrow lesions and frequently identifies tumor months before an abnormality is visible on bone scans (see Chapter 7). However, because total body screening of all marrow with MRI is not practical, general screening is performed with the bone scan. Areas of increased uptake should be compared with clinical symptoms, radiographs, CT, and MRI.

Interpretation of the bone scan (see Fig. 9–17) includes evaluation of the kidneys and the bladder (50% of the agent normally is excreted in 2 to 4 hours), notice of areas in which increased uptake is normal (growth centers, degenerative joint disease, nasal passages), and identification of areas of abnormally increased uptake (hot lesions) or decreased uptake (cold lesions) (Table 9–4).

Several nuclear medicine examinations, obtained for other reasons, show uptake in the bone marrow. Liver-spleen scans show erythropoietic marrow. Myocardial pyrophosphate scans also demonstrate bone uptake. Both may suggest the need for a bone scan. The kidneys occasionally show increased uptake in comparison with the bones. This finding can be a result of irradiation of the kidneys, renal-toxic drugs, renal obstruction, or a general decrease in bone uptake. Alternatively, the renal uptake may be greatly decreased in comparison with the bones (such a finding is called a superscan). Such an appearance is usually attributable to Paget's disease (see Fig. 9–19), metastatic tu-

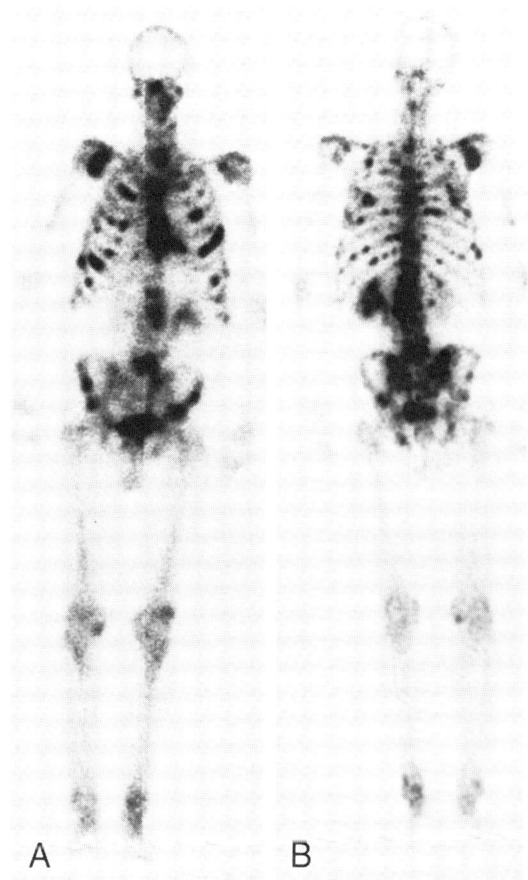

FIGURE 9–18. Metastatic carcinoma of the prostate. Anterior *(A)* and posterior *(B)* whole-body bone scan images show numerous areas of abnormal, increased activity randomly scattered throughout the axial skeleton. They are of different size and intensity. Note also the accumulation of radioactive urine in the left kidney's upper collecting system, which is obstructed by the primary tumor.

FIGURE 9–17. Bone scan. *A.* Diagram. *B.* Whole-body bone scan in the anterior projection shows intense labeling of the left proximal femur in a 20-year-old male with Ewing's sarcoma. (The small dot near the right elbow is an artifact of the intravenous injection.) The increased labeling represents bone formation around the sarcoma. *C.* Radiograph of the left femur shows expansion of the cortical bone and lytic changes characteristic of this primary tumor. The principle utility of the bone scan in this case is to establish whether the tumor is a single- or multiple-site problem.

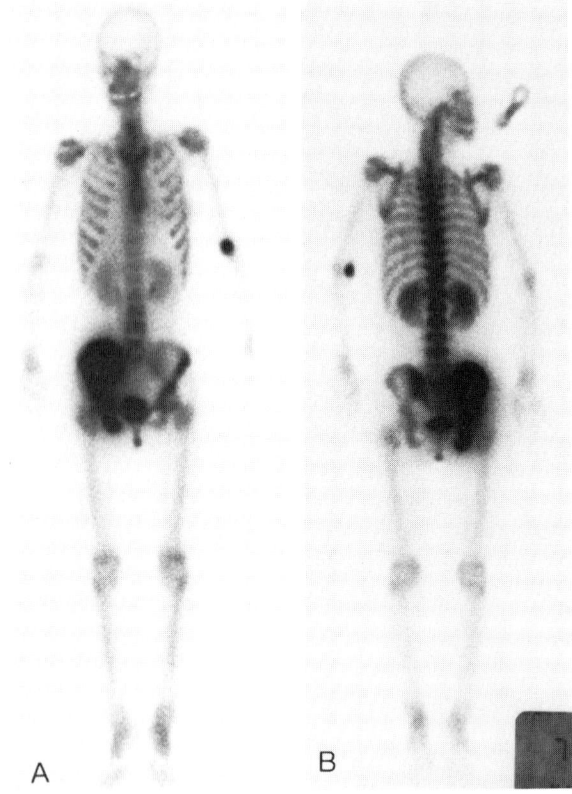

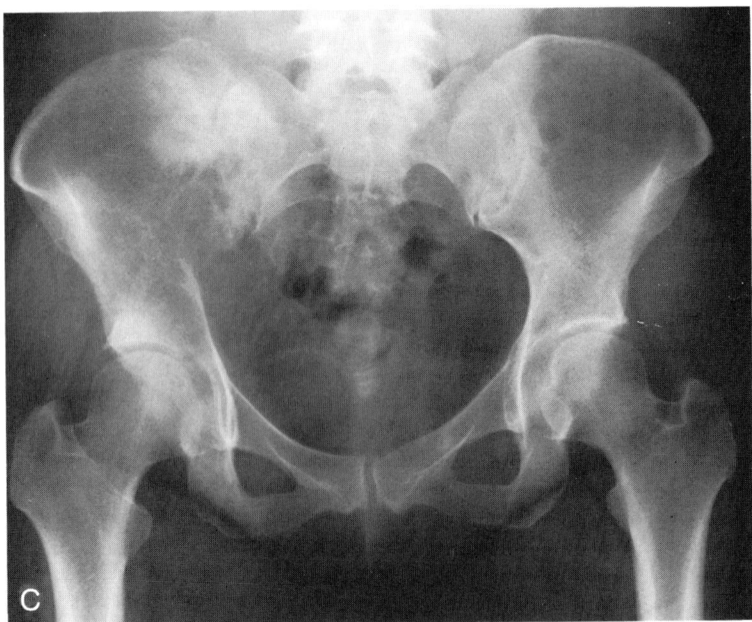

FIGURE 9–19. Paget's disease of the right ilium. Anterior *(A)* and posterior *(B)* whole-body bone scans show uniform intense labeling of the entire right ilium. Pelvic radiograph *(C)* shows sclerotic, thickened trabeculae. A subtle enlargement of the right ilium can be discerned by comparison with the left ilium.

mor (see Fig. 9–18), or renal failure. Other disorders in which bone blood flow is disproportionately increased include those associated with bone marrow hyperplasia (hematological diseases) and increased metabolism (hyperparathyroidism).

Bone Mass Measurement by Dual Photon Absorptiometry

A group of bone disorders collectively discussed as osteoporosis share a characteristic

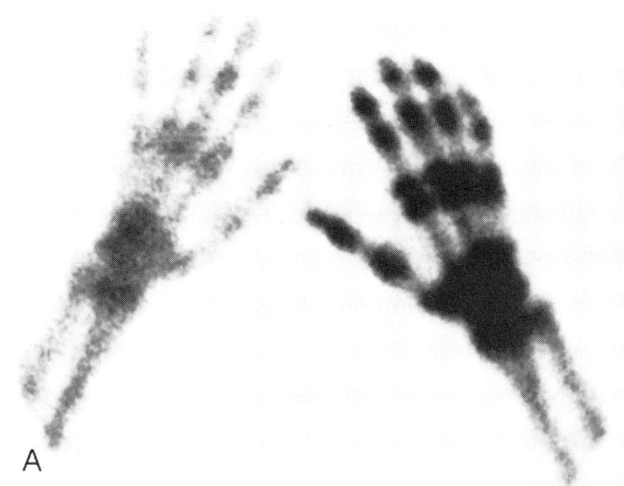

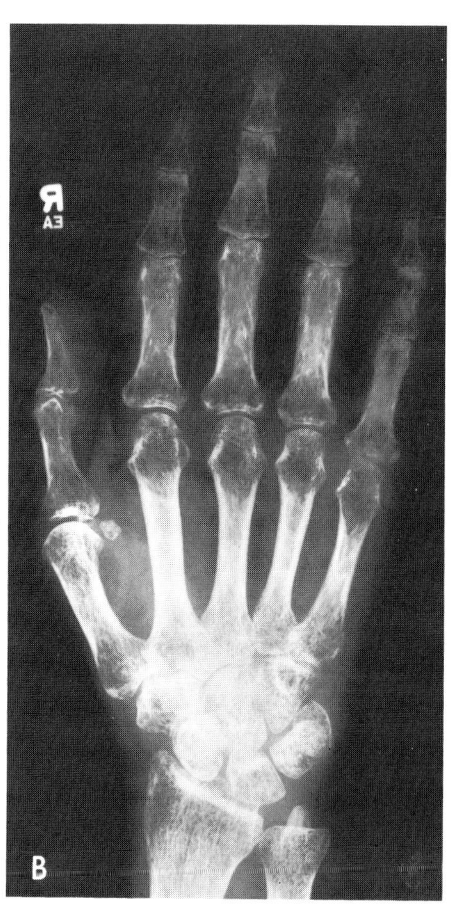

FIGURE 9–20. Reflex sympathetic dystrophy. Bone scan *(A)* of the hands shows abnormally intense labeling of the left hand in a very uniform fashion. When the sympathetic tone of the arteries is lost, increased blood flow promotes both osteoblast *and* osteoclast function. The former is seen on the bone scan; the latter is seen on the radiograph *(B)*. There is severe loss of bone mineral of all the bones. Although both destruction and production of bone are stimulated, bone resorption dominates.

decrease in mineralized bone density. An accurate measurement of bone mass can be made with an instrument called a dual photon absorptiometer. A tightly collimated gadolinium 153 source, mounted in a rectilinear scan device, provides a beam of simultaneous 40- and 100-keV gamma emissions. The differential absorption of these two energies enables calculation of the density of the bone, which indicates the amount of calcium in the path of the beam (Fig. 9–21). Standards for normally aging populations of different ethnic groups

TABLE 9–4. LESIONS SHOWING INCREASED, DECREASED, AND NORMAL UPTAKE ON THE BONE SCAN

Increased Uptake	Decreased Uptake	Normal Uptake
Metastic tumor	Osteonecrosis (early stages)	Simple cyst
Myeloma (80%)	Radiation	Bone island
Osteonecrosis (late stages)	Osteomyelitis	Osteopoikilosis
Inflammation	Photon absorber	Fibrous cortical defect
Fracture (positive for 1 year)	Sickle cell crisis	Myeloma (20%)
Arthritis	Metastases from lung, kidney, breast and melanoma	
Metabolic disease		
Paget's disease		
Soft tissue calcification		
Histiocytosis X		
Fibrous dysplasia		
Melorrheostosis		
Degenerative disease		
Osteoid osteoma		
Aneurysmal bone cyst		

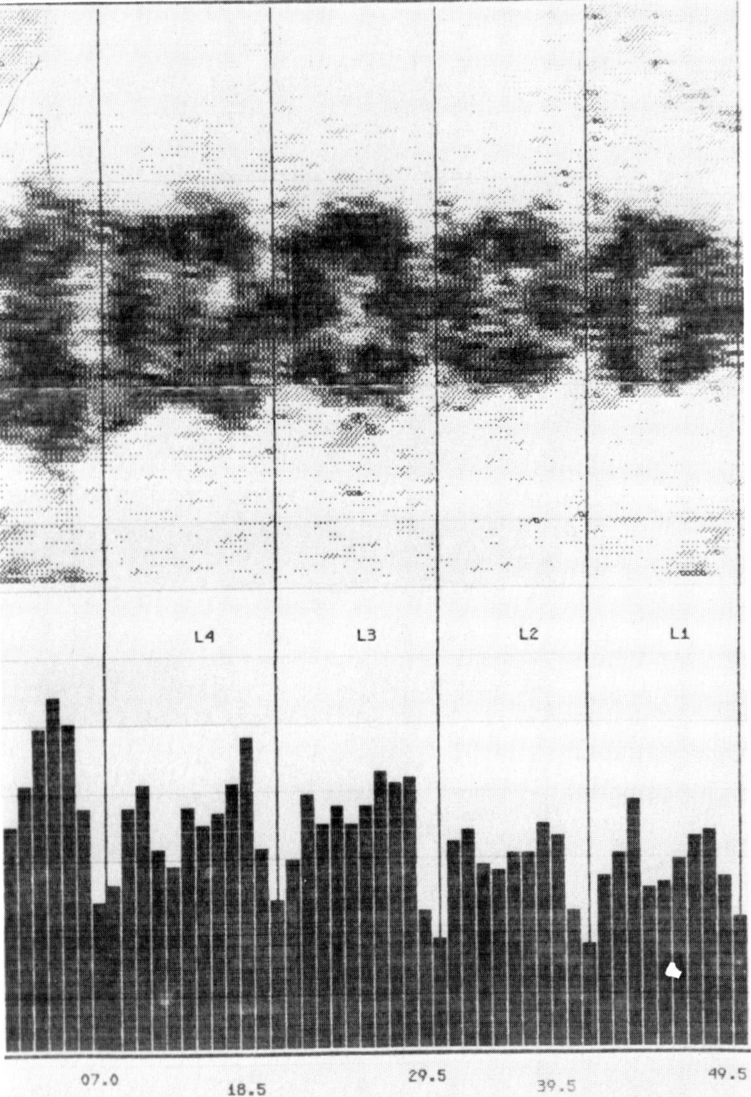

FIGURE 9–21. Dual photon absorptiometry of the lumbar spine in osteoporosis. A 59-year-old white male has a bone mineral density of 1.08 g/cm^2 in the region of L-2 to L-4; this density is 91.5% of that of an age-matched normal control. The display is typical of a coarse rectilinear scan. The histogram below the scan summarizes linear bone mass for each pass of the scanner and helps determine the location of the intervertebral discs.

enable comparison of measurements of bone mass in the lumbar vertebrae and the hips with expected values and with those of young normal people. Single photon absorptiometers, which use a transmission source of ^{125}I, are used to measure the mass of small bones with little overlying soft tissue (such as the distal radius and the ulna). Quantitative CT can be used to make bone mass measurements in the vertebrae with slightly more precision than do dual photon absorptiometers. However, because the loss of skeletal mass as a result of aging is difficult to prevent and even harder to reverse, these measurements are primarily of investigational interest.

CARDIAC EXAMINATION

Cardiovascular nuclear medicine requires knowledge of both cardiovascular disease and imaging techniques of nuclear medicine. Nuclear medicine examinations are used in the evaluation of myocardial infarction, myocardial ischemia, ventricular function, and vascular flow. Because these examinations usually require physiological and image interpretation, they are performed most successfully by a nuclear medicine specialist knowledgeable in cardiovascular physiology and in conjunction with the referring cardiologist.

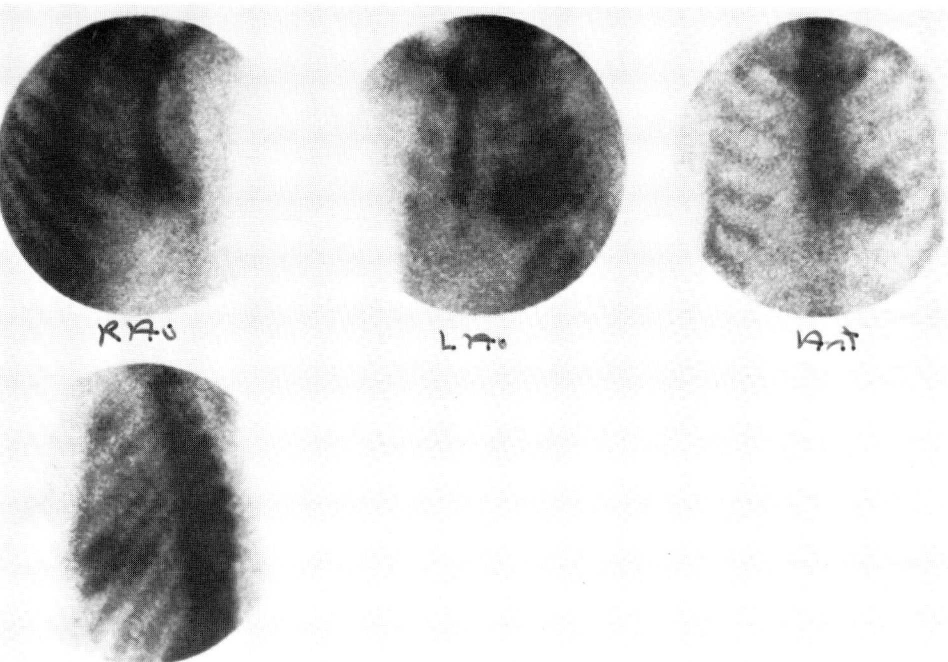

FIGURE 9–22. Pyrophosphate myocardial infarct scan. Three hours after injection of ^{99m}Tc–pyrophosphate, there was intense uptake in a circular area around the apex of the left ventricle in a patient with a 48-hour-old myocardial infarct. Seen best in the anterior projection, this abnormality is as intense as the bone uptake and forms a doughnut around a cold center. The finding indicates a very extensive infarct.

Myocardial Infarction Scan

Although electrocardiographic abnormalities and creatine phosphokinase isoenzyme elevation are usually definitive in the diagnosis of acute myocardial infarction, there are some clinical situations in which a nuclear medicine scan of the heart is needed to establish the diagnosis. These situations include equivocal electrocardiographic or isoenzyme findings, previous electrocardiographic abnormalities or myocardial infarct, suspicion of myocardial infarction after cardiac surgery (when creatine phosphokinase is always elevated), suspicion of right ventricular infarct, cardiac contusion, or suspected extension of previous infarction. Cardiac scanning to detect myocardial infarction is performed with ^{99m}Tc–pyrophosphate which, in addition to being taken up by bone, binds to calcium in infarcted myocardial tissue. Scans are obtained 2 to 4 hours after injection of the agent so as to allow the blood pool background to diminish. The examination is most likely to be positive 48 to 72 hours after myocardial infarction, but it may show an abnormality for 7 days or longer.

Interpretation requires identification of uptake by the infarcted myocardial tissue (Fig. 9–22). The normal myocardium does not take up the radiopharmaceutical. Pyrophosphate is not usually taken up by an old infarct. However, several processes can simulate infarction. These include normal spine and rib uptake (or fracture), calcification in the pericardium, soft-tissue injury, and the presence of free technetium in the stomach. Pyrophosphate is also taken up by muscles elsewhere in the body that are severely ischemic or infarcted from burns, electrical injury, and extreme overuse (e.g., leg muscle damage after marathon running) and in vascular compromise.

Another agent, ^{111}In antimyosin antibody, may be used in place of ^{99m}Tc–pyrophosphate in order to image myocardial tissue. Antimyosin antibodies can be used to label infarcted myocardial tissue or to monitor transplanted hearts for signs of rejection.

Myocardial Perfusion Scan

Cardiac ischemia is usually evaluated by monitored stress testing, and coronary artery stenosis is diagnosed on cardiac angiography.

When symptoms and stress test findings are equivocal, however, a myocardial perfusion scan can be helpful. Thallium 201 chloride (^{201}Tl chloride) is injected intravenously while the patient is strenuously exercising, and scans are obtained immediately (stress phase) and 4 hours later (resting phase). The degree of uptake of thallium, a potassium analog, by the myocardial cells depends on cardiac blood flow or ischemia. When blood flow carries the ^{201}Tl chloride to a viable cell, it is accumulated by sodium-potassium adenosine triphosphatase pumps. After the cessation of exercise, the isotope leaks out of the cell and is reaccumulated in another cell or is excreted by the kidneys. As a result, the measured rate of washout from the myocardium can increase specificity and sensitivity in the diagnosis of reversible myocardial ischemia.

Optimal myocardial evaluation requires single photon emission computed tomography (SPECT) (see Chapter 1) in order to obtain slice images of the myocardium. Images in the short-axis orientation look like doughnuts and provide the clearest depiction of areas of infarction and ischemia. An alternative to the use of physical stress to image with ^{201}Tl chloride is the use of dipyridamole (Persantine) to cause transient dilation of the normal coronary arteries. This drug is most effective when administered intravenously rather than orally. Dilated arteries deliver more blood and more ^{201}Tl chloride to the normal myocardium. Coronary arteries with fixed atherosclerotic disease do not increase in caliber and, consequently, do not distribute the isotope. The dipyridamole method does not require physical exercise but does entail risks similar to those of exercise, including cardiac arrest.

Indications for myocardial perfusion scans are evaluation of coronary artery disease in patients with atypical chest pain, equivocal electrocardiographic findings and a clear clinical history of chest pain, or a physiological evaluation of known coronary artery lesions, including coronary bypass grafts. Interpretation requires evaluation of the distribution of thallium in the heart and the lungs. Poorly perfused areas do not take up the isotope and appear as filling defects. The delayed (resting) scan may show filling in of these defects, indicating exercise-induced ischemia, or it may show a persistent defect, indicating infarction of undetermined age. Ancillary findings, such as cardiac chamber size, lung uptake, and right ventricular uptake, are often helpful in the analysis (Fig. 9–23). The administration of a second injection of ^{201}Tl chloride with the patient at rest before the delayed scan can show deep ischemia (called hibernating myocardium) that is not detected on conventional 4-hour delayed scans. Such lesions may respond to revascularization.

Several ^{99m}Tc-labeled agents are being developed to map myocardial perfusion. Unlike thallium, these radiopharmaceuticals do not have a washout or redistribution phase, and two separate studies are performed, one at rest and one during stress, for comparison.

Radionuclide Cardiac Ventriculography

Ventricular wall motion and mechanics can be studied by labeling the patient's red blood cells with ^{99m}Tc. The labeling is most conveniently accomplished in the patient's blood stream by an intravenous injection of stannous pyrophosphate followed 15 minutes later by pertechnetate Tc 99m.

Imaging the heart's chambers requires computer-gated scanning of multiple (16 or more) time segments of the cardiac cycle. As the labeled red blood cells circulate through the heart, cumulative images of these time segments of the cardiac cycle are generated. Because the total number of counts in each image corresponds to the volume of blood in the heart, comparison of the number of counts during various segments of the cardiac cycle allows computation of the ejection fraction, the average ejection rate, and the maximal ejection rate. Filling rates can also be derived.

The left anterior oblique image is optimally chosen to display the best separation of right and left ventricles. This septal view allows accurate calculation of the change in left ventricular count rate between end diastole (ED) and end systole (ES). After correction for background, the simple calculation is (ED − ES)/ED = ejection fraction. Other images in anteroposterior 70-degree left anterior oblique, and left posterior oblique projections facilitate assessment of left ventricular wall motion. Also, the study can be obtained during exercise-induced (bicycle-pedaling) stress to assess myocardial reserve and stress-induced wall-motion abnormalities.

Indications for ventricular wall-motion scans are concern for generalized or segmental wall-motion abnormalities, including aneurysm and akinesis, and of the regurgitant fraction in patients with aortic and mitral valve disease;

stress-induced abnormalities; and electromechanical conduction defects.

Interpretation of the wall-motion scan is based on subjective evaluation of the contraction of each portion of the left ventricular wall (Fig. 9–24). At rest, focal hypokinesis or akinesis usually indicates infarcted muscle; paradoxical motion suggests aneurysm. The ejection fraction is calculated by computer with the use of operator-drawn or computer-selected boundaries of the left ventricular chamber at systole and diastole. The normal at-rest ejection fraction is between 55% and 75% and should increase with exercise. Statistical images, such as Fourier phase and amplitude maps, can be calculated in order to reinforce or quantify observation of wall-motion abnormalities. These maps show synchrony and amplitude of contraction in patterns characteristic of infarction, cardiomyopathy, aneurysm, and electrical conduction abnormalities.

Other cardiac studies can be performed with pure technetium or technetium-labeled red blood cells in conjunction with computer-gated analysis. These include first-pass right and left ventricular ejection fraction calculations, intracardiac shunt evaluations, and cardiac output determinations. The first-pass right and left ejection fraction studies are performed best with multicrystal cameras (which are no longer manufactured) because they have a rapid count-rate capability, which enables highly accurate measurements to be made quickly. Improvements in computer hardware and software have enabled conventional gamma cameras to function adequately for first-pass measurements.

Left-to-right shunts can be detected with a fast, dynamic acquisition as a single, sharp burst of activity traverses the right side of the heart, the lungs, and the left side of the heart. If there is a left-to-right shunt, early recirculation through the lungs occurs as oxygenated blood passes through the shunt back into the lungs instead of circulating through the systemic arteries. These shunts are quantified with a pulmonary-flow/systemic-flow ratio. In accordance with the science of hydraulics, gamma variate curves are fitted to lung time activity curves. Integration of the areas under

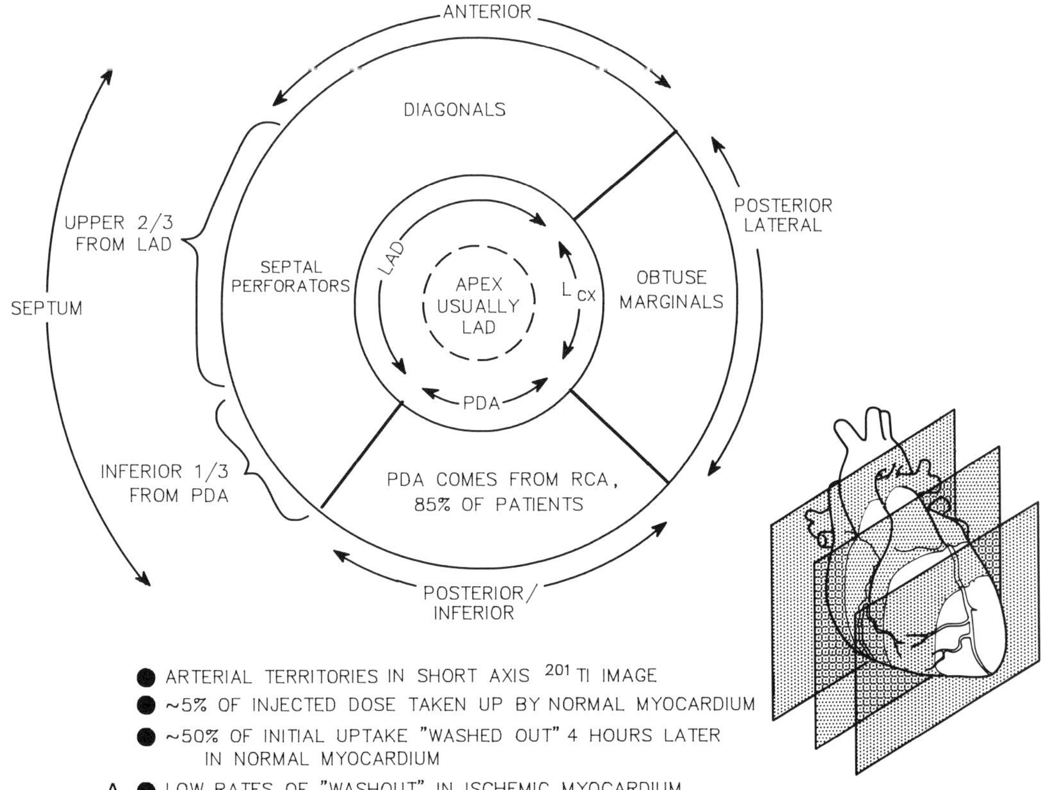

FIGURE 9–23. Thallium myocardial scan: reversible ischemia. *A.* Diagram. Left anterior descending artery; LAD, L_{cx} Left circumflex artery; PDA, Posterior descending artery; RCA, Right coronary artery.

Illustration continued on following page

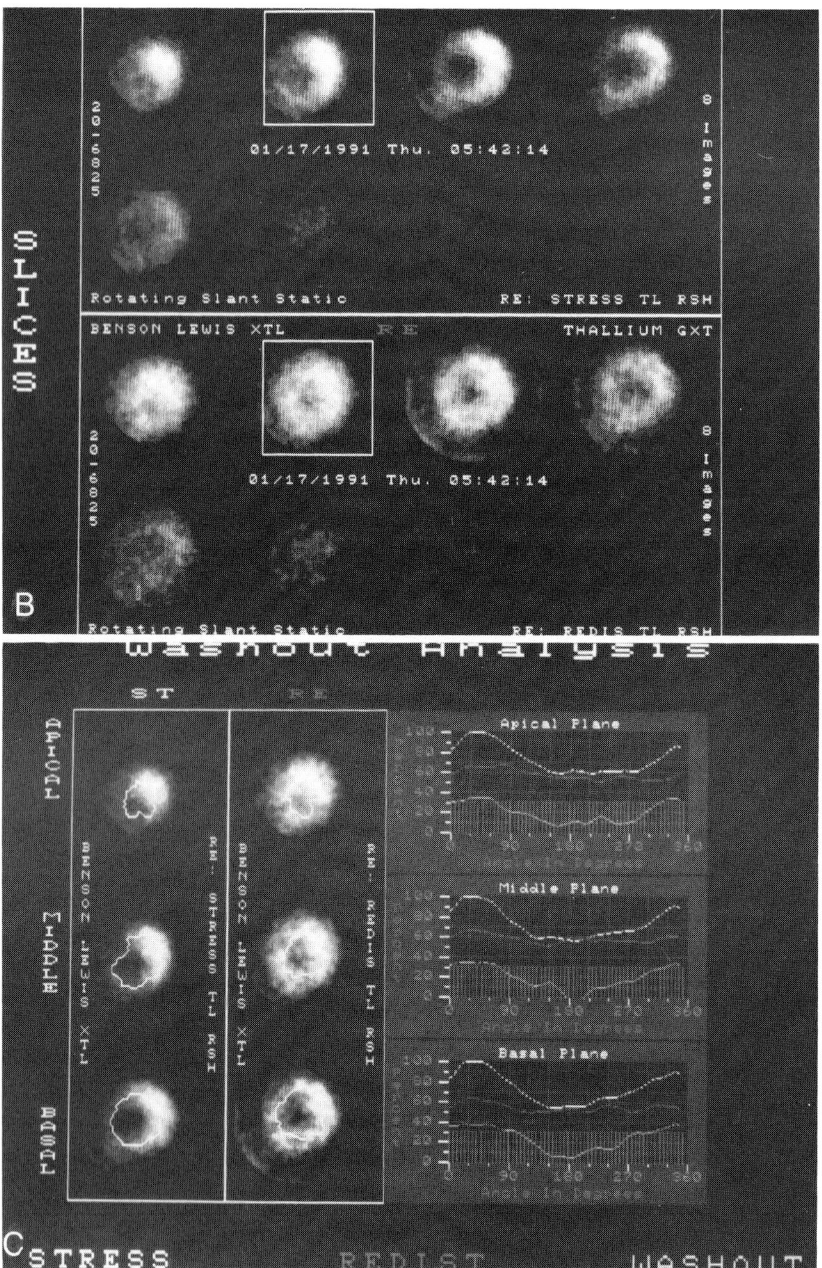

FIGURE 9–23 *Continued B.* Short-axis slices (across the long axis of the left ventricle) from an injection during stress are shown in the upper box. The first slice is near the apex (upper left) and they progress toward the base. The first four slices show an extensive defect from the 12 o'clock position counterclockwise to the 5 o'clock position. The lower box shows matching slices of the left ventricle 4 hours later when the labeling has become more nearly symmetrical around the circumference, indicating all of the defect is viable myocardium that became ischemic with exercise. *C.* Quantitative measurements of the first three slices are displayed side by side in pairs with stress images on the left and images taken 4 hours later on the right. Graphs to the right of each pair show three lines. The upper line on each graph shows the relative labeling around the slice at stress. The graph starts at 0 degrees at the 3 o'clock position and wraps counterclockwise. The highest labeling (set to 100%) is in the circumflex artery distribution (refer to Fig. 9–23*A*). The middle line shows the thallium remaining 4 hours later. The bottom line is a washout line that shows the percentage of thallium that departed the left ventricle during the 4-hour delay period. As seen in the upper and middle curves, and as measured by the lower washout curve, there is relatively good washout of 30% to 40% in the circumflex distribution and remarkably reduced washout in the anterior, septal, and inferior walls. The patient had severe atherosclerotic coronary artery disease in the left anterior descending and posterior descending arteries. Very low washouts indicate the severity of the ischemia.

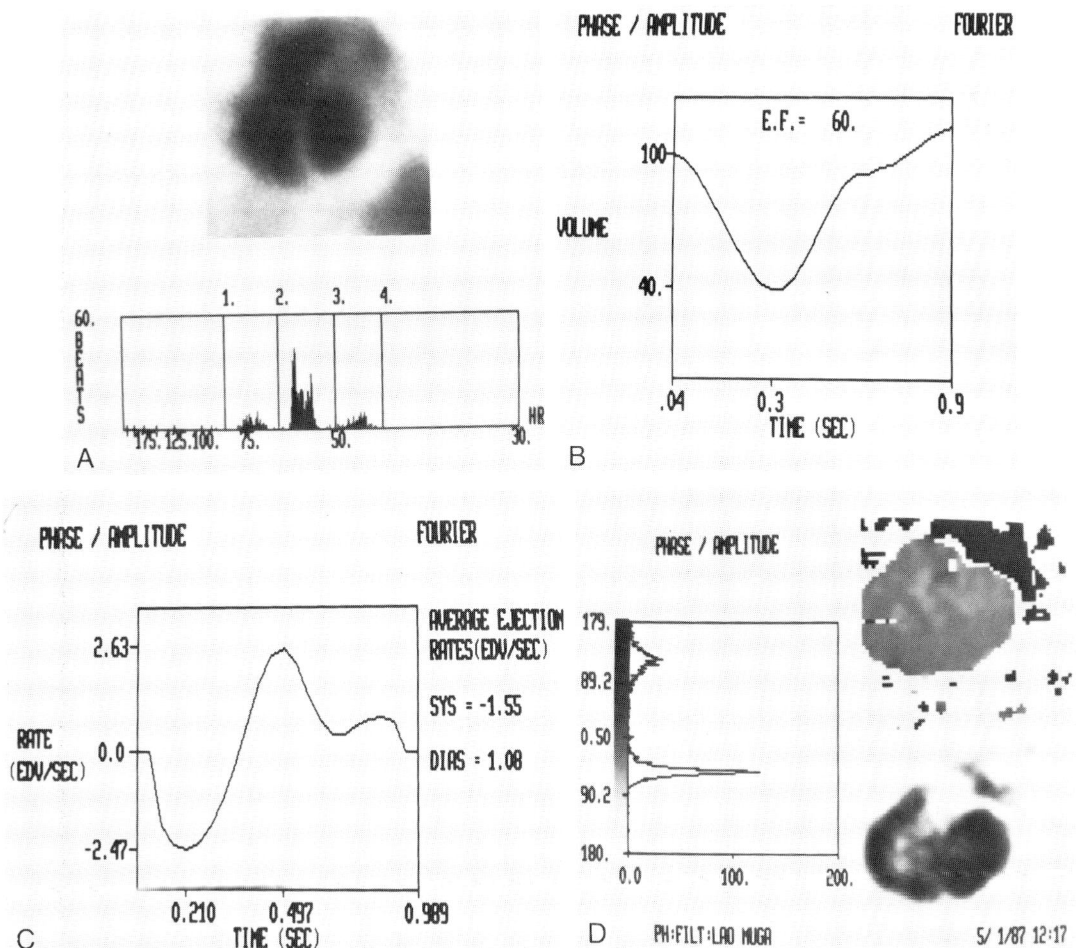

FIGURE 9–24. Multigated radionuclide angiogram. The left anterior oblique projection (*A*, top) shows the side-by-side right and left ventricles as the image of the labeled blood pool. The heart rate histogram (*A*, bottom) shows three windows with recorded heart beat rhythms: section 1, premature; section 2, normal; section 3, compensatory. The time activity curve *(B)* shows the left ventricular volume during the cardiac cycle with an ejection fraction (EF) of 60%. The graph *(C)* is the first derivative of the volume curve and measures systolic (emptying) and diastolic (filling) rates, expressed as end diastolic volumes per second (EDV/SEC). The phase/amplitude images and graph (*D*, left and right) summarize phase angle (upper) and amplitude (lower) values of each pixel derived from Fourier first-harmonic-analysis. The horizontal histogram tallies the number of pixels with a given phase angle value. Note the relatively uniform amplitude and phase angle values in these normal ventricles.

these curves accurately quantifies the amount of blood that is shunted back through the lungs (Fig. 9–25).

The ejection fraction is a relative measurement that can be converted to a measurement of cardiac output in liters per minute, if the left ventricular end-diastolic volume (LVEDV) is known. The LVEDV can be measured with methods in which known radioactivity in sample blood volumes is used and chest wall attenuation of the radioactivity in the end-diastolic blood pool is corrected. In many techniques, this procedure is performed with variable degrees of technical difficulty and accuracy. When the LVEDV is known, cardiac output is calculated as follows:

$$\text{Cardiac output} = \text{ejection fraction} \times \text{heart rate} \times \text{LVEDV}.$$

When the heart is considered as a pump, the cardiac output is an obviously useful measurement.

CENTRAL NERVOUS SYSTEM EXAMINATION

Nuclear medicine examinations of the central nervous system can be used to demonstrate

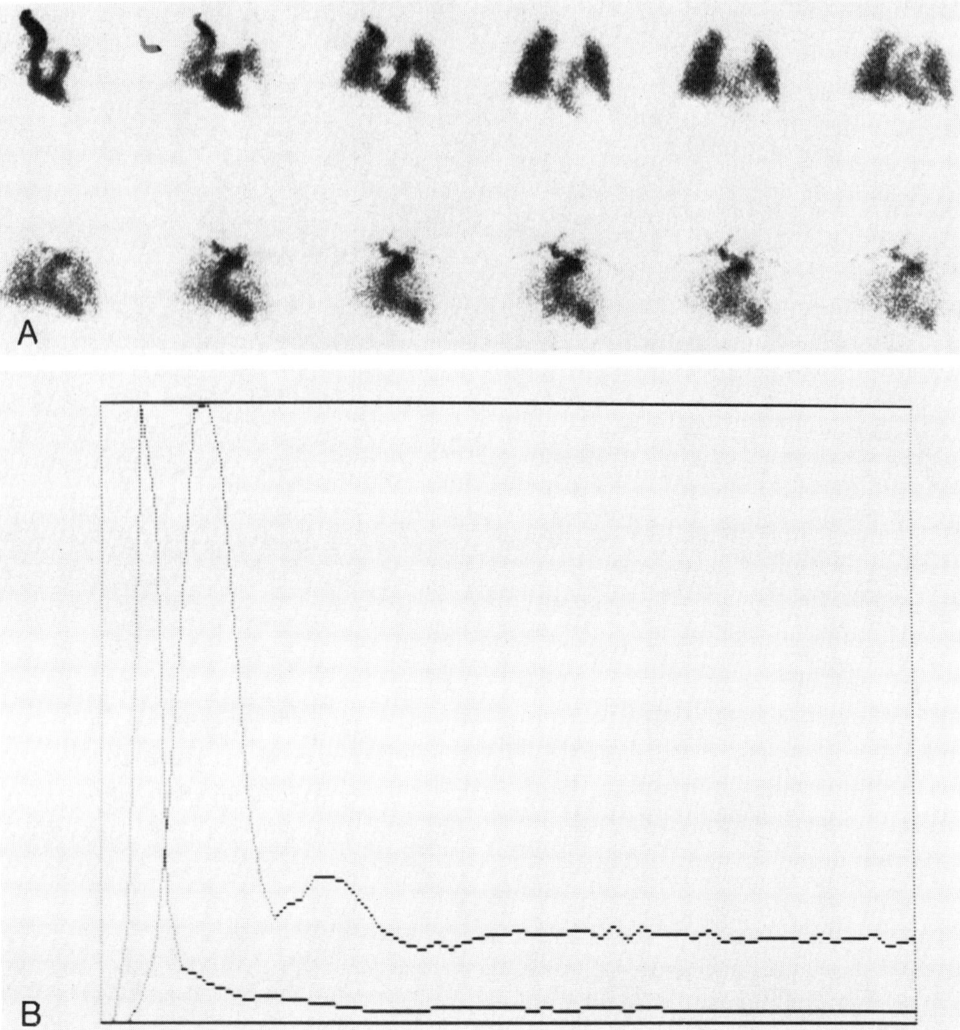

FIGURE 9–25. Left-to-right shunt. *A.* In a patient with posttraumatic (gunshot) fistula between the aortic arch and innominate vein, a sharp bolus of ^{99m}Tc–DTPA was injected into the right external jugular vein. In sequential, 1-second frames, this bolus traverses the superior vena cava, the right side of the heart, and the lungs and returns to the left side of the heart and the aortic arch. There is lung activity late into the study. Because some blood going through the aorta immediately returns to the right side of the heart, it rapidly reappears in the lungs. *B.* Time activity curves for the left-to-right shunt study are conventionally displayed with time (1 to 60 seconds) on the *x*-axis and radioactivity on the *y*-axis. The first curve shows a simple spike of activity at the beginning of the study, recorded in a region of interest over the superior vena cava as a quality control measurement that documents the bolus injection. The second curve is drawn from a region of interest over the lung and shows a spike at the initial time of arrival followed by a shorter, broad spike when shunted blood recirculated into the lungs. The pulmonary-flow/systemic-flow (QP/QS) ratio of the areas under these two curves (1.6 to 1.0) enables calculation of the shunt size.

blood-brain barrier defects, determine flow of cerebrospinal fluid (CSF), assess cerebral shunt function, detect CSF rhinorrhea, and evaluate cerebral blood flow.

Brain Scan

Abnormalities in the brain can be imaged with the use of ^{99m}Tc–DTPA (the same compound used for renal perfusion imaging) injected intravenously. Technetium 99m–DTPA and similar isotopes normally remain within the cerebral capillary vessels. Blood-brain barrier defects around tumors, infections, and healing infarcts allow these radiopharmaceuticals to leak into the brain parenchyma. The scan initially demonstrates the areas of high blood flow in the first minutes after injection (called a cerebral flow examination). Hours later, when the intravascular activity has cleared, blood-brain barrier defects are apparent. The normal brain scan shows no or minimal persistent activity.

The brain scan was formerly used to complement CT evaluation of brain tumor or abscess, particularly as a follow-up examination after surgery, chemotherapy, or radiation therapy. In 75% of patients with cerebral infarcts, follow-up scans show a blood-brain barrier defect during the second and third weeks. This defect generally decreases in size and intensity over the next 5 weeks. Brain scans can be helpful in evaluating patients with contrast allergy or renal failure when intravenous radiographic contrast for CT is contraindicated (Fig. 9–26). They also may be used with exceptionally obese patients who cannot be placed in CT or MRI scanners. However, CT and MRI have nearly ended the use of radionuclide brain scans, and gadolinium-DTPA–enhanced MRI images are preferred in the evaluation of patients with an allergy to iodinated contrast.

Interpretation requires assessment of vascular flow and, on delayed scans, brain uptake.

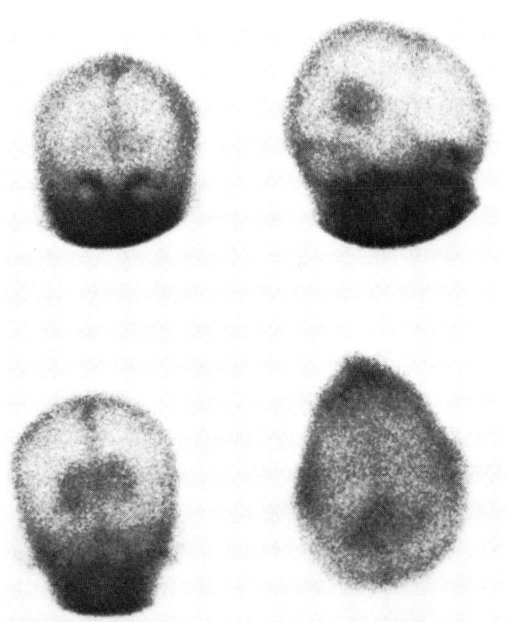

FIGURE 9–26. Brain scan of corpus callosum glioma. Three hours after the administration of ^{99m}Tc–DTPA, images (right to left and top to bottom) were taken in the anterior, right lateral, posterior, and vertex (nose up) projections. There is a bilobed abnormal area of increased activity crossing the midline in the posterior portion of the brain, in which the blood-brain barrier is damaged around the tumor.

Uptake by the paranasal and dural sinuses is normal and can show patency of the sagittal and transverse sinuses in patients with suspected thrombosis. It is historically interesting to note that gadolinium-DTPA is distributed physiologically in the same fashion as ^{99m}Tc–DTPA. This dramatic improvement in imaging technology is the result of taking better advantage of an old idea.

Brain Death Scan

The acquisition of a cerebral flow study in the anterior projection is used as a confirmatory test when brain death is diagnosed clinically. The normal study shows internal carotid circulation converging on the circle of Willis with immediate perfusion of a trident of vessels formed by the paired anterior cerebral arteries and the right and left middle cerebral arteries. Shortly after the arterial phase, the superior sagittal sinus is seen draining the capillary blush. In the abnormal study, the convergent internal cerebral flow is not seen, and the arterial trident is not visible. Instead, there is flow around the scalp in the external carotid circulation. Shunted blood from external to internal circulation may cause intense uptake in the central face, producing the so-called hot nose sign. The superior sagittal sinus is usually not seen in brain death scans. These scans are inexpensive, take only minutes to perform, and, with mobile equipment, can be performed at the patient's bedside to confirm the clinical diagnosis of brain death (Fig. 9–27).

Cerebrospinal Fluid Flow Scan

The ventricular system, the subarachnoid cisterns, the thecal sac, and the shunt tubes within any of these spaces can be imaged with the use of an isotope-labeled large molecule. If the expected imaging time is short (1 day or less), ^{99m}Tc–DTPA can be injected into the desired location and images acquired at the appropriate times to evaluate flow. If the flow must be monitored for longer than 1 day, it is better to use ^{111}In–DTPA because this isotope has a 3-day half-life. These DTPA agents diffuse slowly out of the subarachnoid space, but do not have any adverse clinical effects. Isotope scans of CSF dynamics are used for assessing hydrocephalus and for detecting cysts in the brain, CSF leakage, and spinal lesions.

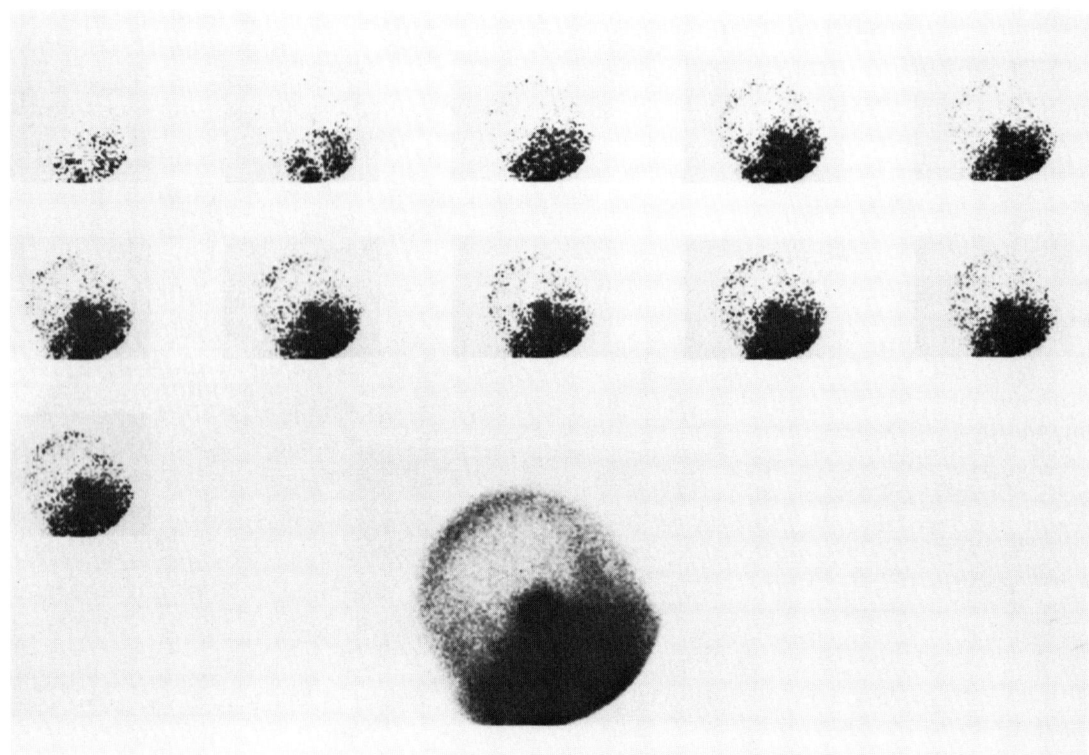

FIGURE 9–27. Brain death. Dynamic scan of a drowning victim was performed in the intensive care unit with a mobile gamma camera. The eleven 1-second images show a bolus intravenous injection of ^{99m}Tc–DTPA arrive in the carotid arteries and then slowly encircle the scalp through the external carotid vessels. Intense activity in the face and the nose continues as shown in the larger, immediate, static image. No perfusion of the anterior or middle cerebral arteries or of the superior sagittal sinus is seen. The patient had no brain perfusion and was therefore dead. The image is rotated counterclockwise about 30 degrees because a ventilator made it difficult to approach the patient's bed directly.

In many of these situations, CT with iodinated contrast better demonstrates the abnormality.

In the assessment of CSF dynamic flow, a normal pattern of ascent is anticipated from the lumbar puncture administration to the basal cisterns and then on to the convexities of the brain; the CSF and the radiopharmaceutical are eventually absorbed through the arachnoid granulations. Entry into the lateral ventricles is not usually seen and can indicate communicating normal-pressure hydrocephalus (Fig. 9–28).

Interpretation of shunt function requires evaluation of the rate of flow after injection of the same radiopharmaceuticals into a CSF shunt reservoir. Exact rates of CSF flow through shunt tubes can be measured if the apparent volume of the injected shunt reservoir is known. The radionuclide study of CSF shunt function is a quick, accurate, and inexpensive test of suspected malfunction.

Metabolic Brain Scan

Radiopharmaceuticals in combination with SPECT techniques can be used to assess cerebral metabolism qualitatively (but not quantitatively) in a manner analogous to that of positron emission tomography imaging (see Chapter 1). Two Food and Drug Administration–approved agents, iodine-labeled iodinated amphetamine (^{123}I–iodinated amphetamine) and technetium-labeled exametazime (^{99m}Tc–exametazime) map functioning cerebral tissue (Fig. 9–29). Both are agents primarily for measuring blood flow and depend on greater flow in gray matter than in white matter (about 4 to 1) in order to distinguish the two tissues. Iodine 123 iodinated amphetamine also binds to ubiquitous amphetamine receptors. Technetium 99m exametazime is a lipid-soluble complex that traverses cell membranes. The image quality of ^{123}I-iodinated ampheta-

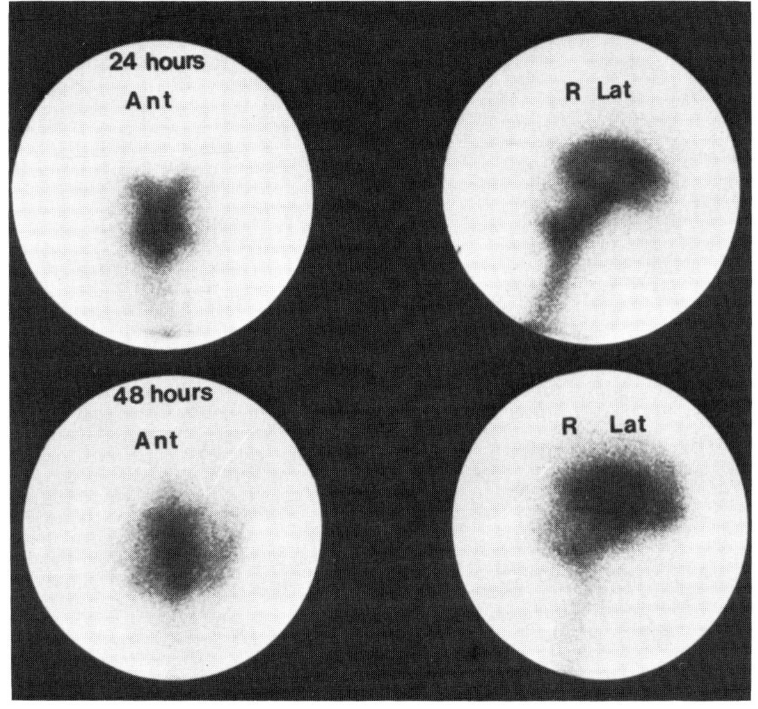

FIGURE 9–28. Normal-pressure hydrocephalus. Anterior and posterior cisternogram images taken 24 and 48 hours after the intrathecal (lumbar puncture) administration of indium 111–labeled DTPA show the paired midline lateral ventricles persistently filled with isotope that has traveled backwards through the fourth and third ventricles.

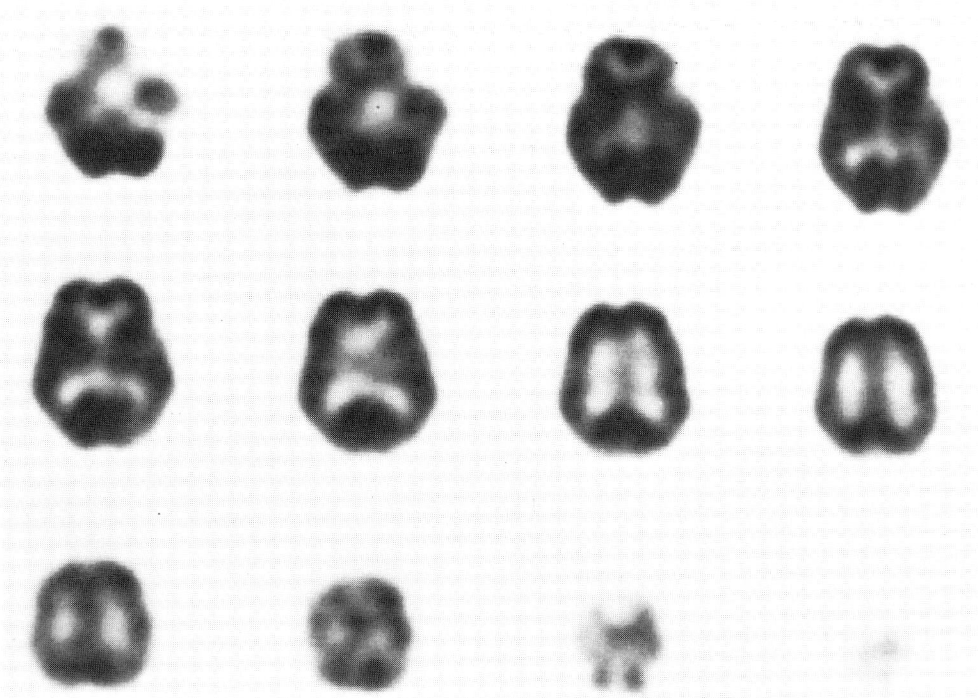

FIGURE 9–29. Brain metabolic scan. Axial slices (left to right, top to bottom) of a single photon emission computed tomographic (SPECT) brain scan with ^{99m}Tc HMPAO. The images map uptake of the isotope through the brain with the highest intensity shown in the cerebral hemispheres. Note the symmetrical side-to-side perfusion in the normal, resting patient.

mine is unfavorably affected by contamination of ^{123}I with high-energy ^{124}I. Because of radiation dose considerations, the presence of this contaminant also limits the amount of this agent that can safely be administered to the patient. If the delivery of this rapidly decaying radiopharmaceutical is delayed or if the patient is unreliable about keeping appointments, it is difficult to use iodinated amphetamine. Technetium 99m exametazime kits can be stored and used whenever the need arises. The higher photon flux available with the ^{99m}Tc label is also a definite advantage in producing good-quality images (see Fig. 9–27).

These brain agents are used for detection of cerebral ischemia and infarct, seizure foci, tumor, and physiological activation of various sites in the cortex (which increases blood flow). They also are used for confirming brain death.

WHOLE-BODY EXAMINATION

Whole-body imaging can be performed with either ^{67}Ga or white blood cells labeled with ^{111}In. These examinations are used primarily to evaluate inflammation.

Inflammation and Tumor Scan: Gallium 67 Citrate

Gallium 67 citrate, when injected intravenously, binds primarily to serum transferrin and is distributed to the liver, the spleen, the lungs, the kidneys, the bones, and the bowel. By 48 hours after injection, lung and kidney uptake have disappeared. Activity in the colon begins to appear 24 hours after injection, and the radionuclide may take days to clear. Gallium is also concentrated in regions of inflammation and tumor. Gallium scans are helpful in locating infections (including abscess, osteomyelitis, and pyelonephritis) and in evaluating and following interstitial lung disease, particularly sarcoidosis. They are also used to assess *Pneumocystis* pneumonia and other opportunistic lung infections of patients who are immunocompromised.

These scans are nonspecific because all pul-

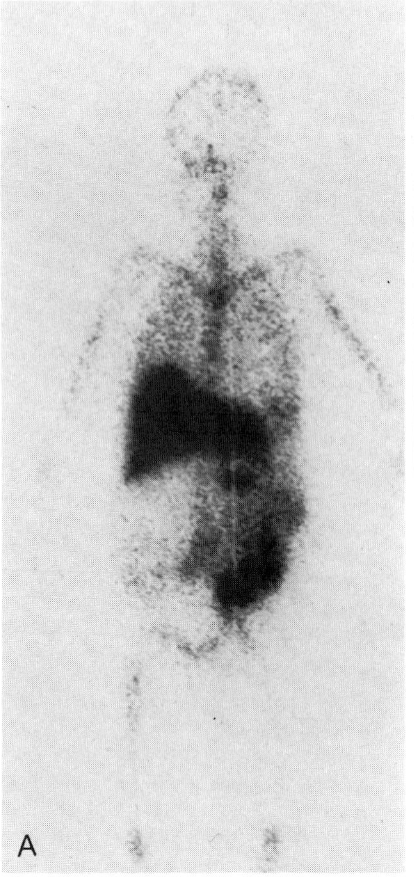

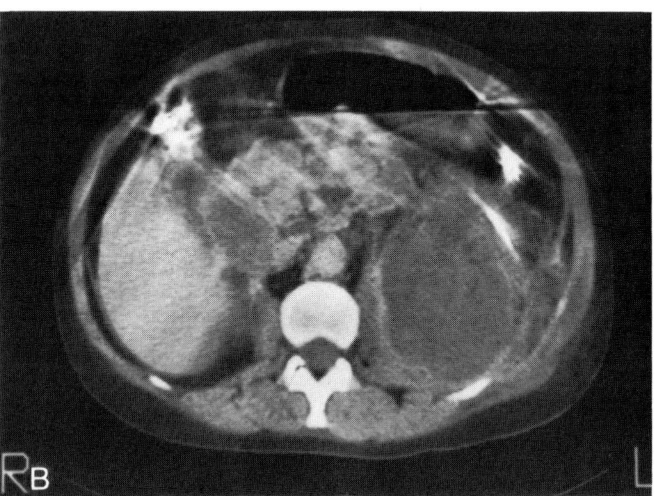

FIGURE 9–30. *A.* Gallium 67 (^{67}Ga) scan of a retroperitoneal abscess. Scan several days after intravenous administration of ^{67}Ga shows normal liver and bone marrow activity and an intense, abnormal collection in the left abdomen. The very intense area in the left lower quadrant could be isotope within the contents of the descending colon. Delayed imaging would answer this question because bowel contents would move but abscess would not. *B.* CT section of the midabdomen shows a large, low-density mass on the left with a bright rim, which corresponds to a walled-off abscess.

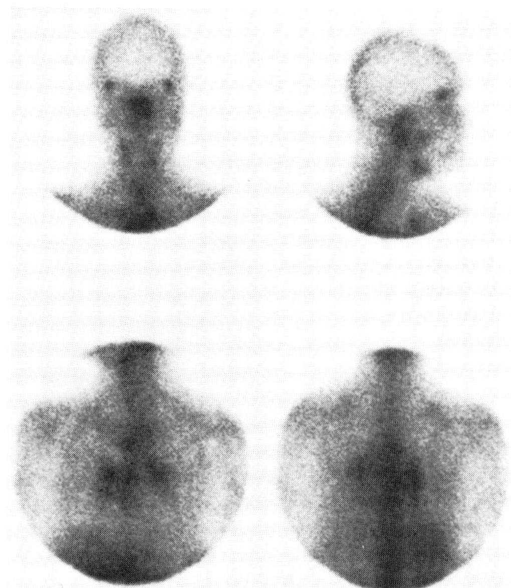

FIGURE 9–31. Gallium 67 scan of sarcoidosis. Twenty-four-hour images from a ^{67}Ga study of the head and the chest show physiological activity in soft tissues, bones, and salivary and lacrimal glands. In the chest, symmetrical areas of increased activity on either side of the mediastinum represent abnormal hilar lymph nodes.

monary inflammations accumulate ^{67}Ga. Lymphomas and, to a lesser degree, many carcinomas may take up ^{67}Ga. Gallium scans are not routinely used for tumor evaluation because they are not sensitive to most tumors and the findings are not specific for most tumors. Tumors and lung disease may coexist with suspected infections and are therefore considered in the differential diagnosis of an abnormal ^{67}Ga scan.

Interpretation of ^{67}Ga scans is based on identification of areas of increased uptake, as distinguished from normal uptake in the liver, the spleen, the bone marrow, and the colon (Fig. 9–30). Usual sites of gallium uptake are the breasts, particularly during lactation; the parotid glands, when affected by sarcoidosis (Fig. 9–31) or radiation therapy; and the lungs, when affected by interstitial processes, such as sarcoidosis and inflammation caused by chemotherapy, pneumonia, and radiation pneumonitis (Figs. 9–32, 9–33).

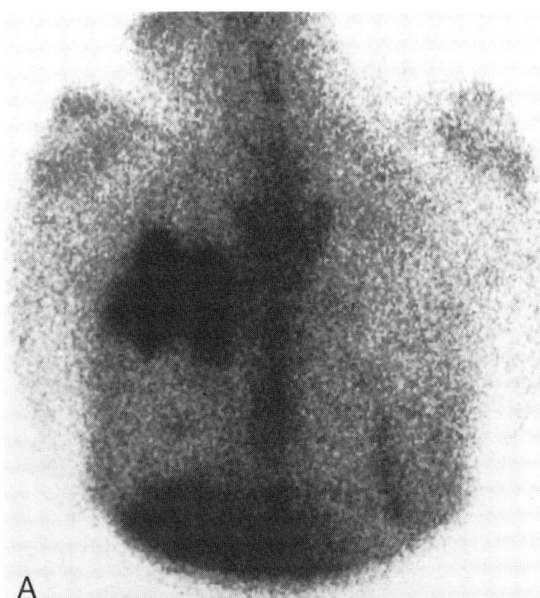

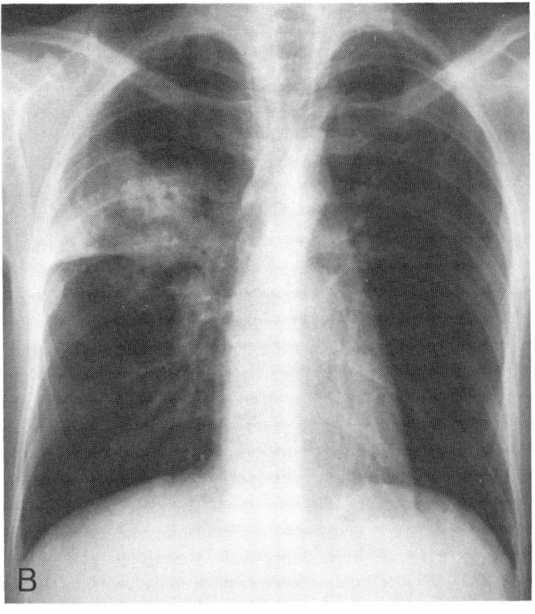

FIGURE 9–32. Gallium 67 scan in pneumococcal pneumonia. Twenty-four-hour ^{67}Ga scan shows an intense abnormality in the right midchest *(A)*, which matches an alveolar opacification in the right upper lobe on the chest radiograph *(B)*.

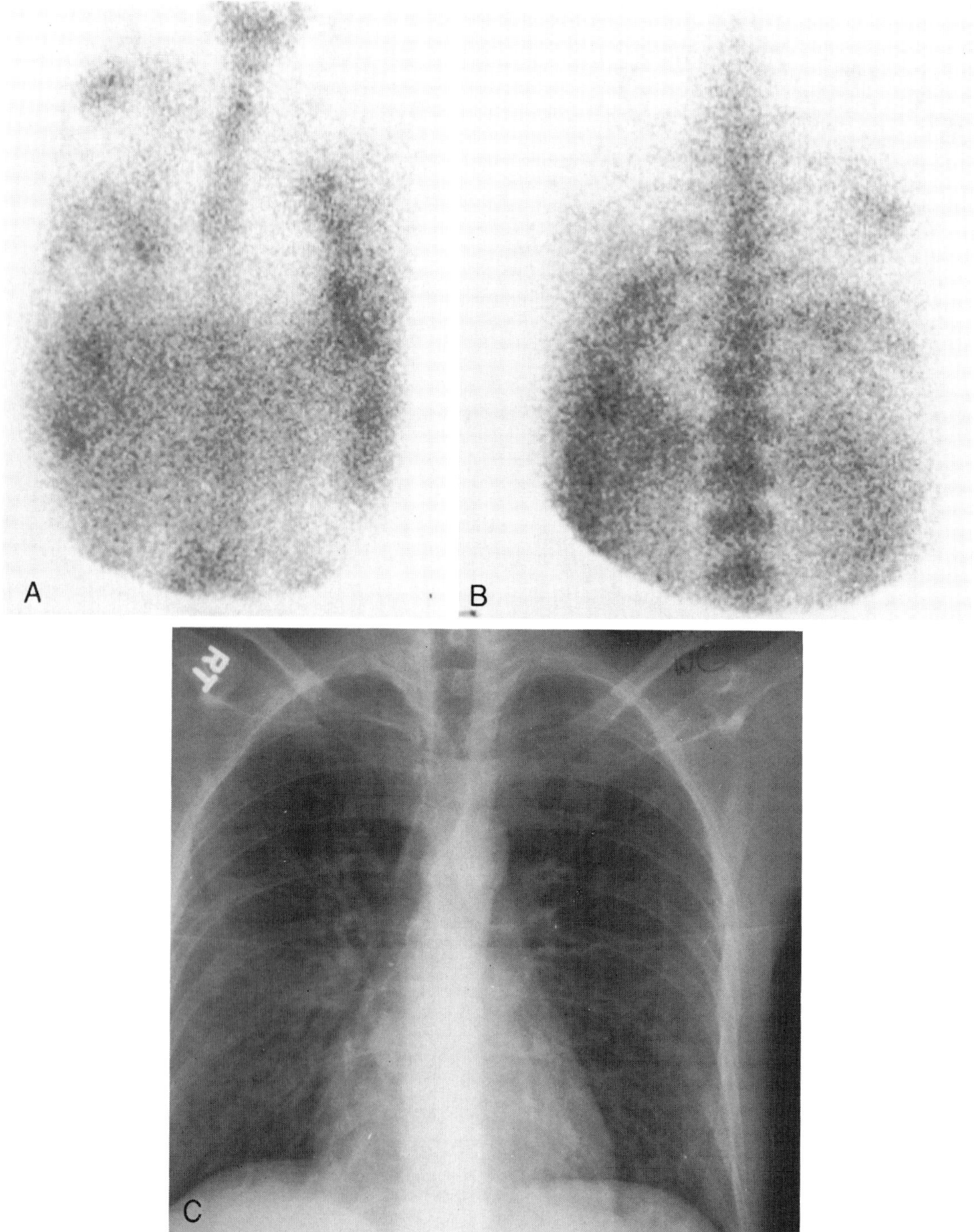

FIGURE 9–33. Gallium 67 scan in *Pneumocystis* pneumonia. Anterior *(A)* and posterior *(B)* ^{67}Ga images in the same patient as in Figure 9–32 were performed 1 year later and show patchy, bilateral areas of mildly increased ^{67}Ga uptake in each lung. The radiograph *(C)* shows only a mild, diffuse increased interstitial pattern. The patient had acquired immunodeficiency syndrome.

Inflammation and Infection Scan: Indium 111–Labeled White Blood Cell Scan

Acute infection is best imaged by labeling a sample of the patient's white blood cells with ^{111}In. In this technique, the leukocytes, which are labeled in vitro, are intravenously injected, respond to chemotactic factors, and migrate to areas of acute inflammation (most readily to areas of acute infection), where they remain. The cells labeled are polymorphonuclear leukocytes, not lymphocytes. Because these leukocytes are sequestered in the spleen, the radiation dose to this organ is higher than that of most nuclear medicine examinations (0.05 to 0.10 Gy). The spleen is not significantly affected by this exposure.

The examination is used exclusively to locate sites of acute infection or inflammation. It is most useful for assessment of areas of the body in which physical examination is difficult (the chest, the abdomen, and the pelvis), when the site of origin of an infection (manifested by fever) is unknown, or when multiple sites of infection are considered (Figs. 9–34, 9–35). Chronic infection, which may be largely mediated by lymphocytes, does not reliably concentrate leukocytes.

Interpretation requires identification of abnormal concentration of the labeled white blood cells in the liver, the spleen, and the bone marrow in relation to normal uptake in these organs.

Caution must be used in the diagnosis of inflammation with ^{111}In–labeled white blood cell scans. Evaluation of hemorrhage in the gut that contains labeled white blood cells and

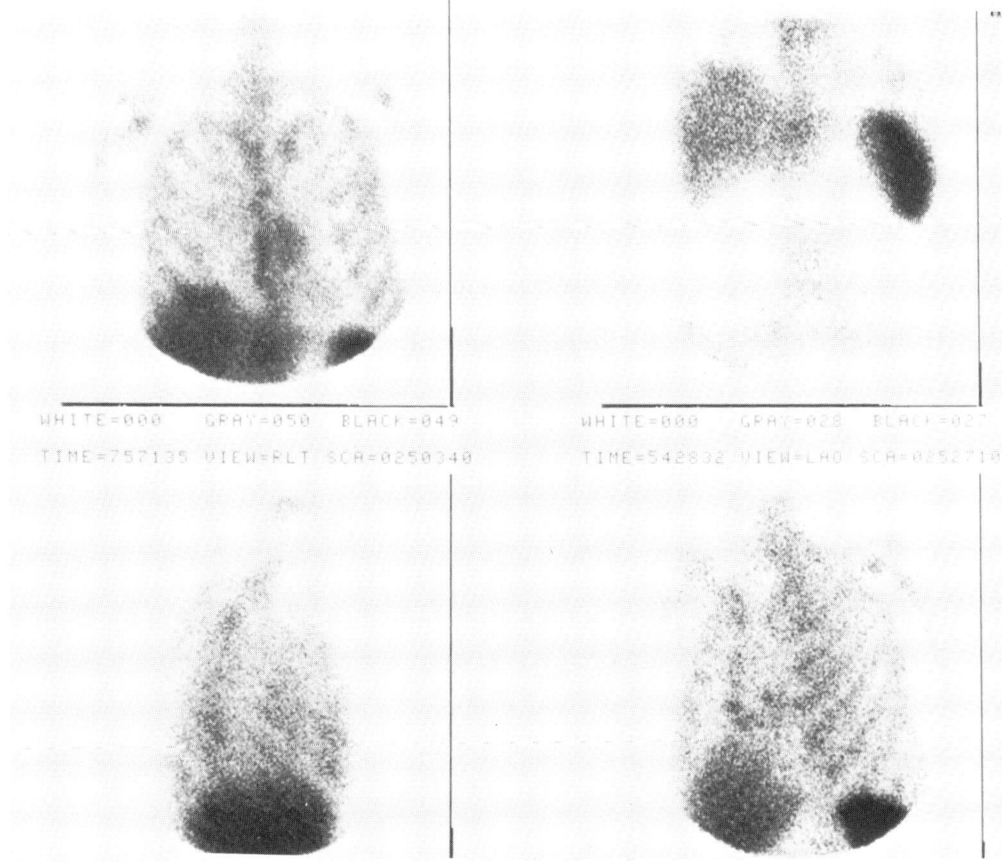

FIGURE 9–34. Mediastinitis shown by ^{111}In–labeled white blood cell scan. Ten days after a coronary artery bypass, the sternal wound is breaking down, and an intense area of abnormal activity is seen to the left of the sternum on the first, anterior view. The next image is an anterior view of the abdomen that shows physiological activity in the liver and the spleen. The bottom left image is a right lateral view that shows that the abnormal chest activity is central in the chest. The bottom right image is a left anterior oblique view that shows the abnormal area projecting between the sternum and the medial ends of the left ribs.

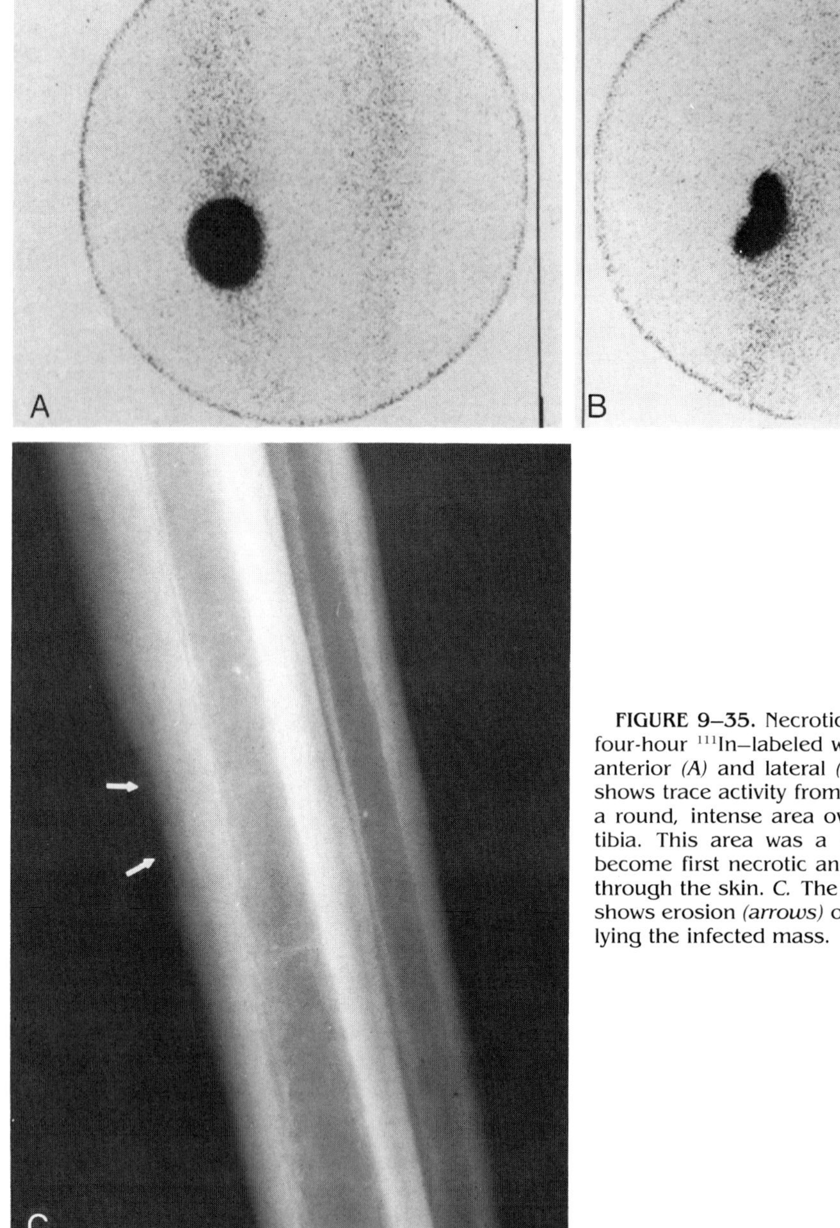

FIGURE 9–35. Necrotic lymphoma mass. Twenty-four-hour ^{111}In–labeled white blood cell scan in the anterior *(A)* and lateral *(B)* views of the lower legs shows trace activity from knees to ankles except for a round, intense area over the middle of the right tibia. This area was a lymphoma mass that had become first necrotic and then infected as it broke through the skin. *C.* The lateral view of the midtibia shows erosion *(arrows)* of the anterior cortex underlying the infected mass.

normal bone marrow with physiological accumulation of the radioisotope in heterotopic bone requires experience in interpretation and correlation with clinical and imaging data.

In the extremities, the limited statistical density and the limited spatial resolution available with ^{111}In–labeled white blood cell scans make it difficult to locate inflammatory lesions precisely. There is controversy over both the sensitivity and specificity, in the detection of osteomyelitis. A small area of infection in the bone may be difficult to distinguish from the inflammation in adjacent soft tissues. A chronic osteomyelitis (particularly one that is being treated with antibiotics) may have a largely lymphocytic response and therefore may not accumulate acute inflammatory cells. It is suggested that an area of osteomyelitis that no longer takes up ^{111}In–labeled white blood cells is completely cured.

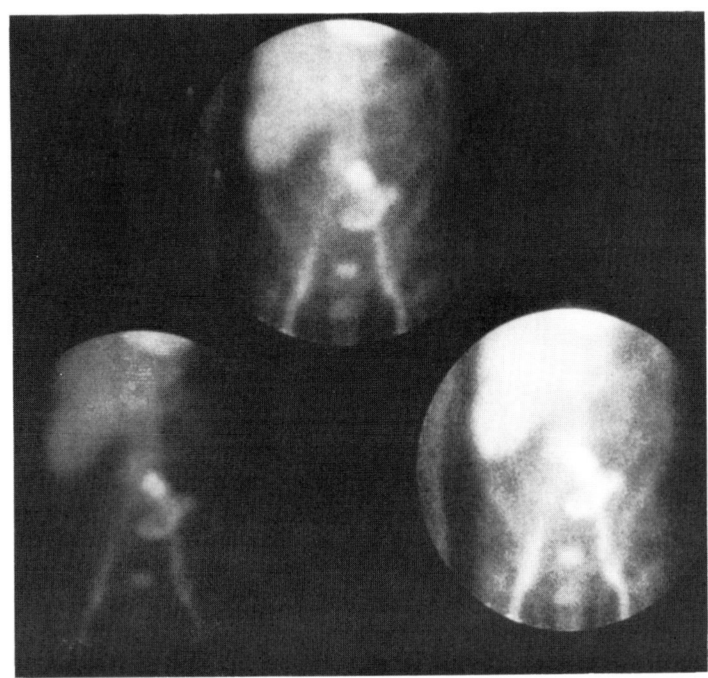

FIGURE 9–36. Small bowel bleeding assessed with a three-image composite study that shows the distribution of ^{99m}Tc–labeled red blood cells. The blood pool in the heart is seen at the top edge of the pictures just above the liver. An inverted "Y" pattern made of the aorta, the inferior vena cava, and the iliac vessels is normally seen. Over the bifurcation on the left is a curled area of intense activity that is accumulating blood in the middle of the small bowel. In order to be sure that this represents bleeding into the bowel, the series of images must demonstrate that the bleeding appears out of the background, becomes more intense with time, and moves through a tube recognizable as a loop of bowel.

VASCULAR EXAMINATION

Gastrointestinal Bleeding Scan

Gastrointestinal bleeding can be evaluated with either technetium–labeled red blood cells or ^{99m}Tc–sulfur colloid (the liver-spleen scanning agent). Active bleeding of 0.05 to 0.10 mL/minute can be demonstrated on these scans, in comparison with angiograms, which demonstrates only more rapid bleeding (1 mL/minute).

Before the gastrointestinal bleeding scan is obtained, upper gastrointestinal bleeding must be ruled out by endoscopy. The nuclear medicine examination is then used to locate a site of gastrointestinal bleeding that is distal to the ligament of Treitz. This type of bleeding is usually intermittent. Gastrointestinal ^{99m}Tc–labeled red blood cell scans assist the angiographer to determine the general site of bleeding (i.e., distal versus proximal small bowel; ascending, transverse, descending, or sigmoid colon). Definitive demonstration (and often treatment) of gastrointestinal bleeding is performed by means of angiography. Angiograms are seldom positive if nuclear medicine scans are negative.

Active hemorrhage is demonstrated by an accumulation of isotope at the bleeding site (Fig. 9–36). This accumulation must be distinguished from normal uptake by the liver, the spleen, and the bone marrow (in ^{99m}Tc–sulfur colloid scans) or from normal circulating red blood cells (with ^{99m}Tc–labeled red blood cell scans). The intense uptake of the upper abdominal organs in ^{99m}Tc–sulfur colloid scans may obscure the likely sites of bleeding. Technetium 99m sulfur colloid scans have a brief window (minutes) during which bleeding must occur in order to be detected. Technetium 99m–labeled red blood cell studies have a much longer window of opportunity (hours) during which the bleeding site can be detected. The ^{99m}Tc–labeled red blood cell study is clearly superior to the ^{99m}Tc–sulfur colloid study, except in the unusual case of continuous bleeding.

Deep Venous Obstruction Scan

Deep venous thrombosis can be evaluated by injecting a ^{99m}Tc agent (pertechnetate Tc 99m or ^{99m}Tc–MAA as used for lung scans) into the veins of the foot and imaging the flow through the deep venous system of the thigh and the pelvis (Fig. 9–37). If normal patency is demonstrated by free flow, deep venous obstruction is ruled out. Obstruction to flow is nonspecific, but in the appropriate clinical setting, it is highly suggestive of deep venous thrombosis. Ultrasonography and contrast venography are usually performed instead of ^{99m}Tc scanning, which is a less specific test for thrombosis. Under ideal conditions, scans performed with ^{111}In–labeled platelets can directly

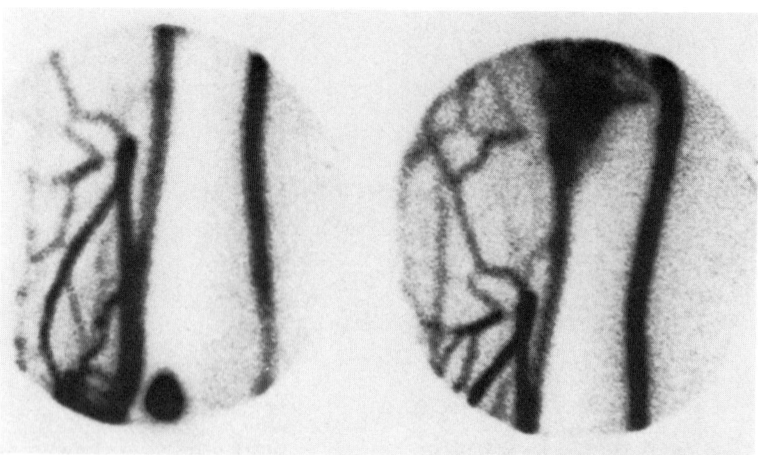

FIGURE 9–37. Deep venous thrombosis. Anterior images taken from the knees down (left) and over the thighs (right) were made immediately after the bilateral, pedal intravenous injection of ^{99m}Tc–DTPA. They show flow up a single vein in the patient's left leg. On the right there are collateral veins weaving past vessels that are obstructed proximally. The flow of isotope ending abruptly at a thrombus and the presence of collaterals are strong evidence of thrombosis.

display forming thromboses as they accumulate by showing the developing uptake.

THYROID EXAMINATION

Evaluation of the thyroid can be performed with three agents, each of which has advantages and disadvantages. Although ultrasonography and CT can demonstrate thyroid lesions, radionuclide scanning is the best overall method for thyroid evaluation because it shows both the anatomy of the gland and its function. The pattern of uptake is the best indicator of the type of lesion. The examination is interpreted in conjunction with thyroid function tests and, if necessary, with thyroid stimulation or suppression tests.

Thyroid Scan: Technetium 99m Pertechnetate

The test with the lowest radiation dose and best image contrast involves the use of intravenously administered free pertechnetate Tc 99m; 2% of the total dose is taken up but not organified (i.e., not incorporated into thyroxine molecules) in the thyroid. Pinhole collimation of the gamma rays produces images of excellent detail and demonstrates the entire thyroid independently of its function. Nodules 4 mm or more in diameter can be detected. This compares favorably to clinical detection; palpable nodules are usually 10 mm or more in diameter.

Technetium 99m pertechnetate scanning is the initial imaging examination for any patient with suspected thyroid abnormalities. The radionuclide is sufficiently accumulated in the thyroid that imaging is possible 15 to 20 minutes after injection. It is usually performed in conjunction with an ^{131}I uptake measurement 24 hours after injection (the 24-hour radioactive iodine uptake) as a measurement of thyroid function. Interpretation requires evaluation of thyroid size and uniformity of uptake. A nonfunctioning (cold) nodule on a pertechnetate Tc 99m scan appears as a focus of diminished uptake against the uniform uptake of the normal gland (Fig. 9–38).

The thyroid scan can be helpful when neonatal hypothyroidism is detected by cord-blood screening. Some of these patients have a transient dysfunction of the gland, some have no gland, and some have a poorly functioning gland in the base of the tongue (Fig. 9–39). Patients in the last two groups require thyroid hormone treatment for life. Because the diagnostic scan requires only a knowledge of the presence and the position of the thyroid, pertechnetate Tc 99m can be ingested orally. It is readily absorbed by the stomach in sufficient quantity to be imaged half an hour later.

Iodine 131 Scan

Iodine 131 was the original thyroid scanning agent. It has a 364-keV gamma ray and abundant beta ray production. This radionuclide is

FIGURE 9–38. Thyroid cold nodule. *A.* Diagram. *B.* Three magnification views followed by an anterior image of the head and neck of the thyroid gland were made with pertechnetate Tc 99m. The gland is of normal size, but there is a small cold defect in the lower pole of the right lobe of the gland. This cold nodule could be a carcinoma, but according to the odds, it is more likely benign.

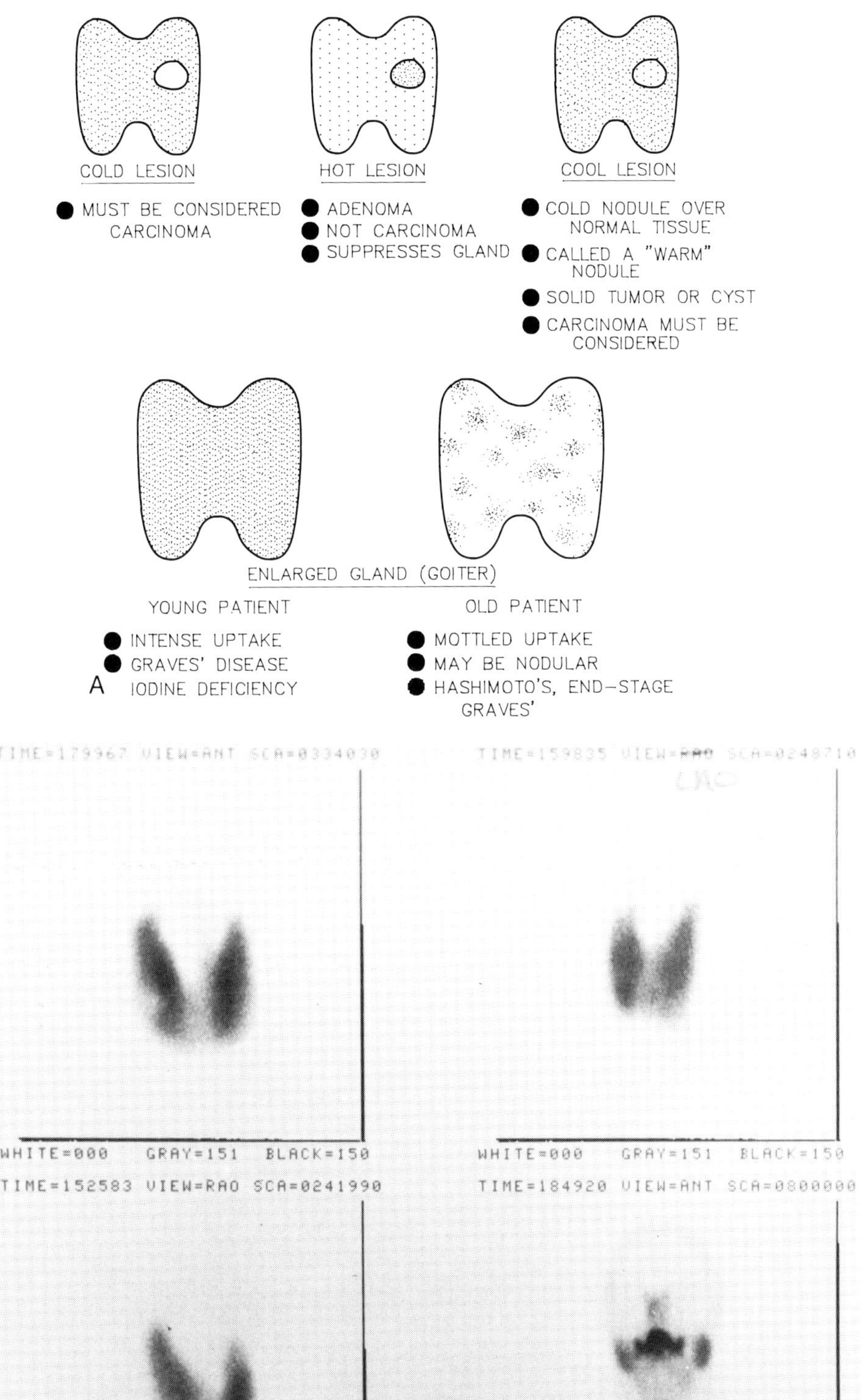

FIGURE 9–38 *See legend on opposite page*

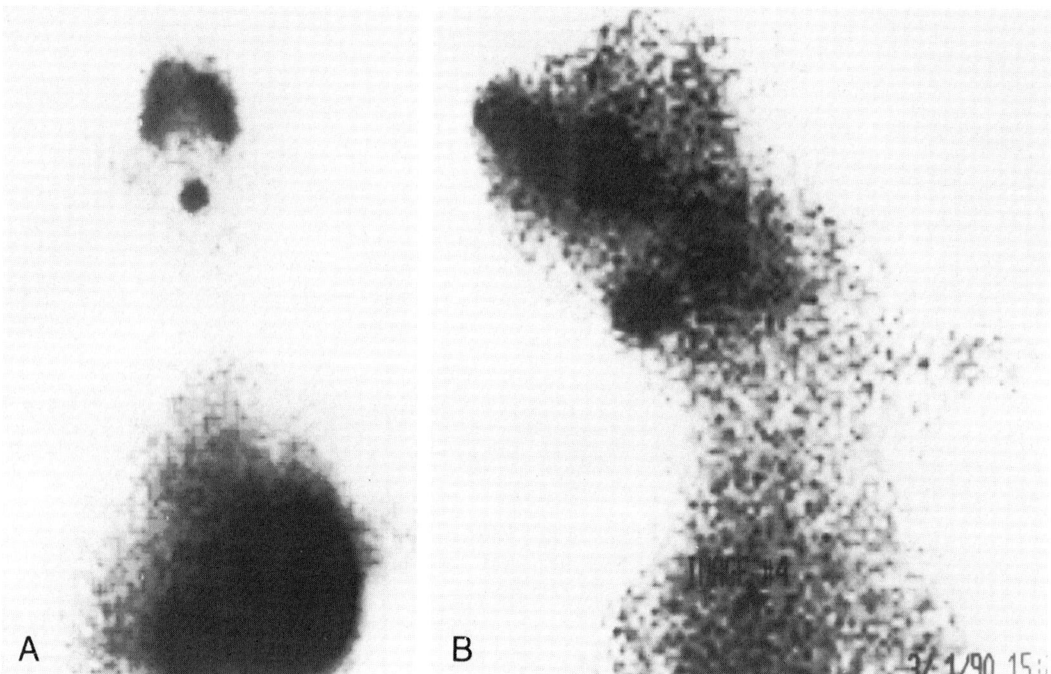

FIGURE 9–39. Sublingual thyroid gland in a newborn. *A.* One half hour after the oral administration of pertechnetate Tc 99m, an anterior image of the head, the neck and the trunk of a 10-day-old shows intense activity in the stomach (of course), in the mouth, and in a single spot in the neck. *B.* The left lateral view of the head and the neck shows activity over the tongue (diagonal intense line) and in a single spot near the base of the tongue. This area is in the vicinity of the thyroglossal duct, is not shaped like a thyroid gland, and is too high for a normal gland.

taken orally and becomes trapped and organified in the thyroid (8% to 30% of the total dose) in the same manner as nonradioactive iodine. The dose to the thyroid is approximately 0.01 Gy/μCi. Scan doses require from 50 to 100 μCi, which results in a dose of 0.50 to 1.00 Gy to the gland. Such doses make it difficult to justify the continued use of this isotope for thyroid diagnosis. In addition, because of its high gamma ray energy, ^{131}I is undesirable as an imaging agent. However, because of its beta ray emissions, ^{131}I is effective as a radiation therapy agent for thyroid carcinomas and for hyperthyroid states (Graves' disease and toxic multinodular goiter) that actively take up iodine.

Iodine 123 Scan

A better isotope for thyroid imaging is ^{123}I, which is ingested orally and delivers a radiation dose similar to that of pertechnetate Tc 99m. Its ideal gamma ray energy (159 keV) makes for excellent image quality with gamma cameras. Because ^{123}I is produced by cyclotron and has a 12-hour half-life, it has no shelf life. It must, therefore, be delivered overnight to the nuclear medicine clinic. Iodine 123 scans can be done either 4 to 6 hours or 24 hours after administration. The radioactive iodine uptake of the thyroid gland can be simultaneously measured. As with pertechnetate Tc 99m, the gland can be examined for nodular disease, and the location of palpable masses can be marked on the scan. The physiological difference between the pertechnetate Tc 99m scan and the ^{123}I scan is due to the difference in how these isotopes are accumulated by the thyroid. Both molecules have the same electric charge (−1) and have about the same radius. The pertechnetate Tc 99m is trapped and released by the gland, whereas the ^{123}I is trapped and then organified; that is, it is incorporated into thyroid hormone, which is stored in the gland.

Interpretation of Thyroid Scans

Interpretation of any thyroid scan consists of evaluation of thyroid size, contour, and homogeneity. Nearly all thyroid nodules (99%, regardless of whether the images are hot or cold) are caused by five conditions (Table 9–5). Cold nodules must be fully investigated

TABLE 9–5. THE MOST COMMON CAUSES OF A THYROID NODULE

Adenoma (25%)
Cyst (30%)
Involution (degeneration of adenoma)
Cancer (15%)
Focal thyroiditis

TABLE 9–6. CAUSES OF COLD THYROID NODULES

Distribution	Cause
50%	Adenomatous hyperplasia (solid or colloid cyst)
20%	Follicular adenoma
20%	Thyroid adenoma
10%	Other (thyroiditis; abscess; hemorrhage; metastases from carcinoma of breast and lung and from melanoma)

because 20% are malignant (Table 9–6). Most of the time, there is no reliable way to tell whether a cold nodule is benign or malignant. Sometimes a pure cyst seen on ultrasonogram can be safely considered benign. The most direct way to evaluate a cold lesion (short of surgery) is needle aspiration and cytological examination. Hot nodules on iodine scans are benign. If a hot nodule is not suppressed by exogenous thyroid hormone (thyroid suppression test), it is almost always a follicular adenoma. If suppression does occur, it may represent a relatively autonomous nodule (also benign) or an area of normal gland surrounded by tissue with subnormal uptake, as occurs in Graves' disease.

Substernal goiter is best evaluated with iodine rather than pertechnetate Tc 99m because of a better target-to-background ratio. Also, substernal goiter usually functions poorly, and so discerning it from the blood pool background in the mediastinum may be difficult if pertechnetate Tc 99m is used. The 364-, 159-, and 140-keV gamma rays of ^{131}I, ^{123}I, and ^{99m}Tc all penetrate the sternum with ease (Fig. 9–40).

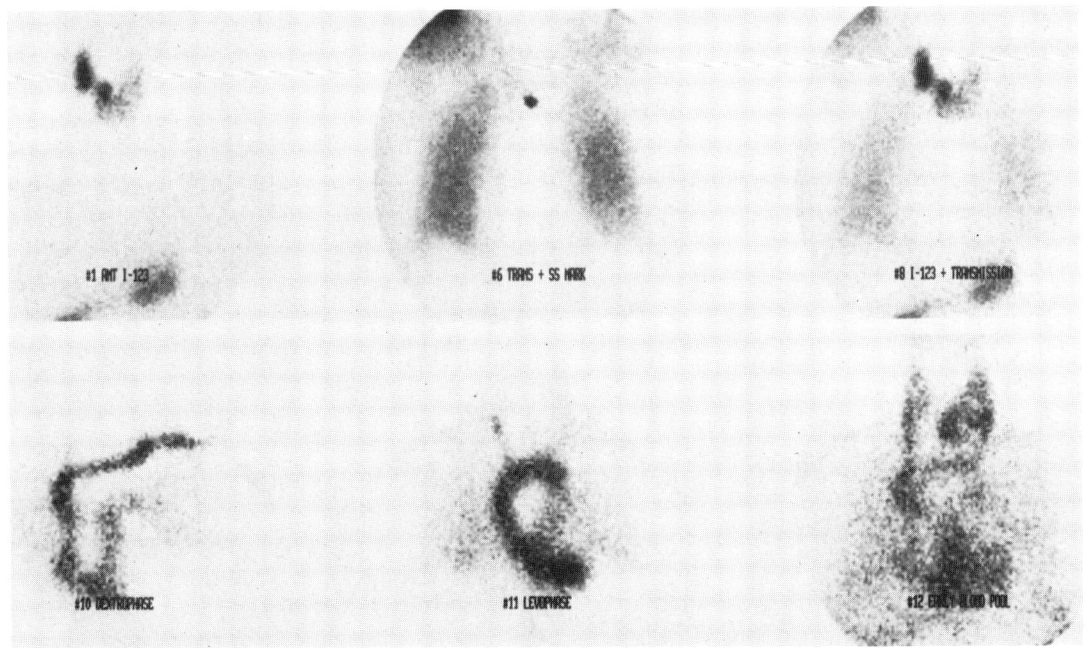

FIGURE 9–40. Substernal goiter. Initial image (top left) shows the thyroid gland and its caudal extension and a physiological accumulation of iodine 123 in the stomach. Center top image is a transmission scan produced by an external radioactive source placed behind the patient. The suprasternal notch is marked by a hot spot. The next image (top right) is a composite of the first two and shows the thyroid extending substernally into the mediastinum between the apices of the lungs. The dextrophase, levophase, and early blood pool images (bottom row) were performed after a bolus of pertechnetate Tc 99m was injected in the left antecubital vein to image the major vessels of the neck and around the mediastinum and in relation to the goiter. Note the prominent blood pool (bottom right) in this goiter.

Suggested Readings

Freeman LM (ed): Freeman and Johnson's Clinical Radionuclide Imaging, 3rd ed, vols 1, 2. Orlando, FL: Grune & Stratton, 1984.

Gottschalk A, Hoffer B, Potchen EJ, Berger HJ (eds): Diagnostic Nuclear Medicine, 2nd ed, vols 1, 2. Baltimore: Williams & Wilkins, 1988.

Mettler FA, Guiberteau MJ: Essentials of Nuclear Medicine, 3rd ed. Philadelphia: WB Saunders, 1991.

Index

Note: Page numbers in *italics* refer to illustrations; page numbers followed by (t) refer to tables.

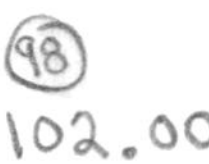